Principles of Frontal Lobe Function

Principles of Frontal Lobe Function

Edited by

DONALD T. STUSS, Ph.D. (C.Psych), O.Ont.
Reva James Leeds Chair in Neuroscience and
    Research Leadership
Vice President, Research, and Director
The Rotman Research Institute
Baycrest Centre for Geriatric Care
Professor, Departments of Medicine (Neurology,
    Rehabilitation Science) and Psychology
University of Toronto

ROBERT T. KNIGHT, M.D.
Evan Rauch Professor of Neuroscience
Director, The Helen Wills Neuroscience Institute
Department of Psychology
University of California, Berkeley

UNIVERSITY PRESS
2002

BS

OXFORD
UNIVERSITY PRESS

Oxford   New York
Auckland   Bangkok   Buenos Aires   Cape Town   Chennai
Dar es Salaam   Delhi   Hong Kong   Istanbul   Karachi   Kolkata
Kuala Lumpur   Madrid   Melbourne   Mexico City   Mumbai   Nairobi
São Paulo   Shanghai   Singapore   Taipei   Tokyo   Toronto

and an associated company in Berlin

Published by Oxford University Press, Inc.
198 Madison Avenue, New York, New York 10016

http://www.oup-usa.org

Oxford is a registered trademark of Oxford University Press

Library of Congress Cataloging-in-Publication Data
Principles of frontal lobe function /
edited by Donald T. Stuss, Robert T. Knight.
p. cm.
ISBN 0-19-513497-4
1. Frontal lobes.
I. Stuss, Donald T.
II. Knight, Robert T.
QP382.F7 .P755 2002   612.8'25—dc21   2001055466

9 8 7 6 5 4 3

Printed in the United States of America
on acid-free paper

4/26/06

To David and Leanne Stuss,
and Tom and Sonia Moser,
for all their support
and love and to D. Frank Benson,
an always remembered mentor,
colleague and friend,
with whom I shared the joys of
initial explorations of the
mysteries of the frontal lobes

D.T.S.

To Donatella Scabini,
whose love and support
made my contribution to this book possible
and to Sara
for all her humor.

R.T.K.

Foreword

MARCUS E. RAICHLE

In the minds of many, an understanding of how the brain works represents the last great frontier in biology, if not in all of science. While a fascination with this agenda concerns brains large and small, the ultimate goal is to understand within the limits of our capacity to do so, the workings of the human brain. For in this knowledge lies not only the potential to understand and ultimately treat, rationally and effectively, some of the most important diseases afflicting humankind but also to address social problems that continue to vex scientists and scholars in fields as diverse as anthropology, political science, psychology, sociology, and economics.

In pursuing a goal of understanding the human brain and, hence, the uniqueness of human behavior it is important to first recognize the ways in which the human brain differs from the brains of other species. While we are only beginning to understand such differences in any detail, the size of the human brain relative to the size of the body in which it is housed is a feature apparent to even the casual observer. The development of the frontal lobes in the human brain in particular accounts for a disproportionate fraction of the increased size of the human brain when compared to the proportion in nonhuman primates. In humans the frontal cortex accounts for 30% of the cortical surface, a fact that has instilled in clinicians and scientists for over two centuries the suspicion that a key to understanding the uniqueness of human behavior will come from an unveiling of the functions of the frontal lobes.

As Marsel Mesulam posits in his superb contribution to this volume (Chapter 2), a seminal event in research on the frontal lobes began at precisely 4:30 PM on Wednesday, September 13, 1848. On that date, in Cavendish, Vermont, exploding dynamite sent an iron tamping rod through the prefrontal cortex of a railroad construction foreman by the name of Phineas Gage. Miraculously surviving this accident, Gage nevertheless was changed for the remainder of his life. Such a profound transformation occurred in his personality that to his friends he was "no longer Gage." Despite the remarkable clinical features of this case and of similar ones that followed, the frontal lobes have, until recently, been slow to yield up their secrets. In fact, they have actually been referred to as the "silent" areas of the brain.

The silence of the frontal lobes has now been broken, as we have learned to ask appropriate questions and have the necessary tools at our disposal to obtain meaningful answers. As a result, much new and important information has been gathered on the functions of the frontal cortex in humans and in nonhuman primates, especially over the past few decades. This volume represents a very timely and important summary of that information. Noteworthy contributions come from the very investigators and laboratories that have led the field through the recent explosive accumulation of knowledge in this area. As such, this volume represents an invaluable resource to all interested in this vitally important area of research, which encompasses human brain function and human behavior at the highest level.

In contemplating the enormous amount of current information on the functions of the frontal lobes and appreciating the impressive array of tools that can help push back the frontier of knowledge even further, several issues come to mind. How is it that the closing decades of the twentieth century have been witness to such an explosion of new information on the frontal lobes? It has been suggested that significant advances in science come when two disparate but potentially complementary disciplines join forces. An apt example here is cognitive neuroscience. This field emerged because of the foresight of the James S. McDonnell Foundation, the Pew Charitable Trusts, and their advisors, who envisioned combining the experimental strategies of cognitive psychology with various techniques to actually examine how the brain functions to support mental activities. The timing was perfect, as the new techniques of functional brain imaging (positron emission tomography [PET] and functional magnetic resonance imaging [fMRI]) had just emerged. Along with the more traditional lesion behavior studies and measurement of event-related potentials, obtained with electroencephalography and magnetoencephalography, these new imaging techniques were placed in the hands of a whole new generation of scientists schooled in sophisticated behavioral techniques as well as in brain science. Studies of the normal human brain moved front and center in brain research.

The availability of a large amount of new information on the human brain, especially from functional brain imaging studies of the normal human brain with PET and fMRI, has presented us with the opportunity to integrate information across multiple levels of investigation in neuroscience. This is a very important opportunity for all concerned. It comes, however, with a challenge, because we lack understanding of the events within the brain surrounding functionally induced changes in activity. For the neurophysiologists these changes are traditionally recorded as changes in the spiking activity of neurons. For them, spiking is the gold standard. However, for those using functional brain imaging, the changes observed occur in the brain circulation and its energy metabolism. Not only does circulation change but also the manner in which additional energy requirements are met. To make matters more complex, spikes are recorded from cell bodies, while the circulatory and metabolic changes occur predominately around axon terminals, dendrites, and their surrounding astrocytes. At the moment, therefore, we cannot, be sure that changes in spiking always coincide spatially with the metabolic and circulatory changes that we observe with functional brain imaging. Both measures reflect important aspects of brain function. Finally, in imaging the whole brain is sampled and imaging almost always reveals widely distributed systems involved in most cognitive activity. The details of activity within a given region of interest are, of course, missing. For neurophysiologists the situation is reversed. In my opinion, both neurophysiologists and cognitive neuroscientists have necessary but not sufficient information to obtain a complete picture of events critical to an understanding of the function of the brain. A balanced perspective, without claims to privileged access to the complete truth, will be most helpful as we seek to understand these issues, and an open and mutually informed dialogue will be critical.

Another issue likely to be of increasing importance to our future understanding of human brain function in general, and frontal lobe function in particular, is the matter of individual differences. From the perspective of cognitive neuroscience and functional brain imaging, an early worry was that individual differences would be sufficiently great that attempts at averaging imaging data across individuals to improve signals and diminish noise would be doomed to failure. These fears were quickly put to rest by the very first attempts to average functional imaging data across individuals—the results were stunning. The approach of averaging data across individuals has dominated the field of cognitive neuroscience, with great success. For all who have examined such data in detail, however, the emergence of individual differences provides exciting prospects for an even deeper understanding of human behavior. Given psychologists' and psychiatrists' long-standing interest in and techniques for the characterization of personality differences, we are poised to make major advances in this area. Our current understanding of frontal lobes functions and connections will play a major role in unraveling the mysteries of each person's individuality.

As exemplified by most of the work in this volume, cognitive neuroscientists have focused largely on the adult human brain, examining how it functions normally and how it changes when focally damaged. In Chapter 29, however, Adele Diamond reminds us of the importance of considering brain function from a developmental perspective. The developmental psychology literature is very rich in details about developmental milestones associated with maturation of the human brain. What is missing, however, is anything remotely approaching a satisfactory understanding of the maturation process within systems of the human brain. Whether it is the development of attention, language, memory, management of distress, or personality development more generally, all of which involve the frontal lobes in some way, we lack information about brain maturation at a systems level. Such information would not only enrich our understanding of development itself but also of the end result of development—that is, the organization of the adult brain. This lack of information reflects not only an inability to safely and accurately acquire the needed data in humans but also a general focus on the cellular and molecular level within developmental neurobiology. Tools are now becoming available to cognitive neuroscientists that will allow safe access to the necessary areas in humans. Various imaging techniques applicable to children can now access not only functional but also anatomical information, including the development of fiber pathways. Data from a small group of pioneering investigators provide exciting glimpses of the future. Parallel studies in nonhuman primates, in which a direct examination of changes at a cellular level are possible, should be encouraged.

Finally, it is important to consider the brain from the perspective of its possible baseline functions. In cognitive neuroscience as well as in the long-standing work of neurophysiologists, the primary focus has been on changes in activity (usually increases; "activations" in the parlance of functional imagers) that are associated with specific mental processes. Evidence is now accumulating that a true baseline level of functionally important activity characterizes the brain. Furthermore, the frontal lobes contribute significantly to this baseline activity, as recognized by researchers such as the late David Ingvar and as more recently detailed by others and us. The important message for investigators probing the functions of the frontal lobes is to view them as operating continuously—enhanced under some circumstances and attenuated under others. As my colleague Debra Gusnard and I have pointed out (Gusnard, D.A. & Raichle, M.E.; [2001] Searching for the baseline: functional imaging and the resting human brain. *Nature Reviews Neuroscience* 2:685–694), this view is consistent with the continuity of a stable, unified perspective of the organism relative to its environment (a 'self'). This unified perspective is generally underappreciated because it largely functions in the background.

In closing, I would like to thank Don Stuss and Bob Knight for the very flattering invitation to contribute a foreword to this important volume on the frontal lobes. They and their contributors are to be congratulated. Studies of the brain, particularly of the human brain, that focus as these do on behaviors at the highest level have broad implications for the integration of the natural and social sciences, as so eloquently discussed by E.O. Wilson (*Consilience: The Unity of Knowledge* [Alfred A. Knopf, 1998, New York]) The end result should be a much better understanding of the human condition.

Preface

Our ultimate hope is that this volume will be the standard reference book on the frontal lobes for at least a decade. We took several steps to achieve this goal. First, we invited those whom we felt are currently the most innovative and prominent researchers in the field of frontal lobe research to contribute to the book. Unfortunately, as is evident from the table of contents of this volume, not everyone in this category is listed there. There were several reasons for this. Some who were invited couldn't participate for various reasons. Certain individuals whom we wanted to invite represented a duplication of content, so we invited the person we considered to have the least overlap with other contributors. The final reason was the limiting one: the envisaged book was already too large to be economically feasible for the publisher.

We encouraged each of the authors to elaborate their chapter in several ways. The chapters were to include information that could be used not only by knowledgeable scientists and clinicians but also by the young, future scientific leaders in frontal lobe research; that is, we wanted history, breadth, depth, practicality, and creativity in each chapter. Where possible, different contributors were encouraged to write chapters together, to enhance cross-fertilization of ideas as well as to foster integration of critical concepts. Each of the authors was encouraged to cross-reference where possible other chapters in the book to add to the integration of ideas. We wanted researchers, clinicians, and particularly students to have a comprehensive picture of current knowledge of the frontal lobe, and to see where not only cohesion but also differences might lie.

This book is intended for virtually anyone interested in the frontal lobes. Just like the song in *A Funny Thing Happened on the Way to the Forum,* there is something for everyone. We wanted to end up with a comprehensive reference book, providing value for the most advanced researcher, the youngest student, and the hands-on clinician. There is no doubt a bias toward the researcher, since active scientists wrote the chapters. Nevertheless, we hope that neuroscientists, neurologists, psychiatrists, psychologists, health-care workers of various professions (including nurses, physiotherapists, and occupational therapists), basic researchers, and clinicians will find the book of value. We are not sure if we will have satisfied all these constituents, since each of the domains covered could be a book unto itself. Moreover, the status of knowledge in certain areas of frontal lobe research was not as well developed as in others, leading to possible inequalities in background and new data. We leave the judgment as to how well we satisfied the variety of potential audiences to these readers.

We are grateful to all the contributors to the book. Their science, their creativity, and the time taken to write the chapters constitute the essence of this volume. Dr. M. Raichle was very gracious in agreeing to write the foreword. Special thanks go to D. Scabini for all her support and encouragement. We are indebted to the following individuals for all their work on the volume: C. Gojmerac, D. Derkzen, and I. Yang for diligent help in preparing the book for submission; C. Copnick, for correspondence and secretarial work; and F. Stevens and J. House of Oxford University Press for their feedback and enthusiasm about the project.

We are personally grateful to those agencies that fund our personal research, without which we would not have been in a position to undertake this effort: for D. T. Stuss, the Canadian Institutes of Health Research and the McDonnell Foundation; and for R.T. Knight, the National Institute of Neurological Disorders and Stroke, the Veterans Administration Research Service, and Varian, Inc. The success of The Rotman Research Institute conference in 2000, which spurred the idea of this volume, was due to the generosity of our academic sponsors—Baycrest Centre for Geriatric Care and the University of Toronto—and our financial sponsors: Sustaining Sponsor, Hong Kong Bank of Canada; Conference Sponsor, Nozomi Hospital, Tokyo Japan; Conference Bag Sponsor, Varian MRI Systems; Contributing Sponsor, Novartis Pharmaceuticals; Sponsor, AstraZeneca pharmaceuticals; and additional support, Fido. We also received two education grants from the Medical Research Council of Canada (now the Canadian Institutes of Health Research) and the Ontario Mental Health Foundation. The abstracts of the presenters' talks and the posters presented at the conference are published in *Brain and Cognition* (H. Whitaker and S. Segalowitz, eds.) 2001, vol. 47 (112), the common practice for The Rotman Research Institute conferences.

The success of the conference was directly due to an outstanding organizing team: conference coordinator, S. Teaves; administration, J. Pagiamtzis, C. Copnick, and S. Ng; registration, H. Roesler and P. Ferreira; audiovisual aids B. Kierdal; and virtually all the other administrative staff of The Rotman Research Institute, and student volunteers.

Toronto, Ontario   D.T.S.
Berkeley, California   R.T.K.

Contents

Contributors

CLAUDE ALAIN, PH.D.
The Rotman Research Institute
Baycrest Centre for Geriatric Care
Department of Psychology
University of Toronto
Toronto, ON, Canada

MICHAEL P. ALEXANDER, M.D.
Departments of Neurology
Beth Israel Deaconess Medical Center
Harvard Medical School and
Boston University School of Medicine (Memory
   Disorders Research Centre)
Boston, MA, USA
Stroke Rehabilitation
Youville Lifecare Hospital
Cambridge, MA, USA

VICKI ANDERSON, PH.D.
Department of Psychology
University of Melbourne
Victoria, Australia
Royal Children's Hospital/
   Murdoch Children's Research Institute
Parkville, Victoria, Australia

AMY F.T. ARNSTEN, PH.D.
Department of Neurobiology
Associate Professor and Director of Graduate
   Studies
Yale University School of Medicine
New Haven, CT, USA

ALAN BADDELEY, PH.D.
Department of Experimental Psychology
University of Bristol
Bristol, UK

DAVID BADRE, PH.D.
Department of Brain and Cognitive Science
Massachusetts Institute of Technology
Cambridge, MA, USA

DEANNA M. BARCH, PH.D
Department of Psychology
Washington University
St. Louis, MO, USA

MALCOLM A. BINNS, M.A.
The Rotman Research Institute
Baycrest Centre for Geriatric Care
Toronto, ON, Canada

SANDRA E. BLACK, M.D.
Sunnybrook and Women's College Health Sciences
   Centre; The Rotman Research Institute
Baycrest Centre for Geriatric Care
Department of Medicine (Neurology)
University of Toronto
Toronto, ON, Canada

TODD S. BRAVER, PH.D.
Department of Psychology
Washington University
St. Louis, MO, USA

YURI L. BRONSTEIN, M.D.
Department of Neurology
UCLA School of Medicine
Los Angeles, CA, USA

PAUL W. BURGESS, PH.D.
Institute of Cognitive Neuroscience
UCL (University College London)
London, U.K.

JONATHAN D. COHEN, M.D., PH.D.
Department of Psychology
Princeton University
Princeton, NJ, USA
Department of Psychiatry
University of Pittsburgh
Pittsburgh, PA, USA

FERGUS I.M. CRAIK, PH.D.
The Rotman Research Institute
Baycrest Centre for Geriatric Care
Department of Psychology
University of Toronto
Toronto, ON, Canada

JEFFREY L. CUMMINGS, M.D.
Departments of Neurology and Psychiatry
  and Biobehavioral Sciences
UCLA School of Medicine
Los Angeles, CA, USA

CLAYTON CURTIS, PH.D.
Department of Psychology
University of California, Berkley
Berkeley, CA, USA

LAUREN DADE, PH.D.
The Rotman Research Institute
Baycrest Centre for Geriatric Care
Department of Psychology
University of Toronto
Toronto, ON, Canada

MARK D'ESPOSITO, M.D.
Professor of Neuroscience and Psychology
Director, Henry H. Wheeler, Jr. Brain
  Imaging Center
Helen Wills Neuroscience Institute and
Department of Psychology
University of California, Berkeley
Berkeley, CA, USA

ADELE DIAMOND, PH.D.
Department of Psychiatry
Professor of Psychiatry
Director, Center for Developmental Cognitive
  Neuroscience
Shriver Center Campus
University of Massachusetts Medical School
Waltham, MA, USA

JOHN DUNCAN, D.PHIL.
MRC Cognition and Brain Sciences Unit
Cambridge, UK

DARLENE FLODEN, M.A.
Department of Psychology
University of Toronto
Toronto, ON, Canada

JOAQUÍN M. FUSTER, M.D., PH.D.
Neuropsychiatric Institute and Brain Research
  Institute
University of California, Los Angeles
Los Angeles, CA, USA

HISAE GEMBA, M.D., PH.D.
Department of Physiology
Kansai Medical University
Moriguchi, Osaka, Japan

ROBBIN GIBB, PH.D.
Canadian Centre of Behavioural Neuroscience
Department of Psychology and Neuroscience
University of Lethbridge
Lethbridge, AB, Canada

PATRICIA S. GOLDMAN-RAKIC, PH.D.
Section of Neurobiology
Yale University School of Medicine
New Haven, CT, USA

CHERYL L. GRADY, PH.D.
The Rotman Research Institute
Baycrest Centre for Geriatric Care
Departments of Psychiatry and Psychology
University of Toronto
Toronto, ON, Canada

JORDAN GRAFMAN, PH.D.
Chief, Cognitive Neuroscience Section
National Institute of Neurological Disorders and
  Stroke
National Institutes of Health
Bethesda, MD, USA

STEPHANIE J. HEVENOR, M.SC.
The Rotman Research Institute
Baycrest Centre for Geriatric Care
Toronto, ON, Canada

RANI JACOBS, PH.D.
Department of Psychology
University of Melbourne
Victoria, Australia
Royal Children's Hospital/
  Murdoch Children's Research Institute
Parkville, Victoria, Australia

JOHN JONIDES, PH.D.
Department of Psychology
University of Michigan
Ann Arbor, MI, USA

DOUGLAS I. KATZ, M.D.
Department of Neurology
Boston University School of Medicine
Boston, MA, USA
Healthsouth Braintree Rehabilitation Hospital
Braintree, MA, USA

ROBERT T. KNIGHT, M.D.
Department of Psychology
Evan Rauch Professor of Neuroscience
Director, The Helen Wills Neuroscience
  Institute
University of California, Berkeley
Berkeley, CA, USA

BRYAN KOLB, PH.D.
Canadian Centre for Behavioural Neuroscience
Department of Psychology and Neuroscience
University of Lethbridge
Lethbridge, AB, Canada

HOI-CHUNG LEUNG, PH.D.
Department of Diagnostic Radiology
Yale University School of Medicine
New Haven, CT, USA

HARVEY S. LEVIN, M.D.
Departments of Physical Medicine and
  Rehabilitation, Neurosurgery, and Psychiatry
  and Behavioral Sciences
Baylor College of Medicine
Houston, TX, USA

BRIAN LEVINE, PH.D.
The Rotman Research Institute
Baycrest Centre for Geriatric Care
Departments of Psychology and Medicine
  (Neurology)
University of Toronto
Toronto, ON, Canada

HELEN S. MAYBERG, M.D., FRCPC
Sandra Rotman Chair in Neuropsychiatry
The Rotman Research Institute
Baycrest Centre for Geriatric Care
Departments of Psychiatry and Medicine
  (Neurology)
University of Toronto
Toronto, ON, Canada

ANTHONY R. MCINTOSH, PH.D.
The Rotman Research Institute
Baycrest Centre for Geriatric Care
Department of Psychology,
University of Toronto
Toronto, ON, Canada

M.-MARSEL MESULAM, M.D.
Dunbar Professor of Neurology and Psychiatry
Director, Cognitive Neurology and Alzheimer's
  Disease Center
Northwestern University Medical School
Chicago, IL, USA

EARL K. MILLER, PH.D.
Center for Learning and Memory
RIKEN-MIT Neuroscience Research Center
Department of Brain and Cognitive Sciences
Massachusetts Institute of Technology
Cambridge, MA, USA

MORRIS MOSCOVITCH, PH.D.
The Rotman Research Institute
Baycrest Centre for Geriatric Care
Department of Psychology
University of Toronto
Toronto, ON, Canada

DEEPAK N. PANDYA, M.D.
Departments of Anatomy and Neurobiology and
  Neurology
Boston University School of Medicine
Harvard Neurological Unit
Beth Israel Hospital
Boston, MA, USA

RICHARD E. PASSINGHAM, PH.D.
Department of Experimental Psychology
University of Oxford
Oxford, UK
Wellcome Department of Cognitive Neurology
Institute of Neurology
London, UK

MICHAEL PETRIDES, PH.D.
James McGill Professor
Director, Cognitive Neuroscience Unit
Montreal Neurological Institute and
Department of Psychology
McGill University
Montreal, PQ, Canada

TERENCE W. PICTON, M.D., PH.D.
The Rotman Research Institute
Baycrest Centre for Geriatric Care
Department of Medicine (Neurology)
University of Toronto
Toronto, ON, Canada

BRADLEY R. POSTLE, PH.D.
Department of Psychology
University of Wisconsin-Madison
Madison, WI, USA

ROBERT RAFAL, M.D.
Professor of Clinical Neuroscience and
Neuropsychology
Centre for Cognitive Neuroscience
School of Psychology
University of Wales, Bangor
Bangor, Wales, UK

NATASHA RAJAH, M.A.
The Rotman Research Institute
Baycrest Centre for Geriatric Care
Toronto, ON, Canada

TREVOR W. ROBBINS, PH.D.
Department of Experimental Psychology
University of Cambridge
Cambridge, UK

IAN H. ROBERTSON, PH.D.
Department of Psychology and Institute of
Neuroscience,
Trinity College
Dublin, Ireland

EDMUND T. ROLLS, D.PHIL., D.SC.
Department of Experimental Psychology
University of Oxford
Oxford, UK

JAMES B. ROWE, PH.D.
Wellcome Department of Cognitive Neurology
Institute of Neurology
London, UK

JEAN A. SAINT-CYR, PH.D.
Departments of Surgery (Neurosurgery and
Anatomy) and Psychology
University of Toronto
Toronto Western Hospital
Toronto, ON, Canada

TIM SHALLICE, PH.D.
Director, Institute of Cognitive Neuroscience
University College London
London, UK

ARTHUR P. SHIMAMURA, PH.D.
Department of Psychology
University of California, Berkeley
Berkeley, CA, USA

EDWARD E. SMITH, PH.D.
Department of Psychology
University of Michigan
Ann Arbor, MI, USA

DONALD T. STUSS, PH.D., O.ONT.
Vice-President Research
Director, The Rotman Research Institute
The Reva James Leeds Chair in Neuroscience
and Research Leadership
Baycrest Centre for Geriatric Care
Departments of Psychology and Medicine
(Neurology, Rehabilitation Science)
University of Toronto
Toronto, ON, Canada

SHARON L. THOMPSON-SCHILL, PH.D.
Department of Psychology
University of Pennsylvania
Philadelphia, PA, USA

DANIEL TRANEL, PH.D.
Department of Neurology
Division of Cognitive Neuroscience
Director, Neuroscience Program
University of Iowa College of Medicine
Iowa City, IA, USA

ENDEL TULVING, PH.D., F.R.S.C., F.R.S.
Tanenbaum Chair in Cognitive Neuroscience
The Rotman Research Institute
Baycrest Centre for Geriatric Care;
University Professor Emeritus
University of Toronto
Toronto, ON, Canada
Clark Way Harrison Distinguished Visiting
  Professor of Psychology and Cognitive
  Neuroscience
Washington University, St. Louis, MO, USA

MASATAKA WATANABE, PH.D.
Department of Psychology
Tokyo Metropolitan Institute for Neuroscience
Tokyo, Japan

GORDON WINOCUR, PH.D.
The Rotman Research Institute
Baycrest Centre for Geriatric Care;
Department of Psychology
Trent University and University of Toronto
Toronto, ON, Canada

Principles of Frontal Lobe Function

1

Introduction

DONALD T. STUSS AND ROBERT T. KNIGHT

The frontal lobes are a toolmaker.

Bob Rafal, Toronto 2000

The title of this book, *Principles of Frontal Lobe Function*, clearly states our emphasis: the functions of the frontal lobes, and frontal systems. Much of the controversy about executive and frontal lobe functions has been the result of inconsistency of operational definitions and limits of discussion. We hope that this treatise will bring clarity to the field as well as raise key issues for future investigation.

As frequently stated in several chapters, the frontal lobes represent a large proportion of the human brain. Although we have tried to cover the roles of all sections, there is a clear emphasis on what is commonly called *prefrontal cortex*, that region antecedent to the motor, premotor and supplementary motor areas. Important information on these latter motor-related structures is provided in Chapter 8, by Gemba, and in Chapter 9, by Rafal.

Our intention in organizing the book was to cover the frontal lobes from birth to death, from biochemistry and anatomy to rehabilitation, from theory to function, and from normal to disrupted function. At first we planned to divide it into sections, such as neuroscience bases, theoretical positions, and so on. It even-

tually became clear that this would be a somewhat arbitrary organization, since so many authors presented material that covered several of these arbitrary distinctions. A second option was to organize the book according to approaches, such as animal research or human research. After some debate, we arranged the chapters more in a logical and conceptual sequence, starting from basic science and ending in more applied work. Although this structure is perhaps still artificial, the attempt was to juxtapose chapters that had some conceptual commonality.

In this introductory chapter, we will present an overview of the different contributions. By highlighting some of the similarities and differences among approaches, we hope to entice the astute reader to consider the diversity of approaches to the same question about the role of the frontal lobes in organized behavior, to advance the field ahead.

We bracketed the book with chapters that introduce and summarize in overarching ways the structure and content of the book. Mesulam, Chapter 2, sets the stage for the rest of the book, and the novice reader of the functions of the frontal lobes should start here. Mesulam's overview imparts the importance of this field of research. His anatomical and clinical distinctions provide organizational and memory "hooks" for reading many of the other chapters. Chapter 34, by Knight and Stuss, is the other bookend, providing an overview of much of the content of the book and forecasting what the future will bring.

The discussion of the anatomy of the frontal lobes was charged to Petrides and Pandya (Chapter 3). In their contribution they extend their previous work on architectonic specificity (see, e.g., Petrides & Pandya, 1994) by presenting how the frontal lobes are interconnected with different brain regions through association pathways and how this is reflected in functional observations. We cannot emphasize enough that the study of frontal lobe functions cannot be done solely by pure localization; the study of systems and pathways in relation to function will continue to be one of the important future initiatives. In this regard, development of novel methods to elucidate white matter pathways in the human brain, such as diffusion tensor analysis, is particularly relevant for future research. Petrides and Pandya wisely state in their concluding paragraph: "Proper knowledge of the course of the different fiber pathways is as important as knowledge of their termination in order to interpret properly the functional deficits resulting from damage to particular regions of the cerebral cortex."

Many other chapters in the book present additional anatomical information related to their particular content. Taken together, these chapters provide a quite astounding amount of information on the anatomy and connectivity of the frontal lobes, and how these relate to different functions. In Chapter 2 Mesulam provides an overview; in Chapter 32 Kolb and Gibb discuss the changes at synaptic levels; in Chapter 29 Diamond discusses maturation at different time points from birth to early adulthood; in Chapter 8 Gemba addresses the role of different subregions in motor control; in Chapter 23 Rolls reviews the anatomy and connections of the orbitofrontal cortex; in Chapter 9 Rafal outlines the cortical and subcortical circuitry for oculomotor control; and in Chapter 26 St. Cyr and colleagues discuss frontal–subcortical circuitry.

If the reader is interested in the neuro-chemistry of brain functioning, either from a purely scientific view or for the purposes of investigating neuropharmacological treatments of prefrontal cortex function, then Chapter 4 by Arnsten and Robbins will be a godsend. The authors review animal and human research on the mechanisms by which dopamine, norepinephrine, serotonin, and acetylcholine may influence prefrontal cortex cognitive functions. It is clear that the brain (usually anatomy) behavior approach to the study of frontal lobe functions must include to a far greater extent the relation of chemical pathways to function as well. In addition to providing information on anatomical development Diamond describes in Chapter 29 the biochemical changes at several developmental periods. In Chapter 26, St. Cyr and colleagues summarize the neurochemistry of frontal–subcortical circuits as a basis for understanding behavioral consequences and treatment.

The controversial issue of segregation versus integration, or the fractionation or homogeneity of the frontal lobes, is discussed in several chapters, reflecting the salience of this question over the past decade. In Chapter 18, Duncan and Miller, in their theory of adaptive coding, argue less for tight regional specificity and more for joint recruitment of different frontal regions in response to different cognitive demands. They base the idea of adaptive functioning on the observation that the same frontal neurons appear to be configured to solve many different cognitive operations (compare this concept with the one postulated by D'Esposito and Postle in Chapter 11). In Chapter 5, Goldman-Rakic and Leung provide a compelling counterpoint to this view and readers are left to draw their own conclusions.

A large number of chapters come down on the side of heterogeneity of frontal lobe functioning. In Chapter 12, Moscovitch and Winocur suggest a component process model for the strategic role of the frontal lobes in memory. In Chapter 25, Stuss and colleagues provide empirical evidence from neuropsychological tests administered to individuals with discrete focal lesions that different regions of the frontal lobes play different roles. Knight's electrophysiological research also suggests regional specificity for different aspects of attention and working memory capacity. This specificity is evident in aging, discussed in Chapter 31 by Craik and Grady, and also at some earlier developmental stages, addressed in Chapter 30 by Anderson and colleagues.

Two chapters even have "fractionation" in their titles. In Chapter 16, Baddeley extends his original working memory model to specify in greater detail the role of the third component, the "central executive." He speculates on what capacities such an executive would need, and uses task performance analysis of patients suffering from early-stage Alzheimer's disease to test the validity of the separation of the proposed executive functions. This chapter presents an important distinction made earlier: the study of executive functions does not necessarily indicate an analysis of frontal lobe function. In Chapter 17, Shallice presents a higher-order model suggested by Fox and Das (2000) to augment the Norman and Shallice model of the supervisory system. In contrast to Baddeley, however, Shallice's thesis on the fractionation of the supervisory system does relate to the frontal lobes, since his supporting data derive from functional imaging and lesion research. The constitutive components of the supervisory system, or central executive, that both authors discuss have notable similarities.

In reviewing primarily animal research, Fuster argues in Chapter 6 that prefrontal lobe functions need to be interpreted as an important part of associative neocortical networks which, while distributed, are overlapping and intersecting. His distinction between operations (e.g., monitoring, planning, attention) and representations (executive memory) may be one way of solving the dilemma over the heterogeneity or homogeneity of functions—that is, it may depend on the level of analysis or the quality of description.

There are levels of complexity in the systems approach to frontal lobe functioning. D'Esposito and Postle conclude in Chapter 11 that different regions within the lateral prefrontal cortex are indeed related to different cognitive operations; yet, at the same time, they suggest, as do Duncan and Miller in Chapter 18, that the same region can also be engaged in different cognitive operations. In Chapter 25, Stuss and colleagues show that different changes in context, illustrated in their discussion of task demands, of what appears to be superficially a very similar task, alter which brain regions appear necessary for that task performance. With a simpler task demand, there is evidence of considerable heterogeneity, although it is *anatomical systems*, not just focal brain regions, that demonstrate this fractionation of function. With different task demands that seem more difficult, there is no evident frontal lobe heterogeneity. In one sense, this latter finding might support Duncan and Miller's findings; it is less obvious how this relates to Fuster's concept of representations. Regardless, in the future of frontal lobe research, context will play an ever-increasing role.

In our view, the controversy over the separation and commonality, and the homogeneity and heterogeneity, of frontal lobe function reflects our comment at the beginning of this chapter on the importance of operational definitions. This controversy must also be seen in light of the importance of dynamic, integrated (and perhaps context-dependent) brain systems.

In Chapter 19, Grafman suggests that the frontal lobes store various representational units, which he calls *structured event complexes*. These elements of memory of higher-level knowledge help guide over time more complex behaviors. Since there is a clear similarity between this proposal and other concepts, Grafman assists the reader by discussing in Chapter 19 the differences and similarities between his approach and similar frameworks. Picton and colleagues, who review human physiological research on frontal lobe functions in Chapter 7, propose a concept that has at least overt similarity to Fuster's representations. They posit that the prefrontal lobes through representational processing are the "theatre of the mind," where options are played out, examined, and understood. A key to Picton and colleagues' model is a return to one of the most important concepts of the 1960s: the Test-Operate-Test-Exit mechanism, to perceive, decode, and respond to information (Miller et al., 1960). This model has also been used to explain different levels of awareness (Stuss, 1991; Stuss et al., 2001). The interactivity of different brain regions is again emphasized in these approaches.

Several contributors have focused on a specific function. In Chapter 8, Gemba summarizes the knowledge of motor control, and in Chapter 9, Rafal reviews visuomotor control. While seemingly lower level, these functions are crucial to understanding the action/active role of the frontal lobes in the final common output pathway. The study of motor programming can be seen as the investigation of voluntary behavior. Gemba outlines how different parts of the frontal lobe and other regions (e.g., limbic, premotor, motor, supplementary motor area) combine for voluntary vocalization and hand movements. Rafal uses eye movements as a model system to investigate how midbrain reflex circuits and frontal and parietal systems for eye movement control combine to produce goal-directed behavior. In both chapters the importance of a systems analysis is again confirmed.

Endel Tulving is known for his ability to synthesize important concepts in memorable terms. More importantly, his elaborations of the concepts are lucid and compelling. "Chronesthesia," as Tulving points out in Chapter 20, has been proposed before—but never in as comprehensive manner as presented here. His idea of mental time travel should be considered by readers in the context of Fuster's temporal integration, and contrasted with the different temporal domains considered in the workings of memory. There is little doubt that the role of the frontal lobes in the integration of the past and present to look into the future is of major importance. In our opinion, this needs to be investigated in a more comprehensive manner, by looking at different aspects of time and comparing the role of the frontal lobes to the temporal functions of other brain areas, such as the cerebellum or basal ganglia, that have been linked to timing control.

In Chapter 10, Alexander provides a comprehensive view of frontal language functions, moving beyond traditional perspectives. In many regards, he is presenting a model for research of the role of frontal lobe in language, since there are not many studies that have pursued some of the less traditional ideas (discourse, scripts, etc.) with well-documented focal frontal lesions. One might wonder if there is any relationship between the scripts proposed for language and Grafman's structured event complexes.

Clearly the study of memory in relation to frontal lobe functions has been a major thrust of research, as evidenced by the number of chapters that have the word "memory" in the title and that cover memory within the text. The connection between working memory in particular and the frontal lobes has generated much interest. D'Esposito and Postle again emphasize (in Chapter 11) that one must consider anatomical and functional systems when attempting to disentangle the role of prefrontal areas in memory. They add a new level of complexity to this area of study.

The question remains, however, whether working memory is a function of maintaining information or of attentional selection. In Chapter 14, Passingham and Rowe suggest that holding information in memory and true selection are dissociable processes, and that it is possible that monkeys with lesions in area 46 fail delayed-response tasks, not because of impaired working memory but because of deficient response selection. Our stated goal of highlighting differences in the theoretical positions of different researchers, and indicating why the differences might exist, is wonderfully highlighted in the comparison of the chapters by Passingham and Rowe (Chapter 14) and Goldman-Rakic and Leung (Chapter 5). The idea that the same cell may be capable of performing a different task under different conditions (see Chapters 11 and 18) may provide another answer to this controversy. Holding information and response selection may both be associated with area 46, depending on the exact nature of the task demands. These new distinctions and concepts are clearly exciting avenues of future research.

Two chapters highlight the active, supervisory, strategic, controlling nature of the frontal lobes in memory functions. At first glance, Chapter 13, by Shimamura, and Chapter 12, by Moscovitch and Winocur appear similar in content. But there are considerable differences in emphases. Moscovitch and Winocur are blatant about how important they feel this role of the frontal lobes is, the medial temporal lobes being viewed as "stupid." Our apologies in advance to our hippocampal colleagues. They describe the role of the frontal lobes as "working with memory," and see this use not just for recovering past experiences but also for directing other activities. Shimamura focuses more on an inhibitory model, which he calls the "dynamic filtering theory." Other processes, such as selecting, maintaining, updating, and rerouting, can be considered in light of this gating function of the frontal lobe.

In Chapter 15, Jonides and colleagues continue the theme of filtering, or selection, but address it independent of memory: they discuss the psychological process of selectively attending to one source of information to the exclusion of others. In a meta-analysis, they review different tasks used to study selective attention, under the construct of conflict resolution, as assessed with functional imaging techniques. Both the anterior cingulate cortex and the dorsolateral prefrontal cortex are involved in some aspect of conflict resolution, which is likely related to different mechanisms. The theme of heterogeneity of function is reflected in these results.

Four chapters provide an excellent overview of the role of orbitofrontal/ventral–medial lobe function in emotional functions and social behavior. In Chapter 21, Watanabe covers the monkey literature related to motivation (orbitofrontal cortex), emotions, and cognition (the latter two being integrated in the lateral prefrontal cortex). The mechanism by which anatomical systems work together is underscored in this chapter: cognition informs motivation and motivation modulates cognition. This chapter again notes the influence of context, this time in the form of the reward expectancy of the monkey.

In Chapter 23, Rolls presents animal and human (lesion and functional imaging) work in his review of the functions of the orbitofrontal cortex. The pivotal point of the reward value of taste and smell demonstrates that there is a very similar base to the behavioral choices made by animals of many species. He proposes the rapid shaping and reversal of reward–punishment contingencies as a key aspect of orbital prefrontal function.

In Chapter 22, Tranel discusses the role of the orbital prefrontal cortex in behavior, with emphasis on the involvement of the ventral–medial prefrontal lobe in emotions and decision making. He demonstrates how use of a "gambling task" has provided the ability to measure decision making and related emotional influences. The somatic marker hypothesis proposed to explain the observed results should be compared with material in all four chapters (21–24) dealing with the emotional changes with frontal lobe damage.

Finally, in Chapter 24, Mayberg takes a common disorder, depression, and shows how limbic–cortical interactions, the play between emotions and cognition, can be so important in depression. This chapter represents the practicality and applied nature of frontal lobe research, and shows the importance of the interrelationships of different approaches. In comparing Chapters 21 with 24, it is clear that Mayberg and Watanabe each approach limbic–cortical relations from quite different perspectives. These studies on the motivational and emotional functions of the frontal lobes announce a return to the early excitement of frontal lobe research—the effect of lesions on personality, emotions, and social behavior. In our view, the story is not yet complete, but rather, unfolding.

Several chapters address how frontal lobe or frontal system damage occurs in specific diseases or disorders. In Chapter 25, Stuss and colleagues summarize the findings of the effects of well-characterized focal frontal lesions, with an emphasis on stroke. In Chapter 28, Levine and colleagues present the effects of traumatic brain injury on frontal lobe functioning. Two practical aspects of this chapter are the critical review of the cognitive and behavioral assessments of traumatic brain injury, and the presentation of a new segmentation approach to assess gray, white, and cerebrospinal fluid compartment volumes. The reader interested in developmental comparisons should read the above two chapters in conjunction with Chapter 30, by Anderson and colleagues, who present interesting (and new) data on the effects of focal lesions and traumatic brain injury in children. It is clear from this work that, when one considers the effects of disease on prefrontal function, children cannot be viewed as just small adults.

Chapter 26, by St. Cyr and colleagues, not only is an excellent review of the consequences of neurosurgical treatment of patients with Parkinson's disease, it epitomizes the value of studying systems and circuitry, particularly the frontal–subcortical circuits. What is new in this chapter is the extension of some of the circuits to include new anatomical regions, and the effect of deep brain stimulation on cognition and motor responses.

In Chapter 27, Braver and colleagues discuss how prefrontal cortex functions change in schizophrenia. This chapter is an example of how a connectionist computational model can be useful in studying psychological constructs.

In our view, the study of frontal lobe functions in different disorders has benefited immensely from new theoretical constructs and advances in anatomy and neurochemistry. This approach needs to be continued and different disorders with supposed frontal system dysfunction also need to be studied in this critical and theoretical manner as well.

There is perhaps no more interesting aspect of frontal lobe function than to see how these functions change developmentally, from birth to old age. Diamond sets the stage for this topic in Chapter 29, by describing how normal development of prefrontal cortex occurs from birth to young adulthood. In this chapter, discussions of anatomy, biochemistry, and function overlap, and the author shows that the functions described and studied in adults unfold in a staged manner in children. If these stages are arrested in some manner, such as by acquired brain damage, what happens? In Chapter 30, Anderson and colleagues contrast the effects of focal lesions and traumatic brain injury as they occur at different developmental stages. In our view, this exciting research is in its infancy—but what a future! Research of frontal lobe functions in adults provides a necessary base for understanding brain–behavior relations; developmental studies have the potential to change education and rehabilitation

for long periods of time. These two chapters should be read in relation to Kolb and Gibb's work in Chapter 32 on frontal brain plasticity.

Currently, there is still evidence for a corresponding staged, peeling away of frontal lobe abilities with aging. Craik and Grady are appropriately cautious in discussing the "frontal lobology" of aging, in Chapter 31. That is what makes their summary of behavioral and imaging changes in memory with aging all the more interesting. Their chapter suggests that memory-performance changes with aging are indeed related to age-related biological changes in the frontal lobes—but not only in the frontal lobes. Brain systems are important at all stages of life, and are perhaps even more important as one adapts to the effects of aging. In Chapter 27, Braver and colleagues apply their modelling approach to the effects of aging in the context of normal and disordered cognitive control.

The success of rehabilitation of frontal lobe dysfunction is dependent on the correct understanding of the functions of this region. The fact that we are still debating what the systems and functions of the frontal lobes are might be one reason for there being only two chapters on this important topic. In Chapter 32, Kolb and Gibb talk about the change over time in the structure of the frontal lobes, according to results in animal research. How the information will apply to clinical rehabilitation is not yet certain. For example, housing animals in complex environments results in increases in spine density in the frontal lobes, but does not affect dendritic length. In contrast, such experiences do increase dendritic length in motor and sensory areas; the relevance of this to rehabilitation presently remains unclear. Nonetheless, there is a sense that this information will some day provide the ultimate measure of rehabilitation efficacy, perhaps indirectly through functional imaging techniques.

In Chapter 33, Burgess and Robertson approach rehabilitation for frontal lobe dysfunction from a somewhat different perspective. Taking different theories they discuss how each theoretical model leads to different implications for research. The result is a very practical set of six principles that direct how rehabilitation should be done. In our opinion, this method has the potential to be transformative in the rehabilitation field.

Through this introduction we hope we have whetted the reader's appetite for an in-depth reading of the individual chapters—not only to gain insight into each chapter's topic but also to see how the different chapters might inform each other. In the last chapter, we provide a summary of much of the recent work on prefrontal cortex and consider what the field might look like in 2010.

REFERENCES

Fox, J. & Das, S.K. (2000). *Safe and Sound: Artificial Intelligence in Hazardous Applications*. Menlo Park, CA: AAAI Press.

Miller, G.A., Galanter, E., & Pribram, K.H. (1960). *Plans and the Structure of Behavior*. New York: Holt, Rinehart and Winston.

Petrides, M. & Pandya, D.N. (1994). Comparative architectonic analysis of the human and the macaque frontal cortex. In: F. Boller & J. Grafman (Eds.), *Handbook of Neuropsychology, Vol. 9* (pp. 17–58). Amsterdam: Elsevier.

Stuss, D.T. (1991). Disturbance of self-awareness after frontal system damage. In: G.P. Prigatano & D.L. Schacter (Eds.), *Awareness of Deficit after Brain Injury: Clinical and Theoretical Issues* (pp. 63–83). New York: Oxford University Press.

Stuss, D.T., Picton, T.W., & Alexander, M.P. (2001). Consciousness, self-awareness, and the frontal lobes. In: S.P. Salloway, P.F. Malloy & J.D. Duffy (Eds.), *The Frontal Lobes and Neuropsychiatric Illness* (pp. 101–109). Washington, DC: American Psychiatric Publishing.

2

The Human Frontal Lobes: Transcending the Default Mode through Contingent Encoding

M.-MARSEL MESULAM

They said, "You have a blue guitar,
You do not play things as they are."
The man replied, "Things as they are
Are changed upon the blue guitar."
Wallace Stevens, The Man with the Blue Guitar

THE LEGACY OF PHINEAS GAGE

Contemporary research on the frontal lobes started at 4:30 P.M. on September 13, 1848, when an accidental explosion at a railroad construction site in Cavendish, Vermont hurled an iron tamping bar through the head of a 25-year-old foreman named Phineas Gage (Harlow, 1848). The tapered end of the 13.25 pound, 3.5 foot–long rod penetrated the head below the left zygomatic arch, passed behind the left eye, and exited through the calvarium, slightly right of the sagittal suture. The reconstruction of the trajectory, as published in 1868, showed that the bar must have pierced and carried away a substantial part of the frontal lobes (Fig. 2–1).

Dr. Edward H. Williams, who reached the scene 25–30 minutes after the accident, reported finding Phineas Gage spitting blood but in no apparent distress, and in the process of describing the event to incredulous bystanders who were amazed that he had walked away from such an accident (Bigelow, 1850). Joseph Adams, a local justice of the peace, submitted written testimony: "I saw him and conversed with him soon after the accident, and am of opinion that he was perfectly conscious" (Bigelow, 1850). Dr. John Harlow, summoned to attend to Gage, arrived approximately an hour later and, with Dr. Edwards' help, shaved the scalp and dressed the wound. The following day, Gage remained quite rational, and displayed an accurate recollection of the events related to the explosion. He subsequently developed a wound infection and lapsed into stupor and delirium for the next month. He then rapidly recuperated to the point where he was deemed physically and intellectually fit for work and, with the exception of blurred vision in the left eye and a slight left facial palsy, appeared none the worse for the wear.

Phineas Gage was examined by the Harvard surgeon Henry Jacob Bigelow in January 1850. Dr. Bigelow concluded that a considerable portion of the brain must have been destroyed and marveled at the sparing of function. Because of Bigelow's eminence in medical circles, Phineas Gage's condition became known as the Boston (rather than Cavendish) Crowbar Case, and the emphasis fell on the recovery. In fact, when the tamp-

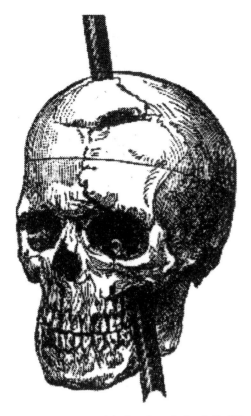

Figure 2–1. Passage of the bar through the skull of Phineas Gage, as reconstructed by Harlow in 1868 (Harlow, 1868).

ing iron was deposited to the museum at Harvard Medical School, it was beautifully engraved with the following inscription: "This is the bar that was shot through the head of M Phinehas P Gage at Cavendish Vermont Sept. 14, 1848. He fully recovered from the injuries."[1]

It appears, however, that Bigelow had been a bit premature in his pronouncements. The recovery might have been complete in the surgical sense, but not in the spiritual. Before the accident, "Gage was an ordinary sober Yankee, intelligent, a home-body, with no peculiar or bad habits."[2] The injury, however, led to a dramatic change, described in a passage that is now a classic in the annals of behavioral neurology (Harlow, 1868):

His contractors, who regarded him as the most efficient and capable foreman in their employ previous to his injury, considered the change in his mind so marked that they could not give him his place again. The equilibrium or balance, so to speak, between his intellectual faculties and animal propensities, seems to have been destroyed. He is fitful, irreverent, indulging at times in the grossest profanity (which was not previously his custom), manifesting but little deference for his fellows, impatient of restraint or advice when it conflicts with his desires, at times pertinaceously obstinate, yet capricious and vacillating, devising many plans of future operation, which are no sooner arranged than they are abandoned in turn for others appearing more feasible.

Harlow added that, to his friends, his patient was "no longer Gage."

In time, Gage became increasingly erratic, moving from one odd job to another, the first being to sit at the entrance of the Boston Museum with the tamping bar between his knees.[3] He "worked" at Barnum where he was displayed as a curiosity. He then moved to Chile and drove a six-horse stagecoach in Valparaiso. All reports comment on his chaotic career and unprovoked profanity. His final destination was San Francisco, where he suffered a fatal epileptic fit in May of 1861, more than 12 years after the accident. Harlow, who had lost contact with Gage, eventually learned of Gage's death, contacted his mother and, with the help of the mayor of San Francisco, had the grave opened in 1868. The skull was removed and delivered to Harvard for safe keeping.[4]

THE SIGNS AND SYMPTOMS

Dozens of reports published since Harlow's 1868 paper have repeatedly confirmed the pivotal lesson taught by the case of Phineas Gage—namely, that massive damage to the frontal lobes can cause dramatic changes in personality and comportment while keeping sensation, movement, consciousness, and most cognitive faculties intact. This dissociation is largely responsible for the sense of enigma and paradox that has permeated research on the human frontal lobes. During the first half of the twentieth century, the "dilemma" of the frontal lobes unfolded in the form of a dialectic between those who considered it the seat of the highest integrative functions of the human mind (Brickner, 1934; Ackerly, 1935; Goldstein, 1936) and those who commented on the paucity of deficits associated with substantial frontal lobe damage (Hebb, 1945; Landis, 1949). This controversy was gradually resolved through the emergence of insightful clinical assessment methods, sophisticated neuropsychological instruments, and a willingness to acknowledge the neurological basis of emotion and personality. By the second half of the twentieth century, the literature on this subject started to reflect a surfeit rather than paucity of deficits linked to frontal lobe damage.

Mounting evidence from comprehensive case reports, for example, began to show that many patients with frontal lobe lesions became puerile, profane, slovenly, facetious, irresponsible, grandiose, and irascible, while others lost spontaneity, curiosity, initiative, and developed an apathetic blunting of feeling, drive, attentive power, and behavior. Frontal lobe damage came to be associated with an erosion of foresight, judgment, and insight, and an inability to delay gratification or experience remorse. Some patients tended to display an impairment of abstract reasoning, hypothesis generation, creativity, problem solving, and mental flexibility; jumped to premature conclusions; and became excessively literal. The orderly planning and sequencing of complex behaviors; the ability to attend to several components simultaneously and then flexibly alter the focus of concentration; the capacity for grasping the context and gist of a complex situation; the resistance to distraction and interference; the ability to follow multistep instructions; the inhibition of immediate but inappropriate response tendencies; and the ability to sustain behavioral output without perseveration could each become markedly disrupted following frontal lobe injury. (Mesulam, 1986).

In keeping with these clinical descriptions, neuropsychological testing of patients with prefrontal damage showed quantifiable deficits in tasks of concentration (as determined by digit span), sustained information retrieval (as determined by the F-A-S task of verbal fluency), and inhibition of inappropriate responses (as determined by the Stroop, go–no go, and Trail Making B tasks). Tests of motor sequencing (Luria), mental flexibility (the Visual-Verbal Test), and hypothesis formation (the Wisconsin Card Sorting Task) were also frequently impaired (Milner, 1963, 1982 Luria, 1966; Benton, 1968; Stuss & Benson, 1984; Leimkuhler & Mesulam, 1985; Weintraub & Mesulam, 1985). In contrast, most tests of perception, construction, language, and spatial attention remained intact. Explicit memory tended to be spared except for difficulties in the organization of retrieval and recall. Many patients displayed a "task difficulty effect," whereby performance in virtually all areas began to decline rapidly when the motivation required of the patient exceeded a certain level.

Despite all these clinical findings, the dilemma of the frontal lobes appeared on the verge of being resurrected by reports of patients with sizeable frontal lobe lesions whose extensive neurological, behavioral, and neuropsychological examinations were quite unremarkable. Such cases started to lose much of their enigma, however, as it became clear that the same patient who gave exemplary answers to questions about social or moral conflicts during neuropsychological assessment could still act with a total lack of judgment when faced with the real situation, and that impeccable conduct in the office was not incompatible with major behavioral impairments in the unstructured setting of daily life.

Is there a unitary "frontal lobe syndrome" encompassing all of these signs and symptoms? Are there regional segregations of function within the frontal lobes? Is it possible to identify a potentially unifying principle of organization which cuts across the heterogeneous specializations attributed to the frontal lobes? The purpose of this review is to offer a very selective introduction to these questions.

SYNOPSIS OF BEHAVIORAL NEUROANATOMY

The 20 billion neurons of the human cerebral neocortex are spread over a surface area of 2–3 square meters which is then folded into the multiple gyri and sulci of the cerebral hemispheres (Tramo et al., 1995; Pakkenberg & Gundersen, 1997). Numerous cytoarchitectonic maps of the cerebral cortex have been published. They vary in complexity from Exner's map of more than 500 zones to the one of Bailey and von Bonin based on only 9 (Exner, 1881; Bailey & Bonin, 1951). The vast majority of investigators agree on the boundaries of primary sensory and motor cortices which, in turn, display a one-to-one correspondence between cytoarchitecture and function. Most investigators disagree on the location of boundaries within association cortex and find exceedingly few one-to-one correspondences between subregions of association cortex and specific behaviors. These are some of the reasons for espousing a functional rather than strictly cytoarchitectonic approach to the mapping of the cerebral cortex. Such an approach allows the subdivision of the cerebral cortex into five zones: primary sensory-motor, unimodal association, heteromodal association, paralimbic, and limbic (Mesulam, 2000b).

The *primary sensory-motor areas* of the cerebral cortex provide the most immediate interface with the extrapersonal environment, whereas the *limbic* areas receive almost no direct visual, auditory, or somatosensory inputs and have their most extensive affiliations with the hypothalamus and internal milieu. *Unimodal* areas provide a site for the modality-specific elaboration of sensory information, and *heteromodal* areas provide a site for the integration of inputs from more than one sensory modality. *Unimodal, heteromodal, and paralimbic* cortices serve as neural bridges between the internal and the external worlds so that the needs of the internal milieu can be discharged according to the opportunities and restrictions that prevail in the outside world. These three zones mediate the associative elaboration and encoding of sensory information, its linkage to motor strategies, and the integration of experience with drive, emotion, and visceral states.

The frontal lobes occupy almost a third of the cortical area in the human cerebral hemispheres. Each frontal lobe can be conceptualized as a pyramid containing an apex at the frontal pole, a base at the level of the central sulcus, and three external surfaces forming the lateral, medial, and orbital walls. All functional types of cortex are represented within the frontal lobes. Limbic cortex is represented in the form of an inconspicuous sliver of pyriform cortex at the most caudal end of the orbital surface; primary motor and motor association cortices are located on the lateral and dorsomedial surfaces; heteromodal cortex covers most of the lateral surface and the anterior parts of the medial and orbital surfaces; and paralimbic cortex is located on the caudal parts of the medial and orbital surfaces (Figure 2–2). The paralimbic component of the frontal lobe is continuous with the cingulate gyrus on the medial surface, and with the insula and temporal pole on the orbital surface.

The terms *prefrontal cortex* and *frontal lobe syndrome* refer almost exclusively to the paralimbic and heteromodal components of the frontal lobes. These are the only two components that will be addressed in this review. The *heteromodal* component of the frontal lobe is characterized by an isocortical architecture (high neuronal density, six layers, granular bands in layers 2 and 4). In contrast, the *paralimbic* component is characterized by a gradual architectonic transition from primitive allocortex to granular isocortex. It tends to have a lower neuronal density, less than six layers, and absent or rudimentary granular bands. The heteromodal component is known as *granular cortex* whereas the paralimbic component is known as *dysgranular* or *agranular cortex* (Mesulam, 2000b). The boundaries between these two components take the form of gradual transitions rather than abrupt shifts.

Orbitofrontal paralimbic cortex is extensively interconnected with the hypothalamus, amygdala, hippocampus, and also with other paralimbic cortices in the temporal pole, insula, parahippocampal gyrus, and cingulate gyrus (Morecraft et al., 1992; Öngür et al., 1998). The major connections of heteromodal prefrontal cortex are with the other heteromodal and unimodal cortices in the brain as well as with orbitofrontal and related paralimbic areas, especially the cingulate gyrus

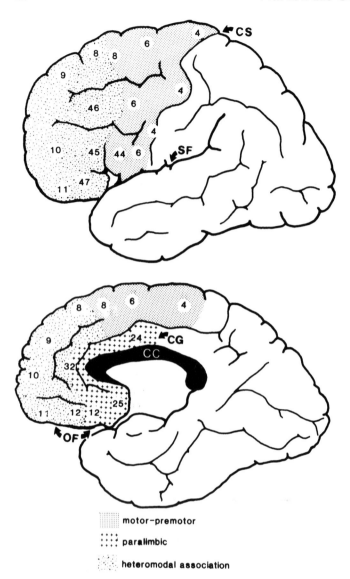

(Chavis & Pandya, 1976; Barbas & Mesulam, 1985). Compared to other heteromodal cortices in the lateral temporal and posterior parietal lobes, prefrontal heteromodal cortex appears to have more pronounced paralimbic connections, a feature that may underlie its distinctive role in integrating extensively preprocessed sensory information with limbic and visceral states.

Prefrontal cortex is also characterized by prominent subcortical projections. Its heteromodal and paralimbic components send axonal projections to the head of the caudate nucleus. With respect to the thalamus, heteromodal prefrontal cortex is interconnected with the parvocellular part of the dorsomedial nucleus, whereas paralimbic orbitofrontal cortex is interconnected mostly with the magnocellular part of the same nucleus. Paralimbic as well as heteromodal components of prefrontal cortex also receive monoaminergic and cholinergic inputs. Interfering with dopaminergic or cholinergic neurotransmission in subregions of prefrontal cortex impairs the functions of the denervated areas, highlighting the importance of these transmitters for frontal lobe function (Brozoski et al., 1979; Dias et al., 1996).

THE CANONICAL FRONTAL SYNDROMES: HETEROMODAL VERSUS PARALIMBIC

Although the literature tends to employ the term *frontal lobe syndrome* as if it referred to a unitary entity, the examination of patients with prefrontal lesions reveals numerous patterns. The specific clinical picture in an individual patient is likely to be influenced by the location of the lesion, its rate of progression, the age of onset, and perhaps even the past personality of the patient. However, two "canonical" subtypes of frontal lobe syndrome can also be identified. One is characterized by a loss of initiative, creativity, and concentration power, with a propensity for apathy and emotional blandness. This pattern can be identified as the *frontal abulic syndrome*. The second subtype is characterized by too much behavior, although the contents of behavior betray a lack of judgment, insight, and foresight. Despite intact retentive memory, patients with this second pattern of prefrontal syndrome do not seem to learn from experience and impulsively stumble from one disastrous situation into another. This can be called the *frontal disinhibition syndrome*. Patients with the *abulic syndrome* are occasionally misdiagnosed as being depressed and those with the *disinhibition syndrome* as being hypomanic.

These canonical syndromes can be illustrated with the help of two clinical vignettes. The magnetic resonance scan in Figure 2–3A belongs to a 50-year-old patent attorney of a Fortune 500 company. He complained of visual blurring and headaches. A left frontal glioma was discovered and removed. The surgery relieved the headaches and visual blurring. As he appeared fit in all physical and mental aspects, he decided to return to work. At work, he displayed his customary mastery of relevant knowledge but seemed to have lost his ability for focused concentration and concern for detail. He started to make careless errors, some of which proved very costly to his company. Reprimands were shrugged off and performance continued to be erratic. He was eventually forced to take early retirement,

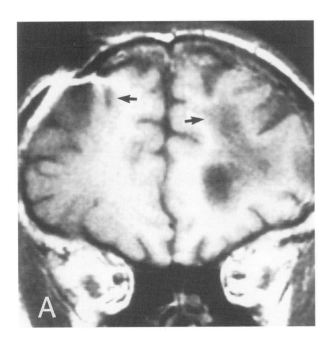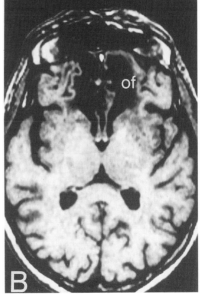

Figure 2–3. Magnetic resonance imaging scans of two patients. *A:* Coronal section through the anterior frontal lobe. The lesions (arrows) are predominantly in the heteromodal component of prefrontal cortex. *B:* Horizontal section through the orbital surface of the brain. The region that should have contained orbitofrontal cortex (of) is occupied by cerebrospinal fluid.

which he did without protesting, and seemed quite content to spend most of his time at home, watching television and helping his wife with household chores. When he last came to the clinic, he casually announced that his wife had just been diagnosed with metastatic breast cancer, but that he was not about to let this news bother him too much. This patient exemplifies the frontal abulic syndrome. His lesion was almost entirely confined to the anterior heteromodal part of the prefrontal cortex. The more posterior orbital and medial surfaces containing the paralimbic components remained quite intact, though undoubtedly disconnected from the damaged parts of heteromodal prefrontal cortex.[5]

A different clinical picture emerges in the case of a widowed woman, in her 50s, who also developed visual blurring (Figure 2–3B). An olfactory groove meningioma was discovered and removed. In the process of the neurosurgical procedure, the orbitofrontal region was extensively destroyed whereas the more dorsal heteromodal part of prefrontal cortex remained almost entirely intact. Prior to surgery, she was a conspicuously conventional woman who had been holding a steady job as an administrative assistant. After surgery, she showed very little neuropsychological impairment, even in "frontal" tests such as the Luria motor sequences, the Stroop Test, or the Wisconsin Card Sorting Test (Mesulam, 2000b). However, she started to encourage intimate encounters with perfect strangers, at least one of whom had just been released from jail. She admitted that her behavior was impulsive, and that it lacked "brakes," but neither the theft of her purse by one of her male guests nor a bout of sexually transmitted disease could curb these inappropriate impulsive behaviors. This patient displays the characteristic traits of the frontal disinhibition syndrome and shares many clinical features with Phineas Gage, whose brain injury must also have involved predominantly the orbital and medial parts of the frontal lobes (Figure 2–1).

These clinicopathological correlations are further supported by observations in nonhuman primates. Orbitofrontal lesions in monkeys, for example, lead to impulsivity and emotional hyperactivity whereas lateral frontal lesions in chimpanzees leave most basic neurological functions intact while inducing a pervasive state of apathy so that the animals spend most of the time in the middle of the cage in a state of indifference (Jacobsen, 1936; Butter & Snyder, 1972).

THE DEFAULT MODE: A STRAIGHT AND NARROW PATH FROM STIMULUS TO RESPONSE

Neither of the two canonical frontal lobe syndromes described above is associated with primary deficits of motility, sensation, or major cognitive domains, supporting the widely expressed contention that prefrontal cortex plays a predominantly "executive" rather than operational role in the control of neural function. Prefrontal lesions do not cause fixed and categorical impairments such as amnesia, prosopagnosia, or alexia. Instead, such lesions seem to promote the resurgence of behavioral tendencies that may occasionally surface in neurologically intact individuals, but that are prepotent only in developmentally more primitive stages of neural integration.

An example of such primitive behavioral tendencies is displayed by turkey hens with newly hatched broods. At this critical stage of motherhood, the hens develop an urge to attack all moving objects that fail to utter the characteristic peep of their chicks, a highly adaptive instinct for discouraging potential predators. If a turkey hen with new chicks is made deaf, however, she will attack her progeny and peck them to death. If a dominant male box turtle is placed before a mirror, it will attack its reflection and fight it from dawn to dusk or until the turtle (and its reflection) collapse from exhaustion. If a herring gull in confinement leaves her nest for momentary relief and her eggs are placed a few feet away on the sand, the returning gull will proceed to incubate the empty nest even though her eggs are in plain sight (Tinbergen, 1951; Schleidt & Schleidt, 1960; Harless, 1979). These three examples of reflexively triggered instinctive behaviors reveal the nature of a hypothetical *default mode*, a realm of neural function where inflexible stimulus-response linkages, sensitive predominantly to the internal milieu, remain impervious to modification by context or experience.

The default mode has several major characteristics. The preferred path from stimulus to response is straight and narrow, triggering automatic reactions and immediate gratification. Options for alternative interpretations or actions are not encouraged, minimizing choice or improvisation. The horizon of consciousness is confined to the here-and-now, leaving little room for hindsight or foresight. Repetitive displays of hard-wired responses are promoted even when they do not fit the prevailing context. Appearance cannot be differentiated from significance: whatever glitters *is* gold. Although the default mode is most conspicuous in submammalian species, the laws of evolution suggest that it should remain represented, perhaps in latent form, in the central nervous system (CNS) of more advanced species as well.

The rest of this review will attempt to show that frontal lobe damage allows a resurgence of the default mode and that the principal physiological function of prefrontal cortex is to suppress and transcend this mode by enabling neuronal responses to become contingent rather than obligatory. This influence of prefrontal cortex is manifested through five core functions: 1) working memory and related attentional processes; 2) the inhibition of distractibility, perseveration and immediate gratification 3) The active pursuit of choice and novelty; 4) the conditional mapping of emotional significance; and 5) the encoding of context, perspective, and mental relativism.

WORKING MEMORY: SELECTIVE EXPANSION OF CONSCIOUSNESS BEYOND THE HERE-AND-NOW

The flow of ambient information greatly exceeds the real-time processing capacity of any CNS (Broadbent, 1958; Baddeley, 1996). It is therefore necessary to postulate the existence of neural systems that selectively focus awareness on behaviorally relevant events while holding potentially distracting stimuli at bay. *Attention* is a generic term used to designate the entire family of neural operations serving this purpose (Mesulam, 2000a). Experiments in monkeys and humans indicate that prefrontal cortex plays a critical role in nearly all such functions, including divided attention, sustained attention, and especially working memory (Pardo et al., 1991; Johannsen et al., 1997; Mesulam, 2000a). *Working memory* constitutes one of the most distinctive specializations of prefrontal cortex. It is an attentional function that enables the on-line holding and mental manipulation of information. Working memory transforms information access from a sequential and disjunctive process, where only one event cluster can be heeded at any given instant, to a conjunctive pattern where several selected clusters can become incorporated into the stream of consciousness (Fig. 2–4).

The critical relevance of the primate prefrontal cortex to working memory was first demonstrated in the course of *delayed-response tasks.* In these experiments, the animal watches food being placed under one of two cups. An opaque screen is then lowered and held there for an interval of seconds to minutes during which the animal has to keep the relevant information in working memory so that it can choose the correct cup when the screen is lifted. Chimpanzees and monkeys with dorsolateral prefrontal lesions are severely impaired in this task (Jacobsen, 1936; Goldman & Rosvold, 1970). In a variant of this task, known as the *delayed matching to sample test,* a monkey is first shown a sample stimulus, exposed to a variable delay, and rewarded for responding to a test stimulus only if it matches the sample. The crucial component is the delay period (up to 20 seconds in these experiments), during which the animal has to maintain a mental, on-line representation of a stimulus that is behaviorally relevant but no longer part of ambient reality. Lateral prefrontal neurons emit sustained responses during delay periods as if prolonging the impact of the stimulus or anticipating its reappearance (Desimone, 1996). These neurons also participate in the on-line maintenance of *convergent* information belonging to different modalities.

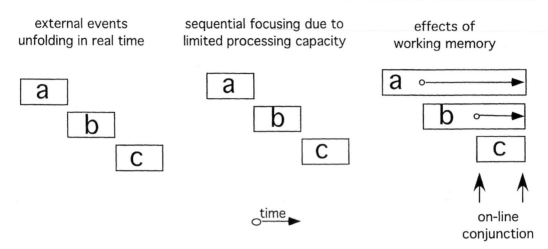

Figure 2–4. Diagrammatic illustration of working memory. The column on the *left* illustrates the real-time unfolding of three events. The *middle* column shows what would have happened to the mental representation of these three events in the absence of working memory. The column on the *right* depicts the contribution of working memory. The horizontal arrows reflect the on-line holding of information.

In one experiment, for example, monkeys were required to retain first the identity of an object and then its location. After having retained object information in the initial delay, many prefrontal neurons switched modes and conveyed spatial information in the second delay (Rao et al., 1997). Prefrontal lesions can disrupt delay activity in the sensory association area corresponding to the modality of stimulus presentation, indicating that prefrontal cortex exerts a top-down (executive) influence on working memory in other parts of the brain (Fuster et al., 1985; Desimone, 1996).

The relevance of the human prefrontal cortex to working memory was confirmed by functional imaging in 1973 when Risberg and Ingvar found that digit span tasks yielded hemodynamic activations in the lateral frontal lobes (Risberg & Ingvar, 1973). Since then, numerous imaging studies have reported lateral prefrontal activation during working memory tasks based on verbal, perceptual, and spatial stimuli (Petrides et al., 1993; D'Esposito et al., 1995; Cohen et al., 1997; LaBar et al., 1999). In the *2-back task*, for example, the subject is shown a string of letters, one letter at a time, and is asked to press a button if the letter is identical to the one that came before the immediately preceding one.

This is a demanding task and requires the on-line holding of at least two bits of information at any given time. Successful performance in this task leads to robust activation in lateral heteromodal prefrontal cortex with a center of gravity in the middle frontal gyrus (LaBar et al., 1999). An even more demanding task, based on the ability to keep one goal in mind while pursuing another, also leads to selective activation within lateral heteromodal prefrontal cortex (Koechlin et al., 1999). As in the case of the monkey, the human lateral prefrontal cortex has also been shown to mediate the convergent on-line holding of multimodal information (Prabhakaran et al., 2000). In keeping with these findings based on functional imaging, patients with lateral prefrontal lesions show profound impairments of working memory—they are impaired in tasks of delayed response (Freedman & Oscar-Berman, 1986), they cannot hold information on-line, and they have difficulty maintaining a coherent stream of thought.

Daily activities that range from keeping a telephone number in mind to considering alternative facets of a moral dilemma rely on working memory. In the clinic, working memory is most readily tested with the *digit span task*. In this task, the ability to hear and then repeat a string of numbers requires the on-line holding of information, while the ability to repeat the numbers in reverse requires a manipulation of the internalized information. The "on-line holding" aspect of working memory is likely to play an important role in shifting the focus of attention from external events to their internal representations. This is an essential ingredient of the phenomenon commonly identified as thinking. The other aspect of working memory, the "manipulation" of the on-line information, is likely to play an important role in the volitional scanning and reorganization of mental content, explaining why patients with prefrontal lesions have prominent difficulties in tasks of verbal fluency and memory retrieval. These two aspects of working memory collectively enable the contents of consciousness to be selected deliberately rather than set reflexively (in a stimulus-bound mode) by events in the environment.

Working memory can be said to enrich the texture of consciousness by prolonging the impact of selected components of experience beyond the here-and-now. It would also seem to play a major role in determining how many channels of information can be handled in parallel. The span of working memory could be likened to the number of balls that a juggler can hold in the air. Simple nervous systems based on the default mode of neural functioning can handle only one ball at a time, and even that one is not thrown very far. In contrast, the working memory capacity of the human brain allows multiple balls to be held up in the air at any given time so that thought can reflect the contributions of multiple processing streams. There are undoubtedly great interindividual variations in the capacity for working memory. A most remarkable example is provided by Julius Caesar, who is said to have had the ability to dictate on different topics to three scribes at the same time (Tucker, 1765).

DISTRACTIBILITY, PERSEVERATION AND DISINHIBITION

An automatic orientation toward salient events, regardless of their relevance to current goals, and a tendency to repeat the same responses even when they have outlived their usefulness are two characteristic features of the default mode. The resultant distractibility and perseveration are ubiquitous in the behavior of animals, children, and adults with brain disease. The inhibition of distractibility and perseveration, appears to require the integrity of prefrontal cortex.

In a delayed matching-to-sample A●B●C●D●A paradigm of working memory, for example, a prefrontal neuron known to emit a selective delay activity following the presentation of A, continues to show high delay activity after B, C, and D and maintains it until the reappearance of A (Desimone, 1996). Prefrontal neurons may therefore play a critical role in protecting on-line information from interference by distractors. In human subjects, the requirement to ignore distractors during target detection leads to the activation of the anterior cingulate, medial prefrontal, and lateral prefrontal cortices (Coull, 1998). Nearly identical areas are activated by the *Stroop Test*, when subjects must state the color in which the word is written while suppressing the distracting tendency to read the word itself (Brown et al., 1999). In keeping with these functional imaging experiments, patients with frontal lobe lesions display a marked increase in distractibility (Chao & Knight, 1995).

The vulnerability to perseveration can be probed through the *go no-go task*, where the subject is asked to respond to one type of stimulus while suppressing responses to another. Tumors in the medial prefrontal region interfere with the inhibition of inappropriate responses during no-go trials, a deficit that can be reversed upon removal of the tumor (Leimkuhler & Mesulam, 1985). Functional imaging in neurologically intact subjects shows that response inhibition in the no go trials is associated with activation in the medial prefrontal cortex as well as in the heteromodal prefrontal cortex of the inferior frontal sulcus (Konishi et al., 1999). This multifocal distribution of activation helps to explain why so many different kinds of prefrontal lesions lead to disinhibition and perseveration. Perseverative tendencies in patients with prefrontal lesions interfere with the acquisition of nonrepetitive sequential behaviors such as those required by the "palm-fist-edge" task of Luria. In other patients, disinhibition undermines the ability to suppress inappropriate behaviors that lead to immediate gratification. In monkeys, inferofrontal/orbitofrontal lesions lead to errors of commission in go–no go tasks and to perseverative errors during reversal learning when previously rewarded and neutral stimuli switch contingencies (Iversen & Mishkin, 1970). In keeping with these results, the suppression of the perseverative tendency to look at a distracting stimulus during an anti-saccade task is associated with lateral prefrontal neuronal activity (Funahashi et al., 1993).

The area of lateral prefrontal cortex activated during the inhibition of responses on no-go trials overlaps with the area activated during category shifts in the Wisconsin Card Sorting Test (Konishi et al., 1999). This finding implies that category shifts may be dependent upon the suppression of perseverative responses so that new hypotheses can be explored. This is in keeping with clinical experience in which patients with prefrontal lesions display major impairments in the Wisconsin Card Sorting Test, mostly because of perseveration and lack of mental flexibility in exploring new sorting criteria (Milner, 1963). This impairment of mental flexibility may also be responsible for the poor performance of such patients in the *Visual–Verbal Test*, where a previously successful sorting strategy must be relinquished and replaced by a partially overlapping alternative.

The relationship of prefrontal cortex to working memory, inhibition, and hypothesis testing underscores the importance of this region for complex reasoning processes such as those that can be probed with *Kuhn's plant problem* (Kuhn & Brannock, 1977). In this problem, the subject is shown pictures of four plants, two of which look healthy and two unhealthy. Each plant has been cared for with one of two different regimens of plant food, watering, and leaf lotion. The goal is to identify which of the three variables is critical for growing a healthy plant. A successful resolution of the problem requires working memory, hypothesis generation, the parallel considera-

tion of multiple variables, the suppression of perseverative inferences, and the inhibition of distractibility by irrelevant cues. Patients with bifrontal lesions acquired early in life have considerable difficulties solving this problem (Price et al., 1990).

NOVELTY, UNCERTAINTY, AND CHOICE

A preference for sameness and uniformity is a property of the default mode and promotes behaviors that can be described as stimulus-bound or stereotyped. The antitheses of this tendency, novelty seeking and playfulness, are inconspicuous in amphibians and reptiles, emerge in birds, and reach their most exuberant expression in advanced mammals, especially primates. Monkeys will work hard in a setting where the only reward is a brief peek through a window, and human subjects who are given a choice between familiar and novel patterns will consistently spend more time viewing the latter (Butler, 1953; Berlyne, 1960). Prefrontal cortex seems to play an essential role in novelty seeking. The P300 elicited by novel, changing, or deviant stimuli, for example, is critically dependent on the integrity of prefrontal cortex, and an N200–P300 response that is maximal over prefrontal cortex appears to determine the attentional resources that will voluntarily be allocated to novel events (Knight, 1984; Daffner et al., 2000). In keeping with these relationships, task-related prefrontal activation decreases significantly as the task becomes more familiar (Raichle et al., 1994). These aspects of frontal lobe function may help to explain why prefrontal lesions lead to apathy and also why patients with such lesions are disproportionately impaired when facing novel situations (Godefroy & Rousseaux, 1997; Daffner et al., 2000).

The default mode of neural function does not tolerate much choice or uncertainty. Prefrontal neurons are sensitive to both of these behavioral parameters. In the monkey, for example, lateral prefrontal neurons can encode the certainty (or uncertainty) with which a cue predicts the outcome of a subsequent response (Quintana & Fuster, 1999). In humans, guessing behaviors, where stimulus–response linkages are maximally unconstrained and where choice and doubt are accentuated, give rise to prominent orbitofrontal activation (Elliott et al., 1999). Furthermore, greater activation of lateral prefrontal cortex has been reported when actions are selected by voluntary choice than when externally specified (Rowe et al., 2000).

These relationships to novelty seeking and choice suggest that prefrontal cortex belongs to a neural circuit that transcends the one-to-one relationship between stimulus and response in favor of a one-to-many setting that tolerates a greater diversity of outcome. In almost all other animals, genetic factors constrain behavioral domains such as those involved in dietary preferences, methods of communication, courting displays, and affiliative interactions. The situation is drastically different in humans, where thousands of languages have been invented to express the same thoughts, thousands of cuisines to satisfy the same hunger, and thousands of diversions to dissipate the same boredom. An ability to tolerate and seek novelty underlies this uniquely human aptitude for discovering multiple solutions to similar problems, a faculty that greatly accelerates adaptation to rapidly changing circumstances (Mesulam, 2000c).

EMOTIONAL COLORING OF ACTION, EXPERIENCE, AND DECISION MAKING

In the reptilian and amphibian CNS, sensory areas are monosynaptically interconnected with the limbic system so that perception becomes colored with emotion at the very initial stages of neural processing. A byproduct of this arrangement, and a chief characteristic of the default mode, is to promote rigid stimulus–response linkages where the salient sensory features of a primary reinforcer trigger automatic responses energized by the prevailing motivational state. The primate CNS introduces a greater degree of flexibility by inserting intervening synapses between sensory and limbic areas, as if to prevent actions from being dominated by limbic imperatives, but then resorts to very complicated multisynaptic

circuitry for integrating experience with emotion, ensuring, however, that one is not overwhelmed by the other (Mesulam, 1998).

Prefrontal cortex appears to play a principal role in this multisynaptic integration of emotion with action and experience. Although all of prefrontal cortex participates in this process, its paralimbic components display a closer affiliation with emotion and related aspects of visceral function. In functional imaging experiments, for example, neural activity in orbitofrontal cortex varies according to the hedonic valence of sensory experience and the magnitude of reward or punishment (Blair et al., 1999; Rolls, 2000). The lateral part of orbitofrontal cortex seems more closely related to punishment whereas its medial part seems more closely related to reward (O'Doherty et al., 2001; Small et al., 2001). Furthermore, attending to the attractiveness or emotional expressiveness of faces yields a relatively selective activation of inferior frontal and orbitofrontal cortex (Nakamura et al., 1999).

In the monkey, single-unit recordings show that the majority of orbitofrontal neurons are sensitive to reward (Hikosaka & Watanabe, 2000). The anticipation of a raisin, for example, elicited brisk orbitofrontal activation during the delay period on trials in which the animal subsequently consumed the reward but not on trials where satiety led to the refusal of the raisin (Hikosaka & Watanabe, 2000). These neurons are thus more responsive to the motivational valence of an anticipated reward than to its identity. In contrast, lateral heteromodal prefrontal cortex contains neurons that are also sensitive to the identity of the reward and the cues with which they have become associated (Watanabe, 1996). It appears, therefore, that orbitofrontal neurons encode the hedonic valence of anticipated experiences, whereas the lateral prefrontal neurons may also encode the cognitive categorization of such experiences and their arbitrary associations (Hikosaka & Watanabe, 2000).

Through its amygdaloid and hypothalamic connections, orbitofrontal cortex can modulate the visceral correlates of emotion. Electrical stimulation of orbitofrontal cortex, for example, causes major changes in blood pressure, heart rate, vascular tone, gastric secretions, and respiratory rate (Kaada et al., 1949; Pool & Ransohoff, 1949; Kaada, 1960; Oppenheimer et al., 1992). These visceral manifestations can mediate the influence of emotions upon thought, experience and action (Mandler, 1962). Patients with damage to the ventromedial components of prefrontal cortex, for example, fail to produce an anticipatory visceral response just prior to making risky decisions in a task in which the winning long-term strategy is based on resisting oversized short-term gains (Bechara et al., 1997). The absence of the anticipatory visceral activation in these patients is associated with a perseverative impulse to seek immediate gratification even when subsequent questioning reveals that they realize this to be a disadvantageous strategy (Bechara et al., 1997). The ventromedial prefrontal damage in these patients presumably disengages decision making from the restraining influence of the anticipatory visceral reaction or "gut feeling." This disengagement seems to allow the short-term imperatives of the default mode to preempt adaptive long-term planning.

Prefrontal damage tends to disrupt the contingent rather than constitutive aspects of emotion and motivation. Thus, patients with frontal lobe damage have no major change in appetite but may become less discriminating in their food preferences; prefrontal lobotomy does not alter the threshold for withdrawing from painful stimuli but blunts the concern for the pain. In monkeys, orbitofrontal or anterior cingulate lesions result in marked alterations of emotional responsivity: the animals do not lose the capacity for the emotion but lose the ability to match its intensity to the significance of the triggering event (Smith, 1944; Butter & Snyder, 1972).

As noted above, heteromodal prefrontal cortex plays a critical role in working memory. The object of working memory need not be confined to numbers, places, or words. Emotion itself could conceivably become the object of working memory for on-line holding and manipulation, allowing the emotional impact of an event to be extended beyond its real-time evolution. Such on-line holding and mental manipulation of an emotion would increase its associative depth and synaptic reverberation. Through such processes, prefrontal cortex would be expected to play an important role in the genesis of complex moral and civic emotions. Prefrontal lesions on the other hand, would be expected to promote a state of emotional shallowness interspersed with stimulus-bound emotional outbursts.

SIGNIFICANCE, CONTEXT AND AMBIGUITY

The behavioral repertoire of primates requires an adaptation to a complex reality where the same cue may signal reward in one context but not in another and where the same stimulus may elicit one response in one setting but a different one in another. This aspect of behavioral flexibility requires neural mechanisms that can encode arbitrary stimulus-response contingencies and their experience-dependent temporal fluctuations. Two pivotal experiments illustrate the relevance of prefrontal cortex to these aspects of encoding.

In one of these, a monkey was first taught to respond to red objects (circles or crosses), but to withhold responding to green objects (circles or crosses). At this stage, some lateral prefrontal neurons gave a much brisker response to the green circles and crosses. The animal was subsequently taught a different contingency in which it had to respond to circles (green or red), but withhold responding to crosses (green or red). At this second stage, the same lateral prefrontal neurons that had previously given a muted response to the red cross (when it was the go signal) gave vigorous responses to the identical cue, now that it had become the no-go signal (Sagakami & Niki, 1994). It appears, therefore, that the primate prefrontal cortex contains the sort of neuron that would be necessary for differentiating appearance from significance, and for realizing that glitter and gold need not overlap. Through the intercession of such neurons, the control of behavior could be liberated from a small set of genetically determined primary reinforcers and transferred to a much larger set of higher-order markers whose relationship to the primary reinforcers can undergo experience-induced modifications.

In another experiment, distinctive visual patterns predicted the delivery of raisin, apple, or cereal rewards. During any given session, the monkey could be receiving one of two types of reward (raisin versus apple or apple versus cereal), each reward being signaled by a specific visual cue. In one animal that fancied raisins the most and cereal the least, the cue that predicted a piece of apple elicited a much brisker response from the same orbitofrontal neuron when the apple reward was paired with the cereal reward than when it was paired with the raisin reward (Tremblay & Schultz, 1999). This sort of neuron appears to encode the way in which context alters the relative significance of a secondary reinforcer, even when its linkage to the primary reinforcer remains unchanged.

An elegant experiment reported in 1974 had already demonstrated the role of the human prefrontal cortex in encoding the influence of context. In this experiment, subjects were shown a set of either three letters or three numbers and were asked to read the members of each set as rapidly as possible. The font was chosen so that one of the stimuli was ambiguous and could be read either as a "B" when it was presented as a letter or as "13" when it was presented as a number. This same stimulus was found to elicit differential evoked potentials in the frontal lobe when it was read as a letter as opposed to a number (Johnston & Chesney, 1974). In contrast, visual cortex in the occipital lobe gave identical responses to this stimulus, regardless of how it was being read. This notable result indicates that occipital cortex is sensitive to the surface sensory properties of visual stimuli, whereas prefrontal cortex is also sensitive to the way in which context alters their meaning.

The encoding of context necessitates the parallel processing of multiple considerations related to the target event and its background. This sort of process becomes particularly critical in guiding behavior under "ambiguous" conditions where there are no absolutely correct choices; When shown "ambiguous" ad-

vertisements that contained literal as well as implied messages, for example, patients with prefrontal lesions could not infer the less obvious nonliteral meaning (Pearce et al., 1998). Furthermore, patients with frontal lobe lesions performed more poorly than control subjects in realworld financial planning tasks in which there were no absolute right or wrong answers and numerous ambiguous variables needed to be considered in concert (Goel et al., 1997). The impairment of humor appreciation that has been described in patients with frontal lobe lesions (Shammi & Stuss, 1999) may also reflect, at least in part, the inability to detect nonliteral inferences and contextual incongruities. Furthermore, certain types of prefrontal lesions can lead to florid confabulations (Moscovitch, 1995), probably because they interfere with the ability to determine contextual plausibility during memory retrieval.

The experiments described in this section also suggest that prefrontal cortex is likely to play a crucial role in abstract thinking in which a literal (stimulus-bound) association needs to be resisted in favor of a less obvious inference implied by the context. Prefrontal damage frequently triggers a stimulus-bound state in which thinking becomes concrete and behavior is guided by the surface properties of events in the environment. One of our patients, for example, slavishly complied with solicitations for magazine subscription she received in the mail, and felt compelled to read aloud all signs and billboards she encountered in the streets. Such stimulus-bound behaviors lead to a phenomenon that has been termed the *environmental dependency syndrome* by Lhermitte (Lhermitte, 1986; Lhermitte et al., 1986). In eliciting the manifestations of this syndrome, Lhermitte employed a less structured setting than is customarily used for neuropsychological assessment. The lack of specific instruction, the ambiguity of the context, and the method of open-ended observation allowed him to show that patients with large prefrontal lesions display a remarkable stimulus-bound tendency to imitate the examiner's gestures and behaviors even when no instruction had been given to do so, and even when this imitation entailed considerable personal embarrassment. Furthermore, the mere sight of an object was shown to elicit the compulsion to use it, although the patient had not been asked to do so and the context was inappropriate—as in the case of the housewife who saw a tongue depressor and proceeded to give Professor Lhermitte a medical checkup. In these patients, an excessive dependency on the immediate environment led to stereotyped responses that ignored the incongruity of context. Prefrontal lesions can thus cause thoughts and actions to fall under the control of external stimuli in ways that interfere with behavioral flexibility and individual autonomy (free will).

SWITCHING PERSPECTIVES AND MENTAL RELATIVISM

In the default mode, events tend to be assessed from an egocentric perspective so that the horizon of consciousness does not extend beyond the here-and-now and the self is the center around which other events revolve. One way to transcend the default mode would be to transpose the effective reference point from self to other, from here to there, and from now to then, so that the same event can be apprehended from multiple vantage points, each generating its own set of considerations. Prefrontal cortex may play a pivotal role in these hypothetical transformations. In *Flavell's role-taking task*, for example, a subject is shown a map and asked to detect ambiguities in directions being given to a fictitious traveler who is trying to reach a specific house on the map (Flavell, 1968). In the first phase of the test, the fictitious traveler and the subject share an identical spatial perspective. In the second, the traveler has a different initial location so that the subject needs to assume the spatial perspective of the traveler. Patients with early-acquired frontal lobe disease do well in the first phase but not in the second, suggesting that the ability to apprehend events from a non-egocentric spatial perspective may be impaired (Price et al., 1990).

Prefrontal cortex could conceivably also mediate shifts in time, rather than space, so that intended actions and their consequences can be apprehended from a vantage point in the future. As noted above, prefrontal neurons in monkeys fire in anticipation of reward, as if a future reality were being previewed (Hikosaka & Watanabe, 2000). In humans, functional imaging shows that premotor (and perhaps prefrontal) cortex participates in the estimation of temporal intervals (Coull & Nobre, 1998), suggesting that this part of the brain may shift awareness into an inferred future. The ability to shift vantage points into the future so as to predict potential consequences of contemplated behaviors would provide the essential ingredients for planning, sequencing, and foresight, faculties that become severely impaired in patients with prefrontal damage.

A third sort of putative shift of perspective entails the ability to enter someone else's shoes and to surmise what that other person might think and feel in response to specific events and actions.[6] Circumstantial evidence implicates prefrontal cortex in the mediation of these "psychological" shifts of perspective as well. For example, the ability to read others' minds or to infer their reactions, intentions, and feelings becomes impaired by prefrontal lesions whereas tasks that require such inferences lead to the activation of medial prefrontal cortex (Stone et al., 1998; Blair & Cipolotti, 2000; Castelli et al., 2000; Gallagher et al., 2000). Interpersonal skills, judgment, socially appropriate comportment, and moral conduct are at least partially dependent on the ability to transcend an egocentric point of view and to regulate behaviors according to their inferred impact on the feelings and reactions of significant others. In the absence of this faculty, compassion, empathy, and conscience may fail to develop, giving rise to the characteristic insensitive behaviors, callous amorality, and sociopathic behaviors of patients with prefrontal disease. Such deficits are particularly pronounced if prefrontal damage is acquired early in life or centered in orbitofrontal cortex (Price et al., 1990; Anderson et al., 1999; Blair & Cipolotti, 2000).

The neural computations that are likely to mediate perspective shifts would be expected to depend on a state of mental relativism where multiple representations of the same event can be tolerated. The capacity for realizing that such multiple representations (for example, the self and its reflection in the mirror) constitute alternative manifestations of the same basic phenomenon is not automatic. Turtles, for example, will attack their own reflection in the mirror; only specially trained monkeys give any sign of rudimentary self-recognition in front of a mirror; and many demented patients will react to their reflections as if they were intruders (Ajuriaguerra et al., 1963; Harless, 1979; Gallup et al., 1980; Hauser et al., 1995). The tolerance of multiple representations may have necessitated the evolution of a critical mass of neurons, such as those in prefrontal cortex, with no obligatory role in routine sensory, skeletomotor, or autonomic function. These neurons would have developed the sort of flexible (discretionary) firing contingencies that could mediate the encoding of multiple representations. One by-product of such a development would be the emergence of an observing self who becomes differentiated from the sensory flux of ambient events and who can therefore intentionally reflect on experience (Mesulam, 1998). Such a capacity for introspection may have generated first the sense of a "commenting self" separate from the experiencing body, then the belief that others also have commenting selves, and, ultimately, that these other commenting selves believe that others also have commenting selves. This is the sort of representational amplification that would be necessary to sustain the shifts of perspective described above, especially those that mediate the ability to experience the world through the eyes, thoughts, and feelings of others.

Is it possible to identify shifts of psychological perspective in nonhuman primates? The premotor cortex of monkeys contains "mirror neurons" that respond both when the animal performs a particular action and when it observes the same action being performed by another animal. The suggestion has been made that these neurons provide precursors of the neural circuitry that allows the reading of other minds (Gallese & Goldman, 1998).

Monkeys are social animals. Their interactions rely on token aggressive and submissive displays, mutual grooming behaviors, and vocalizations. Social success depends on directing the proper behavior to the proper individual in the proper context, presumably based on some awareness of how these behaviors influence conspecifics. Monkeys with orbitofrontal lesions show a severe disruption of these affiliative behaviors and eventually become ostracized into social isolation (Kling & Steklis, 1976). Careful observation in a naturalistic setting is necessary for detecting such alterations since these animals may show few, if any, abnormalities in the structured setting of the laboratory. These experiments provide an animal model for the socially maladaptive behaviors seen after frontal lobe damage and support the contention that these aberrant behaviors are more likely to emerge after damage to the paralimbic component of the frontal lobe. These experiments also support the clinical adage that the consequences of prefrontal lesions become particularly conspicuous in naturalistic settings where behavioral guidelines are ambiguous.

FRONTAL LOBE VERSUS FRONTAL NETWORK SYNDROME

Dorsolateral prefrontal cortex belongs to a neural circuit that includes posterior parietal cortex, the head of the caudate nucleus, and the dorsomedial thalamic nucleus. Orbitofrontal cortex, on the other hand, functions as a component of a paralimbic ring that includes the cingulate gyrus, parahippocampal cortex, the temporal pole, and the insula. Prefrontal cortex could thus be conceptualized as a site of confluence for two partially overlapping and interconnected networks—a ventromedially located limbic system with its well-known relationships to emotion, motivation, memory, and visceral function; and a more dorsolateral frontoparietal system subserving working memory and related cognitive processes.

All complex behavioral domains are coordinated by large-scale distributed networks. The performance of a relevant task engages all components of the pertinent network, and damage to any network component can impair behavior in the relevant domain (Mesulam, 1990). The prefrontal networks follow these principles of organization. In addition to dorsolateral prefrontal cortex, for example, the N-back working memory task also leads to the activation of posterior parietal cortex, the caudate nucleus and the dorsomedial thalamic nucleus (LaBar et al., 1999). Furthermore, working memory tasks modulate the coherence between prefrontal and parietal activity, suggesting that the collaboration of these two areas is essential for performance (Diwadkar et al., 2000). In keeping with this organization, the manifestations of the frontal lobe syndrome, especially those aspects related to abulia, working memory, and other executive functions, can also arise after damage either to the caudate nucleus or to the dorsomedial thalamic nucleus (Richfield et al., 1987; Mendez et al., 1989; Sandson et al., 1991). Although these same signs and symptoms can also result from posterior parietal lesions, the verbal and visuospatial impairments of the parietal syndrome dominate the clinical picture of such patients.

A circumstance of considerable interest is the emergence of the frontal lobe syndrome as a consequence of multifocal white matter disease or metabolic encephalopathy (Wolfe et al., 1990; Mesulam, 2000a). Assuming that a major physiological function of the frontal lobe is the top-down or executive modulation of other networks, the emergence of the frontal lobe syndrome should come as no surprise in these cases, where multifocal partial lesions (none of which are individually severe enough to disrupt specific cognitive domains such as language or memory) collectively undermine internetwork coordination. In clinical practice, multifocal lesions and toxic–metabolic encephalopathies are more frequently encountered causes of the frontal lobe syndrome than lesions directly involving prefrontal cortex. A diagnosis of "frontal network syndrome" rather than "frontal lobe syndrome" may therefore prevent considerable confusion by acknowledging that the responsible lesion could be located anywhere within this distributed network.

OVERVIEW AND SUMMARY

Prefrontal cortex enjoys an exalted ontogenetic and phylogenetic status. It is nearly unidentifiable in subprimate species and reaches its greatest relative size in the human. Even in the human, prefrontal cortex does not fully mature, either physiologically or structurally, until approximately mid-adolescence (Diamond & Doar, 1989; Huttenlocher & Dabholkar, 1997; Luciana & Nelson, 1998). In keeping with these developmental patterns, prefrontal cortex appears to sit at the apex of behavioral hierarchies. Phineas Gage, for example, showed that prefrontal cortex is not all that necessary for enjoying the circus, driving a stagecoach, circumnavigating the globe, recalling yesterday's events, or communicating with others. It would seem that prefrontal cortex assumes a critical role only for behaviors that require the highest levels of mental integration.

Many cortical areas in the human brain are devoted to the modality-specific representation of events, faces, words, and locations. Others mediate the transmodal binding of these representations so that faces can lead to recognition, words to comprehension, intentions to actions, events to memories (Mesulam, 1998). Focal brain lesions that interfere with these processing streams lead to disconnection syndromes such as apraxia, prosopagnosia, color anomia, amnesia, and so on (Geschwind, 1965; Mesulam, 2000b). Prefrontal cortex is not essential for encoding any of these representations and is not implicated in the pathogenesis of any traditional disconnection syndrome. Damage to prefrontal cortex leads to a distinctive set of impairments that are context-dependent (contingent) rather than categorical. The manifestations of prefrontal damage become particularly prominent when the environment contains distractors; when ambiguity and conflict are high; when appearance and significance are at odds; when events must be interpreted in light of contextual peculiarities; when prepotent response tendencies must be restrained for some long-term purpose; when decision trees have multiple branches; and when the egocentric point of view must be transcended.

Prefrontal cortex regulates the selection, timing, monitoring, and interpretation of behavior rather than the formation of the constituent percepts and movements. Prefrontal cortex is consequently said to provide the critical substrate for executive functions through the top-down modulation of other neural systems in the brain. This top-down modulation is exerted through widespread prefrontal connections that are in a position to activate a given network, inhibit another, influence network combinations, and perhaps even allow anticipatory readouts of contemplated actions. Prefrontal cortex could thus enable the highest level of internal representation (of networks rather than of sensory data or motor programs) and provide an arena for the various networks to play out different scenarios.

In most other parts of the brain, regional specializations can be designated by single terms such as *language, vision, spatial attention, face perception,* and so on. No single term is yet available to encompass all the specializations attributed to prefrontal cortex. Perhaps the problem lies in the fact that prefrontal cortex contains different subareas with different specializations; perhaps a unitary functional designation will emerge with more research; or perhaps no unitary designation will be established, even for individual cytoarchitectonic subsectors or topographical regions of prefrontal cortex.

This review has resorted to the pedagogical practice of proposing a unified functional specialization for prefrontal cortex by contrasting it to a hypothetical antithesis designated the *default mode.* The influence of the default mode, as defined in this review, becomes prominent in species that lack prefrontal cortex, during infancy when prefrontal cortex is not yet fully developed, and in adult primates with prefrontal lesions. In this mode of neural function, the path from stimulus to response is short, appearance and significance overlap, familiarity and repetition are promoted, and the horizon of consciousness is confined to the here-and-now of an egocentric perspective. Events in the default mode lead to automatic, predetermined, and obligatory responses without allowing much neuronal space for

thought, foresight, choice, innovation, or interpretation.

Nearly all functional affiliations attributed to prefrontal cortex can be conceptualized as attempts to constrain or transcend the influence of the default mode and its stimulus-bound style of responding to the environment. Working memory allows the contents of awareness to be chosen deliberately rather than set reflexively by ambient events; voluntary shifts of perspective allow the horizon of consciousness to transcend the egocentric vantage point; the suppression of perseveration promotes choice, improvisation, and hypothesis generation; the arbitrary and reversible linkage of emotional valence to secondary reinforcers allows a differentiation of appearance from significance; the ability to inhibit prepotent tendencies helps to establish a state in which the translation of emotions into action and of thoughts into words can be restrained when necessary; and the capacity for the parallel processing of multiple variables enables the encoding of contextual relativity and the realization that things are not always what they seem to be.

One common denominator, if one can be found, is the insertion of a neural buffer between stimulus and response in a way that delays closure so that weaker associations and alternative responses can be considered. The outcome is a mental relativism in which each event can evoke multiple scripts and scenarios that can then compete for access to thought and behavior. These processes rely on contingent rather than obligatory encoding so as to promote the inferential, pragmatic, and interpretive aspects of mental function.

Despite considerable advances in this field of research, it is difficult to dismiss the sense of uniqueness associated with frontal lobe function. It is quite remarkable, for example, that sizeable frontal lobe lesions can remain clinically silent for many years. Even after massive bifrontal lesions in monkeys, chimpanzees, and humans, change can often be detected only in comparison with the previous personality of that individual rather than in reference to any set of absolute behavioral standards. In fact, many of the alterations associated with prefrontal lesions appear to overlap with the range of normal human behavior. For example, while similar behaviors do emerge after frontal lobe lesions, there is also a vast number of improvident, irresponsible, immoral, and facetious individuals who have no evidence of demonstrable brain damage. In contrast, the lack of visible damage to the pertinent cerebral area is a rare occurrence in individuals with aphasia, amnesia, apraxia, or unilateral neglect. This is in keeping with the contention that prefrontal cortex underlies functions that are much less "hard wired" and that it acts predominantly as an orchestrator for integrating other cortical areas and for calling up behavior programs that are appropriate for context. Damage to this part of the brain would thus result in behavioral deficits that are context-dependent rather than static.

There have been numerous attempts to capture the astounding feats of the human brain in comparison to technological artifacts. Hydraulics, switchboards, servo-mechanisms, silicone chips, and massively parallel supercomputer networks have each been invoked to model brain activity. Some of these analogies have been quite helpful in shaping the investigation of movement, perception, attention, language, memory, and even chess playing. Prefrontal cortex has been more resistant to this sort of analysis. With the exception of working memory (where the linkage to random access memory has been made), it is hard to find an adequate technological tool that can model the functions of prefrontal cortex. In the absence of such a model, one could invoke a somewhat fanciful analogy from the field of sculpture. Statues can start either as mounds of clay that are molded into the desired shape or as blocks of marble that change shape as the pieces that occlude the desired form are chipped away. The posterior cortices of the human brain serve the first approach as they synthesize veridical templates of external reality; prefrontal cortex promotes the second approach by chipping away at surface appearance until a deeper "meaning" is uncovered. In a figurative sense, it could be suggested that the dialectic tension between these representative and interpretive approaches to neural encoding help to set the tone of human consciousness.

The phylogenetic emergence of prefrontal cortex may have introduced the capacity for choice, change, and reflection but has not specified the nature of the choices, the contents of the reflections, or the direction of the changes. The mental faculties promoted by prefrontal cortex are thus as likely to lead to the greatest feats of culture and civilization as they are to Hiroshima and Auschwitz. The mechanisms that shape the course of individual actions are currently beyond the scope of neurological analysis. Perhaps this will become possible when a new science is developed for analyzing not only how a single brain reacts to experience but also how brains (and their owners) interact with each other to form social matrices which then influence individual decisions. Such an analysis is likely to show that prefrontal cortex plays a pivotal role in these aspects of social neurology as well.

It is fair to conclude that the sense of enigma surrounding the case of Phineas Gage is rapidly vanishing. It is also clear, however, that much more work needs to be done so that the speculations and metaphors linked to prefrontal cortex can yield to facts and mechanisms. Considering what has already been achieved during the first 150 years of research on the frontal lobes, it would be safe to predict that this field will continue to generate fertile insights into the uniquely human aspects of neural function and mental integration.

ACKNOWLEDGMENTS

This chapter was supported in part by NS-30863 from the National Institute of Neurological Disease and Stroke and AG-13854 from the National Institute on Aging. Sandra Weintraub, Ph.D. offered many helpful suggestions.

NOTES

1. The discrepancy in the date has not been explained. The event definitely occured on September 13.
2. From a 1928 letter, now at the Warren Museum of Harvard Medical School, from Dr. Edward Williams' son, Edward H. Williams, Jr.
3. He became very attached to the iron bar and seems to have kept it until he died.

4. It is now part of the Warren Museum collection at Harvard Medical School.
5. A prototypical example of the frontal abulic syndrome had been reported by Wilder Penfield. He published the effects of a right prefrontal removal (affecting mostly heteromodal cortex) he had performed on his own sister for the treatment of a slowly growing oligodendroglioma. Following the acute postoperative period, Penfield noted that his sister's judgment, insight, social graces, and major cognitive abilities had remained intact. When visiting her home as a dinner guest, however, Penfield noted a diminished capacity for the planning and administration of the meal, decreased initiative, and a slowing of thinking (Penfield & Evans, 1935).
6. This is the mental faculty that is also known by the cumbersome term *theory of mind.*

REFERENCES

Ackerly, S. (1935). Instinctive, emotional and mental changes following prefrontal lobe extirpation. *American Journal of Psychiatry, 92,* 717–729.

Ajuriaguerra, J., Strejilevitch, M., & Tissot, R. (1963). A propos de quelques conduites devant le miroir de sujets atteints de syndromes démentiels du grand âge. *Neuropsychologia, 1,* 59–73.

Anderson, S.W., Bechara, A., Damasio, H., & Damasio, A.R. (1999). Impairment of social and moral behavior related to early damage in human prefrontal cortex. *Nature Neuroscience, 2,* 1032–1037.

Baddeley, A. (1996). The fractionation of working memory. *Proceedings of the National Academy of Science USA, 93,* 13468–13472.

Bailey, P. & Bonin, Gv. (1951). *The Isocortex of Man.* Urbana, Illinois: University of Illinois.

Barbas, H. & Mesulam, M.M. (1985). Cortical afferent input to the principalis region of the rhesus monkey. *Neuroscience, 15,* 619–637.

Bechara, A., Damasio, H., Tranel, D., & Damasio, A.R. (1997). Deciding advantageously before knowing the advantageous strategy. *Science, 275,* 1293–1295.

Benton, A. (1968). Differential behavioral effects in frontal lobe disease. *Neuropsychologia, 6,* 53–60.

Berlyne, D. (1960). *Conflict, Arousal and Curiosity.* New York: McGraw-Hill.

Bigelow, H.J. (1850). Dr. Harlow's case of recovery from the passage of an iron bar through the head. *American Journal of the Medical Sciences, 34,* 2–22.

Blair, R.J.R. & Cipolotti, L. (2000). Impaired social response reversal. A case of 'acquired sociopathy'. *Brain, 123,* 1122–1141.

Blair, R.J.R., Morris, J.S., Frith, C.D., Perret, D.I., & Dolan, R.J. (1999). Dissociable neural responses to facial expressions of sadness and anger. *Brain, 122,* 883–893.

Brickner, R.M. (1934). An interpretation of frontal lobe function based upon the study of a case of partial bilateral frontal lobectomy. *Association for Research in Nervous and Mental Disease Proceedings, 13,* 259–351.

Broadbent, D.E. (1958). *Perception and Communication.* New York: Pergamon Press.

Brodmann, K. (1909). *Vergleichende Lokalisationlehre der Grosshirnrinde in ihren Prinzipien dargestellt auf Grund des Zellenbaues.* Leipzig: J.A. Barth.

Brown, G.G., Kindermann, S.S., Siegle, G.J., Granholm, E., Wong, E.C., & Buxton, R.B. (1999). Brain activation and pupil response during covert performance of the Stroop Color Word task. *Journal of the International Neuropsychological Society, 5,* 308–319.

Brozoski, T.J., Brown, R.M., Rosvold, H.E., & Goldman, P.S. (1979). Cognitive deficit caused by regional depletion of dopamine in prefrontal cortex of rhesus monkey. *Science, 205,* 929–931.

Butler, R.A. (1953). Discrimination learning by rhesus monkeys to visual-exploration motivation. *Journal of Comparative and Physiological Psychology, 46,* 95–98.

Butter, C.M. & Snyder, D.R. (1972). Alterations in aversive and aggressive behaviors following orbital frontal lesions in rhesus monkeys. *Acta Neurobiologiae Experimentalis, 32,* 525–565.

Castelli, F., Happé, F., Frith, U., & Frith, C. (2000). Movement and mind: a functional imaging study of perception and interpretation of complex intentional movement patterns. *NeuroImage, 12,* 314–325.

Chao, L.L. & Knight, R.T. (1995). Human prefrontal lesions increase distractibility to irrelevant sensory inputs. *NeuroReport, 6,* 1605–1610.

Chavis, D.A. & Pandya, D.N. (1976). Further observations on cortico-frontal connections in the rhesus monkey. *Brain Research, 117,* 369–386.

Cohen, J.D., Peristein, W.M., Braver, T.S., Nystrom, L.E., Noll, D.C., Jonides, J., & Smith, E.E. (1997). Temporal dynamics of brain activation during a working memory task. *Nature, 386,* 604–606.

Coull, J.T. (1998). Neural correlates of attention and arousal: insights from electrophysiology, functional neuroimaging and psychopharmacology. *Progress in Neurobiology, 55,* 343–361.

Coull, J.T. & Nobre, A.C. (1998). Where and when to pay attention: the neural systems for paying attention to spatial locations and to time intervals as revealed by both PET and fMRI. *Journal of Neuroscience, 18,* 7426–7435.

Daffner, K.R., Mesulam, M.-M., Scinto, L.F.M., Acar, D., Calvo, V., Fuast, R., Chabrerie, A., Kennedy, B., & Holcomb, P. (2000). The central role of the prefrontal cortex in directing attention to novel events. *Brain, 123,* 927–939.

Desimone, R. (1996). Neural mechanisms for visual memory and their role in attention. *Proceedings of the National Academy of Science USA, 93,* 13494–13499.

D'Esposito, M., Detre, J.A., Alsop, D.C., Shin, R.K., Atlas, S., & Grossman, M. (1995). The neural basis of the central executive system of working memory. *Nature, 378,* 279–281.

Diamond, A & Doar, B. (1989). The performance of human infants on a measure of frontal cortex function, the delayed response task. *Developmental Psychobiology, 22,* 271–294.

Dias, E.C., Compaan, D.M., Mesulam, M.-M., Segraves, M.A. (1996). Selective disruption of memory-guided saccades with injecton of a cholinergic antagonist in the frontal eye field of monkey. *Society of Neuroscience Abstracts, 22,* 418.

Diwadkar, V.A., Carpenter, P.A., & Just, M.A. (2000). Collaborative activity between parietal and dorso-lateral prefrontal cortex in dynamic spatial working memory revealed by fMRI. *NeuroImage, 12,* 85–99.

Elliott, R., Rees, G., & Dolan, R.J. (1999). Ventromedial prefrontal cortex mediates guessing. *Neuropsychologia, 37,* 403–411.

Exner, S. (1881). *Untersuchungen über Localisation der Functionen in der Grosshirnrinde des Menschen.* Vienna: W. Braumuller.

Flavell, J.H. (1968). *The Development of Role-Taking and Communication Skills in Children.* New York and Chichester: John Wiley and Sons.

Freedman, M. & Oscar-Berman, M. (1986). Bilateral frontal lobe disease and selective delayed response deficits in humans. *Behavioral Neuroscience, 100,* 337–342.

Funahashi, S., Chafee, M.V., & Goldman-Rakic, P.S. (1993). Prefrontal neuronal activity in rhesus monkeys performing a delayed anti-saccade task. *Nature, 365,* 753–756.

Fuster, J.M., Bauer, R.H., & Jervey, J.P. (1985). Functional interactions between inferotemporal and prefrontal cortex in a cognitive task. *Brain Research, 330,* 299–307.

Gallagher, H.L., Happé, F., Brunswick, N., Fletcher, P.C., Frith, U., & Frith, C.D. (2000). Reading the mind in cartoons and stories: an fMRI study of 'theory of mind' in verbal and nonverbal tasks. *Neuropsychologia, 38,* 11–21.

Gallese, V. & Goldman, A. (1998). Mirror neurons and the simulation theory of mind reading. *Trends in Cognitive Sciences, 2,* 493–501.

Gallup, G.G.J., Wallnau, L.B., & Suarez, S.D. (1980). Failure to find self-recognition in mother-infant and infant-infant rhesus monkey pairs. *Folia Primatologica, 33,* 210–219.

Geschwind, N. (1965). Disconnection syndromes in animals and man. *Brain, 88,* 237–294.

Godefroy, O. & Rousseaux, M. (1997). Novel decision making in patients with prefrontal or posterior brain damage. *Neurology, 49,* 695–701.

Goel, V., Grafman, J., Tajik, J., Gana, S., & Danto, D. (1997). A study of the performance of patients with frontal lobe lesions in a financial planning task. *Brain, 120,* 1805–1822.

Goldstein, K. (1936). The significance of the frontal lobes for mental performances. *Journal of Neurology and Psychopathology, 17,* 27–40.

Goldman, P.S., & Rosvold, H.E. (1970) Localization of function within the dersolateral prefrontal cortex of the rhesus monkey. *Experimental Neurology, 27,* 291–304.

Harless, M. (1979). Social behavior. In: M. Harless & H. Morlock (Eds.), *Turtles. Perspective and Research* (pp. 475–492). New York: John Wiley and Sons.

Harlow, J.M. (1848). Passage of an iron rod through the head. *Boston Medical and Surgical Journal, 39,* 389–393.

Harlow, J.M. (1868). Recovery after severe injury to the head. *Publication of the Massachusetts Medical Society, 2,* 327–346.

Hauser, M., Kralik, J., Botto-Mahan, C., Garrett, M., & Oser, J. (1995). Self-recognition in primates: phylogeny and the salience of species-typical features. *Proceedings of the National Academy of Science USA, 92,* 10811–10814.

Hebb, D.D. (1945). Man's frontal lobes. *Archives of Neurology and Psychiatry, 54,* 10–24.

Hikosaka, K. & Watanabe, M. (2000). Delay activity of orbital and lateral prefrontal neurons of the monkey varying with different rewards. *Cerebral Cortex, 10,* 263–271.

Huttenlocher, P.R. & Dabholkar, A.S. (1997). Regional differences in synaptogenesis in human cerebral cortex. *Journal of Comparative Neurology, 387,* 167–178.

Iversen, S.D. & Mishkin, M. (1970). Perseverative interference in monkeys following selective lesions on the inferior frontal convexity. *Experimental Brain Research, 11,* 376–386.

Jacobsen, C. (1936). Studies of cerebral function in primates. I. The functions of the frontal association areas in monkeys. *Comparative Psychology Monographs, 13,* 3–60.

Johannsen, P., Jakobsen, J., Bruhn, P., Hansen, S.B., Gee, A., Stødkilde-Jørgensen, H., & Gjedde, A. (1997). Cortical sites of sustained and divided attention in normal elderly humans. *NeuroImage, 6,* 145–155.

Johnston, V.S. & Chesney, G.L. (1974). Electrophysiological correlates of meaning. *Science, 186,* 944–946.

Kaada, B.R. (1960). Cingulate, posterior orbital, anterior insular and temporal pole cortex. In: H.W. Magoun (Ed.),*Neurophysiology* (pp. 1345–1372). Baltimore: Waverly Press.

Kaada, B.R., Pribram, K.H., & Epstein, J.A. (1949). Respiratory and vascular responses in monkeys from temporal pole, insula, orbital surface and cingulate gyrus. *Journal of Neurophysiology, 12,* 348–356.

Kling, A. & Steklis, H.D. (1976). A neural substrate for affiliative behavior in nonhuman primates. *Brain, Behavior and Evolution, 13,* 216–238.

Knight, R.T. (1984). Decreased response to novel stimuli after prefrontal lesions in man. *Electroencephalography and Clinical Neurophysiology, 59,* 9–20.

Koechlin, E., Basso, G., Pietrini, P., Panzer, S., & Grafman, J. (1999). The role of the anterior prefrontal cortex in human cognition. *Nature, 399,* 148–151.

Konishi, S., Nakajima, K., Uchida, I., Kikyo, H., Kameyama, M., & Miyashita, Y. (1999). Common inhibitory mechanism in human inferior prefrontal cortex revealed by event-related functional MRI. *Brain, 122,* 981–991.

Kuhn, D. & Brannock, J. (1977). Development of the isolation of variables scheme in experimental and 'natural experiment' contexts. *Developmental Psychology, 13,* 9–14.

LaBar, K.S., Gitelman, D.R., Parrish, T.D., & Mesulam,

M.-M. (1999). Neuroanatomic overlap of working memory and spatial attention networks: a functional fMRI comparison within subjects. *NeuroImage, 10,* 695–704.

Landis, C. (1949). Psychology. In: F.A. Mettler, (Ed.), *Selective Partial Ablation of the Frontal Cortex* (pp. 492–496). New York: Paul B. Hoeber.

Leimkuhler, M.E. & Mesulam, M.-M. (1985). Reversible go-no go deficits in a case of frontal lobe tumor. *Annals of Neurology, 18,* 617–619.

Lhermitte, F. (1986). Human autonomy and the frontal lobes. II. Patient behavior in complex and social situations. The "environmental dependency syndrome". *Annals of Neurology, 19,* 335–343.

Lhermitte, F., Pillon, B., & Serdaru, M. (1986). Human autonomy and the frontal lobes. I. Imitation and utilization behavior: a neuro-psychological study of 75 patients. *Annals of Neurology, 19,* 326–334.

Luciana, M. & Nelson, C.A. (1998). The functional emergence of prefrontally guided working memory systems in four- to eight-year-old children. *Neuropsychologia, 36,* 273–293.

Luria, A. (1966). *Human Brain and Psychological Processes.* New York: Harper and Row.

Mandler, G. (1962). Emotion. In: R. Brown, E. Galanter, E.H. Hess, & G. Mandler (Eds.), *New Directions in Psychology* (pp. 269–343). New York: Holt, Rinehart and Winston.

Mendez, M.F., Adams, N.L., & Lewandowski, K.S. (1989). Neurobehavioral changes associated with caudate lesions. *Neurology, 39,* 349–354.

Mesulam, M.-M. (1986). Frontal cortex and behavior. *Annals of Neurology, 19,* 320–325.

Mesulam, M.-M. (1990). Large-scale neurocognitive networks and distributed processing for attention, language, and memory. *Annals of Neurology, 28,* 597–613.

Mesulam, M.-M. (1998). From sensation to cognition. *Brain, 121,* 1013–1052.

Mesulam, M.-M. (2000a). Attentional networks, confusional states and neglect syndromes. In: M.-M. Mesulam (Ed.), *Principles of Behavioral and Cognitive Neurology* Second Edition (pp. 174–256). New York: Oxford University Press.

Mesulam, M.-M. (2000b). Behavioral neuroanatomy: large-scale networks, association cortex, frontal syndromes, the limbic system and hemispheric specialization. In: M.-M. Mesulam (Ed.), *Principles of Behavioral and Cognitive Neurology* (pp. 1–120). New York: Oxford University Press.

Mesulam, M.-M. (2000c). Brain, mind, and the evolution of connectivity. *Brain and Cognition, 42,* 4–6.

Milner, B. (1963). Some effects of different brain lesions on card sorting. *Archives of Neurology, 9,* 90–100.

Milner, B. (1982). Some cognitive effects of frontal lobe lesions in man. *Philosophical Transactions of the Royal Society of London B: Biological Sciences, 298,* 211–226.

Morecraft, R.J., Geula, C., & Mesulam, M.-M. (1992). Cytoarchitecture and neural afferents of orbitofrontal cortex in the brain of the monkey. *Journal of Comparative Neurology, 323,* 341–358.

Moscovitch, M. (1995). Confabulation. In: D.L. Schachter, J.T. Coyle, G.D. Fischbach, M.-M. Mesulam, & L.E. Sullivan (Eds.), *Memory Distortion* (pp. 226–251). Cambridge, Massachusetts: Harvard University Press.

Nakamura, K., Kawashima, R., Ito, K., Sugiura, M., Kato, T., Nakamura, A., Hatano, K., Nagumo, S., Kubota, K., Fukuda, H., & Kojima, S. (1999). Activation of the right inferior frontal cortex during assessment of facial emotion. *Journal of Neurophysiology, 82,* 1610–1614.

O'Doherty, J., Kringelbach, M.L., Rolls, E.T., Hornak, J., & Andrews, C. (2001). Abstract reward and punishment representations in the human orbitofrontal cortex. *Nature Neuroscience, 4,* 95–102.

Öngür, D., An, X., & Price, J.L. (1998). Prefrontal cortical projections to the hypothalamus in macaque monkeys. *Journal of Comparative Neurology, 401,* 480–505.

Oppenheimer, S.M., Gelb, A., Girvin, J.P., & Hachinski, V.C. (1992). Cardiovascular effects of human insular cortex stimulation. *Neurology, 42,* 1727–1732.

Pakkenberg, B. & Gundersen, H.J.G. (1997). Neocortical neuron number in humans: effect of sex and age. *Journal of Comparative Neurology, 384,* 312–320.

Pardo, J.V., Fox, P.T., & Raichle, M.E. (1991). Localization of a human system for sustained attention by positron emission tomography. *Nature, 349,* 61–64.

Pearce, S., McDonald, S., & Coltheart, M. (1998). Interpreting ambiguous advertisements: the effect of frontal lobe damage. *Brain and Cognition, 38,* 150–164.

Penfield, W. & Evans, J. (1935). The frontal lobe in man: a clinical study of maximum removals. *Brain, 58,* 115–133.

Petrides, M., Alivisatos, B., Meyer, E., & Evans, A.C. (1993). Functional activation of the human frontal cortex during the performance of verbal working memory tasks. *Proceedings of the National Academy of Science USA, 90,* 878–882.

Pool, J.L. & Ransohoff, J. (1949). Autonomic effects on stimulating rostral portion of cingulate gyri in man. *Journal of Neurophysiology, 12,* 385–392.

Prabhakaran, V., Narayanan, K., Zhao, Z., & Gabrieli, J.D.E. (2000). Integration of diverse information in working memory within the frontal lobe. *Nature Neuroscience, 3,* 85–90.

Price, B.H., Daffner, K.R., Stowe, R.M., & Mesulam, M.-M. (1990). The comportmental learning disabilities of early frontal lobe damage. *Brain, 113,* 1383–1393.

Quintana, J. & Fuster, J.M. (1999). From perception to action: temporal integrative functions of prefrontal and parietal neurons. *Cerebral Cortex, 9,* 213–221.

Raichle, M.E., Fiez, J.A., Videen, T.O., MacLeod, A.M., Pardo, J.V., & Petersen, S.E. (1994). Practice-related changes in human brain functional anatomy during non-motor learning. *Cerebral Cortex, 4,* 8–26.

Rao, S.C., Rainer, G., & Miller, E.K. (1997). Integration of what and where in the primate prefrontal cortex. *Science, 276,* 821–824.

Richfield, E.K., Rwyman, R., & Berent, S. (1987). Neurological syndrome following bilateral damage to the head of the caudate nuclei. *Annals of Neurology, 22,* 768–771.

Risberg, J. & Ingvar, D.H. (1973). Patterns of activation in the grey matter of the dominant hemisphere during memorizing and reasoning—a study of regional cerebral blood flow changes during psychological testing in a group of neurologically normal patients. *Brain, 96,* 737–756.

Rolls, E.T. (2000). The orbitofrontal cortex and reward. *Cerebral Cortex, 10,* 284–294.

Rowe, J.B., Toni, I., Josephs, O., Frackowiak, R.S.J., & Passingham, R.E. (2000). The prefrontal cortex: response selection or maintenance within working memory? *Science, 288,* 1656–1660.

Sagakami, M. & Niki, H. (1994). Encoding of behavioral significance of visual stimuli by primate prefrontal neurons: relation to relevant task conditions. *Experimental Brain Research, 97,* 423–436.

Sandson, T.A., Daffner, K.R., Carvalho, P.A., & Mesulam, M.-M. (1991). Frontal lobe dysfunction following infarction of the left-sided medial thalamus. *Archives of Neurology, 48,* 1300–1303.

Schleidt, W. & Schleidt, M. (1960). Störung der Mutter-Kind-Beziehung bei Truthühnern durch Gehörverlust. *Behaviour, 16,* 3–4.

Shammi, P. & Stuss, D.T. (1999). Humour appreciation: a role of the right frontal lobe. *Brain, 122,* 657–666.

Small, D.M., Zatorre, R.J., Dagher, A., Evans, A.C., & Jones-Gotman, M. (2001). Changes in brain activity related to eating chocolate: from pleasure to aversion. *Brain.* 124, 1720–1733.

Smith, W.K. (1944). The results of ablation of the cingular region of the cerebral cortex. *Federation Proceedings, 3,* 42–43.

Stone, V., Baron-Cohen, S., & Knight, R.T. (1998). Frontal lobe contributions to theory of mind. *Journal of Cognitive Neuroscience, 10,* 640–656.

Stuss, D.T. & Benson, D.F. (1984). Neuropsychological studies of the frontal lobes. *Psychological Bulletin, 95,* 3–28.

Tinbergen, N. (1951). *The Study of Instinct.* Oxford: Oxford University Press.

Tramo, M.J., Loftus, W., Thomas, C.E., Green, R.L., Mott, L.A., & Gazzaniga, M.S. (1995). Surface area of human cerebral cortex and its gross morphological subdivisions: in vivo measurements in monozygatic twins suggest differential hemisphere effects of genetic factors. *Journal of Cognitive Neuroscience, 7,* 292–301.

Tremblay, L. & Schultz, W. (1999). Relative reward preference in primate orbitofrontal cortex. *Nature, 398,* 704–708.

Tucker, A. (1765). *The Light of Nature Pursued.* London: T. Jones (printer).

Watanabe, M. (1996). Reward expectancy in primate prefrontal neurons. *Nature, 382,* 629–632.

Weintraub, S. & Mesulam, M.-M. (1985). Mental state assessment of young and elderly adults in behavioral neurology. In M.-M. Mesulam (Ed.), *Principles of Behavioral Neurology* (pp. 71–123). Philadelphia: FA Davis.

Wolfe, N., Linn, R., Babikian, V.L., Knoefel, J.E., & Albert, M.L. (1990). Frontal systems impairment following multiple lacunar infarcts. *Archives of Neurology, 47,* 129–132.

3

Association Pathways of the Prefrontal Cortex and Functional Observations

MICHAEL PETRIDES AND DEEPAK N. PANDYA

In the primate brain, the posterior boundary of the frontal lobe is the central sulcus (Fig. 3–1). Immediately in front of the central sulcus lies the motor and premotor cortex, which comprises architectonic areas 4 and 6, respectively. Further forward lies the prefrontal cortex, which reaches its highest level of development in the human brain. This large expanse of cortex plays a major role in various executive processes that are critical for the planning of sequences of responses, the selection and formulation of appropriate strategies in complex behavioral situations, the monitoring of the effectiveness of cognitive processing and behavior, and the capacity to make decisions to inhibit or change behavior as environmental circumstances change (see Stuss & Benson, 1986; Petrides, 2000a).

The prefrontal cortical region is not homogeneous but it comprises several architectonically distinct areas in both the human and the monkey brain (Brodmann, 1905, 1908, 1909; Economo & Koskinas, 1925; Walker, 1940; Sarkissov et al., 1955; Barbas & Pandya, 1989; Preuss & Goldman-Rakic, 1991; Petrides & Pandya, 1994). Experimental anatomical investigations in the monkey have shown that these architectonic areas differ in terms of their connections with cortical and subcortical structures (for reviews see Jones, 1985; Pan-

dya & Yeterian, 1985; Alexander et al., 1986; Schmahmann & Pandya, 1997). Afferent connections provide critical information to particular prefrontal areas about perceptual and mnemonic processes occurring in posterior association cortical areas and subcortical structures, while efferent connections provide the means by which the prefrontal cortical areas can regulate selectively information processing in these post-Rolandic cortical association areas and subcortical structures. These afferent and efferent connections are mediated via specific fiber pathways. The technique of autoradiography using anterograde tracers has been particularly useful for identification of these fiber tracts (Cowan et al., 1972). In such material, one can clearly identify the commissural and association fiber pathways, as well as the subcortical connections leading to the striatum, thalamus, pons, reticular formation, tectum, and spinal cord from their point of origin within a particular cortical area (for examples see Fig. 3–2).

The focus of this review is the association pathways linking post-Rolandic cortical areas with particular prefrontal cortical regions, including comments on their possible functional significance. The details concerning the origin, direction, and termination of these association pathways derive from experimental anatomical

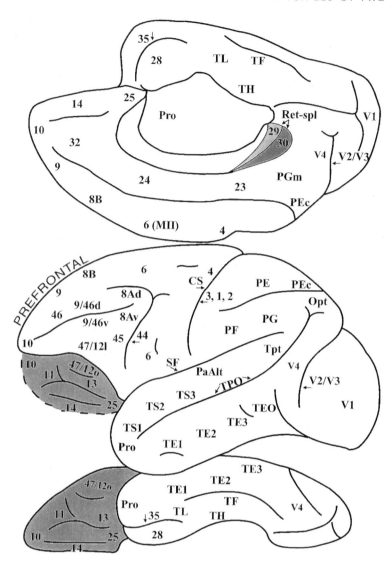

Figure 3–1. Composite diagram of the medial, lateral, and ventral views of the monkey brain to show the architectonic areas of the frontal lobe according to Petrides and Pandya (1994), the parietal lobe according to Pandya and Seltzer (1982), the superior temporal gyrus according to Pandya and Sanides (1973), the inferotemporal cortex according to Seltzer and Pandya (1978), and the posterior parahippocampal gyrus according to Rosene and Pandya (1983). The shaded area highlights the orbital frontal region shown both on the lateral and the ventral views of the brain. Also shaded are the retrosplenial areas (Ret-spl) 29 and 30 that lie in the upper bank of the callosal sulcus. Architectonic areas 44, 3, V2/V3, and TPO lie within the sulci indicated by the arrows. CS, central sulcus; SF, Sylvian fissure.

studies of the monkey brain. In the human brain, the basic direction and the stem of these pathways can be observed from gross dissections and the examination of material stained for fibers (e.g., with myelin stains), but we must rely on monkey data for their precise origin and termination within particular cortical areas.

Although we shall classify and describe these fiber tracts on the basis of their region of origin in post-Rolandic cortex, it must be emphasized that these are bidirectional association systems in the sense that they also contain efferent fibers originating from the target frontal lobe regions and directed back to the same post-Rolandic cortical areas.

PATHWAYS LINKING THE POSTERIOR PARIETAL CORTEX WITH THE FRONTAL CORTEX

The major association pathway that links the parietal cortex with the frontal lobe is the *superior longitudinal fasciculus* (SLF). These fibers course through the central core of the cortical white matter and reach the various regions of the frontal lobe. Experimental anatomical studies in the monkey indicate that the main component of the SLF originates from the parietal cortex (Petrides & Pandya, 1984). We have subdivided the classical tract into three fascicles designated SLF I, SLF II, and SLF III.

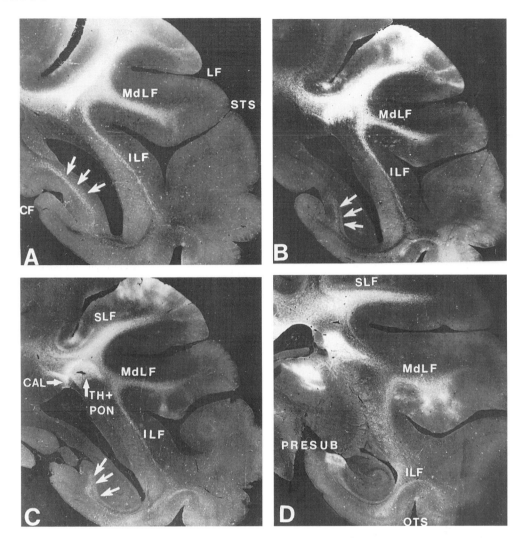

Figure 3–2. Photomicrographs showing labeling in various pathways, following isotope injections in the inferior parietal lobule, at four different caudal–rostral coronal levels (A–D). The three arrows in A, B, and C point to fibers directed towards the presubiculum. CAL, callosal fibers; CF, calcarine fissure; ILF, inferior longitudinal fasciculus; LF, lateral (Sylvian) fissure; MdLF, middle longitudinal fasciculus; OTS, occipitotemporal sulcus; PRESUB, presubiculum; SLF, superior longitudinal fasciculus; STS, superior temporal sulcus; TH+PON, thalamic and pontine fibers.

SLF I originates mainly from the superior parietal region and the adjacent medial parietal cortex (areas PE, PEc, and PGm). These fibers course in the white matter lateral to and above the cingulate sulcus. They terminate in the supplementary motor area (MII), dorsal area 6, and, to a lesser extent, area 8Ad (Fig. 3–3). It should be pointed out that these connections are reciprocal in nature—i.e., not only do the prefrontal areas receive inputs from the above parietal regions but they also (via the same fiber system) give rise to back-

connections that provide the means of regulating the post-Rolandic areas.

Several investigations (Duffy & Burchfield, 1971; Sakata et al., 1973; Mountcastle et al., 1975; Lacquaniti et al., 1995) have shown that the neurons of the cortex of the superior parietal lobule code the location of body parts (e.g., the arm) in a body-centered coordinate system. Thus, the dorsal component of the superior longitudinal fasciculus (SLF I), by virtue of its linking medial and superior parietal regions with the supplementary motor area

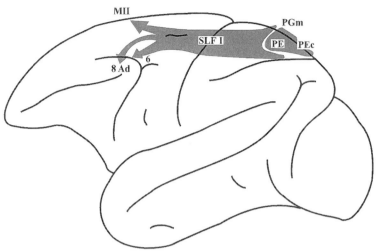

Figure 3–3. Schematic diagram to illustrate the origin, course, and termination of the dorsal component of the superior longitudinal fasciculus (SLF I). Note that this pathway originates in the superior parietal lobule and the adjacent medial parietal cortex. Architectonic areas are according to Figure 3–1.

Superior Longitudinal Fasciculus - SLF I

and the dorsal premotor region, can play a major role in the regulation of higher aspects of motor behavior requiring information on body part location. For instance, lesions of the periarcuate region in the monkey can give rise to severe impairments in conditional associative tasks in which different competing motor acts must be selected on the basis of the appropriate conditional rules (Petrides, 1982; Halsband & Passingham, 1982; see Petrides, 1987, for review). Similar impairments can be ob-

served in human subjects with lesions of the dorsolateral prefrontal region that include the target zone of the SLF I (Petrides, 1985, 1997).

SLF II originates from the caudal part of the inferior parietal lobule (area PG) and the adjacent occipitoparietal region (area Opt). These fibers course in the white matter above the Sylvian fissure and terminate in the posterior dorsolateral frontal lobe in dorsal area 6, area 8 (i.e., 8Ad and 8B), and mid-dorsolateral areas 9/46 and 46 (Fig. 3–4). In

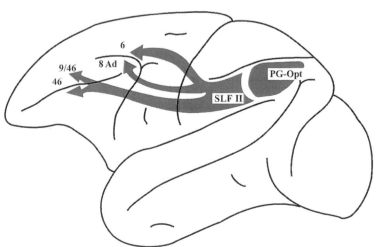

Figure 3–4. Schematic diagram to illustrate the origin, course, and termination of the middle component of the superior longitudinal fasciculus (SLF II). Note that this pathway originates in the caudal inferior parietal lobule. Architectonic areas are according to Figure 3–1.

Superior Longitudinal Fasciculus - SLF II

contrast to the superior parietal lobule, the caudal part of the inferior parietal lobule (areas PG and Opt) plays a major role in visual and oculomotor aspects of spatial function (Mountcastle et al., 1975; Hyvarinen & Shelepin, 1979; Andersen & Gnadt, 1989; Goldberg & Segraves, 1989). Patients with lesions of the parietal region exhibit severe impairments in spatial attention (Mesulam, 1981; Posner et al., 1984). Thus, this pathway can be viewed as a major link providing the prefrontal cortex with information concerning the perception of visual space from the posterior parietal cortex. The fibers originating within the prefrontal cortex and directed back to the posterior parietal region through SLF II provide the means by which the prefrontal cortex can regulate the focusing of attention within different parts of space. For instance, whereas normal subjects can use information provided in advance about the location of an impending stimulus to speed up their detection of it, patients with lateral prefrontal cortical lesions are impaired in using such information (Alivisatos & Milner, 1989; Koski et al., 1998). Another possible functional role of the SLF II pathway may be in the selection between competing locations on the basis of conditional rules. It is known that monkeys with lesions of area 8 are severely impaired in their ability to select between different locations on the basis of conditional rules (see Petrides, 1987). Sim-

ilar deficits can be seen in humans with lesions involving posterior dorsolateral prefrontal cortex (Petrides, 1985).

SLF III originates from the rostral portion of the inferior parietal lobule, which in the human brain constitutes the supramarginal gyrus (i.e., area 40 or PF), and from the adjacent parietal opercular region (Fig. 3–5). These fibers course in the parietal and frontal opercular white matter and terminate in ventral premotor area 6, in adjacent area 44 (pars opercularis in the human brain), in the frontal opercular region (gustatory area), as well as in the ventral part of area 9/46 (Petrides & Pandya, 1984; Cipolloni & Pandya, 1999). SLF III also contains fibers originating in the prefrontal cortex and directed back to the rostral inferior parietal lobule and the adjacent parietal opercular region (e.g., Preuss & Goldman-Rakic, 1989). The rostral portion of the inferior parietal lobule receives input from the ventral postcentral gyrus (Pandya & Seltzer, 1982) and its neurons exhibit complex somatosensory responses related to the face and arm (Hyvarinen & Shelepin, 1979; Leinonen et al., 1979; Robinson & Burton, 1980; Taira et al., 1990). Thus, SLF III provides the ventral premotor region and the rostrally adjacent area 44 with higher-order somatosensory input. It has been shown that neurons in this frontal region respond during specific goal—directed actions and appear to code not the

Figure 3–5. Schematic diagram to illustrate the origin, course, and termination of the rostroventral component of the superior longitudinal fasciculus (SLF III). Note that this pathway originates in the rostral inferior parietal lobule and the adjacent parietal operculum. Architectonic areas are according to Figure 3–1.

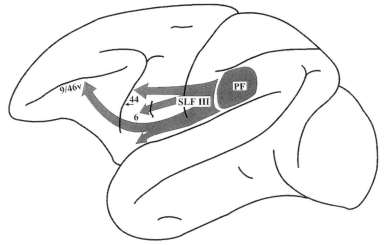

Superior Longitudinal Fasciculus - SLF III

movements per se but rather the action in high-level abstract terms (Rizzolatti et al., 1988; Murata et al., 1997). Furthermore, many neurons in this region of the frontal cortex respond both when the monkey performs a particular movement and also when the monkey observes another animal perform the action coded by these neurons (Rizzolatti et al., 1996). These neurons therefore may be involved in the computation of information necessary for action imitation.

The interactions between rostral inferior parietal cortex and the ventral frontal region made possible by SLF III may be necessary for gestural communication, which may have preceded the evolution of linguistic communication. In this regard, it is interesting to note that the gestural impairments seen in the clinical syndrome of ideomotor apraxia are often the result of lesions of the rostral inferior parietal region or the underlying white matter (De Renzi, 1989). The bidirectional connections between the rostral inferior parietal lobule and ventral area 9/46 via this pathway may be critical for the monitoring of orofacial and hand actions, since this area is part of the mid-dorsolateral prefrontal region that has been shown to play a critical role in the monitoring of information in working memory (Petrides, 1994, 1996).

PATHWAYS LINKING OCCIPITAL AND INFEROTEMPORAL CORTEX WITH THE FRONTAL CORTEX

There are two main streams for the cortical processing of visual stimulation originating in the striate cortex (Ungerleider & Mishkin, 1982). The *occipitotemporal* stream underlying object perception stems mainly from the ventrolateral occipital region serving central vision and is directed through a series of areas to the rostral inferotemporal region. The *occipitoparietal* stream for spatial perception and, in particular, that aspect involved in the control of action (Milner & Goodale, 1995), originates from the medial and dorsal occipital areas that are engaged in peripheral vision and is directed to the posterior parietal region.

Fibers originating in the ventral part of the occipital lobe (area 19) and directed towards the inferotemporal region occupy a position between the optic radiations and the fibers lying immediately subjacent to the temporal cortex. These occipitotemporal fibers, which form the inferior longitudinal fasciculus, descend ventrally and forward in the form of a cascade to terminate in the inferotemporal cortical region (areas TEO, TE3, TE2, and TE1), as well as in the parahippocampal gyrus (areas TF, TL, and TH) (Fig. 3–6) (Tusa &

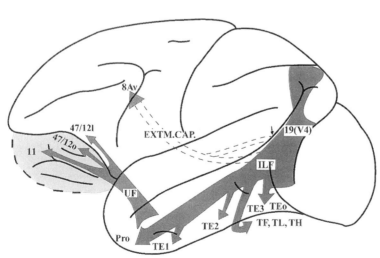

Inferior Longitudinal Fasciculus - ILF

Figure 3–6. Schematic diagram to illustrate the course and termination of the inferior longitudinal fasciculus (ILF) originating in the extrastriate visual region (V4) and directed to the inferior temporal region. Note that fibers from the caudalmost part of the inferior parietal lobule (area Opt) mingle with this pathway. Also, note the origin of a component of the uncinate fasciculus (UF) from the rostralmost part of the inferotemporal cortex and another frontally directed bundle originating from the occipitotemporal region coursing through the extreme capsule (EXTM.CAP.). Architectonic areas are according to Figure 3–1.

Ungerleider, 1985). A contingent of fibers originating from the caudal inferior parietal lobule also courses through this fiber bundle and ends in the parahippocampal region (Seltzer & Pandya, 1984). A few fibers from the occipitotemporal region proceed forward, possibly as a temporofrontal fascicle, to terminate in the ventral part of area 8 (i.e., 8Av) (Fig. 3–6). The occipitotemporal fiber system transmits information originating in the striate cortex and processed in a series of steps all the way to the rostral inferotemporal cortex leading to object identification (Mishkin, 1982). The rostral part of the inferotemporal cortical region (area TE1) and the ventral part of the temporal proisocortex send fibers to the prefrontal cortex via the uncinate fasciculus. These fibers terminate mainly in orbital area 11 and area 47/12 (Fig. 3–6). This component of the uncinate bundle therefore provides critical information about the nature of objects to the orbital and ventrolateral prefrontal region.

As described above, the parietal cortex is bidirectionally linked with the prefrontal cortex by means of the superior longitudinal fasciculus. The question that now arises is the precise course of the pathway that provides direct input to the prefrontal cortex from the occipital region. There has been considerable controversy regarding the pathway connecting the occipital with the frontal region and which

has been called the *occipitofrontal fasciculus* (OFF) (Dejerine, 1895). According to our observations, some of the fibers from the dorsal and medial occipital lobe and the caudal parietotemporal region travel via an ill-defined fiber bundle. This bundle is located in the white matter between the corona radiata and the callosal fibers. These axons follow a horizontal course and terminate predominantly in dorsal and ventral area 8 (i.e., 8Ad and 8Av), with a smaller number terminating in area 8B and caudal area 9/46 (Fig. 3–7). Many of the fibers of the OFF concentrate near a parallel bundle that lies just above the body and head of the caudate nucleus, the subcallosal fasciculus of Muratoff (1893). Although this latter fiber system can easily be confused with the OFF, careful observation reveals that they are in fact two separate fiber tracts. The fibers forming the bundle of Muratoff are derived from posterior parietal, posterior temporal, and occipital cortex, as well as the cortex of the cingulate gyrus and the frontal lobe. These fibers terminate in the striatum, especially the caudate nucleus (Mufson & Pandya, 1984). The OFF, on the other hand, can be viewed as a fiber system that stems from areas serving peripheral vision and may therefore provide the means by which the posterior dorsolateral prefrontal cortex (mainly area 8) receives information from occipital cortex and the caudal-most parietal cortex and can influence, via

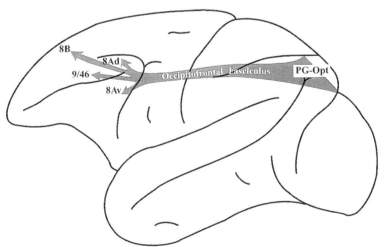

Figure 3–7. Schematic diagram to illustrate the origin, course, and termination of the occipitofrontal fasciculus (OFF). Note that this pathway originates in the dorsal and medial occipitoparietal region. Architectonic areas are according to Figure 3–1.

Occipitofrontal Fasciculus - OFF

feedback connections, visuospatial processing. We must point out that further studies are needed to delineate the exact course and functional contribution of this pathway.

PATHWAYS LINKING THE SUPERIOR TEMPORAL CORTEX WITH THE FRONTAL CORTEX

There are three distinct fiber pathways that arise from the superior temporal gyrus and adjacent superior temporal sulcus (Petrides & Pandya, 1988). One pathway stems from the caudal part of the superior temporal gyrus, i.e., area Tpt (Fig. 3–8). These fibers, which arch around the caudal part of the Sylvian fissure and resume a horizontal course running along the fibers of SLF II, terminate predominantly in area 8Ad (Fig. 3–8). Since these fibers curve around in the parietotemporal junction, as seen in gross dissections of the human brain, this pathway is referred to as the *arcuate fasciculus.* By means of this pathway, the posterior dorsolateral prefrontal cortex may be receiving auditory spatial information. There is evidence that neurons in area Tpt respond selectively to the location of sound source (Leinonen et al., 1980). Like SLF II, which provides the means for visuospatial interactions between prefrontal cortex and the posterior parietal region, this fiber pathway

linking temporal with frontal cortex can be viewed as providing the means by which prefrontal cortex can receive and influence audiospatial information.

The mid-portion of the superior temporal gyrus (areas paAlt and TS3) and the multimodal areas of the adjacent superior temporal sulcus (area TPO) give rise to a distinct fiber system that runs in the extreme capsule. These fibers terminate mainly in area 45 (pars triangularis of the human brain) and, to a lesser extent, in areas 9, 46, and 8Ad (Fig. 3–9). A contingent of fibers originating within the multimodal superior temporal sulcus also runs with this pathway and terminates in frontopolar area 10.

The fiber system arising from the caudal superior temporal region and directed primarily to area 8Ad (Fig. 3–8) is clearly distinct from the pathway arising from the mid-portion of the superior temporal gyrus and directed towards more rostral lateral prefrontal cortex (Fig.3–9) (Petrides & Pandya, 1988; Romanski et al., 1999). These two pathways may be viewed by analogy to the two visual-processing streams specializing for visual spatial and visual object information. Whereas the caudal superior temporal region may be forwarding to the caudal dorsolateral prefrontal cortex (primarily area 8Ad) auditory spatial information, the mid-portion of the superior temporal gyrus may be forwarding auditory object in-

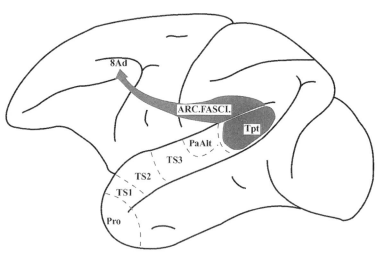

Figure 3–8. Schematic diagram to illustrate the origin, course, and termination of the arcuate fasciculus (ARC.FASCI.). Note that this pathway originates in the caudal superior temporal gyrus. Architectonic areas are according to Figure 3–1.

Arcuate Fasciculus - ARC.FASCI.

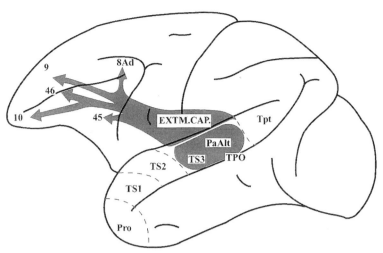

Figure 3–9. Schematic diagram to illustrate the fiber bundle originating in the middle portion of the superior temporal gyrus and adjacent superior temporal sulcus and running through the extreme capsule (EXTM.CAP.). Architectonic areas are according to Figure 3–1.

Extreme Capsule - EXTM.CAP.

formation. There is evidence from work in both monkeys (Colombo et al., 1996) and patients (Zatorre, 1985) that parts of the superior temporal gyrus may operate in a manner analogous to that of the inferotemporal cortex for object vision.

In the human brain, area 45, lying on the pars triangularis of the inferior frontal gyrus, plays a major role in language processing. Indeed, electrical stimulation of both the pars opercularis (area 44) and the caudal part of the pars triangularis (area 45) in the left cerebral hemisphere causes speech disruption (Rasmussen & Milner, 1975; Ojemann, 1979). However, the anatomical connections of these two ventrolateral frontal areas are quite distinct. As pointed out above, area 44 is the recipient of major somatosensory inputs from the supramarginal gyrus via the SLF III (Fig. 3–5), whereas area 45 receives input from the superior temporal region via the extreme capsule (Fig. 3–9). These results suggest that area 44 may be closely involved in the higher-order articulatory control of speech, whereas area 45 may have a role in the non-articulatory control of linguistic processing. The specific role of area 45 in the left hemisphere of the human brain for language may be an adaptation of the more general role of the ventrolateral prefrontal region in primate brains for the top-down regulation of infor-

mation in posterior cortical association areas (Petrides, 1994, 1996). According to this hypothesis, the mid-portion of the ventrolateral prefrontal cortex (areas 45 and 47/12) is critical for the active (i.e., strategic) regulation of information in posterior cortical association areas where information is perceived and coded in short-and long-term form. Thus, various kinds of active selection necessary for encoding and retrieval of specific information held in these posterior cortical regions are regulated by the mid-ventrolateral prefrontal region. This role of the ventrolateral prefrontal cortex can be contrasted with that of the mid-dorsolateral prefrontal cortex (areas 9, 9/46, and 46), which is involved in the monitoring of mnemonic performance on the basis of the subject's current plans (Petrides, 1994, 1996; see below).

Functional neuroimaging studies are generally in agreement with the view that ventrolateral areas 44 and 45 differ in function. For instance, Paulesu et al. (1993), in a positron emission tomography study, have shown the involvement of area 44 in the processing of articulatory information. By contrast, Petrides et al. (1995) have provided evidence that area 45 has a role in the active retrieval of verbal information from memory. In the latter study, when the subjects repeated words spoken by the experimenter (repetition condition), both areas 44 and 45 in the left hemisphere showed increased activity relative to a baseline control condition that involved no speaking. However, when the subjects recalled a list of specific words heard before scanning (recall condition), there was an additional significant increase in activity in area 45 in the left hemisphere compared with that during the repetition condition, indicating that the role of area 45 in verbal information goes beyond the mere articulation of words.

The rostralmost part of the superior temporal gyrus (areas TS2 and TS1) and the temporal proisocortex give rise to fibers that run as part of the uncinate fasciculus (Fig. 3–10). These fibers terminate in areas 13, 47/12, and 11 in the orbital frontal cortex and in areas 14, 25 and 32 in the medial prefrontal cortex (Fig. 3–10). Some of these fibers may be critical for regulating the emotional response to auditory stimuli. This speculation is based on the fact that the orbitofrontal cortex, especially its more caudal part, and the adjacent limbic medial frontal regions are strongly connected with the amygdala (Aggleton et al., 1980; Amaral & Price, 1984; Barbas & De Olmos, 1990; Carmichael & Price, 1995), a structure that is critical for affective responses (see Aggleton, 1992, for review). Furthermore, experiments in monkeys (Ruch

& Shenkin, 1943; Butter et al., 1970) and humans (Hornak et al., 1996; Sarazin et al., 1998; Angrilli et al., 1999) with lesions of the orbitofrontal cortex indicate that this region is important for normal behavioral responses to emotional stimuli. A recent study with positron emission tomography investigated changes in cerebral blood flow in normal human subjects during exposure to unpleasant auditory information, such as the sounds of violent car crashes (Frey et al., 2000). The results indicated a major increase in activity in the caudal orbitofrontal region in relation to unpleasant auditory information (Fig. 3–11). Thus, the connections between the orbitofrontal cortex and the rostral superior temporal region established via the uncinate fasciculus (Fig. 3–10) may be critical for enabling the organism to evaluate and regulate the response to auditory input that has affective quality. The caudal orbitofrontal region via its connections with other frontal areas (Barbas & Pandya, 1989; Carmichael & Price, 1996) is in an ideal position to interact with the lateral prefrontal areas that underlie higher-order cognitive processing (Petrides, 1996). The uncinate fasciculus is a complex system which, in addition to the above-mentioned fibers, comprises fibers from the rostral inferotemporal and parahippocampal gyri (see below).

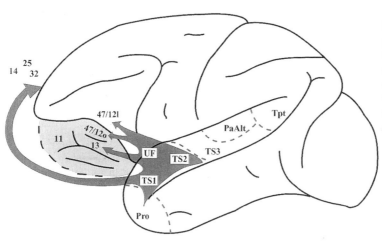

Figure 3–10. Schematic diagram to illustrate the origin, course, and termination of the component of the uncinate fasciculus (UF) arising in the rostral part of the superior temporal gyrus. Architectonic areas are according to Figure 3–1.

Uncinate Fasciculus - UF

Figure 3–11. Summary diagram to illustrate the location of activity peaks in the caudal orbitofrontal region (area 13) in relation to the processing of unpleasant auditory stimuli. IOS, intermediate orbital sulcus; L, left hemisphere; LOS, lateral orbital sulcus; MOS, medial orbital sulcus; OLF, olfactory sulcus; R, right hemisphere; TOS, transverse orbital sulcus.

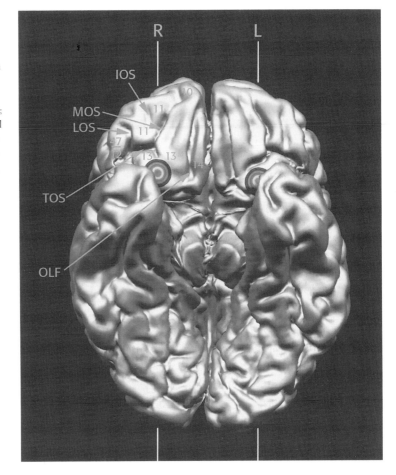

THE LIMBIC PATHWAYS

These pathways link the parahippocampal and cingulate cortical areas with the frontal cortex, and are discussed below.

THE VENTRAL LIMBIC PATHWAYS

The *parahippocampal* region is a complex structure that has been subdivided into several different areas. The anterior part comprises the entorhinal and perirhinal cortex and the posterior part areas TH, TF, and TL (Rosene & Pandya, 1983). This region receives input from visual, auditory, and somatosensory cortical association areas, multimodal cortical areas, the frontal cortex, as well as limbic areas (Van Hoesen 1982; Suzuki & Amaral, 1994). Fibers originating from the parahippocampal region and directed towards the orbital frontal

lobe proceed rostro-dorsally to form a discrete bundle running lateral and ventral to the ventralmost portion of the extreme capsule and the claustrum (Fig. 3–12). These fibers form part of the uncinate fasciculus and course forward through the limen insuli towards the frontal lobe. Some of the fibers leave this bundle and proceed medially to terminate in the medial forebrain region just caudal to the orbital frontal cortex, while others proceed rostrally in the form of a plate in the orbital white matter and terminate in areas 13, 47/12, 11, and 10 (Fig. 3–12). Another contingent of fibers originating in the caudal parahippocampal region enters the extreme capsule and terminates in areas 46, 9/46, and 9 (Fig. 3–12). Finally, a significant number of fibers from the parahippocampal cortex ascend into the white matter dorsally and aggregate in the cingulum bundle, where they course rostrally to

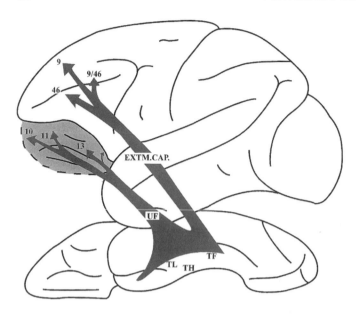

Figure 3–12. Schematic diagram to illustrate the origin, course, and termination of two fiber pathways from the parahippocampal region. The rostral pathway runs through the uncinate fasciculus (UF) towards the orbital frontal region and the medial forebrain region. The caudal pathway originates in the caudal parahippocampal region and runs in the extreme capsule (EXTM.CAP.). Architectonic areas are according to Figure 3–1.

Ventral Limbic Pathway

terminate in area 24 on the medial frontal cortex.

THE DORSAL LIMBIC PATHWAY

The *cingulum bundle* (CB) has two components. It has a central core, which is mainly composed of fibers originating from and directed to the thalamus, surrounded by association fibers (Mufson & Pandya 1984). A component of these association fibers originates in the rostral and caudal cingulate cortex (areas 24 and 23) and the retrosplenial cortex (area 30) and is directed to the prefrontal cortex, forming the dorsal limbic pathway. This component runs as part of the CB and terminates in the mid-dorsolateral prefrontal areas 9, 9/46, and 46 (Mufson & Pandya, 1984; Morris et al., 1999a). Some fibers from this bundle are directed towards the orbitofrontal cortex (area 11), as well as to area 32 on the medial surface of the frontal lobe (Fig. 3–13). This pathway is bidirectional—that is, it also contains fibers originating within the frontal cortex and terminating in the cingulate and retrosplenial cortex (Morris et al., 1999b).

The two limbic pathways described above linking the prefrontal cortex with the limbic medial temporal and cingulate regions are of

particular interest in our understanding of the role of the prefrontal cortex in memory. Bilateral lesions of the medial temporal region, namely the hippocampus and the cortical structures surrounding it (i.e., the entorhinal and perirhinal cortex and the posterior parahippocampal cortex), give rise to a severe amnesic syndrome characterized by an inability to store new information about facts and events (Milner, 1972; Mishkin, 1982; Squire & Zola-Morgan, 1991). Patients with damage restricted to the limbic region of the medial temporal lobe have no difficulty in perceiving and interpreting new information. However, this region is critical if information that has been perceived is to be maintained on a long-term basis when attention is shifted to new information or when the capacity of short-term memory is exceeded.

Recent work in the monkey has shown that the entorhinal and perirhinal region of the medial temporal lobe is critical for recognition memory (Meunier et al., 1993; Suzuki et al., 1993). Interestingly, the entorhinal and perirhinal regions are most strongly connected with the orbital and ventromedial limbic frontal cortex (Barbas & Blatt, 1995). Lesions of this orbitofrontal target zone of the entorhinal and perirhinal cortex in the monkey give rise to

Figure 3–13. Schematic diagram to illustrate the origin, course, and termination of the dorsal limbic pathway running in the cingulum bundle (CB). Architectonic areas are according to Figure 3–1. Ret-Spl, retrosplenial region around the splenium of the corpus callosum.

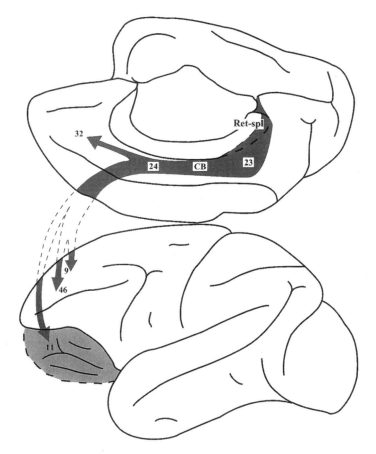

Dorsal Limbic Pathway - CB

impairments in recognition memory, suggesting that it is an important component of the circuit for processing new information (Bachevalier & Mishkin, 1986; Meunier et al., 1997). The role of the orbital prefrontal region in memory may be less direct than that of the limbic medial temporal region. It may lie primarily in the top-down modulation of medial temporal activity, based on the subject's evaluation of the potential interest of incoming information depending on the subject's goals, current motivation, etc. For instance, in a recent study with positron emission tomography, normal human subjects were asked to view a series of novel abstract designs and were told that they should commit to memory these designs (Frey & Petrides, 2000). Relative to the viewing of familiar abstract designs, there was increased activity in the orbitofrontal cortex, specifically in area 11 (Fig. 3–14), and this

area 11 activity was correlated with activity in the entorhinal–perirhinal region of the temporal lobe. These results reinforce the view that the orbitofrontal cortical region is in a close functional interaction with the rostral part of the parahippocampal region during the active encoding of new information.

The role of the orbital and ventral parts of the prefrontal cortex in the self-regulation of behavior is well established (e.g., Bechara et al., 1996). This role is probably mediated largely via the uncinate fasciculus. Support for this derives from a recent case report by Levine et al. (1998) of a patient with traumatic brain injury involving the uncinate fasciculus (temporofrontal disconnection) who had a serious deficit in self-regulatory behavior along with a retrograde amnesia.

Lesions of the lateral prefrontal cortex do not give rise to primary impairments in mem-

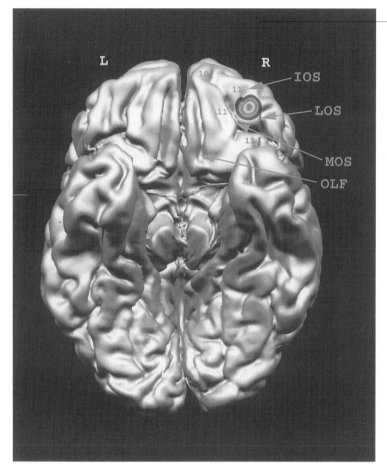

Figure 3–14. Summary diagram to illustrate the location of activity peaks in area 11 of the orbitofrontal region in relation to the encoding of abstract visual information. IOS, intermediate orbital sulcus; L, left hemisphere; LOS, lateral orbital sulcus; MOS, medial orbital sulcus; OLF, olfactory sulcus; R, right hemisphere.

ory, but rather disrupt various executive processes that are necessary to sustain certain aspects of working memory, as well as to encode and retrieve complex information (Petrides, 2000b). For instance, the mid-dorsolateral prefrontal cortical region (areas 46, 9/46, and 9) has been shown to be critical for the monitoring and manipulation of information within working memory. This evidence is based both on lesion work with monkeys (Petrides, 1991, 1995, 2000c) and patients (Petrides & Milner, 1982) as well as functional neuroimaging studies (see Petrides, 2000a). The question that is raised is how the mid-dorsolateral prefrontal cortex interacts with the medial temporal region so that control processes such as monitoring can operate on and influence working memory processing. One such pathway is probably the cingulo-frontal pathway that links the dorsolateral prefrontal cortex with the pos-

terior cingulate and retrosplenial regions, which are in turn linked with the parahippocampal cortex and hippocampus proper. In our recent examination of this pathway (Morris et al., 1999a, 1999b), it was clear that fibers directed to the lateral frontal cortex (or originating from it) were preferentially centered within the mid-dorsolateral prefrontal region, which is the very part of the prefrontal cortex that has been shown to be critical for monitoring information within working memory (Petrides, 1994, 1996). Thus, this bidirectional dorsal limbic association pathway may be the major pathway through which the mid-dorsolateral prefrontal cortex receives critical information about working memory processing from the hippocampal system and modulates this processing.

The importance of the mid-dorsolateral prefrontal cortex together with the posterior

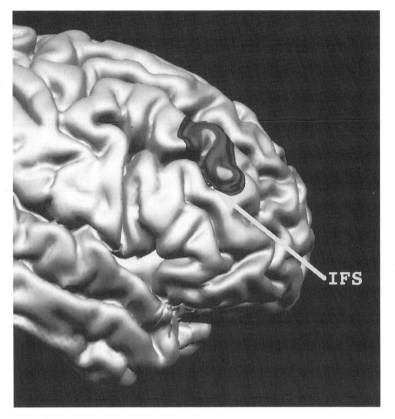

Figure 3–15. Summary diagram to illustrate the location of activity peaks in the mid-dorsolateral prefrontal cortex in relation to the monitoring of visual abstract information in working memory. IFS, inferior frontal sulcus.

cingulate and retrosplenial regions for the mnemonic processing underlying working memory was highlighted in a functional neuroimaging study (Petrides et al., 1993). In this study, local cerebral blood flow was measured with positron emission tomography in normal human subjects while they performed a visual self-ordered memory task requiring monitoring of information in working memory. In this task, which was directly analogous to those previously used with patients (Petrides & Milner, 1982) and monkeys (Petrides, 1991, 1995), the subjects were required to select a different stimulus on each trial from a set of eight stimuli until all had been selected. The subjects were therefore required to monitor carefully what had already been selected and what remained to be selected as they were preparing each new response. Performance of this self-ordered task, in comparison with that of the control task, resulted in significantly greater activity within the mid-dorsolateral frontal cortex (areas 46 and 9/46) (Fig. 3–15). Interestingly, there was also increased activity

in the posterior cingulate region during the performance of this task.

CONCLUSIONS

The fiber pathways described above are reciprocal in nature. The prefrontal cortical areas that receive input from particular post-Rolandic regions give rise to efferent connections that are directed back to the same areas from which they received input. Thus, these pathways provide particular prefrontal areas with sensory-specific or multimodal information and, at the same time, provide the means by which the prefrontal cortical areas can regulate information processing in the posterior cortical areas. Highly processed sensory information in post-Rolandic areas is provided to the orbitofrontal cortical region via the uncinate fasciculus. The orbitofrontal region appears to be critical for the regulation of the emotional significance and the motivational value of stimuli. Thus, via its back-going connections to the areas from which it receives input, the orbitofrontal cortex can exert a modulating influence on cognitive processing and decision making on the basis of current emotional and motivational states.

The post-Rolandic cortical regions provide the lateral prefrontal cortical region with sensory-specific and multimodal information. There is evidence that there is a fundamental distinction between the mid-ventrolateral (areas 45 and 47/12) and mid-dorsolateral (areas 9, 9/46, and 46) prefrontal regions (Petrides, 1994, 1996). The mid-ventrolateral prefrontal region, via its strong bidirectional connections with several post-Rolandic areas, is in a position to exercise a top-down modulation of activity in these areas for the purpose of active (i.e., strategic) judgement, encoding, and retrieval of information. The mid-dorsolateral prefrontal region, on the other hand, is critical for the monitoring of information in working memory, which is necessary for high-level planning and manipulation of information. The interaction between the mid-dorsolateral prefrontal region and the memory system may be exercised via the dorsal limbic pathway that links reciprocally this region of the prefrontal cortex with the hippocampal system via the posterior cingulate–retrosplenial region. In this manner, we can observe distinct levels of control exercised by the prefrontal cortex on posterior cortical processing.

The posterior dorsolateral frontal cortex (i.e., areas 8 and rostral 6) appears to underlie what are sometimes referred to as *attentional* processes. These areas receive input from medial and lateral parieto-occipital cortical regions, as well as from the adjacent caudal superior temporal gyrus via the superior longitudinal, the occipitofrontal, and the arcuate fasciculi. Through these bidirectional connections, the posterior dorsolateral frontal areas are in a position to act upon parieto-occipitotemporal regions for the purpose of selecting on the basis of various operations (e.g., conditional rules) between competing aspects of somatospatial, visuospatial, and audiospatial information. For instance, lesions of rostral area 6 impair the selection between competing motor acts on the basis of condi-

tional rules, whereas lesions of area 8 impair the selection between different locations or different visual stimuli in space (see Petrides, 1987).

Many disease processes involve the white matter per se or in addition to cortical damage. With the current availability of neuroimaging techniques, such as diffusion imaging magnetic resonance, it is possible to discern some of these pathways in vivo in the human brain (Makris et al., 1997). Proper knowledge of the course of the different fiber pathways is as important as knowledge of their termination to interpret properly the functional deficits resulting from damage to particular regions of the cerebral cortex. It should be pointed out that functional loss due to damage of a particular fiber pathway may not necessarily be the same as that resulting from damage to the frontal cortex per se. A clear understanding of the course of the prefrontal pathways will permit the design of experiments to demonstrate their functional contribution.

The possibility of demonstrating foci of increased activation in relation to particular cognitive processing in the human cerebral cortex with modern functional neuroimaging raises the question of where precisely these increases occur. Since there is variability in the gross morphology of the human brain (i.e., its sulcal and gyral parterns), it is necessary in future work to describe and quantify this variability within a standardized proportional stereotaxic space and to investigate its relation to architectonic areas. For instance, if the variability of a given architectonic area in a standardized proportional stereotaxic space were known, the investigator could transform the particular data from an experiment into this space and be able to provide a statistical statement of the probability that a certain activity focus in a group of subjects or an individual case lies within a certain architectonic area. Probability maps describing the variability of different gross morphological structures and architectonic areas within standard stereotaxic space have begun to appear (e.g., Paus et al., 1996; Tomaiuolo et al., 1999; Geyer et al., 2000), but considerably more work will need to be carried out.

REFERENCES

Aggleton, J.P. (1992). *The Amygdala: Neurobiological Aspects of Emotion, Memory, and Mental Dysfunction*. New York: Willey-Liss, Inc.

Aggleton, J.P., Burton, M.J., & Passingham, R.E. (1980). Cortical and subcortical afferents to the amygdala of the rhesus monkey. *Brain Research, 190*, 347–368.

Alexander, G.E., DeLong, M.R., & Strick, P.L. (1986). Parallel organization of functionally segregated circuits linking basal ganglia and cortex. *Annual Review Neuroscience 9*, 357–381.

Alivisatos, B. & Milner, B. (1989). Effects of frontal or temporal lobectomy on the use of advance information in a choice reaction time task. *Neuropsychologia, 27*, 495–503.

Amaral, D.G. & Price, J.L. (1984). Amygdalo-cortical projections in the monkey (Macaca fascicularis). *Journal of Comparative Neurology, 230*, 465–496.

Andersen, R. & Gnadt, J.W. (1989). Role of posterior parietal cortex in saccadic eye movements. In: R. Wurtz & M. Goldberg (Eds.), *The Neurobiology of Saccadic Eye Movements* (pp. 315–335). Amsterdam: Elsevier.

Angrilli, A., Palomba, D., Cantagallo, A., Maietti, A., & Stegagno, L. (1999). Emotional impairment after right orbitofrontal lesion in a patient without cognitive deficits. *NeuroReport, 10*, 1741–1746.

Bachevalier, J. & Mishkin, M. (1986). Visual recognition impairment follows ventromedial but not dorsolateral prefrontal lesions in monkeys. *Behavioral Brain Research, 20*, 249–261.

Barbas, H. & Blatt, G.J. (1995). Topographically specific hippocampal projections target functionally distinct prefrontal areas in the rhesus monkey. *Hippocampus, 5*, 511–533.

Barbas, H. & De Olmos, J. (1990). Projections from the amygdala to basoventral and mediodorsal prefrontal regions in the rhesus monkey. *Journal of Comparative Neurology, 300*, 549–571.

Barbas, H. & Pandya, D.N. (1989). Architecture and intrinsic connections of the prefrontal cortex in the rhesus monkey. *Journal of Comparative Neurology, 286*, 353–375.

Bechara, A., Tranel, D., Damasio, H., & Damasio, A.R. (1996). Failure to respond autonomically to anticipated future outcomes following damage to prefrontal cortex. *Cerebral Cortex, 6*, 215–225.

Brodmann, K. (1905). Beitraege zur histologischen Lokalisation der Grosshirnrinde. III. Mitteilung. Die Rindenfelder der niederen Affen. *Journal für Psychologie und Neurologie (Leipzig), 4*, 177–226.

Brodmann, K. (1908). Beitraege zur histologischen Lokalisation der Grosshirnrinde. VI. Mitteilung: Die Cortexgliederung des Menschen. *Journal für Psychologie und Neurologie (Leipzig), 10*, 231–246.

Brodmann, K. (1909). *Vergleichende Lokalisationslehre der Grosshirnrinde in ihren Prinzipien dargestellt auf Grund des Zellenbaues*. Leipzig: Barth.

Butter, C.M., Snyder, D.R., & McDonald, J.A. (1970). Effects of orbital frontal lesions on aversive and aggressive behaviors in rhesus monkeys. *Journal of Comparative Physiologie Psychology, 72*, 132–144.

Carmichael, S.T. & Price, J.L. (1995). Limbic connections of the orbital and medial prefrontal cortex in macaque monkeys. *Journal of Comparative Neurology, 363*, 615–641.

Carmichael, S.T. & Price, J.L. (1996). Connectional networks within the orbital and medial prefrontal cortex of macaque monkeys. *Journal of Comparative Neurology, 371*, 179–207.

Cipolloni, B. & Pandya, D.N. (1999). Cortical connections of the frontoparietal opercular areas in the rhesus monkey. *Journal of Comparative Neurology, 403*, 431–458.

Colombo, M., Rodman, H.R., & Gross, C.G. (1996). The effects of superior temporal cortex lesions on the processing and retention of auditory information in monkeys (*Cebus apella*). *Journal of Neuroscience, 16*, 4501–4517.

Cowan, W.M., Gottlieb, D.I., Hendrickson, A.E., Price, J.L., & Woolsey, T.A. (1972). Autoradiographic demonstration of axonal connections in the central nervous system. *Brain Research, 37*, 21–51.

Dejerine, J. (1895). *Anatomie des Centres Nerveux, Vol. 1*. Paris: Rueff.

De Renzi, E. (1989). Apraxia. In: F. Boller & J. Grafman (Eds.), *Handbook of Neuropsychology, Vol. 2* (pp. 387–394). Amsterdam: Elsevier Press.

Duffy, F. & Burchfield, J. (1971). Somatosensory system: organizational hierarchy from single units in monkey area 5. *Science, 172*, 273–275.

Economo, C. & Koskinas, G.N. (1925). *Die Cytoarchitektonik der Hirnrinde des erwachsenen Menschen*. Vienna: Springer-Verlag.

Frey, S. & Petrides, M. (2000). Orbitofrontal cortex: a key prefrontal region for encoding information. *Proceedings of the National Academy of Science USA, 97*, 8723–8727.

Frey, S., Kostopoulos, P., & Petrides, M. (2000). Orbitofrontal involvement in the processing of unpleasant auditory information. *European Journal of Neuroscience, 12*, 3709–3712.

Geyer, S., Schormann, T., Mohlberg, H., & Zilles, K. (2000). Areas 3a, 3b, and 1 of human primary somatosensory cortex. 2. Spatial normalization to standard anatomical space. *NeuroImage, 11*, 684–696.

Goldberg, M. & Segraves, M.A. (1989). The visual and frontal cortices. In: R. Wurtz & M. Goldberg (Eds.), *The Neurobiology of Saccadic Eye Movements* (pp. 283–313). Amsterdam: Elsevier.

Halsband, U. & Passingham, R. (1982). The role of premotor and parietal cortex in the direction of action. *Brain Research, 240*, 368–372.

Hornak, J., Rolls, E.T., & Wade, D. (1996). Face and voice expression identification in patients with emotional and behavioural changes following ventral frontal lobe damage. *Neuropsychologia, 34*, 247–261.

Hyvarinen, J. & Shelepin, Y. (1979). Distribution of visual and somatic functions in the parietal associative areas 7 of the monkey. *Brain Research, 169*, 561–564.

Jones, E.G. (1985). *The Thalamus*. New York: Plenum Press.

Koski, L.M., Paus, T., & Petrides, M. (1998). Directed attention after unilateral frontal excisions in humans. *Neuropsychologia, 36,* 1363–1371.

Lacquaniti, F., Guigon, E., Bianchi, L., Ferraina, S., & Caminiti, R. (1995). Representing spatial information for limb movement: role of area 5 in the monkey. *Cerebral Cortex, 5,* 391–409.

Leinonen, L., Hyvarinen, J., Nyman, G., & Linnankoski, I. (1979). Functional properties of neurons in lateral part of associative area 7 in awake monkeys. *Experimental Brain Research, 34,* 299–320.

Leinonen, L., Hyvarinen, J., & Sovijarvi, A.R.A. (1980). Functional properties of neurons in the temporoparietal association cortex of awake monkeys. *Experimental Brain Research, 39,* 203–215.

Levine, B., Black, S.E., Cabeza, R., Sinden, M., Mcintosh, A.R., Toth, J.P., Tulving, E., & Stuss, D.T. (1998). Episodic memory and the self in a case of isolated retrograde amnesia. *Brain, 121,* 1951–1973.

Makris, N., Worth, A.J., Sorensen, A.G., Papadimitriou, G.M., Wu, O., Reese, T.G., Wedeen, V.J., Davis, T.L., Stakes, J.W., Caviness, V.S., Kaplan, E., Rosen, B.R., Pandya, D.N., & Kennedy, D.N. (1997). Morphometry of in vivo human white matter association pathways with diffusion-weighted magnetic resonance imaging. *Annals of Neurology, 42,* 951–962.

Mesulam, M.-M. (1981). A cortical network for directed attention and unilateral neglect. *Annals of Neurology, 10,* 309–325.

Meunier, M., Bachevalier, J., Mishkin, M., & Murray, E.A. (1993). Effects on visual recognition of combined and separate ablations of the entorhinal and perirhinal cortex in rhesus monkeys. *Journal of Neuroscience, 13,* 5418–5432.

Meunier, M., Bachevalier, J., & Mishkin, M. (1997). Effects of orbital frontal and anterior cingulate lesions on object and spatial memory in rhesus monkeys. *Neuropsychologia, 35,* 999–1015.

Milner, A.D. & Goodale, M.A. (1995). *The Visual Brain in Action.* Oxford: Oxford University Press.

Milner, B. (1972). Disorders of learning and memory after temporal lobe lesions in man. *Clinical Neurosurgery, 19,* 421–446.

Mishkin, M. (1982). A memory system in the monkey. *Philosophical Transactions of the Royal Society of London B: Biological Sciences 298,* 85–95.

Morris, R., Petrides, M., & Pandya, D.N. (1999a). Architecture and connections of retrosplenial area 30 in the rhesus monkey (*Macaca mulatta*). *European Journal of Neuroscience, 11,* 2506–2518.

Morris, R., Pandya, D.N., & Petrides, M. (1999b). Fiber system linking the mid-dorsolateral frontal cortex with the retrosplenial/presubicular region in the rhesus monkey. *Journal of Comparative Neurology, 407,* 183–192.

Mountcastle, V.B., Lynch, J.C., Georgopoulos, A., Sakata, H., & Acuna, C. (1975). Posterior parietal association cortex of the monkey: command functions for operations within extrapersonal space. *Journal of Neurophysiology, 38,* 871–908.

Mufson, E.J. & Pandya, D.N. (1984). Some observations on the course and composition of the cingulum bundle in the rhesus monkey. *Journal of Comparative Neurology, 225,* 31–43.

Murata, A., Fadiga, L., & Fogassi, L. (1997). Object representation in the ventral premotor cortex (area F5) of the monkey. *Journal of Neurophysiology, 78,* 2226–2230.

Muratoff, W. (1893). Secundare Degeneration nach Durchschneiden des Corpus Callosum. *Neurologische Zentralblatt 12, 316,* 714–729.

Ojemann, G.A. (1979). Individual variability in cortical localization of language. *Journal of Neurosurgery, 50,* 164–169.

Pandya, D.N. & Sanides, F. (1973). Architectonic parcellation of the temporal operculum in the rhesus monkey and its projection pattern. Zeitschrift für Anatomie und Entwicklungsgeschichte. *139,* 127–161.

Pandya, D.N. & Seltzer, B. (1982). Intrinsic connections and architectonics of posterior parietal cortex in the rhesus monkey. *Journal of Comparative Neurology, 204,* 196–210.

Pandya, D.N. & Yeterian, E.H. (1985). Architecture and Connections of cortical association areas. In: A. Peters & E.G. Jones (Eds.), *Cerebral Cortex: Association and Auditory Cortices, Vol. 4* (pp. 3–61). New York: Plenum.

Paulesu, E., Frith, C.D., & Frackowiack, R.S.J. (1993). The neural correlates of the verbal component of working memory. *Nature, 362,* 342–345.

Paus, T., Tomaiuolo, F., Otaky, N., MacDonald, D., Petrides, M., Atlas, J., Morris, R., & Evans, A.C. (1996). Human cingulate and paracingulate sulci: pattern, variability, asymmetry, and probabilistic map. *Cerebral Cortex, 6,* 207–214.

Petrides, M. (1982). Motor conditional associative learning after selective prefrontal lesions in the monkey. *Behavioral Brain Research, 5,* 407–413.

Petrides, M. (1985). Deficits on conditional associative-learning tasks after frontal- and temporal-lobe lesions in man. *Neuropsychologia, 23,* 601–614.

Petrides, M. (1987). Conditional learning and the primate frontal cortex. In: E. Perecman (Ed.), *The Frontal Lobes Revisited* (pp. 91–108). New York: IRBN Press.

Petrides, M. (1991). Monitoring of selections of visual stimuli and the primate frontal cortex. *Proceedings of the Royal Society of London: Series B 246,* 293–298.

Petrides, M. (1994). Frontal lobes and working memory: evidence from investigations of the effects of cortical excisions in nonhuman primates. In: F. Boller & J. Grafman (Eds.), *Handbook of Neuropsychology, Vol. 9* (pp. 59–82). Amsterdam: Elsevier.

Petrides, M. (1995). Impairments on nonspatial self-ordered and externally ordered working memory tasks after lesions of the mid-dorsal part of the lateral frontal cortex in the monkey. *Journal of Neuroscience, 15,* 359–375.

Petrides, M. (1996). Specialized systems for the processing of mnemonic information within the primate frontal cortex. *Philosophical Transactions of the Royal Society of London B, Biological Science 351,* 1455–1462.

Petrides, M. (1997). Visuo-motor conditional associative learning after frontal and temporal lesions in the human brain. *Neuropsychologia*, 35, 989–997.

Petrides, M. (2000a). Mapping prefrontal cortical systems for the control of cognition. In: A.W. Toga & J.C. Mazziotta (Eds.), *Brain Mapping: The Systems* (pp. 159–176). San Diego: Academic Press.

Petrides, M. (2000b). Frontal lobes and memory. In: F. Boller & J. Grafman (Eds.), *Handbook of Neuropsychology, Second Edition, Vol. 2* (pp. 67–84). Amsterdam: Elsevier.

Petrides, M. (2000c). Dissociable roles of mid-dorsolateral prefrontal and anterior inferotemporal cortex in visual working memory. *Journal of Neuroscience*, 20, 7496–7503.

Petrides, M. & Milner, B. (1982). Deficits on subject-ordered tasks after frontal- and temporal-lobe lesions in man. *Neuropsychologia*, 20, 249–262.

Petrides, M. & Pandya, D.N. (1984). Projections to the frontal cortex from the posterior parietal region in the rhesus monkey. *Journal of Comparative Neurology*, 228, 105–116.

Petrides, M. & Pandya, D.N. (1988). Association fiber pathways to the frontal cortex from the superior temporal region in the rhesus monkey. *Journal of Comparative Neurology*, 273, 52–66.

Petrides, M. & Pandya, D.N. (1994). Comparative architectonic analysis of the human and the macaque frontal cortex. In: F. Boller & J. Grafman (Eds.), *Handbook of Neuropsychology, Vol. 9* (pp. 17–58). Amsterdam: Elsevier.

Petrides, M., Alivisatos, B., Evans, A.C., & Meyer, E. (1993). Dissociation of human mid-dorsolateral from posterior dorsolateral frontal cortex in memory processing. *Proceedings of the National Academy of Science USA*, 90, 873–877.

Petrides, M., Alivisatos, B., & Evans, A.C. (1995). Functional activation of the human ventrolateral frontal cortex during mnemonic retrieval of verbal information. *Proceedings of the National Academy of Science USA*, 92, 5803–5807.

Posner, M.I., Walker, J.A., Friedrich, F.J., & Rafal, R.D. (1984). Effects of parietal injury on covert orienting of attention. *Journal of Neuroscience*, 4, 1863–1874.

Preuss, T.M. & Goldman-Rakic, P.S. (1989). Connections of ventral granular frontal cortex of macaques with perisylvian premotor and somatosensory areas: anatomical evidence for somatic representation in primate frontal association cortex. *Journal of Comparative Neurology*, 282, 293–316.

Preuss, T.M. & Goldman-Rakic, P.S. (1991). Myelo- and cytoarchitecture of the granular frontal cortex and surrounding regions in the strepsirhine primate galago and the anthropoid primate macaca. *Journal of Comparative Neurology*, 310, 429–474.

Rasmussen, T. & Milner B. (1975). Clinical and surgical studies of the cerebral speech areas in man. In: K.J. Zulch, O. Creutzfeldt, & G.C. Galbraith (Eds.), *Cerebral Localization* (pp. 238–257). Berlin: Springer-Verlag.

Rizzolatti, G., Camarda, R., & Fogassi, L. (1988). Func-tional organization of inferior area 6 in the macaque monkey: II. Area F5 and the control of distal movements. *Experimental Brain Research*, 71, 491–507.

Rizzolatti, G., Fadiga, L., & Gallese, V. (1996). Premotor cortex and the recognition of motor actions. *Cognitive Brain Research*, 3, 131–141.

Robinson, C.J. & Burton, H. (1980). Organization of somatosensory receptive fields in cortical areas 7b, retroinsula, postauditory, granular insula of *M. fascicularis*. *Journal of Comparative Neurology*, 192, 69–92.

Romanski, L.M., Tian, B., Fritz, J., Mishkin, M., Goldman-Rakic, P.S., & Rauschecker, J.P. (1999). Dual streams of auditory afferents target multiple domains in the primate prefrontal cortex. *Nature Neuroscience*, 2, 1131–1136.

Rosene, D.L. & Pandya, D.N. (1983). Architectonics and connections of the posterior parahippocampal gyrus in the rhesus monkey. *Society for Neuroscience Abstracts*, 9, 222.

Ruch, T.C. & Shenkin, H.A. (1943). The relation of area 13 on orbital surface of frontal lobes to hyperactivity and hyperphagia in monkeys. *Journal of Neurophysiology*, 6, 349–360.

Sakata, H., Takaoka, Y., Kawarasaki, A., & Shibutani, H. (1973). Somatosensory properties of neurons in the superior parietal cortex (area 5) of the rhesus monkey. *Brain Research*, 64, 85–102.

Sarazin, M., Pillon, B., Giannakopoulos, P., Rancurel, G., Samson, Y., & Dubois, B. (1998). Clinicometabolic dissociation of cognitive functions and social behavior in frontal lobe lesions. *Neurology*, 51, 142–148.

Sarkissov, S.A., Filimonoff, I.N., Kononowa, E.P., Preobraschenskaja, I.S., & Kukuew, L.A. (1955). *Atlas of the Cytoarchitectonics of the Human Cerebral Cortex*. Moscow: Medgiz.

Schmahmann, J.D. & Pandya, D.N. (1997). Anatomic organization of the basilar pontine projections from prefrontal cortices in rhesus monkey. *Journal of Neuroscience*, 17, 438–458.

Seltzer, B. & Pandya, D.N. (1978). Afferent cortical connections and architectonics of the superior temporal sulcus and surrounding cortex in the rhesus monkey. *Brain Research*, 149, 1–24.

Seltzer, B. & Pandya, D.N. (1984). Further observations on parieto-temporal connections in the rhesus monkey. *Experimental Brain Research*, 55, 301–312.

Squire, L.R. & Zola-Morgan, S. (1991). The medial temporal lobe memory system. *Science* 253, 1380–1386.

Stuss, D.T. & Benson, D.F. (1986). *The Frontal Lobes*. New York: Raven Press.

Suzuki, W.A. & Amaral, D.G. (1994). Perirhinal and parahippocampal cortices of the macaque monkey: cortical afferents. *Journal of Comparative Neurology*, 350, 497–533.

Suzuki, W., Zola-Morgan, S., Squire, L.R., & Amaral, D.G. (1993). Lesions of the perirhinal and parahippocampal cortices in the monkey produce long lasting memory impairments in the visual and tactual modalities. *Journal of Neuroscience*, 13, 2430–2451.

Taira, M., Mine, S., Georgopoulos, A.P., Murata, A., &

Tanaka, Y. (1990). Parietal cortex neurons of the monkey related to the visual guidance of hand movement. *Experimental Brain Research, 83*, 29–36.

Tomaiuolo, F., MacDonald, J.D., Caramanos, Z., Posner, G., Chiavaras, M., Evans, A.C., & Petrides, M. (1999). Morphology, morphometry and probability mapping of the pars opercularis of the inferior frontal gyrus: an in vivo MRI analysis. *European Journal of Neuroscience, 11*, 3033–3046.

Tusa, R.J. & Ungerleider, L.G. (1985). The inferior longitudinal fasciculus: a reexamination in humans and monkeys. *Annals of Neurology, 18*, 583–591.

Ungerleider, L.G. & Mishkin, M. (1982). Two cortical visual systems. In D.J. Ingle, M.A. Goodale, & R.J.W. Mansfield (Eds.), *Analysis of Visual Behavior* (pp. 549–586). Cambridge, MA: MIT Press.

Van Hoesen, G.W. (1982). The parahippocampal gyrus. *Trends in Neuroscience, 5*, 345–350.

Walker, A.E. (1940). A cytoarchitectural study of the prefrontal area of the macaque monkey. *Journal of Comparative Neurology, 73*, 59–86.

Zatorre, R. (1985). Discrimination and recognition of tonal melodies after unilateral cerebral excisions. *Neuropsychologia, 23*, 31–41.

4

Neurochemical Modulation of Prefrontal Cortical Function in Humans and Animals

AMY F.T. ARNSTEN AND TREVOR W. ROBBINS

The cognitive functions of the prefrontal cortex (PFC), which include use of working memory to guide behavioral responses and the contents of attentional focus, the inhibition of inappropriate responses, and planning for the future, are among the most fragile in our behavioral repetoire. Deficits in PFC function are evident in every neuropsychiatric disorder (indeed, the term "psychiatric problem" seems synonymous with PFC dysfunction). Abilities carried out by the PFC can also become impaired in so-called "normal" individuals under conditions of uncontrollable stress, fatigue, and with advancing age. Many of these changes clearly result from transient, neurochemical changes in the PFC, and research in animals indicates that the PFC is tremendously sensitive to its neurochemical environment. The ascending monoaminergic and cholinergic systems appear to have marked effects on the cognitive functioning of the PFC as part of their orchestration of cortical arousal. An understanding of the varied mechanisms influencing PFC functioning will be critical for the development of intelligent pharmacological treatments for neuropsychiatric disorders. The following chapter will review research from both animal and human studies on the ways in which dopamine (DA), norepinephrine (NE), serotonin (5HT), and acetylcholine (ACh) may modulate PFC cognitive functions. The anatomical connections of these ascending pathways and the reciprocal connections from the PFC are summarized in Figure 4–1.

STUDIES IN ANIMALS

DOPAMINE

Working Memory Tasks

For more than 20 years, we have known that DA has a critical effect on PFC working memory function. We have learned that either too little or too much DA receptor stimulation impairs spatial working memory performance in monkeys and rodents. Thus, DA receptor stimulation appears to obey an "inverted U-shaped" dose–response function that has been seen in both animals and humans (Fig. 4–2). This section will review data from animal studies.

Catecholamine Depletion. The work of Brozoski et al. (1979) was the first to demonstrate that catecholamines play a critical role in the modulation of the spatial working memory functions of the PFC. Dopamine and NE depletion in the PFC was produced by infusion

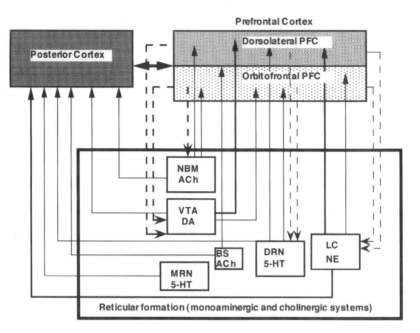

Figure 4–1. Schematic to show main anatomical connections between chemically defined ascending systems of the reticular core and the neocortex (posterior cortex and prefrontal cortex [PFC]; the latter is shown simplistically divided into the dorsolateral and orbitofrontal regions). Projections to the PFC are shown as solid lines; projections from the PFC are shown as dashed lines. The monoamines and acetylcholine (ACh) project to all sectors of the PFC, although there is some variation in the density of innervation for some areas (e.g., for the catecholamines dopamine [DA] and norepinephrine [NE]; see Lewis et al. 1988). There are some differences of innervation in comparison to the posterior neocortex—e.g., the relative lack of strong DA projections. Note also the feedback pathways from the PFC to the vicinity of the cell groups of origin of the ascending systems—e.g., the orbitofrontal cortex to the basal forebrain cholinergic cells (Mesulam, 1995), while the dorsolateral PFC projects to the locus coeruleus (LC) (Arnsten & Goldman-Rakic, 1984). This pattern of projections is intriguing given that the orbital PFC and basal forebrain cholinergic cells often fire on the basis of stimulus relationships to reward (e.g., Richardson & DeLong, 1986; Rolls, 1996), while the dorsolateral PFC and LC are more related to regulation of attention (e.g., Foote et al., 1980; Woods & Knight, 1986). Indeed, one of the special features of the PFC, perhaps unique among cortical areas, is its ability to regulate these chemical systems and thus alter modulation of most brain functions.

This figure is based in part on findings summarized in the following publications: Goldman-Rakic (1987); Lewis et al. (1988); Sesack et al. (1989); Lewis (1990); Williams and Goldman-Rakic (1998); Cavada et al. (2000); and Ongur and Price (2000); BS-ACh, brain stem cholinergic cell groups; DRN, dorsal raphe nuclei; MRN, median raphe nuclei; NBM, nucleus basalis of Meynert; VTA; ventral tegmental area; 5HT, 5-hydroxytrytamine (serotonin).

of the catecholamine neurotoxin 6-hydroxydopamine (6-OHDA) into the dorsolateral PFC of monkeys. Animals with large catecholamine depletion of the PFC were as impaired as those with PFC ablations, which highlights the importance of catecholamine modulatory influences. Animals were not impaired in the performance of a non-PFC task, visual pattern discrimination, implicating an effect of catecholamine depletion on PFC cognitive function rather than nonspecific performance deficits. The Brozoski study focused on the importance of DA to PFC function, as monkeys with large NE depletion and small DA depletion did not show deficits. However, it is now appreciated that both catecholamines are important to PFC function, and it is likely that both must be substantially depleted to produce marked impairment. The landmark Brozoski study has been replicated in rats with 6-OHDA lesions of the medical PFC (Simon, 1981) and in marmosets with 6-OHDA lesions to the dorsolateral PFC (Collins et al., 1998; Roberts et al., 1994).

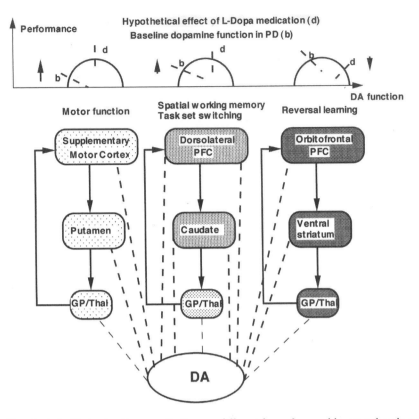

Figure 4–2. Hypothetical effects of L-Dopa medication on cognitive and motor function in Parkinson's disease (PD), interpreted in terms of the differential functioning of frontostriatal loops. *Top:* Inverted U-shaped functions illustrate Yerkes-Dodson principle of optimal levels of arousal for performance; arousal is equated in this case with increased dopaminergic activity in the mesocortical and mesostriatal dopamine (DA) systems. Shown are different baseline levels of DA activity that correspond to the different levels of DA depletion that occur during PD in the putamen and other sectors of the striatum and frontal cortex as a function of disease duration (see text). DA depletion and medication hence differentially affect (arrows) the functioning of hypothetical frontostriatal loops that are preferentially engaged in different forms of motor and cognitive functioning. (b, baseline DA depletion; d, DA receptor stimulation following L-Dopa medication). Thus motor function is improved by L-dopa, as are cognitive functions such as spatial working memory performance and task set-switching (Cools R., Barker R.A., & Sahakian, B.J. & Robbins & 2001). However, a different form of reversal learning thought to depend on the orbitofrontal loop is impaired by L-Dopa medication (see Swainson et al., 2000), as L-Dopa medication may produce excessive levels of DA receptor stimulation in this loop. *Bottom:* Three main loops are shown, in simplified form, each being characterized by topographical projections from several cortical regions (not shown) onto particular striatal structures such as the putamen, caudate nucleus, and ventral striatum. The striatal regions project topographically to different regions of the globus pallidus (GP) and from there to the thalamus (Thal). A feedback projection to a subset of the cortical areas completes the loop (although the loops are open and also project into the brain stem). The putamen forms part of the motor loop and is preferentially depleted of DA in early PD (as indicated by the lighter shading). The caudate and ventral striatum are implicated in cognitive and affective functions and are less depleted of DA in early PD, thus being more susceptible to possible over-dosing effects arising from DA medication. PFC, prefrontal cortex.

Spatial working memory deficits with preserved visual discrimination function have also been observed with global catecholamine depletion. For example, systemic, chronic reserpine treatment impairs delayed response without altering discrimination performance in young adult monkeys (Cai et al., 1993). Furthermore, aged monkeys and rats with naturally occurring catecholamine depletion exhibit prominent spatial working memory deficits and generally spared performance on discrimination tasks (Bartus et al., 1978; Luine et al., 1990). In both young (Sahakian et al., 1985) and aged (Luine et al., 1990) rats, cognitive performance correlated with levels of PFC catecholamines. Pharmacological studies in aged animals and young, depleted animals indicate that both DA and NE facilitate PFC working memory function through actions at D1 and α_2-adrenergic receptors, respectively.

Brozoski et al. (1979) illustrated the importance of DA mechanisms to PFC working memory function by showing that the mixed D1/D2 agonist, apomorphine, could ameliorate delayed alternation deficits in their catecholamine-depleted monkeys (Brozoski et al., 1979). This interpretation was reinforced by electrophysiological findings in monkeys performing a working memory task in which iotophoresis of DA onto PFC neurons enhanced memory-related cell firing during the delay period (Sawaguchi et al., 1988). Dopamine can also excite PFC neurons that respond to the cue signal and/or to the go signal informing the monkey it is time to respond for reward (Sawaguchi et al., 1990). These data are quite consistent with recordings from DA cell bodies in monkeys performing a working memory task, in which DA cells fired to cues associated with reward (Schultz, 1998; Schultz et al., 1993). In highly trained monkeys, the DA neurons fired to the visuospatial cue signal. One thus could speculate that DA release is enhanced in the PFC at the initiation of each trial by the cue signal in time to modulate cue-, delay-and go-related activity. Note that this speculation assumes long-acting effects of DA on PFC cells, i.e., over many seconds, presumably via second messenger actions.

D1 Receptor Stimulation. Research in monkeys and rodents has now established the importance of the D1 receptor family in the regulation of PFC function. Recordings from PFC neurons in monkeys performing a working memory task first suggested that D1 family mechanisms may be more influential than D2 family mechanisms for working memory function, as mixed D1/D2 family antagonists suppressed delay-related activity of PFC neurons, while a more selective D2 family antagonist was ineffective (Sawaguchi et al., 1988). This hypothesis was supported by behavioral studies showing that infusions of selective D1, but not D2/D3 antagonists into the PFC markedly impaired spatial working memory (Sawaguchi & Goldman-Rakic, 1991). Impaired working memory with D1 receptor antagonist infusion has now been replicated in rat PFC, where D1 mechanisms are thought to modulate hippocampal input to PFC (Seamans et al., 1998). Systemic administration of a D1 receptor antagonist can also impair working memory in monkeys (Arnsten et al., 1994) and rats (Murphy et al., 1996a), as can low doses of a D2/D3/D4 agonist that inhibits DA release (Arnsten et al., 1995). Conversely, working memory can be improved by low doses of D1 agonists. For example, systemic administration of low, but not high, doses of D1 agonist improves spatial working memory performance in young monkeys or in aged monkeys with naturally occurring DA depletion (Arnsten et al., 1994; Cai & Arnsten, 1997). Similarly, intra-PFC infusions of low doses of a partial D1 agonist improve attentional performance in rats (Robbins et al., 1998a, see below). Selective, full D1 agonists have only recently become available for research in animals and are not yet available for human usage; thus, less is known about D1 influences on cognitive function in humans. However, the mixed D1/D2 family agonist, pergolide, appears to produce more consistent improvement in spatial working memory in humans than does the D2 family agonist, bromocriptine, suggesting that mechanisms observed with D1 agonists in animals may extend to humans as well (Kimberg et al., 1997; Muller et al., 1998, see below).

High levels of D1 receptor stimulation impair working memory function. Accumulating evidence indicates that high levels of DA receptor stimulation in the PFC impairs working memory function. It has been appreciated for more than 20 years that exposure to even relatively mild, uncontrollable stress greatly increases DA release in the PFC (e.g., Thierry et al., 1976; Deutch & Roth 1990). Recent studies have shown that stress exposure impairs working memory function through excessive stimulation of DA and NE (see below) receptors in the PFC. Studies of neurochemical and cognitive changes in response to stress have particular clinical relevance, as many neuropsychiatric disorders are exacerbated or precipiated by exposure to stress (see, e.g., Mazure, 1995).

Studies in monkeys, rats, and humans have shown that acute exposure to mild uncontrollable stress impairs cognitive functions associated with the PFC. Thus, exposure to either an environmental stress such as loud noise (Arnsten & Goldman-Rakic, 1998) or a pharmacological stressor (Murphy et al., 1996a; Birnbaum et al., 1999a), impairs performance of spatial working memory tasks in monkeys and rats. In contrast, exposure to stress has little effect or actually improves performance of tasks dependent on the inferior temporal cortex (Arnsten & Goldman-Rakic, 1998), parietal cortex (Murphy et al., 1996a), striatum (Selden et al., 1990; J. Kim & M. Packard, personal communication), or cerebellum (Shors et al., 1992). A similar profile has been observed in human studies. The original work of Broadbent, Hockey, and others showed that exposing human subjects to loud noise stress improved reaction time on well-rehearsed or simple tasks, but impaired performance of more complex tasks (Broadbent, 1971), especially when the subjects experienced themselves as having no control over the stressor (Glass et al., 1971). Noise stress impaired the ability to sustain attention (Hockey, 1970) or inhibit prepotent, inappropriate responses on the Stroop Interference Test (Hartley & Adams, 1974).

Accumulating data from animal studies indicate that the cognitive deficits observed during stress result from excessive stimulation of DA D1 receptors in the PFC (and NE α_1-receptors, see below). The working memory deficits induced by stress exposure in rats or monkeys can be blocked by pretreatment with DA receptor antagonists, including the D1 receptor antagonist SCH23390 (Arnsten & Goldman-Rakic, 1990b, 1998; Murphy et al., 1996a). Working memory deficits can also be averted by pretreatment with agents such as clonidine and guanfacine that prevent stress-induced increases in DA turnover (Arnsten & Goldman-Rakic, 1986; Murphy et al., 1996b; Birnbaum et al., 2000). Interestingly, stress-induced working memory deficits correlate with the rise in DA turnover in PFC (NE and its metabolite were not measured, Murphy et al., 1996a). Conversely, stress-induced working memory deficits can be mimicked by the administration of a D1 receptor agonist. Although the systemic administration of low doses of D1 agonists improves working memory performance in young and aged monkeys (Arnsten et al., 1994; Cai & Arnsten, 1997), higher doses impair performance without any evidence of side effects (Arnsten et al., 1994; Cai & Arnsten, 1997). Furthermore, infusion of a full D1 agonist (0.1 µg) directly into the PFC in rats impairs working memory performance and produces a mildly perseverative pattern of response, much as is seen in stressed rats (Zahrt et al., 1997). These deficits can be reversed by treatment with a D1 receptor antagonist (Arnsten et al., 1994; Cai & Arnsten, 1997; Zahrt et al., 1997), consistent with actions at D1 receptors.

Electrophysiological studies of PFC neurons have also shown that high levels of D1 receptor stimulation can erode neuronal function. For example, the iontophoresis of low concentrations of D1 receptor antagonists can *enhance* memory-related neuronal responses in monkeys performing a challenging working memory task (Williams & Goldman-Rakic, 1995). Conversely, intracellular recordings of pyramidal cells from rodent PFC slices have shown that D1 receptor stimulation decreases the n- and p-calcium currents that convey signals from dendrite to soma (Yang & Seamans, 1996). Optimal levels of D1 receptor stimulation appear to focus signal transmission, conveying only large or temporally coincident signals to the cell body (Yang & Seamans, 1996). However, higher concentrations of DA or a D1 agonist abolish calcium currents, effectively "strangling" information transfer from dendrite to soma (Yang & Seamans, 1996; Zahrt et al., 1997; See Fig. 4–3). This interruption of information transfer may underlie the working memory impairment seen at high levels of D1 receptor stimulation (Zahrt et al., 1997). Animals may become perseverative, as no new spatial information can access the soma to change response patterns.

We are currently testing the hypothesis that high levels of D1 receptor stimulation impair PFC cognitive function by activating a cyclic adenosine monophosphate (cAMP)-dependent protein kinase A (PKA) intracellular pathway. Surmeier and colleagues have shown that D1 receptor stimulation decreases n- and p-calcium currents in dendrites of striatal neurons through a cAMP–PKA–protein phosphatase 1 intracellular signalling cascade (Surmeier et al., 1995).

For example, either a D1 agonist or the PKA activator, Sp-cAMPS, decrease n- and p-calcium currents (Surmeier et al., 1995). We examined whether intra-PFC infusion of Sp-cAMPS, like a D1 agonist, would impair working memory performance (Taylor et al., 1999). As predicted, Sp-cAMPS produced a dose-related impairment in delayed alternation performance that could be reversed by the PKA inhibitor Rp-cAMPS (Taylor et al., 1999). The Sp-cAMPS-treated animals exhibited a slightly perseverative pattern of response, as had been observed with D1 agonist infusion or mild stress. These data suggest the exciting possibility that activation of cAMP–PKA intracellular signaling cascades in the PFC contribute to PFC dysfunction. Interestingly, guanfacine is even more potent than clonidine in preventing stress-induced cognitive deficits (Birnbaum & Arnsten, 1996), even though guanfacine is weaker than clonidine in reducing catecholamine release and reducing LC cell firing (Engberg & Eriksson, 1991). These data suggest the intriguing possibility that guanfacine

Figure 4–3. A speculative Model of how moderate levels of catecholamines may enhance, while high levels of catecholamines may impair, working memory function of a layer V pyramidal cell. This model is based on the intracellular recordings of Yang and Seamans (1996) and Marek and Aghajanian (1999). *A:* Moderate levels of norepinephrine (NE) and dopamine (DA) may optimize processing of incoming signals through actions on dendritic spines. Dopamine axons appear to avoid the primary dendritic stem, and there may be little DA receptor stimulation of the stem under these conditions. Thus, robust, calcium-mediated signals would travel from the distal dendritic tree via the primary dendritic stem to the soma. LC, locus coeruleus; VTA, ventral tegmental area. *B:* Schematic representation of the signal at the level of the *(1)* dendritic tree, *(2)* upper portion of the primary dendritic stem, and *(3)* lower portion of the primary dendritic stem. Schematic depiction of an extracellular recording of this neuron *(4)* shows increased firing during the delay period. It is thought that this delay-related activity is used to appropriately guide behavior. *C:* High levels of NE and DA released during stress may erode signal transmission from the dendritic tree to the soma through actions on the dendritic stem. Steroids released during stress may block the extraneuronal catecholamine transporters, thus allowing high levels of catecholamines to build up near the stem. Stimulation of DA D1/D5 receptors on the stem is thought to reduce signals by blocking the n and p calcium channels which normally convey signals to the soma (Yang & Seamans, 1996). This likely involves a protein kinase A (PKA) intracellular mechanism (see text). Stimulation of NE α_1 receptors is thought to increase "noise" by promoting nonspecific glutamate (GLU) release (Marek & Aghajanian, 1999). This likely involves a protein kinase C (PKC) mechanism (see text). *D:* Schematic representation of the signal at the level of the *(1)* dendritic tree, *(2)* upper portion of the primary dendritic stem where high levels of D1/D5 receptor stimulation reduce the signal by closing n and p calcium channels, and *(3)* lower portion of the primary dendritic stem where high levels of NE release induce nonspecific glutamate release, resulting in sodium entry that increases "noise." Thus, the signal-to-noise ratio is reduced. A schematic depiction of an extracellular recording of this neuron *(4)* is also shown. The loss of delay-related activity would impair the ability to appropriately guide behavior; in the absence of new information, the subject may respond perseveratively. (*Source:* Adapted from Birnbaum et al., 1999a and Arnsten, 2000a)

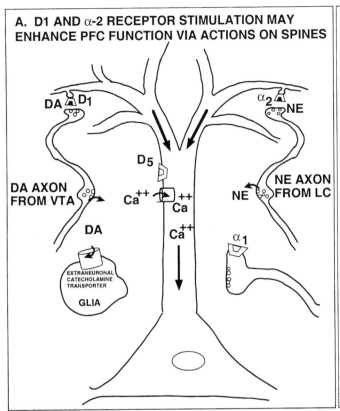

A. D1 AND α-2 RECEPTOR STIMULATION MAY ENHANCE PFC FUNCTION VIA ACTIONS ON SPINES

DA D1

α2 NE

D5

DA AXON FROM VTA

Ca^{++} Ca^{++}

NE

NE AXON FROM LC

DA

Ca^{++}

α1

EXTRANEURONAL CATECHOLAMINE TRANSPORTER

GLIA

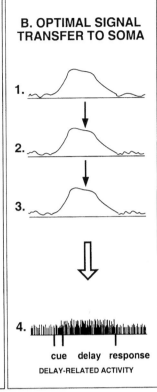

B. OPTIMAL SIGNAL TRANSFER TO SOMA

1.

2.

3.

4.

cue   delay   response

DELAY-RELATED ACTIVITY

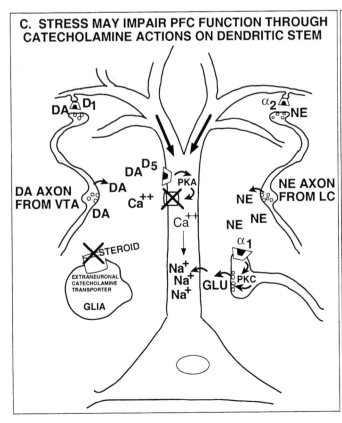

C. STRESS MAY IMPAIR PFC FUNCTION THROUGH CATECHOLAMINE ACTIONS ON DENDRITIC STEM

DA D1

α2 NE

DA D5

PKA

DA AXON FROM VTA

DA

Ca^{++}

NE

NE AXON FROM LC

DA

NE   NE

Ca^{++}

NE

α1

STEROID

Na^+ Na^+ Na^+

GLU   PKC

EXTRANEURONAL CATECHOLAMINE TRANSPORTER

GLIA

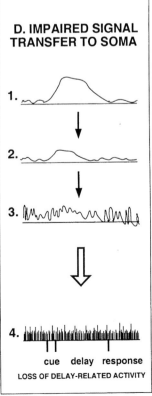

D. IMPAIRED SIGNAL TRANSFER TO SOMA

1.

2.

3.

4.

cue   delay   response

LOSS OF DELAY-RELATED ACTIVITY

may protect cognitive performance by engaging G_i proteins and reducing cAMP–PKA activity in the PFC.

Role of the D2 Family of Receptors. The role of the D2 family of receptors in the modulation of working memory is less well understood. D2/D3 compounds have opposing actions at pre- vs post synaptic receptors, and often produce marked side effects (e.g., dyskinesias, nausea) when administered systemically, which can obscure cognitive changes. Although a D2/D3 antagonist had little effect when infused into the PFC of monkeys, systemic administration of D2/D3/D4 agonists can improve working memory in monkeys (Arnsten et al., 1995) and humans (Kimberg et al., 1997) with working memory impairment (see below). It is possible that D4 receptor mechanisms in PFC contribute to these beneficial drug effects, as high doses of the selective D4 antagonist NGD94-1, can impair an object retrieval task associated with the PFC (Jentsch et al., 1998).

Stimulation of D4 receptors may be involved with stress-induced working memory deficits. Agents with potent D2 or D4 receptor–blocking activity such as haloperidol and clozapine are effective in preventing stress-induced cognitive deficits (Murphy et al., 1996a, 1997; (Arnsten & Goldman-Rakic 1998), but these agents have many other receptor actions, including D1 and α_1-receptor blockade. Recently, we have shown that a selective D4 receptor antagonist can reverse stress-induced cognitive deficits in monkeys (Arnsten et al., 2000), and rat studies have shown that infusion of a D2 receptor family agonist into the PFC impairs working memory in rats (Druzin et al., 2000). These findings suggest that high levels of D2/D3/D4 receptor stimulation may also contribute to cognitive deficits. D4 receptors are concentrated on γ-aminobutyric acid (GABA)ergic interneurons in the primate PFC (Mrzljak et al., 1996), which suggests that modulation of inhibitory mechanisms may contribute to these actions. However, direct infusions of D4 antagonists into the primate PFC and the development of D4 selective agonists are needed to further test the role of D4 receptors in PFC working memory function.

Possible Roles of Prefrontal Cortex Dopamine in Executive and Attentional Functions

When used in the animal literature, the working memory construct generally refers to the capacity to hold information about a stimulus on-line in a period after it is no longer present. However, the more extended concept of working memory in human cognition, introduced by Baddeley (1986), is, as one might expect, more complex, including not only two distinct short-term memory stores—an "articulatory loop," a form of subvocal rehearsal mechanism, and a short-term memory buffer for visuospatial imagery, the "visuospatial sketchpad"—but also a "central executive" system, which coordinates processing between the various dedicated satellite systems. This executive system is commonly related to the functioning of the PFC, although it would be naive to map so simply psychological processes onto anatomical structure. In fact, the 'cental executive' system of Baddeley (1986) has much in common with another possible model of frontal lobe functioning termed the "supervisory attentional system," in which control over instrumental choice behavior is exerted through "attention to action" (Shallice, 1982). This concept is particularly relevant to paradigms such as the spatial delayed-response or delayed-alternation task in which there are other cognitive requirements besides "holding stimuli on-line." For example, the animal has to inhibit making repeated responses to prepotent stimuli (Diamond, 1996). This control is potentially also modulated by PFC DA, as shown by the perseverative behavior elicited in rats by intracortical D1 agonists (Zahrt et al., 1997), regardless of whether one considers the inhibitory function to be a product of working memory processes or a relatively independent form of executive function. Given the possibility that the PFC may mediate "supervisory attentional functions," and the availability of additional approaches to modeling executive functions that also posit attentional mechanisms (Cohen et al., 1998), it is important to study the effects of manipulations of the mesocortical DA system on complex behavior that does not simply reflect the maintenance of stimuli on-line in a short-term store.

This was the approach taken by Collins et al. (1998), who attempted to model the complex aspects of executive control required of marmosets when performing sequences of behavior to achieve a goal. The animals were required to respond to a series of locations on a touch-sensitive screen without repeating responses to particular locations. This task clearly has some working memory requirements, but control experiments found that these were much less important than the capacity to inhibit previously performed responses. The striking result was that, although excitotoxic lesions of the entire PFC produced massive deficits resulting from perseverative responding, mesocortical DA depletion was entirely without effect. The importance of the negative result was confirmed by the usual significant effect of mesocortical DA depletion on spatial delayed-response performance. Thus, whereas prefrontal lesions affected both sequencing and spatial delayed response, mesocortical DA loss affected only the latter. These results suggest indeed a specific role for prefrontal DA in certain aspects of working memory but not in other forms of executive dysfunction. This dissociation has assumed some possible clinical significance from the observation that children with phenylketonuria are impaired in undertaking simple spatial memory tasks, but not in a test of self-ordered working memory (see Chapter 29).

Another commonly used clinical test of prefrontal function in humans, the Wisconsin Card Sorting Test (WCST) (Milner, 1964), often elicits perseverative responding in patients who experience difficulty in shifting one sorting rule to another. We have modelled this complex human paradigm in marmosets, using tests of visual discrimination learning including intradimensional set shifting, extradimensional set shifting, and reversal learning, and have found that reversal learning and extradimensional shift learning (conceptually, the key component of the Wisconsin Card Sort Test) depend on different sectors of the PFC (Dias et al., 1996a,b, 1997). Remarkably, however, prefrontal cortical DA depletion actually appeared to facilitate extradimensional set-

shifting, while having no effect on any other aspect of visual discrimination learning, including reversal and intradimensional set shifting (Roberts et al., 1994). Again, these same DA-depleted animals did exhibit deficits on the classical spatial delayed-response task. Thus, three tasks shown to be sensitive to lesions of the PFC—spatial delayed response, self-ordered sequencing, and a model of the Wisconsin Card Sorting Test—actually exhibit differential effects of prefrontal DA loss: deficit, no effect, and enhancement, respectively. This is important in terms of the inverted U-shaped function relating efficiency of performance to central DA function, as it seems that different tasks have different optimal levels of prefrontal DA activity, according to a Yerkes-Dodson principle. In other words, different operations possibly mediated by distinct regions of the PFC may have differing neurochemical needs in terms of the modulatory functions provided by the midbrain DA system. In theoretical terms, this may reflect the fact that stressful or arousing states probably require different sets of executive operations as a function of the overall level of stress or arousal to enable an adaptive coping with environmental demands (see also Robbins, 2000).

Recent findings have further served to define the nature of the attentional state of marmosets with PFC DA loss. One possible explanation for a facilitation of extradimensional set-shifting might arise from excessive attentional lability (or distractibility), which means that the animals with PFC DA loss may not initially have developed very strong attentional sets, with the result that they find it easier to shift when the reward contingenices are altered. There was no clear evidence of this in the original study (Roberts et al., 1994), but in that case the DA depletion was effected after the initial sets had been established, and this may have served to attenuate attentional problems. In a recent study (Crofts et al., 2000), the PFC DA depletion was effected before attentional set training, and the PFC DA-depleted animals now exhibited deficits at the intradimensional set-shifting stage and also during a special probe test in which novel stimuli irrelevant to the discrimination were introduced, to measure possible disruptive effects on the PFC DA-depleted animals' selective attentional capacities. Therefore, one interpretation of these experiments is that PFC DA-depleted monkeys have problems in the executive control of attention, which may lead to paradoxical improvements in performance under certain circumstances.

The hypothesis of a possible role for PFC DA in attentional function has been bolstered by studies in rats using intracerebral infusions of DA into the PFC in rats performing on a five-choice serial reaction time task in which working memory demands are, again, minimal. Granon et al. (2000) showed that intra-PFC infusions of the partial D1 agonist improved the accuracy of detecting visual targets when baseline performance was at a somewhat low level (about 70% correct) rather than a high level (80%). The D1 receptor antagonist SCH-23390 (but not the D2 receptor antagonist sulpiride) produced almost the opposite pattern of effects: impairment in the high, but not low, baseline rats. These data suggest that engagement of the PFC DA system can be beneficial in performance of an attentional test modelled after tests of continuous performance in humans, which may be relevant to the types of deficit observed in attention deficit hyperactivity disorder (ADHD).

In summary, DA exhibits an inverted "U" dose–response function in regard to PFC working memory and attentional functions through its actions at the D1 family of receptors. Thus, low levels of D1 receptor stimulation are essential for working memory function, but high levels, such as occur during stress, impair working memory function. The role of the D2 family is still being investigated.

NOREPINEPHRINE

Enhancement of Working Memory by α-2 Noradrenergic Receptors

Actions at Post-synaptic Receptors. Function Norepinephrine enhances PFC function via postsynaptic α_2 receptor stimulation. Studies in rodents, monkeys, and humans have all shown that NE has an important beneficial in-

fluence on PFC function through its actions at postsynaptic α_2 receptors. Young monkeys with working memory impairment induced by local PFC (Arnsten & Goldman-Rakic, 1985) or global (Cai et al., 1993) catecholamine depletion are greatly improved by treatment with α_2 agonists such as clonidine and guanfacine. The beneficial effects of α_2 NE agonists have also been observed in aged monkeys (Arnsten & Goldman-Rakic, 1985; Arnsten et al., 1988; Rama et al., 1996) and aged rats (Carlson et al., 1992) with naturally ocurring catecholamine loss. α_2 Agonists also improve working memory performance in intact, young monkeys, but at higher doses than those needed to improve aged or depleted animals (Franowicz & Arnsten, 1998). Indeed, the greater the loss of NE, the lower the dose of α_2 agonist needed to improve PFC performance (Franowicz & Arnsten, 1999), a pattern consistent with drug actions at supersensitive, postsynaptic receptors. Improvements with α_2 agonists can be reversed with α_2, but not α_1, antagonists, and α_2 antagonists by themselves impair PFC function, consistent with an α_2 receptor mechanism (Arnsten & Goldman-Rakic, 1985).

Subtype of α-2 Receptor. Pharmacological profiles further indicate that the α_{2A} receptor subtype may be the most critical for cognitive enhancement (see Arnsten et al., 1996, for review). For example, the α_{2A}-selective agonist, guanfacine, is the most effective compound in enhancing working memory without side effects (Arnsten et al., 1988; Rama et al., 1996). Guanfacine is about ten times weaker than clonidine in inhibiting firing of the NE cell bodies in the locus coeruleus (LC) or in decreasing NE release (Engberg & Eriksson, 1991), but is 10–100 times more potent in improving working memory in aged monkeys (Arnsten et al., 1988). Recent studies in genetically altered mice emphasize the importance of the α_{2A} receptor subtype, as mice with a mutation of the α_{2A} subtype no longer show beneficial effects on working memory (Franowicz et al., 1998), while knockout of the α_{2C} subtype has no effect on drug response (Tanila et al., 1999). Although knockout of the α_{2C} receptor had no effect on working mem-

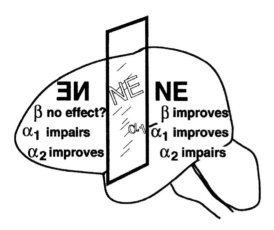

Figure 4-4. The prefrontal cortex (PFC) appears to be modulated in a manner that is "upside and backwards" from the rest of the brain, at least in regard to norepinephrine (NE) mechanisms. Thus, neuromodulation of PFC cognitive functions are the "mirror image" of posterior cortical mechanisms: PFC cognitive functions are improved by α_2 receptor stimulation and impaired by α_1 receptor stimulation, while β receptor stimulation appears to have no effect (these mechanisms are still being investigated). In contrast, α_2 receptor stimulation has no effect or often impairs functions carried out by posterior cortical and subcortical regions, which are improved by β and α_1 receptor stimulation. Because NE has higher affinity for α_2 receptors than for α_1 or β receptors, conditions of modest NE release would favor PFC regulation of behavior, while conditions of high NE release (e.g., stress) would favor posterior cortical and subcortical regulation of behavior. In this way, NE may act as a chemical "switch" to alter the brain systems in control of thoughts and actions. (*Source:* Adapted from Arnsten, 2000b)

ory, it does seem to be related to the modulation of other NE-associated behaviors. Interestingly, knockout of the α_{2C} subtype diminished the response to stress in classic tests of anxiety (Sallinen et al., 1999), which suggests that α_{2C} receptor stimulation contributes to the anxiogenic response.

Second Messenger Actions. The second-messenger mechanisms underlying the beneficial effects of α_2 agonists on PFC function are currently unknown. However, α_2 receptors are commonly coupled to G_i proteins, which inhibit adenylyl cyclase–cAMP pathways (Duman & Nestler, 1995). Because activation of the adenylyl cyclase–cAMP pathway seems to impair PFC function (see above), inhibition of

this intracellular signaling pathway may contribute to the beneficial effects of α_2 agonists on PFC cognitive function.

Effects on non PFC Tasks. α_2 Agonists improve the performance of tasks that challenge the PFC, but often have little benefit under conditions that do not challenge the PFC. α_2 Agonists have been shown to improve working memory for both visuospatial (Arnsten et al., 1988) and visualfeature (Jackson & Buccafusco, 1991) cues, suggesting enhancement of both dorsolateral and ventrolateral PFC function. In contrast, α_2 agonists do not improve, and sometimes impair, cognitive functions associated with parietal and temporal lobe functions (Fig. 4–4). For example, these drugs have no effect on or impair the spatial memory functions of the hippocampus (Sirviö et al., 1991), the visual—feature discrimination memory functions of the inferior temporal cortex (Arnsten & Goldman-Rakic, 1985; Steere & Arnsten, 1997), the visual-feature recognition memory functions of the perirhinal cortex (Arnsten & Goldman-Rakic, 1990a), or the covert visuospatial attention-shifting functions of the parietal cortex (Witte & Marrocco, 1997).

Effects on PFC Neurons. A number of studies in rodents and monkeys have demonstrated that α_2 compounds act directly in the PFC to alter working memory function. As with systemic injection, direct infusion of α_2 antagonists, but not α_1 or β antagonists, into the dorsolateral PFC produces a delay-related impairment in spatial working memory (Li & Mei, 1994), demonstrating that endogenous NE stimulation of α_2 receptors in the PFC is critical to working memory performance. Conversely, intra-PFC infusion of α_2 agonists improves working memory performance in either young (Mao et al., 1999) or aged monkeys (Arnsten, 1997) or aged rats (Tanila et al., 1996). Electrophysiological studies have observed similar findings at the cellular level. Iontophoresis of the α_2 antagonist yohimbine reduces delay-related activity in PFC neurons of monkeys performing spatial working memory tasks (Li et al., 1999; Sawaguchi, 1998). Conversely, systemic clonidine administration enhances delay-related firing in PFC cells, and this effect is reversed by iontophoretic application of yohimbine (Li et al., 1999). Thus, NE actions at α_2 receptors in PFC have powerful effects on delay-related firing, the presumed neuronal substrate of working memory function. It is possible that the beneficial effects of α_2 receptor stimulation occur on dendritic spines (Fig. 4–3), as α_{2A} receptors have been localized on the postsynaptic membranes of spines in monkey PFC (Aoki et al., 1994; Arnsten et al., 1996). However, there are no electrophysiological data to support or refute this hypothesis.

Imaging Data. Imaging studies in monkeys are also consistent with α_2-adrenergic mechanisms enhancing PFC function. We have observed increased regional cerebral blood flow (rCBF) in the dorsolateral PFC of monkeys treated with guanfacine prior to performing a spatial working memory task (Avery et al., 2000). Guanfacine improved working memory performance and increased rCBF in the PFC surrounding the principal sulcus, the same region essential for spatial working memory function (Goldman & Rosvold, 1970). In contrast, guanfacine had no effect on rCBF in the auditory association cortex (superior temporal cortex), a region not involved in task performance (Avery et al., 2000). These results are consistent with imaging studies in humans treated with guanfacine (see below).

Other Prefrontal Cortex Functions. Most studies of NE modulation of PFC function have used working memory tasks, but a few animal studies have shown effects on attention regulation and behavioral inhibition. For example, α_2 agonists are particularly effective in enhancing working memory during distracting conditions (Jackson & Buccafusco, 1991; Arnsten & Contant, 1992), a finding consistent with earlier studies showing that forebrain NE depletion increases distractibility (Carli et al., 1983). Higher doses of guanfacine have also been shown to improve performance of an object reversal task associated with orbital PFC function (Steere & Arnsten, 1997). Clonidine and guanfacine have been shown in humans to improve attentional regulation, behavioral inhibition, and planning as well (see below).

Impairment of Working Memory by α-1 Noradrenergic Receptors.

High Levels of NE Impair Working Memory Function via α_1 Receptor Stimulation. New evidence indicates that high concentrations of NE impair PFC function through activation of α_1 receptors. Norepinephrine has higher affinity for α_{2A} than α_1 receptors (α_{2A} receptors: 56 nM [O'Rourke et al., 1994]; α_1 receptors: 330 nM [Mohell et al., 1983]). Thus it is likely that low levels of NE (e.g., under basal or nonstress conditions) preferentially engage α_2 receptors and improve PFC function, while during conditions of high NE release, α_1 receptors would become engaged and override the effects of α_2 receptor stimulation. It is well established that high levels of NE are released in the PFC during stress exposure (e.g., Finlay et al., 1995; Goldstein et al., 1996), and recent evidence suggests that these high NE levels stimulate α_1 receptors and impair PFC function (Birnbaum et al., 1999a). Thus, stress-induced cognitive deficits were blocked by infusion of the α_1 receptor antagonist urapidil into the PFC prior to cognitive testing (Birnbaum et al., 1999a). Infusions of urapidil had no effect under nonstress conditions (Birnbaum et al., 1999a), presumably because there is little endogenous NE α_1 receptor stimulation during nonstressful conditions.

The effects of stress on working memory performance can be mimicked by infusion of an α_1 receptor agonist into the PFC. Infusions of the α_1 agonist phenylephrine into the PFC in rats markedly impaired working memory performance (Arnsten et al., 1999). This impairment was reversed by co-infusion of the α_1 receptor antagonist urapidil (Arnsten et al., 1999), which is consistent with actions at α_1 receptors. Similar effects have been observed in monkeys, in which infusions of phenylephrine into the dorsolateral PFC produced a marked delay-related impairment in working memory performance (Mao et al., 1999). Infusions were most effective in the caudal two-thirds of the principal sulcal cortex (Mao et al., 1999), the cortical region most tightly associated with spatial working memory performance in monkeys (Goldman & Rosvold, 1970). Thus, high levels of NE release in the

PFC may engage α_1 receptors and impair PFC working memory function. Interestingly, most effective antipsychotic medications, including the new "atypical" neuroleptics, have potent α_1 blocking properties (Baldessarini et al., 1992). Although most previous attention has focused on the sedating effects of these α_1 blocking properties, the current data suggest that α_1 blockade may have therapeutic effects as well.

Second Messenger Actions. α_1 Receptors are commonly coupled to the phosphotidyl inositol–protein kinase C (PKC) intracellular pathway via G_q proteins (Duman & Nestler, 1995). Evidence to date suggests that α_1 receptor stimulation impairs PFC function through activation of this second messenger pathway. For example, the cognitive impairment induced by phenylephrine infusions into the rat PFC can be completely reversed by pretreatment with a dose of lithium known to suppress phosphotidyl inositol turnover (Arnsten et al., 1999). However, lithium can alter other second-messenger pathways; thus current studies in animals are focusing on agents that selectively target molecules in the phosphotidyl inositol–PKC cascade. For example, intra-PFC infusion of the PKC inhibitor chelerythrine appears to block the detrimental effects of α_1 agonists (Birnbaum et al., 1999b). These results are consistent with activation of the phosphotidyl inositol–PKC pathway underlying α_1 receptor–mediated impairment of PFC cognitive function. The finding that excessive activation of PKC impairs PFC function may have direct relevance to the symptoms of disinhibition in mania, a disorder associated with overactivation of PKC and treated by agents such as lithium, which reduce the activity of the phosphotidyl inositol–PKC cascade (Manji & Lenox, 1999).

Model of Actions in Prefrontel Cortex. The intracellular recordings of Marek and Aghajanian (1999) suggest an interesting cellular mechanism by which α_1 receptor stimulation may impair PFC cognitive functioning. Their studies have shown that NE acts at α_1 adrenoceptors to increase glutamate release, which in turn increases excitatory postsynaptic sodium currents in the proximal dendritic stem.

In other words, α_1 receptor stimulation may erode signal transfer by increasing noise in the dendritic stem, as schematically depicted in Figure 4–3. This increase in background noise would obscure signal transmission by decreasing the signal/noise ratio of cell response and would prevent the normal increase in delay-related activity of the soma needed to guide behavior during working memory tasks. In summary, DA D1 receptor stimulation would decrease "signal," while NE α_1 stimulation may increase "noise." It is likely that these NE and DA actions are additive or synergistic, and the signal may be able to survive either modest reduction by DA or modest noise by NE, but could not survive both. This hypothesis is supported by the finding that either a D1 (Murphy et al., 1996a; Arnsten & Goldman-Rakic, 1998) or an α_1-adrenoceptor antagonist (Birnbaum et al., 1999a) can protect performance from the detrimental effects of stress.

The hypothetical model presented in Figure 4–3 implies that it is not only the *level* of catecholamine stimulation that determines beneficial vs. deterimental effects on PFC function, but also the *location* on the neuron where these actions take place. Simply put, the model implies that catecholamine actions on spines and on distal dendrites enhance signal processing and working memory function, while catecholamine actions on the primary dendritic stem erode signal transfer to the soma and impair working memory function. Dopamine fibers generally avoid the primary dendritic stems of pyramidal cells, and extra-neuronal catecholamine transporters on glia may absorb any leakage of catecholamines into the extrasynaptic space, thus maintaining low levels of catecholamine stimulation *near* the dendritic stem. However, during exposure to stress, increases in cortisol would block the extraneuronal catecholamine transporters and allow catecholamine levels to build and engage receptors on or near the stem, reducing signal transmission to the soma. If this model is correct, working memory should be impaired by exogenous administration of cortisol, and recent evidence from human studies suggests this may be true (Lupien et al., 1999). This model may also explain why stimulants such as amphetamine and methylphenidate, which produce high levels of catecholamine release, generally improve rather than impair working memory function in humans (Mehta et al., 2000), as under these nonstressful conditions, the extraneuronal catecholamine transporters would protect the dendritic stem from the high levels of release. The model also predicts that individuals would be more vulnerable to the detrimental effects of catecholamine release during stress if they had either (1) higher cortisol levels (e.g., advanced age) and/or (2) degeneration of distal dendrites and spines (e.g., schizophrenia, advanced age).

In summary, NE has opposing actions on PFC functions: it improves working memory and attention regulation through actions at postsynaptic, α_{2A} receptors, while impairing PFC function through actions at α_1 receptors. Because NE has higher affinity for α_{2A} than α_1 receptors, NE can act as a chemical switch, strengthening PFC function under nonstress conditions and taking PFC off-line during uncontrollable stress when high levels of NE are released in the brain.

SEROTONIN

In comparison with the catecholamines DA and NE, relatively little is known about the precise functions of the indoleamine serotonin (5HT) in cognition in experimental animals, especially with regard to PFC function. This is partly because of the complexity of the distribution of different 5HT receptor types within the neuronal circuitry of the PFC (Goldman-Rakic, 1999). In fact, it may prove to be the case that, in contradistinction to links being made between studies of the functions of PFC catecholamines in experimental animals and hypotheses about the roles of PFC catecholamines in human cognition, the reverse situation is true for PFC 5HT (see section on serotonin effects in humans, below). There are some studies of the effects of 5HT manipulations on spatial working memory processes in rats (Winter & Petti, 1987; Cole et al., 1994; Warburton et al., 1997; see Steckler & Sahgal, 1995, for a review), but these may well involve effects at the level of the hippocampus rather than the PFC. In support of this, the classic study of Brozoski et al. (1979) found no effect of PFC 5HT depletion on spa-

tial delayed response in monkeys. Similarly, systemic administration of 5HT3 receptor antagonists to monkeys had no effect on performance of a working memory task, nor did it impair reversal in object discrimination task (Arnsten et al., 1997). However, these compounds did improve acquisition of the initial object discrimination, suggesting a beneficial effect on inferior temporal cortical function. Although these results suggest that the PFC may be more sensitive to catecholamine than serotonergic influences, the pharmacology of serotonin is immensely complex, and it is likely that important serotonergic influences will be observed when the right pharmacological tools are applied. Recently, electrophysiological studies of PFC neurons have focused on the 5HT2A receptor, given its relevance to schizophrenia. In rat PFC slices, Marek has observed marked increases in the excitatory postsynaptic sodium currents in the proximal dendritic stem of PFC pyramidal cells (Marek & Aghajanian, 1999). These mechanisms are now being studied in the PFC of awake behaving monkeys, in which 5HT2A receptor blockade disrupts spatial tuning of PFC neurons during a spatial working memory task (Williams et al., 1997). However, we still do not know what effects 5HT2A agonist or antagonist infusions into the PFC have on cognitive performance.

In summary, we are still learning about serotonergic influences on PFC function. The complexity of 5HT receptor pharmacology makes this task difficult.

ACETYLCHOLINE

An association of acetylcholine (ACh) with the intellectual deterioration of Alzheimer's disease has become well established from histopathological evidence of degeneration of the basal forebrain cholinergic system projecting to the cerebral cortex and a corresponding reduction of neocortical cholinergic markers such as choline acetyltransferase activity (Perry et al, 1978). More recently, similar relationships have been reported for Parkinson's disease and Lewy Body dementia (Perry et al., 1999). What is less well established is the causal role of ACh in the characteristic deficits in memory and learning as was well as in other domains of cognition shown, for example, in Alzheimer's disease. Pertinent to the present chapter are the effects of cholinergic loss from the PFC itself.

Much of the relevant evidence has derived from work in rats and monkeys after they have either developed lesions of the basal forebrain or received an infusion of cholinergic agents into the prefrontal regions (see Everitt & Robbins, 1997, for a review). The former source of evidence is complicated by the relative lack of specificity of the lesions of the basal forebrain because of the absence at that time of a specific cholinergic neurotoxin. One claim made by our own group has been that basal forebrain lesions in the rat leading to cholinergic depletion of the rat frontal cortex impair the accuracy of discrimination on the same five-choice discrimination task described above (e.g., Granon et al., 2000). These deficits were corrected under certain conditions by administering drugs that boost cholinergic function, such as the anti-cholinesterase physostigmine and nicotine (Muir et al., 1995). This implication of cholinergic systems in attentional functions has recently been substantiated by two lines of evidence: (1) that lesions made using the selective cholinergic immunotoxin saporin mimic to some extent the effects of less specific lesions (McGaughy et al., 2000), and (2) that ACh is released from the frontal cortex as the rat performs this task relative to a suitable control task (Passetti et al., 2000). The hypothesis that ACh has a role in modulating attentional function mediated by the rat frontal cortex is also consistent with evidence from other investigators who have used a variety of approaches (e.g., Sarter & Bruno, 1997).

Other approaches have suggested that ACh contributes to working memory processes within the rat prefrontal cortex. Broersen et al. (1995), for example, have provided evidence for delay-dependent deficits in two rat working memory tasks (delayed matching to position [DMTP] and delayed non-matching to position [DNMTP]) following intra-PFC infusions of the anti-cholinergic drug scopolamine. These effects were much more convincing than those obtained following similar

infusions of D1 antagonists, although intra-PFC scopolamine also impairs performance on the five-choice task (Robbins et al., 1998a), so the precise role of ACh in attention and working memory needs to be determined in the same experimental setting. Intriguingly, Granon et al. (1995) have shown differential effects of intra-PFC infusions of a nicotine receptor antagonist on DMTP and DNMTP working memory tasks for the rat that appear to recruit different degrees of "effortful processing" with detrimental results achieved for the effortful variant but not for the non-effortful one. These data may be related to the observations of Granon et al. (2000) of the effects of intra-PFC infusion of the D1 agonist SKF38393 on rats with relatively low baseline levels of accuracy.

In nonhuman primates, there is less convincing evidence to link frontal cholinergic function with working memory. Classical studies by Bartus and Johnson (1976) seemed to indicate specific delay-dependent impairments in spatial delayed-response performance following systemic scopolamine. However, the behavioral, as well as the neural, specificity of these effects is a little in doubt. For example, scopolamine also certainly impairs attentional performance in monkeys (Witte et al., 1997), but there is no specific evidence to link the delayed-response deficit following administration of scopolamine solely to the PFC and not to other possible contributory structures such as the hippocampus and caudate nucleus.

There have, in fact, been relatively few studies of the role of prefrontal ACh in cognition (see Everitt & Robbins, 1997). One possibly salient result is the demonstration of serial reversal learning deficits but sparing of extradimensional shifting following nonselective excitotoxic lesions of the marmoset basal forebrain that lead to significant reductions of cortical choline acetyltransferase activity (Roberts et al., 1992). Unlike the effects of mesocortical DA depletion (see above), these monkeys also exhibited reductions in distractibility when irrelevant background stimuli were manipulated. The impaired reversal learning but spared extradimensional shift performance is reminiscent of the effects of orbitofrontal, as distinct from lateral, lesions of the marmoset prefrontal cortex (see above, Dias et al., 1996a,). These findings are therefore quite consistent with the existence of strong projections of the orbitofrontal cortex to the basal forebrain, and there may be significant associations of cholinergic activity with orbitofrontal function (Mesulam, 1995). However, these findings need to be reexamined with the more specific lesioning tool of saporin, which has been employed to effect lesions of the marmoset basal forebrain cholinergic neurons sufficient to produce impairments in object discrimination learning (Ridley et al., 1999).

In summary, ACh has a powerful effect on PFC function and may be particularly important for orbital/medial PFC function. Impairment with cholinergic depletion or receptor blockade has been more prominent than improvement with cholinergic agonists. This may be due to the relatively poor availability of cholinergic agonists that can enter the brain. Alternatively, ACh may have rapid, time-dependent actions that are not mimicked well by pharmacotherapies.

STUDIES IN HUMANS

DOPAMINE

Critical evidence for the role of DA in PFC function in humans derives from two main sources: studies of patients with disorders that implicate the DA system, and studies on the effects of dopaminergic drugs in normal subjects. Such work is beginning to be augmented by the use of functional neuroimaging—generally positron emission tomography (PET), but most recently functional magnetic resonance imaging (fMRI)—to measure interactions between task and drug effects on regional cerebral blood flow (rCBF). This latter approach is essential in human studies, as it is the only means at present of resolving whether the primary locus of a DA drug effect is at a striatal or prefrontal cortical level, although anatomical connectivity of the frontostriatal circuitry (Alexander et al., 1986) makes it likely that DA effects within the striatum can

potentially affect prefrontal or, indeed, executive functioning.

Dopamine and Cognition in Clinical Disorders

Restorations of underactive (or alternatively, reductions in overactive) dopaminergic transmission are generally assumed to be beneficial for cognitive function and motivate attempts to treat such diverse disorders as Parkinson's disease (PD), schizophrenia, ADHD, and, more recently, acute brain injury.

A cognitive deficit syndrome occurs in idiopathic PD, even early in its course (Taylor et al., 1986; Owen et al., 1992), and also following MPTP-induced parkinsonism (Stern & Langston, 1985). Many aspects of this syndrome are similar to those seen after PFC dysfunction and include impairments in working memory, planning, and set shifting (Robbins et al., 1998b) in the relatively early stages of the disease, although a range of other memory and learning impairments are also evident (e.g., Knowlton et al., 1996). It is more difficult to be sure which, if any, of these deficits are linked specifically to the loss of PFC DA or even to central DA in general, because of the multivariate nature of the neurochemical pathology of this neurodegenerative disease. Effects of dopaminergic medication for PD would nonetheless appear to implicate DA to some extent. For example, cognitive deficits seen in medicated PD patients with mild clinical disability may be less than those seen in PD patients earlier in the course of the disease who have received no medication (Downes et al., 1989; Owen et al., 1995a). Inferences can also be made on the basis of longitudinal studies in which the effects of medication are assessed prior to and following medication, as long as one assumes that the disease itself pursues an unremitting course of further deficit. In one such large-scale study, Growdon et al. (1998) reported that levodopa improved motor function without impairing cognition in nondemented PD patients with mild disability; in fact, performance in tests of executive function, which were supposed to be sensitive to frontal lobe dysfunction, showed some benefit of medication. However, the most informative evidence may be that in which PD patients have their medication removed in a controlled manner. In one study of this type, Lange et al. (1992) showed that L-Dopa withdrawal from a small group ($n = 10$) of PD patients selectively impaired their performance on tests from the Cambridge Neuropsychological Test Automated Battery (CANTAB) of spatial working memory, planning, and varieties of visual discrimination learning. Of interest was that the latency as well as the accuracy of thinking on the planning task were both affected in this group, which may parallel the beneficial effects of medication on bradykinesia in PD.

However, dopaminergic medication does not always have beneficial effects on cognition in PD. Gotham et al. (1988) provided evidence that certain aspects of cognitive performance in PD could actually be worsened by L-Dopa. They proposed a hypothesis that related the effects of L-Dopa to the pattern and course of DA loss within the striatum in PD. Those regions suffering extensive DA depletion, such as the putamen, would have their functions optimally titrated by DA medication. By contrast, those regions that were relatively spared in the early stages, such as the caudate and ventral striatum, would potentially be disrupted by medication, as the level of DA function would presumably be set supra-optimally by the drug. This hypothesis is schematically represented in Figure 4–2, which invokes the same inverted U-shaped function as that used above to explain the deleterious effects of excessive DA activity in the PFC. Further evidence to support the Gotham et al. (1988) hypothesis comes from a recent study by Swainson et al. (2000), which showed that medicated PD patients with mild disability performed poorly on tests of probability reversal learning, which is likely associated with ventral striatal and orbitofrontal function, while the same PD patients' results were relatively improved on tests of spatial memory function. A recent L-Dopa withdrawal study in Parkinsons disease patients substantiates and extends these findings (Cools et al, 2001, see Fig. 4–2).

The use of dopaminergic medication for other forms of neurological disturbance is more limited, but case study reports and experimental studies (e.g., McDowell et al., 1998) are suggesting possible applications for brain-injured patients. McDowell et al. (1998) examined the effects of a low dose of the DA D2 receptor agonist bromocriptine on working memory and other executive forms of cognitive function in individuals with traumatic brain injury in a double-blind crossover trial with placebo. Consistent with the findings for Parkinson's disease, bromocriptine improved performance on some but not all tasks thought to be subserved by the PFC. Also consistent with results in the Parkinson's disease literature, no effects were observed for control tasks not thought to be subserved by the PFC. More controversially, and seemingly at odds with both the animal literature (see above) and that on normal individuals (to be reviewed below), bromocriptine exerted no effects on working memory tasks, with minimal additional demands placed on executive function. A further puzzle is whether the D2 receptor agonist exerts its beneficial effects on executive performance at the level of the PFC or, indirectly, via the striatum.

Making inferences about the functions of DA in cognition is less promising in the case of schizophrenia, as antipsychotic medication may produce indirect effects on performance by the remediation of disruptive positive symptoms. Additionally, as we have seen above (e.g., Williams et al., 1998) neuroleptic drugs can impair cognitive functioning (King, 1990). In a comprehensive review, Mortimer (1997) concluded that much remained unclear about whether neuroleptic treatment affected the cognitive deficit syndrome present in schizophrenia. The effects of conventional neuroleptics are quite small, often being beneficial and related to the remission of psychosis. The possibility that the so-called atypical neuroleptics such as clozapine exert "cognitive facilitatory" as well as "cognitive sparing" effects needs to be resolved using more sophisticated neuropsychological methods and study designs.

The potential complexity of this area can be gauged from a functional neuroimaging study using PET to measure rCBF in normal and unmedicated schizophrenic subjects following challenge with apomorphine or placebo (Dolan et al., 1995). This study extends an analogously motivated study of the effects of d-amphetamine in schizophrenia (Daniel et al., 1991). Dolan et al. (1995) found that rCBF was enhanced in the anterior cingulate cortex of schizophrenic patients performing a verbal fluency task. One problem in interpreting these results, however, is that it is not known whether the effects of apomorphine depend on an enhancement of DA neurotransmision or, alternatively, on reductions, via its presynaptic action at D2 receptors. Another problem of interpretation is the lack of reported data on verbal fluency performance in that study, so although the therapeutic implications may be evident, the actual impact on cognition of cortical actions of apomorphine in schizophrenic or normal individuals is a little unclear.

Similar uncertainties about whether treatment "damps down" unwanted activity or boosts deficient functioning also hinder our understanding of the basis of the effective strategy of treating ADHD with methylphenidate and amphetamine-like compounds (Mehta et al., 2000, 2001 Solanto et al., 2000). Converging evidence implicates the dopaminergic system and the prefrontal and nigrostriatal regions in the pathophysiology of childhood ADHD and prefrontal catecholaminergic dysfunction in adult ADHD (Ernst et al., 1998), but it remains unclear to what extent the beneficial effects of drugs such as methylphenidate (Ritalin) depend on modulation of dopaminergic or noradrenergic neurotransmission, or both. The neural site of such effects is also unclear. Vaidya et al. (1998) have recently employed fMRI in a go no-go functional imaging paradigm to show that methylphenidate attenuated blood flow in the basal ganglia of normal children but increased blood flow in children with ADHD. Equivalent degrees of frontal activation were seen in both groups, however. Improvements in behavioral performance were also seen in both groups following administration of the drug, but it is difficult to be sure at which neural loci the stimulant is acting to produce these

effects. Studies by Mattay et al. (1996) and Mehta et al. (2000) on the effects of d-amphetamine and methylphenidate, respectively, in normal volunteers implicate cortical networks that include the dorsolateral PFC. In these latter experiments, tasks that normally require PFC functioning (performance on the WCST and self-ordered spatial working memory tasks, respectively) were employed, so the identity of the neural networks upon which stimulant drugs exert their effects on performance—for both normal and clinical populations—may hinge on the nature of the task under study.

Effects of Dopaminergic Drugs on Cognition in Normal Human Volunteers

The early literature showing that amphetamine-like drugs have beneficial effects on vigilance functions has generally been supported by more recent work (Koelega, 1993). Despite the use of methylphenidate in treating ADHD, until recently, the effects of this drug on other aspects of cognition had not been widely investigated. Clark et al. (1986) showed that methylphenidate (0.65 mg/kg p.o.) reversed impairments in a dichotic auditory attention task produced by the neuroleptic droperidol. By itself, however, methyphenidate had little effect except to enhance subjective increases in elation, energy, and alertness. Significant improvements in performance of CANTAB tests of self-ordered spatial working memory and planning functions were produced by a similar oral dose of the drug (Elliott et al. 1997). These improvements were limited mainly to the first test session and so were not correlated with changes in subjective arousal which occurred on both test sessions. Indeed, when taken on a second session, the drug sometimes increased the speed of responding on certain tests at the expense of reduced accuracy. Also evident was an enhanced retrieval of certain aspects of performance, a finding consistent with other data (Evans et al., 1986). A more recent study (Rogers et al., 1999a) has shown that use of methylphenidate in humans (at the same dosage as that employed by Elliott et al.) can improve performance on an extradimensional set shift task, similar to the one employed in a study with monkeys by Roberts et al. (1994), but at the cost of slowing performance and increasing errors in the control test of intradimensional set shifting. These results are important in showing that it is possible to demonstrate improvements in normal individuals treated with methylphenidate as well as in patients with ADHD. However, consistent with the animal and clinical data reviewed above, other functions may also show impairment. Thus, drugs such as methylphenidate (and presumably also amphetamine) seem to place the subject in an altered mode of functioning that is optimal for certain forms of performance, such as working memory, memory retrieval functions, and responding to previously irrelevant stimulus dimensions, but at the cost of other capacities, in a way reminiscent of the effects of manipulations of the PFC in experimental animals. The challenge now is to determine the precise contribution of DA itself to these effects and to identify the neural loci of the drug–task interactions in the intact brain.

The most direct means of taking up this challenge is to study the effects of specific DA agonists and antagonists on human cognition, ideally incorporating a functional imaging approach wherever feasible. Unfortunately, the lack of suitably selective compounds that can be administered to normal human volunteers (e.g., without emetic and dyskinetic side effects) limited in this type of study. Nonetheless, D2 antagonists have been given to normal subjects and have been shown to generally impair cognitive function. The impairments are not simply linked to sedative actions, as, for example, sulpiride produces relatively little effect on tests of sustained attention and associative learning that are sensitive to benzodiazepines such as diazepam (Mehta et al., 1999). In the same study, however, sulpiride (400 mg p.o.) did produce a pattern of impairments that is qualitatively similar to that seen in Parkinson's disease, including deficits in spatial but not visual pattern recognition memory, planning performance, and attentional set shifting—again reflecting capacities mediated by fronto striatal systems.

The greater predominance of D2 receptor binding in striatal as distinct from cortical regions actually implicates the striatum as a probable site of action of many of these effects. This is consistent with evidence of correlations between DA D2 receptor binding in both normal volunteers and neurological patients. For example, Volkow et al. (1998) found several significant correlations between performance measures (on tasks administered outside the scanner) and indices of D2 receptor binding using [^{11}C] raclopride. Although these were greatest for motor tasks such as finger tapping, significant correlations were also found for measures of cognitive function, including performance on Raven's Matrices and the Stroop and WCST tests (categories attained measure), even after correcting for the considerable decline in D2 receptor binding that occurs with normal aging. Additionally, Lawrence et al. (1998) found that several aspects of performance on spatial working memory and planning tasks exhibited significant correlations with indices of striatal D2 receptor binding in patients at various stages of Huntington's disease. An exciting prospect would be to attempt to confirm such findings using functional imaging paradigms to effect DA receptor displacement—in other words, to directly relate DA release to cognitive performance in conscious human subjects. Some progress in attaining this goal has been made in what promises to be a seminal study by Koepp et al. (1998). They were able to show that performance in a motivating video game could be used to reduce binding of raclopride to DA receptors in the region of the ventral striatum, presumably because of striatal DA release engendered by the task. While the nature of the cognitive operations engaged by this task within the striatum could not be identified from this study alone, it nevertheless offers considerable promise for making future advances in this area, particularly if used in combination with the other approaches we have surveyed.

Most impressive of all would be the demonstration of significant facilitation in aspects of cognitive function following administration of specific DA receptor agonists. For the most part, it has only proven feasible to assess performance—altering effects of D2 agents such as bromocriptine or, alternatively, of mixed

D1–D2 agents such as apomorphine and pergolide. Even though only a few studies have emerged so far, significant improvements in some aspects of cognitive performance have been seen in most of these. One exception is that of Grasby et al. (1992), who showed that apomorphine (5 and 10 ug s.c.) impaired learning of an auditory-verbal word list in a PET-scanning paradigm, and that these effects were related to its effects to reduce PFC rCBF.

By contrast, improvements in cognitive function have mainly been observed in visuospatial working memory tasks. Luciana et al. (1992) were the first to demonstrate that bromocriptine (2.5 mg p.o.) enhanced the accuracy of performance in a spatial delayed-response task for humans. Luciana and Collins (1998) extended the result to show improvement of memory for spatial but not object cues at a lower dose of bromocriptine (1.25 mg). Muller et al. (1998) using a rather different delayed matching working memory task in which subjects had to match the location of a complex visual pattern within a spatial frame of reference, failed to find significant improvement with bromocriptine (2.5 mg). They were able, however, to demonstrate significant benefits of the mixed DA agonist pergolide, which they attributed to its D1 receptor agonist properties. Further light has been shed on the possible variables controlling these effects through findings of Kimberg et al. (1997) that the effect of bromocriptine in normal young adults depended on their baseline working memory capacity. After receiving 2.5 mg of bromocriptine, high-capacity subjects performed more poorly on a range of executive and working memory tasks, whereas low-capacity subjects performed better after the same dosage. This finding is reminiscent of the inverted U-shaped Yerkes-Dodson—like functions already shown earlier to be important for influencing the effects of dopaminergic manipulations, although Kimberg et al. (1997) actually invoke more computationally rigorous applications of the sigmoid activation function (Servan-Schreiber et al., 1990).

Kimberg et al. thus failed to replicate Luciana et al.'s (1992) effects with a task that was slightly different from that used by them, in its inclusion of a central distractor condition. While Kimberg et al. suggest that the discrepancy between their results and those of Luciana et al. might reflect differences in the baseline working memory capacities of their subject samples, another plausible explanation is that the less complex visuospatial form of the memory task, requiring memory for only the location of a simple stimulus at a single spatial location, may be more sensitive to improvement than the more complex forms of this task. Mehta et al. (unpublished results, see Mehta et al., 2001) have shown that a lower dose of bromocriptine (1.25 mg) improves performance of the CANTAB spatial span task but not its self-ordered spatial working memory equivalent.

Evidently, the effects of dopaminergic agents such as bromocriptine are quite weak and subtle, depending on both the nature of the task under study as well as the baseline capacities of normal individuals. Nevertheless, the data are exciting in that they help to remove the prospect of "cognitive-enhancing" drugs for normal individuals from the realm of science fiction. It already seems quite clear, however, that enhancement is only likely to be achieved in certain situations and only at the possible cost of inefficiency in other domains. The apparent susceptibility of individuals low in baseline working memory capacity to cognition-enhancing effects of bromocriptine may be a useful portent for the use of D2 agonists in clinical applications.

In summary, altered DA likely contributes to many PFC disorders, including PD, schizophrenia, and ADHD. However, the absence of D1 agonists for human use has greatly hindered the development of DA therapies for these patients. Data from normal volunteers suggest that DA mechanisms likely exhibit an inverted U dose–response curve in humans, just as in animals.

NOREPINEPHRINE

Most research on NE mechanisms and PFC function in humans has focused on α_2 compounds, as agonists at the α_1- and β-adrenergic receptor generally do not cross the blood–brain barrier, and the few that do are usually not approved for human use. Until recently, most of the human research has focused on the α_2 agonist clonidine, a suboptimal drug because of its potent inhibition of LC firing, prominent side-effect profile, and high affinity for imidazoline I1 receptors. Clonidine usually has mixed effects on PFC functions in healthy young adults, presumably because of competing pre- vs. postsynaptic effects and dose limitations from sedative and hypotensive side effects (Coull, 1994; Jakala et al., 1999a). However, the more selective α_{2A} agonist guanfacine has recently been shown to improve working memory, planning, and paired-associates learning tasks in healthy young adults (Jakala et al., 1999a, 1999b).

α_2 Agonists have also been shown to improve performance of PFC tasks, but not non-PFC tasks, in patients with PFC dysfunction. For example, clonidine improved performance of memory recall and the Stroop Interference Task in patients with Korsakoff's amnesia, and was most effective in those with the greatest signs of NE loss (Mair & McEntree, 1986). Clonidine has also been shown to improve memory recall and performance of the Trails B Task in schizophrenic patients (Fields et al., 1988). One recent study has shown that clonidine can even improve working memory in patients with Alzheimer's disease (Riekkinen & Riekkinen, 1999), although previous studies have not shown benefit (Mohr et al., 1989). Interestingly, the α_2 antagonist idazoxan has also been shown to enhance performance of PFC tasks in patients with frontal lobe dementia (Coull et al., 1996). Monkey studies suggest that low doses of α_2 antagonists can improve PFC function by preferentially increasing NE release and enhancing endogenous stimulation of post synaptic α_2 receptors (Arnsten & Cai, 1993). However, it is not known if idazoxan improves performance in demented patients through this same mechanism.

Much research with α_2 agonists has focused on patients with ADHD, a disorder with prominent PFC dysfunction. Early studies demonstrated that clonidine can improve symptoms of ADHD (Hunt el al., 1985), but serious hypotensive and sedative side effects have limited its use. Current studies have turned to the more selective α_{2A} agonist, guanfacine. Guanfacine has been shown to be effective in three open-label trials (Chappell et al., 1995; Horrigan & Barnhill, 1995; Hunt et al., 1995) and now in two placebo-controlled trials as well (in the trial in ADHD adults, guanfacine with dexedrine produced favorable results) [Taylor & Russo, 2000]; in the trial in ADHD children with tics, guanfacine reduced tics and ADHD symptoms [Scahill et al., 2001]). In addition to having therapeutic effects on standard rating scales, guanfacine has been shown to improve performance of PFC tasks such as the Stroop Interference Task (Taylor & Russo, 2000; guanfacine was superior to dexedrine) and the Connors Continuous Performance Task (CPT) which assesses vigilance, working memory, and behavioral inhibition (Scahill et al., 2001). These findings are consistent with clinical reports that guanfacine reduces impulsivity, a sign of improved PFC function. The importance of α_2 mechanisms to PFC function may also be relevant to the recent finding that polymorphisms in α_2 receptors may be linked with ADHD symptoms (Comings et al., 1999). As mutations in the α_{2A} receptor impair PFC function in mice (Franowicz et al., 1998), similar alterations in humans may induce PFC deficits that resemble ADHD.

Imaging Studies of Noradrenergic Function in Humans

Imaging studies in humans generally support findings from animal research. Studies using low doses of clonidine in normal adults generally show a picture of impaired attention and emerging sedation associated with imaging changes in thalamus (Coull et al., 1997) and parietal cortex. These findings are consistent with an older study showing that clonidine impaired attentional orienting (Clark et al., 1987), a function dependent on parietal lobe function (Posner et al., 1984). These findings reinforce the notion that posterior cortex and most subcortical structures are impaired by α_2 receptor stimulation. However, a different picture emerges when higher doses of clonidine are given to patients with presumed NE loss, or when guanfacine is used. For example, administration of higher doses of clonidine to Korsakoff's patients increased rCBF in frontal lobe, and the increased blood flow in the left PFC correlated with improved verbal fluency performance (Moffoot et al., 1994). A more sophisticated analysis also suggests that clonidine can have important modulatory effects on higher cortical function. Clonidine has been shown to increase the effective connectivity between the LC, parietal cortex, and PFC during an attentional task, while decreasing connectivity during rest (Coull et al., 1999). More recently, guanfacine has been shown to increase rCBF in the frontal lobe of healthy adults as measured by PET imaging (Swartz et al., 2000). These studies reinforce the idea that α_2 receptor stimulation often impairs the functioning of most brain regions, and that the PFC is exceptional in its beneficial influence from α_{2A} receptor stimulation.

In summary, research in patients and normal volunteers supports the finding that stimulation of α_{2A} receptors improves PFC functions in humans as well as in animals. The powerful, sedating, and presynaptic effects of clonidine have sometimes obscured this view, but more recent studies with guanfacine have been more successful.

SEROTONIN

There are several methods available for manipulating 5HT function in humans, but pinpointing effects on PFC function necessarily depends on indirect inferences made either concerning effects on cognitive tasks known to be sensitive to PFC damage or from interactions with regional blood flow within the PFC using functional imaging paradigms. As an example of the latter approach, Grasby et al. (1992) have shown that buspirone, a rather nonspecific 5HT1A agonist, impairs verbal learning in a functional neuroimaging context, the deficit correlating, however, with changes in rCBF in the posterior neocortex rather than the PFC, even though changes in blood flow were observed in areas of the PFC, that were associated with this learning task.

As an example of the former approach, employing sensitive tests of PFC dysfunction, Luciana et al. (1998) showed that the indirect

5HT agonist fenfluramine (60 mg, p.o.) impaired delayed visuospatial memory performance selectively at longer delays, in contrast to the mild beneficial effects of the D2 agonist bromocriptine reviewed above. These effects were not simply due to sedative effects reducing arousal levels, but may have been due to actions on 5HT receptors at non-PFC regions. These results of Luciana et al. were extended by a study of effects of fenfluramine (Caycedo et al., 1994), in which 30 mg of the drug disrupted executive functions such as those tapped by the Stroop Test and verbal fluency, while not affecting performance on tests with less executive loading, such as list learning and recognition memory.

We have employed another method to manipulate central 5HT rather more globally, via the tryptophan depletion technique. By giving food-deprived humans or rats a diet deficient in the amino acid tryptophan, it is possible to produce a transient central depletion of the indoleamine 5HT and presumably deficient serotoninergic activity, because tryptophan is a necessary precursor of 5HT synthesized in the brain (Young et al., 1985).

Our initial study of the effects of tryptophan depletion on cognitive function in humans found that there was rather little effect on many tests sensitive to frontal lobe dysfunction. For example, performance on the Tower of London Test of planning and self-ordered spatial working memory were both unaffected (Park et al., 1994) in marked contrast to the effects of sulpiride and methylphenidate, and the noradrenergic agents clonidine and idazoxan (Middleton et al., 1999). Learning of the paired-associates task was retarded, an interesting parallel to the effects seen on verbal learning by Grasby et al. (1992). The paired associates learning deficit may have been due to actions of 5HT in posterior cortical memory circuits, for example, in the parietal or temporal lobe, although the task is also sensitive to frontal cortical damage (Owen et al., 1995b).

The low tryptophan treatment did impair performance on the CANTAB attentional set-shifting paradigm, although the effects were more evident at the extradimensional reversal stage than during the extradimensional shift condition, which immediately precedes it. Reversal learning is another example of shift learning in which the discriminative stimuli remain the same, but identity of the reinforced stimulus (or "object") is switched. Thus, the subject has to desist responding to the previously reinforced stimulus and begin responding to the previously non-reinforced stimulus in order to gain reward. The capacity to show reversal can be divided into two main components: the ability to inhibit responding to the previously reinforced stimulus, and the ability to learn which stimulus is now rewarded. Marmosets with lesions of the lateral and orbitofrontal cortex exhibit differential impairments on reversal learning as compared with extradimensional shift learning. Animals with lateral lesions are impaired in the extradimensional shift-learning task, whereas those with the orbitofrontal lesions are impaired specifically at either simple or extradimensional reversal learning (Dias et al., 1996a). This result can be characterized as a double dissociation of effects of prefrontal lesions on two forms of shift learning: shift learning at the level of single stimuli or objects, and learning at the more abstract level of entire stimulus dimensions. Given the strong anatomical connections of the orbitofrontal cortex with limbic structures such as the anterior cingulate and the amygdala, it is perhaps not surprising that the orbitofrontal lesion should impair the specific stimulus–reward learning required in reversal. Further evidence for a specific role of the orbitofrontal cortex in reversal learning comes from human studies (Rolls et al., 1994; Rahman et al., 1999). Consequently, it appears that there may be functional commonalities between the effects of orbitofrontal lesions and procedures affecting 5HT function in humans.

To test further the hypothesis that reductions in central 5HT may selectively impair reversal learning, Rogers et al. (1999a) used the same three-dimensional discrimination learning and shifting paradigm as that employed to test the effects of methylphenidate (see above). This more difficult form of the two-dimensional version of the task was expected to lead to more clear-cut findings than those apparent in the Park et al. (1994) study, where

effects appeared to be limited largely to the first session in a crossover design. Significantly, the results of Park et al. (1994) were extended and confirmed, reversal learning being much more impaired than nonreversal learning at several of the stages of the task in contrast to the effects of both methylphenidate (described above) and clonidine (Rogers et al., 1999a).

To test the hypothesis that 5HT manipulation might affect functions controlled by the orbitofrontal cortex to a greater extent than those of the dorsolateral PFC, we have compared the effects of the catecholaminergic agent methylphenidate with those of tryptophan depletion on performance in another paradigm that we have shown to be sensitive to orbitofrontal dysfunction. This task is modeled after the "gambling task," which is sensitive to orbitofrontal damage in humans described by Bechara et al. (1998) and described in greater detail in a more recent study (Rogers et al., 1999b). Briefly, subjects are required to make probabilistic decisions and then assign proportions of their previously earned reward to those decisions. This decision-making task is also sensitive to damage of the orbitofrontal cortex, whether produced by lesions (Rogers et al., 1999b) or by neurodegeneration (Rahman et al., 1999). Importantly, in the present context, tryptophan depletion produced effects on performance which mimicked some of those produced by orbitofrontal lesions (Rogers et al., 1999b). On the other hand, the same dose (40 mg p.o.) of methylphenidate previously shown to affect many of the other tasks described above that depended on dorsolateral PFC functioning had no effects on the decision-making task (R.D. Rogers & T.W. Robbins, unpublished findings). Given the relative lack of effect of tryptophan depletion on performance on the self-ordered spatial working memory task and the Tower of London planning task, in relation to its significant effects on reversal learning and the decision-making task, and the opposite effects on these of the indirectly acting catecholaminergic agonist methylphenidate, we appear to have provided evidence for a double dissociation of effects on tasks controlled by different sectors of the PFC. These findings confirm the suggestion made above that operations requiring different regions of the PFC may be modulated optimally by different degrees of activity of the ascending monoaminergic and cholinergic systems.

In summary, 5HT appears to modulate functions controlled by the orbitofrontal cortex to a greater extent than those of the dorsolateral PFC. This finding may explain the importance of 5HT in depression (see Chapter 24).

ACETYLCHOLINE

Despite intense interest in the possible therapeutic efficacy of cholinergic agents in dementia, there has again been relatively little evidence of specific effects on tasks that specifically engage frontal functions in humans, especially when the sedative effects of drugs such as scopolamine are taken into account. Some capacities such as verbal fluency may even be relatively unscathed at doses affecting many other forms of memory and learning functions (Beatty et al., 1986). One important approach has been to examine the relationship between cholinergic drug treatments and changes in rCBF in the context of functional neuroimaging. In one such study (Furey et al., 2000), improvements in the speed of recognizing faces were accompanied by significant task-related reductions in rCBF in the dorsolateral PFC following physostigmine (which prolongs the presence of ACh in the synaptic cleft) while increasing activity in posterior cortical regions such as the extrastriate cortex. Furey et al. (2000) interpret their findings as demonstrating that ACh can reduce the burden on working memory by increasing the visual encoding of the faces. This interpretation is compatible with the finding that nicotine improves performance on a rapid visual information processing test of sustained attention that has a working memory component (Sahakian et al., 1989). How the results of Furey et al. (2000) can be reconciled with the evidence reviewed above in experimental animals that appears to show direct modulation of function by manipulations restricted to the PFC is not yet clear. However, the parallel of

the results of Furey et al. (2000) with the beneficial effects on accuracy of the catecholamine indirect agonist methylphenidate on performance of a self-ordered spatial working memory task, also being associated with reductions in blood flow in the dorsolateral PFC (Mehta et al., 2000), is theoretically interesting, as it suggests that these different systems may be acting on qualitatively distinct aspects of mnemonic processing within the PFC. A definitive comparison of effects of these two drugs, using the same memory task, is now required. Overall, further characterization of the modulation of the cognitive functions of the PFC by cholinergic mechanisms is certainly warranted.

In summary, although scopolamine and Alzheimer's disease have dramatic effects on learning and memory, the relevance of these findings to specific, cholinergic mechanisms in PFC is not known. This remains an area for future investigation.

COMPARISON TO OTHER BRAIN REGIONS

Our emerging picture suggests that the PFC may be modulated differently than other than brain regions. The PFC may be more sensitive to the detrimental effects of DA D1 receptor stimulation than areas such as the amygdala, but this idea remains to be tested within a single lab. Unlike for DA, we were able to observe qualitative differences in the manner in which NE regulates PFC as opposed to posterior cortical functions (reviewed in Arnsten, 2000b). As illustrated in Figure 4–4, NE regulation of the PFC is "upside down and backwards" from much of the rest of the brain. Thus, NE stimulation of α_2 receptors enhances PFC functions but impairs many posterior cortical functions, while stimulation of α_1 and/or β receptors enhances posterior cortical functions but impairs or has no effect on PFC function. As NE has higher affinity for α_2 than α_1 or β receptors (see above), lower levels of NE release during nonstressed conditions may preferentially engage α_2 receptors and facilitate PFC regulation of behavior, while high levels of NE release during stress may engage α_1 and β receptors, taking the PFC "off-line" but providing areas such as the amygdala, hippocampus, sensory/motor cortices, and cerebellum with a more optimal neurochemical environment. This may have survival value, allowing more habitual or reflexive mechanisms to control behavior during dangerous conditions. However, this differential neurochemical regulation may render the PFC particularly vulnerable to dysfunction in our daily lives, and in a wide variety of neuropsychiatric disorders.

TREATMENT OF NEUROPSYCHIATRIC AND NEUROLOGICAL DISORDERS

A critical goal of current research is to develop superior pharmacological treatments for patients with PFC dysfunction. As described above, catecholaminergic agents such as methylphenidate and guanfacine are already being used successfully for disorders such as ADHD with prominent PFC impairments yet intact PFC neurons. These agents are able to strengthen PFC function and thus intelligently inhibit inappropriate behaviors and thoughts. The atypical antipsychotics may also optimize the neurochemical environment in the PFC in schizophrenic patients, for example, by reducing detrimental DA D4 and NE α_1 receptor actions. Similarly, lithium and valproic acid may normalize the intracellular environment of PFC neurons in manic patients by reducing harmful protein kinase C actions. In depression it is conceivable that some of the therapeutic benefit of medication with antidepressant drugs is mediated by effects on serotonin function in ventromedial PFC structures (see Chapter 24). However, it remains to be determined whether these agents can be helpful in patients with lesions of the PFC itself, whether the lesions are due to stroke, tumors, traumatic brain injury, or degenerative disease such as Alzheimer's disease. For example, monkey studies indicate that guanfacine loses efficacy when the PFC is lesioned (Arnsten & van Dyck, 1997), and α_2 agonists do not appear to be helpful in treatment of Alzheimer's disease (Mohr et al., 1989) (although specific

studies of PFC functions do find some improvement [Riekkinen & Riekkinen, 1999]). It may be that extensive PFC lesions leave little substrate for these drugs to work on. There is some evidence that cholinergic agents can improve some aspects of frontal lobe function in patients with Alzheimer's disease. For example, improvements in performance of attentional tasks that depend in part on PFC function have been found following treatment with the AChesterase inhibitor tacrine as well as nicotine (see Sahakian & Coull, 1994, for a review). However, as the degeneration progresses, the benefit of these compounds is often outweighed by the devastation of the disease. In cases of profound frontal lobe damage, alternative and less optimal strategies must be employed, e.g., restricting behavioral output through blockade of striatal D2 receptors with neuroleptic medications or blocking posterior cortical β receptors with compounds such as propranolol. Although these compounds cannot inhibit and guide behavior with the intelligence of the PFC, they may provide a critical, if nonspecific, brake on subcortical and posterior cortical mechanisms.

FUTURE DIRECTIONS

The main theoretical notions advanced in this chapter are that the modulation of cognitive functions depending on the PFC by chemically defined ascending pathways of the reticular core of the brain are quite specific, being determined by (1) the nature of the cognitive task, the operations it requires, and thus the regions of the PFC implicated in those operations, and (2) the particular system involved (i.e., DA, NE, 5HT, or ACh) and the level of activity within that system, both on baseline and in response to demands of the internal and external environment (i.e., stress). It can also be inferred (3) that the precise circumstances evoking changes in activity within the different neurotransmitter systems may well be distinct, providing some further specificity of function for these classical "arousal" systems.

An important future direction will also be to define more precise roles for different receptors and their subtypes in cognitive function. Much progress has already been made on this front, as shown from the work reviewed for the NE and DA systems, but further analysis, for example, of the functional role of the D4 receptor in the prefrontal cortex, may prove to be important. This may be the case especially for the 5HT systems with their multiple receptors. It seems likely that different 5HT receptors, perhaps because of their sometimes quite specific anatomical distributions, will have distinct effects on different aspects of cognitive function. For example, a study by Gomez et al. (1995) reported that the 5HT-1A agonist buspirone produced deficits on tests of verbal learning, which, from the results of Grasby et al. (1992) reviewed above, might be associated with actions in the posterior neocortex. However, performance was enhanced by buspirone on the classical frontal lobe test of verbal fluency, possibly resulting from a release of frontal function from inhibitory actions of the dorsal raphe via somatodendritic 5HT-1A receptors. This intriguing dissociation shows again, as we have seen from the neuromodulatory effects of other neurotransmitters, that cognitive function is not necessarily affected in a global manner by drugs affecting these systems, with evidence of considerable functional specificity at the level of the receptor. It remains to be seen whether this will hold for the 5HT2A receptor, which is particularly implicated in cortical, possibly even anterior cortical, functioning. For example, the 5HT2A agonist psilocybin produces marked cognitive impairments, as well as some hallucinogenic activity, when administered to human volunteers (Hermie et al., 1993); the precise nature of these deficits now warrants further analysis.

In this chapter we have reviewed suggestive evidence of a preferential 5HT-ergic (and possibly also cholinergic) modulation of orbitofrontal function and catecholaminergic modulation of dorsolateral PFC function. Although there are no very clear differences in the manner of innervation of these regions of the PFC by the monoamine systems or in their dynamic modes of operation (Goldman-Rakic, 1999), it is possible that some quantitative variation, e.g., in the density of catecholamine innervation (Lewis et al., 1988; Sesack et al., 1989;

Lewis, 1990), as well as in the feedback projections of the PFC to cells of origin (e.g., orbitofrontal cortex to nucleus basalis [Mesulam, 1995]), will prove to be of functional significance. The functional considerations described above may thus be a stimulus for further neurobiological investigations of these important issues. Consequently, it is most unlikely that there will be qualitatively sharp divisions in the types of function modulated by these systems. Nevertheless, it is possible that the quantitative, differential influences will be significant, not only for understanding normal functioning but also in the study of psychopathology. This may be true in a variety of clinical contexts, ranging from the treatment of depression (see Chapter 24), ADHD (Solanto et al., 2000), schizophrenia, acute brain damage, and neurodegenerative disorders such as Parkinson's disease and frontal lobe dementia.

For the study of both normal cognition and psychopathology, it will be necessary to test these hypotheses by conducting careful studies in which cognitive paradigms are combined in pharmacological and neuroimaging contexts in humans and by relating directly these results to those obtained from the more specific methods available for studying PFC function in experimental animals. It will also be essential to compare rather carefully the precise conditions under which these neurotransmitter systems are regulated in response to environmental demands so that their hypothetically separable functions can be discerned more clearly.

ACKNOWLEDGMENTS

This work was supported by U.S. PHS grant AG06036 (A.F.T.A.) and by the Wellcome Trust and MRC Cooperative in Brain, Behavior and Neuropsychiatry (T.W.R.) We would like to thank our colleagues and students for their invaluable input to this work.

REFERENCES

Alexander, G.E, DeLong, M.R. & Strick P.L. (1986) Parallel organization of functionally segregated circuits linking basal ganglia and cortex. Annual Reviews in Neuroscience 9, 357–381.

Akoki, C., Go, C.G., Venkatesan, C., & Kurose, J. (1994). Perikaryal and synaptic localization of alpha-2A-adrenergic receptor-like immunoreactivity. *Brain Research, 650*, 181–204.

Arnsten, A.F.T. (2000a). Stress impairs PFC function in rats and monkeys: role of dopamine D1 and norepinephrine alpha-1 receptor mechanisms. *Progress in Brain Research, 126*, 183–192.

Arnsten, A.F.T. (2000b). Through the looking glass: differential noradrenergic modulation of prefrontal cortical function. *Neural Plasticity, 7*, 133–146.

Arnsten, A.F.T. & Cai, J.X. (1993). Post-synaptic alpha-2 receptor stimulation improves working memory in aged monkeys: indirect effects of yohimbine vs. direct effects of clonidine. *Neurobiology of Aging, 14*, 597–603.

Arnsten, A.F.T. & Contant, T.A. (1992). Alpha-2 adrenergic agonists decrease distractability in aged monkeys performing a delayed response task. *Psychopharmacology, 108*, 159–169.

Arnsten, A.F.T. & Goldman-Rakic, P.S. (1984). Selective prefrontal cortical projections to the region of the locus coeruleus and raphe nuclei in the rhesus monkey. *Brain Research, 306*, 9–18.

Arnsten, A.F.T. & Goldman-Rakic, P.S. (1985). Alpha-2 adrenergic mechanisms in prefrontal cortex associated with cognitive decline in aged nonhuman primates. *Science, 230*, 1273–1276.

Arnsten, A.F.T. & Goldman-Rakic, P.S. (1986). Reversal of stress-induced delayed response deficits in rhesus monkeys by clonidine and naloxone. *Society of Neuroscience Abstracts, 12*, 1464.

Arnsten, A.F.T. & Goldman-Rakic, P.S. (1990a). Analysis of alpha-2 adrenergic agonist effects on the delayed nonmatch-to-sample performance of aged rhesus monkeys. *Neurobiology of Aging, 11*, 583–590.

Arnsten, A.F.T. & Goldman-Rakic, P.S. (1990b). Stress impairs prefrontal cortex cognitive function in monkeys: role of dopamine. *Society of Neuroscience Abstracts, 16*, 164.

Arnsten, A.F.T. & Goldman-Rakic, P.S. (1998). Noise stress impairs prefrontal cortical cognitive function in monkeys: evidence for a hyperdopaminergic mechanism. *Archives of General Psychiatry, 55*, 362–369.

Arnsten, A.F.T. & van Dyck, C.H. (1997). Monoamine and acetylcholine influences on higher cognitive functions in nonhuman primates: relevance to the treatment of Alzheimer's disease. In: J.D. Brioni & M.W. Decker (Eds.), *Pharmacological Treatment of Alzheimer's Disease: Molecular and Neurobiological Foundations* (pp. 63–86). New York: John Wiley and Sons.

Arnsten, A.F.T., Cai, J.X., & Goldman-Rakic, P.S. (1988). The alpha-2 adrenergic agonist guanfacine improves memory in aged monkeys without sedative or hypotensive side effects. *Journal of Neuroscience, 8*, 4287–4298.

Arnsten, A.F.T., Cai, J.X., Murphy, B.L., & Goldman-Rakic, P.S. (1994). Dopamine D1 receptor mechanisms in the cognitive performance of young adult and aged monkeys. *Psychopharmocology, 116*, 143–151.

Arnsten, A.F.T., Cai, J.X., Steere, J.C., & Goldman-Rakic, P.S. (1995). Dopamine D2 receptor mechanisms contribute to age-related cognitive decline: the effects of quinpirole on memory and motor performance in monkeys. *Journal of Neuroscience, 15*, 3429–3439.

Arnsten, A.F.T., Steere, J.C., & Hunt, R.D. (1996). The contribution of α-2 noradrenergic mechanisms to prefrontal cortical cognitive function: potential significance to attention deficit hyperactivity disorder. *Archives of General Psychiatry, 53*, 448–455.

Arnsten, A.F.T., Lin, C.H., van Dyck, C.H., & Stanhope, K.J. (1997). The effects of 5-HT3 receptor antagonists on cognitive performance in aged monkeys. *Neurobiology of Aging, 18*, 21–28.

Arnsten, A.F.T., Mathew, R., Ubriani, R., Taylor, J.R., & Li, B.M. (1999). Alpha-1 noradrenergic receptor stimulation impairs prefrontal cortical cognitive function. *Biological Psychiatry, 45*, 26–31.

Arnsten, A.F.T., Murphy, B.L., & Merchant, K. (2000). The selective dopamine D4 receptor antagonist, PNU-101387G, prevents stress-induced cognitive deficits in monkeys. *Neuropsychopharmacology, 23*, 405–410.

Avery, R.A., Franowicz, J.S., Studholme, C., van Dyck, C.H., & Arnsten, A.F.T. (2000). The alpha-2A-adenoceptor agonist, guanfacine, increases regional cerebral blood flow in dorsolateral prefrontal cortex of monkeys performing a spatial working memory task. *Neuropsychopharmocology, 23*, 240–249.

Baddeley, A.D. (1986). *Working Memory*. New York: Oxford University Press.

Baldessarini, R.J., Huston-Lyons, D., Campbell, A., Marsh, E., & Cohen, B.M. (1992). Do central antiadrenergic actions contribute to the atypical properties of clozapine? *British Journal of Psychiatry, 160 S17*, 12–16.

Bartus, R.T. & Johnson, H.R. (1976). Short-term memory in the rhesus monkey: disruption from the anticholinergic scopolamine. *Pharmacology, Biochemistry and Behavior, 5*, 39–46.

Bartus, R.T., Fleming, D., & Johnson, H.R. (1978). Aging in the rhesus monkey: debilitating effects on short-term memory. *Journal of Gerontology, 33*, 858–871.

Beatty, W.W., Butters, N., & Janowsky, D.S. (1986). Patterns of memory failure after scopolamine: implications for the cholinergic hypothesis of dementia. *Behavioral Neural Biology, 45*, 196–211.

Bechara, A., Damasio, H., Tranel, D., & Anderson, S.W. (1998). Dissociation of working memory from decision making within the human prefrontal cortex. *Journal of Neuroscience, 18*, 428–437.

Birnbaum, S.G. & Arnsten, A.F.T. (1996). The alpha-2A noradrenergic agonist, guanfacine, reverses the working memory deficits induced by pharmacological stress (FG7142). *Society of Neuroscience Abstracts, 22*, 1126.

Birnbaum, S.G., Gobeske, K.T., Auerbach, J., Taylor, J.R., & Arnsten, A.F.T. (1999a). A role for norepinephrine in stress-induced cognitive deficits: alpha-1-adrenoceptor mediation in prefrontal cortex. *Biological Psychiatry, 46*, 1266–1274.

Birnbaum, S.G., Gobeske, K.T., Auerbach, J., Taylor, J.R., & Arnsten, A.F.T. (1999b). The role of alpha-1-adrenoceptor and PKC activation mediating stress-induced cognitive deficits. *Society of Neuroscience Abstracts, 25*, 608.

Birnbaum, S.G., Podell, D.M., & Arnsten, A.F.T. (2000). Noradrenergic alpha-2 receptor agonists reverse working memory deficits induced by the anxiogenic drug, FG7142, in rats. *Pharmacology, Biochemistry and Behavior, 67,* 397–403.

Broadbent, D. (1971). *Decision and Stress.* San Diego: Academic Press.

Broersen, L.M., Heinsbroek, R.P.W., Debruin, J.P.C., Uylings, H.B.M., & Olivier, B. (1995). The role of the medial prefrontal cortex of rats in short-term-memory functioning—further support for involvement of cholinergic, rather than dopaminergic mechanisms. *Brain Research, 674,* 2, 221–229.

Brozoki, T., Brown, R.M., Rosvold. H.E., & Goldman, P.S. (1979). Cognitive deficit caused by regional depletion of dopamine in prefrontal cortex of rhesus monkey. *Science, 205,* 929–931.

Cai, J.X. & Arnsten, A.F.T. (1997). Dose-dependent effects of the dopamine D1 receptor agonists A77636 or SKF81297 on spatial working memory in aged monkeys. *Journal of Pharmacology and Experimental Therapeutics, 282,* 1–7.

Cai, J.X., Ma, Y., Xu, L., & Hu, X. (1993). Reserpine impairs spatial working memory performance in monkeys: reversal by the alpha-2 adrenergic agonist clonidine. *Brain Research, 614,* 191–196.

Carli, M., Robbins, T.W., Evenden, J.L., & Everitt, B.J. (1983). Effects of lesions to ascending noradrenergic neurons on performance of a 5-choice serial reaction task in rats: implications for theories of dorsal noradrenergic bundle function based on selective attention and arousal. *Behavioral Brain Research, 9,* 361–380.

Carlson, S., Ranila, H., Rama, P., Mecke, E., & Pertovaara, A. (1992). Effects of medetomidine, an alpha-2 adrenoceptor agonist, and atipamezole, an alpha-2 antagonist, on spatial memory performance in adult and aged rats. *Behavioral Neural Biology, 58,* 113–119.

Cavada, C., Company, T., Tejedor, J., Cruz-Rizzolo, R.J., & Reinsoso-Suarez, F. (2000). The anatomical connections of the macaque orbitofrontal cortex. A Review. *Cerebral Cortex, 10,* 220–242.

Caycedo, N., Connell, J., Hellewell, J.S.E., & Deakin, J.F.W. (1994). Effects of fenfluramine on executive and other cognitive functions. Abstract No. 172. *Journal of Psychopharmacology,* Abstract Book Vol. 8 (p. A43).

Chappell, P.B., Riddle, M.A., Scahill, L., Lynch, K.A., Schultz, R., Arnsten, A., Leckman, J.F., & Cohen, D.J. (1995). Guanfacine treatment of comorbid attention deficit hyperactivity disorder and Tourette's Syndrome: Preliminary clinical experience. *Journal of the American Academy of Children and Adolescent Psychiatry, 34,* 1140–1146.

Clark, C.R., Geffen, G.M., & Geffen, L.B. (1986). Role of monoamine pathways in the control of attention: effects of droperidol and methylphenidate in normal adult humans. *Psychopharmacology, 90,* 28–34.

Clark, C.R., Geffen, G.M., & Geffen, L.B. (1987). Catecholamines and attention II: pharmacological studies in normal humans. *Neuroscience and Biobehavioral Reviews, 11,* 353–364.

Cohen, J.D., Braver, T.S., & O'Reilly, R.C. (1998). A computational approach to prefrontal cortex, cognitive control and schizophrenia: recent developments and current challenge. In: A.C. Roberts, T.W. Robbins, & L. Weiskrantz (Eds.), *The Prefrontal Cortex: Executive and Cognitive Functions* Oxford: Oxford University Press. (pp. 195–220).

Cole, B.J., Jobes, G.H., & Turner, J.D. (1994). 5-HT1A receptor agonists improve the performance of normal and scopolamine treated rats in an operant delayed matching to position task. *Psychopharmacology, 116,* 135–142.

Collins, P., Roberts, A.C., Dias, R., Everitt, B.J., & Robbins, T.W. (1998). Perseveration and strategy in a novel spatial self-ordered sequencing task for nonhuman primates: effects of excitotoxic lesions and dopamine depletions of the prefrontal cortex. *Journal of Cognitive Neuroscience, 10,* 332–354.

Collins, P., Wilkinson, L.S., Everitt, B.J., Robbins, T.W., & Roberts, A.C. (2000). The effect of dopamine depletion from the caudate nucleus of the common marmoset (*Callithrix jacchus*) on tests of prefrontal cognitive function. *Behavioral Neuroscience, 114,* 3–17.

Comings, D.E., Gade-Andavolu, R., Gonzalez, N., & MacMurray, J.P. (1999). Additive effect of three noradrenergic genes (*ADRA2A, ADRA2C, DBH*) on attention-deficit hyperactivity disorder and learning disabilities in Tourette syndrome subjects. *Clinical Genetics, 55,* 160–172.

Cools R., Barker R.A., Sahakian, B.J. & Robbins, T.W. (2001) Enhanced or impaired Cognitive function in Parkinson's disease as a function of dopaminergic medication and task demands. *Cerebral Cortex II,* in press.

Coull, J.T. (1994). Pharmacological manipulations of the alpha-2 noradrenergic system: Effects on cognition. *Drugs and Aging, 5,* 116–126.

Coull, J.T., Sahakian, B.J., & Hodges, J.R. (1996). The alpha-2 antagonist idazoxan remediates certain attentional and executive dysfunction in patients with dementia of frontal type. *Psychopharmacology, 123,* 239–249.

Coull, J.T., Frith, C.D., Dolan, R.J., Frackowiak, R.S., & Grasby, P.M. (1997). The neural correlates of the noradrenergic modulation of human attention, arousal and learning. *European Journal of Neuroscience, 9,* 589–598.

Coull, J.T., Buchel, C., Friston, K.J., & Frith, C.D. (1999). Noradrenergically mediated plasticity in a human attentional neuronal network. *Neuroimage, 10,* 705–715.

Crofts HS, Dalley JW, Collins P, Van Denderen JCM, Everitt BJ, Robbins TW & Roberts AC (2001) Differential effects of 6-OHDA lesions of the frontal cortex and caudate nucleus on the ability to acquire an attentional set. *Cerebral Cortex, 11* in press

Daniel, D.G., Weinberger, D.R., Jones, D.W., Zigun, J.R., Coppola, R., Handel, S., Goldberg, T.E., Berman, K.F., & Kleinman, J.E. (1991). The effect of amphetamine on regional cerebral blood flow during cognitive activation in schizophrenia. *Journal of Neuroscience, 11,* 1907–1917.

Deutch, A.Y. & Roth, R.H. (1990). The determinants of

stress-induced activation of the prefrontal cortical dopamine system. *Progress in Brain Research, 8,* 367–403.

Diamond, A. (1996). Evidence for the importance of dopamine for prefrontal cortex functions early in life. *Philosophical Transactions of the Royal Society of London, 351,* 1483–1494.

Dias, R., Roberts, A., & Robbins, T.W. (1996a). Dissociation in prefrontal cortex of affective and attentional shifts. *Nature, 380,* 69–72.

Dias, R., Robbins, T.W., & Roberts, A.C. (1996b). Primate analogue of the Wisconsin Card Sort Test: effects of excitotoxic lesions of the prefrontal cortex in the Marmoset. *Behavioral Neuroscience, 110,* 870–884.

Dias, R., Robbins, T.W., & Roberts, A.C. (1997). Dissociable forms of inhibitory control within prefrontal cortex with an analogue of the Wisconsin Card Sort Test: restriction to novel situations and independence from 'on-line' processing. *Journal of Neuroscience, 17,* 9285–9297.

Dolan, R.J., Fletcher, P., Frith, C.D., Friston, K.J., Frackowiak, R.S.J., & Grasby, P.M. (1995). Dopaminergic modulation of impaired cognitive activation in the anterior cingulate cortex in schizophrenia. *Nature, 378,* 180–182.

Downes, J.J., Roberts, A.C., Sahakian, B.J., Evenden, J.L., & Robbins, T.W. (1989). Impaired extra-dimensional shift performance in medicated and unmedicated Parkinson's disease: evidence for a specific attentional dysfunction. *Neuropsychologia, 27,* 1329–1344.

Druzin, M.Y., Kurzina, N.P., Malinina, E.P., & Kozlov, A.P. (2000). The effects of local application of D2 selective dopaminergic drugs into the medial prefrontal cortex of rats in a delayed spatial choice task. *Behavioural Brain Research, 109,* 99–111.

Duman, R.S. & Nestler, E.J. (1995). Signal transduction pathways for catecholamine receptors. In: F.E. Bloom & D.J. Kupfer (Eds.) *Psychopharmacology: The Fourth Generation of Progress* (pp. 303–320). New York: Raven Press.

Elliott, R., Sahakian, B.J., Matthews, K., Bannerjea, A., Rimmer, J., & Robbins, T.W. (1997). Effects of methylphenidate on spatial working memory and planning in healthy young adults. *Psychopharmacology, 131,* 196–206.

Engberg, G. & Eriksson, E. (1991). Effects of alpha-2-adrenoceptor agonists on locus coeruleus firing rate and brain noradrenaline turnover in EEDQ-treated rats. *Naunyn-Schmiedebergs Archives of Pharmacology, 343,* 472–477.

Ernst, M., Zametkin, A.J., Matochik, J.A., Jons, P.H., & Cohen, R.M. (1998). DOPA decarboxylase activity in attention deficit hyperactivity disorder adults: a (fluorine-18) fluorodopa positron emission tomographic study. *Journal of Neuroscience, 18,* 5901–5907.

Evans, R.W., Gualtieri, T., & Amara, I. (1986). Methyphenidate and memory: dissociated effects in hyperactive children. *Psychopharmacology, 90,* 211–216.

Everitt, B.J. & Robbins, T.W. (1997). Central cholinergic systems and cognition. *Annual Review of Psychology, 48,* 649–684.

Fields, R.B., Van Kammen, D.P., Peters, J.L., Rosen, J.,

Van Kammen W.B., Nugent, A., Stipetic, M., & Linnoila, M. (1988). Clonidine improves memory function in schizophrenia independently from change in psychosis. *Schizophrenia Research, 1,* 417–423.

Finlay, J.M., Zigmond, M.J., & Abercrombie, E.D. (1995). Increased dopamine and norepinephrine release in medial prefrontal cortex induced by acute and chronic stress: effects of diazepam. *Neuroscience, 64,* 619–628.

Foote, S.L., Aston-Jones, G., & Bloom, F.E. (1980). Impulse activity of locus coeruleus neurons in awake rats and monkeys is a function of sensory stimulation and arousal. *Proceeding of the National Academy of Sciences USA, 77,* 3033–3037.

Franowicz, J.C.S. & Arnsten, A.F.T. (1998). The alpha-2A noradrenergic agonist, guanfacine, improves delayed response performance in young adult rhesus monkeys. *Psychopharmacology, 136,* 8–14.

Franowicz, J.S. & Arnsten, A.F.T. (1999). Treatment with the noradrenergic alpha-2 agonist clonidine, but not diazepam, improves spatial working memory in normal young rhesus monkeys. *Neuropsychopharmacology, 21,* 611–621.

Franowicz, J.S., Kessler, L., Morgan, C., & Arnsten, A.F.T. (1998). The alpha-2 noradrenergic agonist, guanfacine, improves spatial working memory in wild-type mice but not mice with point mutations of the gene for the alpha-2A receptor. *Society of Neuroscience Abstracts, 24,* 711.

Furey, M.L., Pietrini, P., & Haxby, J.V. (2000). Cholinergic enhancement and increased selectivity of perceptual processing during working memory. *Science, 290,* 2315–2319.

Glass, D.C., Reim, B., & Singer, J.E. (1971). Behavioral consequences of adaptation to controllable and uncontrollable noise. *Journal of Experimental Social Psychology, 7,* 244–257.

Goldman, P.S. & Rosvold, H.E. (1970). Localization of function within the dorsolateral prefrontal cortex of the rhesus monkey. *Experimental Neurology, 27,* 291–304.

Goldman-Rakic, P.S. (1987). Circuitry of primate prefrontal cortex and the regulation of behaviour by representational memory. In: Plum F, Mountcastle V (eds) *Handbook of Physiology, vol 5.* Amer0ican Physiological Society: Bethesda, MD pp. 373–417

Goldman-Rakic P.S. (1999) The "psychic" neuron of the cerebral cortex. In; Rudy, B. Seeburg, P.H. (Eds.) *Molecular and functional diversity of ion channels and receptors. Annals of the New York Academy of Sciences,* New York, pp 13–26.

Goldstein, L.E., Rasmusson, A.M., Bunney, S.B., & Roth, R.H. (1996). Role of the amygdala in the coordination of behavioral, neuroendocrine and prefrontal cortical monoamine responses to psychological stress in the rat. *Journal of Neuroscience, 16,* 4787–4798.

Gomez, E., Connell, J., Hellewell, J.S.E., & Deakin, J.F.W. (1995). Differential effects of buspirone on executive and memory functions. Abstract No. 59. Journal of *Psychopharmacology Supplement to Vol. 9* (p. A15).

Gotham, A.M., Brown, R.G., & Marsden, C.D. (1988). 'Frontal' cognitive function in patients with Parkinson's disease 'on' and 'off' levodopa. *Brain, 111,* 299–321.

Granon, S., et al. (1995) Granon S., Poucet, B., Thinus-Blanc C., Changeux JP, & Vidal C (1995) Nicotinic and muscarinc receprtors in the rat prefrontal cortex-different roles in working memory, response selection and effortful processing. *Psychopharmacology 119*, 139–144.

Granon, S., Passetti, F., Thomas, K.L., Dalley, J.W., Everitt, B.J., & Robbins, T.W. (2000). Enhanced and impaired attentional performance following infusion of dopamine receptor agents into rat prefrontal cortex. *Journal of Neuroscience, 20*, 1208–1215.

Grasby, P.M., Friston, K.J., Bench, C.J., Frith, C.D., Paulesu, E., Cowen, P.J., Liddle, P.F., Frackowiak, R.S.J., & Dolan, R. (1992). The effect of apomorphine and buspirone on regional cerebral blood flow during the performance of a cognitive task—measuring neuromodulatory effects of psychotropic drugs in man. *European Journal of Neuroscience, 4*, 1203–1212.

Growdon, J.H., Kieburtz, K., McDermott, M.P., Panisset, M., Friedman, J.H., Shoulson, I., et al. (1998). Levodopa improves motor function without impairing cognition in mild nondemented Parkinson's disease patients. *Neurology, 50*, 1327–1331.

Hartley, L.R. & Adams, R.G. (1974). Effect of noise on the Stroop test. *Journal of Experimental Psychology, 102*, 62–66.

Hermie, L., Funfgeld, M., Oepen, G., Botsch, H., Borchard, D., Gouzulis, E., Fehrenbach, R.A., & Spitzer, M. (1993). Mescaline-induced psychopathological, neuropsychological, and neurometabolic effects in normal subjects: experimental psychosis as a tool for psychiatric research. *Biological Psychiatry, 32*, 976–991.

Hockey, G.R.J. (1970). Effect of loud noise on attentional selectivity. *Quarterly Journal of Experimental Psychology, 22*, 28–36.

Horrigan, J.P. & Barnhill, L.J. (1995). Guanfacine for treatment of attention-deficit-hyperactivity disorder in boys. *Journal of Child Adolescent Psychopharmacology, 5*, 215–223.

Hunt, R.D., Mindera, R.B., & Cohen, D.J. (1985). Clonidine benefits children with attention deficit disorder and hyperactivity: reports of a double-blind placebo-crossover therapeutic trial. *Journal of the American Academy of Child Psychiatry, 24*, 617–629.

Hunt, R.D., Arnsten, A.F.T., & Asbell, M.D. (1995). An open trial of guanfacine in the treatment of attention deficit hyperactivity disorder. *Journal of the American Academy of Children and Adolescent Psychiatry, 34*, 50–54.

Jackson, W.J. & Buccafusco, J.J. (1991). Clonidine enhances delayed matching-to-sample performance by young and aged monkeys. *Pharmacology, Biochemistry and Behavior, 39*, 79–84.

Jakala, P., Riekkinen, M., Sirvio, J., Koivisto, E., Kejonen, K., Vanhanen, M., & Riekkinen, P.J. (1999a). Guanfacine, but not clonidine, improves planning and working memory performance in humans. *Neuropsychopharmology, 20*, 460–470.

Jakala, P., Sirvio, J., Riekkinen, M., Koivisto, E., Kejonen, K., Vanhanen, M., & Riekkinen, P.J. (1999b). Guanfa-cine and clonidine, alpha-2 agonists, improve paired associates learning, but not delayed matching to sample, in humans. *Neuropsychopharmology, 20*, 119–130.

Jentsch, J.D., Taylor, J.R., Redmond, D.E.J., Elsworth, J.D., Youngren, K.D., & Roth, R.H. (1998). Dopamine D4 receptor antagonist reversal of subchronic phencyclidine-induced object retrieval/detour deficits in monkeys. *Psychopharmology, 142*, 78–84.

Kimberg, D.Y., D'Esposito, M., & Farah, M.J. (1997). Effects of bromocriptine on human subjects depend on working memory capacity. *NeuroReport, 8*, 3581–3585.

King, D.J. (1990). The effect of neuroleptics on cognitive and psychomotor function. *British Journal of Psychiatry, 157*, 799–811.

Knowlton, B.J., Mangels, J.A., & Squire, L.R. (1996). A neostriatal habit learning system in humans. *Science, 273*, 1399–1402.

Koelega, H.S. (1993). Stimulant drugs and vigilance performance. *Psychopharmacology, 111*, 1–16.

Koepp, M.J., Funn, R.N., Lawrence, A.D., Cunningham, V.J., Dagher, A., Jones, T., Brooks, D.J., Bench, C.J., & Grasby, P.M. (1998). Evidence for striatal dopamine release during a video game. *Nature, 393*, 266–268.

Lange, K.W., Robbins, T.W., Marsden, C.D., James, M., Owen, A.M., & Paul, G.M. (1992). L-dopa withdrawal selectively impairs performance in tests of frontal lobe function in Parkinson's disease. *Psychopharmacology, 107*, 394–404.

Lawrence, A.D., Weeks, R.A., Brooks, D.J., Andrews, T.C., Watkins, L.H.A., Harding, A.E., Robbins, T.W., & Sahakian, B.J. (1998). The relationship between striatal dopamine receptor binding and cognitive performance in Huntington's disease. *Brain, 121*, 1343–1355.

Lewis, D.A. (1990). The organization of chemically identified neural systems in primate prefrontal cortex. *Progress in Neuropsychopharmacology and Biological Psychiatry, 14*, 371–377.

Lewis, D.A., Foote, S.L., Goldsetin. M., & Morrison, J.H. (1988). The dopaminergic innervation of monkey prefrontal cortex: a tyrosine hydroxylase immunohistochemical study. *Brain Research, 449*, 225–243.

Li, B.M. & Mei, Z.T. (1994). Delayed response deficit induced by local injection of the alpha-2 adrenergic antagonist yohimbine into the dorsolateral prefrontal cortex in young adult monkeys. *Behavioral and Neural Biology, 62*, 134–139.

Li, B.M., Mao, Z.M., Wang, M., & Mei, Z.T. (1999). Alpha-2 adrenergic modulation of prefrontal cortical neuronal activity related to spatial working memory in monkeys. *Neuropsychopharmology, 21*, 601–610.

Luciana, M. & Collins, P.F. (1998). Dopaminergic modu0lation of working memory for spatial but not object cues in normal volunteers. *Journal of Cognitive Neuroscience, 9*, 330–347.

Luciana, M., Depue, R.A., Arbisi, P., & Leon, A. (1992). Facilitation of working memory in humans by a D2 dopamine receptor agonist. *Journal of Cognitive Neuroscience, 4*, 58–68.

Luciana, M., Collins, P.F., & Depue, R.A. (1998). Opposing roles for dopamine and serotonin in the modulation of human spatial working memory functions. *Cerebral Cortex, 8,* 218–226.

Luine, V., Bowling, D., & Hearns, M. (1990). Spatial memory deficits in aged rats: contributions of monoaminergic systems. *Brain Research, 537,* 271–278.

Lupien, S.J., Gillin, C.J., & Hauger, R.L. (1999). Working memory is more sensitive than declarative memory to the acute effects of corticosteroids: a dose–response study in humans. *Behavioral Neuroscience, 113,* 420–430.

Mair, R.G. & McEntree, W.J. (1986). Cognitive enhancement in Korsakoff's psychosis by clonidine: a comparison with 1-dopa and ephedrine. *Psychopharmology, 88,* 374–380.

Manji, H.K. & Lenox, R.H. (1999). Protein kinase C signaling in the brain: molecular transduction of mood stabilization in the treatment of manic–depressive illness. *Biological Psychiatry, 46,* 1328–1351.

Mao, Z.M., Arnsten, A.F.T., & Li, B.M. (1999). Local infusion of alpha-1 adrenergic agonist into the prefrontal cortex impairs spatial working memory performance in monkeys. *Biological Psychiatry, 46,* 1259–1265.

Marek, G.J. & Aghajanian, G.K. (1999). 5-HT2A receptor or alpha1-adrenoceptor activation induces EPSCs in layer V pyramidal cells of the medial prefrontal cortex. *European Journal of Pharmacology, 367,* 197–206.

Mattey, V.S., Berman, K.F., Ostrem, J.L., Esposito, G., Van Horn, J.D., Bigelow, L.B., & Weinberger, D.R. (1996). Dextroamphetamine enhances "neural network-specific" physiological signals: a positron-emisson tomography rCBF study. *Journal of Neuroscience, 16,* 4816–4822.

Mazure, C.M. (1995). Does stress cause psychiatric illness? In: D. Spiegel (Ed.), *Progress in Psychiatry* Washington, D.C: American Psychiatric Press.

McDowell, S., Whyte, J., & D'Esposito, M. (1998). Differential effect of a dopaminergic agonist on prefrontal function in traumatic brain injury patients. *Brain, 121,* 1155–1164.

McGaughy J., Dalley, J.W. Everitt, B.J. & Robbins T.W. (2002) Behavioral and Neurochemical effects of Cholinergic Lesions produced by 1921gG-saporin on attentional performance in a 5 choice serial reaction time task. *J Neuroscience,* in press.

McGaughy, J., Everitt, B.J., Robbins, T.W., & Sarter, M. (2000). The role of cholinergic afferent projections in cognition: impact of new selective immunotoxins. *Behavioral Brain Research, 115,* 251–263.

Mehta, M.A., Sahakian, B.J., McKenna, P.J., & Robbins, T.W. (1999). Systemic sulpiride in young adult volunteers simulates the profile of cognitive deficits in Parkinson's disease. *Psychopharmacology, 146,* 162–174.

Mehta, M.A., Owen, A.M., Sahakian, B.J., Mavaddat, N., Pickard, J.D., & Robbins, T.W. (2000). Methylphenidate enhances working memory by modulating discrete frontal and parietal lobe regions in the human brain. *Journal of Neuroscience, 20,* RC651–RC656.

Mehta, M.A., Sahakian, B.J., & Robbins, T.W. (2001). Comparative psychopharmacology of methylphenidate

and related drugs in human volunteers, patients with AD/HD and experimental animals. In: M. Solanto, A.F.T. Arnsten, & F.X. Castellanos (Eds.), *Stimulant Drugs and ADHD: Basic and Clinical Science* (pp. 303–331). New York Oxford University Press.

Mesulam, M.M. (1995). In: F.E. Bloom & D. Kupfer (Eds.), *Psychopharmacology: The Fourth Generation of Progress* (pp. 135–146). New York: Raven Press.

Middleton, H.C., Sharma, A., Agouzoui, D., Sahakian, B.J., & Robbins, T.W. (1999). Idazoxan potentiates rather than antagonizes some of the cognitive effects of clonidine. *Psychopharmacology, 145,* 401–411.

Milner, B. (1964). Some effects of frontal lobectomy in man. In: J.M. Warren and K. Akert (Eds.), *The Frontal Granular Cortex and Behaviour* (pp. 410–444). New York: McGraw-Hill.

Moffoot, A., O'Carroll, R.E., Murray, C., Dougall, N., Ebmeier, K., & Goodwin, G.M. (1994). Clonidine infusion increases uptake of Tc-exametazime in anterior cingulate cortex in Korsakoff's psychosis. *Psychological Medicine, 24,* 53–61.

Mohell, N., Svartengren, J., & Cannon, B. (1983). Identification of [3H] prazosin binding sites in crude membranes and isolated cells of brown adipose tissue as alpha-1 adrenergic receptors. *European Journal of Pharmacology, 92,* 15–25.

Mohr, E., Schlegel, J., Fabbrini, G., Williams, J., Mouradian, M., Mann, U.M., Claus, J.J., Fedio, P., & Chase, N.C. (1989). Clonidine treatment of Alzheimer's disease. *Archives in Neurology, 46,* 376–378.

Mortimer, A. (1997). Cognitive function in schizophrenia—do neuroleptics make a difference? *Pharmacology Biochemistry and Behavior, 56,* 789–795.

Mrzljak, L., Bergson, C., Pappy, M., Levenson, R., Huff, R., & Goldman-Rakic, P.S. (1996). Localization of dopamine D4 receptors in GABAergic neurons of the primate brain. *Nature, 381,* 245–248.

Muir, J.L., Everitt, B.J., & Robbins, T.W. (1995). Reversal of visual attentional dysfunction following lesions of the cholinergic basal forebrain by physostigmine and nicotine but not by the 5HT-3 antagonist, ondansetron. *Psychopharmacology, 118,* 82–92.

Muller, U., von Cramon, D.Y., & Pollmann, S. (1998). D1-versus D2-receptor modulation of visuospatial working memory in humans. *Journal of Neuroscience, 18,* 2720–2728.

Murphy, B., Roth, R., & Arnsten, A.F.T. (1997). Clozapine reverses the spatial working memory deficits induced by FG7142 in monkeys. *Neuropsychopharmacology, 16,* 433–437.

Murphy, B.L., Arnsten, A.F.T., Goldman-Rakic, P.S., & Roth, R.H. (1996a). Increased dopamine turnover in the prefrontal cortex impairs spatial working memory performance in rats and monkeys. *Proccedings of the National Academy of Science USA, 93,* 1325–1329.

Murphy, B.L., Arnsten, A.F.T., Jentsch, J.D., & Roth, R.H. (1996b). Dopamine and spatial working memory in rats and monkeys: Pharmacological reversal of stress-induced impairment. *Journal of Neuroscience, 16,* 7768–7775.

Ongur, D. & Price, J.L. (2000). The organization of networks within the orbital and medial prefrontal cortex of rats, monkeys and humans. *Cerebral Cortex, 10,* 206–219.

O'Rourke, M.F., Blaxall, H.S., Iversen, L.J., & Bylund, D.B. (1994). Characterization of [3H] RX821002 binding to alpha-2 adrenergic receptor subtypes. *Journal of Pharmacology and Experimental Therapeutics, 268,* 1362–1367.

Owen, A.M., James, M., Leigh, P.H., Summers, B.A., Marsden, C.D., Quinn, N.P., Lange, K.W., & Robbins, T.W. (1992). Fronto-striatal cognitive deficits at different stages of Parkinson's disease. *Brain, 115,* 1727–1751.

Owen, A.M., Sahakian, B.J., Hodges, J.R., Summers, B.A., Polkey, C.E., & Robbins, T.W. (1995a). Dopamine-dependent fronto-striatal planning deficits in early Parkinson's disease. *Neuropsychology, 9,* 126–140.

Owen, A.M., Sahakian, B.J., Semple, J., Polkey, C.E., & Robbins, T.W. (1995b). Visuospatial short-term recognition memory and learning after temporal lobe excisions, frontal lobe excisions or amygdala–hippocampectomy in man. *Neuropsychologia, 33,* 1–24.

Park, S.B., Coull, J.T., McShane, R.H., Young, A.H., Sahakian, B.J., Robbins, T.W., & Cowen, P.J. (1994). Tryptophan depletion in normal volunteers produces selective impairments in learning and memory. *Neuropharmacology, 33,* 575–588.

Passetti, F., Dalley, J.W., O'Connell, M.T., Everitt, B.J., & Robbins, T.W. (2000). Increased acetylcholine release in the rat medial prefrontal cortex during performance of a visual attentional task. *European Journal of Neuroscience, 12,* 3051–3058.

Perry, E.K., Tomlinson, B.E., Blessed, G., Bergmann, K., Gibson, P.H., & Perry, R.H. (1978). Correlation of cholinergic abnormalities with senile plaques and mental test scores in senile dementia. *British Medical Journal, 2,* 1457–1459.

Perry, E.K., Walker, M., & Perry, R. (1999). Acetylcholine in mind: a neurotransmitter correlate of consciousness? *Trends in Neuroscience, 22,* 373–380.

Posner, M.I., Walker, J.A., Friedrich, F.J., & Rafal, R.D. (1984). Effects of parietal injury on covert orienting of visual attention. *Journal of Neuroscience, 4,* 1863–1874.

Rahman, S., Sahakian, B.J., Hodges, J.R., Rogers, R.D., & Robbins, T.W. (1999). Specific cognitive deficits in mild frontal variant frontotemporal dementia. *Brain, 122,* 1469–1493.

Rama, P., Linnankoski, I., Tanila, H., Pertovaara, A., & Carlson, S. (1996). Medetomidine, atipamezole, and guanfacine in delayed response performance of aged monkeys. *Pharmacology, Biochemistry and Behavior, 54,* 1–7.

Richardson, R.T. & DeLong, M.R. (1986). Nucleus basalis of Meynert neuronal activity during a delayed response task in a monkey. *Brain Research, 399,* 364–368.

Ridley, R.M., Barefoot, H.C., Maclean, C.J., Pugh, R., & Baker, H.F. (1999). Different effect on learning ability after injection of the cholinergic immunotoxin ME 20.4 IgG-saporin into the diagonal band of Broca, basal nucleus of Meynert, or both in monkeys. *Behavioral Neuroscience, 113,* 303–315.

Riekkinen, P. & Riekkinen, M. (1999). THA improves word priming and clonidine enhances fluency and working memory in Alzheimer's disease. *Neuropsychopharmacology, 20,* 357–364.

Robbins T.W., Owen, A.M. & Sahakian B.J. (1998b) The neuropsychology of basal ganglia disorders: an integrated cognitive and comparative approach. Ed. M Ron and A David, In *Disorders of Mind and Brain,* Cambridge Univ.Press. Cambridge, pp 57–83

Robbins, T.W., Granon, S., Muir, J.L., Durantou, F., Harrison, A., & Everitt, B.J. (1998a) Neural systems underlying arousal and attention. In J.A. Harvey and B.E. Kosofsky (Eds). *Cocaine: Effects on the developing brain,* Annals of the New York Academy of Sciences. Vol. 846. pp 222–237.

Robbins TW (2000) Chemical neuromodulation of frontal-executive function in humans and other animals. *Experimental Brain Research 133:* 130–138.

Roberts, A.C., Robbins, T.W., Everitt, B.J., & Muir, J.L. (1992). A specific form of cognitive rigidity following excitotoxic lesions of the basal forebrain in monkeys. *Neuroscience, 47,* 251–264.

Roberts, A.C., Salvia, M.A., Wilkinson, L.S., Collins, P., Muir, J.L., Everitt, B.J., & Robbins, T.W. (1994). 6-Hydroxydopamine lesions of the prefrontal cortex in monkeys enhance performance on an analog of the Wisconsin Card Sort Test: possible interactions with subcortical dopamine. *Neuroscience, 14,* 2531–2544.

Rogers, R.D., Blackshaw, A.J., Middleton, H.C., Matthews, K., Hawtin, K., Crowley, C., Hopwood, A., Wallace, C., Deakin, J.F.W., Sahakian, B.J., & Robbins, T.W. (1999a). Tryptophan depletion impairs stimulus-reward learning while methylphenidate disrupts attentional control in healthy young adults: implications for the monoaminergic basis of impulsive behaviour. *Psychopharmacology, 146,* 482–492.

Rogers, R.D., Everitt, B.J., Baldacchino, A., Blackshaw, A.J., Swainson, R., Wynne, K., Baker, N.B., Hunter, J., Carthy, T., Booker, E., London, M., Deakin, J.F.W., Sahakian, B.J., & Robbins, T.W. (1999b). Dissociable deficits in the decision-making cognition of chronic amphetamine abusers, opiate abusers, patients with focal damage to prefrontal cortex, and tryptophan depleted normal volunteers: evidence for monoaminergic mechanisms. *Neuropsychopharmacology, 20,* 322–339.

Rolls, E.T. (1996). The orbitofrontal cortex. *Philosophical Transactions of the Royal Society of London, 351,* 1433–1444.

Rolls, E.T., Hornak, J., Wade, D., & McGrath, J. (1994). Emotion-related learning in patients with social and emotional changes associated with frontal lobe damage. *Journal of Neurology Neurosurgery and Psychiatry, 57,* 1518–1524.

Sahakian, B.J. & Coull, J.T. (1994). Nicotine and tetrahydroaminoacridine: evidence for improved attention in patients with dementia of the Alzheimer's type. *Drug Development Research, 31,* 80–88.

Sahakian, B.J., Sarna, G.S., Kantamaneni, B.D., Jackson,

A., Hutson, P.H., & Curzon, G. (1985). Association between learning and cortical catecholamines in non–drug-treated rats. *Psychopharmcology, 86*, 339–343.

Sahakian, B.J., Jones, G., Levy, R., Gray, J.G., & Warburton, D. (1989). The effects of nicotine on attention, information processing and short term memory in patients with dementia of the Alzheimer-type. *British Journal of Psychiatry, 154*, 797–800.

Sallinen, J., Haapalinna, A., MacDonald, E., Viitamaa, T., Lahdesmaki, J., Rybnikova, E., Pelto-Huikko, M., Kobilka, B., & Scheinin, M. (1999). Genetic alteration of the alpha2-adrenoceptor subtype c in mice affects the development of behavioral despair and stress-induced increases in plasma corticosterone levels. *Molecular Psychiatry, 4*, 443–452.

Sarter, M. & Bruno, J. (1997). Cognitive functions of cortical acetylcholine: toward a unifying hypothesis. *Brain Research Review, 23*, 28–46.

Sawaguchi, T. (1998). Attenuation of delay-period activity of monkey prefrontal cortical neurons by an alpha-2 adrenergic antagonist during an oculomotor delayed-response task. *Journal of Neurophysiology, 80*, 2200–2205.

Sawaguchi, T. & Goldman-Rakic. P.S. (1991). D1 dopamine receptors in prefrontal cortex: involvement in working memory. *Science, 251*, 947–950.

Sawaguchi, T., Matsumura, M., & Kubota, K. (1988). Dopamine enhances the neuronal activity of spatial short-term memory task in the primate prefrontal cortex. *Neuroscience Research, 5*, 465–473.

Sawaguchi, T., Matsumura, M., & Kubota, K. (1990). Catecholaminergic effects on neuronal activity related to delayed response task in monkey prefrontal cortex. *Journal of Neurophysiology, 63*, 1385–1400.

Scahill, L., Chappell, P.B., Kim, Y.S., Schultz, R.T., Katsovich, L., Shepherd, E., Arnsten, A.F.T., Cohen, D.J., & Leckman, J.F. (2001). Guanfacine in the treatment of children with tic disorders and ADHD: a placebo-controlled study. *American Journal of Psychiatry, 158*: 1067–1074.

Schultz, W. (1998). The phasic reward signal of primate dopamine neurons. *Advances in Pharmacology, 42*, 686–690.

Schultz, W., Apicella, P., & Ljungberg, T. (1993). Responses of monkey dopamine neurons to reward and conditioned stimuli during successive steps of learning a delayed response task. *Journal of Neuroscience, 13*, 900–913.

Seamans, J.K., Floresco, S.B., & Phillips, A.G. (1998). D1 receptor modulation of hippocampal–prefrontal cortical circuits integrating spatial memory with executive functions in the rat. *Journal of Neuroscience, 18*, 1613–1621.

Selden, N.R.W., Cole, B.J., Everitt, B.J., & Robbins, T.W. (1990). Damage to ceruleo-cortical noradrenergic projections impairs locally cued but enhances spatially cued water maze acquisition. *Behavioral Brain Research, 39*, 29–51.

Servan-Schneider, D., Printz, H., & Cohen, J.D. (1990). A network model of catecholamine effects: gain, signal-to-noise ratio, and behaviour. *Science, 249*, 892–895.

Sesack, S.R., Deutch, A.Y., Roth, R.H., & Bunney, B.S.

(1989). Topographical organization of the efferent projections of the medial prefrontal cortex in the rat: an anterograde tract tracing study with *Phaselous vulgaris* leucoagglutinin. *Journal of Comparative Neurology, 290*, 213–242.

Shallice, T. (1982). Specific impairments of planning. *Philosophical Transactions of the Royal Society Series B: Biological Sciences, 298*, 199–209.

Shors, T.J., Weiss, C., & Thompson, R.F. (1992). Stress-induced facilitation of classical conditioning. *Science, 257*, 537–539.

Simon, H. (1981). Dopaminergic A10 neurons and the frontal system. *Journal de Physiologie, 77*, 81–95.

Sirviö, J., Riekkinen, P., Vajanto, I., Koivisto, E., & Riekkinen, P.J. (1991). The effects of guanfacine, alpha-2 agonist, on the performance of young and aged rats in spatial navigation task. *Behavioral Neural Biology, 56*, 101–107.

Solanto, M., Arnsten A.F.T. & Castellanos F.X. (Eds) (2001) *Stimulant Drugs and ADHD: Basic and Clinical Neuroscience* Oxford, New York, University Press.

Stecker, T. & Sahgal, A. (1995). Serotonergic–cholinergic interactions in the modulation of cognitive behaviour. *Behavioral Brain Research, 67*, 165–199.

Steere, J.C. & Arnsten, A.F.T. (1997). The alpha-2A noradrenergic agonist, guanfacine, improves visual object discrimination reversal performance in rhesus monkeys. *Behavioral Neuroscience, 111*, 1–9.

Stern, Y. & Langston, W. (1985). Intellectual changes in patients with MPTP-induced parkinsonism. *Neurology, 35*, 1506–1509.

Surmeier, D.J., Bargas, J., Hemmings, H.C.J., Nairn, A.C., & Greenguard, P. (1995). Modulation of calcium currents by a D1 dopaminergic protein kinase/phosphatase cascade in rat neostriatal neurons. *Neuron, 14*, 385–397.

Swainson, R., Rogers, R.D., Sahakian, B.J., Summers, B.A., Polkey, C.E., & Robbins, T.W. (2000). Probabilistic learning and reversal deficits in patients with Parkinson's disease or frontal or temporal lobe lesions: possible adverse effects of dopaminergic medication. *Neuropsychologia, 38*, 596–612.

Swartz, B.E., Kovalik, E., Thomas, K., Torgersen, D., & Mandelkern, M.A. (2000). The effects of an alpha-2 adrenergic agonist, guanfacine, on rCBF in human cortex in normal controls and subjects with focal epilepsy. *Neuropsychopharmcology, 23*, 263–275.

Tanila, H., Rama, P., & Carlson, S. (1996). The effects of prefrontal intracortical microinjections of an alpha-2 agonist, alpha-2 antagonist and lidocaine on the delayed alternation performance of aged rats. *Brain Research Bulletin, 40*, 117–119.

Tanila, H., Mustonen, K., Sallinen, J., Scheinin, M., & Riekkinen, P. (1999). Role of alpha-2C-adrenoceptor subtype in spatial working memory as revealed by mice with targeted disruption of the alpha-2C-adrenoceptor gene. *European Journal of Neuroscience, 11*, 599–603.

Taylor, A.E., Saint-Cyr, J.A., & Lang, A.E. (1986). Frontal lobe dysfunction in Parkinson's disease. *Brain, 109*, 845–843.

Taylor, F.B. & Russo, J. (2001). Comparing guanfacine and dextroamphetamine for the treatment of adult attention deficit–hyperactivity disorder. *Journal of Clinical Psychopharmocology, 21,* 223–228.

Taylor, J.R., Birnbaum, S.G., Ubriani, R., & Arnsten, A.F.T. (1999). Activation of protein kinase A in prefrontal cortex impairs working memory performance. *Journal of Neuroscience, 19,* RC23.

Thierry, A.M., Tassin, J.P., Blanc, G., & Glowinski, J. (1976). Selective activation of the mesocortical DA system by stress. *Nature, 263,* 242–244.

Vaidya, C.J., Austin, G., Kirkorian, G., Ridlehuber, H.W., Desmond, J.E., Glover, G.H., & Gabrieli, J.D.E. (1998). Selective effects of methylphenidate in attention deficit hyperactivity disorder: a functional magnetic resonance study. *Proceedings of the National Academy of Sciences USA, 95,* 14494–14499.

Volkow, N.D., Gur, R.C., Wange, C.J., Fowler, J.S., Moberg, P.J., Ding, Y.S., Hitzemann, R., Smith, G., & Logan, J. (1998). Association between decline in brain dopamine activity with age and cognitive and motor impairment in healthy individuals. *American Journal of Psychiatry, 155,* 344–349.

Warburton, E.C., Harrison, A.A., Robbins, T.W., & Everitt, B.J. (1997). Contrasting effects of systemic and intracerebral infusions of the 5-HT$_{1A}$ receptor against 8-OH-DPAT on spatial short-term working memory in rats. *Behavioral Brain Research, 84,* 247–258.

Williams, G.V. & Goldman-Rakic, P.S. (1995). Blockade of dopamine D1 receptors enhances the memory fields of prefrontal neurons in primate cerebral cortex. *Nature, 376,* 572–575.

Williams, G.V., Rao, S.G., & Goldman-Rakic, P.S. (1997). Attenuation of memory fields in primate prefrontal cortical pyramidal cell and interneurons by selective 5-HT2 antagonists. *Society of Neuroscience Abstracts, 23,* 627.7.

Williams, J.H., Wellman, N.A., Geaney, D.P., Cowen, P.J.,

Feldon, J., & Rawlins, J.W.P. (1998). Residual latent inhibition in people with schizophrenia: an effect of psychosis or of its treatment. *British Journal of Psychiatry, 172,* 243–249.

Williams, S.M. & Goldman-Rakic, P.S. (1998). Widespread origin of the primate mesofrontal dopamine system. *Cerebral Cortex, 8,* 321–345.

Winter, J.C. & Petti, D.T. (1987). The effect of 8-hydroxy2-(di-n-propyl-amino) tetralin and other serotonergic agonists on performance in a radial maze: a possible role for 5HT-1A receptors in memory. *Pharmacology, Biochemistry and Behavior, 27,* 625–628.

Witte, E.A. & Marrocco, R.T. (1997). Alterations of brain noradrenergic activity in rhesus monkeys affects the altering component of covert orienting. *Psychopharmacology, 132,* 315–323.

Witte, E.A., Davidson, M.C., & Marrocco, R.T. (1997). Effects of altering cholinergic activity on covert orienting of attention: comparison of monkey and human performance. *Psychopharmacology, 132,* 324–334.

Woods, D.L. & Knight, R.T. (1986). Electrophysiological evidence of increased distractability after dorsolateral prefrontal lesions. *Neurology, 36,* 212–216.

Yang, C.R. & Seamans, J.K. (1996). Dopamine D1 receptor actions in layers V–VI rat prefrontal cortex neurons in vitro: modulation if dendritic–somatic signal integration. *Journal of Neuroscience, 16,* 1922–1935.

Young, S.N., Smith, S.E., Phil, P.O., & Ervin, F.R. (1985). Tryptophan depletion causes a rapid lowering of mood in normal males. *Psychopharmacology, 87,* 173–177.

Zahrt, J., Taylor, J.R., Mathew, R.G., & Arnsten, A.F.T. (1997). Supranormal stimulation of dopamine D1 receptors in the rodent prefrontal cortex impairs spatial working memory performance. *Journal of Neuroscience, 17,* 8528–8535.

5

Functional Architecture of the Dorsolateral Prefrontal Cortex in Monkeys and Humans

PATRICIA S. GOLDMAN-RAKIC AND HOI-CHUNG LEUNG

Working memory is a central concept in the cognitive sciences and today among the most actively studied subjects in cognitive psychology and human imaging. The history and richness of this concept have been elaborated and comprehensively reviewed in a voluminous experimental literature (Baddeley, 1986; Just & Carpenter, 1992; Miyake & Shah, 1999). The focus of cognitive psychologists has naturally been on psychological process rather than on brain mechanisms, although not without awareness that psychological process could be mapped onto brain systems, and indeed, assumptions in the psychological literature have often been made about the cortical or subcortical localization of these systems. A major psychological distinction in the working memory literature is that between the storage and processing components of working memory. Baddeley's model of working memory in particular distinguishes between slave systems (the articulatory loop and visuospatial sketchpad) with strong storage/rehearsal functions and the central executive, a high-level central processor with similarities to the supervisory attentional system of Shallice (1982; 1988).

It is often assumed that the distinct psychological processes of online storage and function are carried out in different areas of cerebral cortex. Some models allocate these distinct processes to posterior parietal and prefrontal cortical areas of the prefrontal cortex (e.g., Courtney et al., 1997; Smith & Jonides, 1997; 1999), respectively, while others have suggested segregation of these functions in different cytoarchitectonic areas of the prefrontal cortex (e.g., Petrides, 1994; Owen, 1997). An alternative hypothesis is that storage and processing are integrally related and dependent on the same neuronal infrastructure. Additionally, on the basis of data from neuropsychological studies and in part from anatomical and electrophysiological research, we have proposed that the prefrontal cortex is topographically organized into informationally constrained domains, each of which is a node in a wider network of sensory, motor, and limbic areas (Goldman-Rakic & Schwartz, 1982; Selemon & Goldman-Rakic, 1985, 1988; Cavada & Goldman-Rakic, 1989). In this framework, each domain-specific network has its own central processor with integrated storage and processing components. Over the past decade, these propositions have driven healthy debate and much research, receiving support from some investigations (McCarthy et al., 1994, 1996; Courtney et al., 1996; 1997; Sweeney et al., 1996; Leung et al., 2000) as well as challenge from other cognitive neuroscience and imaging studies (e.g., Petrides et al.,

1993a; 1993b; Owen et al., 1996; Rushworth et al., 1997; D'Esposito et al., 1999).

Although it is unlikely that these fundamental issues can be easily resolved, knowledge of the functional architecture of the cerebral cortex at a cellular and circuit level can contribute to the development of a comprehensive theory of human cognition and consciousness. Here we argue that convergent findings from neurophysiology, neuroanatomy, and functional magnetic resonance imaging (fMRI) are essential for a comprehensive understanding of the structure of executive processes. In particular, the dorsolateral prefrontal cortex in the nonhuman primate can serve as an unparalleled model system for studying visual memory and examining its properties. Analysis of one system in detail should help to address the larger issues of domain specificity, the neural basis of storage and processing functions, and plasticity within working memory.

CIRCUIT BASIS OF WORKING MEMORY

The method of single-cell recording in awake behaving monkeys as they perform behavioral tasks is at present the most powerful approach to understanding the neural basis of behavior. In contrast to cellular analyses in vitro, e.g., in slice preparations, the *in vivo* approach allows direct correlation of cellular activity and specific processes as they are engaged by behavioral paradigms. In contrast to noninvasive imaging of structure–function relationships in the human or animal brain, the spatial resolution of single-unit recording is on the order of microns and temporal resolution is on the order of microseconds. Furthermore, as cellular activity is coincident with psychological events, inferences about the dynamic basis of information processing are direct. Limitations of this approach include the inability to unequivocally identify the cell under investigation, although the localization of neurons to cytoarchitectonic areas and cortical layers can, with difficulty, be determined. Neurophysiological studies have not only given a dynamic view of neural processing "on-line" but have allowed investigators to examine fundamental issues

about both normal and experimentally altered brain function. However, it should be patently obvious that recording one or a few cells at a time has been a technical necessity and in no way should be taken to imply that any behavior is dependent on a single cell or any one brain area. Rather, the neuron investigated is a representative of a cohort of cells acting in aggregate, including local and long-distance synaptic connections.

Single-neuron recording is and has been a method par excellence for dissecting the neuronal elements involved in perceptual, mnemonic, and motor control processes. Many scientists have applied this method to the investigation of working memory in monkeys trained to perform spatial or nonspatial oculomotor delayed-response (ODR) tasks. Remarkably, the delayed-response format used in nonhuman primate studies has become paradigmatic for probing working memory in human imaging studies (Fig. 5–1). In an oculomotor spatial version of delayed response, the location of a briefly presented visuospatial stimulus is maintained in working memory to provide guidance for subsequent saccadic eye movements (see Fig. 5–1A, upper left). The essential feature of this task is that the item to be recalled has to be updated on every trial in analogous fashion to the moment-to-moment process of human mentation. After training is completed, monkeys are prepared for physiological recording sessions which usually occur on a 5-day-a-week basis. The cortical region that has been most strongly related to spatial processing in nonhuman primates is the dorsolateral region around the posterior third of the principal sulcus corresponding to Walker's mapping of area 46, including tissue adjoining the anterior surface of the frontal eye field in the macaque monkey (Walker, 1940). Area 46 as well as the frontal eye field region of prefrontal cortex is distinguished by its preferential projections to the superior colliculus, which in turn relays cortical signals to oculomotor centers (Fries, 1984).

Because the ODR task requires the registration of information in the stimulus, the on-line maintenance of this information in temporary storage, and its integration with a goal-directed response, *a priori* there would

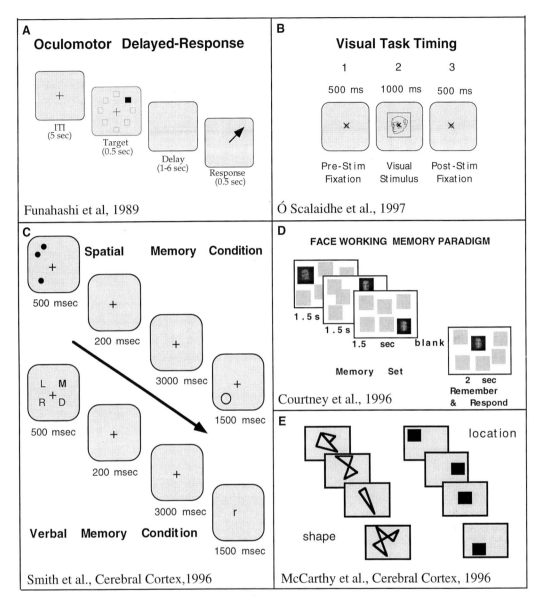

Figure 5–1. Common design of working memory paradigms as employed in studies of nonhuman primates (*A*, *B*) and humans (*C–E*). All tasks employ sequential presentation of the item or items to be recalled (shapes, letters, words, or markers of location), delay periods between items over which items must be recalled, and recall or response epochs. (*Source*: Funahashi et al., 1989; McCarthy et al., 1996; Smith et al., 1996; and O'Scalaidhe et al., 1997, with permission)

be no way of knowing how these real-time events are made operational by the nervous system. Does a single class of neuron carry out this synthesis or is this prospective process decomposed into elemental components, subfunctions, or subroutines? Single-cell recording studies of prefrontal cortex have indicated that separate neurons within a cortical area exhibit elemental processes—i.e., some register information, some hold it "on-line," or respond at the time of the motor response (Fig. 5–2), whereas others within the very same area exhibit remarkable combinatorial properties, often exhibiting all three components

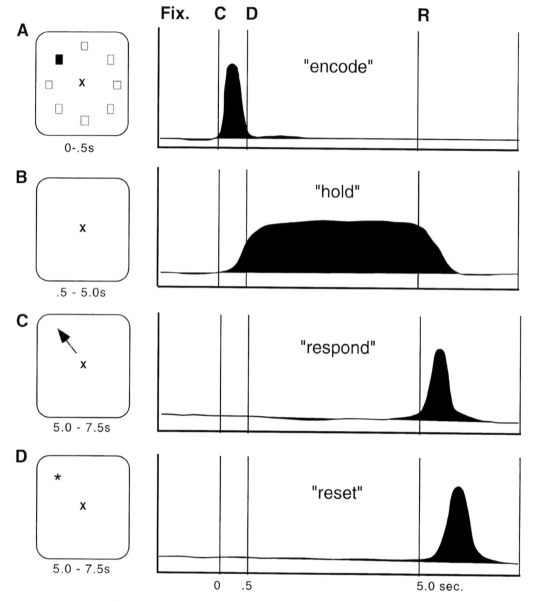

Figure 5–2. Diagrammatic representation of neuronal responses observed in individual neurons recorded from the dorsolateral prefrontal cortex during the oculomotor delayed-response task. A: Some neurons exhibit a phasic response to register or encode a briefly presented stimulus. B: Other neurons show tonic activity during the delay period—i.e., these neurons hold the signal online after the stimulus is withdrawn. Still other neurons exhibit a phasic burst just prior to initiation of a response (presaccadic) (C) or after its completion (postsaccadic) (D). Many neurons exhibit combinations of these "simple" activations. The vertical line marked "R" represents the signal to respond; note that the peak activity in panel c occurs before response initiation. "C," cue period; "D," delay period.

— cue-(sensory), delay- (mnemonic), and response-related activities at different points in a single memory trial (Fig. 5–3). These neurons typically exhibit, relative to baseline, an abrupt, strong phasic increase in rate at the time of the cue, a lower but sustained increase in firing rate throughout the delay period, followed by another strong phasic increase in firing rate at the end of the delay period preceding the animal's response. How do the

PRIMATE SINGLE UNIT RECORDING

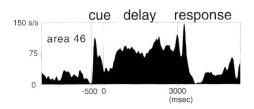

HUMAN HEMODYNAMIC RESPONSE

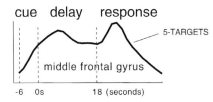

Figure 5–3. *Top*: Example of prefrontal neuronal activity recorded *in vivo* as a monkey performed an oculomotor spatial delayed-response task. The neuron's activity is precisely time locked to the events in the task: the presentation of a spatial cue (500 ms); the delay period interposed between the cue and the response (3000 msec); and the response period after the delay 1000 ms). The raster display above each histogram shows the neuron's firing rate on numerous trials, during which the animal was required to remember the same target location relative to the fixation point trial after trial. The firing rate was consistently enhanced during the delay period whenever the monkey recalled the cue at its preferred target location; such enhancement was not observed for "nonpreferred" locations. The preferential activation of a prefrontal neuron during memory intervals (during which no stimulus is present and no response required) is termed the neuron's *memory field*, in analogy to receptive field properties of neurons in sensory cortices. *Bottom*: Average percent of hemodynamic signal change in the middle frontal gyrus during trials in which human subjects were asked to recall five sequentially indicated locations over an 18-second interval. The x-axis represents time in terms of image frames (a total of 30 frames or 45 seconds). The first vertical line marks the end of the cue presentation, and the second line marks the onset of the probe presentation, followed by responses. (*Source of top panel*: Goldman-Rakic, 1996, with permission from the publisher of *Philosophical Transactions of the Royal Society of London*)

neurons that appear to have separate cue-, delay- or response-related responses coordinate their function? A likely way is for these neurons to form a microcircuit in which cue information is passed to a "delay" cell, which

in turn is terminated by a "go" signal from a third neuron with presaccadic activity. Alternatively or additionally, in analogy with visual cortical cells, elemental or "simple" process neurons might converge on higher-order neurons which combine some or all elemental signals provided by the single-process neurons. A still third scenario is that neurons with cue-, delay-, or response-related activities might be interconnected in a completely re-entrant neural net—i.e., with mutual interconnections between all elements. In any case, these elemental neurons would form a local network that binds real-time events together in the service of comprehension, willed action, updating of information, etc. Recent studies in this laboratory with multiple electrodes are beginning to decipher the rules of microcircuit functional connectivity that form the structure of a microcolumn (Constantinidis et al., 2001).

SIMILAR PROFILES OF INFORMATION PROCESSING EVENTS IN NONHUMAN PRIMATES AND HUMANS

In the human prefrontal cortex, area 46 has been mapped by cytoarchitectonic criteria to the anterior portion of the middle frontal gyrus (MFG). It should be mentioned that such mapping can only be approximate. Recent event-related fMRI studies carried out in collaboration with Hoi-Chung Leung and John Gore at Yale University have shed new light on the functional localization of this area in humans and have aided in isolating the component processes of visuospatial working memory in humans. The findings reveal a remarkable similarity to the component analysis from neuronal recordings in monkeys and also establish grounds for functional homology between the MFG and caudal principal sulcus region in nonhuman primates. In the fMRI studies, we asked normal human subjects to perform an ODR task in which a varied number of locations, presented serially, were to be recalled after a delay. The number of items varied from 1 to 5 and were either pictures or simple geometric stimuli such as circles or dots. The delay period in our studies lasted either 18 or 24 seconds for different cohorts of subjects. Because of the long latencies of hemodynamic responses, the extended delay periods allowed us to better resolve the hemodynamic response to sensory, mnemonic, and response events in these tasks. We found that the MFG was activated transiently when subjects recalled three locations but showed sustained activations through 18 seconds when the number of memoranda was elevated to 5. Moreover, the MFG exhibited the strongest activations of any prefrontal area, including the inferior and superior prefrontal regions (Fig. 5–4). This result is in keeping with previous studies showing load effects for verbal (Cohen et al., 1997) and spatial (Carlson et al., 1998) processing in the dorsolateral pre-

frontal cortex. Importantly, as illustrated in Figure 5–3, in the five-item condition, the profile of signal change resembles that observed in single-unit activity in nonhuman primates—there are stronger signals to the response events of a trial than during the mnemonic episode itself. It should be noted in the single-unit profile that although the firing rate of the cell is sustained over the duration of the delay interval, the firing rate is usually *lower* than at the time of response. This lower signal is likely to be more difficult to detect in fMRI studies than the phasic bursts of neuronal activity in conjunction with motor- and sensory-related signals and could account for negative results in some studies. The selective activation of the human prefrontal region corresponding to the dorsolateral region in monkeys where cells with visuospatial memory fields are located (Fuster and Alexander, 1971; Kubota and Niki, 1971; Niki, 1974; Funahashi et al., 1989), where lesions selectively impair visuospatial delayed-response performance (Goldman et al., 1971), and where cytoarchitectonic analysis reveals anatomical homology to area 46 in monkeys (Walker, 1940; Rajkowska and Goldman-Rakic, 1995a; 1995b) provides a compelling argument for the conservation of a strong structure–function relationship in cortical specialization during primate evolution.

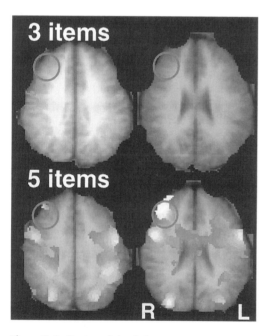

Figure 5–4. Percent of signal change in group composite maps of 11 subjects, based on contrasts between the memory and baseline of three-item (*upper*) and five-item spatial (*lower*) working memory tasks. Mean percent signal differences for areas above a threshold of $P < 0.005$ (uncorrected) are shown for the last 6 seconds of the 18-second delay period. Middle frontal gyrus (MFG) activation was observed in the three-item task, but this activation did not persist throughout the delay period. The MFG is indicated by circles. Positive signals are indicated by the light patches and negative signals are not visible in this black and white figure. R, right; L, left.

RESOLVING DISCREPANCIES IN THE LITERATURE

How do we explain inconsistencies in the literature regarding the location of the visuospatial memory domain within the frontal lobe? Although MFG activations have been found in numerous studies of visuospatial working memory (McCarthy et al., 1994, 1996; Baker et al., 1996; Smith et al., 1996; Sweeney et al., 1996; Leung et al., 2000), other studies have contested this localization and indicated that other frontal lobe areas might be more important for the maintenance function of visuospatial memoranda. Courtney et al. (1997), for example, found strong activations in the precentral cortices in a spatial working memory task identical to our three-item task (with similar face memoranda), except that they used a 9-second delay period rather than 18 seconds. Their report also included evidence of significant activations in the MFG, corresponding to the transient activation we saw in our three-item task. We also found the same strong activations in the precentral cortex as did Courtney et al. in their three-item task. Thus, the results of the two studies would appear to be in quite good agreement. However, we have shown that sustained MFG activations rises above threshold only with higher memory demands, as in our five-item tasks, and that denial of a role for this region in storage (or processing) is unwarranted.

The same argument can apply to the visuospatial working memory task developed by Rowe et al. (2000), in which three red dots were presented in random locations at the start of a trial, and both shorter to longer (9.5–18.5 seconds) delays followed before the subjects were required to make a response. As in the Leung et al. (2000) study described above, the virtue of this design is that subjects cannot prepare a response during the delay period. Similar to Rowe and Passingham (see Chapter 14), we used 18- and 24-second delays to segregate the cue, mnemonic, and response activations. Like Rowe and Passingham we observed significant activation in area 46 at the time of response selection. We also saw transient activation during a three-item task for the first 12 seconds of the 18-second delay interval. We then repeated our study with five items and also found stronger responses at the response period, but now we obtained a mnemonic response that lasted throughout the 18–24 seconds in individual subjects. Thus, in our view, the failure to activate area 46 in Rowe and Passingham's visuospatial memory tasks is explicable in terms of the inadequate load imposed in their fMRI study.

There remains the issue of why Rowe and Passingham observed area 8 activity in their three-item working memory task. It seems possible that this could be due to the residual stimulus-related activity present in the delay period (they did not statistically evaluate duration of response within the delay period), to

eye movements that occurred during the delay period, or to a mnemonic process, as claimed. In any case, it is evident from the above results that low-load working memory functions can be supported by areas outside of area 46 itself and, although we did not observe activations in area 8 in our own study, it is a possible locus for supporting visuospatial working memory. We and others have reported evidence that area 8A neurons exhibit robust activity in delay periods of oculomotor delayed-response tasks (e.g., Funahashi et al., 1989). What is at issue is not the involvement of area 8 in working memory processes, but the denial of this function for area 46.

Passingham and Rowe have also attempted to harmonize electrophysiological data in the nonhuman primate with that in humans, on the premise that the basic mechanisms of cognition are conserved among mammals (see Chapter 14). However, their references to the behavioral deficits that follow lesions of the prefrontal cortex are incomplete. Certain other findings should be recalled. Bilateral lesions of area 8a do not produce deficits on the classical delayed-response task, as would be predicted from the Passingham and Rowe study (Goldman et al., 1971); bilateral area 46 lesions do not produce deficits on tasks requiring only response selection such as visual discrimination, conditional position tasks, or object alternation, all of which involve response selection but none of which are impaired by full lesions of the principal sulcus Mishkin & Pribram, 1955; (Goldman et al., 1971). The lesion findings do not therefore support the thesis that area 46 is critical for response selection from memory as a generic proposition; they do support the thesis that this area is involved in using "short-term representational memory (i.e., internalized knowledge) *to guide behavior* in the absence of informative external cues" (Goldman-Rakic, 1987). It should also be recalled that one of the most important properties of neurons in area 46 and in area 8a is that they are spatially tuned in their delay-period activations—i.e., they have memory fields, analogous to sensory receptive fields. What purpose would this property serve if not to provide direction to response choice? Furthermore, it has been shown that delay-period activity predicts whether an animal will make a correct response or an error; when a neuron's memory-related activity falters in the middle of a delay or does not arise at all, an error inevitably occurs (Funahashi et al., 1989). Thus, the same neuron codes the same location and guides the same directional response, trial after trial, and different locations in the visual field are remembered by different neurons. Further, temporary inactivation of one or a few modules results in the loss of memory-guided responses to visuospatial cues while sparing sensory-guided responses (Sawaguchi & Goldman-Rakic, 1991). The disruption of other prefrontal domains has either been shown or can be expected to cause the loss of memory for faces, names, subjects of sentences, ideas, and goals. Indeed, we have already observed such processing in the form of face and object responsive cells as well as vocalization responsive neurons in inferior portions of the nonhuman primate prefrontal cortex (O'Scalaidhe et al., 1997; 1999; Romanski & Goldman-Rakic, 1999).

TERMINOLOGICAL OR CONCEPTUAL DISCREPANCIES?

We have proposed that prefrontal neurons in area 46 with their distinct sensory, mnemonic, and response-related activations provide a neural basis for *guiding behavior* in visuospatial working memory tasks. According to this view, the mnemonic neural component is the link between sensation and response choice. Passingham and Rowe argue on the basis of the study described earlier that area 8, not area 46, is engaged by the mnemonic process *per se*. In this volume and in previous publications, these authors have proposed that area 46 is activated when working memory tasks require "attentional selection" between items within memory. We see little difference between this construct and working memory constructs other than terminology. Both are referent to the same capacity and the same area of the dorsolateral prefrontal cortex.

WORKING MEMORY, DORSOLATERAL PREFRONTAL CORTEX, AND SCHIZOPHRENIA

Recent advances in integrative and cognitive neuroscience now allow penetration into the neural circuits and cellular processes that underlie human cognition and provide insights into the pathophysiology of diseases such as schizophrenia. Nonhuman primates share with humans the capacity for working memory, the ability to hold items of information transiently in mind to meld together separate events and ideas into coherent lines of thought and communications. Metaphors for working memory include "blackboard of the mind," "mental sketch-pad" (Baddeley, 1986), and "on-line memory" (Goldman-Rakic, 1987). When we listen to human speech, we are using working memory to hold the segments of sentences "on-line" millisecond by millisecond. We employ working memory to carry forward, in real time, the subject of a sentence and associate it with verbs and objects to comprehend the sense and meaning of sentences. When we perform a mental arithmetic problem, recall a phone number, plan a hand of bridge or chess move, or follow a verbal instruction, we use working memory. In fact, it is difficult to think of a cognitive function that does not engage the working memory systems of the brain. It is not surprising, therefore, that the dorsolateral prefrontal cortex has become a major focus of intense investigation of schizophrenia with noninvasive neuroimaging analyses and with morphologic and biochemical analyses of postmortem brains (for reviews, see Goldman-Rakic & Selemon, 1997; McCarley et al., 1999). Using stereologic methods, findings in this laboratory have shown that neuronal density is elevated in areas 9 and 46 in schizophrenic patients (Selemon et al., 1995, 1998), without loss of neurons, and these findings have led to the hypothesis that a reduction in cortical neuropil may be the neuropathologic substrate for cognitive dysfunction of the prefrontal cortex in schizophrenia (Selemon & Goldman-Rakic, 1999). Numerous postmortem studies of pre- and postsynaptic elements support the hypothesis that neuronal connectivity is compromised in the dorsal areas of prefrontal cortex in schizophrenic brains (e.g., Garey et al., 1998; Glantz & Lewis, 2000). The neuropathological findings in the dorsolateral prefrontal cortex provides a biological basis for visuospatial working memory impairments, including eye-tracking deficits, that are reliably observed in schizophrenic patients (Park & Holzman, 1992) and can account as well for numerous reports of aberrant activation of this region in position emission tomographic (PET) and fMRI studies of cognitive processing (e.g, Weinberger et al., 1988; Manoach et al., 2000). Early psychiatrists designated this condition as *schizophrenia* (translated from the Greek *schizein* and *phren* as split-mind). Because the working memory functions of the prefrontal cortex are essential for keeping the thought process on track, deficiency of prefrontal circuitry can be expected to lead to the derailed and fragmented mental state of the schizophrenic patient (Goldman-Rakic, 1987, 1991).

WORKING MEMORY NETWORKS

The data described above identify the dorsolateral prefrontal cortex as a critical element in a neural system that utilizes working memory to hold specific items of spatial information on-line. Nevertheless, it is clear that the neural system supporting working memory capacity cannot reside wholly within prefrontal cortex, but extends beyond it to involve and, in fact, require interactions with other distant cortical areas. Among these are the posterior parietal cortex, the inferotemporal cortex, the cingulate gyrus, and hippocampal formation, all of which have connections with dorsolateral prefrontal cortex (Petrides & Pandya, 1984; Schwartz & Goldman-Rakic, 1984; Barbas, 1988; Selemon & Goldman-Rakic, 1988; Cavada & Goldman-Rakic, 1989; Stanton et al., 1995). These long-tract connections form interactive networks; how information is integrated within networks is the subject of much discussion and theorizing in the imaging literature, the computational literature, and the neuropsychological fields. Analysis of how networks are formed and how they work is fundamental to diagnosis and treatment in neurology and psychiatry and to an understanding of higher brain function in academic science.

REFERENCES

Baddeley, A. (1986). *Working Memory*. New York: Oxford University Press.

Baker, S.C., Frith, C.D., Frackowiak, R.S.J., & Dolan, R.J. (1996). Active representation of shape and spatial location in man. *Cerebral Cortex, 6,* 612–619.

Barbas, H. (1988). Anatomic organization of basoventral and mediodorsal visual recipient prefrontal regions in the rhesus monkey. *Journal of Comparative Neurology, 276,* 313–342.

Carlson, S., Martinkauppi, S., Rama, P., Salli, E., Korvenoja, A., & Aronen, H.J. (1998). Distribution of cortical activation during visuospatial n-back tasks as revealed by functional magnetic resonance imaging. *Cerebral Cortex, 8,* 743–752.

Cavada, C. & Goldman-Rakic, P.S. (1989) Posterior parietal cortex in rhesus monkey: II. Evidence for segregated corticocortical networks linking sensory and limbic areas with the frontal lobe. *Journal of Comparative Neurology, 287,* 422–445.

Cohen, J.D., Perlstein, W.M., Braver, T.S., Nystrom, L.E., Noll, D.C., Jonides, J., & Smith, E.E. (1997). Temporal dynamics of brain activation during a working memory task. *Nature, 386,* 604–608.

Constantinidis, C., Franowicz, M.N., & Goldman-Rakic, P.S. (2001). Coding specificity in cortical microcircuits: a multiple-electrode analysis of primate prefrontal cortex. *Journal of Neuroscience, 21,* 3646–3655.

Courtney, S.M., Ungerleider, L.G., Keil, K., & Haxby, J.V. (1996). Object and spatial visual working memory activate separate neural systems in human cortex. *Cerebral Cortex, 6,* 39–49.

Courtney, S.M., Ungerleider, L.G., Keil, K., & Haxby, J.V. (1997). Transient and sustained activity in a distributed neural system for human working memory. *Nature, 386,* 608–611.

Courtney, S.M., Petit, L., Maisog, J.M., Ungerleider, L.G., & Haxby, J.V. (1998). An area specialized for spatial working memory in human frontal cortex. *Science, 279,* 1347–1351.

D'Esposito, M., Postle, B.R., Ballard, D., & Lease, J. (1999). Maintenance versus manipulation of information held in working memory: an event-related fMRI study. *Brain and Cognition, 41,* 66–86.

Fries, W. (1984). Cortical projections to the superior colliculus in the macaque monkey: a retrograde study using horseradish peroxidase. *Journal of Comparative Neurology, 230,* 55–76.

Funahashi, S., Bruce, C.J., & Goldman-Rakic, P.S. (1989). Mnemonic coding of visual space in the monkey's dorsolateral prefrontal cortex. *Journal of Neurophysiology, 61,* 1–19.

Fuster, J.M. & Alexander, G.E. (1971). Neuron activity related to short-term memory. *Science, 173,* 652–654.

Garey, L.J., Ong, W.Y., Patel, T.S., Kannai, M., Davis, A., Mortimer, A.M., Barnes, T.R.E., & Hirsh, S.R. (1998). Reduced dendritic spine density on cerebral cortical pyramidal neurons in schizophrenia. *Journal of Neurology, Neurosurgery and Psychiatry, 65,* 446–453.

Glantz, L.A. & Lewis, D.A. (2000). Decreased dendritic spine density on prefrontal cortical pyramidal neurons in schizophrenia. *Archives of General Psychiatry, 57,* 65–73.

Goldman, P.S., Rosvold, H.E., Vest, B., & Galkin, T.W. (1971). Analysis of the delayed-alternation deficit produced by dorsolateral prefrontal lesions in the rhesus monkey. *Journal of Comparative Physiology and Psychology, 77,* 212–220.

Goldman-Rakic, P.S. (1987). Circuitry of primate prefrontal cortex and regulation of behavior by representational memory. In:F. Plum (Ed.), *Handbook of Physiology, The Nervous System, Higher Functions of the Brain,* Section I, Vol. V., Part 1, Chapter 9 (pp. 373–417). Bethesda, MD: American Physiological Society.

Goldman-Rakic, P.S. (1991). Prefrontal cortical dysfunction in schizophrenia: the relevance of working memory. In: Carroll, B.J. & Barrett, J.E. (Eds.), *Psychopathology and the Brain* (pp. 1–23). New York: Raven Press.

Goldman-Rakic, P.S. (1996). The prefrontal landscape: implications of functional architecture for understanding human mentation and the central executive. *Philosophical Transactions of the Royal Society of London B: Biological Sciences, 351,* 1445–1453.

Goldman-Rakic, P.S. & Schwartz, M.L. (1982). Interdigitation of contralateral and ipsilateral columnar projections to frontal association cortex in primates. *Science, 216,* 755–757.

Goldman-Rakic, P.S. & Selemon, L.D. (1997). Functional and anatomical aspects of prefrontal pathology in schizophrenia. *Schizophrenia Bulletin, 23,* 437–458.

Just, M.A. & Carpenter, P.A. (1992). A capacity theory of comprehension: individual differences in working memory. *Psychological Review, 99,* 122–149.

Kubota, K. & Niki, H. (1971). Prefrontal cortical unit activity and delayed alternation performance in monkeys. *Journal of Neurophysiology, 34,* 337–347.

Leung, H.C., Gore, J.C. & Goldman-Rakic, P.S., (2002). Sustained mnemonic response in the human middle frontal gyrus during online storage of spatial memoranda. *Journal of Cognitive Neuroscience* (in press).

Manoach, D.S., Gollub, R.L., Benson, E.S., Searl, M.M., Goff, D.C., Halpern, E., Saper, C.B., & Rauch, S.L. (2000). Schizophrenic subjects show abberant fMRI activation of dorsolateral prefrontal cortex and basal ganglia during working memory performance. *Biological Psychiatry, 48,* 99–109.

McCarley, R.W., Wible, C.G., Frumin, M., Hirayasu, Y., Levitt, J.J., Fischer, I.A., & Shenton, M.E. (1999). MRI anatomy of schizophrenia. *Biological Psychiatry, 45,* 1099–1119.

McCarthy, G., Blamire, A.M., Puce, A., Nobre, A.C., Bloch, G., Hyder, F., Goldman-Rakic, P., & Shulman, R.G. (1994). Functional magnetic resonance imaging of human prefrontal cortex activation during a spatial working memory task. *Proceeding of the National Academy of Sciences USA, 91,* 8690–8694.

McCarthy, G., Puce, A., Constable, R.T., Krystal, J.H., Gore, J.C., & Goldman-Rakic, P.S. (1996). Activation of human prefrontal cortex during spatial and object working memory tasks measured by functional MRI. *Cerebral Cortex, 6,* 600–611.

Mishkin, M. & Pribram, K.H. (1955). Analysis of the effects of frontal lesions in object alternation. *Journal of Comparative Physiology and Psychology, 48,* 492–495.

Miyake, A. & Shah, P. (1999). In: A. Miyake & P. Shah (Eds.), *Models of Working Memory: Mechanisms of Active Maintenance and Executive Control* (pp. 1–27). Cambridge, UK: Cambridge University Press.

Niki, H. (1974). Prefrontal unit activity during delayed alternation in the monkey. I. Relation to direction of response. *Brain Research, 68,* 185–196.

O'Scalaidhe, S.P., Wilson, F.A.W., & Goldman-Rakic, P.S. (1997). A real segregation of face-processing neurons in prefrontal cortex. *Science, 278,* 1135–1138.

O'Scalaidhe, S.P., Wilson, F.A.W., & Goldman-Rakic, P.S. (1999). Face-selective neurons during passive viewing and working memory performance of rhesus monkeys: evidence for intrinsic specialization of neuronal coding. *Cerebral Cortex, 9,* 459–475.

Owen, A.M. (1997). The functional organization of working memory processes within human lateral frontal cortex: the contribution of functional neuroimaging. *European Journal of Neuroscience, 9,* 1329–1339.

Owen, A.M., Evans, A.C., & Petrides, M. (1996). Evidence for a two-stage model of spatial working memory processing with the lateral frontal cortex: a positron emission tomography study. *Cerebral Cortex, 6,* 31–38.

Park, S. & Holzman, P.S. (1992). Schizophrenics show spatial working memory deficits. *Archives of General Psychiatry, 49,* 975–982.

Petrides, M. (1994). Frontal lobes and behaviour. *Current Opinion in Neurobiology, 4,* 207–211.

Petrides, M. & Pandya, D.N. (1984). Projections to the frontal cortex from the posterior parietal region in the rhesus monkey. *Journal of Comparative Neurology, 228,* 105–116.

Petrides, M., Alivisatos, B., Evans, A.C., & Meyer, E. (1993a). Dissociation of human mid-dorsolateral from posterior dorsolateral frontal cortex in memory processing. *Proceedings of the National Academy of Sciences U.S.A, 90,* 873–877.

Petrides, M., Alivisatos, B., Meyer, E., & Evans, A.C. (1993b). Functional activation of the human frontal cortex during the performance of verbal working memory tasks. *Proceedings of the National Academy of Sciences U.S.A, 90,* 878–882.

Rajkowska, G. & Goldman-Rakic, P.S. (1995a). Cytoarchitectonic definition of prefrontal areas in the normal human cortex: I. Remapping of areas 9 and 46 using quantitative criteria. *Cerebral Cortex, 5,* 307–322.

Rajkowska, G. & Goldman-Rakic, P.S. (1995b). Cytoarchitectonic definition of prefrontal areas in the normal human cortex: II. Variability in locations of areas 9 and 46 and relationship to the Talairach coordinate system. *Cerebral Cortex, 5,* 323–337.

Romanski, L.M. & Goldman-Rakic, P.S. (1999). Physiological identification of an auditory domain in the prefrontal cortex of the awake behaving monkey. *Society for Neuroscience Abstracts, 25,* 620.1.

Rowe, J.B., Toni, I., Josephs, O., Frackowiak, R.S., & Passingham, R.E. (2000). The prefrontal cortex: response selection of maintenance within working memory? *Science, 288,* 1656–1660.

Rushworth, M.F., Nixon, P.D., Eacott, M.J., & Passingham, R.E. (1997). Ventral prefrontal cortex is not essential for working memory. *Journal of Neuroscience, 17,* 4829–4838.

Sawaguchi, T. & Goldman-Rakic, P.S. (1991). D1 dopamine receptors in prefrontal cortex: involvement in working memory. *Science, 251,* 947–950.

Schwartz, M.L. & Goldman-Rakic, P.S. (1984). Callosal and intrahemispheric connectivity of the prefrontal association cortex in rhesus monkey: relation between intraparietal and principal sulcal cortex. *Journal of Comparative Neurology, 226,* 403–420.

Selemon, L.D. & Goldman-Rakic, P.S. (1985). Longitudinal topography and interdigitation of corticostriatal projections in the rhesus monkey. *Journal of Neuroscience, 5,* 776–794.

Selemon, L.D. & Goldman-Rakic, P.S. (1988). Common cortical and subcortical target areas of the dorsolateral prefrontal and posterior parietal cortices in the rhesus monkey: evidence for a distributed neural network subserving spatially guided behavior. *Journal of Neuroscience, 8,* 4049–4068.

Selemon, L.D. & Goldman-Rakic, P.S. (1999). The reduced neuropil hypothesis: a circuit based model of schizophrenia. *Biological Psychiatry, 45,* 17–25.

Selemon, L.D., Rajkowska, G., & Goldman-Rakic, P.S. (1995). Abnormally high neuronal density in the schizophrenic cortex: a morphometric analysis of prefrontal area 9 and occipital area 17. *Archives of General Psychiatry, 52,* 805–818.

Selemon, L.D., Rajkowska, G., & Goldman-Rakic, P.S. (1998). Elevated neuronal density in prefrontal area 46 in brains from schizophrenic patients: application of a 3-dimensional, stereologic counting method. *Journal of Comparative Neurology, 392,* 402–412.

Shallice, T. (1982). Specific impairments in planning. *Philosophical Transactions of the Royal Society of London B: Biological Sciences, 298,* 199–209.

Shallice, T. (1988). *From Neuropsychology to Mental Structure.* Cambridge, UK: Cambridge University Press.

Smith, E.E. & Jonides, J. (1997). Working memory: a view from neuroimaging. *Cognitive Psychology, 33,* 5–42.

Smith, E.E. & Jonides, J. (1999). Storage and executive processes in the frontal lobes. *Science, 283,* 1657–1661.

Smith, E.E., Jonides, J., & Koeppe, R.A. (1996). Dissociating verbal and spatial working memory using PET. *Cerebral Cortex, 6,* 11–20.

Stanton, G.B., Bruce, C.J., & Goldberg, M.E. (1995). Topography of projections to posterior cortical areas from the macaque frontal eye fields. *Journal of Comparative Neurology, 353,* 291–305.

Sweeney, J.A., Mintun M.A., Kwee, M.B., Wiseman, D.L., Brown, D.R., Rosenberg, D.R., & Carl, J.R. (1996). Positron emission tomography study of voluntary saccadic eye movements and spatial working memory. *Journal of Neurophysiology, 75,* 454–468.

Walker, A.E. (1940). A cytoarchitectural study of the prefrontal area of the macaque monkey. *Journal of Comparative Neurology, 73,* 59–86.

Weinberger, D.R., Berman, K.F., & Illowsky, B.P. (1988). Physiological dysfunction of dorsolateral prefrontal cortex in schizophrenia. III. A new cohort and evidence for a monoaminergic mechanism. *Archives of General Psychiatry, 49,* 609–615.

6

Physiology of Executive Functions: The Perception–Action Cycle

JOAQUÍN M. FUSTER

In this chapter, the executive functions of the prefrontal cortex are discussed against the background of its position in the neocortical map of cognitive representations. Lateral prefrontal areas constitute the highest stage in the cortical hierarchy of executive memories. Their neuronal networks represent schemas of sequential action, past or planned. The enactment of a goal-directed sequence of actions is a continuous process of temporal integration. At the root of this process is the mediation of cross-temporal contigencies between the action plan, the goal, and the acts leading to the goal. The lateral prefrontal cortex controls at least four cognitive operations that mediate those contingencies: selective attention, working memory, preparatory set, and monitoring. Microelectrode data obtained by the author and collaborators provide evidence for the following: (a) temporal integration takes place in prefrontal cortex through local transactions between cells active in working memory and cells active in preparatory set; (b) working memory essentially consists of the temporary activation, for prospective action, of a wide cortical network of long-term memory; and (c) working memory is maintained by reverberating activity within that network.

The study of the functions of the prefrontal cortex requires a clear distinction between cortical *representation* and cortical *operation*. In much of the prefrontal literature, the two are confounded, and the first commonly ignored. The emphasis of most studies is on the operations of the prefrontal cortex—that is, on what the prefrontal cortex *does*, commonly disregarding this cortex as part of the permanent cortical store of memory and knowledge. As a consequence, certain functions of the prefrontal cortex, such as its role in attention, monitoring, working memory, and planning, which intimately depend on that permanent substrate, are construed and tested as if they could be isolated from it. This separation of operation from representation is not only implausible but leads to artificious and often phrenological views of prefrontal functions.

In this chapter, I attempt to place prefrontal functions within the broad framework of the cortical substrate of long-term memory, which is formed by a complex array of widely distributed, overlapping, and intersecting neuronal networks in neocortex of association. The prefrontal networks, which in the aggregate constitute what we call *executive memory*, are part of that vast array of associative neocortical networks. It is only within that broader context that the executive functions of the prefrontal cortex can be understood. For this reason, I shall preface the discussion of those functions with a conceptual model of the distribution of long-term memory in the neocortex. The chapter concludes with a brief discussion of microelectrode data from the lateral prefrontal cortex that not only reaffirm the anchoring of its functions in long-term memory but also provide insight into the mechanisms of temporal integration, which is cardinal among those functions.

EXECUTIVE MEMORY IN THE CORTICAL COGNITIVE MAP

The neocortex of the primate is, anatomically and physiologically, divided by the central or rolandic fissure into two major regions, posterior and frontal. Generally, the cortex behind the fissure, namely the cortex of the occipital, parietal, and temporal lobes, is dedicated to the representations and functions related to perception. Broadly speaking, it is cortex devoted to the processing of information acquired through the senses. By contrast, the frontal cortex in its entirety is broadly devoted to the processing of actions. Whereas the orbital and medial regions of the frontal lobe are critically involved in emotional actions, the lateral frontal cortex—that is, the cortex of the convexity of the frontal lobe—is essential for the temporal organization of actions in the domains of behavior, speech, and reasoning.

Following that line of thinking, and from a large body of neuropsychological, anatomical, and physiological evidence (reviewed in Fuster, 1995), it can be concluded that the permanent or long-term memory of the individual is distributed in wide networks of the neocortex of association. Accordingly, the two large categories of long-term memory, perceptual and executive, are distributed in posterior and frontal cortex, respectively. This distribution has been best substantiated in the human (Fig. 6–1). Also on the basis of a large body of evidence, it seems reasonable to infer that in both sectors of the cortex long-term memory is formed under influences from structures of the medial temporal lobe, notably the hippocampus and the amygdala (Amaral, 1987; Squire & Zola-Morgan, 1988). The two

broad categories of cortical memory, perceptual and executive, are hierarchically organized. The connections between successive areas in either cortical hierarchy are bidirectional, and have been anatomically well substantiated, especially in the nonhuman primate (Pandya & Yeterian, 1985; Mesulam, 1998).

Perceptual memory is memory acquired through the sensory organs. At its most basic level, it includes the memory of elementary sense perceptions, in sensory and parasensory cortices. At higher and more general levels, perceptual memory comprises multimodal sensory memories, in "trans-modal" cortex (Mesulam, 1998). Above those levels, in higher cortex of association, perceptual memory includes episodic and semantic memories, which in the aggregate constitute the so-called declarative memory. The highest cognitive level, also in posterior association cortex, is *conceptual memory*, the most general and abstract form of perceptual knowledge.

Although the different categories of perceptual memory are in general terms hierarchically organized, individual items of memory are essentially heterarchical. An autobiographic memory, for example, contains semantic as well as well as episodic and sensory elements. This implies that the network representing that memory spans several levels of the mnemonic hierarchy in posterior cortex. Consequently, a local cortical lesion of that cortex may produce selective amnesia for certain aspects of the memory but not for others.

The counterpart of the hierarchy of perceptual memory in posterior cortex is a hierarchy of executive memory in frontal cortex. Its lowest level is the primary motor cortex (phyletic motor memory), which represents the most elementary aspects of movement, as defined by the contraction of particular muscles and muscle groups. Above that layer of elementary representations, the premotor cortex stores the memory of motor programs defined by goal and trajectory. Elementary structures of language are also represented in certain areas of premotor cortex (e.g., Broca's area).

The lateral prefrontal cortex constitutes the highest level of the frontal cortical hierarchy

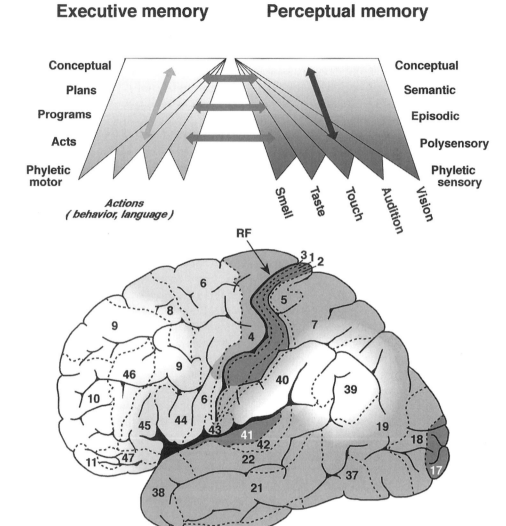

Figure 6–1. Cognitive representation in the neocortex of the human. *Top:* Schema of memory hierarchies. *Bottom:* General distribution of memory networks. RF, rolandic fissure.

for the representation of executive memory. Judging by the neuropsychological evidence from the human, neuronal networks of the lateral prefrontal cortex harbor representations of plans and schemas of behavior and language (Fuster, 1997). This cortical region appears most clearly implicated in the representation of novel and complex schemas of action. It also appears important for the representation of old schemas that contain uncertainties or ambiguities to be resolved by temporal integration of environmental signals. This is the

case, for example, in delay tasks (e.g., delayed response, delayed matching). The highest levels of prefrontal representation include the rules and contingencies for the execution of those plans and schemas of behavior and language, in addition to the most general and abstract concepts of action.

In sum, my model stipulates that the cortex of the lateral convexity of the frontal lobe provides the structural substrate for long-term executive memory. Both the structure and contents of long-term memory consist of hierarchically organized neuronal networks. The representations of action increase in generality and abstraction from the bottom up, from the elementary motor networks of primary motor cortex to the most general and abstract representations of action in lateral prefrontal cortex. There seems to be a hierarchical order in frontal cortex for each separate domain of action (e.g., locomotion, eye movement, speech), though there also appears to be considerable interaction between domains in the representation of complex schemas and plans of action. In any event, as in the case of the perceptual memory networks of posterior cortex, individual executive networks are probably mixed and heterarchical, made of representations at various levels of the frontal hierarchy.

TEMPORAL INTEGRATION AND ITS ANCILLARY FUNCTIONS

The most general function of the lateral prefrontal cortex is the temporal organization of behavior, speech, and reasoning. This inference is based mainly on neuropsychological data from the human (Luria, 1966, 1970; Fuster, 1997). Humans with extensive lesions of this cortex have well-documented difficulties in executing plans of behavior, sequences of propositional language, and complex mental operations. These deficits are attributable to impairments in the representation and execution of goal-directed sequences of actions.

A critical element of the role of the lateral prefrontal cortex in both the representation and the execution of goal-directed actions is the capacity to integrate information in the time domain. Temporal integration is essential to temporal organization. Temporal order derives directly from the mediation of cross-temporal contingencies—that is, from the integration of temporally separate units of perception, action and cognition into a sequence toward a goal (Fig. 6–2). Because temporal integration is necessary for all goal-directed tasks (e.g., delay tasks), the functional integrity of the lateral prefrontal cortex is necessary for their performance. In accord with this view, a large variety of tasks activate a vast region of this cortex in common (Duncan & Owen, 2000).

Temporal integration is the result of the functional cooperation of the prefrontal cortex with subcortical structures and with other areas of the neocortex, notably the association cortex of the parietal, occipital, and temporal lobes. That cooperation serves at least four cognitive functions that are essential for temporal integration: attention, working memory, set, and monitoring. All four are under some degree of prefrontal control, at least inasmuch as they serve the temporal organization of behavior. There does not appear to be conclusive evidence for the areal segregation of these functions; the four are closely intertwined and

Figure 6–2. Sequencing of actions toward a goal. *Top:* Overlearned or routine sequence of acts ($a_1 \ldots a_n$), each leading to the next, in chain-like fashion, with contingencies (two-way arrows) only between successive acts. *Bottom:* A new and complex sequence, where acts are contingent across time on the plan, on the goal, and on other acts; the lateral prefrontal cortex mediates cross-temporal contingencies and organizes the sequence.

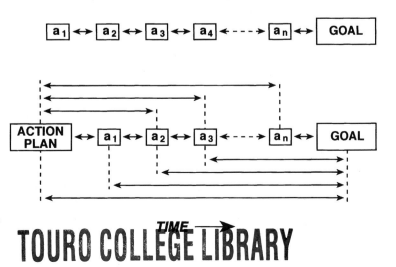

operate in all lateral prefrontal areas. However, both in the monkey and in the human, there is evidence, reviewed elsewhere (Fuster, 1997), for the areal segregation of the representational contents of those cognitive functions, in other words, of the material in long-term memory with which they operate. Furthermore, there appear to be separate groups of hierarchically organized frontal areas for different sectors of executive representation (e.g., locomotion, eye motility, linguistic expression).

ATTENTION

The structuring of behavior requires the selective and orderly activation of cortical networks that are highly specific in terms of the information they represent, their inputs, and their outputs. That selective and orderly activation is critical for the performance of any novel and complex form of goal-directed behavior. It must take place in a cortex-wide system of intersecting and overlapping networks that profusely share neurons and pathways. The available evidence indicates that the prefrontal cortex plays a crucial role in ensuring both selectivity and order in the recruitment of cortical networks for temporal integration, and thus for temporal organization. That role is the essence of what has been called "the supervisory attentional control" of the prefrontal cortex (Shallice, 1988).

Neurophysiology and neuroimaging provide ample evidence of the participation of prefrontal areas in the cortical control of attention. Humans with prefrontal injury have difficulties in holding and shifting attention on sensory material. A neuroelectric manifestation of these difficulties is the loss of attention-related modulation of sensory evoked potentials in posterior cortex (Knight, 1984; Barcelo et al., 2000; Daffner et al., 2000). Functional imaging (Pardo et al., 1990; Posner & Petersen, 1990; Corbetta et al., 1993; Kastner et al., 1999) reveals that cognitive tasks with important attentional requirements activate three major parts of the prefrontal cortex: the anterior cingulate region, the orbital region, and the lateral region.

From neuropsychological evidence it is reasonable to infer that each of those activations reflects a different aspect of attention. The cingulate activation probably reflects drive and motivation; for that, the anterior cingulate cortex receives profuse afferents from limbic brain structures. The orbital activation may reflect mainly the exclusionary aspects of attention—that is, the inhibitory control and filtering out of material unrelated to the task at hand (see Chapter 13). The lateral activation has to do, most likely, with the selective and orienting aspects of attention—that is, the focus of attention. Especially relevant in this respect is the activation of lateral areas, notably area 8, that play a role in gaze and receptor orientation control. Some of that lateral activation may also have to do, however, with motor attention or set (below).

WORKING MEMORY

Of all the temporal integrative functions of the prefrontal cortex, working memory is the best substantiated physiologically. It was the first to be supported by neuronal data (Fuster & Alexander, 1971; Fuster, 1973). So-called memory cells were first discovered in the prefrontal cortex of monkeys performing delayed-response tasks. They were characterized by sustained elevated discharge during the delay period (memory period) of delayed-response trials; that discharge was higher than intertrial baseline (the phenomenon cannot be evinced in delayed alternation for lack of such a baseline).

The memory-related delay discharge of memory cells, now demonstrated in many laboratories on various types of delay tasks, has some important properties: (*a*) it only occurs when the signal preceding the delay calls for a motor act; (*b*) it does not occur in the mere expectation of reward; (*c*) it is correlated with the animal's performance (efficacy of short-term memory); and (*d*) it can be disrupted by the distraction of the animal.

Functional neuroimaging has now amply substantiated the activation of prefrontal regions in working memory for visual information (Jonides et al., 1993; Cohen et al., 1994; Swartz et al., 1995) and for verbal information (Grasby et al., 1993; Petrides et al., 1993b, Smith, et al., 1996). Characteristically in the human, as in the nonhuman primate, the lateral prefrontal areas are especially activated during working memory. Imaging studies challenge the segregation of these areas in terms of the kind of information that the subject must retain in working memory (Owen et al., 1998; Postle & D'Esposito, 1999; Prabhakaran et al., 2000; see Chapter 11). Furthermore, imaging studies substantiate the activation of lateral prefrontal areas in other than delay tasks. Temporal integration, that is, the mediation of cross-temporal contingencies, seems to be the common element of all the paradigms that have been used to demonstrate lateral prefrontal activation. In many of the relevant studies, the subject's requirement to temporally integrate the tester's instructions with subsequent behavior or cognitive operations is curiously ignored. A recent meta-analysis by Duncan and Owen (2000) illustrates the commonality of temporal integration to the paradigms with which lateral prefrontal activation has been demonstrated in the human.

PREPARATORY SET

Whereas working memory serves temporal integration retrospectively, by retention of recent sensory information, preparatory set serves it prospectively; it prepares the organism for anticipated signals to act and for action itself. Preparatory set is clearly another function of the lateral prefrontal cortex. The original evidence came from human neuropsychology. That evidence was the deficit that frontal patients had in preparing for and initiating serial actions; it was a deficit obviously related, if not identical, to the well-documented planning deficit of those patients (Ackerly & Benton, 1947; Lhermitte, et al., 1972; Eslinger & Damasio, 1985). That deficit reflects the underlying difficulty in mediating contingencies between present events and their anticipated consequences, between the image of a goal and the acts that will lead to it. It is a failure of prospective memory or "memory of the future" (Ingvar, 1985). Electrophysiology (Singh & Knight, 1990) and imaging (Partiot et al., 1995; Baker et al., 1996) substantiate the activation of lateral prefrontal cortex of humans in prospective preparation and planning.

In the prefrontal cortex of monkeys performing a delay task with double cross-temporal contingencies, Quintana and Fuster (1999) obtained cellular evidence of both working memory and preparatory set. On every trial, the animal had to first attend to a color in a central disk at eye level. A period of 12-second delay ensued, at the end of which a second visual signal appeared. Depending on the combination of the color and the second signal, the animal had to move its hand to a right or a left location. Both the first and the second signal changed at random from trial to trial. Thus, every choice of location at the end of the trial was based on the double contingency between the two signals separated by the delay. In the fully trained animal, the first signal (color) predicted the second—and the location of choice—with some degree of probability; some colors predicted location with 100% certainty and others with 75%.

Cells were found in lateral prefrontal cortex that responded specifically to the color (first signal). Their discharge diminished in the course of the delay (Fig. 6–3). Such cells behaved like conventional working memory cells. Conversely, other cells' discharge augmented gradually in the delay period, and after that period they reacted differentially to the side of the response (right or left). Furthermore, the degree of acceleration of their delay activity was proportional to the certainty with which the monkey could anticipate the specific movement that the second signal would call for. Thus, these cells were attuned to the movement (motor-coupled), and appeared to anticipate it and participate in its preparation. It was not possible to separate topographically the two types of cells. Both working memory cells and set cells were found intermingled in the lateral prefrontal cortex (upper prefrontal convexity and upper bank of the sulcus principalis) and seemed to participate in the temporal integration of visual information with consequent action.

RESPONSE MONITORING

For methodological reasons, the prefrontal functions that serve temporal integration are discussed here separately, even though there is no clear separate anatomy for any of them.

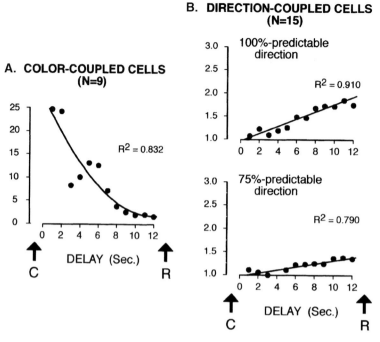

Figure 6–3. Discharge of prefrontal units during the delay period of a double-contingency task (see text for details). *A:* Working memory cells for color (color-coupled). *B:* Preparatory set cells (direction-coupled). Note the opposite temporal firing trends of the two cell types; in set cells, note the relation between accelerating trend and predictability of response direction.

It would be reasonable, however, to put all the prefrontal functions discussed thus far under the heading of the first—attention. *Attention,* which is physiologically a process of selective allocation of neural resources, is inseparable from working memory and from set. Thus, the prefrontal cortex can be assumed to control three forms of content-defined selective attention—that means, physiologically, there are three forms of selective recruitment and activation of cortical cognitive networks. First, the prefrontal cortex facilitates the activation of networks involved in the reception of sensory signals and in the execution of motor actions that are part of a behavioral sequence. Second, the prefrontal cortex, by its role in working memory, ensures the sustained attention to the representation of recent signals. Third, by preparatory set or motor attention, the prefrontal cortex activates the representation of forthcoming actions that depend on those signals. Working in tandem, those two forms of internal and temporally symmetric attention, one retrospective (working memory) and the other prospective (set), ensure the mediation of cross-temporal contingencies between signals and actions that is key to the

temporal integration and organization of behavior.

A fourth aspect of attention, the monitoring of responses, should also be considered a prefrontal function that serves temporal integration. All goal-directed behavior is performed within the broad context of the perception–action cycle (Fuster, 1997), which is grounded on a basic biological principle: the circular cybernetic flow of cognitive information that links the organism to its environment (Fig. 6–4). Sensory inputs are processed in sensory structures. The result of that processing leads to actions, which induce changes in the environment. These, in turn, generate new sensory signals, which feed back into the cycle and help control new action. That feedback control has been termed *monitoring.*

The notion of a role of the prefrontal cortex in monitoring originated with the old concept of "corollary discharge" (Teuber, 1972). From neuropsychological observations in the human, it was inferred that the prefrontal cortex was essential for the integration of information resulting from the organism's own actions. That information derived,

Figure 6–4. Schematic diagram of cortical interactions in the perception–action cycle (unlabeled rectangles signify intermediate areas or subareas). All arrows signify general pathways identified anatomically in the monkey.

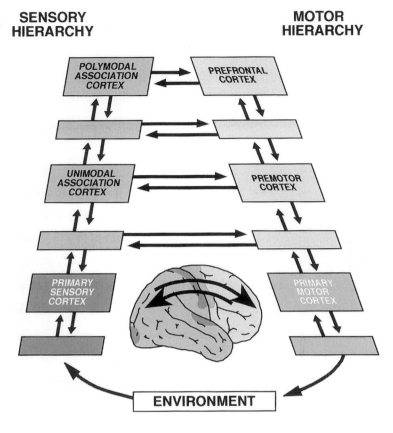

in part, from efferent copies of the actions, and in part from sensory inputs (including proprioceptive) resulting from them. Based on that information, the prefrontal cortex would generate corollary discharge, which would flow upon motor and sensory systems and prepare them for further actions and percepts. Lesion experiments in the monkey (Petrides, 1991) support the monitoring role of the prefrontal cortex and provide it with some topography in the lateral region. Neuroimaging in the intact human brain (Petrides et al., 1993a; Fletcher et al., 1998; McDonald et al., 2000) and electrophysiology in patients with lateral lesions (Gehring & Knight, 2000) further support the involvement of lateral prefrontal cortex in response monitoring. The same methodologies appear to support a parallel or subsidiary role of the anterior cingulate cortex in the monitoring of response errors (Carter et al., 1999; Gehring & Knight, 2000; McDonald et al., 2000; see Chapter 27).

MECHANISMS OF TEMPORAL INTEGRATION

The neural mechanisms of temporal integration are the mechanisms of the prefrontal cognitive functions that serve it. These mechanisms are only sketchily understood. Among the four functions outlined, working memory is the one that has been most intensely explored physiologically and, consequently, the best substantiated from the point of view of mechanisms.

From microelectrode studies in the monkey, the concept is emerging of working memory as the temporary activation, under prefrontal control, of a neocortical network for the execution of prospective actions. As these actions are contingent on recent, commonly sensory, events, the activation of that network has the function of retaining the memory of those events and thus integrating them with subsequent actions. If this assumption is correct, the activated network

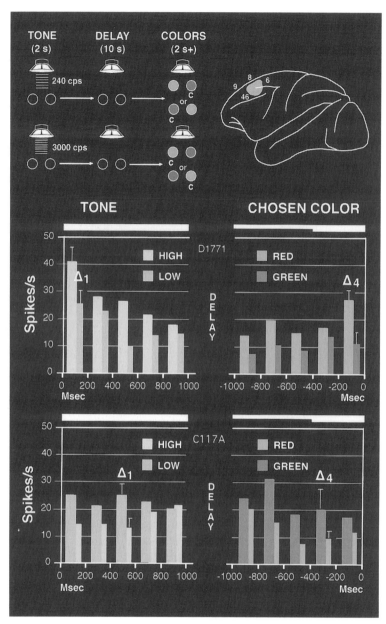

Figure 6–5. Frontal cells in a cross-modal delay task (*top left*): for 10 seconds the animal must remember a tone in order to choose a color. Low-pitched tone calls for green choice, high-pitched tone calls for red (*c* indicates correct choice). *Top right:* Diagram of monkey's brain indicating the area from which tone- and color-discriminating cells were recorded (numbers indicate cytoarchitectonic areas). *Bottom:* Frequency histograms of two cells discriminating tones and colors according to the task rule (upper cell prefers high tone and red; lower cell, low tone and green). (*Source:* Modified from Fuster et al., 2000)

also has the function of mediating that contingency across time. In this light it is reasonable to assume that prefrontal memory cells "remember for action."

What are the neuronal constituents of a working memory network? How does it stay active? It is now clear, from 30 years of physiological research, that the prefrontal cortex is not the only cortex involved in working memory, and, as we have seen, working memory is not the only function of the prefrontal cortex.

We know, from use of memory tasks, that visual working memory activates inferotemporal units (Fuster & Jervey, 1982; Miller, et al., 1993) as well as frontal units. Tactile working memory activates somatosensory units (Zhou & Fuster, 1996) as well as frontal units (Romo et al., 1999). It seems, therefore, that a working memory network spans both posterior and frontal regions and includes elements of perceptual memory as well as executive memory. Indeed, on the basis of microelectrode and imaging studies it appears increasingly plausible that a working memory network is an activated long-term memory network with perceptual as well as executive components. This does not exclude new percepts or new actions from working memory; these can be easily incorporated into active networks of long-term memory by similarity, categorization, and perceptual or executive constancy.

A recent study (Fuster, et al., 2000) supports the structural identity of working and long-term memory. Monkeys were trained to perform a cross-modal delayed matching task (Fig. 6–5). The animal had to listen to a brief tone in order to choose a color 12 seconds later. A high-pitched tone called for red choice, a low-pitched tone for green. In dorsolateral frontal cortex, cells reacted with different firing rates to the two tones and, then again, to the two colors. Those cellular reactions were correlated according to the task

rule: some cells reacted more to low tone and green than to high tone and red, while others did the reverse. Those correlations disappeared when the monkey failed to perform the task correctly. Furthermore, in correct performance the correlations persisted through the delay or working memory period (Fig. 6–6). Thus, in conclusion, neurons of lateral frontal cortex integrate information across time and across modalities—in our case, sound and vision. The discharge of the neurons in working memory is not only related to sound and to color but also to the *association* between the two, which is in the long-term memory of the trained animal. This observation can be best understood by assuming that those frontal neurons are constituents of a network of long-term memory temporarily activated, in working memory, for the temporal integration of information of two separate modalities.

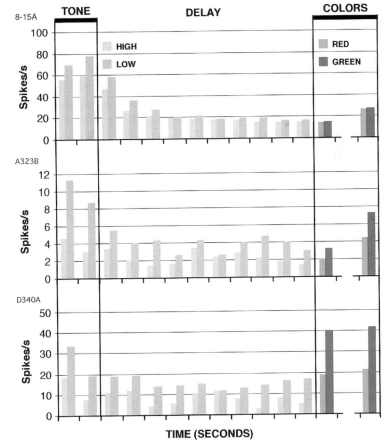

Figure 6–6. Three cells that prefer the low tone in the task of Figure 6–5. The average frequency histograms of the second and third cells show, in addition to sustained working memory activity for the low tone during the delay, marked preference for green, the matching color. (*Source:* Modified from Fuster et al., 2000)

The results of the study just described also imply that the frontal component cells of the working memory network—that is, an activated long-term memory network—receive associative, task-related sensory inputs from posterior association cortex. Furthermore, the firing of frontal memory cells is attuned to those inputs during the working memory period. There is experimental and computational evidence that working memory is sustained by recurrent excitation, through re-entrant circuits, between the constituent neuronal components of an active memory network (Fuster, 2001). In working memory as in other executive functions of the frontal lobe, the prefrontal cortex cooperates not only with subcortical structures (e.g., thalamus, basal ganglia) but also with posterior cortices (Hasegawa et al., 1998; Kastner et al., 1999; Tomita et al., 1999; Daffner et al., 2000). In monkeys performing a visual delayed matching task (Fuster, et al., 1985), the reversible inactivation of lateral prefrontal or inferotemporal cortex has two correlated effects: *(1)* a behavioral deficit in working memory for color, and *(2)* a decrease in the ability of cells in either cortex to discriminate colors in the working memory period. These observations indicate that the inactivation of either cortex, prefrontal or inferotemporal, interrupts loops of reverberating discharge between them that are engaged in working memory and critical for its maintenance.

The results of experiments such as the one just described indicate that the reverberation through recurrent neuronal circuits is a likely mechanism of working memory, and therefore of temporal integration. Computer modeling supports this concept further. Zipser et al. (1993), in a fully recurrent network trained to perform working memory, observed "cells" (hidden units) that behaved like real cortical cells in working memory tasks. Consequently, working memory appears to be a mechanism of temporal integration based on the recurrent activation of cell assemblies in cortical long-term memory networks.

CONCLUSIONS

Neuropsychological studies document the role of the prefrontal cortex in the representation and execution of plans and schemas of behavior. From results of these studies derives the notion of a critical involvement of the prefrontal cortex in the temporal organization of speech and behavior. The temporal organizing function of the prefrontal cortex rests on its ability to integrate information in the time domain—that is, its ability to mediate contingencies across time. With its role of temporally integrating new and complex behavior at the summit of neural hierarchies, the prefrontal cortex implements the perception–action cycle, which is the cortical exponent of a basic biological principle. Temporal integration is served by at least four prefrontal functions: attention, working memory, preparatory set, and monitoring. In all four, the lateral prefrontal cortex cooperates physiologically with subcortical structures and with posterior association cortex. Working memory appears essentially based on the activation of neuronal cortical networks of long-term memory, and maintained by reverberation of activity between prefrontal and posterior cortical components of those networks. Future progress in frontal lobe research should be aimed at gaining a better understanding of the basic mechanisms of prefrontal cognitive functions. Promising methodologies include the use of electrophysiological techniques, reversible lesions, and neuroimaging, singly or in combination. Neuroimaging, which appears in the vanguard of progress, is still encumbered by the serious and unresolved problem of adjusting its spatial and temporal scales to those of cognition in the cerebral cortex.

REFERENCES

Ackerly, S.S. & Benton, A.L. (1947). Report of case of bilateral frontal lobe defect. *Research Publications—Association for Research in Nervous and Mental Disease, 27,* 479–504.

Amaral, D.G. (1987). Memory: anatomical organization of candidate brain regions. In: F. Plum (Ed.), *Handbook of Physiology; Nervous System, Vol. V: Higher Functions of the Brain, Part 1* (pp. 211–294). Bethesda, MD: American Physiological Society.

Baker, S.C., Rogers, R.D., Owen, A.M., Frith, C.D., Dolan, R.J., Frackowiak, R.S.J., & Robbins, T.W. (1996). Neural systems engaged by planning: a PET study of the Tower of London task. *Neuropsychologia, 34,* 515–526.

Barcelo, P., Suwazono, S., & Knight, R.T. (2000). Prefrontal modulation of visual processing in humans. *Nature Neuroscience, 3,* 399–403.

Carter, C.S., Botvinick, M.M., & Cohen, J.D. (1999). The contribution of the anterior cingulate cortex to executive processes in cognition. *Reviews in the Neurosciences, 10,* 49–57.

Cohen, J.D., Forman, S.D., Braver, T.S., Casey, B.J., Servan-Schreiber, D., & Noll, D.C. (1994). Activation of the prefrontal cortex in a nonspatial working memory task with functional MRI. *Human Brain Map, 1,* 293–304.

Corbetta, M., Miezin, F.M., Shulman, G.L., & Petersen, S.E. (1993). A PET study of visuospatial attention. *Journal of Neuroscience, 13,* 1202–1226.

Daffner, K.R., Mesulam, M.-M., Scinto, L.F.M., Acar, D., Calvo, V., Faust, R., Chabrerie, A., Kennedy, B., & Holcomb, P. (2000). The central role of the prefrontal cortex in directing attention to novel events. *Brain 123,* 927–939.

Duncan, J. & Owen, A.M. (2000). Common regions of the human frontal lobe recruited by diverse cognitive demands. *Trends in Neurosciences, 23,* 475–483.

Eslinger, P.J. & Damasio, A.R. (1985). Severe disturbance of higher cognition after bilateral frontal lobe ablation: patient EVR. *Neurology, 35,* 1731–1741.

Fletcher, P.C., Shallice, T., Frith, C.D., Frackowiak, R.S.J., & Dolan, R.J. (1998). The functional roles of prefrontal cortex in episodic memory. II. Retrieval. *Brain, 121,* 1249–1256.

Fuster, J.M. (1973). Unit activity in prefrontal cortex during delayed-response performance: neuronal correlates of transient memory. *Journal of Neurophysiology, 36,* 61–78.

Fuster, J.M. (1995). *Memory in the Cerebral Cortex: An Empirical Approach to Neural Networks in the Human and Nonhuman Primate.* Cambridge, MA: MIT Press.

Fuster, J.M. (1997). *The Prefrontal Cortex: Anatomy, Physiology and Neuropsychology of the Frontal Lobe.* Philadelphia: Lippincott-Raven.

Fuster, J.M. (2001). The prefrontal cortex—an update: time is of the essence. *Neuron, 30,* 319–333.

Fuster, J.M. & Alexander, G.E. (1971). Neuron activity related to short-term memory. *Science, 173,* 652–654.

Fuster, J.M. & Jervey, J.P. (1982). Neuronal firing in the inferotemporal cortex of the monkey in a visual memory task. *Journal of Neuroscience, 2,* 361–375.

Fuster, J.M., Bauer, R.H., & Jervey, J.P. (1985). Functional interactions between inferotemporal and prefrontal cortex in a cognitive task. *Brain Research, 330,* 299–307.

Fuster, J.M., Bodner, M., & Kroger, J. (2000). Cross-modal and cross-temporal association in neurons of frontal cortex. *Nature, 405,* 347–351.

Gehring, W.J. & Knight, R.T. (2000). Prefrontal–cingulate interactions in action monitoring. *Nature Neuroscience, 3,* 516–520.

Grasby, P.M., Frith, C.D., Friston, K.J., Bench, C., Frackowiak, R.S.J., & Dolan, R.J. (1993). Functional mapping of brain areas implicated in auditory–verbal memory function. *Brain, 116,* 1–20.

Hasegawa, I., Fukushima, T., Ihara, T., & Miyashita, Y. (1998). Callosal window between prefrontal cortices: cognitive interaction to retrieve long-term memory. *Science, 281,* 814–818.

Ingvar, D.H. (1985). "Memory of the future": An essay on the temporal organization of conscious awareness. *Human Neurobiology, 4,* 127–136.

Jonides, J., Smith, E.E., Koeppe, R.A., Awh, E., Minoshima, S., & Mintun, M.A. (1993). Spatial working memory in humans as revealed by PET. *Nature, 363,* 623–625.

Kastner, S., Pinsk, M.A., De Weerd, P., Desimone, R., & Ungerleider, L.G. (1999). Increased activity in human visual cortex during directed attention in the abscence of visual stimulation. *Neuron, 22,* 751–761.

Knight, R.T. (1984). Decreased response to novel stimuli after prefrontal lesions in man. *Electroencephalography and Clinical Neurophysiology, 59,* 9–20.

Lhermitte, F., Deroulsne, J., & Signoret, J.L. (1972). Analyse neuropsychologique du syndrome frontal. *Revista de Neurologia, 127,* 415–440.

Luria, A.R. (1966). *Higher Cortical Functions in Man.* New York: Basic Books.

Luria, A.R. (1970). *Traumatic Aphasia.* The Hague: Mouton.

McDonald, A.W., Cohen, J.D., Stenger, V.A., & Carter, C.S. (2000). Dissociating the role of the dorsolateral prefrontal and anterior cingulate cortex in cognitive control. *Science, 288,* 1835–1838.

Mesulam, M.-M. (1998). From sensation to cognition. *Brain, 121,* 1013–1052.

Miller, E.K., Li, L., & Desimone, R. (1993). Activity of neurons in anterior inferior temporal cortex during a short-term memory task. *Journal of Neuroscience, 13,* 1460–1478.

Owen, A.M., Stern, C.E., Look, R.B., Tracey, I., Rosen, B.R., & Petrides, M. (1998). Functional organization of spatial and nonspatial working memory processing within the human lateral frontal cortex. *Proceedings of the National Academy of Sciences USA, 95,* 7721–7726.

Pandya, D.N., & Yeterian, E.H. (1985). Architecture and connections of cortical association areas. In: A. Peters & E.G. Jones (Eds.), *Cerebral Cortex,* Vol. 4 (pp. 3–61). New York: Plenum Press.

Pardo, J.V., Pardo, P.J., Janer, K.W., & Raichle, M.E. (1990). The anterior cingulate cortex mediates processing selection in the Stroop attentional conflict paradigm. *Proceedings of the National Academy of Sciences of the USA, 87,* 256–259.

Partiot, A., Grafman, J., Sadato, N., Wachs, J., and Hallett, M. (1995). Brain activation during the generation of non-emotional and emotional plans. *NeuroReport, 6,* 1269–1272.

Petrides, M. (1991). Monitoring of selections of visual stimuli and the primate frontal cortex. *Proceedings of the Royal Society of London, Series B, 246,* 293–306.

Petrides, M., Alivisatos, B., Evans, A.C., & Meyer, E. (1993a). Dissociation of human mid-dorsolateral from posterior dorsolateral frontal cortex in memory processing. *Proceedings of the National Academy of Sciences of the USA, 90,* 873–877.

Petrides, M., Alivisatos, B., Meyer, E., & Evans, A.C.

(1993b). Functional activation of the human frontal cortex during the performance of verbal working memory tasks. *Proceedings of the National Academy of Sciences of the USA, 90*, 878–882.

Posner, M.I. & Petersen, S.E. (1990). The attention system of the human brain. *Annual Review of Neuroscience, 13*, 25–42.

Postle, B.R. and D'Esposito, M. (1999). "What"-then-"where" in visual working memory: an event-related fMRI study. *Journal of Cognitive Neuroscience, 11*, 585–597.

Prabhakaran, V., Narayanan, K., Zhao, Z., & Gabrieli, J.D.E. (2000). Integration of diverse information in working memory within the frontal lobe. *Nature Neuroscience, 3*, 85–90.

Quintana, J. & Fuster, J.M. (1999). From perception to action: temporal integrative functions of prefrontal and parietal neurons. *Cerebral Cortex, 9*, 213–221.

Romo, R., Brody, C.D., Hernández, A., & Lemus, L. (1999). Neuronal correlates of parametric working memory in the prefrontal cortex. *Nature, 399*, 470–473.

Shallice, T. (1988). *From Neuropsychology to Mental Structure*. New York: Cambridge University Press.

Singh, J. & Knight, R.T. (1990). Frontal cortex contribution to voluntary movements in humans. *Brain Research, 531*, 45–54.

Smith, E.E., Jonides, J., & Koeppe, R.A. (1996). Dissociating verbal and spatial working memory using PET. *Cerebral Cortex, 6*, 11–20.

Squire, L.R. & Zola-Morgan, S. (1988). Memory: brain systems and behavior. *Trends in Neurosciences, 11*, 170–175.

Swartz, B.E., Halgren, E., Fuster, J.M., Simpkins, F., Gee, M., & Mandelkern, M. (1995). Cortical metabolic activation in humans during a visual memory task. *Cerebral Cortex, 3*, 205–214.

Teuber, H.-L. (1972). Unity and diversity of frontal lobe functions. *Acta Neurobiologiae Experimentalis, 32*, 625–656.

Tomita, H., Ohbayashi, M., Nakahara, K., Hasegawa, I., & Miyashita, Y. (1999). Top-down signal from prefrontal cortex in executive control of memory retrieval. *Nature, 401*, 699–703.

Zhou, Y. & Fuster, J.M. (1996). Mnemonic neuronal activity in somatosensory cortex. *Proceedings of the National Academy of Sciences USA, 93*, 10533–10537.

Zipser, D., Kehoe, B., Littlewort, G., & Fuster, J. (1993). A spiking network model of short-term active memory. *Journal of Neuroscience, 13*, 3406–3420.

7

The Theatre of the Mind: Physiological Studies of the Human Frontal Lobes

TERENCE W. PICTON, CLAUDE ALAIN, AND
ANTHONY R. McINTOSH

What's Hecuba to him, or he to her,
That he should weep for her?

Hamlet, II: 2

In the epigraph, Hamlet considers what he should do by comparing his own behavior to what he imagines someone else might do. The situation has many levels: we imagine the character of Hamlet as played by an actor; Hamlet considers how the lead player pretends to be Aeneas; and Aeneas remembers the events of the fall of Troy and Hecuba's grief at her husband's death. Hamlet goes on to evaluate his own "motive and cue for passion" in light of these other characters. The proposal of this chapter is that the frontal lobes, and in particular the prefrontal cortices, enact the "theatre of the mind." They provide the "representational processing" that allows the human subject to entertain alternative interpretations of reality, to understand past causes and predict future effects, and to fit individual data to abstract concepts. This requires making comparisons between two or more concurrently active representations using a variety of criteria, and operating at multiple levels. Representational processing works in the realm of both the subjunctive and the subjective, looking at what is possible and how

it affects the self. Its goal is to discover meaning and purpose. A sense of this creative process is captured by an old word—apprehension—used by Hamlet earlier in this scene of the play ("in apprehension how like a god"), and by Baddeley in Chapter 16.

The processing is cybernetic, involving multiple feedback loops. Although the frontal regions are essential to representational processing, the actual processing involves interactions between multiple areas of the brain. Figure 7–1 is one of many diagrams deriving from the Test-Operate-Test-Exit, or TOTE, of Miller and colleagues (1960). In terms of incoming information, the system generates a model to fit the information, and adapts the model based on the goodness of fit and the stringency of the fitting criteria. The diagram differs from the original TOTE, in that it also includes an output system. A model of activity is constructed and the output is adjusted to fit that model. The key to these processes—what we propose as the essential prefrontal function—is the generative activity (Picton & Stuss, 2000). This is necessary for constructing an interpretation of a perceived reality or adjusting a behavior towards an intended goal. The modeling process can go on at many different levels (Stuss et al., 2001). The generation of the model depends on the error signal,

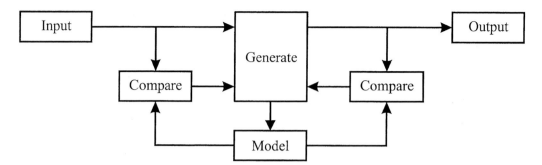

Figure 7–1. Model making in the nervous system. This diagram illustrates how the brain might evaluate incoming information and monitor outgoing behavior. A generator mechanism creates a model and adjusts this model until the fit with the incoming information reaches some cri-terion. Once the fit is accepted, the model becomes the perception of the input. On the output side, the central mechanism generates a model for the desired behavior and then initiates output until it fits with this model. This diagram has been adapted from Picton and Stuss (2000).

which itself depends on the discrepancy between the model and the information, and on some selected criteria for discrepancy. This error signal may itself relate to various subjective experiences depending upon the level of the hierarchy at which the modeling occurs. At lower levels it may indicate a perceived fuzziness and at higher levels it may relate to anxiety.

PHYSIOLOGICAL MEASUREMENTS OF COGNITION

The functioning of the human brain can be measured using two main methods: electromagnetic and hemodynamic. Figure 7–2 presents the temporal and spatial resolution of these human techniques using a diagrammatic convention first employed by Churchland and Sejnowski (1991) to show the various experimental techniques used in animal and human neuroscience. The details are similar to those presented by Churchland and Sejnowski, except for the division of the positron emission tomography (PET) studies into hemodynamic (oxygen) and metabolic (using 2-deoxy-glucose, or 2DG), and the addition of functional magnetic resonance imaging (fMRI) (Menon & Kim, 1999). Hemodynamic methods such as PET and fMRI show greater anatomical precision but less temporal precision than the electric and magnetic recordings, which are necessary for investigating the time course of perceptual and cognitive functions. The combination of data from both hemodynamic and electromagnetic techniques can provide a full spatiotemporal analysis. Electroencephalography (EEG) is less precise in terms of spatial resolution than the other techniques. Nevertheless, it is inexpensive and has good temporal resolution. Furthermore, since it can be recorded simultaneously with any of the other techniques, EEG can serve as a go-between to ensure that paradigms are providing consistent data in the different recording environments. Despite being fuzzy, EEG is frugal, fast, and friendly.

Electromagnetic recordings look at the electrical or magnetic fields that are generated at the scalp by the activity of neurons within the brain. The recorded fields occur at the same time as the neurons are active, and reflect the summed activities of many neurons. Since electromagnetic activity is bipolar, superimposed fields of different neurons may cancel themselves out. Larger fields are therefore created when the fields of the active neurons are parallel, such as the pyramidal cells of the cortex, and when their activation is synchronized. Transient bursts of activity are associated with the transfer of information from one cerebral region to another. Sustained activity is associated with the processing of information or the maintenance of that information in working memory. Rhythmic activity is less clearly understood. Some rhythms such as the alpha rhythm may reflect decreased in-

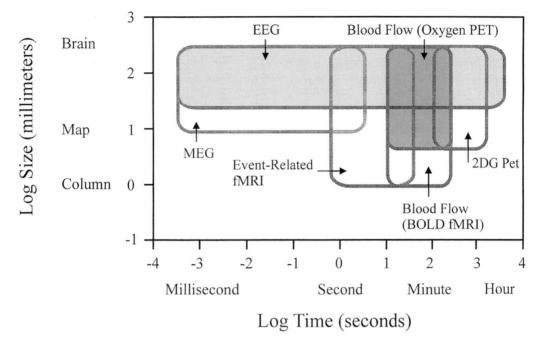

Figure 7–2. Spatial and temporal resolution. This diagram shows the resolution of different techniques used to evaluate the function of the human brain. The spatial resolution is shown on the y-axis, using a logarithmic scale such that value 0 equals 1 mm, value 1 equals 10 mm, etc. The temporal resolution is given on the x-axis, again using a logarithmic scale such that the number 0 equals 1 second, the number 1 equals 10 seconds, etc. In order to disentangle the overlap, two of the procedures (EEG and blood flow with oxygen PET) have been shaded. Techniques using electroencephalography (EEG) and magnetoencephalography (MEG) show better temporal resolution than the blood flow techniques or the metabolic technique using labeled 2-deoxyglucose (2DG). Functional magnetic resonance imaging with the blood oxygenation level–dependent (BOLD) effect shows a better spatial resolution than positron emission tomography (PET).

formation processing, and are attenuated or desynchronized when the cortex is active (Pfurtscheller & Lopes da Silva, 1999). Other rhythms—gamma rhythms—may be associated with binding together information being processed in separate areas of the cortex (Llinas et al., 1998; Singer, 2000). Analyses of the coherency of EEG or magnetoencephalographic (MEG) activity between different regions of the brain demonstrate the flow of information between these regions. These measurements are powerful because of the accurate time dimension. However, care must be taken when using scalp recording to ensure that field spread is distinguished from neuronal transmission (Nunez et al., 1999).

Hemodynamic studies of the human brain look at the changes in blood flow that follow the activation of neurons. Since these changes occur several seconds after the neuronal activation, the temporal resolution of the analysis is limited. However, the anatomical resolution is much better than for the electromagnetic techniques, particularly for fMRI. Correlational analysis of hemodynamic data is well justified since the measurements do not change polarity. However, they are limited since they cannot easily be done over time.

Three general principles are helpful in evaluating physiological measurements (either electromagnetic or hemodynamic) during cognition. First, multiple areas of the brain are simultaneously active. Neuronal activity in the frontal lobes does not occur without simultaneous activity elsewhere. This may make it difficult to study. Neuronal firing patterns at one location cannot be understood independently of neuronal activity in other locations. At the

level of the scalp-recorded potentials there is
the added problem that the fields generated
by neurons in one area may significantly overlap with those generated in other areas. Second, when processing depends on networks of
interacting neurons (McIntosh, 1999, 2000),
the localization of functions to specific areas is
difficult. Lesion studies have complex effects.
Third, the most informative measurements of
neuronal networks may involve correlational
studies. All begin with *c*: *c*oncurrent activation
of different areas, *c*omplex effects of lesions,
and *c*orrelational measurements of activity.

Our chapter looks at the functions of the
frontal lobes of the human brain from the perspective of physiology. The development of
the chapter will follow the general model of
representational processing. We shall make
some working hypotheses about the workings
of the frontal lobes and see how well they fit.
These hypotheses are speculative—the generating process is active and the fitting criteria
are loose. This mode of thinking is necessitated by the general lack of knowledge about
how the human frontal lobes work.

PERCEPTION

PROCESSING SENSORY INFORMATION

Although sensory stimulation primarily activates the sensory cortices, the frontal regions of
the brain are often activated in parallel with the
more specifically sensory areas. In the auditory
system, the sensory response generates a large
electrical P1–N1–P2 complex. These potentials
are largely generated in the auditory cortices of
the supratemporal plane, and picked up over
the frontal scalp because of the spread of the
electrical fields through volume conduction.
However, the frontal lobes are active at the
same time or slightly later than the temporal
lobes. Figure 7–3 shows a simplified source
analysis of the late auditory evoked potentials
(Picton et al., 1999). The sources are shown in
only one hemisphere. Activation of the supratemporal plane is quickly followed by activation
of the lateral temporal lobe and several regions
of the frontal lobe. Similar results have been
suggested by analysis of the current source
densities of these responses (Giard et al., 1994)

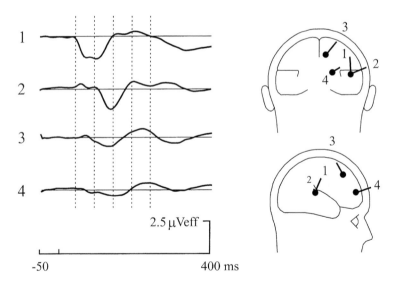

Figure 7–3. Source analysis of the auditory evoked potentials. This figure shows the source waveforms active
during the period of the auditory evoked potentials (P1–
N1, P2–N2). In order to make the analysis more easily
understood, only those sources active in the right hemisphere in response to left ear stimulation are shown. A
full analysis is presented in Picton et al. (1999). In general,
the source waveforms are reasonably symmetrical between homologous areas in the two hemispheres, with
some slight asymmetry such that the contralateral temporal regions are more active in response to a monaural
sound than the ipsilateral temporal regions. The vertical
dashed lines represent timing at 50-ms intervals after the
onset of the tone. The source waveforms illustrate a flow
of activation from the temporal regions to the anterior and
midfrontal regions.

The overlap between the different source components makes it difficult to recognize the effects of frontal lesions. Lesions to the temporoparietal regions significantly attenuate the N1 wave of the auditory evoked potential, whereas lesions to the frontal lobe do not (Knight et al., 1980; Alain et al., 1998). Source analysis indicates that the temporal lobe is clearly the dominant generator and that removing one of the frontal sources would have only little effect on the scalp measurements. Intracerebral recordings (Alain et al., 1989; Baudena et al., 1995) have not shown evidence of frontal generators, but this may be related to the limited locations of the electrodes.

Although blood flow studies of passive listening usually show activation that is limited to the temporal lobes, regions of the frontal lobe are recruited during active listening as well (Hall et al., 2000; Pedersen et al., 2000). It is difficult to determine from these studies whether the frontal regions are continuously active in terms of general attention or whether there are more specific stimulus-by-stimulus interactions. The electrical source analysis suggests that the interactions occur for each stimulus.

Rapid activation of the frontal lobes also occurs during the processing of visual information. During attention to visual stimuli, a frontal negative wave occurs slightly later (120 ms) than the posterior P1 wave at about 100 ms (Luck & Hillyard, 1994). Target detection is similarly associated with a posterior N2pc wave that is quickly followed by an anterior N2 wave (Luck et al., 1994). In an intriguing study, Thorpe et al. (1996) showed early changes in the event-related potential at frontal regions when subjects have to decide whether complex photographs contain an animal or not. The frontal differences beginning at approximately 150 ms likely represent an interaction between the visual areas and the response–selection system.

Concurrent activation of frontal and sensory cortices may relate to conscious awareness. Koch and Crick (2000) have postulated that connections between the sensory cortices and the prefrontal cortex are essential to awareness. In general, lesions to the frontal lobes do not impair awareness, but this may not be true when the sensory input is complex. A large lesion of the right frontal lobe impaired perception of auditory temporal patterns (Griffiths et al., 2000). This suggests that the auditory system up to and including the primary auditory cortex is not sufficient for the normal perception of temporal pattern without additional frontal processing. This vital interplay of prefrontal cortex and sensory regions in awareness was also shown in an fMRI study of Lumer and Rees (1999). Subjects participated in a binocular rivalry task, in which distinct stimuli were presented to the left and right visual fields. Under normal circumstances, subjective percepts switch between the two stimuli. A significant covariation existed between peristriate, ventral occipitotemporal, and superior prefrontal cortices during rivalry conditions. Presumably, the coactivation of these areas carried the information on the dominant percept. Such a distributed pattern of coactivation in perceptual rivalry has also been reported in steady-state MEG recordings (Tononi et al., 1998; Srinivasin et al., 1999).

The rapid rhythms of the EEG probably play a crucial role in the interactions between the prefrontal regions and the rest of the brain. One possibility (Singer & Gray, 1995; Singer, 2000) is that synchronized rhythmic firing of the neurons in various regions of the brain might bind sensory attributes into perceived objects. The networks might function through synchronized gamma rhythms (with frequencies of 30 Hz or greater). Gamma rhythms may be recorded in the human EEG. They must be analyzed in the frequency domain on each trial, since trial-to-trial variations in their frequency or phase may cancel out the activity in an averaged recording. Furthermore, care must be taken to distinguish brain activity from muscle artifacts. Tallon-Baudry and colleagues (1997) showed that the perception of an object in a camouflaged background was associated with a burst of gamma activity. Rodriguez and colleagues (1999) had subjects view abstract figures that were sometimes recognizable as faces and sometimes not. When the subject perceived a face there was a high correlation between gamma activities recorded over anterior and posterior regions of the scalp. Meaningful perception thus occurred when the frontal and posterior regions became synchronized.

NOTICING CHANGES

The *mismatch negativity* (MMN) is a small negative wave that can be recorded from the scalp when a repeating auditory stimulus changes (Picton et al., 2000). The MMN reflects a process in sensory memory that detects a deviation from some regularity. The MMN occurs regardless of whether the subject is attending to the deviant stimuli. Although it is mainly generated in the auditory cortices of the supratemporal plane, the scalp-recorded MMN also receives some contribution from the right frontal cortex (Giard et al., 1990). The MMN process might represent a call to attention—something has changed and this may be important. Concurrent activation

of sensory and frontal cortex therefore occurs both during the sensory response (something has happened) and during the mismatch response (something has changed).

Lesions to the temporal lobe unilaterally attenuate the MMN to stimuli that are presented contralaterally to the lesion, whereas lesions to the frontal lobe cause bilateral attenuation (Alain et al., 1998). Figure 7–4 illustrates these findings (lesions to the hippocampus do not affect the response). The MMN is therefore mainly generated in the temporal lobe with the hemisphere contralateral to the side of stimulation playing the dominant role. The role of the frontal lobes is less clear. Bilateral frontal generators may contribute to the scalp-recorded MMN (regardless of the ear of stimulation) and these generators may interact such that a lesion to one frontal region impairs the function of the other, or the frontal lobes may facilitate the MMN generators in both temporal lobes. Whatever the ex-

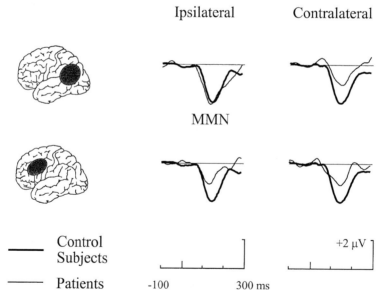

Figure 7–4. Effects of brain lesions on mismatch negativity (MMN). This figure shows the average deviant–standard difference waveforms for a group of patients with temporoparietal lesions (*upper*) and a group of patients with frontal lesions (*lower*). The patient waveforms are compared to those of normal control subjects. Responses are shown when the stimulus was presented ipsilaterally and contralaterally to the lesioned hemisphere. For the

control subjects, the ipsilateral and contralateral responses are identical and represent the mean of the right and left ear responses. A clear mismatch negativity began at about 50 ms after the stimulus and peaked at about 150 ms. Unilateral frontal lesions decrease the MMN to either right or left ear stimulation bilaterally, whereas temporoparietal lesions only decrease the response when the stimuli are contralateral.

planation, the frontal and temporal lobes interact in the generation of the MMN. A complex network underlies sensory memory.

If the subject attends to the discrepant stimulus in order to detect it as a target, the MMN is followed by a large complex of waves, usually consisting of N2, P3, and slow wave. The largest of these is the late positive wave, called *P3* from its location in the P1–N1–P2–N2–P3 sequence or *P300* because of its typical latency in milliseconds in young subjects (Picton, 1992). Determination of the brain regions generating this wave has long been a source of controversy. Several recent fMRI studies have looked at the cerebral locations of increased blood flow during target detection (Menon et al., 1997; Linden et al., 1999; Yoshiura et al., 1999; Downar et al., 2000). Increased blood flow occurs in the temporoparietal regions and in several other areas of the brain, including the frontal cortex. This fits with intracranial recordings in human subjects, which show simultaneous activity in multiple regions of the brain (Halgren et al., 1998) during the time of the scalp-recorded late positive wave. The P300 is likely a network response with no dominant focal generator. The late positive wave occurs in a variety of circumstances in addition to the detection of an improbable target—in go/no-go tasks, in feedback, and in the detection of novelty ("beep, beep, beep, bark"). In all of these contexts, the frontal lobes contribute more significantly to the scalp-recorded wave.

Many researchers have recognized two main types of P300 wave, the P3a and P3b (Squires et al., 1975; He et al., 2001). The *P3b* occurs when an expected target is detected and is maximally recorded from the parietal scalp; the *P3a* occurs when a novel stimulus—a dog bark or other strange noise—is noticed and is maximally recorded more frontally. Prefrontal lesions cause a significant reduction in the P3a amplitude (Knight, 1984). Hippocampal lesions also significantly affect the novelty P3a but spare the target P3b (Knight, 1996; Knight & Scabini, 1998). The networks underlying these two late positive waves are set up differently. Novelty detection involves the medial temporal regions and the prefrontal

cortex much more than routine target detection, which is handled in the temporoparietal association areas. These results fit well with hemodynamic studies of novelty detection which indicate significant activation of the medial temporal regions (Tulving et al., 1996).

HYPOTHESES CONCERNING PERCEPTION

Sensory information reaching the cortex may or may not reach consciousness. Much of what comes in is disregarded or handled automatically. Paying attention to some part of the incoming information probably involves interactions between the prefrontal cortices and the sensory regions of the brain. These interactions may be initiated top-down or bottom-up, and are probably associated with facilitated transmission of information from one region of cortex to another and by rapid oscillations in the electrical activity of interacting neurons. When such interactions occur, the information becomes conscious.

Changes can be expected or novel. When an expected change in the input occurs that requires a routine response, it is handled mainly through the sensorimotor association areas of the parietal regions. These are the focus of a network of activity that may also involve motor activation, memory updating, sensory tuning, and other procedures. When something novel occurs, the medial temporal regions and the prefrontal cortex are much more involved.

CONTROL OF BEHAVIOR

INHIBITING RESPONSES

If the usual target-detection task is inverted so that the subject responds to the standard stimuli and withholds response from the target, the N2 wave to the no-go stimulus is increased in amplitude (Eimer, 1993) and the P300 is more frontally distributed (Hillyard et al., 1976; Simson et al., 1977; Roberts et al., 1994; Falkenstein et al., 1995). A similar set of potentials is associated with the presentation of a stop signal in a paradigm in which an ongoing discriminative response must be prevented if a stop signal occurs just after the stimulus to be discriminated (Pliszka et al., 2000). Here, the N2 wave is larger over the right frontal regions than over the left.

Source analyses of the cerebral activity underlying the no-go response indicates a complex set of overlapping generators in the inferior prefrontal regions, cingulate, and premotor regions (Kiefer et al., 1998). The role of the right inferior regions of the frontal cortex in response inhibition has also been implicated in fMRI studies (Casey et al., 1997).

MONITORING OF ERRORS

At times the subject may make a mistake during target discrimination and respond to a no-go stimulus. This situation is often set up by making the no-go stimulus improbable (Robertson et al., 1997). The subjective error experience in this task is sometimes described as "Oops" (and often with more expletive terms). If the event-related potentials (ERP)

are recorded using the error response as a trigger, we can see the cerebral concomitants of this experience (Falkenstein et al., 1991, 1994; Gehring et al., 1993; Scheffers et al., 1996). The event-related potentials recorded when the response was correct are subtracted away from the potentials recorded when an error was made to give an "error-related" ERP. This contains an Ne–Pe complex that is maximally recorded over the midfrontal scalp (Fig. 7–5).

When feedback on a task is given after the response, the ERP to the feedback stimulus that denotes that the response was incorrect contains an increased N2 wave (Miltner et al., 1997). Source analysis of this wave shows a similar generator to the anterior cingulate source underlying the Ne wave for an incorrect response to a no-go stimulus. In the no-go task, the subjects are immediately aware of their errors and provide their own feedback.

Several studies have implicated the anterior cingulate cortex in the generation of these error-related potentials. Source analysis of the

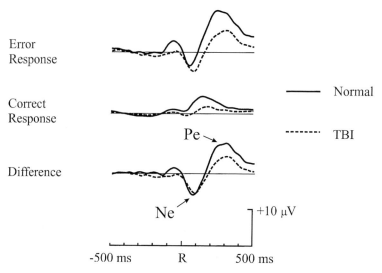

Figure 7–5. Error-related responses. This figure shows the event-related potentials synchronized to the motor response in a paradigm in which the subject was required to withhold a response to an improbable no-go stimulus while responding as rapidly as possible to all other stimuli. Sometimes the subject was unable to withhold the response and committed an error. The difference between the response-related potentials for the error and for the correct response shows the error-related potentials at the bottom. The major components of this response are the Ne and Pe waves. This figures shows the difference in these waves between a group of 10 patients who had suffered from traumatic brain injury (TBI) and a group of age-matched control subjects. Unpublished data are from M.L. Armilio, I.H. Robertson, D.T. Stuss, and T.W. Picton.

error-related negativity shows focal activity in the anterior cingulate region (Dehaene et al., 1994; Holroyd et al., 1998). If one looks at these error responses using event-related fMRI, one finds a significant activation in the medial prefrontal cortex (Kiehl et al., 2000). Several processes are going on during the recognition of an error. The error must be detected, the guilt or frustration must be acknowledged, and compensatory behavior must be initiated. Other regions of the brain probably interact with the anterior cingulate during such error processing.

The Ne wave recorded from individuals with lateral prefrontal damage is significantly reduced (Gehring & Knight, 2000). The lateral prefrontal cortex must therefore interact with the anterior cingulate cortex in monitoring behavior and in guiding compensatory systems. Interestingly, both the correct response and the error elicited large negative waves. It is possible that the patients did not properly discriminate errors from correct responses in terms of how they reacted to them. As shown in Figure 7–5, the error-related response is also abnormal after head injury. These patients may notice errors—the Ne is not significantly different from normal—but not be

able to cope with them—the Pe wave is significantly reduced.

Errors often result from a lapse in intention or goal neglect (Duncan et al., 1996). A slow positive shift can be observed over the frontal pole in the event-related potentials preceding an error in a Stroop paradigm (West & Alain, 2000). This slow wave inverts in polarity from the frontal pole to the frontocentral region, suggesting a dipole source in the anterior frontal regions. This likely represents the decline in a sustained frontal negativity associated with maintaining task goals in mind.

SWITCHING TASKS

Figure 7–6 represents some data recorded in a paradigm that required the subject to switch from one task to another (Moulden, 1999). One task was to respond on the basis of whether a stimulus was on the left or right of a grid; the other was to respond whether it was at the top or the bottom. Two types of visual cues indicated which task to perform when the target stimulus occurred. Following the cue, a negative preparatory wave occurred in the frontal regions of the scalp as the subject prepared for the upcoming task. If the cue

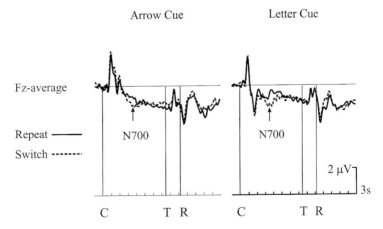

Figure 7–6. Event-related potentials associated with task switching. In this paradigm, a cue (C) stimulus came on 1500 ms before a target stimulus (T). The target stimulus was a red circle located in one sections of a 2 × 2 grid. The cue informed the subject whether to respond on the basis of whether the circle was on the left or the right or whether it was in the upper or lower half of the grid. Both the cue and the target persisted until the response. The

task changed randomly from trial to trial. Two types of cue, were used, one using arrows and one using letters. When the task was switched from the previous trial, there was an increased negative wave at around 700 ms after the cue, compared to when the task was the same as previously. This negativity was recorded maximally from the midfrontal regions. Unpublished data are from J.A. Moulden (1999).

indicated that the required responses would be different from that on the preceding trial, the subject had to switch. In this case, there was an additional mid-frontal negative wave, the N700 wave, which appears to indicate the revising of the stimulus–response rules.

Hemodynamic studies of task switching have shown increased activation in many brain regions, particularly the lateral prefrontal cortex and the parietal lobes (Dove et al., 2000; Kimberg et al., 2000; Sohn et al., 2000). Studies of patients with lesions indicated that the right hemisphere is more involved in task switching than the left, but patients with frontal lesions did not show the expected deterioration in switching efficiency (Mecklinger et al., 1999). Switching between tasks is necessarily complex since it must involve the schemata (or stimulus–response rules) for each of the tasks as well as the executive process of switching between them. The electrical recordings are important because the timing of the switch likely occurs before the activation and inactivation of the task schemata. We might therefore speculate that the dorsolateral prefrontal regions might initiate the switching of the stimulus rules that are perhaps set up in the sensory and motor regions of the cortex.

HYPOTHESES CONCERNING BEHAVIORAL CONTROL

The frontal lobes are intimately related to the control of behavior, with the main motor outflow from the cerebral cortex deriving from the precentral gyrus. Areas anterior to this gyrus are involved in initiating behavior, overseeing complicated behavioral patterns, and stopping behavior. The most exciting recent results concern the implication of inferior frontal regions in stopping behavior and the existence of an error-processing network linked to the anterior cingulate region.

Switching between tasks is a complex process that requires initiating new task rules and withdrawing others. The cerebral processes responsible for switching therefore involve many areas of the brain. The dorsolateral prefrontal regions seem crucial to these switching networks, although the parietal regions likely

maintain representations of the active stimulus–response rules.

LEARNING AND MEMORY

BECOMING AWARE OF CONTINGENCIES

Understanding the relationships between stimuli is the domain of the contingent negative variation (CNV), initially reported by Walter et al. (1964). This is a negative baseline shift that occurs between two stimuli (S1 and S2) when a subject recognizes a meaningful association, or contingency, between the stimuli (McCallum, 1988). In most CNV paradigms, S1 warns of the upcoming occurrence of S2, which requires a motor response. Multiple different processes likely contribute to the CNV: an early orientation to the first stimulus, a late preparation of the response to the second stimulus, and an overriding process that organizes behavior according to the contingencies of the task. The amplitude of the CNV in a simple response task is related to neuropsychological tests of executive function in patients with traumatic brain injury (Segalowitz et al., 1992). Prefrontal lesions significantly reduce the amplitude of the later portions of the CNV (Rosahl & Knight, 1995).

Figure 7–7 shows some data recorded during a paradigm involving associations between stimuli (Proulx, 1981; Proulx & Picton, 1984). Four different pairs of tones occurred, with only one of these pairs occurring right before a buzzer that the subject had to turn off. Some subjects recognized the association between the buzzer and the particular tone pair that preceded it, and others did not. For the subjects who became aware of the rules, a CNV occurred during the tone pair that indicated an upcoming response, and not during a tone pair that was unrelated to the response. The wave was significantly affected by anxiety. The subjects had to discover the contingencies for themselves. A relaxed subject had no difficulty recognizing the stimulus association, developing a CNV to the relevant stimulus and responding quickly. If the subject was anxious by nature, there were two possibile results. The subject could become involved in the task, de-

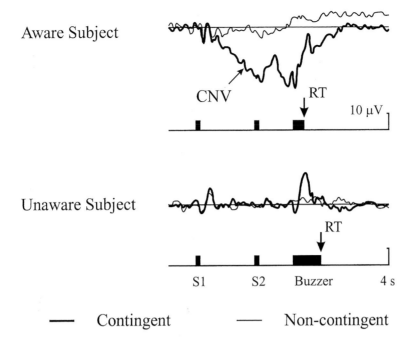

Aware Subject

CNV RT

10 μV

Unaware Subject

RT

S1 S2 Buzzer 4 s

—— Contingent —— Non-contingent

Figure 7–7. Contingent negative variation. In this paradigm, multiple different pairs of stimuli (S1–S2) occurred. If the two tones were high pitched, the pair of stimuli was then followed by a buzzer. The instructions were to turn off the buzzer as quickly as possible. Some of the subjects, such as the subject whose event-related potentials are shown in the upper part of the figure, recognized the association between the high-pitched tones and the buzzer and developed a contingent negative variation (CNV) after the initial stimulus. The responses when the two stimuli were high pitched are shown by the thick lines. The responses when the two stimuli were low pitched are shown by the thin lines. Other subjects, such as the one whose waveforms are shown in the lower part of the figure, did not recognize the association between the tones and the buzzer, did not show any changes in their baseline EEG level, and responded to the buzzer with a slow reaction time (RT).

velop a large CNV, perform well, but suffer from high levels of anxiety. Or the subject could decide not to become involved, not develop a CNV, perform poorly, and feel fine.

What is happening in the brain during this CNV? Figure 7–8 shows some PET data obtained during an analogous task (McIntosh et al., 1999). At the beginning, the subjects were not aware of the contingencies. Some subjects became aware that one stimulus predicted the upcoming task and the others did not. A region of the left dorsolateral cortex became highly related to behavioral performance and to other active regions of the brain, either positively or negatively. Subjects who did not become aware of the association did not show this pattern of correlations. These results are analogous to those discussed earlier in the chapter in relation to perceptual awareness. The prefrontal regions are essentially involved

in becoming aware of both what something is and what it means. The proper interpretation of the world requires communication between the prefrontal regions and the rest of the brain.

Rhythmic gamma activity also occurs in these tasks (Miltner et al., 1999). As an association between a visual stimulus and an upcoming somatosensory stimulus was made, gamma activity increased at occipital and parietal sites and a CNV developed between the stimuli. In addition, the gamma activity showed increased coherence between the occipital areas (subserving vision) and the central areas (subserving somatic sensation).

SHORT-TERM MEMORIES

Tallon-Baudry and colleagues (1998) looked at the neurophysiological concomitants of short-term memory. Their task was to determine

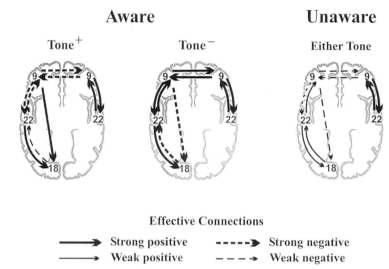

Figure 7–8. Awareness of contingencies. This figure shows the functional networks derived by path analysis of PET blood flow data during late phases of training in a differential sensory conditioning task (adapted from McIntosh, et al., 1999). Two different tones differentially signaled the upcoming occurrence (or not) of a visual stimulus that the subject had to discriminate. Some subjects became aware of the association between the tones and the visual stimuli and some did not. Separate network analyses were performed from the two groups. The arrows represent the effect one region has on another, with the size and sign of the effect indicated in the legend. Aware subjects showed strong difference in effective connections involving left prefrontal area 9 and other regions that distinguished between the two tones. Conversely, the network for the unaware subjects did not differ between tones and showed no strong left prefrontal involvement.

whether a second visual shape was the same as the first. A control task used the same first stimulus but the subject only responded to a dimming of the foveal fixation cross at the time of the second stimulus. During the first stimulus the slower rhythms were significantly reduced; this is termed *event-related desynchronization* (Pfurtscheller & Lopes da Silva, 1999). Bursts of gamma rhythm occurred at the onset and the offset of the stimulus. If the stimulus had to be maintained in working memory, a further burst of gamma rhythm occurred to set up this representation.

When information is held in working memory, hemodynamic studies show complex interactions between frontal cortex, hippocampus, anterior cingulate, and sensory cortices (McIntosh, 1999). In a delayed match-to-sample task for faces, these interactions changed with changes in the interval between the sample and the matching-task. In particular, the frontal regions became more involved

as the delay increased and memory moved from short- to long-term.

LONG-TERM MEMORY

Encoding into long-term memory involves complex interactions between different brain regions with the frontal regions, playing an important role (Mangels et al., 2001). In a simple learning paradigm subjects learn a list of words and then are tested for recall and recognition. At the time of encoding, what determines whether the word will be later recalled? This was studied by selectively averaging the event-related potentials recorded during encoding on the basis of later recall (Fig. 7–9).) The main findings were sustained potentials in both the posterior and frontal scalp. The combined activation of frontal and posterior cortex set up the episodic context that allows later recall. The frontal activity was larger over the right hemisphere, which does not fit with the

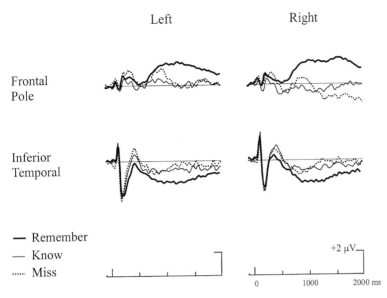

Figure 7–9. Encoding information into episodic memory. In this paradigm, subjects were requested to learn lists of words. The event-related potentials recorded during each word were then separately averaged on the basis of whether the word was later recognized or not ("missed"). The recognized words were separated into those that the subjects "remembered" seeing on the learning list and those which they "knew" were on the list without any clear memory of learning them. The words that were remembered were associated with increased sustained potentials both frontally and posteriorly. These were particularly evident over the right frontal regions.

usual hemispheric recording-retrieval asymmetry. Generally, the left prefrontal regions are activated during encoding and the right prefrontal regions are activated during retrieval (Tulving et al., 1994; Cabeza & Nyberg, 2000). One suggested explanation for this is that, although left-hemisphere semantic processing is necessary for encoding, processing the words in terms of a specific personal context (mediated more by the right prefrontal regions) facilitates later episodic recall.

A major ERP finding in recognition tasks is an increased amplitude of the late positive wave recorded over the parietal regions following old stimuli compared to that following new stimuli—the "old–new effect" (Rugg, 1995). Swick and Knight (1999) examined behavioral and ERP measures of recognition in patients with dorsolateral prefrontal lesions. In normal subjects, recognition accuracy and the ERP old–new effect declined with increasing retention intervals. Although frontal patients showed a higher false-alarm rate to new words, their hit rate to old words and ERP old–new effect were intact, suggesting that recognition processes were not fundamentally altered by prefrontal damage. The opposite

behavioral pattern was observed in patients with hippocampal lesions: a normal false-alarm rate and a precipitous decline in hit rate at long lags. The intact ERP effect and the change in response bias during recognition suggest that frontal patients exhibited a deficit in strategic processing or postretrieval monitoring, in contrast to the more purely mnemonic deficit shown by hippocampal patients.

Düzel and colleagues looked at the human event-related potentials and PET measurements of blood flow during an episodic retrieval task (Düzel et al., 1999). Subjects were presented with a list of four words and were asked to decide whether each of the words had been present on a prior list or not. The task was associated with increased blood flow in the right frontal lobe and a slowly developing positive shift recorded from the right frontopolar scalp. Episodically retrieved old items were associated with increased blood flow in the left medial temporal lobe and an increased amplitude of the transient late positive wave in the ERP. These results suggest that the right frontal cortex is continuously active during an episodic retrieval task, whereas the left medial temporal lobe is intermittently active as item-

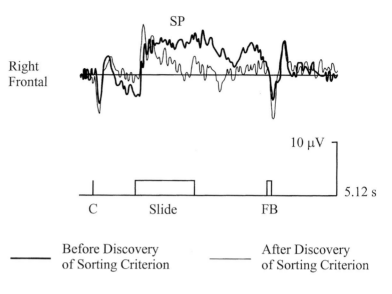

Figure 7–10. Problem solving. In this paradigm, subjects were presented with a slide showing visual information that could be categorized according to multiple criteria. The subjects' task was to decide which was the correct criteria for categorizing the stimuli. A cue (C) preceded the slide and feedback (FB) was given after the response. Before the discovery of the correct sorting criterion, while the subject was trying to figure out the correct response, there was an increased positive sustained potential (SP) recorded over the frontal regions, particularly on the right, compared to when the subject knew how to respond.

specific information is retrieved. The prefrontal cortex monitors the information retrieved through the medial temporal regions.

PROBLEM SOLVING

Figure 7–10 shows some ERP data recorded in a paradigm derived from the Wisconsin Card Sort Task (Stuss & Picton, 1978). In this test paradigm, a click warned of an upcoming visual stimulus that had to be categorized according to several possible criteria. Feedback was given after the response. Negative expectancy waves occurred in preparation for the visual stimulus and for the feedback. A sustained right frontal positive wave occurred during the visual stimulus in the trials in which a subject was still trying to determine the sorting criterion. On these trials the subject considered all the possible ways to categorize the stimuli and then chose one. The sustained frontal positive wave may represent the prefrontal cortex generating the possibilities.

Hemodynamic studies of the Wisconsin Card Sorting Paradigms have shown increased activation of the prefrontal regions, in association with activation of several other regions of the brain (Berman et al., 1995). This suggests that a network of activity underlies these pro-

cesses of working memory, and would be compatible with the idea of the prefrontal regions controlling operations in other areas of the brain. When performance on the sorting task was impaired by having the subjects perform a second task, the amount of prefrontal activation decreased (Goldberg et al., 1998). The efficiency of working memory therefore seems to depend on the amount of prefrontal activation.

HYPOTHESES CONCERNING LEARNING AND MEMORY

New knowledge is attained through experience and through the reorganization of past experience. The prefrontal regions of the brain become involved when the brain recognizes associations between stimuli or the implications of these stimuli for response. Such involvement can be manifest by activation of the frontal regions, increased coherence between these regions and those processing or maintaining the information, and increased rapid electrical rhythms.

The medial temporal regions are crucial to encoding information into long-term memories and later retrieving this information. The frontal regions, however, determine which information is encoded—we learn what we attend to. Furthermore, the frontal regions supervise the retrieval process and evaluate the information that is retrieved. Activation of the frontal lobes during memory shows up with increased blood flow and sustained electrical potentials.

Problem solving uses information available in both short- and long-term memory. The manipulation of this information involves extensive interactions between different regions of the brain, with the prefrontal regions being crucial to setting up and maintaining these networks.

CONCLUDING COMMENTS

CHECKING THE MODEL

It is an exciting time for studying human cognition. Hemodynamic techniques can show us clearly which regions of the brain are involved in cognitive processing. Electromagnetic techniques can give us some idea of when these regions are involved. One definite conclusion that comes from these studies is that cognition involves multiple activities in multiple regions of the brain. This is particularly true when the frontal lobes are involved. Activity in the frontal lobes cannot occur independently of simultaneous activity in other regions of the brain. Cognition should be conceived in terms of interacting networks (McIntosh, 1999). There is likely no specific role of the prefrontal regions other than to initiate and tie together these interacting networks.

Although we are gaining a better knowledge of where and when processes are active in the human brain, our model of cognition contains little information about how they are active. Here we must have recourse to animal studies and neuronal models. To understand the processes of cognition, we shall need to know the actual neuronal mechanisms—not just that neurons are active, but also what they are doing.

THE THEATRE OF THE MIND

This chapter has selectively considered the neurophysiology of the human frontal lobes under the rubric of the "theatre of the mind." The neurophysiological findings suggest that the frontal regions of the human brain are crucial elements in the interacting networks that instantiate representational processing. A representational processor interprets what is occurring by making explanatory models, and adjusts behavior to fit with desired goals. At its highest levels the representational processor can be separated from reality and can operate on hypothetical contents. This is not the passive Cartesian theatre of the philosophers but the active cortical theatre of the human brain.

The processing involves simultaneous activities in multiple regions of the brain, which are essentially linked through prefrontal neurons. The concurrence of these activities makes it difficult to disentangle the individual processes. The neuropsychology of the frontal lobes must consider the disruption of networks rather than the localization of function.

Neurophysiology must develop new ways to measure the activity of networks. This will probably involve correlational studies and attention to rhythms as well as to isolated potentials.

The prefrontal regions function by interacting with all the other regions of the brain. They attempt to find meaning and purpose by fitting the possible to the actual, the future to the past, and the individual to the universal. An example is when Hamlet remembers Yorick from his graveyard skull. Yorick was a "fellow of infinite jest, and most excellent fancy," who would have appreciated the idea that Hamlet is performing a decayed match-to-sample paradigm. Hamlet imagines how the skull might have appeared before death, remembers the past and predicts his own future, seeing in all this the universal principles of mortality. His prefrontal cortex is enacting the theatre of the mind. How this occurs remains to be discovered. It is the play's unfolding we must probe, to catch the function of the frontal lobe.

ACKNOWLEDGMENTS

The research reviewed in this chapter has been supported by the Canadian Institutes for Health Research. We thank several colleagues—Maria Armilio, Jeni Mangels, Drew Moulden, Guy Proulx, and Don Stuss—for allowing us to present some of their unpublished data. Libby Duke and Patricia Van Roon helped in the preparation of the manuscript.

REFERENCES

Alain, C., Richer, F., Achim, A., & Saint Hilaire, J.M. (1989). Human intracerebral potentials associated with target, novel, and omitted auditory stimuli. *Brain Topography, 1*, 237–245.

Alain, C., Woods, D.L., & Knight, R.T. (1998). A distributed cortical network for auditory sensory memory in humans. *Brain Research, 812*, 23–37.

Baudena, P., Halgren, E., Heit, G., & Clarke, J.M. (1995). Intracerebral potentials to rare target and distractor auditory and visual stimuli. III. Frontal cortex. *Electroencephalography and Clinical Neurophysiology, 94*, 251–264.

Berman, K.F., Ostrem, J.L., Randolph, C., Gold, J., Goldberg, T.E., Coppola, R., Carson, R.E., Herscovitch, P., & Weinberger, D.R. (1995). Physiological activation of a cortical network during performance of the Wisconsin Card Sorting Test: a positron emission tomography study. *Neuropsychologia, 33*, 1027–1046.

Cabeza, R. & Nyberg, L. (2000). Imaging cognition II: an empirical review of 275 PET and fMRI studies. *Journal of Cognitive Neuroscience, 12*, 1–47.

Casey, B.J., Trainor, R.J., Orendi, J.L., Schubert, A.B., Nystrom, L.E., Giedd, N.J., Castellanos, F.X., Haxby, J.V., Noll, D.C., Cohen, J.D., Forman, S.D., Dahl, R.E., & Rapoport, J.L. (1997). A developmental functional MRI study of prefrontal activation during performance of a go-no-go task. *Journal of Cognitive Neuroscience, 9*, 835–847.

Churchland, P.S. & Sejnowski, T.J. (1991). Perspectives on cognitive neuroscience. In: R.G. Lister & H.J. Weingartner (Eds.), *Perspectives on Cognitive Neuroscience* (pp. 3–23). New York: Oxford University Press.

Dehaene, S., Posner, M.I., & Tucker, D.M. (1994). Localization of a neural system for error detection and compensation. *Psychological Science, 5*, 303–305.

Dove, A., Pollmann, S., Schubert, T., Wiggins, C.J., & von Cramon, D.Y. (2000). Prefrontal cortex activation in task switching: an event-related fMRI study. *Cognitive Brain Research, 9*, 103–109.

Downar, J., Crawley, A.P., Mikulis, D.J., & Davis, K.D. (2000). A multimodal cortical network for the detection of changes in the sensory environment. *Nature Neuroscience, 3*, 277–283.

Duncan, J., Emslie, H., Williams, P., Johnson, R., & Freer, C. (1996). Intelligence and the frontal lobe: the organization of goal-directed behavior. *Cognitive Psychology, 30*, 257–303.

Düzel, E., Cabeza, R., Picton, T.W., Yonelinas, A.P., Scheich, H., Heinze, H.J., & Tulving, E. (1999). Task- and item-related processes during memory-retrieval: a combined PET and ERP study. *Proceedings of the National Academy of Sciences of the U.S.A., 96*, 1794–1799.

Eimer, M. (1993). Effects of attention and stimulus probability on ERPs in a Go/Nogo task. *Biological Psychology, 35*, 123–138.

Falkenstein, M., Hohnsbein, J., Hoormann, J., & Blanke, L. (1991). Effects of crossmodal divided attention on late ERP components. II. Error processing in choice reaction tasks. *Electroencephalography and Clinical Neurophysiology, 78*, 447–455.

Falkenstein, M., Koshlykova, N.A., Kiroj, V.N., Hoormann, J., & Hohnsbein, J. (1995). Late ERP components in visual and auditory Go/Nogo tasks. *Electroencephalography and Clinical Neurophysiology, 96*, 36–43.

Gehring, W.J. & Knight, R.T. (2000). Prefrontal–cingulate interactions in action monitoring. *Nature Neuroscience, 3*, 516–520.

Gehring, W.J., Goss, B., Coles, M.G.H., Meyer, D.E., & Donchin, E. (1993). A neural system for error detection and compensation. *Psychological Science, 4*, 385–390.

Giard, M.H., Perrin, F., Pernier, J., & Bouchet, P. (1990). Brain generators implicated in the processing of auditory stimulus deviance: a topographic event-related potential study. *Psychophysiology, 27*, 627–640.

Giard, M.H., Perrin, F., Echallier, J.F., Thevenet, M., Froment, J.C., & Pernier, J. (1994). Dissociation of temporal and frontal components in the human auditory N1 wave: a scalp current density and dipole model analysis. *Electroencephalography and Clinical Neurophysiology, 92*, 238–252.

Goldberg, T.E., Berman, K.F., Fleming, K., Ostrem, J., Van Horn, J.D., Esposito, G., Mattay, V., Gold, J.M., & Weinberger, D.R. (1998). Uncoupling cognitive workload and prefrontal cortical physiology: a PET rCBF study. *Neuroimage, 7*, 296–303.

Griffiths, T.D., Penhune, V., Peretz, I., Dean, J.L., Patterson, R.D., & Green, G.G. (2000). Frontal processing and auditory perception. *NeuroReport, 11*, 919–922.

Halgren, E., Marinkovic, K., & Chauvel, P. (1998). Generators of the late cognitive potentials in auditory and visual oddball tasks. *Electroencephalography and Clinical Neurophysiology, 106*, 156–164.

Hall, D.A., Haggard, M.P., Akeroyd, M.A., Summerfield, A.Q., Palmer, A.R., Elliott, M.R., & Bowtell, R.W. (2000). Modulation and task effects in auditory processing measured using fMRI. *Human Brain Mapping, 10*, 107–119.

He, B., Lian, J., Spencer, K.M. Dien, J., & Donchin, E. (2001). A cortical potential imaging analysis of the P300 and novelty P3 components. *Human Brain Mapping, 12*, 120–130.

Hillyard, S.A., Courchesne, E., Krausz, H.I., & Picton, T.W. (1976). Scalp topography of the P3 wave in different auditory decision tasks. In W.C. McCallum (Ed.), *The Responsive Brain* (pp. 81–87). Bristol: John Wright and Sons Limited.

Holroyd, C.B., Dien, J., & Coles, M.G. (1998). Error-related scalp potentials elicited by hand and foot movements: evidence for an output-independent error-processing system in humans. *Neuroscience Letters, 242,* 65–68.

Kiefer, M., Marzinzik, F., Weisbrod, M., Scherg, M., & Spitzer, M. (1998). The time course of brain activations during response inhibition: evidence from event-related potentials in a go/no go task. *Neuroreport, 9,* 765–770.

Kiehl, K.A., Liddle, P.F., & Hopfinger, J.B. (2000). Error processing and the rostral anterior cingulate: an event-related fMRI study. *Psychophysiology, 37,* 216–223.

Kimberg, D.Y., Aguirre, G.K., & D'Esposito, M. (2000). Modulation of task-related neural activity in task-switching: an fMRI study. *Cognitive Brain Research, 10,* 189–196.

Knight, R. (1996). Contribution of human hippocampal region to novelty detection. *Nature, 383,* 256–259.

Knight, R.T. (1984). Decreased response to novel stimuli after prefrontal lesions in man. *Electroencephalography and Clinical Neurophysiology, 59,* 9–20.

Knight, R.T. & Scabini, D. (1998). Anatomic bases of event-related potentials and their relationship to novelty detection in humans. *Journal of Clinical Neurophysiology, 15,* 3–13.

Knight, R.T., Hillyard, S.A., Woods, D.L., & Neville, H.J. (1980). The effects of frontal and temporal-parietal lesions on the auditory evoked potential in man. *Electroencephalography and Clinical Neurophysiology, 50,* 112–24.

Koch, C. & Crick, F. (2000). Some thoughts on consciousness and neuroscience. In: M.S. Gazzaniga (Ed.), *The New Cognitive Neurosciences,* Second Edition (pp. 1285–1294). Cambridge, MA: MIT Press.

Linden, D.E., Prvulovic, D., Formisano, E., Vollinger, M., Zanella, F.E., Goebel, R., & Dierks, T. (1999). The functional neuroanatomy of target detection: an fMRI study of visual and auditory oddball tasks. *Cerebral Cortex, 9,* 815–823.

Llinas, R., Ribary, U., Contreras, D., & Pedroarena, C. (1998). The neuronal basis for consciousness. *Philosophical Transactions of the Royal Society (London) B Biological Sciences, 353,* 1841–1849.

Luck, S.J. & Hillyard, S.A. (1994). Electrophysiological correlates of feature analysis during visual search. *Psychophysiology, 31,* 291–308.

Luck, S.J., Hillyard, S.A., Mouloua, M., Woldorff, M.G., Clark, V.P., & Hawkins, H.L. (1994). Effects of spatial cuing on luminance detectability: psychophysical and electrophysiological evidence for early selection. *Journal of Experimental Psychology: Human Perception and Performance, 20,* 887–904.

Lumer, E.D. & Rees, G. (1999). Covariation of activity in visual and prefrontal cortex associated with subjective visual perception. *Proceedings of the National Academy of Sciences USA, 96,* 1669–1673.

Mangels, J.A., Picton, T.W., & Craik, F.I.M. (2001). Attention and successful episodic encoding: an event-related potential study. *Cognitive Brain Research, 11,* 77–95.

McCallum, W.C. (1988). Potentials related to expectancy, preparation and motor activity. In Picton, T.W. (Ed.) *Handbook of Electroencephalography and Clinical Neurophysiology* (Revised series) *Vol. 3: Human Event-Related Potentials* (pp. 427–534). Amsterdam: Elsevier.

McIntosh, A.R. (1999). Mapping cognition to the brain through neural interactions. *Memory, 7,* 523–548.

McIntosh, A.R. (2000). Towards a network theory of cognition. *Neural Networks, 13,* 861–870.

McIntosh, A.R., Rajah, M.N., & Lobaugh, N.J. (1999). Interactions of prefrontal cortex in relation to awareness in sensory learning. *Science, 284,* 1531–1533.

Mecklinger, A., von Cramon, D.Y., Springer, A., & Matthes-von Cramon, G. (1999). Executive control functions in task switching: evidence from brain injured patients. *Journal of Clinical and Experimental Neuropsychology, 21,* 606–619.

Menon, R.S. & Kim, S. (1999). Spatial and temporal limits in cognitive neuroimaging with fMRI. *Trends in Cognitive Sciences, 3,* 207–216.

Menon, V., Ford, J.M., Lim, K.O., Glover, G.H., & Pfefferbaum, A. (1997). Combined event-related fMRI and EEG evidence for temporal-parietal cortex activation during target detection. *NeuroReport, 8,* 3029–3037.

Miller, G.A., Galanter, E., & Pribram, K.H. (1960). *Plans and the Structure of Behavior.* New York: Holt, Rinehart and Winston.

Miltner, W.H.R., Braun, C.H., & Coles, M.G.H. (1997). Event-related brain potentials following incorrect feedback in a time-estimation task: evidence for a "generic" neural system for error detection. *Journal of Cognitive Neuroscience, 9,* 788–798.

Miltner, W.H., Braun, C., Arnold, M., Witte, H., & Taub, E. (1999). Coherence of gamma-band EEG activity as a basis for associative learning. *Nature, 397,* 434–436.

Moulden, J.A. (1999) Physiological Mechanisms of Task-switching in Human Subjects. Ph.D. Thesis, University of Ottawa.

Nunez, P.L., Silberstein, R B., Shi, Z., Carpenter, M.R., Srinivasan, R., Tucker, D M., Doran, S.M., Cadusch, P.J., & Wijesinghe, R.S. (1999). EEG coherency II: experimental comparisons of multiple measures. *Clinical Neurophysiology, 110,* 469–486.

Pedersen, C.B., Mirz, F., Ovesen, T., Ishizu, K., Johannsen, P., Madsen, S., & Gjedde, A. (2000). Cortical centres underlying auditory temporal processing in humans: a PET study. *Audiology, 39,* 30–37.

Pfurtscheller, G. & Lopes da Silva, F.H. (1999). Event-related EEG/MEG synchronization and desynchronization: basic principles. *Clinical Neurophysiology, 110,* 1842–1857.

Picton, T.W. (1992). The P300 wave of the human event-related potential. *Journal of Clinical Neurophysiology, 9,* 456–479.

Picton, T.W. & Stuss, D.T. (2000). Consciousness. In: Bittar, E.E. & Bittar, N. (Eds.), *Biological Psychiatry (Principles of Medical Biology, Vol. 14)* (pp. 1–25). Stamford, Ct: JAI Press.

Picton, T.W., Alain, C., Woods, D.L, John, M.S., Scherg, M., Valdes-Sosa, P., Bosch-Bayard, J. & Trujillo, N.J. (1999). Intracerebral sources of human auditory evoked potentials. *Audiology and Neuro-Otology, 4,* 64–79.

Picton, T.W., Alain, C., Otten, L., Ritter, W., & Achim, A. (2000). Mismatch negativity: different water in the same river. *Audiology and Neuro-Otology, 5,* 111–139.

Pliszka, S.R., Liotti, M., & Woldorff, M.G. (2000). Inhibitory control in children with attention-deficit/hyperactivity disorder: event-related potentials identify the processing component and timing of an impaired right-frontal response-inhibition mechanism. *Biological Psychiatry, 48,* 238–246.

Proulx, G.B. (1981). The Effects of Anxiety on Event-related Potentials during a Learning Task. Ph.D. Thesis, University of Ottawa.

Proulx, G.B. & Picton, T.W. (1984). The effects of anxiety and expectancy on the CNV. *Annals of the New York Academy of Sciences, 425,* 617–622.

Roberts, L.E., Rau, H., Lutzenberger, W., & Birbaumer, N. (1994). Mapping P300 waves onto inhibition:go/no-go discrimination. *Electroencephalography and Clinical Neurophysiology, 92,* 44–55.

Robertson, I.H., Manly, T., Andrade, J., Baddeley, B.T., & Yiend, J. (1997). 'Oops!': performance correlates of everyday attentional failures in traumatic brain injured and normal subjects. *Neuropsychologia, 35,* 747–758.

Rodriguez, E., George, N., Lachaux, J.P., Martinerie, J., Renault, B., & Varela, F.J. (1999). Perception's shadow: long-distance synchronization of human brain activity. *Nature, 397,* 430–433.

Rosahl, S.K. & Knight, R.T. (1995). Role of prefrontal cortex in generation of the contingent negative variation. *Cerebral Cortex, 5,* 123–34.

Rugg, M.D. (1995). ERP studies of memory. In: M.D. Rugg & M.G.H. Coles (Ed.), *Electrophysiology of Mind: Event-Related Brain Potentials and Cognition* (pp. 132–170). New York: Oxford University Press.

Scheffers, M.K., Coles, M.G., Bernstein, P., Gehring, W., & Donchin, E. (1996). Event-related brain potentials and error-related processing: an analysis of incorrect responses to go and no-go stimuli. *Psychophysiology, 33,* 42–53.

Segalowitz, S.J., Unsal, A., & Dywan, J. (1992). CNV evidence for the distinctiveness of frontal and posterior neural processes in a traumatic brain-injured population. *Journal of Clinical and Experimental Neuropsychology, 14,* 545–565.

Simson, R., Vaughan, H.G., Jr., & Ritter, W. (1977). The scalp topography of potentials in auditory and visual Go/NoGo tasks. *Electroencephalography and Clinical Neurophysiology, 43,* 864–875.

Singer, W. (2000). Response synchronization: a universal coding strategy for the definition of relations. In: M.S. Gazzaniga (Ed.), *The New Cognitive Neurosciences,* Second Edition, (pp. 325–338). Cambridge, MA: MIT Press.

Singer, W. & Gray, C.M. (1995). Visual feature integration and the temporal correlation hypothesis. *Annual Review of Neuroscience 18,* 555–586.

Sohn, M.S., Ursu, S., Anderson, J.R., Stenger, V.A., & Carter, C.S. (2000). The role of prefrontal cortex and posterior parietal cortex in task switching. *Proceedings of the National Academy of Science USA, 97,* 13448–13454.

Squires, N.K., Squires, K.C., & Hillyard, S.A. (1975) Two varieties of long-latency positive waves evoked by unpredictable auditory stimuli in man. *Electroencephalography and Clinical Neurophysiology, 38,* 387–401.

Srinivasan, R., Russell, D.P., Edelman, G.M., & Tononi, G. (1999). Increased synchronization of neuromagnetic responses during conscious perception. *Journal of Neuroscience, 19,* 5435–5448.

Stuss, D.T. & Picton, T.W. (1978). Neurophysiological correlates of human concept formation. *Behavioral Biology, 23,* 135–162.

Stuss, D.T., Picton, T.W., & Alexander, M.P. (2001). Consciousness, self-awareness and the frontal lobes. In: S. Salloway, P. Malloy, & J. Duffy (Eds.), *The Frontal Lobes and Neuropsychiatric Illness* (pp. 101–109). Bethesda, MD: American Psychiatric Press.

Swick, D. & Knight, R.T. (1999). Contributions of prefrontal cortex to recognition memory: electrophysiological and behavioral evidence. *Neuropsychology, 13,* 155–170.

Tallon-Baudry, C., Bertrand, O., Delpuech, C., & Permier, J. (1997). Oscillatory gamma-band (30–70 Hz) activity induced by a visual search task in humans. *Journal of Neuroscience, 17,* 722–734.

Tallon-Baudry, C., Bertrand, O., Peronnet, F., & Pernier, J. (1998). Induced gamma-band activity during the delay of a visual short-term memory task in humans. *Journal of Neuroscience, 18,* 4244–4254.

Thorpe, S., Fize, D., & Marlot, C. (1996). Speed of processing in the human visual system. *Nature, 381,* 520–522.

Tononi, G., Srinivasan, R., Russell, D.P., & Edelman, G.M. (1998). Investigating neural correlates of conscious perception by frequency-tagged neuromagnetic responses. *Proceedings of the National Academy of Sciences USA, 95* 3198–203.

Tulving, E., Kapur, S., Craik, F.I., Moscovitch, M., & Houle, S. (1994). Hemispheric encoding/retrieval asymmetry in episodic memory: positron emission tomography findings. *Proceedings of the National Academy of Sciences USA, 91,* 2016–2020.

Tulving, E., Markowitsch, H.J., Craig, F.I.M., Habib, R., & Houle, S. (1996). Novelty and familiarity activations in PET studies of memory encoding and retrieval. *Cerebral Cortex, 6,* 71–79.

Walter, W.G., Cooper, R., Aldridge, V., McCallum, W.C., & Winter, A.L. (1964). Contingent negative variation: and electric sign of sensorimotor association and expectancy in the human brain. *Nature, 203,* 380–384.

West, R. & Alain, C. (2000). Evidence for the transient nature of a neural system supporting goal-directed action. *Cerebral Cortex, 10,* 748–752.

Yoshiura, T., Zhong, J., Shibata, D.K., Kwok, W.E., Shrier, D.A., & Numaguchi, Y. (1999). Functional MRI study of auditory and visual oddball tasks. *NeuroReport, 10,* 1683–1688.

8

Motor Programming for Hand and Vocalizing Movements

HISAE GEMBA

How the brain works in a person behaving voluntarily is an attractive scientific theme and has been studied by many scientists for more than 100 years. Motivation to willingly initiate any act or stop any ongoing act comes from (1) inward information related to instinct or homeostasis, or (2) outward information received by a sensory organ. Sensory information is transmitted to the prefrontal cortex from a peripheral sensory receptor via different neural pathways from inward information. The frontal lobe, including the prefrontal, premotor, and motor cortices, is thought to be at least partly related to a motor program that is involved from the time of decision making of movement initiation up to motor execution.

Many neural connections involving the prefrontal or motor cortex have been revealed by morphological studies using tracer methods and by physiological studies using electrical stimulation. It seems rather difficult to assess what neural connections are activated during volitional movements from cell recording experiments with monkeys performing tasks, and functional magnetic resonance imaging (fMRI) or positron emission tomography (PET) studies of humans performing tasks. However, simultaneous recording of field potentials on the surface and at 2.0–3.0 mm depth in a particular cortex is a very useful

method for finding out functional neuronal circuits on voluntary movement, which in turn enables us to predict which kind of synaptic input will be activated. In this chapter, I shall present a study in which a monkey was trained for hand movement and vocalization, and cortical field potentials were recorded during the movement by a pair of electrodes implanted in the cerebral cortex in the monkey. The potentials were analyzed in connection with behavioral observations.

METHODS

Excitatory postsynaptic potentials (EPSPs) generated in apical dendrites of pyramidal cells in the cerebral cortex mainly contribute to cortical field potentials. Afferent synaptic inputs into the cerebral cortex are conveyed by thalamocortical and corticocortical projections. Synaptic inputs into the superficial part of the apical dendrite of the pyramidal cell are due to superficial thalamocortical projections (Fig. 8–1, I). Inputs into the deeper part of the apical dendrite are due to deep thalamocortical and corticocortical projections. When superficial thalamocortical projections are activated, negative and positive potentials can be recorded with electrodes implanted on the

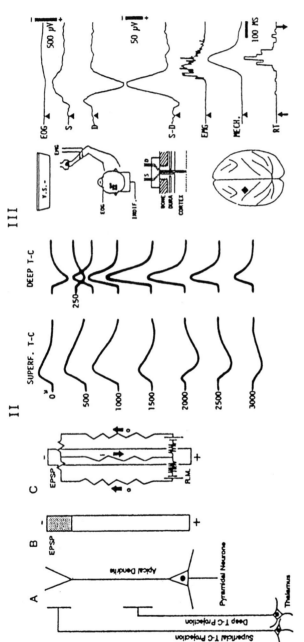

Figure 8–1. *I:* Origin of cortical field potentials. *A:* Thalamocortical (T-C) projection. *B:* Excitatory postsynaptic potential (EPSP) generated in the apical dendrite of a pyramidal neuron by superficial thalamocortical projection. +, positive potential in a deeper part outside the dendrite; −, negative potential in a superficial part outside the dendrite. *C:* Current flow (arrow) generated inside (i) and outside (o) the dendrite by EPSP (shown in B). *II:* Depth profiles of cortical field potentials in superficial (SUPERF. T-C) and deep (DEEP T-C) thalamocortical projections respectively (negativity upward). *III:* Arrangements for recording cortical field potentials (top left) and specimens (right side of diagram) obtained by electrodes (middle left) chronically implanted in the forelimb motor area (bottom left) in a monkey performing visual-initiated hand movements. Potentials were averaged 100 times by stimulus onset pulse (triangles and upward arrow) with electrooculogram (EOG), electromyogram (EMG), and mechanogram (MECH.). The 500 μV amplitude scale is for EOG; the 50 μV amplitude scale is for cortical potentials. V.S., diode for visual stimulus; INDIF, indifferent electrodes implanted in the bone; S, surface potential; D, depth potential; S − D, surface minus depth potential; RT, reaction time histogram. See text for further discussion. (*Source:* Reprinted from Gemba, 1996, with permission)

surface and at 2.0–3.0 mm depth in the cortex, respectively. When deep thalamocortical or corticocortical projections are activated, positive and negative potentials can be recorded with electrodes implanted on the surface and at 0.5–3.0 mm depth in the cortex, respectively (Fig. 8–1, II) (Sasaki, 1979; Sasaki et al., 1981b; Sasaki & Gemba, 1993a). This technique was applied to chronic experiments with monkeys in the present study.

An example in which these methods were used is shown in Figure 8–1, III. A monkey was fully trained to lift a lever quickly and properly in response to a visual stimulus (visual-initiated hand movement). Field potentials were recorded with electrodes implanted chronically on the surface and at 2.0–3.0 mm depth in the forelimb motor cortex, and these were referred to indifferent electrodes buried in the bone behind both ears. Surface (S), depth (D), and surface-minus-depth (S−D) potentials, were measured. Electomyomyographic (EMG) data were recorded bipolarly with surface electrodes on the wrist extensor muscle. The mechanogram was recorded through a transducer attached to the lever. The histogram of reaction times (RT) from the stimulus onset to the movement onset was also recorded. These were averaged 100 times by stimulus onset pulse. Surface-positive, depth-negative (s-P, d-N) potential appeared at a latency of about 50 ms after the stimulus onset, and was followed by surface-negative, depth-positive (s-N, d-P) potential. This late component is thought to be due to superficial thalamocortical projection (Gemba et al., 1981; 1982).

HAND MOVEMENT

MOTOR EXECUTION

Monkeys were trained for lever lifting at self-pace. Potentials recorded in the forelimb motor area, contralateral to the moving hand are shown in Figure 8–2 with EMG. Surface, middle, depth, and surface-minus-depth potentials were averaged 100 times by the movement onset pulse. Surface-negative, depth-positive (s-N, d-P) slow potentials started about 1 sec-

ond before the movement. The slow potentials were considered to be readiness potential for hand movements. The readiness potential was recorded in the premotor, forelimb motor, and somatosensory areas, contralateral to the moving hand, and in the premotor area on the ipsilateral side, and also in the supplementary motor area (SMA) on the contralateral side (not shown here) (Gemba et al., 1979; 1980; 1982; Gemba & Sasaki, 1984b).

The effect of cerebellar hemispherectomy upon the readiness potential is shown in Figure 8–3. The cerebellum was resected on the right side. The left (PREOP.) and right (POSTOP.) columns show the potentials recorded before and after the hemicerebellectomy, respectively. Potentials averaged 100 times by the movement onset pulse are shown in S−D potentials. Mechanograms are shown below the potentials. After the operation, the upward (s-N, d-P) potential, the readiness potential, in the motor cortex was almost completely eliminated (POSTOP., D) (Sasaki et al., 1979). Other areas were unaffected. From these results, together with those of the other study, the readiness potential in the motor cortex was inferred to be the cerebelloventrolateral thalamic nuclei–motor cortical response (Sasaki, 1979).

MOTOR LEARNING

To study motor learning, cortical field potentials were recorded in various cortical areas in a naive monkey learning to lift a lever in response to a visual stimulus (green with 0.5–1.0 seconds duration) appropriately and quickly (visual-initiated hand movement). The monkey was rewarded for hand movements performed within the duration of the stimulus.

Figure 8–4 shows changes in field potentials during the learning processes of visual-initiated hand movements in a single monkey. Columns I to IV show learning stages I to IV, respectively. Data are from the prefrontal (A–C), premotor (D), motor (E), prestrite (F), and striate (G) cortices, contralateral to the moving hand. Upward and downward arrows show the onset and end times of stimuli, respectively. The potentials were averaged 100 times by the stimulus onset pulse and are

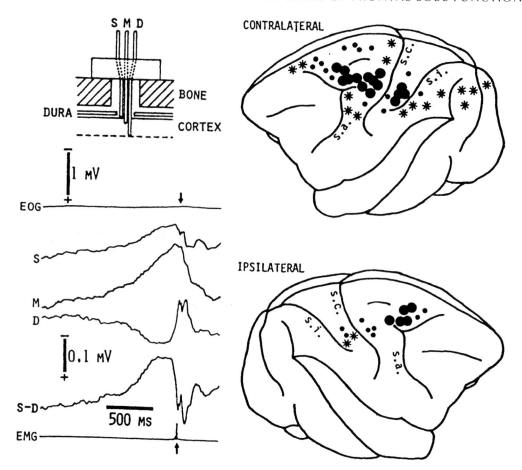

Figure 8–2. Distribution of premovement slow cortical potentials summarized from the data of seven monkeys with self-paced hand movements. Surface (S), middle (M), depth (D), and surface minus depth (S − D) potentials were averaged 100 times by movement onset pulse (upward and downward arrows) with electrooculogram (EOG) and electromyogram (EMG). The 1 mV amplitude scale is for EOG; the 0.1 mV amplitude scale for cortical potentials. Sites of large and small potentials are indicated with large and small circles, respectively; sites of no potential are indicated with asterisks. s.a., arcuate sulcus; s.c., central sulcus; s.i., intraparietal sulcus. See text for further discussion. (*Source:* Reprinted from Gemba et al. 1980, with permission from Elsevier Science)

shown in S−D. The data at stage I were recorded on the first training day, when the monkey elevated the lever regardless of stimuli, as seen in the RT histogram. At stage II, recorded on the 21st training day, an upward (s-N, d-P) potential appeared in the prefrontal (C) and prestriate (F) areas, although the monkey still lifted the lever independent of stimuli. As the upward potential became bigger along with further training, the monkey came to respond to stimuli with the hand movements, as seen at stage III (III, C, F, and RT). We called the early learning period stages, I to III, *recognition learning*. As an up-

ward (s-N, d-P) potential occurred and became bigger in the motor cortex (E) in connection with further intensive training, the monkey came to lift the lever appropriately and quickly, as seen at stage IV. We called the late learning period stages, III to IV, *skill learning*. Figure 8–5 shows that the upward potential in the motor cortex originates in the cerebellum, and that skill learning is due to cerebrocerebellar interactions (Sasaki and Gemba, 1981a; 1981b; 1982; 1983; 1989a; 1993a; 1993b; Gemba & Sasaki, 1984a; Sasaki et al., 1982; Tsujimoto et al., 1993). Neuroimaging studies in human subjects have indicated

Figure 8–3. Cortical field potentials (S − D) associated with self-paced hand movements before (PREOP.) and after (POSTOP.) cerebellar hemispherectomy. Potentials were averaged 100 times by movement onset pulse (broken line and upward arrows). Negativity of potentials is upward. See further text for further discussion.

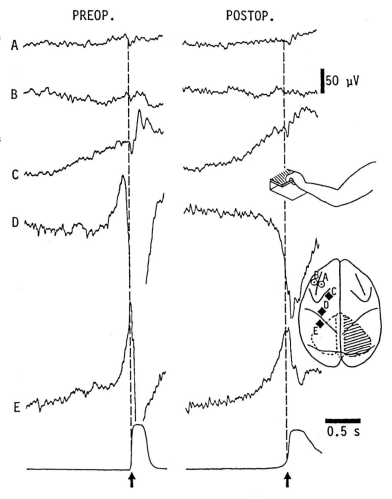

that the cerebellum is related to visuomotor skill learning (Doyon et al., 1996).

Left (PREOP.) and right (POSTOP.) columns in the left part in Figure 8–5 show data before and after the cerebellectomy (A). The potentials averaged 100 times by the stimulus onset pulse are shown in S–D in the upper part (diode for visual stimulus [V.S.]). The same data were aligned 100 times by the movement onset pulse, shown in the lower part (lever elevation [L.E.]). After the cerebellum was resected on the side, ipsilateral to the moving hand, the upward potential was almost completely eliminated in the motor cortex (FM), and was associated with more irregular and longer reaction times than before (A: FM and RT). The data after the operation are similar to data in learning stage III in Figure 8–4.

It can also be seen that the cerebellar hemispherectomy induced enhancement of the upward potential in the forelimb somatosensory cortex (FS) (Fig. 8–5 A: V.S.). In fact, the area of upward potential prior to the movement, marked by arrows with a broken line in L.E. averages, increased after the hemispherectomy to almost three times as much as before the operation. The postoperative increase of the FS premovement potential (area in S–D record) is plotted on the ordinate against days after the operation on the abscissa for three monkeys in the right part of the figure (B). The premovement potential increased to 250%–300% of the preoperative value several days after the operation, but declined steeply within 30–40 days after the operation. Such enhancement of premovement potentials was not in the other cortical areas other than the

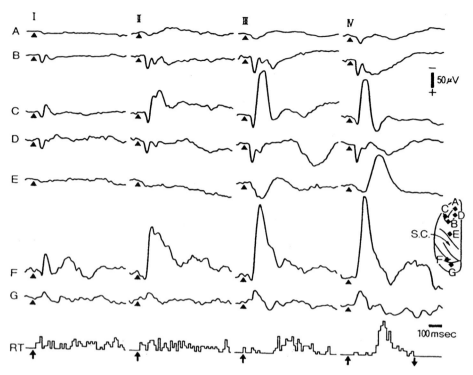

Figure 8–4. Changes of cortical field potentials (S − D) in learning processes of visual-initiated hand movements in same monkey. Potentials were averaged 100 times by stimulus onset pulse (triangle and upward arrows). Columns I–IV: Learning stages I–IV. Data are from the pre- frontal (A–C), premotor (D), motor (E), prestriate (F), and striate (G) cortices, contralateral to the moving hand. S.C., central sulcus; downward arrows, end times of stimuli. See text for further discussion. (*Source*: Reprinted from Sasaki and Gemba, 1982, with permission)

SMA, which showed a slight increase of the premovement potential component (Gemba & Sasaki, 1984b; Sasaki & Gemba, 1984a; 1991a; 1991b). The increased premovement activity of the somatosensory cortex after cerebellar hemispherectomy suggests a motor function of the somatosensory cortex to compensate for the motor cortex dysfunction caused by lack of cerebellar influence (Sasaki & Gemba, 1984b).

To study audio-initiated hand movement, a monkey was trained to lift the lever by hand in response to auditory stimulus. When a pure tone (1000 or 2000 Hz) was used as auditory stimulus, it took more training days for monkeys to learn audio-initiated hand movements than it did to learn visual-initiated hand movements. One monkey did not lift the lever in response to the auditory stimulus of pure tone, despite continued intensive training over more than 2 months, whereas the monkey

could respond to the visual stimulus with hand movement after the usual training of 3 weeks (Gemba & Sasaki, 1987, 1988). However, it took almost the same number of training days for monkeys to learn the audio-initiated hand movements with a complex tone (monkey call or buzzer) as it did to learn visual-initiated hand movements. It appeared to be easier for monkeys to learn audio-initiated hand movements with complex tone than with pure tone (Gemba & Sasaki, 1993; Gemba et al., 1995a). Natural stimuli, being mostly complex tones, as in animal vocalizations, rather than pure tones, are of general significance to monkeys.

Figure 8–6 shows changes in cortical field potentials during learning processes of audio-initiated hand movements with complex tone. Columns Ia to III show recognition learning, while columns III to IV show skill learning. A new auditory stimulus elicited a bigger cortical response than a familiar one. Learning stage I

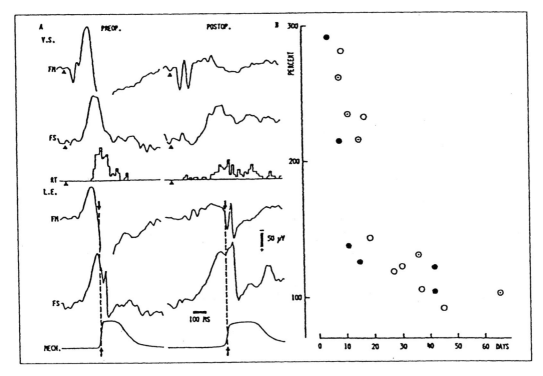

Figure 8–5. *A:* Cortical field potentials (S−D) from the forelimb motor (FM) and somatosensory (FS) cortices associated with visual-initiated hand movements before (PREOP.) and after (POSTOP.) cerebellar hemispherectomy. The same data were aligned 100 times by stimulus (triangle: upper half, visual stimulus [V.S.]) and movement (arrows with broken line: lower half, lever elevation [L.E.]) onset pulses respectively. *B:* Enhancement of pre-movement component (premovement area of S−D potential [ordinate]) of the somatosensory potentials after the cerebellar hemispherectomy is plotted against days after the operation [abscissa]. The three different symbols show data from three different monkeys. See text for further discussion. (*Source*: Reprinted from Sasaki and Gemba 1984b, with permission).

is divided into Ia and Ib, and is different from visual-initiated hand movement. Potentials were averaged 100 times by the stimulus onset pulse. When an upward (s-N, d-P) potential appeared and increased in the rostral bank of the inferior limb of the arcuate sulcus (A) in the left hemisphere, the monkey could associate the auditory stimulus with lever lifting (Ia–III, A and RT). As an upward (s-N, d-P) potential appeared and gradually increased in the motor cortex, the monkey gradually came to lift the lever appropriately and quickly (III–IV, C and RT). In the rostral bank of the inferior limb of the arcuate sulcus (A), the upward potential became larger at stage IV than at stage III. Such upward potential was scarcely recorded in the other prefrontal cortical areas (B, D, E) during the learning process. The upward potential in the motor cortex

was eliminated by the cerebellar hemispherectomy (not shown here); this potential is considered to be the same cerebellar-mediated potential as that in the visual-initiated hand movement. This suggests that skill learning is due to cerebrocerebellar interactions in conjuction with audio-initiated hand movements, as with visual-initiated hand movements (Gemba & Sasaki, 1987).

Analyses of cortical field potentials during learning processes of visual- and audio-initiated hand movements in monkeys showed that activities of the prefrontal cortex gradually increased during the early learning period of associating stimulus with movement (recognition learning) for both types of movement. Even if monkeys moved either their right or left hands, marked cortical activities were recorded in the rostral bank of the inferior limb

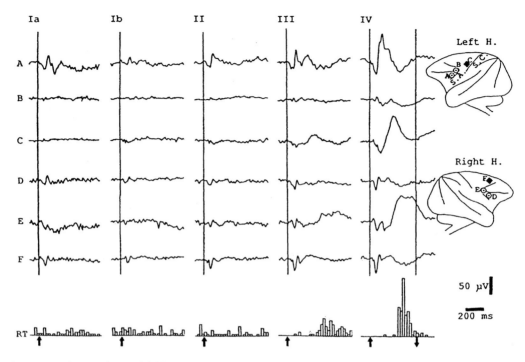

Figure 8–6. Changes of cortical field potentials (S–D) in learning processes of audio-initiated hand movements with complex tone in same monkey. Potentials were averaged 100 times by stimulus onset pulse (vertical line and upward arrows). Columns *Ia–III*: recognition learning; *III–IV*: skill learning. A–F: Cerebral cortical areas as indicated in diagrams (right). RT, reaction time histogram; S.A., arcuate sulcus; S.C., central sulcus; filled diamond, electrode loci in cerebral gyrus; circle with dot in center, electrode loci in bank of cerebral sulcus. See text for further discussion. (*Source*: Reprinted from Gemba et al., 1995a, with permission from Elsevier Science)

of the arcuate sulcus in the left cerebral hemisphere during recognition learning, whereas significant activities did not take place in the right hemisphere.

JUDGEMENT OR DECISION MAKING

To study the neural process of decision making, cortical field potentials were recorded and analyzed while monkeys learned go/no-go reaction time hand movements with tone discrimination. Tones of 1000 Hz and 2000 Hz with a duration of 500 ms were used as go and no-go stimuli. The go and no-go stimuli were given to the monkey in random order and at random intervals of 5.0–10.0 seconds. When the monkey lifted the lever by hand within 500 ms after the onset of the go stimulus, it was rewarded, whereas it was not rewarded after the no-go stimulus, regardless of whether it lifted or did not lift the lever. Changes in cortical field potentials in a single monkey while

it learns go/no-go reaction time hand movements with tone discrimination are shown in Figure 8–7.

Columns I, II, III, and IV show learning stages I, II, III, and IV, respectively. Potentials were averaged 100 times by onset pulses of go and no-go stimuli, respectively. The upper rows show go trials, and the lower rows show no-go trials. Data at stage I were recorded on the first training day. At stage I, the monkey responded to both go and no-go stimuli, and similar potentials were recorded on both stimuli, as in the case of simple-task, audio-initiated hand movements. Six days after stage I, an upward (s-N, d-P) potential emerged in the dorsal bank of the principal sulcus (II, B, lower row) on no-go trials, although the monkey still lifted the lever to both go and no-go stimuli (II, MECH., upper and lower rows). The upward potential started at about 100 ms after the onset of no-go stimuli (II, B, lower row). In the auditory association cortex (A),

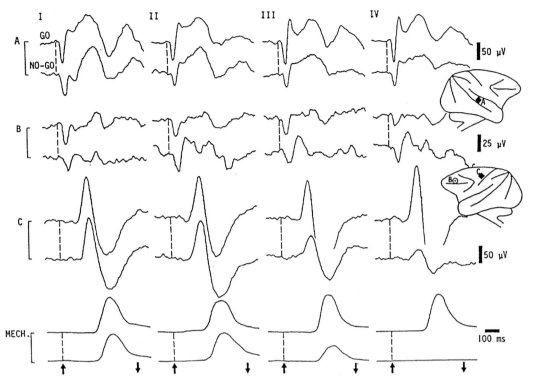

Figure 8–7. Changes of cortical field potentials (S−D) in a single monkey while it learns go/no-go reaction time hand movements with tone discrimination. Potentials were averaged 100 times by respective onset pulses of go (tone of 1000 Hz) and no-go (tone of 2000 Hz) stimuli. The onset and the end of auditory stimulus are shown by upward arrow and broken lines, and by downward arrow respectively. Columns *I–IV*: Learning stages I–IV. *A*: au-ditory association cortex; *B*: dorsal bank of principal sulcus; *C*: motor cortex. MECH., mechanogram; filled diamond, electrode loci in cerebral gyrus; circle with dot in center, electrode loci in bank of cerebral sulcus. The 50 μV amplitude scale is for *A* and *C*; the 25 μV amplitude scale is for *B*. See text for further discussion. (*Source*: Reprinted from Gemba 1993, with permission from Elsevier Science)

the upward (s-N, d-P) potential at a latency of about 50 ms became larger during stage II than at stage I on go as well as no-go trials (I and II, A, upper and lower rows). As respective upward potentials in the auditory association cortex (A) and in the dorsal bank of the principal sulcus (B) became more marked at stage III than in stage II, with further training for a week (II and III, A and B), the monkey began to stop the hand movement on no-go stimuli (MECH. rows in III). By the end of additional training for 6 days, the monkey had almost completely discriminated between go and no-go stimuli, as seen in the MECH. rows in IV. The upward potential in the motor cortex (C) on no-go trials became much smaller by stage IV than in stage III (III and IV, C, lower rows).

Sasaki and Gemba have termed the upward potential recorded only in no-go trials in the dorsal bank of the principal sulcus (B) the *no-go potential*, which is related to the judgement (or decision) not to move (Gemba & Sasaki, 1990; Gemba, 1993). Changes in upward potential in the auditory association cortex (A) during the process of learning the tone discrimination task may, however, reflect a scenario in which information about tone stimuli is processed in the auditory association cortex more carefully and attentively on the discrimination task than on the simple-task, audio-initiated hand movement, so that the go and no-go stimuli could be discriminated and judged in the prefrontal cortex.

Monkeys were also trained for go/no-go reaction time hand movement with color discrimination between green and red, and cortical field potentials were recorded in various cortices. The potentials were averaged 50 times by the onset pulses of go and no-go stimuli, respectively. An upward (s-N, d-P) potential at about 70 ms latency from stimulus was recorded in the dorsal bank of the principal sulcus and in the rostroventral corner of the prefrontal cortex in no-go trials only. The upward potential was assumed to be the no-go potential, related to the decision not to move (Sasaki & Gemba, 1986, 1989b, 1991a, 1991b, 1993c, Gemba et al., 1990; Sasaki et al., 1992). The electrodes chronically implanted in various cortical areas, for recording cortical field potentials, were also used for bipolar stimulation of the cortical area. A train of brief electrical pulses was delivered to the loci producible of the no-go potential at different times after the onset of go visual stimulus. The stimulation suppressed the go movement by cancelling and delaying it. The grade of the suppressor effect depended on the timing of electrical stimulation after the onset of visual stimulus, and was maximal at around the time of the appearance of the no-go potential. It was suggested that the no-go potential represented the suppressor action of the prefrontal areas by revoking and deferring the motor command initiated by the visual stimulus (Sasaki et al., 1989, 1994).

No-go potentials for visual stimuli have been recorded in the caudal part of the dorsal bank of the principal sulcus and the rostroventral corner in the prefrontal cortex on both sides. No-go potentials for auditory stimuli have been recorded in the rostral part of the principal sulcus (Fig. 8–8); Gemba & Sasaki, 1990). No-go potentials have also been recorded in humans (Gemba & Sasaki, 1989; Sasaki et al., 1993).

MOTIVATION-DEPENDENT ACTIVITY

It is generally known that the medial and ventral parts of the prefrontal cortex are mostly involved in affective and motivational functions and in the inhibitory control of both external influences and internal tendencies that interfere with purposive behavior and provoke inappropriate motor acts in monkeys. The dorsolateral part of the prefrontal cortex is, on the other hand, considered to be primarily involved in cognitive aspects of behavior. I have found motivation-dependent activity in the dorsolateral part of the prefrontal cortex in monkeys, as described below (Gemba & Sasaki, 1993, 1996; Gemba et al., 1997b).

Figure 8–9 shows data from monkeys that were well trained for visual-initiated hand movement. The left column (I, early) shows data from the first session of a day, and the right (I, late), data from the last session of the same day for the same monkey. Potentials are presented here only in S−D. In the first session, the monkey appeared to be thirsty and to lift the lever eagerly with intensive desire for a reward of juice, because the monkey had been given no water the day before the experiment. In this session, a large upward (s-N, d-P) potential at a latency of about 80 ms was recorded in the rostral bank of the arcuate sulcus (I, Early, A). A little later, cerebellar-mediated potential appeared markedly in the motor cortex along with short reaction times (I, Early, B and RT). In the last session, the monkey appeared to be tired of drinking the juice and lifting the lever. The upward potential in the prefrontal cortex decreased to about half the size of that in the first session (I, Late, A). The cerebellar-mediated potential in the motor cortex also became later in starting and smaller in size, with longer reaction times, than in the early session (I, Late, B and RT).

The relationship between the amplitude of the upward potential in the prefrontal cortex (closed circles) and the reaction time (open circles) is shown in Figure 8–9, part II. The data, obtained from a different monkey from the one in Figure 8–9, part I, were plotted for every session during a 4–day experiment. When the monkey eagerly lifted the lever with intensive motivation for reward early in the morning, the potential was large in amplitude with a short reaction time. As one session succeeded another, the potential gradually became smaller in amplitude with a longer reaction time. The results suggest that the upward potential in the prefrontal cortex is motivation-dependent activity. Such motivation-dependent activity was not re-

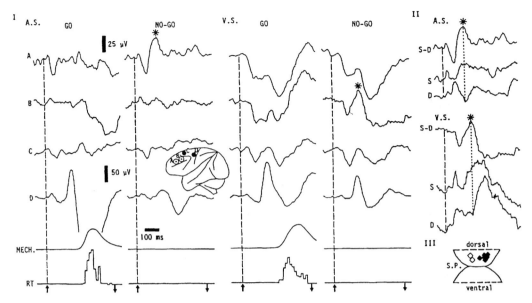

Figure 8–8. *I:* cortical field potentials (S−D) on go/no-go discriminative movements with auditory (A.S.) and visual (V.S.) stimuli in same monkey. Data are from the rostral (*A*) and caudal (*B*) parts of the dorsal bank of the principal sulcus, and the premotor (*C*) and forelimb motor (*D*) cortices, contralateral to the moving hand. Tones of 1000 Hz and 2000 Hz were used for go and no-go auditory stimuli respectively, while green and red colors were used for go and no-go visual stimuli respectively. Potentials were averaged 100 times by respective onset pulses of go (1000 Hz or green) and no-go (2000 Hz or red) stimuli. Onset and end of stimulus are shown by upward arrow and broken line, and by downward arrows, respectively. Note that no-go potentials (marked by asterisk) were recorded in the rostral (*A*) and caudal (*B*) parts of the dorsal bank of the principal sulcus, respectively on auditory and visual stimuli. S.P., principal sulcus; MECH., mechanogram; RT, reaction time histogram; filled circle, electrode loci in cerebral gyrus; circle with dot in center, electrode loci in bank of cerebral sulcus. The 25 μV amplitude scale is for A–C; the 50 μV amplitude scale is for D. *II:* The same surface minus depth (S−D) potentials as in the rostral (*A*) and caudal (*B*) parts of the dorsal bank of the principal sulcus respectively on no-go auditory and visual stimuli in I are shown together with the cortical surface (S) and depth (D) potentials. Note the s-N, d-P no-go potentials (marked by dotted lines with asterisks) respectively on auditory and visual stimuli. *III:* Distribution of the no-go potential in the dorsal bank of the principal sulcus, which is schematically unfolded. Broken lines (dorsal and ventral) should be together in composing the outer line of the principal sulcus when folded. Open diamond, no-go potential on auditory stimuli; filled diamond, no-go potential on visual stimuli. (*Source:* Reprinted from Gemba and Sasaki, 1990, with permission from Elsevier Science)

corded in the rostral bank of the inferior limb of the arcuate sulcus in the left hemisphere, which was reported to be related to recognition learning of associating a stimulus with movement in the learning processes of the visual- or audio-initiated hand movements. It appears probable that the motivation-dependent activity modulates motor responses through prefrontal cortico-cerebello-thalamo-motor cortical projections. Morphological studies have suggested that the nucleus ventralis anterior pars magnocellular (VAmg) thalamic nuclei are related to the initiation of motivation-dependent activity (Miki & Gemba, 1994).

Motivation-dependent potentials were also recorded in the monkey performing mouth movement at self-pace. Data from the session with the reward of apple juice are shown in the first and third columns in Figure 8–10; data from another session with a reward of water are in the second and fourth columns. The potentials were averaged 100 times by the onset pulse of mouth opening movement, and shown in S−D. In the rostral bank of the arcuate sulcus of the right hemisphere (D, E),

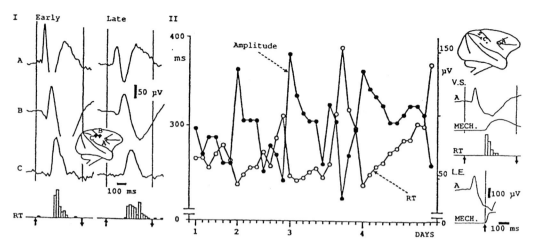

Figure 8–9. *I:* Cortical field potentials (S−D) in visual-initiated hand movements in a monkey. Potentials were averaged 100 times by stimulus onset pulse (vertical line and upward arrows). Data in the *Early* column are from the first session of the day; data in the *Late* column, from the last session. *A:* rostral bank of the arcuate sulcus; *B:* motor cortex; *C:* somatosensory cortex. RT, reaction time histogram; filled diamond, electrode loci in cerebral gyrus; circle with dot in center, electrode loci in bank of cerebral sulcus. *II:* Main diagram, relationship between peak amplitude of upward potential in the rostral bank of the arcuate sulcus (A) and mean reaction time. Note inverse relationship. Filled circle, upward potential in the prefrontal cortex; open circle, reaction time; V.S., visual stimulus; L.E., lever elevation; S.C., central sulcus; MECH., mechanogram. See text for further discussion. (*Source:* Reprinted from Gemba et al., 1997b, with permission from Elsevier Science)

an upward (s-N, d-P) potential occurred markedly in the session with a reward of juice, but it did not appear in the session with a reward of water. This suggests that the upward potential in the prefrontal cortex (D, E) is motivation-dependent activity. Such a potential did not occur at all in the loci of the left hemisphere (A, B).

The distribution of motivation-dependent potentials in monkeys performing visual-initiated and self-paced hand (and mouth-opening) movements in the cerebral hemisphere is shown in Figure 8–11. The motivation-dependent potential was mainly recorded in the rostral bank of the arcuate sulcus on both sides, except for the inferior limb of the arcuate sulcus in the left hemisphere and in the cingulate cortex in the left hemisphere.

SUMMARY

The rostral bank of the inferior limb of the arcuate sulcus in the left hemisphere was found to be related to recognition learning of associating stimulus with movement in the learning processes of visual- or audio-initiated hand movements, while the other rostral banks of the arcuate sulcus showed motivation-dependent activity. The dorsal bank of the principal sulcus, however, was related to deciding not to move. Neuroimaging studies in normal human subjects and patients with focal brain lesions have shown that the left dorsolateral prefrontal cortex is of significance for visuomotor learning (Toni & Passingham, 1999), and that the dorsolateral prefrontal cortex is related to inhibitory control of sensory processing (Chao & Knight, 1998). These activities in the prefrontal cortex seem to modulate hand movements through neuronal connections between the prefrontal cortex, cerebellum, ventrolateral thalamic nuclei, and the forelimb motor cortex.

VOCALIZATION

MOTOR EXECUTION AND MOTIVATION-DEPENDENT ACTIVITY

It is generally said that animal vocalization differs fundamentally from human speech—namely in that a major pattern of human vocal

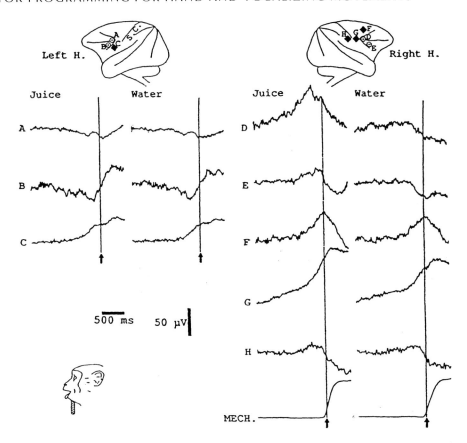

Figure 8–10. Cortical field potentials (S–D) associated with self-paced mouth movements in a monkey. Data are from 100 mouth movements with reward of juice (Juice) and 100 movements with reward of water (Water). Potentials were averaged 100 times by movement onset pulse (vertical line and upward arrows). MECH., mechanogram; S.C., central sulcus; filled diamond, electrode loci in cerebral gyrus; circle with dot in center, electrode loci in bank of cerebral sulcus. See text for further discussion.

behavior is be acquired by learning. Animal vocalization is largely considered to be genetically preprogrammed utterances, relating simply to internal states or courses of action and being similar to emotional vocal manifestation in humans (Robinson, 1967; Sutton et al., 1974; Aitken, 1981; Kirzinger & Jürgens, 1982). Physiological studies have reported that the hypothalamus and the limbic system are related to generation and control of animal vocalization, but not the neocortical areas. Some ethological studies have reported, however, that primate utterances could provide evidence of communicative intentionality, convey specific information concerning environmental referents to conspecific animals, and display a syntactical organization. To study which cortices are activated in association with monkey vocalization, and how, monkeys were trained to vocalize at self-pace many times, and cortical field potentials were recorded in various cortical areas and analyzed. It was found that the neocortical area homologous to the human speech area took part in the generation and control of monkey vocalization, as described below (Gemba et al., 1995b).

Cortical field potentials associated with self-paced vocalization are shown in Figure 8–12. Vocalization was recorded through a microphone near the monkey's mouth, and then amplified. A vocalization sample and its sonagram are shown in Figure 8–12, part III. Data are from the cingulate gyrus (A), the SMA (B), the caudal bank of the arcuate sulcus (homolog of the Broca's area) (C), and the face motor (D) and somatosensory (E) cortices. Field potentials and vocalizations were averaged 100 times, respectively, by the vocalization onset

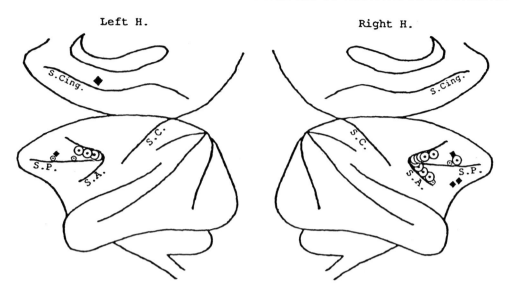

Figure 8–11. Cortical areas of motivation-dependent activity in the dorsal and mesial aspects of the left and right cerebral hemispheres in seven monkeys are marked by two different symbols. S.P., principal sulcus; S.A., arcuate sulcus; S.C., central sulcus; S. Cing., cingulate sulcus; filled diamond, electrode loci in cerebral gyrus; circle with dot in center, electrode loci in bank of cerebral sulcus. See text for further discussion.

pulse. Surface-negative, depth-positive (s-N, d-P) potentials started about 1 second before the vocalization in all of the cortical loci. To further study how significant the s-N, d-P, premovement potentials are for monkeys to vocalize, field potentials were recorded in connection with various emotional states and then analyzed.

In Figure 8–13, data in the left (I, motivated) and middle (II, less-motivated) columns were recorded in the first and last sessions of the same day, respectively. The monkey was seen to vocalize 100 times eagerly with intense motivation for reward of juice in the first session (I), because the monkey had been given no water the day before the experiment. But in the last session (II), the monkey might have been less motivated for reward because it had already drunk a lot of juice as reward for more than 700 vocalizations. The right column (III, irritated) shows data from a session on another day. In this session, the monkey was not rewarded for vocalization. In this session, the monkey seemed to vocalize with irritation and anger. The potentials were averaged 100 times by movement onset pulse, and are shown in S−D. There were not so clear changes in the upward (s-N, d-P) premove-

ment potentials in the SMA and the premotor and motor, somatosensory cortices among the three sessions of different emotional states. In the cingulate and prefrontal cortices, however, the upward (s-N, d-P) premovement potentials in the less-motivated session decreased to about half the size of that in the motivated session, and no potentials were recorded prior to vocalization in the irritated session. Similar results were obtained from five monkeys. It was found that readiness potentials for vocalization were recorded in the premotor, motor, and somatosensory cortices in both hemispheres and in the SMA in the left hemisphere. The motivation-dependent potentials were, however, recorded in the rostral bank of the arcuate sulcus in both hemispheres (except for the inferior limb of the arcuate sulcus in the left hemisphere) as well as in the cingulate cortex in the left hemisphere.

Some influences of right hemicerebellectomy on the potentials and vocalization were also studied. The left (I, motivated) and middle (II, irritated) columns in Figure 8–14 show data from before cerebellectomy, and the right (III, motivated) column shows data from after cerebellectomy. The readiness potentials in the caudal bank of the arcuate sulcus (homo-

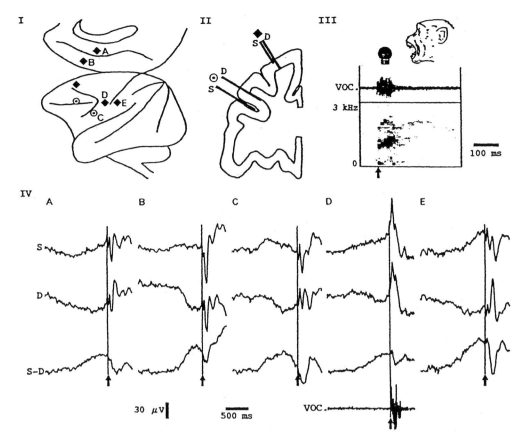

Figure 8–12. Cortical field potentials associated with self-paced vocalization. *I:* Electrode loci of recording specimens in panel IV. Filled diamond, electrode loci in cerebral gyrus; circle with dot in center, electrode loci in bank of cerebral sulcus. *II:* Recording electrodes in the dorsolateral cortex (marked by filled diamond) and in the dorsal bank of the principal sulcus (marked by circle with dot in center) are schematically illustrated in the frontal section. *III:* A vocalization sample (top) (VOC.) and its sonagram (bottom) are shown. *IV:* Cortical field potentials associated with self-paced vocalization. Potentials were averaged 100 times by vocalization onset pulse (vertical lines and upward arrows). *A:* cingulate gyrus; *B:* supplementary motor area; *C:* caudal bank of arcuate sulcus; *D:* face motor cortex; *E:* face somatosensory cortex. S, surface potential; D, depth potential; S–D, surface minus depth potential; filled diamond, electrode loci in cerebral gyrus; circle with dot in center, electrode loci in bank of cerebral sulcus. See text for further discussion. (*Source:* Reprinted from Gemba et al., 1995b, with permission from Elsevier Science)

log of the Broca's area) (B) and motor cortex (C) were almost entirely eliminated after the hemicerebellectomy, as seen in the upper part of the figure. After the operation, the tone of vocalization came to have fewer different frequencies, and its duration varied much more than before, as seen in sonagrams in the lower part. These results suggest that the neocortical area homologous to the human speech area and the cerebellum take part in the generation and control of monkey vocalization, possibly through cerebrocerebellar interac-

tions (Gemba et al., 1995b, 1997a, 1998a). From morphological and electrical stimulation study it appears that the cerebello–nucleus ventralis posterior pars oralis (VPLC)–motor area and cerebello–area x–premotor area neuronal connections are probably active during monkey vocalization (Kyuhou et al., 1997).

MOTOR LEARNING

Studies on cortical involvement in monkey vocal communication have seemed to be helpful

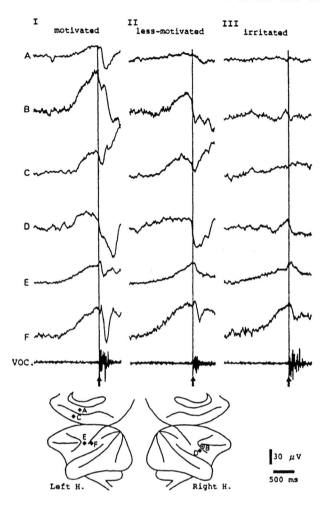

Figure 8–13. Cortical field potentials (S−D) associated with self-paced vocalization in various emotional states in same monkey. *A:* cingulate gyrus; *B:* rostral bank of arcuate sulcus; *C:* supplementary motor area; *D:* premotor cortex; *E:* face motor cortex; *F:* face somatosensory cortex. Potentials were averaged 100 times by vocalization onset pulse (vertical line and upward arrows). VOC., vocalization sample; filled diamond, electrode loci in cerebral gyrus; circle with dot in center, electrode loci in bank of cerebral sulcus. See text for further discussion. (*Source:* Reprinted from Gemba et al. 1995b, with permission from Elsevier Science)

for clarifying the brain mechanism in human speech. Therefore, I attempted to make an experimental model of vocal communication using monkeys. I started to train a monkey to respond to auditory stimulus (monkey's coo call with 400 msec duration) with vocalization (audio-initiated vocalization). After intimate and intensive training over a long period (6 days a week for 3–6 months), five of seven monkeys vocalizing at self-pace came to vocalize in response to an auditory stimulus, whereas the remaining two monkeys could not. This indicated that it was more difficult for monkeys to learn audio-initiated vocalizations, than to learn audio-initiated hand movements. The five monkeys were further trained for audio-initiated vocalization for more than 2 months, then recording electrodes were implanted in various cortices. Cortical field po-

tentials associated with audio-initiated and self-paced vocalizations in a single well-trained monkey are shown in Figure 8–15.

The first (I, aud-init) and second (II, aud-init) columns show data on audio-initiated vocalization, while the third (III, self-pac) shows data on self-paced vocalization. The fourth column shows vocalization samples and their sonagrams of audio-initiated and self-paced vocalizations. Potentials were averaged 100 times by the stimulus onset pulse in the first column, while the second and third columns show data averaged 100 times by the vocalization onset pulse. Potentials are shown in S−D. In the rostral bank of the inferior limb of the arcuate sulcus (A), no significant potential occurred in association with self-paced vocalizations, whereas an upward (s-N, d-P) potential at 70 msec latency after the stimulus

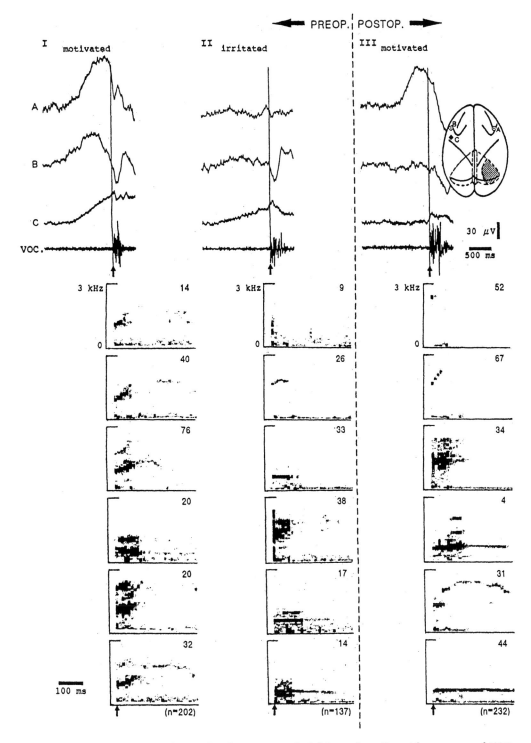

Figure 8–14. Cortical field potentials (S−D) and sonagrams of vocalization calls associated with self-paced vocalization in same monkey. Columns *I* and *II* show data in motivated and irritated states, respectively, before the resection of the cerebellum on the right side, while column *III* shows data of a motivated state after the operation. Data are from the rostral bank (*A*) of the arcuate sulcus in the right cerebral hemisphere, and the caudal bank (*B*) of the arcuate sulcus and face motor cortex (*C*) in the left hemisphere. Potentials were averaged 100 times by vocalization onset pulse (vertical line and upward arrows). The 500 ms time scale is for cortical potentials; the 100 ms time scale for sonagrams. VOC., vocalization sample; filled diamond, electrode loci in cerebral gyrus; circle with dot in center, electrode loci in bank of cerebral sulcus. See text for further discussion. (*Source:* Reprinted from Gemba et al. 1995b, with permission from Elsevier Science)

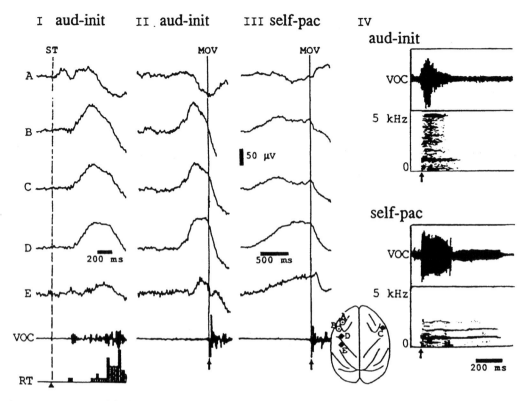

Figure 8–15. *I:* Cortical field potentials (S−D) in audio-initiated vocalization (aud-init) in a single monkey. Potentials were averaged 100 times by stimulus onset pulse (broken line and triangles). *II:* Data in column I were averaged 100 times by vocalization start (vertical line and upward arrows). *III:* Cortical field potentials (S−D) during self-paced vocalization (self-pac) in same monkey. Potentials were averaged 100 times by vocalization start. The 200 ms time scale for all records in column I; the 500 ms time scale is for those in columns II–III. *IV:* Vocalization sample (VOC) and its sonagram associated with audio-initiated vocalization in column I (top) and with self-paced vocalization in column III (bottom). Data are from the rostral *(A)* and caudal *(B)* banks of the arcuate sulcus, and the face motor *(D)* and somatosensory *(E)* cortices in the left cerebral hemisphere, and the premotor cortex *(C)* in the right hemisphere. RT, reaction time histogram; filled diamond, electrode loci in cerebral gyrus; circle with dot in center, electrode loci in bank of cerebral sulcus. See text for further discussion. (*Source:* Reprinted from Gemba et al., 1999a, with permission from Elsevier Science)

was associated with audio-initiated vocalizations (I and III, A). This potential appears to be related to associating stimuli with vocalizing movements, as in audio-initiated hand movements. In the motor cortex (C), an upward (s-N, d-P) potential in association with audio-initiated vocalizations was recorded at about 200 msec latency from the stimulus and 700 msec before the vocalization onset (I and II, C). The potential was almost the same as the readiness potential on self-paced vocalizations. Reaction times were irregular, but averaged about 0.9 seconds (I, RT) (Gemba et al., 1998a; 1999a).

Changes in field potentials during relearning processes of audio-initiated vocalization in a single monkey that had forgotten the vocalization task after not performing it for more than 2 months were also recorded and analyzed (not shown here). Relearning stages were divided into three. Relearning stages I to III corresponded to learning stages I to III, respectively, in learning processes of audio- or visual-initiated hand movements. When an upward (s-N, d-P) potential at 70 msec latency after the stimulus emerged, at stage II in the rostral bank of the inferior limb of the arcuate sulcus, and increased, the monkey came to vocalize in response to the stimulus. The reaction times at stage III were rather irregular, but averaged about 0.9 seconds. The relearning processes were similar to those of recognition learning in visual- or audio-initiated hand movements. Further intensive training of audio-initiated vocalizations did not make the monkey perform the task more appropriately and quickly. This finding indicates that there is no skill learning in audio-initiated vocalization, in contrast with audio-initiated hand movement. As for reaction time hand movements, skill learning elicited marked differences between audio-initiated and self-paced hand movements in the upward (s-N, d-P) potentials in the motor cortex (see Figs. 8–4, 8–5 and 8–6). Moreover, reaction times were gradually shortened during the skill learning of audio- and visual-initiated hand movements, while longer and more variable reaction times were recorded in the monkey fully trained for audio-initiated vocalization. This result shows that there is a big contrast between audio-initiated vocalizations and hand movements (Gemba et al., 1998b, 1999b).

The influence of right hemicerebellectomy on cortical field potentials and vocalizations was studied in the monkey on audio-initiated vocalization. It was found that the hemicerebellectomy eliminated the upward potential in the motor cortex and changed vocal tone in the audio-initiated vocalization (not shown here). But there was hardly any change in reaction time before and after the operation. This finding suggests that there is a great difference between cerebellar actions during audio-initiated vocalizations and those during hand movements (Gemba et al., 1999b).

It took 10 to 20 times longer for a monkey to be trained for audio-initiated vocalization than for audio-initiated hand movement, as described above. The correct response rate (correct response number divided by stimulus number) was very different for audio-initiated hand movements and audio-initiated vocalization. The rate of audio-initiated vocalizations varied greatly from day to day, even after the accomplishment of the task, whereas the rate of audio-initiated hand movements increased in connection with the learning processes of the task. This suggests that vocalization is more easily influenced by motivation to perform (or not) than by hand movement.

Cerebrocerebellar interactions—that is, the prefrontal cortex–pontein nucleus–cerebellum–thalamus–motor cortex neural circuits are activated to skillfully perform audio-initiated hand movements. These neural circuits are also activated to perform audio-initiated vocalizations, but a separate neural circuit may break into these circuits and hinder the skillfulness of the movement. From morphological and lesion studies on the frontal lobe in monkeys, a possible candidate for such a circuit is the reciprocal neural circuit between the prefrontal cortex and the rostral cingulate gyrus. Through this circuit, information concerning emotion or instinctive behaviors may intrude into the cerebrocerebellar interactions in audio-initiated vocalizations. The limbic system seems to be more significant in vocalization than in hand movement in the monkey.

SUMMARY

The neocortical area homologous to the human speech area takes part in the generation and control of monkey vocalization through neuronal connections between the prefrontal cortex, cerebellum, VPLo thalamic nuclei (or area x thalamic nuclei), and the face motor cortex (or the premotor cortex). In fact, clinical and neuroimaging studies of patients with neurological disorders have shown that the left prefrontal cortex is significant for word generation (Stevens et al., 1998; Stuss et al., 1998; Thompson Schill et al., 1998). I also found that central nervous mechanisms in audio-initiated vocalization differed from those for audio-initiated hand movements.

CONCLUSION

The prefrontal cortex continuously receives information on emotion or internal states from the limbic system, while outward information is transmitted into the prefrontal cortex from a sensory organ through the sensory cortex. Through the studies presented in this chapter, it is suggested that the specific response to information—i.e., to move or not to move, and to move willingly or reluctantly, is judged and decided on in the prefrontal cortex. It is also suggested that the limbic system is more significant in vocalization than in hand movements. If information is properly managed in the prefrontal cortex so that it is prepared for the SMA and the premotor, motor, and somatosensory cortices, where it will be used to ensure reasonable behavior, we can expect to live together pleasantly—many persons, in harmony with nature, on the earth.

REFERENCES

Aitken, P.G. (1981). Cortical control of conditioned and spontaneous vocal behavior in rhesus monkeys. *Brain and Language, 13,* 171–184.

Chao, L.L. & Knight, R.T. (1998). Contribution of human prefrontal cortex to delay performance. *Journal of Cognitive Neuroscience, 10,* 167–177.

Doyon, J., Owen, A.M., Petrides, M., Sziklas, V., & Evans, A.C. (1996). Functional anatomy of visuomotor skill learning in human subjects examined with positron emission tomography. *European Journal of Neuroscience, 8,* 637–648.

Gemba, H. (1993). Changes in cortical field potentials during learning processes of go/no-go reaction time hand movement with tone discrimination in the monkey. *Neuroscience Letters, 159,* 21–24.

Gemba, H. (1996). Intellect, emotion and will and the frontal lobe. In: T. Itakura & T. Maeda (Eds.), *The Frontal Lobe* (pp. 39–59). Tokyo: Burenn Shuppann (translated from Japanese).

Gemba, H. & Sasaki, K. (1984a). Studies on cortical field potentials recorded during learning processes of visually initiated hand movements in monkeys. *Experimental Brain Research, 55,* 26–32.

Gemba, H. & Sasaki, K.(1984b). Distribution of potentials preceding visually initiated and self-paced hand movements in various cortical areas of the monkey. *Brain Research, 306,* 207–214.

Gemba, H. & Sasaki, K. (1987). Cortical field potentials associated with audio-initiated hand movements in the monkey. *Experimental Brain Research, 65,* 649–657.

Gemba, H. & Sasaki, K. (1988). Changes in cortical field potentials associated with learning processes of audio-initiated hand movements in monkeys. *Experimental Brain Research, 70,* 43–49.

Gemba, H. & Sasaki, K, (1989). Potentials related to no-go reaction in go/no-go hand movement task with color discrimination in human. *Neuroscience Letters, 101,* 263–268.

Gemba, H. & Sasaki, K. (1990). Potential related to no-go reaction in go/no-go hand movement with discrimination between tone stimuli of different frequencies in the monkey. *Brain Research, 537,* 340–344.

Gemba, H. & Sasaki, K. (1993). Functional differences between the prefrontal cortices of left and right cerebral hemispheres in the monkey. *Japanese Journal of Physiology (Suppl.), 43,* S250.

Gemba, H. & Sasaki, K. (1996). Cortical field potentials and emotion in the monkey. In: C. Ogura, et al. (Eds.), *Recent Advances in Event-Related Brain Potential Research* (pp. 327–333). Amsterdam: Elsevier.

Gemba, H., Hashimoto, S., & Sasaki, K. (1979). Slow potentials preceding self-paced hand movements in the parietal cortex of monkeys. *Neuroscience Letters, 15,* 87–92.

Gemba, H., Sasaki, K., & Hashimoto, S. (1980). Distribution of premovement slow cortical potentials associated with self-paced hand movements in monkeys. *Neuroscience Letters, 20,* 159–163.

Gemba, H., Hashimoto, S., & Sasaki, K. (1981). Cortical field potentials preceding visually initiated hand movements in the monkey. *Experimental Brain Research, 42,* 435–441.

Gemba, H., Sasaki, K., & Ito, J. (1982). Different cortical potentials preceding self-paced and visually initiated hand movements and their reciprocal transition in the same monkey. *Brain Research, 306,* 207–214.

Gemba, H., Sasaki, K., & Tsujimoto, T. (1990). No-go potential in monkeys and human subjects. In C.H.M. Brunia, et al. (Eds.), *Psychophysiological Brain Research* (pp. 133–136). Tilburg: Tilburg University Press.

Gemba, H., Miki, N., & Sasaki, K. (1995a). Field potential change in the prefrontal cortex of the left hemisphere during learning processes of reaction-time hand movement with complex tone in the monkey. *Neuroscience Letters, 190,* 93–96.

Gemba, H., Miki, N., & Sasaki, K. (1995b). Cortical field potentials preceding vocalization and influences of cerebellar hemispherectomy upon them in monkeys. *Brain Research, 697,* 143–151.

Gemba, H., Miki, N., & Sasaki, K. (1997a). Cortical field potentials preceding vocalization in monkeys. *Acta Oto-Laryngologica, Supplement, 532,* 96–98.

Gemba, H., Miki, N., Sasaki, K., Kyuhou, S., Matsuzaki, R., & Yoshimura, H. (1997b). Motivation-dependent activity in the dorsolateral part of the prefrontal cortex in the monkey. *Neuroscience Letters, 230,* 133–136.

Gemba, H., Kyuhou, S., Matsuzaki, R., & Amino, Y. (1998a). Cortical field potentials preceding vocalization in monkeys. *Proceedings of the Australian Physiological and Pharmacological Society, 29,* 24.

Gemba, H., Kyuhou, S., Matsuzaki, R., & Amino, Y. (1998b). Different central nervous mechanisms in audio-initiated vocalizations from audio-initiated hand movements in the monkey. *Japanese Journal of Physiology (Suppl.), 48,* S162.

Gemba, H., Kyuhou, S., Matsuzaki, R., & Amino, Y. (1999a). Cortical field potentials associated with audio-initiated vocalization in monkeys. *Neuroscience Letters, 272,* 49–52.

Gemba, H., Kyuhou, S., Matsuzaki, R., & Amino, Y.

(1999b). Cortical field potentials associated with audio-initiated vocalization and influences of cerebellar nuclei resection upon them in monkeys. *International Journal of Psychophysiology, 33,* S66.

Kirzinger, A., & Jürgens, U. (1982). Cortical lesion effects and vocalization in the squirrel monkey. *Brain Research, 233,* 299–315.

Kyuhou, S., Matsuzaki, R., & Gemba, H. (1997). Cerebello-cerebral projections onto the ventral part of the frontal cortex of the macaque monkey. *Neuroscience Letters, 230,* 101–104.

Miki, N. & Gemba, H. (1994). Thalamocortical projections from the anterior thalamus onto layer 1 of the prefrontal cortex in monkeys. *Japanese Journal of Physiology (Suppl.), 44,* S229.

Robinson, B. (1967). Vocalization evoked from forebrain in Macaca mulatta. *Physiology and Behavior, 2,* 345–354.

Sasaki, K. (1979). Cerebro-cerebellar interconnections in cats and monkeys. In J. Massion, et al. (Eds.), *Cerebro-cerebellar Interactions* (pp. 105–124). Amsterdam: Elsevier, North-Holland.

Sasaki, K. & Gemba, H. (1981a). Changes of premovement field potentials in the cerebral cortex during learning processes of visually initiated hand movements in the monkey. *Neuroscience Letters, 27,* 125–130.

Sasaki, K. & Gemba, H. (1981b). Cortical field potentials preceding self-paced and visually initiated hand movements in one and the same monkey and influences of cerebellar hemispherectomy upon the potentials. *Neuroscience Letters, 25,* 287–292.

Sasaki, K. & Gemba, H. (1982). Development and change of cortical field potentials during learning processes of visually initiated hand movements in the money. *Experimental Brain Research, 48,* 459–473.

Sasaki, K. & Gemba, H. (1983). Learning of fast and stable hand movement and cerebro-cerebellar interactions in the monkey. *Brain Research, 277,* 41–46.

Sasaki, K. & Gemba, H. (1984a). Compensatory motor function of the somatosensory cortex for the motor cortex temporarily impaired by cooling in the monkey. *Experimental Brain Research, 55,* 60–68.

Sasaki, K. & Gemba, H. (1984b). Compensatory motor function of the somatosensory cortex for dysfunction of the motor cortex following cerebellar hemispherectomy in the monkey. *Experimental Brain Research, 56,* 532–538.

Sasaki, K. & Gemba, H. (1986). Electrical activity in the potential cortex specific to no-go reaction of conditioned hand movement with colour discrimination in the monkey. *Experimental Brain Research, 64,* 603–606.

Sasaki, K. & Gemba, H. (1989a). Motor Programme for voluntary movement in the cerebro-cerebellar neuronal circuit. In: M. Ito (Ed.), *Taniguchi Symposia on Brain Science No. 12: Neural Programming* (pp. 67–76), Basel: S. Karger Publishing.

Sasaki, K. & Gemba, H. (1989b). "No-go potential" in the prefrontal cortex of monkeys. In: E. Basar, et al. (Eds.), *Springer Series in Brain Dynamics* (pp. 290–301). New York: Springer-Verlag.

Sasaki, K. & Gemba, H. (1991a). How do the different cortical motor areas contribute to motor learning and compensation following brain dysfunction? In: D.R. Humphrey, et al. (Eds.), *Motor Control: Concepts and Issues* (pp. 445–461). New York: John Wiley & Sons.

Sasaki, K. & Gemba, H. (1991b). Cortical potentials associated with voluntary movements in monkeys. In: C.H.M. Brunia, et al. (Eds.), *Event-related Brain Reserch,* Electroenceph. clin. Neurophysiol, suppl 42, 80–96.

Sasaki, K. & Gemba, H. (1993a). Action of the cerebello-thalamo-cortical projection upon visually initiated reaction-time hand movements in the monkey. *Stereotactic and Functional Neurosurgery, 60,* 104–120.

Sasaki, K. & Gemba, H. (1993b). Cerebro-cerebellar interactions: For fast and stable timing of voluntary movement. In: N. Mano, et al. (Eds.), *Role of the Cerebellum and Basal Ganglia in Voluntary Movement* (pp. 41–50). Amsterdam: Elsevier.

Sasaki, K. & Gemba, H. (1993c). Prefrontal cortex in the organization and control of voluntary movement. In: T. Ono, et al. (Eds.), *Brain Mechanism of Perception and Memory: From Neuron to Behavior* (pp. 473–496). New York: Oxford University Press.

Sasaki, K., Gemba, H., Hashimoto, S., & Mizuno, N. (1979). Influences of cerebellar hemispherectomy on slow potentials in the motor cortex preceding self-paced hand movements in the monkey. *Neuroscience Letters, 15,* 23–28.

Sasaki, K., Gemba, H., & Hashimoto, S. (1981a). Influences of cerebellar hemispherectomy upon cortical potentials preceding visually initiated hand movements in the monkey. *Brain Research, 205,* 425–430.

Sasaki, K., Gemba, H., & Hashimoto, S. (1981b). Premovement slow cortical potentials on self-paced hand movements and thalamo-cortical and cortico-cortical responses in the monkey. *Experimental Neurology, 72,* 41–50.

Sasaki, K., Gemba, H., & Mizuno, N. (1982). Cortical field potentials preceding visually initiated hand movements and cerebellar actions in the monkey. *Experimental Brain Research, 46,* 29–36.

Sasaki, K., Gemba, H., & Tsujimoto, T. (1989). Suppression of visually initiated hand movement by stimulation of the prefrontal cortex. *Brain Research, 495,* 100–107.

Sasaki, K., Gemba, H., Nambu, A., Jinnai, K., Yamamoto, T., & Llinas, R. (1992). Cortical activity specific to no-go reaction in go/no-go reaction time hand movement with colour discrimination in monkeys and human subjects. *Biomedical Research (Suppl.), 13,* 5–9.

Sasaki, K., Gemba, H., Nambu, A., & Matsuzaki, R. (1993). No-go activity in the frontal association cortex of human subjects. *Neuroscience Research, 18,* 249–252.

Sasaki, K., Gemba, H., Nambu, A., & Matsuzaki, R. (1994). Activity of the prefrontal cortex on no-go decision and motor suppression. In: A.M. Thierry, et al. (Eds.), *Motor and Cognitive Functions of the Prefrontal Cortex* (pp. 139–159). Berlin: Springer-Verlag.

Stevens, A.A., Goldman-Rakic, P.S., Gore, J.C., Fulbright, R.K., & Wexler, B.E. (1998). Cortical dysfunction in schizophrenia during auditory word and tone working memory demonstrated by functional magnetic resonance imaging. *Archives of General Psychiatry, 55,* 1097–1103.

Stuss, D.T., Alexander, M.P., Hamer, L., Palumbo, C., Dempster, R., Binns, M., Levine, B., & Izukawa, D. (1998). The effects of focal anterior and posterior brain lesions on verbal fluency. *Journal of the International Neuropsychological Society, 4,* 265–278.

Sutton, D., Larson, C., & Lindeman, R.C. (1974). Neocortical and limbic lesion effects on primate phonation. *Brain Research, 71,* 61–75.

Thompson-Schill, S.L., Swick, D., Farah, M.J.,

D'Esposito, M., Kan, I.P., & Knight, R.T. (1998). Verb generation in patients with focal frontal lesions: a neuropsychological test of neuroimaging findings. *Proceedings of the National Academy of Sciences USA, 95,* 15855–15860.

Toni, I. & Passingham, R.E. (1999). Prefrontal–basal ganglia pathways are involved in the learning of arbitrary visuomotor associations: a PET study. *Experimental Brain Research, 127,* 19–32.

Tsujimoto, T., Gemba, H., & Sasaki, K. (1993). Effect of cooling the dentate nucleus of the cerebellum on hand movement of the monkey. *Brain Research, 629,* 1–9.

9

Cortical Control of Visuomotor Reflexes

ROBERT RAFAL

In 1973, Easton published an essay in the *American Scientist* entitled "The Normal Use of Reflexes" (Easton, 1973). Its theme was that the neural circuits that subserve reflexes are the building blocks for more complex behavior, and that the nervous system routinely goes about its business through an orchestration of those circuits by cortical processes that activate or inhibit them. With regard to the frontal lobes, I've come to think of this as the Apollo 13 framework.

You may recall that three astronauts were on their way to the moon when something went seriously wrong. Finding themselves stranded between the earth and the moon they reported to mission control, "Houston, we have a problem." In the movie made about their plight, one particular scene made an impression on me. Their CO_2 scrubber was dying, and they would too if they couldn't get a new one. The mission control boss called the engineers into a room and, showing them an item in his hand, he said, "this is a CO_2 scrubber." Then pointing to a bunch of junk on a table, he said, "this is everything they have with them up there." The survival of the astronauts required that they figure out how to make a CO_2 scrubber out of all that junk.

The predicament of the Apollo 13 astronauts is, of course, exactly that of a species confronting evolutionary pressures. To meet new demands and survive it has to make use of those circuits that have been bequeathed to it by its own evolutionary history. In this regard the frontal lobes can be thought of as a toolmaker; they use old circuits to solve new problems. Reflex circuitry provides the tools that the toolmaker uses to make new tools. This job may require putting these circuits to uses quite different from those that they originally evolved for, holding them online in working memory to be integrated with other circuits, and inhibiting their "default mode."

This chapter will explore this framework by examining eye movements as a model system. We will first take a look at eye movement reflexes, and the midbrain circuits that mediate them. I'll then review studies that have examined the cortical systems of the frontal and parietal lobe that put this oculomotor machinery to use in the service of goal-directed behavior.

THE VISUAL GRASP REFLEX: MIDBRAIN MECHANISMS FOR REFLEXIVE ORIENTING

Our neural machinery for visual orienting is the product of a long evolutionary history (Ingle, 1973). All vertebrates have primitive mid-brain circuits for reflexively orienting the eyes toward salient events occurring in the visual periphery. In foveate mammals, including humans, these archetypal pathways function to align high-acuity regions of the retina with objects of potential interest; but their activity must be coordinated with a phylogenetically new visual cortex that receives its dominant input from the retina through the lateral geniculate nucleus of the thalamus. The demands of increasingly complex visual cognition presumably generated the evolutionary pressures leading to the development of a completely new, parallel visual pathway in mammals. What function does the phylogenetically older midbrain pathway serve in humans?

Two converging strands of research in neurological patients have been used to investigate human extrageniculate pathways for mediating visuomotor reflexes. One approach has been to study the effects of midbrain lesions on orienting behavior. Another has been to study heminaopic patients in order to identify what visuomotor reflexes are present when only subcortical visual pathways are available. Patients with degeneration of the midbrain from progressive supranuclear palsy (PSP) were shown to be impaired not only in moving their eyes but also in shifting covert attention (Rafal et al., 1988). We also showed that midbrain circuits damaged in PSP are involved in the generation of an inhibitory spatial tag, called *inhibition of return* (IOR) (Posner et al., 1985). This inhibitory tag has been shown to serve an important function as a "foraging facilitator" that optimizes the efficiency of visual search by favoring novelty (Klein & MacInnes, 1999). More recent studies have provided converging evidence for midbrain mediation of IOR. Sapir and colleagues reported that IOR was abolished in the visual field contralateral to a unilateral lesion of the colliculus (Sapir et al., 1999). Furthermore, we have shown that IOR could be generated in the blind field of a hemianopic patient, even in the absence of awareness of the stimuli that evokes it (Danziger et al., 1997).

We live in a world of moving objects and so, while IOR may be generated in the colliculus, if this inhibitory tag is to be useful in regulat-ing visual search, it might be expected that the tag would be transmitted to a cortical object-based reference frame. Tipper and colleagues have shown that IOR can tag and follow moving objects. We showed in split-brain patients that interhemispheric transmission of this tag requires an intact corpus callosum (Tipper et al., 1997). When an object tagged by a cue moved within a hemifield, IOR was observed, but not when the object crossed the midline and had to be represented in the opposite hemisphere. It seems likely, then, that IOR is generated and maintained in a corticocollicular circuit. As this example of the inhibitory tagging illustrates, the phylogenetically older and the newer cortical systems must be integrated to provide a coherence of goal-directed behavior and a continuity of perceptual experience. The remainder of this chapter will review some of what has been learned about interactions between midbrain and cerebral cortex in humans.

CORTICOCOLLICULAR INTERACTIONS

Frontal and parietal cortex both have regions involved in oculomotor control. They are connected to one another and both are connected to the superior colliculus. The frontal eye fields are located just anterior to the motor hand area of each hemisphere, at the junction of the superior frontal sulcus and the precentral sulcus. It projects to the superior colliculus both directly and via the basal ganglia through the caudate nucleus and the substantia nigra pars reticulata (see Fig.9–1). The substantia nigra has inhibitory, GABAnergic projections to the colliculus on the same side, and crossed projections to the contralateral colliculus. The parietal eye fields are located in the intraparietal sulcus. They receive input from the colliculus through the pulvinar nucleus of the thalamus; and they can influence the colliculus, in part through connections to primary visual cortex.

In the following sections, I will first summarize the pioneering work of Jim Sprague in cats that first revealed the dynamic interactions of cortical and subcortical systems for the control of orienting behavior. I'll then sum-

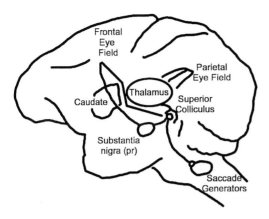

Figure 9–1. Some of the cortical and subcortical circuitry for oculomotor control. (*Source:* Adapted from Goldberg & Segraves, 1989, with permission)

sions the colliculus looses this tonic activation (Hovda & Villablanca, 1990). At the same time, the opposite (contralesional) colliculus becomes hyperactive. This imbalance is sustained and aggravated by the mutually inhibitory connections between the two colliculi themselves. The more active contralesional superior colliculus is released from inhibition and produces disinhibited reflexive orienting to signals in the field ipsilateral to the cortical lesion. If the contralesional superior colliculus is then removed (or the fibers of passage from the substantia nigra *pars reticulata* to the opposite colliculus), the ipsilesional hyperorienting is eliminated and contralesional orienting is restored.

marize work, mostly from my own laboratory, demonstrating the role of frontal and parietal lobes in regulating midbrain visuomotor reflexes.

PARIETAL LESIONS AND THE SPRAGUE EFFECT

Sprague first demonstrated that visual orienting is mediated by a dynamic interaction between the cerebral cortex and the midbrain pathways for reflexive orienting (Sprague, 1966). In a classic experiment, cats were rendered blind in one visual field by unilateral extirpation of occipital and parietal cortex. It was then shown that orienting toward the contralesional field was restored if the *opposite* superior colliculus was removed. A similar result was obtained if the inhibitory connections were severed between the contralesional substantia nigra pars reticulata and the ipsilesional colliculus (Wallace et al., 1989; 1990). Converging evidence for midbrain mediation of the Sprague effect was also demonstrated by Sherman (1974), who sectioned the interhemispheric commisure in cats and showed that the Sprague effect was restricted to the temporal hemifield.

The Sprague effect is thought to work in the following way. Parieto-occipital projections to the ipsilateral superior colliculus normally exert a tonic facilitation on it. After parietal le-

EFFECTS OF FRONTAL EYE FIELD LESIONS ON VISUALLY GUIDED AND VOLUNTARY SACCADES

Acute lesions in the superior part of the dorsolateral prefrontal cortex—including the frontal eye field (FEF)—can cause hemispatial neglect. However, the neglect is typically transient. There are extensive direct and indirect projections from this part of cortex, especially from the FEF, to the midbrain, including the superior colliculus and the substantia nigra pars reticulata. An acute lesion to the FEF causes a kind of shock to connected regions, called *diaschesis*, that can be measured experimentally as hypometabolism in remote structures including the superior colliculus (Deuel & Collins, 1984). So the acute neglect seen after FEF lesions may result, in part, because the ipsilesional superior colliculus is transiently dysfunctional. In the chronic, compensated state, however, lesions restricted to the FEF do not result in persistent neglect or any evident impairments of eye movement in daily life, or on clinical examination of eye movements at the bedside. This recovery reflects the reorganized state of frontocollicular circuitry.

We have investigated the reorganization of dynamic interactions between the FEF and the midbrain by examining the effects of chronic unilateral lesions of the human FEF on the latencies of eye movements. In one experiment, we compared visually guided saccades and voluntary saccades (Henik et al., 1994). The patients in this study were part of a group of individuals who have suffered brain injuries, mostly from strokes, and who have been gracious in helping us to investigate the consequences of these injuries. Each was selected for having a single, unilateral lesion restricted to the dorsolateral frontal cortex. All had recovered from the acute phase of the illness, during which diaschesis can have a major affect on remote structures; most were studied several years after the ictus. All were competent and independent individuals, and have been active participants in neurobehavioral research over a number of years.

For us to make inferences about FEF function, we used the following approach. We compared the nine patients in this frontal lesion group in whom the lesion included the FEF, with seven neurological control patients who had frontal lesions that spared the FEF. The region involved in these patients included that area believed to be the FEF, based on positron emission tomography (PET) studies (Paus, 1996). This includes the most posterior part of the middle frontal gyrus where it joins the precentral sulcus.

The patients were tested on their performance of two saccade tasks: visually guided saccades to targets that appeared 10° to the left or right; and voluntary saccades from a symbolic arrow cue at the center of the display that pointed to a marker target, 10° to the left

or right. The results are shown in Figure 9–2.

For the neurological control patients whose frontal lesions spared the FEF, the latencies of voluntary saccades were, as for normal individuals, longer than for visually guided saccades. Moreover, the frontal lesions did not produce an asymmetry of eye movements. Saccade latencies were not different for contralesional and ipsilesional fields for either kind of eye movement.

In patients with FEF lesions, voluntary saccades were slower to the contralesional field. In contrast, visually guided saccades were slower to the ipsilesional field. In the ipsilesional field the patients' visually guided saccade latencies were, quite abnormally, no faster than their latencies for voluntary saccades to that field. These results indicate that FEF lesions have two separate effects on eye movements: *(1)* the frontal eye fields are involved in generating endogenous saccades to the contralateral field, and lesions in this region therefore increase their latency; and *(2)* FEF lesions also influence the *opposite* superior colliculus. It seems not to generate a visual grasp reflex, and saccades made toward signals in the field ipsilesional to it must be made voluntarily without the usual advantage of this midbrain reflex.

Thus, unilateral lesions of the FEF, in the chronic state, can produce a kind of reverse Sprague effect. One explanation of this apparent reversed Sprague effect is that FEF lesions disinhibit the ipsilesional substantia nigra *pars reticulata*, resulting in inhibition of

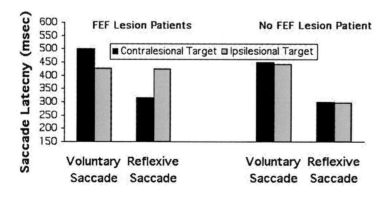

Figure 9–2. Saccade latencies to the ipsilesional and contralesional field for voluntary and visually summoned saccades in patients with lesions of the dorsolateral frontal cortex. A group of patients in whom the lesion involved the frontal eye field (FEF) are compared with a group of patients in whom the lesion spared that region of the frontal lobe. (*Source:* From Henik et al., 1994, with permission)

the superior colliculus opposite to the FEF lesion.

MAPPING THE FRONTAL EYE FIELD WITH TRANSCRANIAL MAGNETIC STIMULATION

To determine whether the reverse Sprague effect reflects a plastic reorganization following recovery from brain injury or the immediate effect of FEF inactivation, we investigated the effect of single-pulse transcranial magnetic stimulation (TMS) of the FEF in normal subjects. In this technique, a transient magnetic field is generated on the scalp to induce a very brief electrical stimulation that inactivates the underlying cortex for a few hundred milliseconds—in essence, an ultra-temporary lesion is produced. When TMS was applied over the FEF, there was an increase in latency for voluntary saccades to the contralateral field—the same pattern as seen in patients with chronic focal lesions. However, unlike the results in the patient study, TMS had no effect on ipsilateral visually guided saccades (Ro et al., 1997). Since TMS of the FEF did not have the effect on ipsilesional visually guided saccades that occurs with chronic lesions of the FEF, we concluded that the reverse Sprague effect after chronic FEF lesions is the result of plastic reorganization after brain injury.

More recently, we have combined structural magnetic resonance imaging (MRI) and TMS to map the FEF (Ro et al., 1999). The hand area of the motor cortex was identified by locating the area where TMS produced visible twitches in the contralateral hand. This location served as a physiological landmark for mapping the FEF. Figure 9–3 shows that the MRI scan confirmed the location of the motor hand area. The site at which finger movements were elicited was over the precentral gyrus. The figure also shows those sites, anterior to this landmark, where TMS prolonged the latency of contralateral voluntary saccades. The FEF was localized to a region 2 cm anterior to the hand area of the motor cortex.

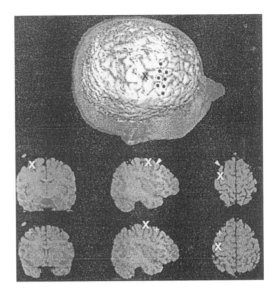

Figure 9–3. Colocalization of frontal eye fields (FEF) using structural magnetic resonance imaging (MRI) and transcranial magnetic stimulation (TMS). The X indicates the location of the motor hand area where TMS evoked finger movements. The dark circles on the top panel indicate the sites where TMS increased the latencies for contralateral endogenous saccades. (*Source*:From Ro et al., 1999, with permission)

EFFECT OF FRONTAL EYE FIELD AND PARIETAL LESIONS ON ANTISACCADES

The antisaccade task, in which a saccade must be made *away* from a peripheral target, demands both that the visual grasp reflex be inhibited and that a voluntary saccade be generated toward the opposite field. In a recent study using the antisaccade task, we confirmed that chronic, unilateral FEF lesions cause disinhibition of the visual grasp reflex mediated by the ipsilesional superior colliculus (Rafal et al., 2000). Figure 9–4 shows the number of reflexive glances, that is, errors in which saccades were made toward instead of away from the target, in patients with FEF lesions, patients with parietal lesions, and normal controls. In the FEF lesion patients, reflexive glances were increased toward contralesional targets, whereas in the parietal patients, fewer reflexive glances were made toward the contralesional field than were made by control

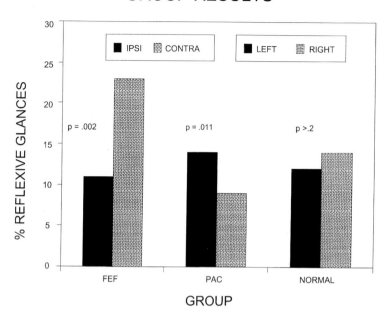

Figure 9–4. Effects of frontal eye field (FEF) lesions and parietal lesions on errors in the antisaccade task. The number of reflexive glances toward the contralesional and ipsilesional fields is shown for patients with frontal lesions involving the FEF, frontal lesions sparing the FEF and patients with parietal lesions (PAC), as well as normal controls. (*Source:* From Rafal et al., 2000, with permission)

subjects. These results confirm that FEF lesions result in disinhibition of the ipsilesional colliculus, whereas parietal lesions result in inhibition of the ipsilesional colliculus.

SACCADIC BIAS: A STUDY OF FRONTAL AND PARIETAL LESIONS

In a recent study, we examined the effects of chronic unilateral lesions of the inferior parietal lobe and the frontal eye fields on oculomotor bias (Ro et al., 2001). Two visual events were presented for each trial, one in each hemifield at various stimulus onset asynchronies. The patients were tested in their performance of two tasks. In the saccade task, patients moved their eyes to whichever stimulus attracted their gaze first. In the perceptual task, they pressed a button to indicate which stimulus was perceived first. Patients with lesions of the FEF showed no bias in either the saccade or perceptual task. That is, when the two signals appeared simultaneously, these patients were just as likely to judge the contralesional stimulus as having occurred first, or to make a saccade toward the contralesional stimulus, as they were to report the ipsile-

sional stimulus as occurring first or to make a saccade toward it. Patients with parietal lesions also showed no bias in the perceptual task. However, their saccades tended to be ipsilesional unless the contralesional target led substantially. This result reveals a bias in saccade choice after parietal damage that cannot be attributed to deficient visual perception.

Why did the patients with FEF lesions not show an oculomotor bias in this task? The saccadic task requires a decision on which way to move the eyes. An impairment in generating contralesional voluntary eye movements might be expected to have resulted in an ipsilesional bias. However, as we have seen, FEF lesions also cause disinhibited orienting toward contralesional signals. Therefore, it is possible that the bias to choose an ipsilesional saccade may have been counteracted by a disinhibition of reflexive orienting toward the contralesional target.

STRATEGIC CONTROL OF OCULAR FIXATION

So far we have considered the neural control of saccadic eye movements. Their purpose is to bring objects of interest onto the fovea so that they can be fixated for identification and analysis. Oculomotor control requires that the neural systems controlling saccades and fixation be coordinated. Part of this coordination is implemented within the superior colliculus itself (Munoz & Wurtz, 1992; Munoz & Istvan, 1998). In the rostral pole of each colliculus are cells that are active during fixation (even in the dark) and whose activity is further increased by a visual signal at fixation. These fixation, or pole, neurons help keep the eyes from moving. Caudal to the fixation neurons, and inhibited by them, are cells (commonly referred to as *movement cells*) whose activity helps the eyes move to a new position. Eye movements, then, are controlled by an opponent process involving intrinsic collicular circuits: there is mutual inhibition between the visual grasp reflex (VGR), activated by abrupt signals in the visual periphery and mediated by more caudal movement cells, and the fixation reflex, activated by visual signals at fixation and mediated by rostral pole neurons. Together, the activity of these two types of cells determine when and where the eyes will move.

The offset of a fixated stimulus prior to, or simultaneous with, the onset of a peripheral target disinhibits the VGR and speeds reaction time to initiate an eye movement to a peripheral target. The benefit of fixation offset on saccadic latencies was first reported by Saslow (1967), and has been termed the *fixation offset effect* (FOE) (Klein & Kingstone, 1993). Fixation offset paradigms are used to compare latencies to make eye movements when a fixation stimulus remains present at target onset to those when the fixation stimulus offsets.

The FOE is thought to result from changes in cellular activity in local inhibitory circuits within the superior colliculus that are triggered by the offset of a fixated stimulus (Munoz & Istvan, 1998). When a fixated stimulus offsets, the activity of fixation neurons in the rostral pole decreases and eye movement latency is reduced (Munoz & Wurtz, 1992; Dorris & Munoz, 1995). Conversely, stimulating fixation neurons just prior to or during an eye movement can delay or arrest the eye movement (Munoz & Istvan, 1998). This finding is consistent with the demonstration that unilat-

eral microstimulation of the rostral superior colliculus inhibits movement cells in both colliculi (Munoz & Wurtz, 1993; Munoz & Istvan, 1998). Together, these neurophysiological findings suggest that when fixation cell activity decreases in response to fixation offset, movement cell activity increases, disinhibiting the VGR and speeding reaction time to initiate an eye movement to a peripheral target.

The difference in saccade latency between fixation offset and fixation overlap conditions (the FOE) is a measure of the degree to which rostral pole neurons are *under external control by the fixation point*. Manipulations of strategic set that bring these neurons under voluntary control, and thereby reduce the influence of the external stimulus at fixation, will decrease the size of the FOE. The magnitude of the FOE thereby provides a measure of the degree to which collicular circuitry is under cortical control rather than under the control of external stimuli. The magnitude of the FOE can therefore be used experimentally as a measure of cortical control over intrinsic collicular circuits.

Voluntary control over collicular circuitry increases during infant development. The VGR is quite brisk in newborns (Mauer & Lewis, 1997). The fixation reflex, in which a visual signal at the point of fixation reflexively activates fixation neurons that inhibit the VGR to eccentric events, becomes quite strong during the first 2 months (Johnson, 1990). At about 2 months of age, the colliculi come under unopposed inhibitory influence of the basal ganglia (substantia nigra *pars reticulata*). This uninhibited fixation reflex may serve to facilitate paternal bonding by maintaining eye contact between infants and parents. However, infants presented with something like a checkerboard pattern may become distressed because they are unable to break the lock of a visual stimulus in order to move their eyes. The FOE decreases during infancy (Hood et al., 1997; Johnson & Gilmore, 1997), marking a maturation of fronto-basal ganglia-collicular circuits that brings the fixation reflex under voluntary control and permit efficient visual search with alternating saccades and fixations.

We have recently shown that normal adults can modulate the FOE on the basis of strategic set. The FOE decreased as the proportion of catch trials (i.e., in which no target was presented and no eye movement was made) decreased (Machado & Rafal, 2000b), suggesting that increasing oculomotor readiness reduces the inhibitory effect of the fixation point on rostral pole neurons. We have also shown that the FOE decreases when a voluntary saccade is prepared (Rafal et al., 2000).

Another experiment demonstrated that the FOE can be modified differentially by strategic set for visually triggered and voluntary saccades (Machado & Rafal, 2000b). Saccades were made either to a peripheral target (visually triggered) or were generated voluntarily in response to an auditory tone to look right or left. On half the trials the fixation point remained present (overlap condition); on the other half it offset when the target was presented (offset condition). In one block of trials endogenous saccades were more frequent (80%); in the other, saccades to peripheral targets were required on 80% of trials. Table 9–1 shows the effects on saccade latency of manipulating strategic set for voluntary or reflexive eye movements on the FOE. When reflexive saccades were frequent and voluntary saccades were infrequent, the FOE was attenuated for reflexive saccades. When voluntary saccades were frequent and reflexive ones infrequent, the FOE was attenuated for voluntary saccades. We concluded that cortical processes related to task strategy are able to decrease fixation neuron activity even in the presence of a fixation stimulus, resulting in a smaller FOE, and that there are separate neural mechanisms for modulation of fixation cell activity for the two types of saccades.

Our most recent work in normal individuals has examined strategic modulation of the FOE under conditions in which subjects must inhibit the VGR. An example is the antisaccade task which requires that the VGR be inhibited and a saccade be made in the opposite direction. The FOE is typically reduced in the antisaccade task (Reuter-Lorenz et al., 1991; Forbes & Klein, 1996). In our experiments, we compared the FOE in antisaccade and go no-go paradigms (Machado & Rafal, 2000a). Peripheral targets were, unpredictably and with equal probability, either red or green. In the antisaccade task, subjects made prosaccades toward green targets and away from red targets. In the go no-go task, they made saccades toward green targets and held fixation if a red target appeared. In both tasks, the fixation point offset when targets appeared on half the trials, and overlapped target onset of the other half. As expected, there was a small FOE when antisaccades were made. Moreover, there was a small FOE for prosaccades in the antisaccade–prosaccade task, indicating that the strategic requirements to inhibit the VGR in the antisaccade task also determined the FOE on prosaccade trials. By contrast, in the go no-go task, the FOE was found to be increased compared to blocks in which only prosaccades were made. Thus, although there

Table 9–1. Latencies for saccades to peripheral targets and for endogenous saccades in response to auditory cues[*]

Block	Peripheral Target Trials			Tone Target Trials		
	Overlap ms (SD)	Offset ms (SD)	FOE	Overlap ms (SD)	Offset ms (SD)	FOE
20% peripheral target/ 80% tone target	359 (58)	300 (55)	59	424 (85)	411 (89)	13
80% peripheral target/ 20% tone target	277 (48)	251 (39)	26	557 (132)	518 (123)	39

[*]Results are from two tasks that differed in strategic set to make reflexive or voluntary eye movements. FOE, fixation offset effect; SD, standard deviation.

(*Source:* From Machado & Rafal, 2000b).

is a requirement to inhibit the VGR in both antisaccade and go no-go tasks, we observed opposite effects on the FOE in these two paradigms. The requirement, in the antisaccade task, that some eye movement be made on every trial obliges subjects to adopt a different strategy for inhibiting the VGR than that which they adopt in the go no-go task, in which oculomotor inhibition may be used as the default mode.

The strategic modulation of fixation demonstrated in the experiments reviewed here is presumably mediated by cortical influences on the superior colliculus, either direct or via the basal ganglia. Future research will focus on determining the specific cortical substrates and the circuitry involved.

SUMMARY AND CONCLUSIONS

Converging evidence from patients with midbrain lesions and from hemianopic patients reveals that midbrain pathways are responsible for reflexive orienting in humans. The VGR mediated by the colliculus is modulated by a dynamic interaction between cortical and subcortical systems. Chronic lesions of the FEF cause a slowing of visually guided saccades toward the ipsilesional field; whereas parietal lesions cause a bias against making voluntary saccades toward the contralesional field. Similarly, in the antisaccade task, the VGR was disinhibited toward the contralesional field in patients with FEF lesions, and inhibited toward the contralesional field in patients with parietal lesion. Thus, the FEF and parietal lobes appear to normally have opposing influences on collicular function: the parietal lobe facilitates the VGR and the FEF inhibits it.

REFERENCES

Danziger, S., Fendrich, R., & Rafal, R.D. (1997). Inhibitory tagging of locations in the blind field of hemianopic patients. *Consciousness and Cognition, 6*, 291–307.

Deuel, R.K. & Collins, R.C. (1984). The functional anatomy of frontal lobe neglect in monkeys: behavioral and 2-deoxyglucose studies. *Annals of Neurology, 15*, 521–529.

Dorris, M.C. & Munoz, D.P. (1995). A neural correlate for the gap effect on saccadic reaction times in monkey. *Journal of Neurophysiology, 73*, 2558–2562.

Easton, T.A. (1973). On the normal use of reflexes. *American Scientist, 60*, 591–599.

Forbes, K. & Klein, R.M. (1996). The magnitude of the fixation offset effect with endogenously and exogenously controlled saccades. *Journal of Cognitive Neuroscience, 8*, 344–352.

Goldberg, M.E., & Segraves, M.A. (1989) The visual and frontal cortices. In R.H. Wurtz & M.E. Goldberg (Eds.) *The Neurobiology of Saccadic Eye Movements* (pp. 283–214). Amsterdam: Elserier Science Publishers BV.

Henik, A., Rafal, R., & Rhodes, D. (1994). Endogenously generated and visually guidedsaccades after lesions of the human frontal eye fields. *Journal of Cognitive Neuroscience, 6*, 400–411.

Hikosaka, O. & Wurtz, R.H. (1989). The basal ganglia. In: R.H. Wurtz & M.E. Goldberg (Eds.), *The Neurobiology of Saccadic Eye Movements* (pp. 257–282). Amsterdam: Elsevier Science Publishers.

Hood, B.M., Atkinson, J., & Braddick, O.J. (1997). Selection-for-action and the development of visual selective attention. In: J.E. Richards (Ed.), *Cognitive Neuroscience of Attention: A Developmental Perspective*. Hillsdale, NJ.: Lawrence Erlbaum Associates.

Hovda, D.A. & Villablanca, J.R. (1990). Sparing of visual field perception in neonatal but not adult cerebral hemispherectomized cats. Relationship with oxidative metabolism in the superior colliculus. *Behavioral Brain Research, 37*, 119–132.

Ingle, D. (1973). Evolutionary Perspectives on the function of the optic tectum. *Brain Behavior and Evolution, 8*, 211–237.

Johnson, M.H. (1990). Cortical maturation and the development of visual attention in early infancy. *Journal of Cognitive Neuroscience, 2*, 81–95.

Johnson, M.H. & Gilmore, R.O. (1997). Toward a computational model of the development of saccade planning. In: J.E. Richards (Ed.), *Cognitive Neuroscience of Attention: A Developmental Perspective*. Hillsdale, NJ.: Lawrence Erlbaum Associates.

Klein, R. & Kingstone, A. (1993). Why do visual offsets reduce saccadic latencies. *Behavioral and Brain Science, 16*, 583–584.

Klein, R.M. & MacInnes, W.J. (1999). Inhibition of return is a foraging facilitator in visual search. *Psychological Science, 10*, 346–352.

Machado, L. & Rafal, R. (2000a). Control of eye movement reflexes. *Experimental Brain Research, 135*, 73–80.

Machado, L. & Rafal, R. (2000b). Strategic control over the visual grasp reflex: studies of the fixation off set effect. *Perception and Psychophysics, 62*, 1236–1242.

Mauer, D. & Lewis, T.L. (1997). Overt orienting toward peripheral stimuli: normal development and underlying mechanisms. In: J.E. Richards (Ed.), *Cognitive Neuroscience of Attention: A Developmental Perspective*. Hillsdale, NJ: Lawrence Erlbaum Associates.

Munoz, D.P. & Istvan, P.J. (1998). Lateral inhibitory interactions in the intermediate layers of the monkey superior colliculus. *Journal of Neurophysiology, 79*, 1193–1209.

Munoz, D.P. & Wurtz, R.H. (1992). Role of the rostral superior colliculus in active visual fixation and execution of express saccades. *Visual Neuroscience, 9*, 409–414.

Munoz, D.P. & Wurtz, R.H. (1993). Fixation cells in monkey superior colliculus. I. Characteristics of cell discharge. *Journal of Neurophysiology, 70*, 559–575.

Paus, T. (1996). Location and function of the human frontal eye field: a selective review. *Neuropsychologia, 34*, 475–484.

Posner, M.I., Rafal, R.D., Choate, L., & Vaughn, J. (1985). Inhibition of return: neural basis and function. *Cognitive Neuropsychology, 2*, 211–228.

Rafal, R., Machado, L., Ro, T., & Ingle, H. (2000). Looking forward to looking: saccade preparation and control of the visual grasp reflex. In: S. Monsell & J. Driver (Eds.), *Control of Cognitive Operations: Attention and Performance XVIII* (pp. 155–174). Cambridge, MA: MIT Press.

Rafal, R.D., Posner, M.I., Friedman, J.H., Inhoff, A.W., & Bernstein, E. (1988). Orienting of visual attention in progressive supranuclear palsy. *Brain, 111*, 267–280.

Reuter-Lorenz, P.A., Hughes, H.C., & Fendrich, R. (1991). The reduction of saccadic latency by prior offset of the fixation point: an analysis of the gap effect. *Perception and Psychophysics, 50*, 383–387.

Ro, T., Henik, A., Machado, L., & Rafal, R.D. (1997). Transcranial magnetic stimulation of the prefrontal cortex delays contralateral endogenous saccades. *Journal of Cognitive Neuroscience, 9*, 433–440.

Ro, T., Cheifet, S., Ingle, H., Shoup, R., & Rafal, R. (1999). Localization of the human frontal eye fields and motor hand area with transcranial magnetic stimulation and magnetic resonance imaging. *Neuropsychologia, 37*, 225–232.

Ro, T., Rorden, C., Driver, J., & Rafal, R. (2001). Ipsilesional biases in saccades but not perception after lesions of the human inferior parietal lobule. *Journal of Cognitive Neuroscience, 13*, 920–929.

Sapir, A., Soroker, N., Berger, A., & Henik, A. (1999). Inhibition of return in spatial attention: direct evidence for collicular generation. *Nature Neuroscience, 2*, 1053–1054.

Saslow, M.G. (1967). Effects of components of displacement-step stimuli upon latency for saccadic eye movements. *Journal of the Optical Society of America, 57*, 1024–1029.

Sherman, S.M. (1974). Visual fields of cats with cortical and tectal lesions. *Science, 185*, 355–357.

Sprague, J M. (1966). Interaction of cortex and superior colliculus in mediation of peripherally summoned behavior in the cat. *Science, 153*, 1544–1547.

Tipper, S., Rafal, R., Reuter-Lorenz, P.A., Starreveld, Y., Ro, T., Egly, R., Weaver, B., & Danziger, S. (1997). Object-based facilitation and inhibition from visual orienting in the human split brain. *Journal of Experimental Psychology: Human Perception and Performance, 23*, 1522–1532.

Wallace, S.F., Rosenquist, A.C., & Sprague, J.M. (1989). Recovery from cortical blindness mediated by destruction of nontectotectal fibers in the commissure of the superior colliculus in the cat. *Journal of Comparative Neurology, 284*, 429–450.

Wallace, S.F., Rosenquist, A.C., & Sprague, J.M. (1990). Ibotenic acid lesions of the lateral substantia nigra restore visual orientation behavior in the hemianopic cat. *Journal of Comparative Neurology, 296*, 222–252.

10

Disorders of Language after Frontal Lobe Injury: Evidence for the Neural Mechanisms of Assembling Language

MICHAEL P. ALEXANDER

When asked by a friend about a recent vacation, one is likely to immediately break into a complex tale of travel problems, sites visited, meals eaten, and local color, all woven together with complex syntax: "After the airline finally found our bags—what a mess! I don't ever want to fly again—and we found a cab that wasn't too disgusting to touch, we got so lost looking for the hotel, which turned out to be practically a brothel, that we thought, 'Why have we done this?' " This description is filled with rich vocabulary, and is interwoven with recognition of what the friend already knows about the trip, sensitivity to how much detail he can abide and his tolerance for off-color asides, and humor to keep his interest. This narrative is guided by the narrator's knowledge of the script that the listener will expect the teller of the tale to follow—"the vacation story script." There are many ways to weave this story within the accepted script, and one will have to form a plan for unfolding the one version appropriate for the setting and the friend. The frontal lobes will be the active agents in this endeavor.

Damage to the frontal lobes, particularly on the left, will impair this capacity. Depending on the location, the impairment may be at different levels of the narrative. This chapter will review these impairments at four discrete, although overlapping, levels of clinical phenomena. (1) *transcortical motor aphasia* (TCMA), the classical aphasic syndrome of left posterior frontal injury; (2) *dynamic aphasia*, which is the core impairment of (TCMA) and a disturbance of complex, open—ended sentence assembly; (3) *discourse impairments*, which are disturbances in the assembly of complex narratives; and (4) *disrupted action planning*, the fundamental impairment of complex, goal-directed, intentional behavior. Dynamic aphasia and discourse impairment should be seen as action planning deficits specific to language use.

TRANSCORTICAL MOTOR APHASIA

Damage restricted to the posterior, lateral portion of the left frontal lobe causes language impairment. The precise form of the impairment depends, as always in clinical phenomenology, on several factors beyond coarse lobar localization: the exact location of the injury, the depth of injury, the time post—onset if onset was acute, the condition of the brain prior to injury, and the age of the patient if a child, allowing for variances through all of these mechanisms. The usual result of posterior, lateral frontal damage is TCMA (Mega et al., 2000).

Transcortical motor aphasia is defined first by nonfluent output, although usually not the markedly restricted, telegraphic and agrammatical output of classic Broca's aphasia (Goodglass, 1993). The output is more typically grammatical but simplified, repetitive, and delayed, with quite variable severity of anomia. Many responses are echolalic, sometimes completely so, and other times only a portion of the examiner's question or statement is made into a response, termed *incorporation echolalia*. It is an absolute defining characteristic of TCMA that repetition is intact, regardless of the grammatical or syntactic complexity (Goodglass, 1993). Failure to inhibit repetition underlies the echolalic responses. Oral reading is also usually intact. Auditory and written comprehension are normal, at least at the relatively unchallenging level of most clinical aphasia tests. In the acute phases, pervasive deficits in response set may simulate a comprehension deficit, and it is not unusual for large frontal lesions to initially appear as mixed transcortical aphasia. Writing is the most variable aspect of TCMA, and no profile of writing abnormality is useful in defining TCMA.

Since initial descriptions by Lichtheim (1885) and initial theory of neural mechanism by Wernicke, it has been asserted that TCMA is caused by lesions in the lateral left frontal lobe, variously anterior or superior to Broca's area (Goldstein, 1948; Goodglass, 1993; Alexander, 1997). This definition, of course, hedges the definition of Broca's area. Norman Geschwind often told his students that "Broca's area is that area, which, when damaged, produces a permanent Broca's aphasia." By that definition, Broca's area could be very large. Numerous neuroimaging studies in the last 25 years have demonstrated that chronic Broca's aphasia is generally associated with a large lesion of frontal operculum, middle frontal gyrus, lower motor and sensory cortices, often supramarginal gyrus, much subcortical white matter, and often the dorsal caudate. Some of the same studies have also demonstrated that permanent Broca's aphasia could occur without any damage to frontal cortex. In these cases, there was usually extensive damage to subcortical white matter, paraventricular white matter, and caudate.

With my colleagues at the Boston Veteran's Administration Medical Center, we have described three clinical–anatomical bases of TCMA. First, lesions restricted to the frontal operculum, an anatomically conservative definition of Broca's area and the area where most reviews place the "B," produce TCMA (Freedman et al., 1984). Thus, lesions in "Broca's area" do not cause Broca's aphasia, and Broca's aphasia does not require a lesion in "Broca's area." Second, lesions in the white matter deep to frontal operculum down to the paraventricular white matter produce an identical clinical aphasia picture (Fig. 10–1). Most of these lesions also involve the dorsal caudate (Mega & Alexander, 1994). In either case, in

Figure 10–1. As described in the text, transcortial motor aphasia (TCMA) can be seen with a wide variety of lesion locations. This figure is a schematic of perhaps the most typical lesion site: dorsal midfrontal above and involving the anterior operculum. The white matter portion of this lesion alone (cross-hatched area) is also a common finding in TCMA.

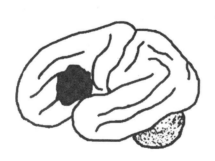
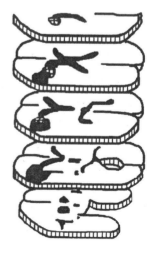

the initial phase, there may be transient mutism. If the lesion involves lower motor cortex or its descending white matter pathways, there may be considerable dysarthria (Freedman et al., 1984). Larger lesions produce transient agrammatism and/or phonemic paraphasias (acute Broca's aphasia), but with recovery, overt agrammatism clears.

Third, lesions of the medial frontal lobe involving supplementary motor area (SMA) produce a form of TCMA (Alexander & Schmitt, 1980; Freedman et al., 1984). The modifier "a form" is required because with recovery it may not always be convincing that patients are actually aphasic so much as unable to speak at length (Von Stockert, 1974). Either right or left medial frontal lesions may produce initial mutism with evolution over hours or days to simplified language with frequent pauses and blocks (Rubens, 1976; Masdeu et al., 1978; Freedman et al., 1984). When a left-sided lesion also involves medial white matter, including the anterior corpus callosum, mutism may be more prolonged and recovery of lengthy, fluid language utterances much more delayed and even incomplete (Rubens, 1976).

At the boundaries of these three lesions lies the paraventricular white matter adjacent and superior to the left frontal horn of the lateral ventricle. A lesion in this region represents the overlap of the systems relevant to TCMA. This region is a key intersection of several neural networks of language and speech output: ascending pathways from the mesencephalic ventral tegmental area (VTA) to the medial frontal lobes (see below) (Lindvall et al., 1974), lateral and oblique pathways from both medial frontal lobes to the left lateral frontal lobe and dorsal caudate and to the contralateral cerebellum (Baleydier & Mauguiere, 1980; Jürgens, 1984), and long, bidirectional association pathways between the left lateral and polar frontal lobe and posterior cortex (Nauta & Freitag, 1986). It is the involvement of these systems that produces TCMA. Extension of a lesion to adjacent structures may cause agrammatism, dysarthria, or even right hemiparesis. Thus, TCMA, like all aphasia syndromes, may be modified, atypical, or overlap with other syndromes depending on the exact lesion boundaries. These variations from

being prototypical are in addition to variance caused by biological factors such as gender or the forms of anomalous language organization more common in left-handers than right-handers.

There is ongoing controversy about the possible role of cortical injury in regions that appear on structural imaging to be restricted to subcortical regions (Godefrey et al., 1992). When caused by infarction, there is always associated reduced perfusion of the overlying frontal cortex on positron emission tomography (PET) studies (Nadeau & Crosson, 1995), and the cases with aphasia are more likely than those without aphasia to have demonstrable severe ipsilateral carotid occlusive disease (Olsen et al., 1986). The perfusion deficits have been variously interpreted as diaschisis, deafferentation of cortex (Alexander, 1992), or evidence of hypoxic neuronal injury without frank infarction (Olsen et al., 1986; Nadeau & Crosson, 1995). Some of the language abnormalities may be due to this microscopic cortical injury, but there are also reasons to believe that the subcortical lesion itself may be the cause of aphasia. First, subcortical lesions can certainly produce remote effects on neuronal function. The same patients have equally significant perfusion deficits in contralateral cerebellum that cannot be accounted for as hypoxic injury (Alexander, 1992). Second, identical language disorders are seen after deep, lobar hemorrhages in which there is no a priori mechanism for sufficient cortical neuronal injury to account for aphasia (D'Esposito & Alexander, 1995). Third, there are numerous examples of critical white matter lesions producing cognitive impairments so there is no need to discover a cortical explanation for all cognitive deficits.

Mutism without any overt language abnormalities, as best as can be judged in patients who rarely speak, is also caused by damage to the ascending dopaminergic systems originating in the VTA of the upper midbrain and terminating in the SMA and anterior cingulate gyrus (Ross & Stewart, 1981). When lesions of these pathways or their terminal cortical targets are bilateral, full akinetic mutism results (Freemon, 1971). When unilateral, less striking speech reductions and contralateral akinesia occur (Alexander & Schmitt, 1980). Thus, as noted above, when lesions are restricted to the SMA and anterior cingulate gyrus, it is arguable that there is no aphasia, just a reduced propensity to speak (Von Stockert, 1974; Devinsky et al., 1995). With larger medial cortical lesions, overt language impairment does appear.

SUMMARY

Transcortical motor aphasia is a syndrome defined by minimal speech output, word selection deficits, reduced grammatical complexity, and variable tendencies to echo, perseverate, or just not respond when any complex or novel language is called for. Mutism and its lesser forms may be a factor independent of any actual language impairment.

DYNAMIC APHASIA

So what is the core of TCMA, stripped of mild agrammatism and articulation impairment, that might be seen in some, or most, patients? There is a long history of answers to this question, and they all revolve around the same key claims. Goldstein (1948) and Luria (Luria & Tsevtkova, 1967; Luria, 1973), in particular, are credited with asking the correct questions and providing provisional answers. Luria coined the term that best captures the core impairment: *dynamic aphasia*. Those two original observers and others since have variously held that dynamic aphasia represents an impairment of *translating* or *transforming* or *mapping* of *concepts* or *intentions* or *verbal plans* or *thought* on to linguistic forms. Luria devoted much effort to demonstrating that these patients had two deficits that defined dynamic aphasia, and his observations have subsequently been more empirically elaborated by modern cognitive neuropsychologists. Luria asserted that one deficit is a failure of predication—that is, an inability to define the critical predicate, or action that determines an utterance's intention (Luria, 1973). The second deficit is an inability to produce a linear structure for an intended utterance (Luria & Tse-

vtkova, 1967). These hypotheses remained largely unexplored for several years after Luria's studies, but recently detailed analysis of individual cases have specified the nature of dynamic aphasia much beyond the evocative, but only metaphorical, assertions of disconnections of thought from language.

In sum, dynamic aphasia represents the core impairment of TCMA. It is characterized by a severe reduction in spontaneous speech but accurate responses to direct questions, a poverty of responses or even a complete incapacity to respond to open-ended questions, and a severe reduction in capacity to carry the flow of standard conversational exchanges. The limited number of fully elaborated utterances are grammatically and syntactically correct. Paraphasias are uncommon but uniformly semantic. Speech is normally articulated and prosodic. The few modern, well-studied cases have had lesions in left dorsolateral frontal lobe including deep white matter (Fig. 10–2). The same language disturbance has been described in patients with frontal lobe dementia and with progressive supranuclear palsy, which, in turn, is often accompanied by frontal lobe dementia.

Patients with dynamic aphasia often have accompanying deficits in other executive tasks, but dynamic aphasia is not simply due to general executive deficits. It is a very specific deficit in the execution of complex language. There are many routes to executive impairment. Focal injury in various frontal structures, right or left, causes cognitive manifestations of varying degrees of specificity, depending on the precise lesion site. Widespread injury, such as diffuse axonal injury from trauma, can cause executive impairments; whether they should be considered frontal or not is controversial. Often executive impairments are transient because of metabolic encephalopathies. Some are transient because functional disturbances, such as anxiety or depression, have occurred. None of these causes dynamic aphasia.

There have been a few painstaking single case analyses to determine the precise cognitive mechanism of dynamic aphasia. Careful control of each element required in complex

Figure 10–2. Dynamic aphasia has not been systematically correlated with any particular lesion site, but following Sirigu et al. (1998) and various single case studies, it appears that a more anterior location with more extension anterior to that frontal horn is most typical.

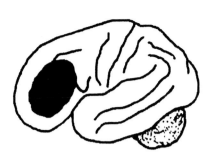

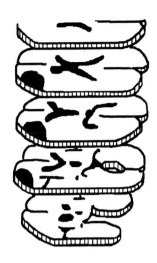

language construction was essential for each study. Costello and Warrington (1989) demonstrated that their patient had intact syntactic capacities allowing for normal language production when construction of an utterance was guided by context. When presented with elements of an utterance of unambiguous form and intent, capacity was preserved. Only when the utterance required that the patient form a plan out of several possible plans was the patient unable to carry this out. These investigators concluded that the patient had deficient verbal planing prior to actual sentence construction or syntactic form decision. . . . Fletcher et al. (1996) phrased their conclusion differently after analysis of their patient, focusing on the patient's inability to establish the arrangement of semantic elements in an utterance when the elements did not imply a specific concrete linkage. Robinson and colleagues (1998) concluded that their patient was unable to generate well-formed propositional utterances when the context did not provide a constrained option among multiple possible constructions. All of these investigations define more precisely what might be meant by an inability to *translate* or *transform* into or *map* onto linguistic forms, *concepts, intentions, verbal plans*, or *thought*.

This account of dynamic aphasia receives support from other directions. Price and colleagues (1999) reported on the mechanisms of translation between languages in bilingual patients, as opposed to simple speech or oral reading in one language or the other. They asserted that moving between languages required language-specific "task schemas," described as "effectively action sequences in the domain of language." These schemas are "external to the lexical semantic system," and the schemas unique to each language "compete to control outputs from the lexical semantic system." These action output control schemas would be the sites of impairment in dynamic aphasia.

Many years ago, Luria (1973) and Rubens (1976) demonstrated that patients with TCMA could produce intact utterances around a single target noun but were markedly impaired when the sentence also had to include a modifier for the target word. Mega and Alexander (1994) demonstrated that patients with mild TCMA from subcortical strokes were impaired at generation of a sentence from specified verbs. In modern research it has frequently been demonstrated with PET or functional magnetic resonance imaging (FMRI) that in normal subjects, generation of a modifier or associated word to a target produces blood flow activation in the left ventrolateral frontal cortex (Petersen et al., 1988, 1989). Thompson-Schill et al. (1998) recently analyzed this generative task when the response could come from multiple unconstrained choices. They found that the left lateral frontal lobe modulates the selection and assembly of output when context and external constraints do not define that output.

SUMMARY

Dynamic aphasia is the core impairment of TCMA. It is an action planning disturbance at the level of production of complex, novel sentences. The apparatus of grammar and of syntax is intact. It is the recruitment to fit a particular intention that is defective. The more unconstrained the intention, the more difficult it is to produce a sentence structure in a coherent and timely manner.

DISCOURSE

Discourse is another level of language assembly. *Discourse* refers to the production of structured, complex outputs that follow an anticipated form (Chapman et al., 1992). The forms may be very culture-specific. Discourse has different structured forms: telling a story, describing a procedure, giving directions, and telling a joke. Anyone who has raised children is aware of the gradual development of discourse capacity as children learn the expectations of the speaker and the rules of discourse unique to the ambient culture. Allowing for cultural differences, discourse has a set of procedural rules: use of reference, story grammars, requirements for linear coherence, use of indirection, allowance for humor or surprise, and so on. Some forms of discourse are very rule bound, such as pleading a court case or the structure of a scientific report. Others are much freer: describing a vacation and similar narratives. Many forms of discourse require some knowledge of what the listener knows, expects, or will tolerate—that is, that the narrator have a "theory of mind" (Stone et al., 1998). Thus, the forms of discourse are "verbal schemas" of considerable complexity. They are plans of action in the verbal domain, on a much large scale than that of the individual sentence.

Analysis of discourse is extremely time consuming, and there are relatively few studies of discourse after development of focal lesions. The available studies demonstrate prominent deficits after frontal lesions and different forms of deficit after left or right frontal injury (Kaczmarek, 1984; Novoa & Ardila, 1987; Levelt, 1989; Chapman et al., 1992). Left frontal lesions result in reduced number of words and themes, i.e., key elements of the narrative. In patients with left frontal lesions there is a reduction in variation in sentence structure with a tendency to reuse or repeat sentence structures. This simplification and perseveration of sentence forms were previously described in TCMA. The overall narratives are generally coherent. They have preserved structure and gist, but with a poverty of specific references. Right frontal lesions produce narrative with poor coherence—i.e., the structural framework is poorly maintained. There may be intrusion of thematic elements that are unrelated or at least inessential to the overall narrative goal. Some examples of poor semantic plausibility are frankly confabulatory. The patients with right frontal lesions may have reduced theory of mind, omitting elements that the listener requires to understand the narrative. The social aspects of discourse may be abused with inappropriate humor, language selection, or informality.

It should be apparent that there is no strict boundary between the language formulation deficits of dynamic aphasia and those of discourse impairment. If the language abnormality emerges out of a transient period of overt aphasia, is associated with any degree of straightforward anomia, and is sufficiently severe to impede conversation or preclude well-formed responses to questions, it is likely to be recognized as an aphasia disorder (acute Broca's aphasia becoming TCMA, TCMA becoming dynamic aphasia). If it begins with a period of mutism and continues to be defined by terse, unelaborated utterances, it is also likely to be heard as TCMA becoming dynamic aphasia. If there is no overt aphasia at onset and language is relatively readily produced except in open-ended utterances, it is likely to be viewed as a discourse impairment. Sirigu et al. (1998) described a small number of patients with lesions in the left dorsolateral frontal lobe (areas 9, 44, and 46), the left posterior frontal lobe (areas 44, 45, 6, and 4), or in both. The first group was impaired at assembling elements of a story script into a coherent narrative but was able to assemble words into a grammatical sentence. The second group had the opposite profile. The third group was impaired at both tasks. A fourth group that was not studied by Sirigu et al. could assemble simple, familiar scripts but could not assemble more complex ambiguous scripts. These groups represent nested levels in a hierarchy of capacities to mobilize complex mental procedures for use of language when the phonetic, phonemic, lexical, semantic, and grammatical functions of language are preserved.

SUMMARY

The parallels between discourse and other complex behaviors should be apparent, but the following example may illuminate the relationship. Presenting a medical report is a very complex discourse type. It has an expected form—a script. It requires considerable coherence, complex ordering of elements, and a specialized vocabulary that must be precisely recruited. This is an example of action planning in the verbal domain. Performing the medical examination that leads to the report also follows a form, or script. It requires coherence, complex ordering of elements, and the precise, but flexible, recruitment of specialized motor and perceptual skills. This is action planning in a specialized cognitive domain. The cognitive architecture of either one should inform us about the other.

ACTION PLANNING

The notion that dynamic aphasia and discourse impairments represent disturbances in action planning restricted to the verbal domain has received support from the analysis of other forms of impaired action planning, for example, through study of the routine performance of learned tasks (Shallice, 1982) and study of patients who were unable to organize a procedure for carrying out complex, multistep activities that might be performed in a variety of ways (Schwartz et al., 1991; Shallice

& Burgess, 1991). The example studied by Schwartz et al. was eating a meal. The "semantics" of movement and the operations (themes) necessary to organize a meal are preserved: slicing, pouring, stirring, mixing, and salting. The "lexical" elements are recognized for their place in the overall action: coffee is drunk, sugar is mixed, spoons are for stirring and for soup, straws are for sipping, butter is spread, and so on. The order is not fixed, as the various elements can be acted on in numerous orders. A plan for ordering the actions must be created: for example, the sugar goes in the coffee before it is drunk, and the bread is buttered before it is eaten. Impaired production of an action plan is to praxis and object recognition what dynamic aphasia is to language—an inability to generate and keep in mind a complex task that will unfold in the near future.

CONCLUSION

There are layers of language impairment that may result from frontal injuries. The first is a reduction in the activation to speak or to use language at all. This problem ranges from frank mutism to delayed speech/language initiation to terse, poorly sustained output. This deficit revolves around injury to the medial frontal lobes, the left more than the right. The damage can be in different projections to medial frontal lobes from dopaminergic neurons in the upper brain stem, in medial frontal structures directly, or to the efferent projections from medial frontal lobes to left lateral frontal lobe.

The second layer of language impairment is faulty generative, intentional language use at the level of impoverished open-ended, unconstrained language, with restricted and repetitive structure and even poor word choice (TCMA). This pattern follows left frontal injury focused on the dorsolateral cortex. The third layer is unelaborated conversational output with restricted capacity for complex discourse procedures. This deficit follows development of anterior left frontal lesions. A complementary discourse deficit with dilapidated organization and socially inappropriate or frankly confabulatory output follows right lateral and anterior frontal lesions. The second and third frontal language disorders are not strictly aphasic. They are impairments in the use of learned mental procedures (action plans) for mobilization of complex, functional language.

REFERENCES

Alexander, M.P. (1992). Speech and language deficits after subcortical lesions of the left hemisphere: a clinical, CT and PET study. In:G. Vallar, S.F. Cappa, & C.-W. Wallesch (Eds.), *Neuropsychological Disorders Associated with Subcortical Lesions* (pp. 455–477). Oxford: Oxford University Press.

Alexander, M.P. (1997). Aphasia: clinical and anatomic aspects. In: T.E. Feinberg & M.J. Farah (Eds.), *Behavioral Neurology and Neuropsychology* (pp. 133–149). New York: McGraw-Hill.

Alexander, M.P. & Schmitt, M.A. (1980). The aphasia syndrome of stroke in the left anterior cerebral artery territory. *Archives of Neurology, 37*, 97–100.

Baleydier, C. & Mauguiere, F. (1980). The duality of the cingulate gyrus in monkey: neuroanatomical study and functional hypothesis. *Brain, 103*, 525–554.

Chapman, S.B., Culhane, K.A., Levin, H.S., Harward, H., Mendelson, D., Ewing-Cobbs, L., Fletcher, J.M., & Bruce, D. (1992). Narrative discourse after closed head injury inchildren and adolescents. *Brain and Language, 43*, 42–65.

Costello, A.L. & Warrington, E.K. (1989). Dynamic aphasia. The selective impairment of verbal planning. *Cortex, 25*, 103–114.

D'Esposito, M. & Alexander, M.P. (1995). Subcortical aphasia: distinctprofiles following left putaminal hemorrhages. *Neurology, 45*, 33–37.

Devinsky, O., Morrell, M.J., & Vogt, B.A. (1995). Contributions of anterior cingulate cortex to behaviour. *Brain, 118*, 279–306.

Fletcher, P.C., Shallice, T., Frith, C.D., Frackowiack, R.S., & Dolan, J. (1996). Brain activity during memory retrieval: the influence of imagery and semantic cueing. *Brain, 119*, 1587–1596.

Freedman, M., Alexander, M.P., & Naeser, M.A. (1984). Anatomic basis of transcortical motor aphasia. *Neurology, 34*, 409–417.

Freemon, F.R. (1971). Akinetic mutism and bilateral anterior cerebral artery occlusion. *Journal of Neurology, Neurosurgery and Psychiatry, 34*, 693–698.

Godefrey, O., Rousseaux, M., Leys, D., Desteé, A., Scheltens, P., & Pruvo, J.P. (1992). Frontal lobe dysfunction in unilateral lenticulostriate infarcts: prominent role of cortical lesions. *Archives of Neurology, 49*, 1285–1289.

Goldstein, K. (1948). *Language and Language Disorders*. New York: Grune & Stratton.

Goodglass, H. (1993). *Understanding Aphasia*. San Diego: Aademic Press.

Jürgens, U. (1984). The efferent and afferent connections of the supplementary motor area. *Brain Research, 300*, 63–81.

Kaczmarek, B.L.J. (1984). Neurolinguistic analysis of verbal utterances in patients with focal lesions of frontal lobes. *Brain and Language, 21*, 52–58.

Levelt, W.J.M. (1989). *Speaking: From Intention to Articulation*. Cambridge, MA: MIT Press.

Lichtheim, L. (1885). On aphasia. *Brain, 7*, 433–484.

Lindvall, O., Bjorkland, A., Moore, R.Y., & Stenevi, U. (1974). Mesencephalic dopamine neurons projecting to neocortex. *Brain Research, 81*, 325–331.

Luria, A.R. (1973). *The Working Brain*. New York: Basic Books.

Luria, A.R. & Tsevtkova, L.S. (1967). Towards the mechanism of "dynamic aphasia". *Acta Neurologica Psychiatrica Belgica, 67*, 1045–1067.

Masdeu, J.C., Schoene, W.C., & Funkenstein, H.H. (1978). Aphasia following infarction of the left supplementary motor area. *Neurology, 28*, 1220–1223.

Mega, M.S., & Alexander, M.P. (1994). The core profile of subcortical aphasia. *Neurology, 44*, 1824–1829.

Mega, M.S., Alexander, M.P., Cummings, J.L., & Benson, D.F. (2000). The Aphasias and Related Disorders. In R.J. Joynt & R.C. Griggs (Eds.), *Baker's Clinical Neurology on CD-ROM*. Philadelphia: Lippincott, Williams and Wilkins.

Nadeau, S. & Crosson, B. (1995). Subcortical aphasia. *Brain and Language, 58*, 355–402.

Nauta, W.J.H. & Freitag, M. (1986). *Fundamental Neuroanatomy*. New York: W.H. Freeman and Company.

Novoa, O.P., & Ardila, A. (1987). Linguistic abilities in patients with prefrontal damage. *Brain and Language, 30*, 206–225.

Olsen, T.S., Bruhn, P., & Öberg, R.G.W. (1986). Cortical hypoperfusion as a possible cause of 'subcortical aphasia'. *Brain, 109*, 393–410.

Petersen, S.E., Fox, P.T., Posner, M.I., Mintun, M.A., & Raichle, M.E. (1988). Positron emission tomographic studies of the cortical anatomy of single-word processing. *Nature, 331*, 585–589.

Petersen, S.E., Fox, P.T., Posner, M.I., Mintun, M.A., & Raichle, M.E. (1989). Positron emission tomographic studies of the processing os single words. *Journal of Cognitive Neuroscience, 1*, 153–170.

Price, C.J., Green, D.W., & von Studnitz, R. (1999). A functional imaging study of translation and language switching. *Brain, 122*, 2221–2235.

Robinson, G., Blair, J., & Cipolotti, L. (1998). Dynamic aphasia: an inability to select between competing verbal responses? *Brain, 121*, 77–89.

Ross, E.D. & Stewart, R.M. (1981). Akinetic mutism from hypothalamic damage: successful treatment with dopamine agonists. *Neurology, 31*, 1435–1439.

Rubens, A.B. (1976). Transcortical motor aphasia. *Studies in Neurolinguistics, 1*, 293–306.

Schwartz, M.F., Reed, E.S., Montgomery, M.W., Palmer, C., & Mayer, N.H. (1991). The quantitative description of action disorganization after brain damage: a case study. *Cognitive Neuropsychology, 8*, 381–414.

Shallice, T. (1982). Specific impairments of planning. *Phil-

osophical Transactions of the Royal Society of London, *298,* 199–209.

Shallice, T. & Burgess, P.W. (1991). Deficits in strategy application folowing frontal lobe damage in man. *Brain,* *114,* 727–741.

Sirigu, A., Cohen, L., Zalla, T., Pradat-Diehl, P., Van Eeckhout, P., Grafman, J., & Agid, Y. (1998). Distinct frontal regions for processing sentence syntax and story grammar. *Cortex, 34,* 771–778.

Stone, V.E., Baron-Cohen, S., & Knight, R.T. (1998). Frontal lobe contributions to theory of mind. *Journal of Cognitive Neuroscience, 10,* 640–656.

Thompson-Schill, S.L., Swick, D., Farah, M.J., D'Esposito, M., Kan, I.P., & Knight, R.T. (1998). Verb generation in patients with focal frontal lesions: a neuropsychological test of neuroimaging findings. *Proceedings of the National Academy of Sciences USA 95,* 15855–15860.

Von Stockert, T.R. (1974). Aphasia sine aphasie. *Brain and Language, 1,* 277–282.

11

The Organization of Working Memory Function in Lateral Prefrontal Cortex: Evidence from Event-Related Functional MRI

MARK D'ESPOSITO AND BRADLEY R. POSTLE

The prefrontal cortex (PFC) is a heteromodal association area interconnected with a widely distributed network of cortical and subcortical regions. Thus, the PFC is in a privileged position to make critical contributions to many cognitive functions. An early glimpse into this role was the landmark observation by Jacobsen (1935) that monkeys with PFC lesions were impaired on delayed-response tasks. In these tasks, the monkey had to keep "in mind," or actively maintain, a representation of the target stimulus over a short delay. Decades later, the ability to record from individual neurons in lateral PFC cortex led to the observation that some of these neurons activated exhibit sustained, elevated levels of activity during the delay period when the monkey is maintaining information in memory prior to a making a motor response that is contingent on this information (Funahashi et al., 1989; Fuster, 1997; see Fig. 11–1). This type of activity is consistent with that predicted by models of the neurophysiological mechanisms that may support the maintenance of items in short-term memory (Hebb, 1949). More recently, our conception of short-term memory has evolved to encompass not only the temporary maintenance "in mind" of information that is not accessible in the environment but also the set of processes that permit the manipulation

and transformation of this information in the service of planning and guiding behavior, and the term *working memory* (Miller et al., 1960 Baddeley & Hitch, 1974) has been adopted to connote this richer concept. Working memory is believed to make important contributions to many cognitive functions such as reasoning, language comprehension, planning, and spatial processing (Baddeley, 1986; Jonides, 1995).

Hypotheses about the critical role of the PFC in supporting working memory function were first prompted by syntheses of the results from experimental lesion studies (Pribram et al., 1964). These data were soon supplemented and extended with results from electrophysiological studies of sustained delay-period activity such as those described above. Such studies in monkeys performing delayed-response and delayed-recognition tasks have revealed that PFC neurons can also respond in a selective way to many non-delay portions of the task, such as to target (or cue) presentation, and to probe presentation and response (Fuster et al., 1982; Funahashi et al., 1989; Chafee & Goldman-Rakic, 1998), properties also observed in human PFC (Rypma & D'Esposito, 1999; Jha & McCarthy, 2000; Rowe et al., 2000). Thus, in addition to active maintenance of temporarily stored information, the PFC appears to support processes

A MONKEY

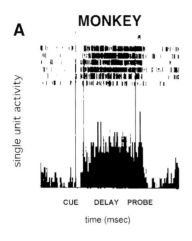

B HUMAN

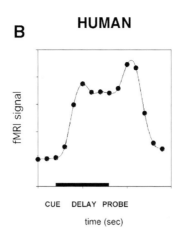

Figure 11–1. Delay-period activity in lateral prefrontal cortex during single-unit recording in a monkey (*A*) (adapted from Funahashi et al., 1989) and during an event-related functional magnetic resonance imaging (fMRI) experiment in a human subject (*B*) (adapted from Zarahn et al., 1997), while both performed a spatial delayed-response task.

that may include stimulus encoding, sustaining of attention to stimuli, manipulation of working memory representations, decision about a probe, preparation for a motor response, and execution of the motor response itself. According to one influential view, these manifold properties of lateral PFC can be understood as supporting the temporal integration of behavior (Fuster, 1997; also see Chapter 6).

In this chapter, we will focus much of our attention on methods, data, and interpretation of delay-specific activity in human PFC. After reviewing important neuroimaging methods, we will assess two influential models of the organization of working memory function in lateral PFC. Then we will review evidence of the hypothesis that many discrete regions of the PFC each support multiple discrete working memory–related processes.

FUNCTIONAL NEUROIMAGING OF WORKING MEMORY FUNCTION IN HUMAN PREFRONTAL CORTEX

Attributing delay-period activity to PFC function in humans analogous to that measured electrophysiologically in the monkey was not feasible until the advent of functional neuroimaging methods such as positron emission tomography (PET) and functional magnetic resonance imaging (fMRI). The first generation of functional neuroimaging investigations of working memory behavior could only assess delay-period activity in an indirect way, em-

ploying blocked experimental designs that required the integration of neuroimaging signal across entire blocks of trials (Posner et al., 1988). For a delayed-recognition task, the rationale of a block design is that "cognitive" subtraction of images obtained during sensorimotor control trials (i.e., not requiring memory) from images obtained from the memory trials will reveal brain regions that support the maintenance of information during the delay period of the task (see, for example, Jonides et al., 1993). This approach deviates methodologically in important ways from monkey electrophysiological experiments that can attribute unequivocally neural activity to particular epochs of a task.

First, the temporal resolution of blocked PET or fMRI designs is inherently poor, typically on the order of tens of seconds, and is thus ill suited to measure directly cognitive processes that evolve on the order of seconds or milliseconds.

Second, this approach often requires application of the logic of "cognitive subtraction" (Posner et al., 1988) and the companion assumption of "additivity" of discrete components of a task. These assumptions, also called *pure insertion*, posit that a cognitive process can be added to a preexisting set of cognitive processes without affecting them (Sternberg, 1969). For example, delayed-response tasks are characterized by a target-presentation epoch (entailing perceptual and encoding processes), a delay epoch (entailing the mnemonic processes of storage and maintenance), and a probe epoch (entailing stimulus evaluation, decision, response selection, and motoric output processes). A block-designed functional neuroimaging experiment of such a task seeks to uncover the neural substrates of its mnemonic processes via the subtraction of the integrated (i.e., averaged, summed, or totaled) neuroimaging signal derived from a block of trials lacking the delay epoch from that derived from a block of trials containing a delay epoch. Interpretation of the results of such an experiment, however, is conditioned on the possibility of a failure of the assumption of pure insertion. This could happen, for example, if the "inserted" delay epoch interacts with any of the processes associated with the probe epoch, such that the neuroimaging signal evoked by the probe epoch is greater when this stage is preceded by a delay than when it is not. In this example, the cognitive subtraction would yield a greater signal in memory trials than in sensorimotor control trials even if there was no signal change evoked by the delay epoch itself (for an empirical example of such a failure of the assumption of pure insertion in PFC, see Zarahn et al., 1997).

A third potential limitation of block designs that applies to fMRI may explain one reason for failures of pure insertion. To yield nonartifactual results, the function defining the transform from neural signal to neuroimaging signal must be linear. Several reports, however, have described some nonlinearities associated with fMRI data (Boynton et al., 1996; Vazquez & Noll, 1998; Huettel & McCarthy, 2000). A systematic pattern of diminution of the magnitude of the evoked blood oxygen–level dependent (BOLD) response to noninitial stimuli in a serial train of stimuli, for example, might explain why a probe epoch fMRI signal might be greater when preceded immediately by a (stimulus-free) delay epoch than when preceded immediately by the target-presentation epoch. This and many other such conceivable nonlinear interactions among BOLD responses to trial epochs would be undetectable in a blocked experiment.

The fourth limitation of inference, the last one that we will consider in detail here, is associated with tasks of a "continuous performance" nature, as opposed to tasks that are administered as a series of discrete trials. The most widely used of such tasks in working memory investigations is the n-back task, in which subjects monitor a serial presentation of stimuli and judge, for each one, whether or not it matches the stimulus that appeared n positions previously. This demanding task requires several computational operations, including (a) encoding a stimulus into a memory store; (b) maintaining the representation of this stimulus in memory despite the subsequent presentation of additional interfering and attentionally salient stimuli; (c) shifting attention back to this mnemonic representation when necessitated by task contingencies; (d) making a discrimination between this mnemonic representation and the stimulus on the screen and (e) guiding behavior with the outcome of this discrimination; and (f) actively discarding this mnemonic representation so that it won't interfere with subsequent operations to be performed with other mnemonic representations (Postle et al., 2000b). It is impossible in a blocked administration of a continuous performance task to dissociate activity that is, in principle, attributable to each of the many discrete mental processes engaged by these tasks. For example, to anticipate an issue that we will revisit later, is the greater activity seen when comparing a spatial 2-back task to its control task due to the increased encoding demands of the former, to its memory storage demands, to its increased attention shifting demands, to the increased difficulty of the decision about each stimulus, or to some combination of these?

To overcome these limitations, a new class of "event-related" designs for fMRI have been developed (for review, see D'Esposito et al., 1998; Rosen et al., 1998). This second generation of fMRI designs allows one to detect changes in fMRI signal that are attributable to neural events that are associated with discrete epochs within behavioral trials, as contrasted with a signal that can only be attributed to entire blocks of trials. Most event-related fMRI designs are analogous to event-related potential (ERP) designs of electroencephalographic studies in that the evoked responses attributed to different temporal epochs of the task can be sorted and analyzed separately.

Event-related fMRI represents an important methodological advance, because it permits direct measurement of PFC activity associated with each of the theoretically dissociable mental processes engaged by a task. In this sense, it is analogous to the methods employed in extracellular electrophysiological studies of awake, behaving monkeys. In the context of working memory studies, event-related designs permit direct assessment of delay-period activity, an important advantage over blocked designs. Using event-related fMRI designs, for example, several groups have confirmed that lateral PFC in humans is active during the maintenance of information across short-delay epochs of delayed-recognition tasks (e.g., Courtney et al., 1997; Zarahn et al., 1997; 1999; see Fig. 11–1). A more detailed consideration of different types of functional neuroimaging experimental designs can be found in Aguirre and D'Esposito (1999). What follows is a review of the application of these event-related fMRI methods to investigations of the functional organization of PFC.

THE LABELED-LINE MODEL OF PREFRONTAL CORTEX FUNCTION

Goldman-Rakic (1987) has proposed that discrete regions of the PFC are critical for the temporary maintenance of different domains of information. Particularly influential has been the hypothesis that lateral PFC is organized into discrete dorsal and ventral systems that support the temporary storage of spatial or object information, respectively. This hypothesis has the appeal of parsimony because it represents a rostral extension of the "what/where" organization of the visual system (Ungerleider & Haxby, 1994). It is also consistent with anatomical evidence from monkeys for the "labeled lines" that could carry this information about "where" and "what": parietal cortex (i.e., spatial vision regions) projects predominantly to a dorsal region of lateral PFC (Petrides & Pandya, 1984; Cavada & Goldman-Rakic, 1989), and temporal cortex (i.e., object vision regions) projects more ventrally within lateral PFC (Barbas, 1988). Goldman-Rakic and colleagues have recorded from

neurons in the caudal third of the principal sulcus of dorsolateral PFC and in the inferior convexity of ventrolateral PFC while monkeys performed spatial-delayed response tasks, and found that a greater proportion of neurons responded in a stimulus-selective way during the delay period in the former than in the latter region (Funahashi et al., 1990). Conversely, they have also found that more neurons in the inferior convexity than in principal sulcus demonstrated stimulus-selective delay-period activity during a pattern delayed-response task (Wilson et al., 1993). Goldman-Rakic and colleagues have also proposed that a third, more ventral area of lateral PFC may selectively support face working memory (O'Scalaidhe et al., 1997). Neuropsychological corroboration of these results has been seen in the fact that lesions of the dorsolateral PFC can impair spatial working memory performance (Gross, 1963; Funahashi et al., 1993; Levy & Goldman-Rakic, 1999), whereas lesions of more ventral areas of lateral PFC can impair nonspatial working memory performance (Passingham, 1975; Mishkin & Manning, 1978).

Shortly after the introduction of the cognitive subtraction methodology to functional neuroimaging, investigators began using this method to address this question in humans by determining the pattern of PFC activity during spatial and nonspatial working memory tasks. And although several early reports of neuroimaging studies of visual working memory described anatomical segregation for working memory for "what" and "where" in lateral PFC, there is very little consistency among them: one study reported spatial activity in right ventrolateral PFC but no object activity in the PFC (Smith et al., 1995); a second reported spatial activity in right dorsolateral PFC and object activity in dorsolateral PFC bilaterally (McCarthy et al., 1996); a third found greater spatial activity in dorsolateral and ventrolateral PFC bilaterally and greater object activity in left ventrolateral PFC (Baker et al., 1996); a fourth reported greater spatial activity in the superior frontal sulcus in premotor cortex and greater object (face stimuli) working memory activity in right inferior and orbital frontal cortex (Courtney et al.,

1996a); and a fifth reported greater spatial activity in medial superior frontal gyrus and greater object activity in middle and inferior frontal gyri bilaterally (Belger et al., 1998). (Note that the foci of spatially related superior frontal cortex activation reported by the fourth (Courtney et al., 1996a) and fifth [Belger et al., 1998] studies did not overlap, as the former did not find spatial activation in the PFC, and the latter did not acquire data from the premotor cortex.)

Confronted with this heterogeneity in the literature, we performed a critical examination of these first-generation studies of spatial and nonspatial working memory to see if a common trend toward segregation by stimulus type would emerge when data from different studies were compared directly. Our meta-analysis, however, found no evidence for a clear dorsal/ventral dissociation of PFC activity by stimulus domain (D'Esposito et al., 1998). In this meta-analysis we plotted the locations of activations from all reported functional neuroimaging studies of spatial and nonspatial working memory on a standardized brain. The labeled-line model predicted that the human homologue of the principal sulcal region of lateral PFC, the middle and superior frontal gyrus (Brodmann's area 9/46), would subserve spatial working memory, whereas the inferior frontal gyrus (Brodmann's areas 47, 44, 45) would preferentially subserve nonspatial working memory. As illustrated in Figure 11–2, however, numerous block design studies of spatial working memory have demonstrated activation within ventrolateral PFC, and, con-

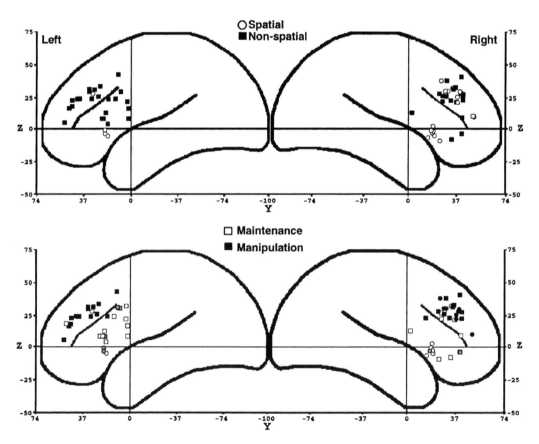

Figure 11–2. Meta-analysis of published functional neuroimaging studies of working memory (D'Esposito et al., 1998). Each square or circle represents a significant activation reported in a standardized atlas (Talairach & Tournoux, 1988). *Top*: Activations from either spatial or nonspatial studies. *Bottom*: Activations from the same studies reclassified as requiring maintenance or manipulation processes.

versely, numerous block design studies of non-spatial working memory have demonstrated activation within dorsolateral PFC.

Most of the studies incorporated in the above analysis examined either spatial or non-spatial working memory, but not both. We therefore performed an accompanying fMRI study in which we scanned subjects performing 2-back working memory tasks with stimuli drawn from two different domains of information during fMRI. The spatial task featured identical squares appearing in different locations and the verbal task featured different letters all appearing centrally. Paired with each 2-back task was a control task in which subjects monitored serially presented stimuli for a single, predetermined item. Group and individual subject analyses revealed activation in right middle frontal gyrus that did not differ between spatial and nonspatial working memory conditions. Since this study there have been several other first-generation studies that have also not found a clear segregation of function between dorsal and ventral PFC—e.g. locations versus abstract patterns (Owen et al., 1998); location versus abstract shapes (Postle et al., 2000b); and location versus letters versus abstract shapes (Nystrom et al., 2000).

Results from one laboratory stand out as an exception to all the studies presented above (Courtney et al., 1996b, 1998). In an initial blocked design PET study of delayed recognition that used face identity and face location as nonspatial and spatial memoranda, respectively (Courtney et al., 1996b), a direct comparison of the two memory conditions revealed that the spatial working memory task was associated with greater activation within left superior frontal sulcus (Brodmann's areas 8/6), whereas the face working memory task was associated with greater activation in right ventral PFC (areas 9/45/46). An unintended finding of this study was that the spatial working memory task did not produce PFC activation relative to its matched control task. In a follow-up study using an event-related fMRI design, this group reported a double dissociation of the neural loci of sustained (i.e., delay period) activity between face and spatial work-

ing memory–related activity: significantly more sustained activity occurred during spatial than during face trials within superior frontal sulcus, bilaterally, and significantly more sustained activity occurred during face than during spatial trials in left ventral PFC (Courtney et al., 1998). A subset of subjects also performed a visually guided saccade task, and it was determined that the spatial sustained activity in these subjects extended anteriorly and superiorly (by approximately 8.5 mm) beyond the region activated by the saccade task. This result was interpreted as evidence for an area "specialized" for spatial working memory that is discrete from the frontal eye fields, a hypothesis that we will revisit later in this chapter.

There are two salient methodological features of the Courtney et al. (1998) study that may contribute to the qualitative difference between its results and those of many other studies of working memory for different domains of information. First, it is likely that the measures of "sustained" activity reported in this study were contaminated by activity that preceded and followed the delay period. This is because sustained delay-period activity was modeled in the regression model as a square wave (or "boxcar") spanning the entire length of the delay period, and then convolved with a gaussian smoothing kernel. In any linear modeling approach to fMRI analysis, independent variables, or regressors or covariates, in the model must be convolved with a filter that approximates the low-pass filtered qualities of the fMRI signal—the fMRI response to neural activity is "smeared out" in time with respect to the underlying neural activity. The choice of modeling the entire delay period of a task necessarily resulted in an estimate of delay period activity that was influenced by activity that immediately preceded and immediately followed the delay period (Zarahn et al., 1997), because, in essence, encoding activity will "smear" into the delay period, and delay-period activity will "smear" into the probe/response epoch. In statistical terms, choosing to model the entire delay period with a boxcar regressor results in a situation in which the coefficient (or the parameter estimate) corresponding to this regressor likely reflects stimulus/encoding- and/or response-evoked activity as well as delay-period activity. This problem haunts any experiment in which events of interest occur in a temporally dependent manner (e.g., delay periods always follow a stimulus presentation epoch, and are always followed by a probe/choice/response epoch). For such experiments, randomization of events of interest (e.g., Burock et al., 1998; Clark et al., 1998) is not feasible. To achieve more reliable results in such experiments, which are central to working memory research, modeled epochs of a trial should be spaced out by at least 4 seconds, the minimum gap that permits theoretically distinct epochs of an fMRI time series to be measured without concern of contamination by events that precede or follow them (Zarahn et al., 1997). Second, visual working memory studies by this group are the only "what" versus "where" studies that we know of in which faces have been employed as the nonspatial stimuli. The nature of the stimuli used in this study may have been an important determinant contributing to the dissociation that was found.

We have performed a study using event-related fMRI that examined the neural correlates of the maintenance of spatial versus shape information. Our study differed from that of Courtney et al. (1998) in that our nonspatial stimuli were difficult-to-verbalize shapes (Attneave & Arnoult, 1956; Vanderplas & Garvin, 1959), and we employed a task with a "what-then-where" design that incorporated an object and a spatial delay period in each trial. This task was adapted from a monkey electrophysiology study by Miller and colleagues that provided evidence that there was extensive overlap in the topography of delay-active neurons tuned for spatial and object stimuli within lateral PFC (indeed, many neurons carried both kinds of signal) and no clear segregation (Rao et al., 1997). Similar to the results in the monkey, we found that identical regions of lateral PFC were activated when subjects maintained either spatial or object information. Reliable spatial/object differences in delay period activity were observed, however, in posterior cortical regions of the dorsal

and ventral visual streams (Postle & D'Esposito, 1999).

In a second study (Postle et al., 2000a), we tested directly the hypothesis that a region immediately anterior to the frontal eye fields in the vicinity of superior frontal sulcus in superior frontal cortex (SFC) is "specialized for spatial working memory" (Courtney et al., 1998, p. 1347). This hypothesis was an important claim, because it represented the only published evidence consistent with the original labeled-line model of a dorsal–ventral segregation of spatial versus object working memory in human frontal cortex. Our study featured variations of a delayed-recognition task that permitted comparison of memory for unpredictable locations on a two-dimensional display screen with saccades performed in two behavioral contexts: (*a*) repetitive, predictable horizontal (i.e., one-dimensional) saccades; and (*b*) unpredictable two-dimensional saccades. (The Courtney et al. (1998) study had only employed saccades of the former type.) When we compared delay-evoked activity to one-dimensional saccades (the type used by Courtney et al. [1998], we observed greater delay-evoked than saccade evoked activity in the SFC. However, when we compared delay-evoked activity to (memory-free) saccades made in the same unpredictable, two-dimensional circumstances as were the memory encoding–related saccades, there was no difference in fMRI activity. This result suggests that the memory-related function of this area is no more important than its saccade-related function, and that it is not specialized for memory function (Postle et al., 2000a). Thus, we failed to find support for a model that is critical to the labeled-line view of the organization of working memory function in the PFC.

Most of the evidence drawn from the human neuroimaging studies reviewed here is inconsistent with one particular labeled-line model of the organization of working memory function in PFC (Goldman-Rakic, 1987). It is important to emphasize, however, that although this model is derived from monkey studies, there are many reported monkey electrophysiological studies of dorsal and ventral regions of lateral PFC in which neither region exhibits delay-active neurons clearly segregated by domain specificity (Rosenkilde et al., 1981; Fuster et al., 1982, 2000; Quintana et al., 1988; Rainer et al., 1998; Rao et al., 1997). Additional evidence from monkey studies that is inconsistent with the labeled-line model of PFC is that (a) cooling (Fuster & Bauer, 1974; Bauer & Fuster, 1976; Quintana & Fuster, 1993) and lesions (Mishkin et al., 1969; Petrides, 1995) of a dorsal region of lateral PFC cause impairments on nonspatial working memory tasks, and (b) lesions in ventrolateral PFC cause spatial impairments (Mishkin et al., 1969; Iversen & Mishkin, 1970; Butters et al., 1973); whereas (c) ventrolateral PFC lesions do not cause delay-dependent defects on visual pattern association and color matching (Rushworth et al., 1997).

In several of the first-generation neuroimaging studies discussed above, there was a suggestion of a hemispheric dissociation between spatial and nonspatial working memory (e.g., greater right PFC activation in spatial paradigms and greater left PFC activation in nonspatial paradigms), although, as we noted, there was marked heterogeneity across studies. These hemispheric differences were found during performance of delayed-recognition tasks of comparing spatial and nonspatial stimuli (letters: Smith et al., 1996; objects; (Smith et al., 1995; Baker et al., 1996; Belger et al., 1998) in an N-back task comparing spatial and object stimuli (Smith et al., 1996), and in a repetition detection working memory task comparing spatial and object stimuli (McCarthy et al., 1996). However, lateralization by stimulus domain was not always reported in block design studies (Postle et al., 2000b; D'Esposito et al., 1998; Owen et al., 1998).

Prompted by the equivocalness of the corpus of first-generation neuroimaging studies on this question, we reanalyzed data from several event-related fMRI studies to address directly the question of lateralization by stimulus type of maintenance-related (i.e., delay-period) activity (Postle & D'Esposito, 2000). A reanalysis of spatial-versus object-delayed recognition revealed no evidence for lateralization of delay-period activity in dorsal PFC

(i.e., areas 9 and 46). It did suggest, however, a trend toward lateralization of delay-period activity in anterior ventral PFC (area 47), with object delay-period activity being stronger in the left hemisphere and spatial delay-period activity being stronger in the right. A reanalysis of delayed recognition of letter (i.e., verbal) stimuli also found no evidence for laterality differences in dorsolateral PFC nor, for these stimuli, in area 47. This reanalysis did, however, yield strong evidence for greater letter delay-period activity in the left hemisphere than in the right hemisphere in posterior ventral PFC (areas 44/45). This result is thus consistent with models positing an important role for Broca's area in the working memory rehearsal and maintenance of verbal stimulus material (Paulesu et al., 1993; Awh et al., 1996; Gabrieli, 1998; Smith & Jonides, 1998, 1999; Henson et al., 2000).

In this section, we have reviewed the human neuroimaging data investigating the principle of labeled-line organization of working memory function in lateral PFC. On the basis of this review, our working hypothesis is that there do exist varying degrees of segregation of function by stimulus domain (e.g., strongly so for verbal stimuli, more weakly for visual stimuli), but that the topographical patterns of segregation are not those that would be predicted by interpolation from the functional organization of the visual system. Most importantly, rather than being segregated in a dorsal–ventral fashion, spatial and object visual working memory functions appear to be broadly overlapping, and perhaps weakly segregated by hemisphere in anterior ventral PFC.

PROCESSING MODELS OF PREFRONTAL CORTEX FUNCTION

In some behavioral contexts, information must be maintained in a state analogous to that in which it was encoded (as when one remembers a telephone number when walking from the phone book to the telephone). Other circumstances require the manipulation of this remembered information (as when one performs mental calculations and must first generate, then retain, the intermediate products). Presumably, these manipulations or additional operations entail the recruitment of additional cognitive processes not required for simple maintenance of information. Petrides (1994) has proposed a processing model in which the ventrolateral PFC (primarily the inferior frontal gyrus) is the site where information is initially received from posterior association areas and where organization of information held in working memory is performed, whereas dorsolateral PFC (primarily the middle frontal gyrus) is additionally recruited only when monitoring and manipulation of information within working memory is required. The emphasis of this and other processing models, then, is that the fundamental factor along which lateral PFC function is organized is cognitive process (in contrast with the factor of information content, the organizing principle of labeled-line models). Note, however, that most processing models of the organization of working memory function of the PFC are, in principle, orthogonal to and mutually compatible with at least some versions of the labeled-line models described in the previous section.

Empirical support for such a dorsal–ventral organization-by-process in human PFC came first from a block design PET study contrasting PFC activation associated with several different spatial working memory tasks that were designed to vary in terms of manipulation and monitoring demands (Owen et al., 1996). The results were consistent with Petrides' processing model, and have been replicated in subsequent block design experiments employing fMRI (Owen et al., 1998) and PET (Owen et al., 1999). Interpretation of these results was complicated, however, by the complex set of subtractions and comparisons required to parcel out the relative contributions of the tasks that they employed—delayed-response, span, self-ordered choosing, and N-back, and of the control task associated with each—to measures of PFC activation. As with most first-generation neuroimaging studies relying on cognitive subtraction logic, the blocked designs of these studies also prevented direct inference as to whether the additional neuroimaging signal was attributable to neural activity arising during encoding, delay, or probe portions of such tasks. Thus, although these studies represent important initial tests of this processing model of the anatomical organization of working memory function in the PFC, they left many important questions unresolved.

We have performed three event-related fMRI studies designed to investigate the proposed neural dissociation between processes required for the active maintenance of information in working memory and the processes engaged when this information is manipulated. In the first study (D'Esposito et al., 1999a), the behavioral paradigm was a delayed-recognition task in which a set of five letters was presented simultaneously, in a randomly determined order, followed immediately by an instruction cue ("Forward" or "Alphabetize"), followed by an 8-second delay during which only a fixation cross appeared on the screen, followed by a probe that prompted the subject to make a motor response. Thus, subjects were presented with two types of trials (in random order) in which they were required either to (1) maintain a randomly ordered sequence of five letters across a delay period or (2) manipulate a comparable sequence of letters by arranging them into alphabetical order during the delay period. In both conditions, the probe consisted of a letter and number. In the forward condition, subjects were instructed to determine whether the letter was in the ordinal position represented by the number. This condition, therefore, simply required retention of the letters in the same format as presented at the beginning of the trial. In the alphabetize condition, subjects were instructed to determine whether that letter would be in the ordinal position represented by the number if the items in the memory set were rearranged into alphabetical order. This condition, therefore, required subjects to transpose the encoded order of the five items during the delay period.

In each subject, activity during the delay period was found in both dorsolateral and ventrolateral PFC in both types of trials. Additionally, in each subject dorsolateral PFC activity was significantly greater in trials during which information held in working memory was manipulated (see Fig. 11–3). A second study also employing letter stimuli, whose results will be considered in more detail below, replicated these results (Postle et al., 1999), and a third study confirmed that this property of dorsolateral PFC generalizes to spatial stimuli (Postle et al., 2000a). Thus, our results were broadly consistent with a two-stage processing model of the organization of working memory function in lateral PFC, in that they revealed a consistently greater contribution of dorsal than ventral PFC to manipulation processes.

The results of our event-related studies differed importantly, however, from those of previous block design studies of maintenance in working memory (Awh et al., 1996; Owen et al., 1996, 1998; Smith & Jonides, 1998) in that they provided evidence that dorsolateral PFC is also active during working memory maintenance trials. Thus, our model of organization-by-process of PFC is a nested, hierarchical one, in which all of lateral PFC can be recruited to support maintenance requirements of a working memory task, but only dorsolateral regions are recruited to an additional extent when manipulation of mnemonic representations is required. We believe that the discrepancy between our results and those of Owen and colleagues, for example, are more likely attributable to neuroimaging task design (i.e., blocked versus event-related) than to differences in behavioral tasks. Although

our maintenance task differed procedurally from some of those of Owen and colleagues in that it may not have required "monitoring" operations to the same extent, this difference would only be expected to lessen the extent to which our tasks would recruit dorsolateral PFC. The results from our group that were summarized in the previous paragraph are consistent with those of several other event-related fMRI studies that have shown, with several different types of stimuli, that active maintenance in working memory can recruit dorsolateral PFC (e.g., Cohen et al., 1997; Courtney et al., 1997; Zarahn et al., 1999). The finding that dorsolateral PFC can be engaged during maintenance-requiring as well as during manipulation-requiring delay periods is the first piece of evidence that we have marshaled in support of our view that lateral PFC supports several discrete working memory–related cognitive processes.

The second event-related fMRI study of maintenance versus manipulation of letters (Postle et al., 1999), mentioned briefly above, replicated the results of the first study (D'Esposito et al., 1999a), providing corroborative evidence for dorso- and ventrolateral PFC activity during the delay period of working memory maintenance trials, and consistently greater activity during alphabetization trials only in dorsolateral PFC (Postle et al., 1999). This second study also extended our earlier results in two important ways. First, it

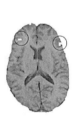
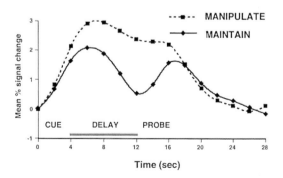

Figure 11–3. Trial-averaged functional magnetic resonance imaging (fMRI) time series from voxels in lateral prefrontal cortex that were significant in the direct contrast between manipulation and maintenance in a representative normal subject. Note that the two peaks in the maintenance condition correspond to the stimulus presentation (cue) and the probe periods of the trial. In the manipulation condition, the voxels displayed maintained a high level of activity throughout the delay period. The solid bar represents the duration of the delay period.

established that the maintenance/manipulation organization of dorsolateral PFC is not confounded by differences in difficulty, because performance on forward and alphabetize trials (each presenting five letters) was equivalent. Second, the inclusion of a condition requiring maintenance of two letters permitted investigation of working memory load effects. We did not find consistent delay-specific load effects in dorsolateral PFC, and, importantly, there was no evidence of delay-period load effects in any voxels that evinced greater manipulation than maintenance activity (Postle et al., 1999). (We did find, in contrast, consistent delay-period load effects in left posterior perisylvian cortex.) This result, therefore, provides the first evidence that the manipulation-related processes ascribed to dorsolateral PFC are fundamentally extramnemonic in nature. That is, whereas they play an important role in the exercise of executive control of working memory, they operate independently of the processes responsible for the storage of information in working memory. Indeed, the alphabetization-related processes required by our manipulation working memory trials are likely the same as those that would be required were one to alphabetize a string of letters that were present throughout the trial (i.e., in a task that did not require working memory).

This result has implications not only for hierarchical processing models of the organization of working memory function in PFC but also for the interpretation of "load effects" observed in the PFC in experiments that manipulate parametrically the number of items maintained in an N-back task (Braver et al., 1997; Cohen et al., 1997; Jonides et al., 1997). This result suggests that these effects may be attributable to processes contributing to performance of these tasks that are not storage or maintenance related. Examples of such processes include encoding-specific processes, and control processes such as attention shifting and inhibition of prepotent responses. This idea received support from the results of the next study we will describe, an examination of load effects in item-recognition working memory.

PREFRONTAL CORTEX SUPPORTS MANY WORKING MEMORY–RELATED PROCESSES

The findings from the studies reviewed in this section will reveal an apparent paradox regarding the organization of working memory–related functions of lateral PFC: functional subdivisions clearly exist in that different regions within lateral PFC are engaged by different cognitive operations, yet any one region of lateral PFC may be engaged by multiple theoretically discrete cognitive operations. In the previous section we have already noted one example of this phenomenon: dorsolateral PFC is engaged in both the maintenance and manipulation of information in working memory (D'Esposito et al., 1999a); although no single voxel within this region seems to support both (Postle et al., 1999). As we shall now see, the advent of event-related fMRI designs has led to the discovery of many more such examples of the multifunctionality of this region.

Recently, two first-generation neuroimaging studies have shown that activity in dorsolateral PFC increases in concert with increased memory load during performance of tasks with no overt requirements to manipulate information held in working memory (Manoach et al., 1997; Rypma et al., 1999). For example, Rypma and colleagues (1999) observed activation in dorsolateral PFC in a Sternberg (1966)-type item-recognition task in which subjects were required to maintain one, three, or six letters in working memory for 5 seconds. In the three-letter condition, relative to one letter, activation in the PFC was limited to left ventrolateral PFC (Brodmann's area 44). However, in the six-letter condition, relative to one letter, the additional activation of dorsolateral PFC was observed. Rypma and colleagues proposed that dorsolateral PFC may be recruited during maintenance tasks in which subjects must actively maintain information loads that approach or exceed short-term memory capacity. According to this view, the same dorsolateral PFC circuits important for manipulation of information in working memory may be recruited for the mediation of strategic processes necessary for the maintenance of a high load of information. Alternative interpretations of the Rypma et al. (1999) and Manoach et al. (1997) results were possible, however, because both featured blocked designs that made identification of the specific component processes that were sensitive to varying load impossible.

In an event-related fMRI study intended to elucidate the relative contributions of cue, delay, and probe task periods to PFC activation in item-recognition working memory performance, Rypma and D'Esposito (1999) asked subjects to maintain either two or six letters across an unfilled delay period and found that the effects of increased memory load were observed only in dorsolateral PFC and only in the encoding period of the task. Consistent with the result described earlier (Postle et al., 1999), delay-period load effects were seen only in left posterior cortex. These results suggest that the load-sensitive effects in dorsolateral PFC that were identified in earlier block design studies (Manoach et al., 1997; Rypma et al., 1999) may have been due to encoding-related processes, rather than to the maintenance of information in working memory. It may be that initial encoding of information requires cognitive operations (e.g., monitoring the contents of working memory, and updating and coordination of multiple memory buffers) that are similar to those required in the manipulation tasks described previously. It is also possible, however, that the same brain region that supports delay-related manipulation processes also supports distinct encoding-related processes. This possibility constitutes a second example of how dorsolateral PFC can support several discrete working memory–related processes. Additional experiments are required to adjudicate between the "manipulation" and "encoding" alternatives.

Because we observed considerable inter-subject variability in fMRI signal magnitude and activation extent in this event-related study of item recognition (Rypma & D'Esposito, 1999), we performed additional analyses to explore possible relations between individual differences in PFC physiological measures and task performance. For these analyses we measured performance of each in-

dividual subject in terms of his or her memory retrieval rate, the interpolated slope being obtained when plotting reaction time against memory load (two- vs. six-letter trials). This reaction time slope is believed to index memory retrieval rate when subjects must make a yes/no judgment about the membership of a probe stimulus in the memory set (Sternberg, 1966). This memory retrieval rate may vary with the efficiency of memory scanning processes. We measured PFC activity as the number of voxels identified with a load-independent contrast selective for voxels evincing delay-period activity during two- and six-letter trials. Linear regression analyses were then applied to data from each trial component (i.e., cue, delay, and probe) and from two PFC regions of interest (dorsolateral and ventrolateral) to test for relationships between performance and activity. The results of these analyses of individual differences showed a significant effect only in the dorsolateral PFC, whereas the retrieval rate was positively correlated with activity during only one trial epoch, the probe epoch (see Fig. 11–4). Because this epoch encompasses decision- and response-related processes, these results suggest two conclusions. First, because a slower retrieval rate corresponds to less efficient working memory scanning, poorer performers on this task may have recruited broader networks within dorsolateral PFC to compensate for inefficient working memory scanning processes. Second, the finding of a significant brain–behavior link only in dorsolateral PFC, and only during response, suggests that this region of the PFC represents an important substrate of memory scanning, a retrieval process that is initiated with the onset of the probe stimulus. Here, then, is the third example of a discrete working memory–related process being supported by dorsolateral PFC.

Although the previously described study characterized the neural substrate of one component process (or set of processes) that is recruited in association with the onset of the probe stimulus in a delayed-recognition task, there are certainly many other processes engaged during this portion of the task, candidates among them including shifting attention

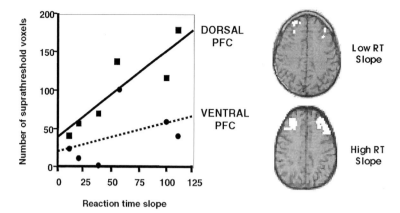

Figure 11–4. Scatter plot of the numbers of suprathreshold voxels during the response period of a delayed response task in dorsal prefrontal cortex (PFC) (squares) and ventral PFC (circles) plotted against reaction time (RT) slopes. The linear relationship between PFC activity and RT is significant in dorsal, but not ventral PFC. Also shown are axial slices of activation patterns in the two representative subjects with the lowest (fastest memory scanning rate) and highest (slowest scanning rate) RT slopes.

among items held in working memory (McElree & Dosher, 1987; Garavan et al., 2000); inhibition of prepotent responses (Diamond, 1990); mediation of proactive interference (Jonides et al., 1998); coordination of multiple task performance (D'Esposito et al., 1995); response selection and preparation (D'Esposito et al., 2000; Rowe et al., 2000; Schumacher & D'Esposito, 2000); and motor execution. An important empirical question is the extent to which each of these theoretically dissociable probe-related processes relies on the same neural substrate. To begin to approach this problem we chose to focus on another working memory–related phenomenon, proactive interference, whose effects are measured by reaction times (RTs).

Using event-related fMRI, we scanned subjects as they performed a four-letter item-recognition task in which two types of trials were of greatest interest: those with recent negative probes that matched a letter from the target set of the two previous, but not the present, trial; and those with nonrecent negative probes that did not match a target letter from any of these trials. A previous imaging study indicated that recent negative trials are associated with an RT cost believed to reflect the operation of a process or set of processes that detects and resolves proactive interfer-

ence (Jonides et al., 1998), and behavioral results from our study also revealed a small but reliable RT effect. The physiological data from our task confirmed that there were no differences between the two trial types anywhere in the PFC during target presentation and delay-period epochs, but that there was significantly greater probe-related activation for recent negative than for nonrecent negative trials within left ventrolateral PFC (but not in other regions of the PFC). These findings characterized spatially and temporally a physiological proactive interference effect that was reliable across subjects and that correlated with the mean RT cost of 32 ms produced by our proactive interference manipulation.

An additional study has established that this left ventral region of PFC is also sensitive to proactive interference that is generated within, in contrast to across, trials (Postle et al., 2001). In a running span, or "updating" task, subjects viewed letter stimuli as they were presented in groups of one, two, or three, and they were instructed to maintain a memory of the four most recently presented items. The fMRI correlates of the probe-related *intratrial* proactive interference (PI) effect were found reliably only in Brodmann's area 45, and thus were anatomically specific, and were consistent with the results obtained with *intertrial* proactive interference in delayed item-recognition tasks (Jonides et al., 1998, 2000), D'Esposito et al., 1999b).

Note that the left ventral PFC region associated with this proactive interference effect is the same region associated with delay-specific activity (perhaps attributable to rehearsal) in verbal working memory (Paulesu et al., 1993; Awh et al., 1996; Gabrieli, 1998; Smith et al., 1998; Smith & Jonides, 1999; Henson et al., 2000; Postle & D'Esposito, 2000). Further investigation of these effects needs to be carried out to determine whether the process(es) indexed by these effects are best characterized as response inhibition (Jonides et al., 1998), selection among candidate memoranda (Thompson-Schill et al., 1997), probe discrimination (Monsell, 1978; McElree & Dosher, 1987), or an as yet unarticulated alternative. But regardless of what subsequent studies tell us about the computational nature of the processes underlying this PI effect, we have already established that it is supported by a different region of PFC than that which supports memory scanning–related processes that are also associated with the probe/response component of working memory–task performance. Thus, we have also characterized a fourth discrete working memory–related process that is supported by lateral PFC—in this case, by the same region associated with the maintenance of verbal stimulus material.

Finally, this same study of updating in working memory (Postle et al., 2001) revealed a fifth and sixth working memory–related process associated with lateral PFC: an item-accumulation effect and a trial-length effect. We assumed that updating comprises (1) discarding items from, (2) repositioning items in, and (3) adding items to a running working memory span. The item-accumulation effect, observed in updating-sensitive voxels in the PFC, was manifested by a monotonic increase in signal with the number of items presented during a trial, despite the insensitivity of behavioral measures to the trial-length factor. The trial-length effect, in contrast, was a probe-specific effect corresponding to signal intensity differences between 4- and 12-item

trials. This effect was only significant in left dorsolateral PFC. Note that this effect is likely different from the memory scanning–related probe effects seen in tests that vary memory load (e.g., Rypma et al., 1999), because the memory load in the updating task is held constant at four items, regardless of trial length.

CONCLUSION

Lateral PFC in humans is clearly recruited during many discrete cognitive processes that are engaged by the performance of delayed-recognition tasks. Figure 11–5 summarizes schematically the findings of the event-related fMRI studies from our laboratory that were reviewed in this chapter. One strong conclusion that can be drawn from these data is that lateral PFC activity cannot be ascribed to the function of a single, unitary cognitive operation. Consistent with the picture that has emerged from the monkey electrophysiological literature, we have seen that human PFC is involved in several encoding- and response-related processes as well as in the mnemonic and extramnemonic processes that can be engaged during the delay periods of working memory tasks.

When the amount of to-be-remembered information presented at the beginning of a delayed-response trial approaches or exceeds short-term memory capacity (e.g., Waugh & Norman, 1965), dorsolateral PFC is engaged, suggesting that processes supported by this region may facilitate the efficient encoding of information. During the subsequent delay interval, when no information is accessible to the subject, both ventro- and dorsolateral PFC are recruited. Our data indicate that maintenance-related processes engaged by all stimulus types are distributed broadly across both hemispheres of PFC. Maintenance of verbal stimuli is strongest, however, in left posteroinferior PFC, and maintenance of spatial and nonspatial visual stimuli may exhibit weak lateralization within right and left anteroinferior PFC, respectively. If manipulation of this information (regardless of type) is additionally required during the delay period, dor

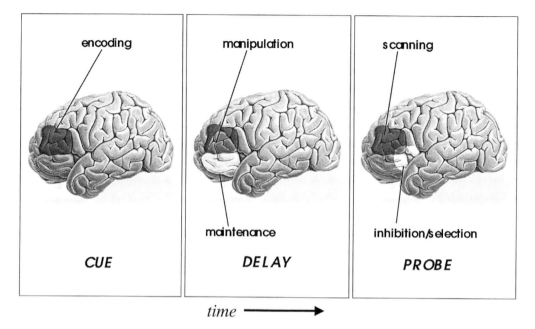

time ⟶

Figure 11–5. Schematic illustration that summarizes the findings from the functional magnetic resonance imaging (fMRI) studies presented in this chapter. Each panel il- lustrates dorsal and ventral prefrontal cortex areas that were active during different stages of delayed-response tasks.

solateral PFC is engaged to a significantly greater extent. Upon the presentation of the probe stimulus, when a subject is required to make a response based on what was presented at the beginning of the trial, dorsolateral PFC is again engaged, presumably as the subject scans the information that was retained across the trial and chooses an appropriate motor re- sponse. Furthermore, the extent of activation of dorsolateral PFC is inversely correlated with the efficiency of this scanning process. That is, faster memory scanning is associated with less PFC activation, and vice versa. If at the time of the probe there is proactive inter- ference from previously remembered infor- mation, a more ventral region of left PFC is engaged to adjudicate the conflict caused by this interference. Also at the time of the probe, activity in left dorsolateral PFC is sen- sitive to the number of items that have been presented during a trial, regardless of the ac- tual memory load required by that trial. Or- thogonal to all these effects, the accumulation of items during an updating task is indexed broadly across PFC in the item accumulation effect. Together, the results of these studies

reveal a temporally and topographically com- plex pattern of PFC function in the service of working memory task performance.

Our data have provided evidence for func- tional subdivisions within lateral PFC and we propose that lateral PFC is organized both by content (right/left) and process (dorsal/ventral) (see Fig. 11–6). However, it is clear that any one region within lateral PFC can be engaged by distinctly different cognitive operations in different contexts. For example, dorsal, and not ventral, PFC is preferentially engaged when encoding a large number of items, when information being maintained must be manip- ulated, when the presentation of a probe stim- ulus prompts a scan of the contents of working memory, and during the selection of a re- sponse based on the remembered informa- tion. Yet, presumably very different cognitive operations are engaged during each of these processing stages. And whereas many of these processing stages are engaged during different task epochs, some are associated with the same epochs. For example, maintenance and manipulation of information, two different cognitive operations, can recruit the same re-

Figure 11–6. Proposed hybrid model of the organization of lateral prefrontal cortex.

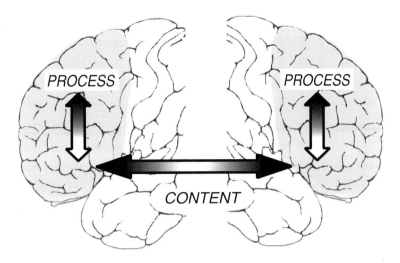

Figure 11–6. Proposed hybrid model of the organization of lateral prefrontal cortex.

gion of dorsolateral PFC (although apparently, not the same voxels within this subregion).

A priority of future research will be to determine if the two subregions of lateral PFC that we have concentrated on in this chapter, the dorsal and ventral portions, can be further subdivided on functional grounds, or whether each of these regions truly has the adaptive capacity to be engaged by different cognitive operations in different contexts. The latter possibility would suggest that the functional significance of activity in a particular subregion of lateral PFC may depend on the posterior and subcortical brain regions with which it is interacting at that moment (McIntosh et al., 1996; Fuster, 2001) and/or on the current tonus set by subcortical modulatory systems (Kimberg et al., 1997).

It is important to emphasize the limits of inferences that can be drawn from our review of functional neuroimaging studies of PFC function. It is the nature of all physiological studies of the nervous system (including single- and multiunit electrophysiology, electroencephalograpy, magnetoencephalography, and measures of glucose metabolism, as well as hemodynamic measures such as fMRI) that they support inferences about the association of a particular brain system with a cognitive process. Thus, functional neuroimaging is an observational, correlative method (Sarter et al., 1996). The inference of necessity of a brain region to a given cognitive function cannot be made without a demonstration that the inac-

tivation of this region disrupts the function in question. But interpretation of neuropsychological data is subject to a different set of caveats. Among them, lesion localization is difficult in human studies, and the interruption of fibers of passage by a brain insult is difficult to assess, as are compensation, plasticity, and other recovery processes. Additionally, strong inferences about structure–function relationships can be complicated by the possibility that the lesioned area contributes in a nonspecific way to the normal functioning of a distal region that is itself the true neural substrate of the function in question. When lesion and functional neuroimaging studies are combined, however, a stronger level of inference can result.

Few human studies of patients with focal lesions of PFC performing delayed-response or recognition tasks have been reported. In a recent review of such studies, we found that some groups of patients with PFC lesions can show impairment, and that these deficits tend to be more prominent when patients perform tasks that include distraction during the delay period (D'Esposito & Postle, 1999). Several transcranial magnetic stimulation studies have shown that stimulation over lateral PFC during the delay period of a delayed-response task degrades performance (Pascual-Leone & Hallett, 1994; Muri et al., 1996; Brandt et al., 1998). These findings, coupled with the finding that patients with PFC lesions are generally not impaired on tests of working memory span (i.e., digit span and spatial [Corsi block] span (D'Esposito & Postle, 1999), are consistent with the idea that lateral PFC is especially critical for the extramnemonic executive control processes investigated by many of the fMRI studies presented in this review. Because patients with focal lesions of the PFC are rare, and their lesions are not typically restricted to small subdivisions, the neuropsychological evidence for functional subdivisions within lateral PFC is scant. It is our hope that future neuropsychological studies guided by functional imaging studies, such as those presented in this chapter, will lead to new insight regarding the functional organization of the frontal lobes.

REFERENCES

Aguirre, G.K. & D'Esposito, M. (1999). Experimental design for brain fMRI. In: C.T.W. Moonen & P.A. Bandettini (Eds.), *Functional MRI* (pp. 369–380). Berlin: Springer-Verlag.

Attneave, F. & Arnoult, M.D. (1956). Methodological considerations in the quantitative study of shape and pattern perception. *Psychological Bulletin*, 53, 221–227.

Awh, E., Jonides, J., Smith, E.E., Schumacher, E.H., Koeppe, & R.A. Katz, S. (1996). Dissociation of storageand rehearsal in verbal working memory: evidence from PET. *Psychological Science*, 7, 25–31.

Baddeley, A. (1986). *Working Memory*. New York: Oxford University Press.

Baddeley, A. & Hitch, G.J. (1974). Working memory. In: G.A. Bower (Ed.), *Recent Advances in Learning and Motivation*, Vol. 8 (pp. 47–89). New York: Academic Press.

Baker, S.C., Frith, C.D., Frackowiak, R.S.J., & Dolan, R.J. (1996). Active representation of shape and spatial location in man. *Cerebral Cortex*, 6, 612–619.

Barbas, H. (1988). Anatomic organization of basoventral and mediodorsal visual recipient prefrontal regions in the rhesus monkey. *Journal of Comparative Neurology*, 276, 313–342.

Bauer, R.H. & Fuster, J.M. (1976). Delayed-matching and delayed-response deficit from cooling dorsolateralprefrontal cortex in monkeys. *Journal of Comparative and Physiological Psychology*, 90, 293–302.

Belger, A., Puce, A., Krystal, J.H., Gore, J.C., Goldman-Rakic, P., & McCarthy, G. (1998). Dissociation of mnemonic and perceptual processes during spatial and nonspatial working memory using fMRI. *Human Brain Mapping*, 6, 14–32.

Boynton, G.M., Engel, S.A., Glover, G.H., & Heeger, D.J. (1996). Linear systems analysis of functional magnetic resonance imaging in human V1. *Journal of Neuroscience*, 16, 4207–4221.

Brandt, S.A., Ploner, C.J., Meyer, B.U., Leistner, S., & Villringer, A. (1998). Effects of repetitive transcranial magnetic stimulation over dorsolateral prefrontal and posterior parietal cortex on memory-guided saccades. *Experimental Brain Research*, 118, 197–204.

Braver, T.S., Cohen, J.D., Nystrom, L.E., Jonides, J., Smith, E.E., & Noll, D.C. (1997). A parametric study of prefrontal cortex involvement in human working memory. *NeuroImage*, 5, 49–62.

Burock, M.A., Buckner, R.L., Woldorff, M.G., Rosen, B.R., & Dale, A.M. (1998). Randomized event-related experimental designs allow for extremely rapid presentation rates using functional MRI. *NeuroReport*, 9, 3735–3739.

Butters, N., Butter, C., Rosen, J., & Stein, D. (1973). Behavioral effects of sequential and one-stage ablations of orbital prefrontal cortex in monkey. *Experimental Neurology*, 39, 204–214.

Cavada, C. & Goldman-Rakic, P.S. (1989). Posteriorparietal cortex in rhesus monkey: II. Evidence for segregated corticocortical networks linking sensory and limbic areas with frontal lobe. *Journal of Comparative Neurology*, 287, 422–445.

Chafee, M.V. & Goldman-Rakic, P.S. (1998). Matching patterns of activity in primate prefrontal area 8a and parietal area 7ip neurons during a spatial working memory task. *Journal of Neurophysiology*, 79, 2919–2940.

Clark, V.P., Maisog, J.M., & Haxby, J.V. (1998). fMRI study of face perception and memory using random stimulus sequences. *Journal of Neurophysiology*, 79, 3257–3265.

Cohen, J.D., Perlstein, W.M., Braver, T.S., Nystrom, L.E., Noll, D.C., Jonides, J., & Smith, E.E. (1997). Temporal dynamics of brain activation during a working memory task. *Nature*, 386, 604–607.

Courtney, S.M., Ungerleider, L.G., Keil, K., & Haxby, J. (1996a). Object and spatial visual working memory activate separate neural systems in human cortex. *Cerebral Cortex*, 6, 39–49.

Courtney, S.M., Ungerleider, L.G., Keil, K., & Haxby, J.V. (1996b). Object and spatial visual working memory activate separate neural systems in human cortex. *Cerebral Cortex*, 6, 39–49.

Courtney, S.M., Ungerleider, L.G., Keil, K., & Haxby, J.V. (1997). Transient and sustained activity in a distributed neural system for human working memory. *Nature*, 386, 608–611.

Courtney, S.M., Petit, L., Maisog, J.M., Ungerleider, L.G., & Haxby, J.V. (1998). An area specialized for spatial working memory in human frontal cortex. *Science*, 279, 1347–1351.

D'Esposito, M. & Postle, B.R. (1999). The dependence of span and delayed-response performance on prefrontal cortex. *Neuropsychologia*, 37, 89–101.

D'Esposito, M., Detre, J.A., Alsop, D.C., Shin, R.K., Atlas, S. & Grossman, M. (1995). The neural basis of the central executive system of working memory. *Nature*, 378, 279–281.

D'Esposito, M., Aguirre, G.K., Zarahn, E., & Ballard, D. (1998). Functional MRI studies of spatial and nonspatial working memory. *Cognitive Brain Research, 7,* 1–13.

D'Esposito, M., Postle, B.R., Ballard, D., & Lease, J. (1999a). Maintenance versus manipulation of information held in working memory: an event-related fMRI study. *Brain and Cognition, 41,* 66–86.

D'Esposito, M., Postle, B.R., Jonides, J. & Smith, E.E. (1999b). The neural substrate and temporal dynamics of interference effects in working memory as revealed by event-related functional MRI. *Proceedings of the National Academy of Sciences USA, 96,* 7514–7519.

D'Esposito, M., Ballard, D., Zarahn, E. & Aguirre, G.K. (2000). The role of prefrontal cortex in sensory memory and motor preparation: an event-related fMRI study [see comments]. *NeuroImage, 11,* 400–408.

Diamond, A. (1990). The development and neural bases of memory functions as indexed by the A-not-B and delayed response tasks in human infants and infant monkeys. In: A. Diamond (Ed.), *The Development and Neural Bases of Higher Cognitive Functions* (pp. 267–317). New York: The New York Academy of Sciences.

Funahashi, S., Bruce, C.J., & Goldman-Rakic, P.S. (1989). Mnemonic coding of visual space in the monkey's dorsolateral prefrontal cortex. *Journal of Neurophysiology, 61,* 331–349.

Funahashi, S., Bruce, C.J., & Goldman-Rakic, P.S. (1990). Visuospatial coding in primate prefrontal neurons revealed by oculomotor paradigms. *Journal of Neurophysiology, 63,* 814–831.

Funahashi, S., Bruce, C.J., & Goldman-Rakic, P.S. (1993). Dorsolateral prefrontal lesions and oculomotor delayed-response performance: evidence for mnemonic "scotomas". *Journal of Neuroscience, 13,* 1479–1497.

Fuster, J. (1997). *The Prefrontal Cortex: Anatomy, Physiology, and Neuropsychology of the Frontal Lobes,* 3rd ed. New York: Raven Press.

Fuster, J.M. (2001). The prefrontal cortex—an update: time is of the essence. *Neuron, 30,* 319–333.

Fuster, J.M. & Bauer, R.H. (1974). Visual short-term memory deficit from hypothermia of frontal cortex. *Brain Research, 81,* 393–400.

Fuster, J.M., Bauer, R.H., & Jervey, J.P. (1982). Cellular discharge in the dorsolateral prefrontal cortex of the monkey in cognitive tasks. *Experimental Neurology, 77,* 679–694.

Fuster, J.M., Bodner, M., & Kroger, J.K. (2000). Cross-modal and cross-temporal association in neurons of frontal cortex. *Nature, 405,* 347–351.

Gabrieli, J.D. (1998). Cognitive neuroscience of human memory. *Annual Review of Psychology, 49,* 87–115.

Garavan, H., Ross, T.J., Li, S.J., & Stein, E.A. (2000). A parametric manipulation of central executive functioning. *Cerebral Cortex, 10,* 585–592.

Goldman-Rakic, P.S. (1987). Circuitry of the prefrontal cortex and the regulation of behavior by representational memory. In: F. Plum & V. Mountcastle (Eds.), *Handbook of Physiology, Section 1. The Nervous System, Vol. 5.* (pp. 373–417). Bethesda, MD: American Physiological Society.

Gross, C.G. (1963). A comparison of the effects of partial

and total lateral frontal lesions on test performance by monkeys. *Journal of Comparative and Physiological Psychology, 56,* 41–47.

Hebb, D.O. (1949). *Organization of Behavior.* New York: John Wiley & Sons.

Henson, R.N.A., Burgess, N., & Frith, C.D. (2000). Recoding, storage, rehearsal and grouping in verbal short-term memory: an fMRI study. *Neuropsychologia, 38,* 426–440.

Huettel, S.A. & McCarthy, G. (2000). Evidence for a refractory period in the hemodynamic response to visual stimuli as measured by MRI. *NeuroImage, 11,* 547–553.

Iversen, S.D. & Mishkin, M. (1970). Perseverative interference in monkeys following selective lesions of the inferior prefrontal convexity. *Experimental Brain Research, 11,* 376–386.

Jacobsen, C.F. (1935). Functions of frontal association areas in primates. *Archives of Neurology and Psychiatry, 33,* 558–560.

Jha, A. & McCarthy, G. (2000). The influence of memory load upon delay interval activity in a working memory task: an event-related functional MRI study. *Journal of Cognitive Neuroscience, 12,* 90–105.

Jonides, J. (1995). Working memory and thinking. In: E.E. Smith & D.N. Osherson (Eds.), *An Invitation to Cognitive Science* (pp. 215–265). Cambridge, MA: MIT Press.

Jonides, J., Smith, E.E., Koeppe, R.A., Awh, E., Minoshima, S., of Mintun, M.A. (1993). Spatial working memory in humans as revealed by PET. *Nature, 363,* 623–625.

Jonides, J., Smith, E.E., Marshuetz, C., Koeppe, R.A., & Reuter-Lorenz, P.A. (1998). Inhibition of verbal working memory revealed by brain activation. *Proceedings of the National Academy of Sciences USA 95,* 8410–8413.

Jonides, J., Schumacher, E.H., Smith, E.E., Lauber, E., Awh, E., Minoshima, S., & Koeppe, R.A. (1997). Verbal working memory load affects regional brain activation as measured by PET. *Journal of Cognitive Neuroscience, 9,* 462–475.

Jonides, J., Marshuetz, C., Smith, E.E., Reuter-Lorenz, P.A., & Koeppe, R.A. (2000). Age differences in behavior and PET activation reveal differences in interference resolution in verbal working memory. *Journal of Cognitive Neuroscience, 12,* 188–196.

Kimberg, D., D'Esposito, M., & Farah, M. (1997). Effects of bromocriptine on human subjects depend on working memory capacity. *NeuroReport, 8,* 3581–3585.

Levy, R. & Goldman-Rakic, P.S. (1999). Association of storage and processing functions in the dorsolateral prefrontal cortex of the non-human primate. *Journal of Neuroscience, 19,* 5149–5158.

Manoach, D.S., Schlaug, G., Siewert, B., Darby, D.G., Bly, B.M., Benfield, A., Edelman, R.R., & Warach, S. (1997). Prefrontal cortex fMRI signal changes are correlated with working memory load. *NeuroReport, 8,* 545–549.

McCarthy, G., Puce, A., Constable, R.T., Krystal, J.H., Gore, J.C., & Goldman-Rakic, P.S. (1996). Activation of human prefrontal cortex during spatial and nonspatial working memory tasks measured by functional MRI. *Cerebral Cortex, 6,* 600–611.

McElree, B. & Dosher, B.A. (1987). Serial position and set size in short-term memory: the time course of recognition. *Journal of Experimental Psychology: General, 118,* 346–373.

McIntosh, A.R., Grady, C.L., Haxby, J.V., Ungerleider, L.G., & Horwitz, B. (1996). Changes in limbic and prefrontal functional interactions in a working memory task for faces. *Cerebral Cortex, 6,* 571–584.

Miller, G.A., Galanter, E., & Pribram, K.H. (1960). *Plans and the Structure of Behavior.* New York: Henry Holt and Company.

Mishkin, M. & Manning, F.J. (1978). Non-spatial memory after selective prefrontal lesions in monkeys. *Brain Research, 143,* 313–323.

Mishkin, M., Vest, B., Waxler, M., & Rosvold, H.E. (1969). A re-examination of the effects of frontal lesions on object alternation. *Neuropsychologia, 7,* 357–363.

Monsell, S. (1978). Recency, immediate recognition memory, and reaction time. *Cognitive Psychology, 10,* 465–501.

Muri, R.M., Vermersch, A.I., Rivaud, S., Gaymard, B., & Pierrot-Deseilligny, C. (1996). Effects of single-pulse transcranial magnetic stimulation over the prefrontal and posterior parietal cortices during memory guided saccades in humans. *Journal of Neurophysiology, 76,* 2102–2106.

Nystrom, L.E., Braver, T.S., Sabb, F.W., Delgado, M.R., Noll, D.C., & Cohen, J.D. (2000). Working memory for letters, shapes and locations: fMRI evidence against stimulus-based regional organization of human prefrontal cortex. *NeuroImage, 11,* 424–446.

O'Scalaidhe, S.P., Wilson, F.A., & Goldman-Rakic, P.S. (1997). Areal segregation of face-processing neurons in prefrontal cortex. *Science, 278,* 1135–1138.

Owen, A.M., Evans, A.C., & Petrides, M. (1996). Evidence for a two-stage model of spatial working memory processing within the lateral frontal cortex: a positron emission tomography study. *Cerebral Cortex, 6,* 31–38.

Owen, A.M., Stern, C.E., Look, R.B., Tracey, I., Rosen, B.R., & Petrides, M. (1998). Functional organization of spatial and nonspatial working memory processing within the human lateral frontal cortex. *Proceedings of the National Academy of Sciences USA 95,* 7721–7726.

Owen, A.M., Herrod, N.J., Menon, D.K., Clark, J.C., Downey, S.P., Carpenter, T.A., Minhas, P.S., Turkheimer, F.E., Williams, E.J., Robbins, T.W., Sahakian, B.J., Petrides, M., & Pickard, J.D. (1999). Redefining the functional organization of working memory processes within human lateral prefrontal cortex. *European Journal of Neuroscience, 11,* 567–574.

Pascual-Leone, A. & Hallett, M. (1994). Induction of errors in a delayed response task by repetitive transcranial magnetic stimulation of the dorsolateral prefrontal cortex. *NeuroReport, 5,* 2517–2520.

Passingham, R. (1975). Delayed matching after selective prefrontal lesions in monkeys. *Brain Research, 92,* 89–102.

Paulesu, E., Frith, C.D., & Frackowiak, R.S. (1993). The neural correlates of the verbal component of working memory. *Nature, 362,* 342–345.

Petrides, M. (1994). Frontal lobes and working memory: evidence from investigations of the effects of cortical excisions in nonhuman primates. In: F. Boller & J. Grafman (Eds.), *Handbook of Neuropsychology* (pp. 59–84). Amsterdam: Elsevier Science.

Petrides, M. (1995). Impairments on nonspatial self-ordered and externally ordered working memory tasks after lesions of the mid-dorsal lateral part of the lateral frontal cortex of monkey. *Journal of Neuroscience, 15,* 359–375.

Petrides, M. & Pandya, D.N. (1984). Projections to the frontal cortex from the posterior parietal region in the rhesus monkey. *Journal of Comparative Neurology, 228,* 105–116.

Posner, M.I., Petersen, S.E., Fox, P.T., & Raichle, M.E. (1988). Localization of cognitive operations in the human brain. *Science, 240,* 1627–1631.

Postle, B.R. & D'Esposito, M. (1999). "What"—then—"where" in visual working memory: an event-related fMRI study. *Journal of Cognitive Neuroscience, 11,* 585–597.

Postle, B.R. & D'Esposito, M. (2000). Evaluating models of the topographical organization of working memory function in frontal cortex with event-related fMRI. *Psychobiology, 28,* 132–145.

Postle, B.R., Berger, J.S., & D'Esposito, M. (1999). Functional neuroanatomical double dissociation of mnemonic and executive control processes contributing to working memory performance. *Proceedings of the National Academy of Sciences USA, 96,* 12959–12964.

Postle, B.R., Berger, J.S., Taich, A.M., & D'Esposito, M. (2000a). Activity in human frontal cortex associated with spatial working memory and saccadic behavior. *Journal of Cognitive Neuroscience, 12,* 2–14.

Postle, B.R., Stern, C.E., Rosen, B.R., & Corkin, S. (2000b). An fMRI investigation of cortical contributions to spatial and nonspatial visual working memory. *NeuroImage, 11,* 409–423.

Postle, B.R., Berger, J.S., Goldstein, J.H., Curtis, C.E., & D'Esposito, M. (2001). Behavioral and neurophysiological correlates of episodic encoding, proactive interference, and list length effects in a span verbal working memory task. *Cognitive, Affective and Behavioral Neuroscience, 1,* 10–21.

Pribram, K.H., Ahumada, A., Hartog, J., & Roos, L. (1964). A progress report on the neurologicalprocesses disturbed by frontal lesions in primates. In J.M. Warren & K. Akert (Eds.), *The Frontal GranularCortex and Behavior* (pp. 28–55). New York: McGraw-Hill.

Quintana, J. & Fuster, J.M. (1993). Spatial and temporal factors in the role of prefrontal and parietal cortex in visuomotor integration. *Cerebral Cortex, 3,* 122–132.

Quintana, J., Yajeya, J., & Fuster, J. (1988). Prefrontal representation of stimulus attributes during delay tasks. I. Unit activity in cross-temporal integration of motor and sensory-motor information. *Brain Research, 474,* 211–221.

Rainer, G., Asaad, W.F., & Miller, E.K. (1998). Memory-fields of neurons in the primate prefrontal cortex. *Proceedings of the National Academy of Sciences USA, 95,* 15008–15013.

Rao, S.C., Rainer, G., & Miller, E.K. (1997). Integration of what and where in the primate prefrontal cortex. *Science, 276,* 821–824.

Rosen B.R., Bucker R.L., & Dale A.M. (1998) Event-related functional MRI: past, present, and future. *Proceedings of the National Academy of Sciences 3,* 773–780.

Rosenkilde, C.E., Bauer, R.H., & Fuster, J.M. (1981). Single cell activity in ventral prefrontal cortex of behaving monkeys. *Brain Research, 209,* 375–394.

Rowe, J.B., Toni, I., Josephs, O., Frackowiak, R.S.J., & Passingham, R.E. (2000). The prefrontal cortex: response selection or maintenance within working memory? *Science, 288,* 1656–1660.

Rushworth, M.F.S., Nixon, P.D., Eacott, M.J., & Passingham, R.E. (1997). Ventral prefrontal cortex is not essential for working memory. *Journal of Neuroscience, 17,* 4829–4838.

Rypma, B. & D'Esposito, M. (1999). The roles of prefrontal brain regions in components of working memory: effects of memory load and individual differences. *Proceeding of the National Academy of Sciences USA, 96,* 6558–6563.

Rypma, B., Prabhakaran, V., Desmond, J.E., Glover, G.H., & Gabrieli, J.D. (1999). Load-dependent roles of frontal brain regions in the maintenance of working memory. *NeuroImage, 9,* 216–926.

Sarter, M., Bernston, G., & Cacioppo, J. (1996). Brain imaging and cognitive neuroscience: toward strong-inference in attributing function to structure. *American Psychologist, 51,* 13–21.

Schumacher, E.H., D'Esposito, M. (2000). Neural mechanisms for stimulus encoding and response selection processes in the performance of a perceptual-motor task. *Journal of Cognitive Neuroscience, 31E,* Suppl., S 2000.

Smith, E.E. & Jonides, J. (1998). Neuroimaging analyses of human working memory. *Proceeding of the National Academy of Sciences USA, 95,* 12061–12068.

Smith, E.E. & Jonides, J. (1999). Storage and executive processes of the frontal lobes. *Science, 283,* 1657–1661.

Smith, E.E., Jonides, J., Koeppe, R.A., Awh, E., Schumacher, E.H., & Minoshima, S. (1995). Spatial versus object working memory: PET investigations. *Journal of Cognitive Neuroscience, 7,* 337–356.

Smith, E.E., Jonides, J., & Koeppe, R.A. (1996). Dissociating verbal and spatial working memory using PET. *Cerebral Cortex, 6,* 11–20.

Smith, E.E., Jonides, J., Marshuetz, C., & Koeppe, R.A. (1998). Components of verbal working memory: evidence from neuroimaging. *Proceedings of the National Academy of Sciences USA, 95,* 876–882.

Sternberg, S. (1966). High-speed scanning in human memory. *Science, 153,* 652–654.

Sternberg, S. (1969). The discovery of processing stages: extensions of Donders' method. *Acta Psychologica, 30,* 276–315.

Talairach, J. & Tournoux, P. (1988). *Co-planar Stereotaxic Atlas of the Human Brain.* New York: Thieme.

Thompson-Schill, S.L., D'Esposito, M., Aguirre, G.K., & Farah, M.J. (1997). Role of left inferior prefrontal cortex in retrieval of semantic knowledge: a reevaluation. *Proceedings of the National Academy of Sciences USA, 94,* 14792–14797.

Ungerleider, L.G. & Haxby, J.V. (1994). 'What' and 'where' in the human brain. *Current Opinion in Neurobiology, 4,* 157–165.

Vanderplas, J.M. & Garvin, E.A. (1959). Theassociation of random shapes. *Journal of Experimental Psychology, 57,* 147–163.

Vazquez, A.L. & Noll, D.C. (1998). Nonlinear aspectsof the BOLD response in functional MRI. *NeuroImage, 7,* 108–118.

Waugh, N.C. & Norman, D.A. (1965). Primary memory. *Psychological Review, 72,* 89–104.

Wilson, F.A., Scalaidhe, S.P., & Goldman-Rakic, P.S. (1993). Dissociation of object and spatial processing domains in prefrontal cortex. *Science, 260,* 1955–1958.

Zarahn, E., Aguirre, G.K., & D'Esposito, M. (1997). A trial-based experimental design for functional MRI. *NeuroImage, 6,* 122–138.

Zarahn, E., Aguirre, G.K., & D'Esposito, M. (1999). Temporal isolation of the neural correlates of spatial mnemonic processing with fMRI. *Cognitive Brain Research, 7,* 255–268.

12

The Frontal Cortex and Working with Memory

MORRIS MOSCOVITCH AND GORDON WINOCUR

In numerous attempts to characterize the functional significance of the frontal cortex (FC), investigators have emphasized the structure's role in episodic memory and various memory-related processes such as working memory, temporal ordering, and metamemory. There is little doubt that the FC is involved in memory, but it is equally clear that its role is different from that associated with structures in the medial temporal lobe (e.g., hippocampus) and diencephalon (e.g., anterior and dorsomedial thalamus). While the latter regions differ in terms of their specific contributions, there is no question as to their fundamental importance to memory processes. Damage to medial temporal lobe and diencephalic regions reliably produces profound, global anterograde amnesia that is manifested as impaired recall and recognition. By comparison, damage to the FC does not typically produce generalized memory loss and, indeed, when it comes to remembering salient or distinctive events, patients with FC damage often experience little or no difficulty. Such patients also typically perform within normal limits on tests of cued recall or recognition memory unless some organizational component is needed to facilitate performance (Moscovitch & Winocur, 1995; Wheeler et al., 1995). They are severely handicapped, however, when success-

ful recall depends on self-initiated cues or when targeted information is relatively inaccessible (Moscovitch & Winocur, 1995). In other words, the FC is required if accurate memory depends on organization, search, selection, and verification in the retrieval of stored information. The important point that emerges is that the FC is less involved in memory recollection per se, than it is in mediating the strategic processes that support memory encoding, recovery, monitoring, and verification.

An equally important point, in terms of understanding FC function, is that its participation in strategic processes is not restricted to the recovery of past experiences. Indeed, there is considerable evidence that the structure uses established memories to direct other activities, such as new learning, problem solving, and behavioral planning. In previous publications, we have referred to medial temporal lobe and diencephalic systems as "raw memory" structures, because of their close and direct links to basic memory processes. By comparison, we have argued that the FC must work *with* memory to perform its diverse strategic functions by either influencing input to medial temporal lobe–diencephalic systems or by acting on output from these regions.

We have chosen the term *working-with-*

memory (WWM) to distinguish our notion from that of *working memory*, which we believe has different, and more restrictive, connotations in the literature on both human and animal memory (see Moscovitch & Winocur, 1992a, 1992b). Our idea is that strategic contributions to long-term memory are of the same type as those made to other functions, such as short-term or working memory, problem solving, attention, and response planning. Our approach to FC involvement in memory fits into a broader framework in which the FC is viewed as a central-system structure that operates on many domains of information, rather than as a domain-specific module (Moscovitch & Umiltà, 1990, 1991; Moscovitch, 1992, 1994a; Moscovitch & Winocur, 1992a, 1992b). The various central-system functions of the FC are localized in different regions. Thus, localization of function is as much a characteristic of central, frontal systems as of posterior neocortical modular systems. What distinguishes one from the other is that *modules* are defined in terms of their *content* or nature of the *representation*, such as faces, phonemes, objects, and so on, whereas *central, frontal systems* are defined in terms of their *function*, such as monitoring, searching, verification, and so on.[1]

In our framework, the medial temporal lobes, which include the hippocampus and related neocortical structures, as well as the diencephalic structures associated with them (Aggleton & Brown, 1999), are modules whose domain is conscious or explicit memory (Moscovitch, 1992, 1994a, 1995; Moscovitch & Winocur, 1992a, 1992b). They mandatorily encode and retrieve information that is consciously apprehended, and the information is stored randomly with no organizing principle except that of short-latency, temporal contiguity. As WWM structures, regions of the FC operate strategically on information delivered to the medial–temporal/diencephalic system and recovered from it, thereby conferring "intelligence" to what essentially is a "stupid" medial temporal lobe/diencephalic system. The FC is needed to implement encoding and retrieval strategies. The latter includes initiating and directing search in accordance with the demands of the task, monitoring and verifying

recovered memories, and placing them in the proper temporal–spatial context.

In our research program, we have addressed issues related to this theoretical framework from different perspectives, using human subjects as well as animal models and a variety of experimental paradigms. As part of our ongoing testing of specific hypotheses that follow from our theoretical position, we attempt to show that the FC works with other structures in performing various tasks, and that the contributions of the respective brain regions can be functionally dissociated. This chapter will focus on studies from our animal- and human-based research that reflect our general approach and provide converging evidence in support of the WWM model.

As useful as our WWM framework has been for guiding research on memory in humans and animals, in its original version it lacked the specificity that is required for subsequent developments on localization of function within the FC. When we first proposed the model (Moscovitch, 1989; Moscovitch & Winocur, 1992a), little was known about the localization of the various strategic encoding and retrieval functions, in part because the FC was not thought to play a prominent role in episodic memory. The situation has changed markedly since then, and we now have a better idea of the distribution of these functions within the FC, and the prefrontal cortex (PFC) in particular. Accordingly, in the concluding section we briefly review recent evidence regarding the localization of function within the PFC and present a revised version of our model that takes the new evidence into account.

ANIMAL STUDIES

Our overall research strategy is guided by the premise that, for the most part, cognitive tasks are multidimensional, and successful performance depends on the effective recruitment and integration of various component processes (Witherspoon & Moscovitch, 1989; Moscovitch, 1992; Winocur, 1992b; Roediger et al., 1999). For example, when presented with a complex new problem, we tend to learn specific features of that problem which, if remembered, will be useful when confronted again with the same problem. We and others associate this function with the hippocampus and related structures. We also learn conceptually related information that can be abstracted and strategically applied when dealing with variations of the problem, a process likely mediated by the FC (see also Miller, 2000; Chapter 18). In the normal course of events, these distinct processes are combined as part of an efficient cognitive operation, but undoubtedly they are controlled by different neural structures, and, theoretically at least, they are separable and amenable to independent measurement.

MAZE LEARNING

Our component process approach was tested in a rat model (Winocur & Moscovitch, 1990). In a test of complex maze learning, hungry rats had to avoid blind alleys in learning a specific route to a goal area where food was available. For this study, rats were subjected, in approximately equal numbers, to lesions of the FC or hippocampus, or to a control procedure in which no brain tissue was destroyed. Half the rats in each group received initial training on maze A, while the other half received no maze training. Subsequently, half the rats in each training condition were tested on maze A, while the other half were tested on a different maze (maze B). Thus, in the training condition (T), half the rats were re-tested on maze A, while the other half were tested on a

new but similar maze. In the non-training (NT) condition, all the rats experienced a maze for the first time at test.

The results, which are summarized in Table 11–1, reveal a clear dissociation between the effects of FC and hippocampal lesions. As expected, at test, control rats in the T condition performed better than NT controls, and they also did better on maze A than on maze B. On the familiar maze A, the controls were able to benefit from specific as well as general task-related information, whereas on maze B, they were able to draw only on general information.

Lesions to hippocampus or FC generally disrupted maze performance, relative to controls, but the patterns of deficit were quite different. Rats with hippocampal lesions and in the T condition made fewer errors than those in the NT condition, but within the T condition, they performed equally on mazes A and B. Thus, rats with hippocampal lesions, trained on maze A, appear to have acquired a maze-learning strategy that they were able to transfer to a similar problem. However, their failure to display additional savings when tested on maze A suggests that they remembered general information about this type of maze that would support a learning set but that, essentially, they had forgotten the specifics of their maze A training experience.

As for the groups with FC lesions, there was no significant difference between T and NT rats on the unfamiliar maze B, but rats in the T condition performed better than in the NT

Table 12–1. Errors at testing for all groups in training and no-training conditions during 60 trials of maze learning.

Maze	Hippocampal Lesion		Frontal Cortex Lesion		Control	
	T	NT	T	NT	T	NT
A (familiar)						
Mean	105.3	142.6	82.7	103.8	52.3	80.8
SE	4.6	3.8	2.8	2.6	1.8	2.3
B (unfamiliar)						
Mean	112.3	133.1	99.6	101.6	64.2	81.6
SE	4.6	5.7	3.3	2.7	2.0	2.0

T, training; NT, no training; SE, standard error.

condition rats in the NT condition on maze A. Clearly, rats with FC lesions benefited from training on maze A only when they were re-tested on the same task. This shows that, whereas rats with FC lesions were able to recognize the familiar maze A, this memory did not help them on maze B.

These results are consistent with the WWM notion of FC function. Bilateral lesions to the hippocampus selectively affected rats' memory for the specific and contextually defined experience associated with maze A learning, but spared procedural learning and memory that could be applied when subsequently tested on either maze A or B. In contrast, the FC-lesioned group had good memory for the salient maze A-learning experience, but were unable to use that memory in a flexible, strategic way that would enable savings on another task, even one that was closely related to the original one.

Related work (Winocur, 1992b) has emphasized that the impairment of FC-lesioned rats in transfer of learning is, in fact, a WWM deficit and not simply a failure of procedural or rule learning. In one experiment, rats with hippocampus, FC, or sham lesions were trained on a problem in which they were required to discriminate between circles of different sizes. The groups did not differ in learning or remembering the original discrimination. However, the FC lesioned-group was severely impaired at transferring the learned discrimination to a new set of stimuli (triangles). Although relatively simple on the surface, there was a substantial strategic component to this problem in that, to transfer learning successfully, rats had to compare training and test conditions, attend to critical similarities while ignoring irrelevant differences and, of course, apply previous learning to the new discrimination. All these operations required the animal to work with memory.

In the same experiment, rats with FC or hippocampus lesions, and control rats were administered a size-discrimination problem in which the stimulus pairs changed on every trial. All groups learned the rule at the same rate and showed excellent retention several weeks later. This outcome is instructive because, although rats had to apply the rule to different stimuli on each trial, the requirements quickly became routine and predictable. In this case, the transfer of information required little in the way of planning or strategic operations, and no comparisons between experiences separated in time; as such, this transfer placed no demands on WWM processes.

CONDITIONAL ASSOCIATIVE LEARNING

The maze-learning and transfer studies demonstrate the importance of FC for transferring information to new learning situations that require the effective integration of past experience with current task demands over extended time periods. While such tasks draw on what may be considered long-term memory, similar processes are involved in other tasks in which accurate responding depends on short-term memory. For example, in conditional associative learning (CAL), in which different stimuli are associated with different responses, on each trial the subject must select, from among several alternatives, the response that is appropriate to the most recently presented stimulus. The delay between stimulus presentation and the opportunity to respond is brief and often on the order of seconds. Variations of this task have been developed for humans and nonhuman primates, with the consistent finding that lesions to the FC, particularly areas 6 and 8, impair performance (see Petrides & Milner, 1982, Milner & Petrides, 1984; Petrides, 1990; 1995; chapter 3).

Impairment of CAL following FC damage has been characterized as a working memory deficit resulting from a lesion-induced inability to retain trial-specific information over the stimulus–response delay period. However, when we compared the effects of FC and hippocampal lesions on a rat version of CAL, the results suggested other interpretations (Winocur, 1991; Winocur & Eskes, 1998). In this task, one wall of a Skinner box was outfitted with a display panel, consisting of six lights placed above two retractable levers that were located on either side of the food chamber. Rats were reinforced for pressing the left lever in response to a light on the left side of the panel, and the right lever, to a light on the right side. Initially, rats were trained with the conditional stimulus and both levers presented together on each trial. The lights were extinguished and the levers withdrawn after a response was made to allow for a 30-second intertrial interval. When responding stabilized in the 0-delay training condition, rats received five additional days of training with a 5-second stimulus–response delay, and five more days of training in which the delay was increased to 15 seconds. For the delay trial, the conditional stimulus was presented for 10 seconds and then turned off while the rats waited the prescribed delay period for the levers to reappear.

There was no difference between hippocampus-lesioned and control groups in learning the conditional rule in the 0-delay condition, but the group with FC lesions improved at a much slower rate and, as can be seen in Figure 12–1, failed to reach the performance level of the other groups even after 30 training sessions. Since there was no stimulus–response delay during training, this result shows that the FC group's deficit was not linked to the requirement that critical information be retained over a period of time. Similar patterns of performance have also been observed in FC- and hippocampus-lesioned groups in tests of delayed alternation and delayed matching-to-sample (Winocur, 1991, 1992a, 1992b).

These data argue that the deficit cannot be attributed to memory loss or to the retention components of working memory. This conclusion is reinforced by the results of the delay conditions (see Fig. 12–1). Here, we see a rapid decline in performance of the hippocampus-lesioned group, indicating that these animals were unable to remember each trial's signal even after a brief period of time. Of particular interest was the finding that increasing the stimulus–response delay did not adversely affect the performance of rats with FC lesions. As the delays increased, the performance of this group declined at the same rate as that of the control group. It should be noted that an alternative working memory interpretation of these results is that rats had to coordinate, in working memory, the signal and the response, as well as the interfering effects of past experiences, and those with FC lesions did not have the capacity to do that.

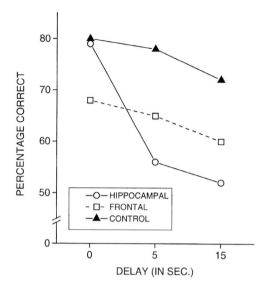

Figure 12–1. Percentage correct on the conditional associative learning test for hippocampus-lesioned, frontal cortex–lesioned, and control groups.

These results indicate that impairments on conditional learning tasks following FC lesions are neither time-dependent nor due to a straightforward memory failure, as might be argued for hippocampus-lesioned rats. More likely, the effects of FC damage were on conditional rule learning or on the process of response selection. We are not prepared to dismiss a rule-learning deficit, although, as we have seen in the transfer studies, FC lesions do not necessarily disrupt rule learning. In a recent experiment, Winocur & Eskes (1998) showed that modifying the CAL task to reduce demands on response-selection processes resulted in a significant improvement in performance in FC-lesioned rats. Our interpretation is that lesions to the FC interfered with the animal's ability to use critical information in the context of a learned rule for the purposes of accurate response selection. We view this as another expression of WWM. The CAL results highlight the point that the WWM function applies to the strategic use of specific and nonspecific memories at short as well as long delays.

RECENT AND REMOTE MEMORY

The FC, as a WWM structure, is also involved in the recovery of remote memories. There is growing evidence that damage to the FC in humans produces a severe retrograde amnesia that can extend back many years. This pattern contrasts with the temporally graded retrograde amnesia that has often been reported for humans and animals (Winocur, 1990; Zola-Morgan & Squire, 1990; Squire, 1992; Squire & Alvarez, 1995) with incomplete medial temporal lobe/hippocampal damage (but see Nadel & Moscovitch, 1997; Nadel et al., 2000; Rosenbaum et al., 2001).

Investigations of memory function in animals with FC damage have been concerned mainly with anterograde memory, but recently we examined the effects of FC lesions in rats on a test of anterograde and retrograde memory for a learned food preference (Winocur & Moscovitch, 1999). In this test, a subject-rat acquires the preference by interacting with a demonstrator-rat that has just eaten a particular food. Memory for the preference is indicted when the subject later prefers that food to an unfamiliar food that is presented alongside it.

In previous work with this paradigm (Winocur, 1990), rats with lesions to hippocampus or dorsomedial thalamus were tested following pre- and postoperative acquisition of the food preference. There was no effect of thalamic lesions on anterograde or retrograde memory, but the groups with hippocampal lesions exhibited clear impairment. On the anterograde test, rats with hippocampal lesions learned normally but forgot the acquired preference at an abnormally rapid rate. In the retrograde test, they suffered a temporally graded retrograde amnesia in which preferences, acquired well before surgery, were remembered better than more recently acquired ones.

When rats with FC lesions were tested on this task, there were no differences between FC and control groups in either memory condition (Winocur & Moscovitch, 1999). Although surprising at first, on further reflection, the failure of FC lesions to affect memory performance made sense. In the food-preference task, memory is assessed in what is essentially a two-choice recognition memory test, and it is well known that FC damage does not affect performance on standard tests of recognition memory (Wheeler et al., 1995;

Mangels et al., 1996). In our experience, however, aged animals with frontal lobe dysfunction (Winocur & Gagnon, 1998; Winocur & Moscovitch, 1999) and patients with Parkinson's disease (Ergis et al., 2000) who exhibit frontal symptoms do exhibit impaired recognition memory when interference is introduced by increasing the number of response alternatives and their similarity to the target. Accordingly, in a second experiment, the number of food choices was increased from two to three, so that rats had to select the sample food from three equally desirable diets.

As can be seen in Figure 12–2, in the three-choice test, rats with FC lesions, in contrast to the control groups, exhibited poor memory for the acquired food preference. The effect was especially marked in the retrograde memory test, where the FC groups showed no gradient over the delay period, and at no time did their average intake of the sample food exceed 50% of the total amount consumed. In the anterograde memory test, the group with FC lesions showed declining memory for the food preference with increased delays.

These results are interesting for several reasons. First, they represent the first clear demonstration in FC-lesioned animals of patterns of anterograde and retrograde memory loss that correspond to those reliably observed in patients with comparable damage on context-free (semantic) tests of memory (see discussion in Rosenbaum et al., 2001). Second, they confirm that the FC does not mediate basic processes related to the acquisition and retention of new information, but that the structure does play a role when the tasks are more complex and greater effort is required to perform them. Thus, in experiment 2, the increased number of alternatives placed greater demands on search and selection operations and that clearly put the group with FC lesions at a disadvantage. Third, the results provide further evidence that, under certain conditions, even recognition memory, which typically resists the effects of FC damage, can be compromised. Finally, an important finding was that anterograde amnesia at long delays correlated significantly with retrograde amnesia in rats with FC damage. This result was undoubtedly related to the fact that the antero-

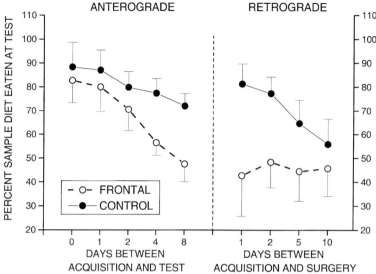

Figure 12–2. Amount of sample diet consumed by frontal cortex–lesioned and control groups, expressed as a percentage of the total amount of food consumed, at the various delays in the (three-choice) retrograde and (three-choice) anterograde amnesia tests. (*Source:* From Winocur & Moscovitch, 1999)

grade and retrograde tests were similar, and that they drew on similar FC-mediated processes.

This study provides an important example of how the FC directs goal-oriented strategies that lead to the recovery of relatively inaccessible information. In the absence of sufficient external cues, the FC is recruited to initiate appropriate search operations aimed at finding specific memory traces. Factors such as the passage of time, the number of competing associations, and difficulty in placing events in spatial–temporal context add to the complexity of the process, and place additional demands on FC. The three-choice version of the food-preference task incorporates all these factors, and its sensitivity to the effects of FC lesions, on both anterograde and retrograde measures, offers strong support for the WWM hypothesis.

SUMMARY

In this section we reviewed the results of several experiments, each involving different paradigms and each revealing deficits in rats with FC lesions that are broadly consistent with deficits seen in patients with FC damage. Although very different in terms of their cognitive demands, they all had a memory component that, in itself, posed no problems for the groups with FC lesions. They also re-

quired the animals to work *with* specific memories—whether in acquiring new responses, retrieving old ones, or in using memory in a strategic way. The results consistently show that it was the WWM function that was impaired in the FC-lesioned rats.

HUMAN STUDIES

Our studies on FC and memory in humans parallel those conducted with animal models. In both cases we try to distinguish between the contribution of the FC and other brain regions to performance on tests that have a WWM component. The studies on humans and animal were not intended to be analogous in the sense that they would resemble one another in surface structure, but rather they were designed to share processing components with each other. In fact, this approach was necessitated by the different evolutionary histories and adaptations of the organisms.

Our comparative approach is illustrated most clearly in our studies of remote memory. Because rats rely so much on olfaction, we used socially transmitted olfactory learning to examine their remote memory. In humans, it was more appropriate to rely on verbal and pictorial information to test memory for personal and public events and personalities. We used neuroimaging and lesion studies to identify the regions that are implicated in retrieval of recent and remote memories. By comparing frontal and medial temporal contributions to memory in animals and humans, as measured by corresponding tests, we hoped to develop a better appreciation of the processes mediated by these structures.

In this section on human studies, we will focus on lesion studies on memory distortion because we believe that these provide the most compelling evidence of the contribution of the FC to memory. The studies we review show that the FC contributes to acquisition of new memories and to retrieval of both recent and remote memories. In line with our view that frontal lobes make a similar contribution in all domains, we will also show that damage to the FC leads to distortion of both autobiographical memory and general knowledge. We then will turn to neuroimaging studies of recent and remote memory to identify the contribution of different regions of the FC to retrieval.

LESION STUDIES: REMOTE MEMORY AND MEMORY DISTORTION

The contribution of the frontal lobes to retrieval of remote memory was noted by Kopelman (1989, 1991), who found that performance on tests of remote memory in amnesia was correlated with the severity of deficits on tests of frontal lobe function. More recent studies by Levine et al. (1998) have shown that loss of remote autobiographical memories, particularly the ability to re-experience them as elements of one's personal past, is associated with damage to the inferior, right FC and the uncinate fasciculus that connects it to the anterior temporal lobe. This same region was found by Levine (personal communication) to be activated when re-experiencing or remembering an event, as opposed to "knowing" that it occurred. By comparison, performance is relatively preserved on recognition tests that are mediated primarily by the medial temporal lobes.

In contrast to Levine et al.'s patient who finds his own past unfamiliar, there are patients with the opposite disorder: they find familiarity even in novel events and stimuli

(Schacter et al., 1996a; Rapcsak et al., 1999). This overextended sense of familiarity, most noticeable when novel items belong to the same category as recently studied targets, is also observed when these patients encounter people, faces, and words for the very first time, presumably because at some level they resemble familiar stimuli. The lesion associated with this disorder has not yet been localized to a particular region in the frontal lobes, although it occurs more often with damage in the right hemisphere (but see Parkin et al., 1999, next section). There are a number of possible interpretions of this disorder, which we consider below. The overextended sense of familiarity resembles a common feature of confabulation, although the latter is a more complex form of memory distortion in which elements of old memories may be combined with one another, and with current perceptions and thoughts, to create new memories that the individual truly believes to be veridical and experiential (Dalla Barba, 1993a, 1993b). Overextended familiarity in confabulating people is apparent on tests of recognition. Correct responses to targets may be normal, but there are more false alarms either to new, related items (see Moscovitch, 1989) or to items that had once served as targets but now act as lures (Schnider et al., 1996; Schnider & Ptak, 1999). In line with their performance on laboratory tests, many confabulating patients will claim to be familiar with people and places encountered for the first time. With very good retrieval cues, FC-damaged patients are able to provide correct answers and their confabulations are diminished and even eliminated (Moscovitch, 1989).

It was observations such as these that led us to conclude that confabulations arise in conditions in which search is faulty but not empty, and in which the erroneous products of that search are not monitored well (Moscovitch, 1995). The FC is needed both to initiate and guide search and to monitor the product of that search at different levels (see Gilboa and Moscovitch, in press, for review).

Most of our knowledge of remote memory and confabulation is based on informal observation and reports of spontaneously occurring confabulation. To bring confabulation for remote memory under some experimental control, Moscovitch and Melo (1997) administered an autobiographical and historical/semantic version of the Crovitz cue-word test (Crovitz & Schiffman, 1974) to confabulating and nonconfabulating amnesic patients and to their matched controls. In these tests, participants were asked to use a cue word, such as *broken* for the autobiographical version, and *assassinations* for the historical/semantic version, to retrieve, and describe in detail, either a personal memory related to that word or an historical event that also occurred before the participant was born. There are a number of interesting aspects to the results, which are noted in Figure 12–3.

First, the Crovitz test proved to be effective in eliciting confabulations under laboratory conditions, but only in people prone to confabulation outside the laboratory. Nonconfabulating amnesics and controls produced few confabulations. Second, consistent with

our idea that the FC is a central system structure that works with memory across all domains, we found that confabulation was not restricted to autobiographical memory but included knowledge of the historical events that belong to the domain of semantic memory (but see Dalla Barba, 1993a, 1993b).

A third aspect of the results is that confabulating amnesics recalled far less information, whether veridical or otherwise, than other amnesics or controls, and benefited disproportionately from prompting. It should be noted that prompts increased veridical and confabulating responses equally.

These findings indicate that although the final, proximal cause of confabulation may be defective postretrieval monitoring and verification of recovered memories, deficits in a number of preretrieval components are associated with the disorder and in all likelihood contribute to it. They include impairments in formulating the retrieval problem and in spec-

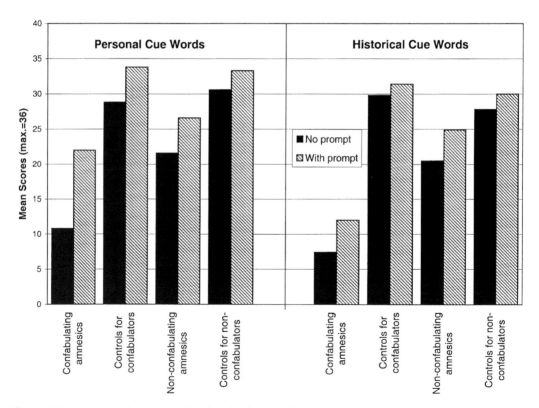

Figure 12–3. Mean score (maximum 36), with and without prompt, for confabulating and non-confabulating patients and their respective controls on the Crovitz personal and historical cue word test. (*Source:* From Moscovitch & Melo, 1997)

ifying appropriate cues. Other components that may be deficient are those guiding search and selection among alternative memory candidates and responses. Similar proposals for fractionating the retrieval process into a number of subcomponents have been advanced by Burgess and Shallice (1996) (see chapter 17), by Schacter et al. (1998a), and by Kopelman (1999). This view suggests that the nature of the confabulation errors that are observed will depend on which and how many of the subcomponents are affected. The idea is consistent with our WWM model, which assigns different components of encoding and retrieval to the FC, and raises the possibility that they are mediated by different regions in the FC (see Localization of function in Frontal Cortex and chapter 17).

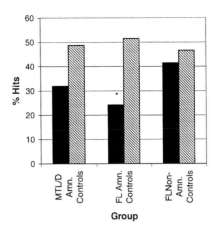

Figure 12–4. Proportion of study list words produced by patients ▨ and controls ■ °$P < 0.05$. Amn., amnesia; FL, frontal lesion; MTL/D, medial temporal lobe/diencephalon (*Source:* From Melo et al., 1999).

LESION STUDIES: MEMORY ACQUISITION AND MEMORY DISTORTION

If memory is a reconstructive process (Bartlett, 1932), confabulation and an overextended sense of familiarity may be caused by deficits at encoding as much as by deficits at retrieval in people with FC lesions. Parkin et al. (1999) provide compelling evidence that a defect in encoding the target distinctively, rather than by its general characteristics, can lead to exaggerated false recognition in a patient with left frontal lesions. To study the effects of frontal lesions on distortion of newly acquired memories, Melo, Winocur and Moscovitch 1999) induced distortions in the laboratory. They used the Deese-Roediger-McDermott paradigm (Deese, 1959; Roediger & McDermott, 1995) to examine memory distortion in amnesic people with and without FC damage, as well as in people with FC damage without amnesia. In this paradigm, people try to remember lists of related words, such as *bed, nap, pillow, snooze,* all of which are associated to a common word, which, in this particular example, would be *sleep.* The word *sleep,* however, is not presented and serves as a *critical lure* at test. Following each list presentation, participants are asked to recall as many of the items as they can remember. Once all the lists are presented and recalled,

a break ensues, after which participants are asked to recognize the target items and distinguish them from unrelated lures and from the critical lure.

The controls behaved as normal people did in most published studies: they recalled and recognized as high a proportion of the critical lures as that of the target items, and very few of the unrelated lures (see Figs. 12–4 and 12–5). Although there are a number of explanations for this outcome, the one we prefer is that participants base their responses both on their specific (verbatim) memory for the tar-

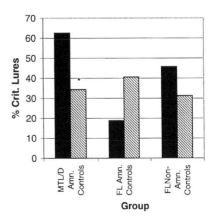

Figure 12–5. Proportion of critical lures intruded by patients ▨ and controls ■ °$P < 0.05$. Amn., amnesia; FL, frontal lesion; MTL/D, medial temporal lobe/diencephalon (*Source:* From Melo et al., 1999)

gets as well as on the gist that they extracted from them, which, in most cases, was exemplified best by the critical lure (Brainerd et al., 1995, 2000; Reyna & Brainerd, 1995; Schacter et al., 1996c, 1998b). Monitoring at retrieval for perceptual qualities of the recovered memory can be helpful in distinguishing targets from critical lures (Schacter et al., 1999), but is not a major factor unless participants are trained or instructed to attend to the relevant features.

On the basis of this analysis and our WWM framework, we predicted that amnesic patients, whose memory for the targets is poor but who can still retain the gist if tested immediately after the list is presented, will respond with a higher than normal proportion of critical lures, and a lower proportion of targets, at recall. When recognition is delayed, their memory for both targets and gist will be poor, and so they will show poorer than normal recognition of both. Patients with only lateral, FC lesions will be impaired at monitoring and so are expected to show a slight increase in recalling and recognizing critical lures, although their memory for targets will be normal. The increase should be slight because monitoring plays a minimal role in normal performance on this test (see above). Amnesics with medial temporal lobe/diencephalic (MTL/D) and FC damage suffer from a compound deficit. Their lesions typically include the ventromedial frontal lobes and basal forebrain. Consequently, their memory for the targets will be as poor as that of amnesics. Their frontal damage may not only impair their ability to monitor but may even prevent them from extracting the gist at encoding or using it to guide retrieval. As a result, their memory for targets and critical lures should be disproportionately low even when tested immediately.

The findings were consistent with our predictions (see Fig. 12–4 and 12–5). Though providing general support for the WWM model, showing different effects of MTL/D and FC lesions on performance, our results do not distinguish clearly whether the distortion in patients with FC lesions arises at encoding or retrieval. This is an issue that has yet to be resolved in all studies employing the Deese-Roediger-McDermott (DRM) paradigm. In addition, our study also suggests a degree of specialization within the FC in that patients with primarily lateral frontal lesions do not show as much distortion as those whose lesions are more medial and implicate the basal forebrain. These differences will need to be taken into account in developing the model further (see Components of Retrieval and Frontal Cortex).

LOCALIZATION OF FUNCTION IN FRONTAL CORTEX

Our initial intent in developing the WWM model was to establish its basic principles with respect to the broad range of FC functions, such as initiating and guiding retrieval of memories (which may involve cue specification and maintenance), monitoring memories, evaluation, and response selection, that are implicated in tests of episodic memory. (In addition to the studies reported here, the model was supported by studies of aging [Moscovitch & Winocur, 1992b, 1995], word fluency, [Troyer, et al., 1997; 1998a, 1998b]; and of divided attention [Moscovitch, 1994b; Troyer et al., 1999; Fernandes & Moscovitch, 2000; Moscovitch et al., in press]. Each of these component functions of the FC is likely mediated by different regions of the FC. There is growing evidence in the literature that a comprehensive model of frontal function must take regional specialization into account—and this clearly is the direction in which the field is heading. Although our research has not addressed the issue of localization of function in the FC directly, our findings indicate its importance. For example, as noted above, there is a clear dissociation of function between the lateral and ventromedial aspects of the FC in memory distortion.

One of the difficulties of the traditional neuropsychological approach to this issue is that patients rarely present with sufficiently circumscribed lesions to allow precise localization of function in large-scale studies (but see Milner and Petrides, 1984; Chapter 3; Stuss, this volume, Chapter 25). Sophisticated neuroimaging and controlled animal studies, however, can be used to address this issue more effectively. Our neuroimaging work on recovery of recent and remote autobiographical memory illustrates the benefits of this approach.

NEUROIMAGING STUDIES: RECENT AND REMOTE AUTOBIOGRAPHICAL MEMORY

We conducted a functional magnetic resonance imaging (fMRI) study on remote memory for autobiographical events to identify structures associated with the various component processes that are activated during retrieval (Ryan et al., 2001). We asked participants to recollect (re-experience) in as much detail as possible a personal episode that occurred either recently (within the last couple of years) or long ago (20 or more years earlier). Activation in the autobiographical memory test was compared to two baseline conditions: rest and a sentence completion test.

Two important results emerged from this study. The first was that retrieval of autobiographical memory was associated with increased hippocampal and diencephalic activity, as compared to the control conditions, regardless of whether the memory was recent or remote. Second, we also found greater activation in a number of neocortical regions, most particularly in the FC. Here, too, the extent of activation was no different for retrieval of recent memories than for that of remote memories, although Maguire (2001), in her review of this literature, has noted greater activation in the region of left, posterior ventrolateral PFC.

One interpretation of these results is that retention and retrieval of autobiographical memories, both recent and remote, depend on the interaction of medial temporal/diencephalic regions with the FC. This interpretation is consistent with the WWM model, and also supports the multiple trace theory (MTT) of memory proposed by Nadel and Moscovitch (1997, 1998).[2]

Within the FC, areas 6 (premotor cortex), 9, 46 (mid-dorsolateral FC), and 47 (ventrolateral FC) were activated, as well as areas 44

and 45, indicating widespread FC involvement in the retrieval of autobiographical memories. These results are consistent with those of Fink et al. (1996) Levine (personal communication), and Gilboa, Winocur, Grady & Moscovitch (in preparation) who found greater right PFC activation in some of these regions during recognition of personal autobiographical memory than of semantic memories or information associated with another person. In the WWM model, we assume that each of these activated regions serves a different function. We are drawing on the human and animal literature to speculate about the function of each of these regions and are attempting to develop the model further. We are doing so with the knowledge that the function of some of these regions is understood better than that of others, and that even for those that are relatively well understood, there is some debate as to how best to characterize the functions, as is obvious by comparing most of the chapters in this volume. We also hope that this model will serve as a useful guide for future research.

COMPONENTS OF RETRIEVAL AND FRONTAL CORTEX

One of the core ideas of WWM is that regions of the FC that are implicated in memory retrieval are described best in terms of their function or general cognitive operation, rather than in terms of information content or the domain in which they operate. Thus, when the same functions are performed, the same general regions of FC that are activated during retrieval of recent and remote memory are also activated during tests of working memory, problem solving, or even during tests of perception. There is some dispute, however, as to whether smaller, local, or lateralized regions within the more general area are activated differentially depending on whether the material is spatial, verbal, or pictorial (see Moscovitch & Umiltà, 1990; Footnote 1; and Chapters 3, 5, 11, 15, and 18).

In considering the components of retrieval, we deliberately made little reference to lateralization of function in the frontal lobes. Doing so enabled us to focus on the function of the various subregions without entering the debate concerning lateralization.

Area 6 (Premotor Cortex): Response Selection and Inhibition

The area that was most consistently activated in our neuroimaging study was area 6 (premotor cortex), the likely homologue of the FC lesion that led to equal deficits in remote and recent memory in rats (Winocur & Moscovitch, 1999). Activation of area 6 is likely associated with memory-based response selection. Damage to this region leads to deficits on tests of CAL in monkeys (Petrides, 1982; see Chapter 3). and in humans (Petrides & Milner, 1982; Milner & Petrides, 1984) and is activated during tests of CAL in normal people (Petrides, 1995; see Chapter 3). In a series of studies, Winocur found that lesions to the FC that consistently destroyed all or most of the premotor area disrupted performance on a variety of conditional learning tasks (CAL, delayed alternation: Winocur, 1991; matching-to-sample; Winocur, 1992a) that required accurate response selection from among competing alternatives. Of particular importance is Winocur and Eskes' finding (1998, see Conditional Associative Learning, above) that deficits in CAL are reduced in rats with FC lesions in the region of the premotor cortex when response selection is not an overriding factor. Similarly, on the socially acquired food preference-test (Winocur & Moscovitch, 1999), remote and recent memory were impaired only when the number of alternatives was increased from two to three. Response selection clearly is an important factor in retrieval of autobiographical memory in which the appropriate event and corresponding details must be selected from a variety of other similar items.

Response selection (or inhibition of alternative responses) also seems to play a role in performing some implicit tests of memory, such as stem completion, whose performance is related to frontal function in older adults (Winocur et al., 1996). The correlation between tests of stem completion and frontal function are found only when there are many multiple solutions to the stems (Nyberg et al., 1997) and not on tests of fragment completion with only one solution (see also Gabrieli et al., 1999). Consistent with this interpretation is some suggestive evidence that the premotor area is one of several FC structures activated when normal subjects select primed responses in tests of word-stem completion (e.g., Buckner et al., 1995).

Areas 9 and 46 (Mid-dorsolateral Frontal Cortex): Monitoring and Manipulation of Information Held in Mind (Working Memory)

The mid-dorsolateral PFC (areas 9 and 46) is implicated in tests that require manipulation of information that is being actively maintained such as in animal and human tests of working memory (Petrides, 1995). Thus, activation of this region is associated with increasing complexity of operations in tests of memory and problem solving (Christoff & Gabrieli, 2000; Duncan & Owen, 2000; Petrides, 2000; Postle & D'Esposito, 2000; see Chapters 3 and 18). This area is also implicated in tests of long-term memory such as free recall, in which one must keep track of responses in order not to repeat them (Stuss et al., 1994; Fletcher et. al., 1998; Henson et al., 2000). As might be expected, area 9 is also activated on tests of temporal order in humans (Cabeza et al., 1997). It is very likely that manipulation of information, which relies on monitoring and maintaining temporal order, is also crucial for recounting events that have a narrative structure, such as autobiographical memories, which may explain why this region was activated during retrieval in our neuroimaging study.

Work with animals provides converging evidence that areas 9 and 46 play a crucial role in monitoring information that derives from temporally ordered events. Damage to this region in monkeys and its homologue in rats (dorsomedial prefrontal cortex) reliably produces deficits on tests of working memory (Becker et al., 1980; Petrides, 1991, 2000; Granon & Poucet, 1995) and self-ordered pointing (Petrides, 1989), as well as on ordering item and spatial information (Kesner & Holbrook, 1987). All of these studies have ordering and response-selection components, but a study by Delatour and Gisquet-Verrier (2001) showed that lesions to this area affect response selection only when tasks place high demands on ordering processes. These investigators compared rats with lesions to dorsomedial prefrontal cortex on two response alternation tasks—one in which correct behavioral sequencing required the use of temporally ordered information and a second in which explicit cues specified the correct response on each trial. Both tasks required the selection of a correct response but the lesioned rats were impaired only on the former task where response selection was directly linked to temporal patterning.

Ventrolateral Frontal Cortex (Area 47): Cue Specification and/or Maintenance at Retrieval and at Encoding

The mid-ventrolateral FC (area 47) has been implicated in tests of recognition independently of the number of items held in memory or the operations performed on them (Henson et al., 2000; Fletcher & Henson, 2001). A number of investigators have proposed that this region is crucial for using distinctive retrieval cues to specify information that needs to be recovered from long-term memory (Wagner, 1999; Henson et al., 2000; Fletcher & Henson, 2001), as in detailed recall of specific autobiographical events, and possibly also for encoding information distinctively enough to discriminate targets from similar lures (Brewer et al., 1998; Wagner et al., 1998; Parkin et al., 1999). Thus, poor cue specification, with an overreliance on gist as seen in our memory distortion study (Melo et al., 1999), may be responsible for the overextended sense of familiarity observed in some patients with ventral FC lesions, with lesions on the left being associated with encoding deficits (Parkin et al., 1999) and lesions on the right with deficits at retrieval (Schacter et al., 1996a). This disorder may also be linked to dysfunction in the ventromedial area, which is adjacent to area 47 and often difficult to isolate functionally in lesion or activation studies (see next section). Sufficiently poor cue specification also leads to errors of omission on tests of re-

call, a common feature of frontal lobe amnesias (Moscovitch & Melo, 1997). Such an impairment, associated with lesions to area 47 and the uncinate fasciculus, which projects from this region to the temporal lobes, could also account for the loss of a sense of recollection that accompanies autobiographical memory (see Levine et al., 1998). This disorder is opposite the one associated with confabulation in which subjects experience a sense of recollection that is virtually indistinguishable for true and false memories and is likely related to damage to ventromedial PFC (see next section). Thus, cue specification is a necessary early step in accessing stored memories.

Consistent with the idea that the function of area 47 is cue specification, monkeys with lesions to the ventrolateral cortex, like humans, have difficulty choosing between novel and familiar items (Petrides, 2000). In rats, the deficit manifests itself on tests that require flexibility in response to cues that change their significance within the same context. For example, in a test of alternation behavior conducted in a cross-maze, rats were able to alternate on the basis of spatial location or on the basis of their own prior response. However, having learned one rule for alternation, lesioned animals were unable to shift to another one in the same context (Ragozzino et al., 1999). This deficit is similar to one Schnider et al., (2000) proposed to account for confabulation (discussed in next section) and may also be associated with ventromedial lesions.

Ventromedial Frontal Cortex (Areas 11, 13, 25): Felt-Rightness for Anomoly or Rejection

The lesions most commonly associated with confabulation are found in the ventromedial FC and basal forebrain, which include areas 11, 13, and 25 (and possibly 32, although its role seems to be associated more with conflict resolution), so it is puzzling that they were not activated in our neuroimaging study on retrieval of recent and remote memories. One possibile explanation is that the location of the areas makes them difficult to observe on neuroimaging studies, particularly those studies using fMRI. We should note, however, that on PET scans, the comparison sentence-completion task may also activate the same or adjacent regions of FC (see Elliot et al., 2000), thus even if this region could have been imaged on fMRI, no difference would have been detected between the memory and baseline, sentence-completion task. We will return to this point shortly.

In a PET study, Schnider and colleagues (2000) showed that the ventromedial FC is crucial for temporal segregation (see also Pribram & Tubbs, 1967; Schacter, 1987), so that currently relevant memories can be differentiated from memories that may have been relevant once but are no longer. Temporal confusion, however, may not be the primary cause of confabulation but secondary to some other aspect of strategic retrieval mediated by the ventromedial FC (see Moscovitch 1989, 1995).

The hypothesis we favour is derived from studies on the effects of ventromedial FC lesions on emotion, risk taking, and social awareness and interaction (Bechara et al., 2000a, 2000b). Patients with ventromedial FC lesions have difficulty taking into account the emotional and social consequences of their actions so that they can plan appropriately and maximize their rewards in the long run. They are described as being "cognitively [but not motorically] impulsive," as not being able to appreciate the *"felt-rightness,"* of a response in relation to the goals of a task, regardless of whether the domain is social (Bechara et al., 2000a, 2000b) or cognitive (Elliot et al., 2000).

From the point of view of memory retrieval, felt-rightness is an intuitive, rapid endorsement or rejection of recovered memories with respect to the goals of the memory task. "Cognitive impulsivity" in the memory domain, manifested as the absence of a mechanism for felt-rightness, leads to the hasty acceptance of any strong, recovered memory as appropriate to the goals of the memory task, even if it is not. The extensive, direct connections of the ventromedial PFC to the hippocampus, amygdala, and adjacent structures in the medial temporal lobes, and to the temporal pole, make it ideally situated to play a prominent role in the first, postecphoric stages of memory retrieval from the MTL. Both elements,

the content of the memory and the overall context in which it is made, are crucial. This early, rapid (intuitive) decision to reject an item as incorrect is necessarily a first stage of retrieval that likely precedes the more thorough, cognitive check on the memory's plausibility, which occurs under conditions of uncertainty or when the initial response is incompatible with other knowledge or memories.

This hypothesis receives some support from a PET study (Moroz 1999) on memory for words coded in relation to oneself and in relation to another person. In this study, an investigator might ask, for example, "Does the word *modest* apply to you" (self)? "Does it apply to the current Prime Minister of Canada" (other)? Moroz (1999), working with us, found that different regions of the FC were activated depending on whether a target item elicited a "remember" or a "know" response at retrieval, regardless of whether it was related to the self or to another (Craik et al., 1999). "Remember" responses are associated with a contextually rich memory for an item, an indication that the person re-experienced the event at retrieval. A "know" response indicates only familiarity that the event occurred. Typically, "remember" responses are much faster and of higher confidence than "know" responses, which are more tentative, as they were in our study. "Remember" responses were positively correlated with activation in a neural network that included the anterior cingulate, which is part of the ventromedial PFC, and related limbic structures. "Know" responses, on the other hand, being less certain and requiring more monitoring, were correlated with activation in the mid-dorsolateral PFC [left (Brodmann's area 6/9/46) > right (Brodmann's area 9, 47)]. Similar results were reported by Henson et al (1999) in their study on remembering and knowing.

Area 10 (Anterior Prefrontal Cortex): Felt-Rightness for Acceptance or Endorsement

This region is also often implicated during retrieval of episodic memory, but its function has yet to be determined with any great degree of confidence. Some investigators equate activation of area 10 on the right with retrieval mode (LePage et al., 1998) or with recovery of episodic memories (Tulving et al., 1994). In a recent review of the literature, Henson et al. (2000; Fletcher & Henson, 2001) suggested that area 10 is activated during successful (correct) retrieval of episodic (Henson et al., 2000; Fletcher & Henson, 2001) or semantic (Rugg et al., 1998) information. If their conjecture is correct, area 10 may work in concert with the ventromedial PFC to set *context-dependent* criteria of felt-rightness for correct acceptance (area 10) or rejection (ventromedial) of retrieved information, be it episodic or semantic. That area 10 may be activated equally by retrieval of episodic and semantic memory may also explain why we did not observe greater activation in this area during retrieval of autobiographical memories than during retrieval of semantic memories in the baseline, sentence-completion task.

There is no dearth of alternative proposals for the function of area 10. Fletcher and Henson (2001) have proposed that area 10 may act as a superordinate supervisory system needed to maintain complex plans in mind for coordinating retrieval operations handled by other regions such as the ventrolateral FC and dorsolateral FC. That may account for evidence that activation of this region is task-sensitive. Our own proposal of *context dependent criterion setting* would provide an equally plausible explanation of these effects. Yet another alternative is Christoff and Gabrieli's (2000) suggestion that this region is concerned with monitoring of self-generated, as opposed to externally generated, information, which is the province of the dorsolateral FC. The latter proposal seems at variance with evidence of dorsolateral FC involvement on tests of monitoring such as free recall and random number generation, all of which involve self-generated information. A final possibility is that this region implicated the "sense of self," which is a crucial component of episodic (autobiographical) memory that underlies the ability to re-experience the past (Craik et al., 1999; Levine et al., 1998; Moroz, 1999; Mosocovitch, 2000; Wheeler et al., 1997). All of these proposals, have some merit, and although all, including ours, are frankly speculative at this stage of investigation, they are useful in that they provide clear hypotheses that can be tested in future studies.

SEQUENCE OF INTERACTION AMONG COMPONENTS

As yet, we know little about the sequence of interaction among the various regions of the FC at encoding and retrieval. By considering the functions we have assigned to these regions in the previous section, it is possible to derive some suggestions about the processing sequence at retrieval (see Fig. 12–6).

Retrieval is initiated with the establishment of a retrieval mode, which includes setting the goals of the task and initiating a retrieval strategy if external or internal cues cannot elicit a memory directly. Assuming that the function of the dorsolateral PFC is manipulation of information in working memory, then it is more suited than any of the other areas to coordinate these strategic activities and to monitor their outcome. In animal models, this process would involve learning the goals of the task and coordinating the activities necessary to achieve them.

Once the retrieval strategy is in place and initiated, the ventrolateral PFC is recruited. As noted earlier, its role is to specify and describe the cues needed to gain access to the MTL and maintain the information until the memory is recovered. The involvement of the ventrolateral PFC in this process begins at encoding and is reiterated at retrieval, where cue distinctiveness is a crucial factor in performance (Moscovitch & Craik, 1976). This cue information is transmitted to the MTL where it interacts with a code or index that elicits a (consciously apprehended) memory trace. If the cue is not specific or distinctive enough to interact with the MTL code and activate a memory trace, the process is repeated until an adequate cue is found and a memory is recovered, or the process is terminated.

It is also possible that a cue can activate the MTL directly, rather than via the ventrolateral PFC, if the cue is highly specific and strongly related to the information represented in the MTL code. In our component process model,

Figure 12–6. Flow diagram for interactions among medial temporal cortex and regions of frontal cortex during retrieval of episodic memories. DLPFC, dorsolateral prefrontal cortex; VLPFC, ventrolateral prefrontal cortex; VMPFC, ventromedial prefrontal cortex. The DLPFC is represented twice in the diagram to indicate its involvement in different processes at different points in the sequence.

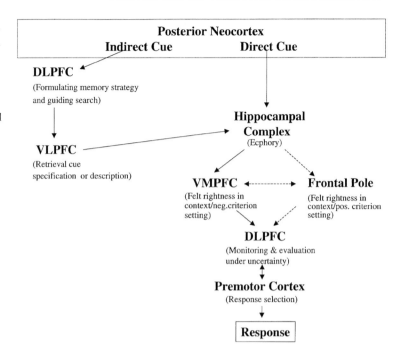

we refer to this direct process as *associative-cue dependent* (Moscovitch, 1992; Moscovitch & Winocur, 1992a, 1992b).

Once a memory is recovered, the information it represents is delivered to the ventromedial PFC. Although it is difficult to distinguish between the contribution of the ventrolateral and ventromedial regions to memory in lesion and neuroimaging studies, we have assigned different functions to them. Based on information about the goals of the task from dorsolateral PFC and about cues from ventrolateral PFC (and possibly context from Area 10), the ventromedial cortex automatically and immediately signals whether recovered memory traces satisfy those goals and are consistent with the cues in that particular context. It signals the felt-rightness of the recovered memory rather than the results of a considered evaluation. Because damage to ventromedial cortex leads to indiscriminate acceptance of recovered memories, its likely role is inhibitory in setting criteria (rejection).

In cases of uncertainty, the setting criteria may also implicate area 10, where it plays a reciprocal role of signaling acceptance or endorsement (excitatory) rather than rejection (inhibitory) before the recovered memory is subjected to further processing. In those latter circumstances, the dorsolateral PFC is recruited to engage strategic verification processes, that would involve a host of regions in the FC, including the ventrolateral region, and posterior neocortex. These regions would then supply relevant information about the recovered memory, such as its perceptual characteristics (Johnson et al., 1996; Schacter et al., 1996b) and its compatibility with other knowledge about the event in question, that would influence the decision to accept or reject the recovered memory.

Response selection, mediated by area 6 (premotor motor cortex) is a crucial element in the retrieval process, although it is difficult to know where to place it in the sequence. It can either operate early in the process to help select among alternative strategies or cues with which to probe memory, or later to select among possible responses to memories that were recovered, or both. If the required information is not recovered or accepted, the retrieval processing sequence may be repeated or the search terminated.

We have focused on retrieval, but some of the same regions likely also operate at encoding. In particular, areas 9 and 46 (DLPFC) are implicated at encoding to direct attention and establish encoding strategies (area 46) that will make the target distinctive (area 47, ventro-lateral), thereby influencing its stored representation in MTL and, ultimately, making it more easily retrievable via specific cues laid down at encoding.

CONCLUSION

When we first proposed our WWM model, our goal was to provide a framework for distinguishing medial temporal from frontal contributions to memory (Moscovitch, 1989, 1992; Moscovitch & Winocur, 1992a, 1992b; Winocur, 1992b). In particular, we wished to place studies on memory in the context of a more general framework of modules and central systems (Moscovitch & Umiltà, 1990, 1991). In reviewing the literature at the time, we noted that there was ample evidence that the FC was crucial for performance on some tests of long-term, episodic memory, but with one or two exceptions (Shallice, 1988; Petrides, 1989), there was no theoretical framework that integrated those observations. Most of the focus in memory research was still on the medial temporal lobes. On the basis of our review, we proposed that the medial temporal lobes are "stupid" modules that obligatorily, and relatively automatically, encode and retrieve information that is consciously apprehended, whereas the frontal lobes act as "intelligent" central system structures that work with memory delivered to the medial temporal lobes or recovered from it. We proposed that as central system structures, the frontal lobes are needed for strategic aspects of encoding and retrieval. These include organizing input at encoding and initiating and directing search at retrieval, as well as monitoring and verifying the memories to see that they fit with the goals of the task and to place the recovered memories in their proper temporal–spatial context. At the time of that initial proposal, there was little evidence to assign each of these strategic operations to different regions of the FC, and we thought we had gone far enough in distinguishing between the strategic

function of the FC and the modular functions of the medial temporal lobes. The decade of research since our proposal has generally supported our idea that the frontal lobes are WWM structures and we have extended it by attempting to identify the regions in the FC that mediate the different components of WWM. Although a consensus has yet to be reached about what the various components are and where they are localized, there is sufficient evidence to formulate, as we did in the previous section, hypotheses about the function of different regions of the FC, in general, and more particularly, about their role in memory encoding and retrieval. Recognizing that some of the hypotheses are more speculative than others, and that further work is necessary, particularly with respect to developing animal models, we offer an updated version of the WWM model, based on these hypotheses. Like the previous version, the new version is a component process model that is concerned as much with the interaction among the components as it is with assignment, and localization, of function. We believe the model helps integrate the findings we reviewed and provides a framework for future research.

ACKNOWLEDGMENTS

The preparation of this chapter and the research reported here were supported by grants to Morris Moscovitch and Gordon Winocur from the Canadian Institutes of Health Research and the Natural Sciences and Engineering Research Council. The authors gratefully acknowledge the technical assistance of Heidi Roesler, Marilyne Ziegler, and Doug Caruana during various stages of the research and preparation of the manuscript.

NOTES

1. Given the specificity of connections from other structures to the FC, there may well be some domain specificity at a very local level within each region of the FC (see Moscovitch & Umiltà, 1990, p 21; Miller, 2000; Petrides, 2000).
2. The multiple trace theory (MTT) argues against the traditional view that, as memories become consolidated, the role of the hippocampal complex in memory retention and retrieval diminishes with time whereas that of the neocortex increases. According to the MTT and the results we obtained, the hippocampal complex is impli-

cated regardless of the age of the memory. However, supported by evidence such as that obtained in the food-preference study (see Recent and Remote Memory, above), proponents of the traditional view have offered alternative interpretations. Indeed, the question as to whether the hippocampal complex is needed for retention and recovery of remote memories is currently under intensive debate in both the human and animal literature (Moscovitch & Nadel, 1998, 1999; Rosenbaum et al., 2001).

REFERENCES

Aggleton, J.P. & Brown, M.W. (1999). Episodic memory, amnesia, and the hippocampal-anterior thalamic axis. *Behavioral and Brain Sciences, 22,* 425–489.

Bartlett, F.C. (1932). *Remembering: A Study in Experimental and Social Psychology.* New York: Cambridge University Press.

Bechara, A., Damasio, H., & Damasio, A.R. (2000a). Emotion, Decision Making and the Orbitofrontal Cortex *Cerebral Cortex, 10,* 295–307.

Bechara, A., Tranel, D., & Damasio, H. (2000b). Characterization of the decision-making deficit of patients with ventromedial prefrontal cortex lesions. *Brain, 123,* 2189–2202.

Becker, J.T., Walker, J.A., & Olton, D.S. (1980). Neuroanatomical bases of spatial memory. *Brain Research, 200,* 307–321.

Brainerd, C.J., Reyna, V.F., & Brandes, E. (1995). Are children's false memories more persistent than their true memories? *Psychological Science, 6,* 359–364.

Brainerd, C.J., Wright, R., Reyna, V.F., & Mojardin, A.H. (2000). Conjoint recognition and phantom recollection. *Journal of Experimental Psychology: Learning, Memory and Cognition, 27,* 307–327.

Brewer, J.B., Zhao, Z., Desmond, J.E., Glover, G.H., & Gabrieli, J.D.E. (1998). Making memories: brain activity that predicts how well visual experience will be remembered. *Science, 281,* 1185–1187.

Buckner, R.L., Raichle, M.E., & Petersen, S.E. (1995). Dissociation of human prefrontal cortical areas across different speech production tasks and gender groups. *Journal of Neurophysiology, 74,* 2163–2173.

Burgess, P.W. & Shallice, T. (1996). Confabulation and the control of recollection. *Memory, 4,* 359–411.

Cabeza, R., Mangels, J., Nyberg, L., Habib, R., Houle, S., McIntosh, A.R., & Tulving, E. (1997). Brain regions differentially involved in remembering what and when: a PET study. *Neuron, 19,* 863–870.

Christoff, K. & Gabrieli, J.D.E. (2000). The frontopolar cortex and human cognition: evidence for a rostrocaudal hierarchical organization within the human prefrontal cortex. *Psychobiology, 28,* 168–186.

Craik, F.M., Moroz, T.M., Moscovitch, M., Stuss, D.T., Winocur, G., Tulving, E., & Kapur, S. (1999). In search of self: a PET investigation of self-referential information. *Psychological Science, 10,* 26–34.

Crovitz, H.F. & Schiffman, H. (1974). Frequency of epi-

sodic memories as a function of their age. *Bulletin of the Psychonomic Society, 4,* 517–518.

Dalla Barba, G. (1993a). Confabulation: knowledge and recollective experience. *Cognitive Neuropsychology, 10,* 1–20.

Dalla Barba, G. (1993b). Different patterns of confabulation. *Cortex, 29,* 567–581.

Deese, J. (1959). On the prediction of occurrence of particular verbal intrusions in immediate recall. *Journal of Experimental Psychology, 58,* 17–22.

Delatour, B. & Gisquet-Verrier, P. (2001). Involvement of the dorsal anterior cingulate cortex in temporal behavioral sequencing: subregional analysis of the medial prefrontal cortex in rat. *Behavioral Brain Research, 126,* 105–114.

Duncan, J. & Owen, A.M. (2000). Common regions of the human frontal lobe recruited by diverse cognitive demands. *Trends in Neuroscience, 23,* 475–483.

Elliot, R., Dolan, R.J., & Frith, C.D. (2000). Dissociable functions in the medial and lateral orbitofrontal cortex: evidence from human neuroimaging studies. *Cerebral Cortex, 10,* 308–317.

Ergis, A.M., Winocur, G., Saint-Cyr, J., Van der Linden, M., Melo, B., & Freedman, M. (2000). Troubles de la reconnaisance dans de la maladie de Parkinson. In: M.C. Gely-Nargeot, L. Ritchiek, & L. Touchon (Eds.), Actualites sur la maladie d'Alzheimer et les syndromes apparentes (pp. 481–489). Marseille: Jolal.

Fernandes, M.A. & Moscovitch, M. (2000). Divided attention and memory: evidence of substantial interference effects at retrieval and encoding. *Journal of Experimental Psychology: General, 129,* 155–176.

Fink, G.R., Markowitsch, H.J., Reinkemeier, M., Bruckbauer, T., Kessler, J., & Heiss, W.D. (1996). Cerebral representation of one's own past: neural networks involved in autobiographical memory. *Journal of Neuroscience, 16,* 4275–4282.

Fletcher, P.C. & Henson, R.N.A. (2001). Frontal lobes and human memory. Insights from functional neuroimaging. *Brain, 124,* 849–881.

Fletcher, P.C., Shallice, T., Frith, C.D., Frackowiak, R.S., & Dolan, R.J. (1998). The functional roles of prefrontal cortex in episodic memory. II. Retrieval. *Brain, 121,* 1249–1256.

Gabrieli, J.D.E., Vaidya, C.J., Stone, M., Francis, W.S., Thompson-Schill, S.L., Fleischman, D.A., Tinklenberg, J.R., Yesavage, J.A., & Wilson, R.S. (1999). Convergent behavioral and neuropsychological evidence for a distinction between identification and production forms of repetition priming. *Journal of Experimental Psychology: General, 128,* 479–498.

Gilboa, A., Moscovitch, M. (in press). The cognitive neuroscience of confabulation: A review and a model. In A. Baddeley, B.A. Wilson, & M. Kapelman (Eds.) *Handbook of memory disorders: 2nd Edition.* Oxford: Oxford University Press.

Gilboa, A., Winocur, G., Grady, C., Moscovitch, M. (in preparation) Recent and remote memory for autobiographical events elicited by family photographs.

Granon, S. & Poucet, B. (1995). Medial prefrontal lesions

in the rat and spatial navigation: evidence for impaired planning. *Behavioral Neuroscience, 109,* 474–484.

Henson, R.N.A., Rugg, M.D., Shallice, T., Josephs, O., & Dolan, R.J. (1999). Recollection and familiarity in recognition memory: an event-related functional magnetic resonance imaging study. *Journal of Neuroscience, 19*(10), 3962–3972.

Henson, R., Shallice, T., Rugg, M., Fletcher, P., & Dolan, R. (2000). Functional imaging dissociations within right prefrontal cortex during episodic memory retrieval. Presented at the Frontal Lobe Conference, Toronto, March 20–24, 2000.

Johnson, M.K., Kounios, J., & Nolde, S.F. (1996). Electrophysiological brain activity and source memory. *NeuroReport, 7,* 2929–2932.

Kesner, R.P. & Holbrook, T. (1987). Dissociation of item and order spatial memory in rats following medial prefrontal cortex lesions. *Neuropsychologia, 25,* 653–664.

Kopelman, M.D. (1989). Remote and autobiographical memory, temporal context memory and frontal atrophy in Korsakoff and Alzheimer patients. *Neuropsychologia, 27,* 437–460.

Kopelman, M.D. (1991). Frontal dysfunction and memory deficits in the alcoholic Korsakoff syndrome and Alzheimer-type dementia. *Brain and Cognition, 114,* 117–137.

Kopelman, M.D. (1999). Varieties of false memory. *Cognitive Neuropsychology, 16,* 197–214.

Lepage, M., Habib, R., & Tulving, E. (1998). Hippocampal PET activations of memory encoding and retrieval: the HIPER model. *Hippocampus, 8,* 313–322.

Levine, B., Black, S.E., Cabeza, R., Sinden, M., McIntosh, A.R., Toth, J.P., Tulving, E., & Stuss, D.T. (1998). Episodic memory and the self in a case of isolated retrograde amnesia. *Brain, 121,* 1951–1973.

Maguire, E.A. (2001). Neuroimaging studies of autobiographical event memory. *Philosophical Transactions of the Royal Society of London, B, Biological Sciences, 356,* 1441–1452.

Mangels, J.A., Gershberg, F.B., Knight, R.T., & Shimamura, A.P. (1996). Impaired retrieval from remote memory in patients with frontal lobe damage. *Neuropsychology, 10,* 32–41.

Melo, B., Winocur, G., & Moscovitch, M. (1999). False recall and false recognition: An examination of the effects of selective and combined lesions to the medial temporal lobe/diencephalon and frontal lobe structures. *Cognitive Neuropsychology, 16,* 343–359.

Miller, E.K. (2000). The prefrontal cortex and cognitive control. *Nature Reviews: Neuroscience, 1,* 59–65.

Milner, B. & Petrides, M. (1984). Behavioural effects of frontal-lobe lesions in man. *Trends in Neurosciences, 7,* 403–407.

Moroz, T. (1999). Memory for Self-referential Information: Behavioural and Neuroimaging Studies in Normal People. Doctoral thesis, University of Toronto, Toronto, Ontario.

Moscovitch, M. (1989). Confabulation and the frontal systems: strategic versus associative retrieval in neuropsychological theories of memory. In: H.L. Roediger, III

& F.I.M. Craik (Eds.), *Varieties of Memory and Consciousness: Essays in Honour of Endel Tulving* (pp. 133–160). Hillsdale, NJ: Lawrence Erlbaum Associates.

Moscovitch, M. (1992). Memory and working-with-memory: a component process model based on modules and central systems. *Journal of Cognitive Neuroscience, 4,* 257–267.

Moscovitch, M. (1994a). Memory and working-with-memory: evaluation of a component process model and comparisons with other models. In: D.L. Schacter and E. Tulving (Eds.), *Memory Systems* (pp. 269–310). Cambridge, MA: MIT/Bradford Press.

Moscovitch, M. (1994b). Interference at retrieval from long-term memory: the influence of frontal and temporal lobes. *Neuropsychology, 4,* 525–534.

Moscovitch, M. (1995). Confabulation. In: D.L. Schacter, J.T. Coyle, G.D. Fischbach, M.M. Mesulum, & L.G. Sullivan (Eds.), *Memory Distortion,* (pp. 226–251). Cambridge, MA: Harvard University Press.

Moscovitch, M. (2000) Theories of memory and consciousness. In E. Tulving & F.L.M. Craik (Eds.), *The Oxford handbook of memory* (pp. 609–628). Oxford: Oxford University Press.

Moscovitch, M. & Craik, F.I.M. (1976). Depth of processing, retrieval cues and uniqueness of encoding as factors in recall. *Journal of Verbal Learning and Verbal Behavior, 15,* 447–458.

Moscovitch, M. & Melo, B. (1997). Strategic retrieval and the frontal lobes: evidence from confabulation and amnesia. *Neuropsychologia, 35,* 1017–1034.

Moscovitch, M. & Nadel, L. (1998). Consolidation and the hippocampal complex revisited: in defence of the multiple-trace model. *Current Opinion in Neurobiology, 8,* 297–300.

Moscovitch, M. & Nadel, L. (1999). Multiple-trace theory and sematnic dementia: a reply to K.S. Graham. *Trends in Cognitive Neuroscience, 3,* 87–89.

Moscovitch, M. & Umiltà, C. (1990). Modularity and neuropsychology. In: M.F. Schwartz (Ed.), *Modular Deficits in Alzheimer's Disease* (pp. 1–59). Cambridge, MA: MIT Press/Bradford.

Moscovitch, M. & Umiltà, C. (1991). Conscious and nonconscious aspects of memory: a neuropsychological framework of modular and central systems. In: R.G. Lister & H.J. Weingartner (Eds.), *Perspectives on Cognitive Neuroscience.* New York: Oxford University Press.

Moscovitch, M. & Winocur, G. (1992a). Frontal lobes and memory. In: L.R. Squire (Ed.). *The Encyclopedia of Learning and Memory: A Volume in Neuropsychology* (D.L. Schacter, Ed.). New York: Macmillan.

Moscovitch, M. & Winocur, G. (1992b). The neuropsychology of memory and aging. In: F.I.M. Craik, and T.A. Salthouse (Eds.). *The Handbook of Aging and Cognition* (pp. 315–372). Hillsdale, NJ,: Lawrence Erlbaum Associates.

Moscovitch, M. & Winocur, G. (1995). Frontal lobes, memory and aging. *Annals of the New York Academy of Sciences, 769,* 119–150.

Moscovitch, M., Fernandes, M.A., Troyer, A.K. (in press)

Working-with-memory and cognitive resources: A component process account of divided attention. In M. Naveh-Benjamin, R.L. Roediger, M. Moscovitch (Eds.). *Perspectives on human memory and cognitive aging: Essays in honor of F.I.M. Craik*. New York: Psychology Press.

Nadel, L. & Moscovitch, M. (1997). Memory consolidation, retrograde amnesia and the hippocampal complex. *Current Opinion in Neurobiology, 7*, 217–227.

Nadel, L. & Moscovitch, M. (1998). Hippocampal contributions to cortical plasticity. *Neuropharmacology, 37*, 431–439.

Nadel, L., Samsonovich, A., Ryan, L., & Moscovitch, M. (2000). Multiple trace theory of human memory: computational, neuroimaging, and neuropsychological results. *Hippocampus, 10*, 352–368.

Nyberg, L., Winocur, G., & Moscovitch, M. (1997). Correlation between frontal-lobe functions and explicit and implicit stem completion in health elderly. *Neuropsychology, 11*, 70–76.

Parkin, A.J., Ward, J., Bindschaedler, C., Squires, E.J., & Powell, G. (1999). False recognition following frontal lobe damage: the role of encoding factors. *Cognitive Neuropsychology, 16*, 243–265.

Petrides, M. (1982). Motor conditional associative-learning after selective prefrontal lesions in the monkey. *Behavioural Brain Research, 5*, 407–413.

Petrides, M. (1989). Frontal lobes and memory. In: F. Boller & J. Grafman (Eds.), *Handbook of Neuropsychology, Vol. 3.* (pp. 75–90). Amsterdam: Elsevier.

Petrides, M. (1990). Nonspatial conditional learning impaired in patients with unilateral frontal but not unilateral temporal lobe excisions. *Neuropsychologia, 28*, 137–149.

Petrides, M. (1991). Monitoring of selections of visual stimuli in the primate frontal cortex. *Proceedings of the Royal Society of London Series B, 246*, 293–298.

Petrides, M. (1995). Functional organization of the human frontal cortex for mnemonic processing: evidence from neuroimaging studies. *Annals of the New York Academy of Sciences, 769*, 85–96.

Petrides, M. (2000). The role of the mid-dorsolateral prefrontal cortex in working memory. *Experimental Brain Research, 133*, 44–54.

Petrides, M. & Milner, B. (1982). Deficits on subject-ordered tasks after frontal- and temporal-lobe lesions in man. *Neuropsychologia, 20*, 249–262.

Postle, B.R. & D'Esposito, M. (2000). Evaluating models of the topographical organization of working memory function in frontal cortex with event-related fMRI. *Psychobiology, 28*, 132–145.

Pribram, K.H. & Tubbs, W.E. (1967). Short-term memory, parsing, and the primate frontal cortex. *Science, 156*, 1765–1767.

Ragozzino, M.E., Detrick, S., & Kesner, R.P. (1999). Involvement of the prelimbic-infralimbic areas of the rodent prefrontal cortex in behavioral flexibility for place and response learning. *Journal of Neuroscience, 19*, 4585–4594.

Rapcsak, S.Z., Reminger, S.L., Glisky, E.L., Kaszniak, A.W., & Comer, J.F. (1999). Neuropsychological mechanisms of false facial recognition following frontal lobe damage. *Cognitive Neuropsychology, 1*, 267–292.

Reyna, V.F. & Brainerd, C.J. (1995). Fuzzy-trace theory: an interim synthesis. *Learning and Individual Differences, 1*, 1–75.

Roediger, H.L., III & McDermott, K.B. (1995). Creating false memories: remembering words not presented in lists. *Journal of Experimental Psychology: Learning, Memory, and Cognition, 21*, 803–814.

Roediger, H.L., III, Buckner, R.L., & McDermott, K.B. (1999). In: J.K. Foster and M. Jelicic (Eds.), *Memory: Systems, Process, or Function? Debates in Psychology* (pp. 31–65). New York: Oxford University Press.

Rosenbaum, R.S., Winocur, G., & Moscovitch, M. (2001). New views on old memories: reevaluating the role of the hippocampal complex. *Behavioural Brain Research, 127*, 183–198.

Rugg, M.D., Fletcher, P.C., Allan, K., Frith, C.D., Frackowiak, R.S., & Dolan, R.J. (1998). Neural correlates of memory retrieval during recognition memory and cued recall. *NeuroImage, 8*, 262–273.

Ryan, L., Nadel, L., Keil, K., Putnam, K., Schnyer, D., Trouard, T. & Moscovitch, M. (2001). The hippocampal complex and retrieval of recent and very remote autobiographical memories: evidence from functional magnetic resonance imaging in neurologically intact people. *Hippocampus, 11* 707–714.

Schacter, D.L. (1987). Memory, amnesia, and frontal lobe dysfunction. *Psychobiology, 15*, 21–36.

Schacter, D.L., Curran, T., Galluccio, L., Milberg, W., & Bates, J. (1996a). False recognition and the right frontal lobe: a case study. *Neuropsychologia, 34*, 793–808.

Schacter, D.L., Reiman, E., Curran, T., Yun, L.S., Brandy, D., McDermott, K.B., & Roediger, H.L., III. (1996b). Neuroanatomical correlates of veridical and illusory recognition memory: evidence from positron emission tomography. *Neuron, 17*, 267–274.

Schacter, D.L., Verfaellie, M., & Pradere, D. (1996c). The neuropsychology of memory illusions: false recall and recognition in amnesic patients. *Journal of Memory and Language, 35*, 319–334.

Schacter, D.L., Norman, K.A., & Koutstaal, W. (1998a). The cognitive neuroscience of constructive memory. *Annual Review of Psychology, 49*, 289–318.

Schacter, D.L., Verfaellie, M., Anes, M.D., & Racine, C. (1998b). When true recognition suppresses false recognition: evidence from amnesic patients. *Journal of Cognitive Neuroscience, 10*, 668–679.

Schacter, D.L., Israel, L., & Racine, C. (1999). Suppressing false recognition in younger and older adults: the distinctiveness heuristic. *Journal of Memory and Language, 40*, 1–24.

Schnider, A. & Ptak, R. (1999). Spontaneous confabulators fail to suppress currently irrelevant memory traces. *Nature Neuroscience, 2*, 677–681.

Schnider, A., von Daniken, C., & Gutbrod, K. (1996). The mechanisms of spontaneous and provoked confabulations. *Brain, 119*, 1365–1375.

Schnider, A., Ptak, R., von Daeniken, C., & Remonda, L. (2000). Recovery from spontaneous confabulations parallels recovery of temporal confusion in memory. *Neurology, 55,* 74–83.

Squire, L.R. (1992). Memory and the hippocampus: a synthesis from findings with rats, monkeys, and humans. *Psychological Review, 99,* 195–231.

Squire, L.R. & Alvarez, P. (1995). Retrograde amnesia and memory consolidation: a neurobiological perspective. *Current Opinion in Neurobiology, 5,* 169–177.

Stuss, D.T., Alexander, M.P., Palumbo, C.L., Buckle, L., Sayer, L., & Pogue, J. (1994). Organizational strategies with unilateral or bilateral frontal lobe injury in word learning tasks. *Neuropsychology, 8,* 355–373.

Troyer, A., Moscovitch, M., & Winocur, G. (1997). Clustering and switching as two components of verbal fluency: evidence from younger and older healthy adults. *Neuropsychology, 11,* 138–146.

Troyer, A.K., Moscovitch, M., Winocur, G., Leach, L., & Freedman, M. (1998a). Clustering and switching on verbal fluency tests in Alzheimer's and Parkinson's disease. *Journal of the International Neuropsychological Society, 4,* 137–143

Troyer, A.T., Moscovitch, M., Winocur, G., Alexander, M.P., & Stuss, D.T (1998b). Clustering and switching on verbal fluency: the effects of focal frontal- and temporal-lobe lesions. *Neuropsychologia, 36,* 499–504.

Troyer, A.K., Winocur, G., Craik, F.I.M., & Moscovitch, M. (1999). Source memory and divided attention: reciprocal costs to primary and secondary tasks. *Neuropsychology, 13,* 467–474.

Tulving, E., Kapur, S., Craik, F.I.M., Moscovitch, M., & Houle, S. (1994). Hemispheric encoding/retrieval asymmetry in episodic memory: positron emission tomography findings. *Proceedings of the National Academy of Sciences USA, 91,* 2016–2020.

Wagner, A.D. (1999). Working memory contributions to human learning and remembering [review]. *Neuron, 22,* 19–22.

Wagner, A.D., Schacter, D.L., Rotte, M., Koutstaal, W., Maril, A., Dale, A.M., Rosen, B.R., & Buckner, R.L. (1998). Building memories: remembering and forgetting of verbal experiences as predicted by brain activity. *Science, 281,* 1188–1191.

Wheeler, M.A., Stuss, D.T., & Tulving, E. (1995). Frontal lobe damage produces episodic memory impairment. *Journal of the International Neuropsychological Society, 1,* 525–536.

Wheeler, M.A., Stuss, D.T., & Tulving, E. (1997) Toward a theory of episodic memory: The frontal lobes and autonoetic consciousness. *Psychological Bulletin, 121,* 331–354.

Winocur, G. (1990). Anterograde and retrograde amnesia in rats with hippocampal or thalamic lesions. *Behavioural Brain Research, 38,* 145–154.

Winocur, G. (1991). Functional dissociation of the hippocampus and prefrontal cortex in learning and memory. *Psychobiology, 19,* 11–20.

Winocur, G. (1992a). A comparison of normal old rats and young adult rats with lesions to the hippocampus or prefrontal cortex on a test of matching-to-sample. *Neuropsychologia, 30,* 769–781.

Winocur, G. (1992b). Dissociative effects of hippocampal and prefrontal cortex damage on learning and memory. In: L.R. Squire and N. Butters (Eds.), *Neuropsychology of Memory,* 2nd Ed. (pp. 191–201). New York: Guilford Press.

Winocur, G. & Eskes, G. (1998). The prefrontal cortex and caudate nucleus in conditional associative learning: dissociated effects of selective brain lesions in rats. *Behavioral Neuroscience, 112,* 89–101.

Winocur, G. & Gagnon, S. (1998). Glucose treatment attenuates spatial learning and memory deficits of aged rats on tests of hippocampal function. *Neurobiology of Aging, 19,* 233–241.

Winocur, G. & Moscovitch, M. (1990). Hippocampal and prefrontal cortex contributions to learning and memory: analysis of lesion and aging effects on maze learning in rats. *Behavioral Neuroscience, 104,* 544–551.

Winocur, G. & Moscovitch, M. (1999). Anterograde and retrograde amnesia after lesions to frontal cortex. *Journal of Neuroscience, 19,* 9611–9617.

Winocur, G., Moscovitch, M., & Stuss, D.T. (1996). A neuropsychological investigation of explicit and implicit memory in institutionalized and community-dwelling old people. *Neuropsychology, 10,* 57–65

Witherspoon, D. & Moscovitch, M. (1989). Independence of the repetition effects between word fragment completion and perceptual identification. *Journal of Experimental Psychology: Memory, Learning, and Cognition, 15,* 22–30.

Zola-Morgan, S. & Squire, L.R. (1990). The primate hippocampal formation: evidence for a time-limited role in memory storage. *Science, 250,* 288–290.

13

Memory Retrieval and Executive Control Processes

ARTHUR P. SHIMAMURA

When was the last time you went to the movies? What movie did you see? Where were you? Who went with you? Unless you have seen a movie very recently, the answers to these questions require a strategic search through your memory. Such searches place significant demands on *executive control*—that is, the ability to select, manipulate, and update retrieved memories. For example, you may have generated several movies that were recently seen and then updated the information to determine which one was the most recent. When you retrieved what you thought was the most recent movie, further monitoring and control was necessary to retrieve answers to the other questions, such as when and where you saw the movie. In this example, your ability to retrieve memory embedded within a spatial-temporal context was tapped.

Executive control is particularly required when retrieval depends on recollecting memories within a specific context. The context may be episodic in nature, as in the example above, or the context may be semantic, as in answering an essay question (e.g., describe the role of executive control in memory retrieval). Findings from cognitive neuroscience suggest that the prefrontal cortex contributes significantly to memory retrieval. For example, neuropsychological studies show that patients with

frontal lobe lesions exhibit significant deficits in retrieving both semantic and episodic memory. Functional neuroimaging findings (i.e., positron emission tomography [PET] and functional magnetic resonance imaging [fMRI]) have corroborated and extended findings from patients with frontal lobe lesions. In particular, neuroimaging studies have located specific regions within the prefrontal cortex that appear to mediate different aspects of retrieval.

Theories have been developed to characterize the role of the prefrontal cortex in memory and cognition. Indeed, this volume is a testament to the variety of views on, and empirical approaches toward, the analysis of frontal lobe function. With respect to memory retrieval, theorists have drawn attention to the importance of the prefrontal cortex in accessing, updating, and monitoring retrieved information. There is some general agreement concerning the importance of the prefrontal cortex in executive control processes associated with working memory. Baddeley's seminal description of the "dysexecutive" syndrome characterizes well the cognitive disorder associated with frontal lobe damage (Baddeley, 1986). Moscovitch described the role of the prefrontal cortex as "working with memory" and emphasized the importance of the prefrontal cortex in strategic memory searches (Moscovitch, 1992). Finally, neuroimaging results have implicated aspects of executive control, such as memory maintenance, updating, and manipulation, in the service of memory retrieval (in particular, see Chapters 3, 11, 15, and 17).

EXECUTIVE CONTROL AND DYNAMIC FILTERING THEORY

Shimamura (2000) developed a theoretical framework called *dynamic filtering theory*. By this view, the prefrontal cortex monitors and controls information processing by a filtering or gating mechanism. Four aspects of executive control can be characterized in terms of dynamic filtering of information processing— selecting, maintaining, updating, and rerouting. *Selecting* refers to the ability to focus attention on perceptual features or on activated memory representations. *Maintaining* refers to the ability to keep active any selected information. Short-term memory tasks, such as the digit span task, assess the ability to maintain information in working memory. *Updating* refers to processes involved in modulating and rearranging activity in working memory. For example, in a backward digit span task, subjects report the string of digits backwards, from the last one presented to the first. In this case, subjects must rearrange or update the order of digits in working memory before responding. *Rerouting* refers to the ability to switch from one cognitive process or response set to another. Tasks that require rerouting involve an entire shift from one stimulus–response path to another. Set shifting tasks, such as the Wisconsin Card Sorting Test (Milner, 1964), tap rerouting of information processing.

The dynamic filtering theory suggests that these four aspects of executive control can be described in terms of the interplay between regions within the prefrontal cortex and regions in the posterior cortex. This dynamic interplay involves feedforward and feedback activations between prefrontal and posterior regions. In cognitive terms, prefrontal regions monitor posterior activity and then control these activations by recurrent circuits back to posterior regions. These feedback circuits act

to select and maintain certain activations and filter (i.e., inhibit) others. By this view, posterior cortical activations at any given moment consist of a cacophony of neural signals in response to sensory information and memory activations. The prefrontal cortex orchestrates these signals by maintaining certain activations and inhibiting others. As such, the prefrontal cortex refines cortical activity by increasing signal-to-noise ratios.

Shimamura (2000) proposed that the four aspects of executive control can be construed in terms of different filtering properties, such as engaging a filter (selecting), keeping a filter active (maintaining), or switching between filters (updating or rerouting). These aspects are arranged by level of complexity, from the most rudimentary, selecting, to the most demanding, rerouting. The dynamic filtering theory was initially proposed to account for deficits in patients with frontal lobe lesions (Shimamura, 1995, 1996). A recent extension of this view (Shimamura, 2000) draws heavily on functional neuroimaging findings and conceptualizations developed by others, such as those of D'Esposito et al. (1998), Knight et al. (1999), Shallice and Burgess (1998), Petrides (1998), and Smith and Jonides (1999).

It is presumed that the four aspects of executive control are essential for successful memory retrieval. That is, when asked to recollect information, such as remembering the last movie you saw, memory representations must be selected, maintained, and updated. To the extent that some memory activations become irrelevant (e.g., determining that a retrieved movie was not the last one seen), activations must be inhibited and processing rerouted. Thus, strategic memory searches place significant demands on executive control. If relevant information cannot be selected and maintained or if irrelevant information cannot be inhibited, memory retrieval will be hampered.

The following sections review neuropsychological findings from patients with frontal lobe lesions. These patients incurred unilateral damage of the frontal lobe that centered on the dorsolateral prefrontal cortex. Findings from these patients suggest problems in aspects of executive control as the source of impairment in memory retrieval (see also Chapter 34). In a variety of test paradigms, such as retrieval of semantic knowledge, retrieval of public events, word list recall, and source recollection, patients with frontal lobe lesions exhibit significant impairment. In these tasks, a strategic search of memory is critical.

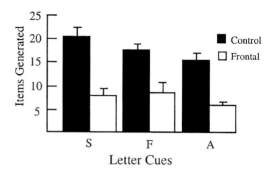

RETRIEVING SEMANTIC KNOWLEDGE

Semantic knowledge refers to one's expanse database of factual information. Such information is generally viewed as well-integrated knowledge structures accessed by inter-item associations. Consider a semantic retrieval task, such as the verbal fluency task, in which subjects are given 1 minute to retrieve as many words as they can that begin with a letter (e.g., F, A, and S) (Milner, 1964; Benton & deHamsher, 1976). This task requires the retrieval of semantic or lexical knowledge and can be facilitated by cuing inter-item associations. Such tasks also require the ability to monitor previously responded items and to update retrieved items after each response. That is, after a successful retrieval has been made, subjects must keep in mind prior responses so that they will not be repeated. Failure to update this set will lead to repetition errors (i.e., perseverations).

Patients with frontal lobe lesions exhibit significant impairment on fluency tasks (Milner, 1964; Benton & deHamsher, 1976; Jones-Gottman & Milner, 1977; Baldo & Shimamura, 1998). In one study (Baldo & Shimamura, 1998), verbal fluency was assessed using letters ("F," "A," "S") and semantic categories as cues ("animals," "occupations," "fruits"). In both cases, retrieval was impaired in patients with frontal lobe lesions (see Fig. 13–1). As in many studies of verbal fluency, a concomitant of impaired retrieval in patients with frontal lobe lesions is an inordinate number of response repetitions or perseverations. This failure to inhibit or gate prior responses contributes to a problem in updating information during retrieval. Impaired retrieval and perserverative responses can also be observed in studies using nonverbal material as well (Jones-Gottman & Milner, 1997; Baldo et al.,

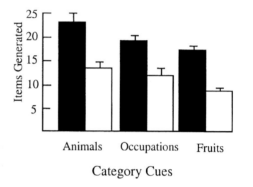

Figure 13–1. Performance by control subjects and patients with frontal lobe lesions on tests of verbal fluency. On these tests, subjects were given 1 minute to retrieve as many items as possible using either letter cues, such as "S," "F," and "A" (top graph) or category cues, such as "animals," "occupations," and "fruits." Patients with frontal lobe lesions exhibited significant impairment in the retrieval of such well-learned semantic knowledge. (*Source:* Data from Baldo & Shimamura, 1998)

2001). Moreover, neuroimaging studies have shown increased activation in prefrontal regions during the generation and retrieval of semantic knowledge (Frith et al., 1991; Gabrieli et al., 1996; Thompson-Schill et al., 1998).

To the extent that prefrontal cortex is involved in *controlling* retrieval, it is necessary to substantiate that semantic information was initially encoded and stored in a normal fashion. That is, poor encoding or degradation of semantic representations can also lead to impairment on memory tests. It is particularly important to address the status of encoding and memory storage in patients with frontal lobe lesions, because it is well documented that such patients do exhibit problems in some aspects of learning and organizing information at the time of encoding Hirst & Volpe, 1988; Gershberg & Shimamura, 1995; Baldo & Shimamura, 2000). To substantiate a retrieval deficit, as opposed to an encoding deficit, Mangels et al. (1996) administered tests of remote public knowledge, such as memory for public events or memory for famous faces. These tests have been used previously to assess retrograde amnesia in patients with severe memory disorders (Albert et al., 1979; Squire, et al., 1989).

For the public events tests, test questions assessed knowledge about specific incidences (e.g., "Who shot John Lennon?" [answer: "Chapman"]). Both recall and four-alternative, forced-choice recognition tests were administered. For the famous faces test, photographs of public figures (e.g., Anwar Sadat, Meryl Strepp) were shown, and subjects were asked to name the individual. If the name could not be retrieved, semantic and phonemic cues were provided (e.g., "This movie actress starred in *Sophie's Choice*; her initials are M.S."). Both the public events and famous faces tests assessed very remote knowledge (from as early as the 1940s), and exposure to these events and people occurred well before the onset of neurological damage (which occurred during the late 1980s or early 1990s in the patients). Thus, it can be presumed that deficits in performance on these tests are likely due to problems in retrieval rather than encoding.

Patients with prefrontal lesions exhibited impairment on free recall measures of remote public events and famous faces. Free recall impairment was significant and comparable across all decades tested. On the famous faces test, cued recall was also impaired (see Fig. 13–2). Recognition memory, however, was not reliably impaired. The disproportionate impairment on tests of recall compared to recognition memory tests suggests that the prefrontal cortex is involved in searching through semantic memory. That is, selecting, updating, and rerouting play a significant role in strategic retrieval of information, such as recalling the name of a famous individual. Such retrievals require searching through semantic knowledge, accessing relevant information, and disregarding irrelevant information. Item familiarity, as measured by recognition tests, does not require such a detailed search of memory. Recognition memory can be more easily based on familiarity judgments—that is, on recognition tests it is simply necessary to determine which choice seems more closely associated (i.e., familiar) with the question (e.g., "Who killed John Lennon: Mark Chapman or David Roth?").

Sylvester and Shimamura (in press) used another technique to address the status of semantic knowledge in patients with frontal lobe

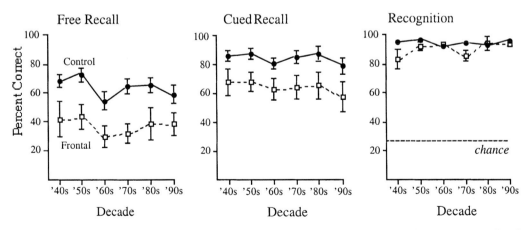

Figure 13–2. Control subjects and patients with frontal lobe lesions were given tests of remote memory. Subjects were presented photographs of individuals who became famous during various time periods between 1940 and 1995. Free and cued recall performance was significantly impaired in patients with prefrontal lesions, whereas recognition memory was less affected. (*Source:* Data from Mangels et al., 1996)

lesions. In that study, semantic relationships of animals were assessed. Multidimensional scaling techniques were applied as a way to assess semantic knowledge of animals. Subjects were presented all possible triplets of 12 animal names (e.g., "giraffe," "dog," "cat") and were asked to determine on each trial which two animals were most similar. On the basis of these similarity judgments, a map of "semantic space" could be constructed. Such maps have been used to describe the degree to which items are related to each other. For example, during the experiment, "dog" and "cat" were presented in 10 different triplets. If "dog" and "cat" were always judged to be the most similar pair in a triplet, then these two animals would be represented very close to each other in semantic space. To obtain the similarity relationships among the entire set of 12 animals, multidimensional scaling techniques were applied.

Previous studies using multidimensional scaling methods have shown that patients with mild to moderate Alzheimer's disease exhibit abnormal semantic representations (Chan et al., 1993). Such findings suggest that posterior cortical atrophy can significantly disrupt semantic knowledge. Using the same method employed to demonstrate impaired semantic representations in patients with Alzheimer's disease, Sylvester and Shimamura (in press) found no impairment of semantic space in patients with frontal lobe lesions; both patients and control subjects produced nearly identical similarity relationships. Figure 13–3 displays a two-dimensional representation of similarity judgments. The semantic relations suggested that both groups categorized animals in terms of physical and conceptual dimensions, such as size and domesticity. Importantly, the category used to demonstrate intact semantic knowledge (i.e., animals) was the same one used to demonstrate impaired semantic retrieval on fluency tests (Baldo & Shimamura, 1998).

In summary, retrieval of items from well-learned semantic categories and retrieval of very remote public events are impaired in patients with frontal lobe lesions. In these studies, recall performance is disproportionately impaired compared to recognition memory. Moreover, the ability to make semantic similarity judgments, as measured by semantic relationships using multidimensional scaling methods, suggests that patients with frontal lobe lesions perform well when the demands of retrieval search are minimized. It is suggested that the selecting, maintaining, updat-

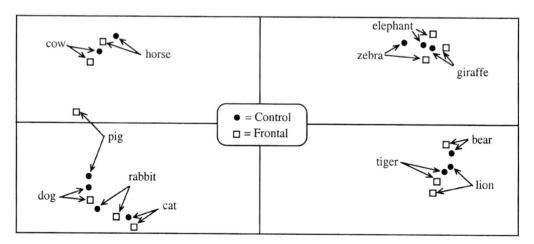

Figure 13–3. Two-dimensional representation of semantic space using similarity judgments and multidimensional scaling methods. Control subjects (circles) and patients with frontal lobe lesions (squares) were presented all possible triplets of 12 animal names and asked to determine which two were more similar. Controls and frontal pa-tients exhibited very similar semantic representation of animals. Note that these findings suggest that patients with frontal lobe lesions exhibit intact representation for semantic knowledge, despite impairment in the ability to retrieve such information on verbal fluency tasks. (*Source:* Data from Sylvester & Shimamura, 2001)

ing, and rerouting of memory play a significant role in searching and retrieving information through semantic memory. The next section suggests that these same executive control processes play a prominent role in retrieving episodic memory.

EPISODIC MEMORY RETRIEVAL AND SOURCE RECOLLECTION

Episodic memory refers to autobiographical memories that are embedded within a time and place context (see Tulving, 1983; Tulving & LaPage, 2000). Searching through episodic memory often involves selecting and filtering memories of life events. The opening exercise of remembering the last time you went to the movies is an example of retrieving episodic memory. Closely related to episodic memory is the notion of *source recollection* (see Johnson, et al., 1993), in which individuals are asked to recollect specific features of an episode, such as the color of a stimulus or the voice of the person who presented some information.

Recent findings from functional neuroimaging studies suggest a prominent role of the prefrontal cortex in both episodic retrieval and source recollection. In many PET and fMRI studies, the right prefrontal cortex is particularly active during tasks that involve the retrieval of recently presented information (see Buckner & Peterson, 1996; Henson et al., 1999). Various aspects of retrieving information have been associated with prefrontal activation, such as indicating a successful memory retrieval or setting a general mode of retrieval (see Kapur et al., 1995; Rugg et al., 1996; Buckner et al., 1998). Moreover, neuroimaging studies have identified three distinct subregions within the right prefrontal cortex that appear particularly active during memory retrieval. These subregions include *(1)* a ventral region (Brodmann's area 45/47), *(2)* a mid-dorsolateral region (Brodmann's area 9/46), and *(3)* a frontal polar region (Brodmann's area 10) (see Henson et al., 1999).

Neuropsychological studies have also demonstrated a prominent role of the prefrontal cortex in mediating some aspects of episodic memory. Although patients with frontal lobe lesions do not exhibit severe amnesia, they are impaired on tests of free and cued recall for recently presented material (Hirst & Volpe, 1988; Janowsky et al., 1989; Stuss et al., 1994; Gershberg & Shimamura, 1995). As in the retrieval of remote memories, patients with frontal lobe lesions exhibit a disproportionate impairment of recall compared to recognition memory performance (Janowsky et al., 1989 Gershberg & Shimamura, 1995; Wheeler, et al., 1995). This finding suggests that patients with frontal lobe lesions have minimal problems in making familiarity judgments for recently presented material. Their recall impairment during learning appears to be related to poor semantic organization during learning (Hirst & Volpe, 1988; Gershberg & Shimamura, 1995). Such executive control deficits during learning of episodic material stand in contrast to patients with severe amnesia, as in patients with medial temporal lobe damage. Patients with severe amnesia exhibit impairment in the storage of recently learned information, which affects both recall and recognition memory (see Gershberg & Shimamura, 1998; Squire & Knowlton, 2000).

To the extent that retrieval deficits in patients with frontal lobe lesions are attributed to problems in executive control, it should be possible to degrade memory performance by taxing executive processes. The dynamic filtering theory purports that a prominent feature of executive control is the filtering of extraneous information processing. The occurrence of extraneous or distracting information places heavy demands on updating and rerouting. Shimamura et al. (1995) demonstrated increased susceptibility to extraneous information in patients with frontal lobe lesions. Three study-test learning trials of a list of 12 paired-associates (e.g., "thief–crime;" "lion–hunter") were presented. Memory was tested by presenting the first word in each pair and asking subjects to report the second word (e.g., "thief–?"). For the initial list, performance by patients with frontal lobe lesions was not different from that of control subjects. Subjects were then presented a second list in which the same cue words were paired with different target words (e.g., "thief–bandit;" "lion–cir-cus"). On this second set, patients with frontal lobe lesions exhibited significant impairment (see Fig. 13–4). Moreover, they made many intrusion errors, using words from the first set during testing of the second set. Thus, patients with frontal lobe lesions incurred impairment when memory retrieval required the executive control of recent associations, such as updating recent associations and inhibiting prior ones. The importance of the prefrontal cortex in mitigating interference effects has also been demonstrated in a similar fMRI study (Dolan & Fletcher, 1997).

Early neuropsychological studies of source recollection implicated the importance of the frontal lobe in this aspect of episodic memory (Schacter et al., 1984; Shimamura & Squire, 1987; Janowsky et al., 1989b). That is, patients with frontal lobe lesions exhibit particular impairment in remembering details of a learning event, such as where and when some information was presented (Janowsky et al., 1989b). Such findings have been associated with disorders in memory for temporal order (Shimamura et al., 1990; Milner et al., 1991; Mangels, 1997). In neuroimaging studies, the left prefrontal cortex is particularly active during retrieval of source information (Nolde et al., 1998; Rugg et al., 1999; Ranganath et al., 2000).

From findings of source memory, it is rea-

sonable to suggest that the frontal lobes contribute specifically to the encoding and representation of temporal information. Such a view would be consistent with the general role of the prefrontal cortex in episodic memory. That is, a failure to store temporal information, such as a time tag to stimulus events, would significantly affect episodic memory. Yet, according to the dynamic filtering theory, the prefrontal cortex does not directly represent or store any specific form of memory, such as a temporal tag or other time-based forms of episodic memory. Instead, the prefrontal cortex is presumed to be involved in the on-line control of memory activations. Efficient monitoring and control facilitate the processing of memory activations both at the time of encoding and retrieval.

To the extent that the prefrontal cortex is involved in the control of source information, rather than in the actual storage of such information, it is necessary to demonstrate that source recollection happens to place particular demands on executive control. That is, selecting, maintaining, updating, and rerouting information must be particularly important for retrieval of specific details of one's past experiences (such as remembering the order of events or who presented some information). McAndrews and Milner (1991) addressed this issue by using a task that facilitated executive control in patients with frontal lobe lesions.

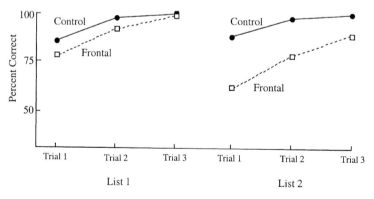

Figure 13–4. Control subjects and patients with frontal lobe lesions were administered memory tests in which they were presented word pairs (e.g., "lion–hunter") and then tested for the second word when cued with the first (e.g., "lion–?"). The two groups performed similarly on the first list. However, patients performed poorly when given a second set of word pairs involving the same cue words but different response words (e.g., "lion-circus"). Findings suggest that the patients with frontal lobe lesions were particularly susceptible to interference from prior associations. (*Source:* Data from Shimamura et al., 1995)

Subjects were presented objects and were asked to perform an action with each one (e.g., bounce the ball). This manipulation was presumed to increase sensorimotor activation during encoding and thereby increase the distinctiveness of stimuli. Memory for temporal order was assessed by presenting pairs of objects on test trials and asking subjects to determine which of the two were presented more recently. Performance by patients with frontal lobe lesions did not differ from performance by control subjects on tests of temporal order when study objects were manipulated. However, the patients exhibited significant impairment on a control task in which they were presented the objects but did not manipulate them. This benefit appeared to be rather selective to patients with frontal lobe lesions because performance by amnesic patients with temporal lobe lesions was not facilitated by the manipulation condition. These findings suggest that frontal lobe function is more associated with attentional processes than with processes associated specifically with memory for temporal order.

Executive control was manipulated during encoding in a study of source memory (Jurica & Shimamura, 1999). In that study, the task involved a simulated social conversation in which subjects "conversed" with various "people" (i.e., faces on a computer screen). During a study phase, subjects were asked questions ("Where do you think the most scenic spot in California is located?") or read statements ("Bicycles are a common means of transportation these days") presented by one of three sources (faces). Questions were used to focus attention on the conceptual information by having subjects generate an answer. The facilitation of memory for items that are generated is a well-known phenomenon and is called the *generation effect*. Jurica and Shimamura (1999) wondered whether a generation effect for item information would extend to a facilitation of source memory.

A rather surprising effect was observed. Although topics presented as questions were remembered better than topics presented as statements (i.e., the standard generation effect), a *negative* generation effect was observed for source memory. Whereas subjects were better able to remember the content of information presented as a question, they were less able to remember who asked the question. Thus, source memory for items presented as questions was poorer than source memory for items presented as statements. These findings suggest a tradeoff of attentional control for item and source information; directing attentional control to item information reduced encoding of source information. With respect to patients with frontal lobe lesions, such patients may have only enough attentional control (i.e., selecting, maintaining, updating) to implement encoding of item information. This interpretation would explain why such patients often perform well on item memory but fail to remember source information.

Another study suggests that executive control during the time of retrieval can also hamper source recollection (Dodson & Shimamura, 2000). Subjects were presented words spoken in one of two voices (female or male voice). Typically, subjects are tested by presenting a word visually (without any voice) and asking them to determine whether the word had been originally presented by a male or female voice. Dodson and Shimamura (2000) modified this standard paradigm by presenting test words spoken by irrelevant voices. These test voices had been used during the study phase and either matched or mismatched the original voice used to present a word. The voices at test were presented as a way to introduce extraneous information during source recollection. For this test, efficient source recollection depended on successful filtering of the test voice. The results demonstrated a significant impairment of source recollection when a mismatched voice was used to present a test item. Interestingly, item memory, as measured by old/new recognition performance, was not affected by presenting matched or mismatched voices during the test phase.

Taken together, these findings suggest that episodic retrieval and source recollection are associated with frontal lobe function. Moreover, the role of the prefrontal cortex in such retrieval tasks appears to be related to on-line control of memory activations. That is, extraneous information at the time of recollection can significantly interfere with episodic retrieval and source recollection. Indeed, such interference effects appear more significant for source recollection than for the recollection of item information. Boosting or supporting executive control can improve source memory performance in patients with frontal lobe lesions (McAndrews & Milner 1991). According to the dynamic filtering theory, the prefrontal cortex facilitates executive control of episodic memories by monitoring and controlling activation in working memory. The prefrontal cortex does not house or represent specific knowledge about episodic memory. Indeed, episodic memory, like semantic knowledge, is presumed to be represented in widely distributed networks involving many regions within posterior cortex.

CONCLUSION

The dynamic filtering theory offers a useful framework within which to conceptualize the role of prefrontal cortex in executive control. With respect to memory retrieval, strategic searches of either semantic or episodic memory place heavy demands on selecting, maintaining, updating, and rerouting information processing. It is likely that different regions within the prefrontal cortex are associated with different aspects of executive control. That is, rerouting may activate different (and perhaps more) prefrontal regions than selecting or maintaining. It is also likely that different prefrontal regions control different aspects of memory. Thus, control of semantic representations will likely involve prefrontal regions that are different from those involved in control of episodic representations. Currently, it is unclear what the contributions of specific prefrontal regions are in the service of memory retrieval. Importantly, it is likely that prefrontal areas involved in the control of memory retrieval are also involved in other cognitive tasks that place heavy demands on aspects of memory control (problem solving, conceptual analysis). Clearly, further advances in functional neuroimaging will strengthen our understanding of regional specificity within the prefrontal cortex in the service of memory retrieval and executive control.

REFERENCES

Albert, M.S., Butters, N., & Levin, J. (1979). Temporal gradients in the retrograde amnesia of patients with alcoholic Korsakoff's disease. *Archives of Neurology, 36*, 211–216.

Baddeley, A. (1986). *Working Memory.* Oxford: Oxford University Press.

Baldo, J.V. & Shimamura, A.P. (1998). Letter and category fluency in patients with frontal lobe lesions. *Neuropsychology, 12*, 259–226.

Baldo, J.V. & Shimamura, A.P. (2000). Spatial and color working memory in patients with lateral prefrontal cortex lesions. *Psychobiology, 28*, 156–167.

Baldo, J.V., Shimamura, A.P., & Delis, D. (2001). Design and verbal fluency in patients with frontal lobe lesions: effects of task switching. *Journal of the International Neuropsychological Society, 7*, 586–596.

Benton, A. & de Hamsher, K. (1976). *Multilingual Aphasia Examination.* Iowa City: University of Iowa Press.

Buckner, R.L. & Petersen, S.E. (1996). What does neuroimaging tell us about the role of prefrontal cortex in memory retrieval? *Seminars in Neuroscience, 8*, 47–55.

Buckner, R.L., Koutstaal, W., Schacter, D.L., Wagner, A.D., & Rosen, B.R. (1998). Functional-anatomic study of episodic retrieval using fMRI: I. Retrieval effort versus retrieval success. *NeuroImage, 7*, 151–162.

Chan, A.S., Butters, N., Paulsen, J.S., Salmon, D.P., Swenson, M.R., & Maloney, L.T. (1993). An assessment of the semantic network in patients with Alzheimer's disease. *Journal of Cognitive Neuroscience, 5*, 254–261.

D'Esposito, M., Aguirre, G.K., Zarahn, E., & Ballard, D. (1998). Functional MRI studies of spatial and nonspatial working memory. *Cognitive Brain Research, 7*, 1–13.

Dodson, C.S. & Shimamura, A.P. (2000). Differential effects of cue dependency on item and source memory. *Journal of Experimental Psychology: Learning, Memory, and Cognition, 26*, 1023–1944.

Dolan, R.J. & Fletcher, P.C. (1997). Dissociating prefrontal and hippocampal function in episodic memory encoding. *Nature, 388*, 582–585.

Frith, C., Friston, K., Liddle, P., & Frackowiak, D. (1991). A PET study of word finding. *Neuropsychologia, 29*, 1137–1148.

Gabrieli, J.D., Desmond, J.E., Demb, J.B., Wagner, A.D., Stone, M.V., Vaidya, C.J., & Glover, G.H. (1996). Functional magnetic resonance imaging of semantic memory processes in the frontal lobes. *Psychological Science, 7*, 278–283.

Gershberg, F.B. & Shimamura, A.P. (1995). The role of the frontal lobes in the use of organizational strategies in free recall, *Neuropsychologia, 13*, 1305–1333.

Gershberg, F.B. & Shimamura, A.P. (1998). The neuro-psychology of learning and memory in humans. In: J.L. Martinez, Jr. & R.P. Kesner (Eds.), *Learning and Memory: A Biological Perspective* (pp. 333–359). New York: Academic Press.

Henson, R.N.A., Shallice, T., & Dolan, R.J. (1999). Right prefrontal cortex and episodic memory retrieval: a functional MRI test of the monitoring hypothesis. *Brain, 122,* 1367–1381.

Hirst, W. & Volpe, B.T. (1988). Memory strategies with brain damage. *Brain and Cognition, 8,* 379–408.

Janowsky, J.S., Shimamura, A.P., Kritchevsky, M., & Squire, L.R. (1989a). Cognitive impairment following frontal lobe damage and its relevance to human amnesia. *Behavioral Neuroscience, 103,* 548–560.

Janowsky, J.S., Shimamura, A.P., & Squire, L.R. (1989b). Source memory impairment in patients with frontal lobe lesions. *Neuropsychologia, 27,* 1043–1056.

Johnson, M.K., Hashtroudi, S., & Lindsay, D.S. (1993). Source monitoring. *Psychological Bulletin, 114,* 3–28.

Jones-Gotman, M. & Milner, B. (1977). Design fluency: the invention of nonsense drawings after focal cortical lesion. *Neuropsychologia, 15,* 653–674.

Jurica, P.J. & Shimamura, A.P. (1999). Monitoring item and source information: evidence for a negative generation effect in source memory. *Memory and Cognition, 27,* 648–656.

Kapur, S., Craik, F.I.M., Jones, C., Brown, G.M., Houle, S., & Tulving, E. (1995). Functional role of the prefrontal cortex in retrieval of memories: a PET study. *NeuroReport, 6,* 1880–1884.

Knight, R.T., Staines, W.R., Swick, D., & Chao, L.L. (1999). Prefrontal cortex regulates inhibition and excitation in distributed neural networks. *Acta Psychologia, 101,* 159–178.

Mangels, J.A. (1997). Strategic processing and memory for temporal order in patients with frontal lobe lesions. *Neuropsychology, 11,* 207–221.

Mangels, J.A., Gershberg, F.B., Shimamura, A.P., & Knight, R.T. (1996). Impaired retrieval from remote memory in patients with frontal lobe lesions, *Neuropsychology, 10,* 32–41.

McAndrews, M.P. & Milner, B. (1991). The frontal cortex and memory for temporal order. *Neuropsychologia, 29,* 849–859.

Milner, B. (1964). Some effects of frontal lobectomy in man. In: J. Warren & K. Akert (Eds.), *The Frontal Granular Cortex and Behavior* (pp. 313–331). New York: McGraw-Hill.

Milner, B., Corsi, P., & Leonard, G. (1991). Frontal-lobe contribution to recency judgements. *Neuropsychologia, 29,* 601–618.

Moscovitch, M. (1992). Memory and working-with-memory: a component process model based on modules and central systems. *Journal of Cognitive Neuroscience, 4,* 257–267.

Nolde, S.F., Johnson, M.K., & D'Esposito, M. (1998). Left prefrontal activation during episodic remembering: an event-related fMRI study. *NeuroReport, 9,* 3509–3514.

Petrides, M. (1998). Specialized systems for the process-ing of mnemonic information within the primate frontal cortex. In: A.C. Roberts, T.W. Robbins, & L. Weiskrantz (Eds.), *The Prefrontal Cortex: Executive and Cognitive Function* (pp. 103–116). Oxford: Oxford University Press.

Ranganath, C., Johnson, M.K., & D'Esposito, M. (2000). Left anterior prefrontal activation increases with demands to recall specific perceptual information. *Journal of Neuroscience, 20* (RC108), 1–5.

Rugg, M.D., Fletcher, P.C., Frith, C.D., Frackowiak, R.S. & R.J. Dolan (1996). Differential activation of the prefrontal cortex in successful and unsuccessful memory retrieval. *Brain, 19,* 2073–2083.

Rugg, M.D., Fletcher, P.C., Chua, P.M., & Dolan, R.J. (1999). The role of the prefrontal cortex in recognition memory and memory for source: an fMRI study. *NeuroImage, 10,* 520–529.

Schacter, D.L., Harbluck, J., & McLaughlin, D. (1984). Retrieval without recollection: An experimental analysis of source amnesia. *Journal of Verbal Learning and Verbal Behavior, 23,* 593–611.

Shallice, T. & Burgess, P. (1998). The domain of supervisory processes and temporal organization of behaviour. In: A.C. Roberts, T.W. Robbins, & L. Weiskrantz (Eds.), *The Prefrontal Cortex: Executive and Cognitive Functions* (pp. 22–35). New York: Oxford University Press.

Shimamura, A.P. (1995). Memory and frontal lobe function. In: M.S. Gazzaniga (Ed.), *The Cognitive Neurosciences* (pp. 803–813). Cambridge, MA: MIT Press.

Shimamura, A.P. (1996). The control and monitoring of memory functions. In: L. Reder (Ed.), *Metacognition and Implicit Memory* (pp. 259–274). Mahwah, NJ: Lawrence Erlbaum Associates.

Shimamura, A.P. (2000). The role of the prefrontal cortex in dynamic filtering. *Psychobiology, 28,* 207–218.

Shimamura, A.P. & Squire, L.R. (1987). A neuropsychological study of fact memory and source amnesia. *Journal of Experimental Psychology: Learning, Memory, and Cognition, 13,* 464–473.

Shimamura, A.P., Janowsky, J.S. & Squire, L.R. (1990). Memory for the temporal order of events in patients with frontal lobe lesions and amnesic patients. *Neuropsychologia, 28,* 803–813.

Shimamura, A.P., Jurica, P.J., Mangels, J.A., Gershberg, F.B., & Knight, R.T. (1995). Susceptibility to memory interference effects following frontal lobe damage: findings from tests of paired-associate learning, *Journal of Cognitive Neuroscience, 7,* 144–152.

Smith, E.E. & Jonides, J. (1999). Storage and executive processes in the frontal lobes. *Science, 283,* 1657–1661.

Squire, L.R. & Knowlton, B.J. (2000). The medial temporal lobe, the hippocampus, and the memory systems of the brain. In: M.S. Gazzaniga (Ed.) *The New Cognitive Neurosciences,* 2nd ed. (pp. 765–779). Cambridge, MA: MIT Press.

Squire, L.R., Haist, F., & Shimamura, A.P. (1989). The neurology of memory: quantitative assessment of retrograde amnesia in two groups of amnesic patients. *Journal of Neuroscience, 9,* 828–839.

Stuss, D.T., Alexander, M.P., Palumbo, C.L., Buckle, L., Sayer, L., & Pogue, J. (1994). Organizational strategies of patients with unilateral or bilateral frontal lobe injury in word list learning tasks. *Neuropsychology 8,* 355–373.

Sylvester, C.Y. & Shimamura, A.P. in Press Intact semantic representations in patients with frontal lobe lesions. *Neuropsychology.*

Thompson-Schill, S.L., Swick, D., Farah, M.J., D'Esposito, M., Kan, I.P., & Knight, R.T. (1998). Verb generation in patients with focal frontal lesions: a neuropsychological test of neuroimaging findings. *Proceedings of the National Academy of Sciences USA, 95,* 15855–15860.

Tulving, E. (1983). *Elements of Episodic Memory.* Oxford: Clarendon Press.

Tulving, E. & Lepage, M. (2000). Where in the brain is the awareness of one's past? In: D.L. Schacter & E. Scarry (Eds.), *Memory, Brain, and Belief* (pp. 208–228). Cambridge, MA: Harvard University Press.

Wheeler, M.A., Stuss, D.T., & Tulving, E. (1995). Frontal lobe damage produces episodic memory impairment. *Journal of the International Neuropsychological Society, 1,* 525–536.

14

Dorsal Prefrontal Cortex: Maintenance in Memory or Attentional Selection?

RICHARD E. PASSINGHAM AND JAMES B. ROWE

It has long been known that monkeys with prefrontal lesions are unable to perform a simple memory task (Jacobsen, 1935). All that they are required to do is to remember the location of a peanut for a few seconds. It was later demonstrated that the critical region is the principal sulcus (Mishkin, 1957). More specifically, a focal lesion in the middle third of this sulcus alone is sufficient to cause the impairment (Butters & Pandya, 1969). The middle and anterior third correspond to area 46, whereas the posterior third includes area 8A, and a transitional area for which Petrides and Pandya (1995) suggest the term 9/46.

It was natural to suppose that the problem was that the monkeys could not remember what they had seen. And this hypothesis was strengthened when it was discovered that there were cells in sulcus principalis (area 46) that continued to fire during the delay period (Fuster & Alexander, 1971; Niki, 1974; Koshima & Goldman-Rakic, 1984; Funahashi et al., 1989). This view was formalized as the working memory hypothesis by Goldman-Rakic (1987). The suggestion is that the dorsal prefrontal cortex maintains information during the delay. This hypothesis has been of enormous influence in the field, and has proved to be very fruitful in generating important experiments. Studies using functional brain im-

aging have been much influenced by the working memory hypothesis, and there are now several functional magnetic resonance imaging (fMRI) studies showing prefrontal activity during the delay on complex working memory tasks (Cohen et al., 1997; Courtney et al., 1997; Postle et al., 1999).

However, there are results that are not easy to explain through this view. For example, many imaging studies have shown that there is activation in the anterior middle frontal gyrus (area 46) when human subjects freely select among movements (Deiber et al., 1991; Frith et al., 1991; Hyder et al., 1997; Jueptner et al., 1997). The subjects are required to make movements to pacing cues, and to choose freely on each trial which movement to make. One possibility is that on such 'free-selection' tasks the subjects remember the last few moves, and that they vary their current moves accordingly. But rapid rate transcranial magnetic stimulation (TMS) over the left dorsal prefrontal cortex delays freely selected responses even when there is no memory load; whereas stimulation has no effect on responses to external stimuli (Hadland et al., 2001). This suggests that this area plays a genuine role in selection.

We have therefore directly compared the effects of maintenance of items in memory and the selection of them. We have used a task in which the subjects were required to maintain spatial cues during a delay period, but could neither prepare their response nor manipulate the information in memory during the delay (Rowe et al., 2000). In previous studies using the N-back task, such as that by Cohen et al. (1997), the subjects could update the list of items during the delay, rejecting items in memory that were no longer relevant. On our task the subjects were not required to do this. We used event-related fMRI to chart activity, and decorrelated activity during the delay with activity at the time of response by varying the length of the delays. This method was introduced in a functional imaging study by Toni et al. (1999).

MAINTAINING SPATIAL LOCATIONS VERSUS SELECTING BETWEEN LOCATIONS

The task is illustrated in Figure 14–1. During working memory trials, the subjects saw three red dots presented briefly in random locations (solid circles). There followed a variable delay of 9.5 to 18.5 seconds, during which the subjects were instructed to remember exactly the location of the dots. In the figure the locations in memory are indicated by dotted circles; these were not actually presented to subjects. A line then appeared briefly across the screen, running through the location of just one of the dots. This indicated which of the remembered dots was the target for response, without specifying the location directly. The line was then replaced by a central cursor identical in appearance to the dots and the subjects moved the cursor to the remembered target location using a joystick. This ended the trial. Thus, during the delay the subjects maintained the items in memory, but were not able to prepare their response. The subjects could only select the appropriate remembered location at the end of the working memory delay. Overall, 218/253 (86%) responses were made to the correct target location.

The visual and motor components of the control task were similar to those of memory

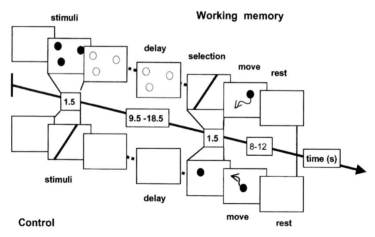

Figure 14–1. Schematic representation of the first spatial working memory task and control task. For a memory trial, the subjects saw three red dots presented simultaneously for 1.5 seconds on a screen, in random locations (solid circles). There followed a delay of 9.5 to 18.5 seconds (in steps of 1 seconds, randomly ordered), during which the subjects remembered the exact location of the dots. A line then appeared for 1.5 seconds across the screen, running through the location of just one of the previous red dots. This indicated which of the remembered dots now became the target for response, *without specifying the location* directly. The line was then replaced by a central cursor identical in appearance to the red dots. The subjects moved the cursor to the remembered target location using a joystick. After the response, the trial ended and was followed by a rest period of 8–12 seconds. For control trials the visual and motor components of the task were similar to those of memory trials, but the stimuli were presented in reverse order such that there were no spatial cues to remember during the prolonged delay (nominal "non-memory" period). The target for the cursor response in the control trials was the location of the single red dot, with no intervening delay.

trials, but the stimuli were presented in reverse order, so that there were no spatial cues to remember during the delay. In the analysis this formed the nominal "non-memory" period. The target for the cursor response in the control trials was the location of the single dot, with no intervening delay. Statistical parametric mapping was used to identify brain regions that were activated by maintenance of the spatial location in memory, by the selection of a location from memory, or both (P < 0.05 corrected for multiple comparisons).

We were able to dissociate the regions in which the activation was associated with the sustained maintenance of items from those in which the activation was transient and associated with the selection of an item from within memory. Relative to the equivalent non-memory periods on control trials, maintenance in working memory on the experimental trials was associated with bilateral activation in prefrontal area 8 (Fig. 14–2A) and the intraparietal cortex, but not in the anterior middle frontal gyrus (area 46). Reducing the significance level (0.001 uncorrected) revealed activations posteriorly in the superior frontal sulcus and in the inferior frontal gyrus. Figure 14–2B shows the time course of activity during the working memory trials as best fitted to the data for each length of memory delay. In frontal area 8 there were sustained increases in (the blood oxygen level–dependent (BOLD) signal throughout the course of the working memory delay, seen as a plateau for which the length was in direct proportion to the duration of the maintenance delay (Fig. 14–2B). Activation dorsally and anterior to the frontal eye fields has been reported in previous studies of spatial working memory (Belger et al., 1998; Courtney et al., 1998; Owen et al., 1999).

The selection of the target location from memory was associated with activations of the right anterior middle frontal gyrus (area 46) (Fig. 14–3A) and the tissue immediately posterior to it, but not in area 8 itself. There were additional activations in the right ventral and orbital frontal cortex, as well as in the posterior intraparietal cortex and medial parietal cortex. The time course of activity is presented in Figure 14–3B for working memory trials as best fitted by the model. Associated with the selection event there was a transient increase in the BOLD signal in the anterior middle frontal gyrus (area 46). From Figure 14–3B it can be seen that for this peak there was no

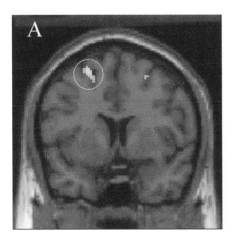

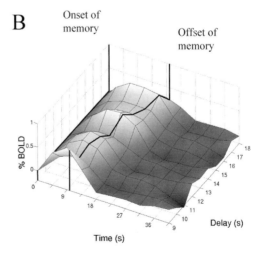

Figure 14–2. *A:* Voxels in left area 8 were significantly more active during working memory delay periods than during the non-memory delay periods in control trials (*t* > 4.91, P < 0.05), shown here superimposed on a coronal slice from a representative T1 image in standard anatomic space. *B:* The fitted data from the voxels in right area 8 have been temporally realigned to the onset of working memory trials, and are shown as changes in blood oxygen level–dependent (BOLD) signal (*z*-axis) over time (*x*-axis) for each delay length of working memory (*y*-axis). The gray scale indicates the relative change in BOLD signal from the start of each trial. The plots demonstrate the sustained activity that lasts as long as the working memory delay.

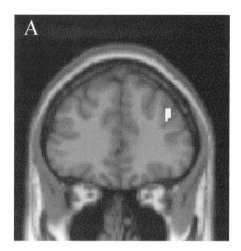

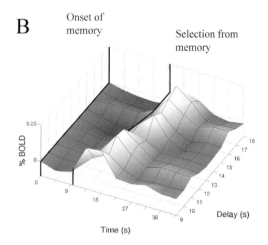

Figure 14–3. *A:* Voxels in prefrontal area 46 were significantly activated by selection from memory, shown here superimposed on a coronal slice from a representative T1 image in standard anatomic space. *B:* The fitted data from these voxels have been temporally realigned to the onset of working memory trials that preceded selection, and are shown as changes in blood oxygen level–dependent (BOLD) signal (*z*-axis) over time (*x*-axis) for each delay length of working memory (y-axis). The thick black line indicates the offset of the working memory delays, and the gray scale indicates the relative change in BOLD signal from the start of each trial. In this area, there is no activation during the working memory interval, but a peak of activation following selection of the item at the end of the memory period.

sustained activity here associated with the maintenance of the locations during the memory delay. In summary, the prefrontal activation associated with the maintenance of the locations in memory lay posteriorly (area 8A), and the activation associated with selection between the locations in memory lay anteriorly (area 46).

MAINTAINING THE ORDER OF PRESENTATION VERSUS SELECTING

It could be argued that this experiment did not make sufficient demands on working memory. In the N-back task, for example, there is the extra demand to maintain the order in which the items were presented. In a second experiment we therefore modified the procedure so as to require the subjects to remember the order in which three locations were presented (Rowe & Passingham, 2001). The task is shown in Figure 14–4. On all trials three dots were presented in order and during the delay the subjects remembered both the locations and the order. On half the trials, a

number was presented at the end of the delay, and the subjects moved the cursor to the location of the dot at that point in the sequence. On the other half of trials, an X was presented and the subjects had to simply move the cursor to the location of the X. The increase in the number of memory trials had the advantage that we could plot the actual (adjusted) rather than just the fitted data.

As in the previous experiment, there were regions of brain activation associated with sustained maintenance of items rather than selection among items. Relative to the intertrial interval as baseline, the maintenance of items was associated with the bilateral activation of prefrontal area 8 (Fig. 14–5A) and intraparietal cortex, but not of the anterior middle frontal gyrus (area 46). Figure 14–5B shows that in prefrontal area 8 there were sustained increases in activity throughout the course of the working memory delay, seen as a plateau, the length being in direct proportion to the duration of the maintenance delay.

As in the previous experiment (Rowe et al., 2000), the selection of the target location from memory was associated with activations of an-

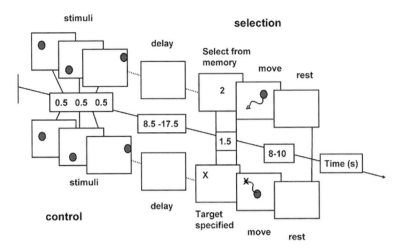

Figure 14–4. Schematic representation of the second working memory task. In all trials, the subjects saw three red dots presented sequentially for 0.5 seconds each on a screen, in random locations (solid circles). There followed a delay of 8.5 to 17.5 seconds (in steps of 1 seconds, randomly ordered), during which the subjects remembered the exact location of the dots and their temporal order. In selection trials, a number, 1, 2, or 3, then appeared for 1.5 seconds centrally. This indicated whether the first, second, or third dot now became the target for response, without specifying the location. The number was then replaced by a central cursor identical in appearance to the red dots. The subjects moved the cursor to the remembered target location using a joystick. After the response, the trial ended and was followed by a rest period of 8–12 seconds. For control trials the working memory period was identical to selection trials, but the target for the cursor response was indicated by a cross, and subjects did not select the location for response from memory.

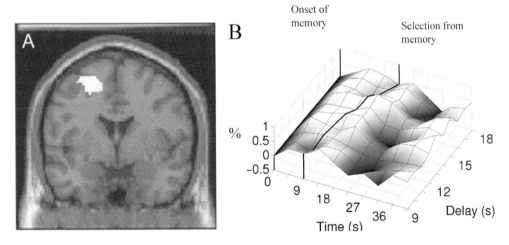

Figure 14–5. *A:* Voxels in area 8 were significantly more active during working memory delays than baseline ($t >$ 4.91, $P < 0.05$), shown here superimposed on a coronal slice from a representative T1 image in standard anatomic space. *B:* The blood oxygen level–dependent (BOLD) data (bandpass filtered) from the peak voxel in right area 8 have been temporally realigned to the onset of working memory trials, and are shown as changes in BOLD signal (z-axis) over time (x-axis) for each delay length of working memory (y-axis). The gray scale indicates the relative change in BOLD signal from the start of each trial. It can be seen that maintenance of the dots' positions and order is associated with sustained activation, which lasts as long as the delay period.

terior middle frontal gyrus (area 46); in this experiment the activation was bilateral (Fig.14–6A). The activity also extended posteriorly along the middle frontal gyrus into the transitional area 9/46. There was additional activation of the orbital frontal cortex and the anterior cingulate cortex. Finally, there was bilateral activation of the intraparietal and medial parietal cortex. There was some overlap in the prefrontal and parietal cortex between areas associated with selection and areas associated with maintenance. However, Figure 14–6B shows that in the anterior middle frontal gyrus (area 46) there was no significant activity associated with maintenance. Thus, the activations are more widespread when the subjects are required to remember the order in which locations were presented rather than the locations alone, but the pattern is similar.

COMPARISON WITH OTHER DATA

At first sight these results appear not to agree with those from single-unit recording. Many electrophysiological studies report activity in sulcus principalis during the delay (Fuster & Alexander, 1971; Niki, 1974; Koshima & Goldman-Rakic, 1984; Funahashi et al., 1989). However, a proper comparison of the data requires that the tasks be similar. In our first

experiment (Rowe et al., 2000), we compared activity during a delay when the subjects had to maintain items with a delay during which they did not. Koshima and Goldman-Rakic (1984) also did this with monkeys, and only 19% of the cells fired differentially in the two delay periods. Secondly, we ensured that the subjects could not prepare a response during the delay period so that we could isolate activity related only to the maintenance of items in memory. This was also done by Sawaguchi and Yamane (1999), and the cell activity related to maintenance was found in area 8A, as in the present experiments. Indeed, most of the cells that fire during the delay on spatial delayed-response tasks are to be found in the posterior third of sulcus principalis (area 8A) and the convexity of area 8 (Funahashi et al., 1989; Chafee & Goldman-Rakic, 1998). Thus, when the imaging and electrophysiological results are examined in detail, they can be seen to be less discrepant.

It could still be argued that our results do not agree with those from other recent imaging experiments. Activity in areas 9 and 46 has been reported previously during delay periods in working memory studies of spatial (Postle et al., 1999), visual (Courtney et al., 1997) and verbal material (D'Esposito et al., 1999; 2000; Postle et al., 1999; Rypma and D'Esposito, 1999, 2000), even when there was no demand

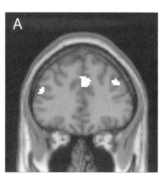
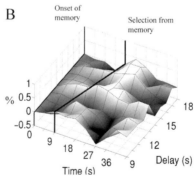

Figure 14–6. *A:* Voxels in prefrontal area 46 were significantly more active during selection from memory than during the externally specified target ($t > 4.91$, $P < 0.05$), shown here superimposed on a coronal slice from a representative T1 image in standard anatomic space. *B:* The blood oxygen level–dependent (BOLD) data (bandpass filtered) from the peak voxel in area 46 have been temporally realigned to the onset of working memory trials that preceded selection, and are shown as changes in BOLD signal (z-axis) over time (x-axis) for each delay length of working memory (y-axis). The gray scale indicates the relative change in BOLD signal from the start of each trial. The thick black line indicates the time of selection from memory.

for manipulation of the items in memory. There may be several reasons for the apparent difference in results. First, we used a spatial task, and in a recent single-unit study (Hoshi et al., 2000) there was suggestive evidence that spatial material was maintained more posteriorly than visual material. But Postle et al. (1999) also used a spatial task. A second possibility is that the methods we used are not as sensitive as those used in that study (Postle et al., 1999; Zarahn et al., 1999;). However, even if this were so, and sensitive methods can detect some activation in area 46 related to the maintenance of spatial items, our findings clearly show that activation in this region is *dominated* by the requirement for selection. Using verbal material, Rypma and D'Esposito (1999) also found that in dorsal prefrontal cortex the activity at the time of the response was much greater than the activity during the delay period.

There is another possibility. In the study by Courtney et al. (1997) the subjects were specifically instructed to actively rehearse the visual material (faces) during the delay. Furthermore, when subjects remember verbal material (letters or digits), as in the studies by D'Esposito and colleagues (D'Esposito et al., 1999, 2000; Postle et al., 1999; Rypma and D'Esposito, 1999, 2000), they do so by a process of covert articulation (Baddeley 1986; Paulesu et al., 1993). In our study, the subjects were not instructed to actively rehearse the spatial items during the delay. It is possible that the mechanisms for the continuous rehearsal of items are related to the mechanisms for active retrieval.

ATTENTIONAL SELECTION

In previous studies we have proposed that area 46 is only activated when working memory tasks require the "attentional selection" between items within memory (Rowe et al., 2000; Rowe & Passingham, 2001). Consider three tasks. First, on the N-back task the subjects must use the N-back rule to select between the items in recent memory, and must update the list of items in memory, retaining some and dropping others. Second, on the

"self-ordered" task (Petrides et al., 1993), the subjects make a series of responses, obeying the rule that they must not make the same response more than once. On each trial they must select items from the list of possible responses. Finally, on tasks requiring the "manipulation" of items in memory (D'Esposito et al., 1999; Owen et al., 1999), the subjects are required to produce them in an order that differs from the order in which they were presented. Here the re-ordering requires the subject to select out items so as to arrive at the new order.

The term *attentional selection* has two advantages over alternative proposals. The first is that it can be applied to the performance of monkeys on the delayed response task. The proposal that area 46 is critical for the manipulation of items in memory (Owen et al., 1996; D'Esposito et al., 2000) cannot be extended to the performance of monkeys on delayed-response tasks in which no such manipulation is required. The alternative proposal by Petrides (1998) is that area 46 is crucial for monitoring items in memory. By this he means that "each selection must be marked in the subject's mind." It is clear that this formulation is very close to that of attentional selection. We prefer the terminology of *attentional selection* because it makes the direct link between the selection between items on memory tasks and the free selection of actions. As already noted, area 46 is activated when subjects are required to freely select among actions such as finger movements (Frith et al., 1991; Jueptner et al., 1997).

To further strengthen this link, we have recently used fMRI to image the prefrontal cortex while subjects are required to selectively attend to their fingers. In the control condition the subjects were required to make sequential finger movements in a simple overlearned sequence (1, 2, 3, 4, 1, 2, 3, 4); the movements were paced at one every 3 seconds. In the experimental condition the subjects were required to perform the same sequence of movements, but to attend to each finger in turn. The instruction was to "think about the next move." Figure 14–7 shows that when a comparison was made between the attended and non-attended condition there was activa-

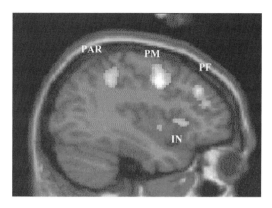

Figure 14–7. The prefrontal area 46 (PAR), dorsal premotor cortex, (PM), and intraparietal cortex (IN) were more activated when the subjects specifically attended to action than when the subjects performed the simple motor sequence alone. The SPM {*t*} for this contrast is shown at P < 0.001 (uncorrected) superimposed on a left parasaggital section from a representative T1 image in standard anatomic space. The dorsal activations were all significant (P < 0.05 corrected) within prespecified regions of interest.

tion in prefrontal area 46. We suggest that on a free-selection task the subjects select among fingers by temporarily attending to the relevant finger or key.

CONCLUSION

The evidence that we have reviewed suggests an alternative reason why monkeys with lesions in the middle of sulcus principalis (area 46) fail delayed-response tasks: they may fail, not because they do not remember what they have seen, but because they are impaired at selecting among items in memory. It has been shown that there is interference among trials on delayed-response tasks (Mishkin & Delacour, 1975). The monkey sees each side baited several times, and on any particular trial must select the side that has been baited *most recently*. As on the N-back task, the cues are tagged by the time at which they are presented. Diamond and Goldman-Rakic (1989) have shown that monkeys with dorsal prefrontal lesions make errors when they must choose the side opposite the one that was baited on the previous trial. On such trials they fail to

choose the location that was most recently presented.

While it is true that there are many cells in this sulcus that are active during the delay period, most of these are in the posterior third of the sulcus (area 8A) (Funahashi et al., 1989; Chafee & Goldman-Rakic 1998; Sawaguchi & Yamane, 1999). Yet permanent (Butters & Pandya, 1969) or temporary lesions (Hoshi et al., 2000) in the posterior third have little effect on performance. It is lesions in the middle third of the sulcus (area 46) that lead to a severe impairment (Butters & Pandya, 1969; Hoshi et al., 2000). The data presented in this chapter suggest that the impairment on delayed response may occur at the stage of response selection.

INVITED COMMENTARY

In Chapter 5, Goldman-Rakic and Leung comment on the data presented in this chapter. The following comments have been added so as to clarify the differences between the position outlined in this chapter and in Chapter 5.

POSTERIOR PREFRONTAL CORTEX AND THE INTRA-PARIETAL CORTEX

We have reported activation posteriorly in prefrontal cortex when subjects perform spatial working memory tasks (Rowe et al., 2000; Rowe & Passingham, 2001), whereas Goldman-Rakic and Leung (Chapter 5) have not. It appears from Figure 5–4 that there was posterior activation in frontal cortex: presumably Goldman-Rakic and Leung attributed this to premotor area 6, whereas others (Belger et al., 1998, Courtney et al., 1998, Rowe et al., 2000; Rowe & Passingham, 2001) have attributed it to posterior prefrontal cortex. The activity in the study by Rowe and Passingham (2001) probably extends into the transitional area 9/46 identified in the recent cytoarchitectonic analysis by Petrides (1999). Chafee and Goldman-Rakic (1998) refer to this area as 8A, and this is where they recorded delay-related activity. In their chapter Goldman-Rakic and Leung point to the older cytoarchitectonic classification of Walker (1940) who included this transitional region in area 46.

Goldman-Rakic and Leung (Chapter 5) question whether the activity in this region is mnemonic. They cite the paper by Goldman et al. (1971) in which lesions of area 8 produced a lesser effect on spatial delayed response than lesions of sulcus principalis. In the companion paper (Goldman & Rosvold, 1970) animals with lesions of the arcuate cortex were impaired on spatial delayed alternation compared with animals with premotor lesions, and one animal failed to learn within the limits of testing. Chafee and Goldman-Rakic (1998) recorded similar delay-related activity in both area 8A and the intra-parietal sulcus. It is possible that only a combined lesion of the intra-parietal cortex and area 8 would consistently cause a severe impairment.

AREA 46

The critical issue raised by Goldman-Rakic and Leung (Chapter 5) is why they found delay-related activity more anteriorly in the human middle frontal gyrus, whereas we failed to do so (Rowe et al., 2000; Rowe & Passingham, 2001). Goldman-Rakic and Leung argue that the negative results in our studies may be due to the fact that only three items were presented. But Pochon et al. (2001) also included a condition in which subjects were required to maintain spatial items without being able to prepare their response. Like Goldman-Rakic and Leung (Chapter 5), Pochon et al. (2001) presented five items, but unlike Goldman-Rakic and Leung they found no significant activity during the delay. It could be argued that in the study by Pochon et al (2001) the delay of 6 seconds was too short, but the same study found significant activity during this delay in another condition where the subjects could *prepare* their response. Furthermore, in our own studies on some trials the delays were as long as 17.5 seconds.

It may be that it is the *interaction* between the number of items and the delay length that is crucial. This raises the question as to why there should be activation in area 46 with many items and long delays. One possibility is that the attentional load is high in this condi-

tion and subjects must engage in *active rehearsal* to hold the items in memory against distraction. Under some conditions (e.g., few items, short delay) the subject may not have to attend to the task of maintaining the items in memory. Here the maintenance might be said to be "passive." Under other conditions (e.g., many items and a long delay) the subject may have to attend closely, actively rehearsing the items so as to preserve them against distraction.

The distinction between passive maintenance and active rehearsal is suggested by a recent study from our laboratory by Sakai et al. (2001). The subjects were presented with a sequence of five locations, which they had to remember for between 8 and 16 seconds. On half the trials a spatial distractor task followed at the end of the delay to prevent further rehearsal, and on half the trials no distractor task was given. Memory of the sequence was then tested by a probe technique. Delay-related activations were measured using the same methodology as in the previous studies by Rowe and colleagues (Rowe et al., 2000, Rowe & Passingham, 2001). However, the studies differed in that in this one the subjects knew that on half the trials they would be given a distraction task at the end of the delay. There was significant activation during the delay in prefrontal areas 46 as well as in the more posterior prefrontal cortex and in the intra-parietal cortex.

When memory was tested after distraction, the subjects sometimes made errors. On these error trials, delay-related activation in areas 8 and parietal cortex was normal, whereas there was no significant delay-related activation in area 46. The crucial observation, however, is that the subjects made very few errors if memory was tested on trials with no distraction. Yet the subjects did not know in advance whether there was going to be a distractor task or not on that trial. This means that on non-distractor trials the subjects were able to remember the items in working memory irrespective of whether there was or was not delay-related activity in prefrontal area 46. Goldman-Rakic and Leung (Chapter 5) question whether the activity in prefrontal area 8 is mnemonic. The above result suggests that activity in area 8 and the intra-parietal sulcus may be adequate for correct working memory performance, so long as there is no distraction task.

WORKING MEMORY AND RESPONSE SELECTION

There are many points of agreement between what is said here and in Chapter 5. There is agreement that the reason for maintaining information in the short term is to guide action from moment to moment so that it is adapted to the current context. There is agreement that it is possible under some conditions to record activations in prefrontal area 46 during a delay period. There is also agreement that area 46 is only involved in the selection of responses when that selection is based on an *internal* representation and is not guided by external cues.

Finally, there is agreement that attentional load may be a factor. However, this effect is interpreted differently in this chapter and in Chapter 5. There it is suggested that there is activity in human area 46 during the delay under conditions of low load, but fMRI is not sensitive enough to detect it. Here it has been argued that there may only be activity when active rehearsal is required. Active rehearsal can be viewed as the repeated selection of the items for retrieval or the recoding of the items to protect them against distraction. However, even if it were agreed that it might be possible, during a maintenance delay, to detect some single cell activity in human area 46 using microelectrodes, the critical issue is whether that activity is *necessary* for the maintenance of spatial items in working memory. We take it to be an important observation that patients with dorsal prefrontal lesions can maintain five spatial items for 10 seconds in working memory as tested by recognition, but are severely impaired at reproducing the sequence (Teixeira-Ferreira et al., 1998). This strongly suggests that the critical role for the dorsal prefrontal cortex is not the maintenance of items but the preparation and selection of responses. Whereas Goldman-Rakic (1987) argued that area 46 in monkeys was critical for the maintenance of items in memory, we have

emphasized that imaging studies suggest that activity in area 46 in the human brain is related to response preparation (Pochon et al., 2001) and to the period at which subjects retrieve the items and select their response (Rowe et al., 2000, Rowe & Passingham, 2001).

ACKNOWLEDGMENTS

This work has been supported by the Wellcome Trust.

REFERENCES

Baddeley, A. (1986). *Working Memory.* Oxford: Oxford University Press.

Belger, A., Puce, A., Krystal, J.H., Gore, J.C., Goldman-Rakic, P., & McCarthy, G. (1998). Dissociation of mnemonic and perceptual processes during spatial and nonspatial working memory using fMRI. *Human Brain Mapping, 6,* 14–32.

Butters, N. & Pandya, D. (1969). Retention of delayed-alternation: effect of selective lesions of sulcus principalis. *Science, 165,* 1271–1273.

Chaffe, M.V. & Goldman-Rakic, P.S. (1998). Matching patterns of activity in primate prefrontal area 8 and panikal are a spatial working memory task. J. Neurophysical. p. 72, 2919–2940.

Cohen, J.D., Perlstein, W.M., Braver, T.S., Nystrom, L.E., Noll, D.C., Jonides, J., & Smith, E.E. (1997). Temporal dynamics of brain activation during a working memory task. *Nature, 386,* 604–607.

Courtney, S.M., Ungerleider, L.G., Keil, K., & Haxby, J.V. (1997). Transient and sustained activity in a distributed neural system for human working memory. *Nature, 386,* 608–611.

Courtney, S.M., Petit, L., Maisog, J.M., Ungerleider, L.G., & Haxby, J.V. (1998). An area specialized for spatial working memory in human frontal cortex. *Science, 279,* 1347–1351.

Deiber, M.P., Passingham, R.E., Colebatch, J.G., Friston, K.J., Nixon, P.D., & Frackowiak, R.S.J. (1991). Cortical areas and the selection of movement: a study with positron emission tomography. *Experimental Brain Research, 84,* 393–402.

D'Esposito, M., Postle, B.R., Ballard, D., & Lease, J. (1999). Maintenance versus manipulation of information held in working memory: an event-related fMRI study. *Brain and Cognition, 41,* 66–86.

D'Esposito, M., Postle, B.R., & Rypma, B. (2000). Prefrontal cortical contributions to working memory: evidence from event-related fMRI studies. *Experimental Brain Research,* 3–11.

Diamond, A. & Goldman-Rakic, P.S. (1989). Comparison of human infants and rhesus monkeys on Piaget's AB task: evidence for dependence on dorsolateral prefrontal cortex. *Experimental Brain Research, 74,* 24–40.

Frith, C.D., Friston, K., Liddle, P.F., & Frackowiak, R.S.J.

(1991). Willed action and the prefrontal cortex in man: a study with PET. *Proceedings of the Royal Society of London, Series B 244*, 241–246.

Funahashi, S., Bruce, C.J., & Goldman-Rakic, P.S. (1989). Mnemonic coding of visual space in monkey dorsolateral prefrontal cortex. *Journal of Neurophysiology, 61*, 331–349.

Fuster, J.M. & Alexander, G.E. (1971). Neuron activity related to short term memory. *Science, 173*, 652–654.

Goldman, P.S., & Rosvold, H.E. (1970). Localization of function within the dorsolateral prefrontal cortex of the rhesus monkey. *Experimental Neurology, 27*, 291–304.

Goldman, P.S., Rosvold, H.E., Vest, B., & Galkin, T.W. (1971). Analysis of the delayed-alternation deficit produced by dorsolateral prefrontal lesions in the rhesus monkey. *Journal of Comparative Physiology and Psychology, 77*, 212–220.

Goldman-Rakic, P. (1987). Circuitry of primate prefrontal cortex and regulation of behaviour by representational memory. In: F. Plum & V. Mountcastle (Eds.), *Handbook of Physiology: The Nervous System, Vol. 5* (pp. 373–417). Bethesda, MD: American Physiological Society.

Hadland, K.A., Rushworth, M.F.S., Passingham, R.E., Jahanshahi, M., & Rothwell, J. (2001). Interference with performance of a response selection task that has no working memory component: an rTMS comparison of the dorsolateral prefrontal and medial frontal cortex. *Journal of Cognitive Neuroscience, 13*, 1097–1138.

Hoshi, E., Shima, K., & Tanji, J. (2000). Neuronal activity in the primate prefrontal cortex in the process of motor selection based on two behavioral rules. *Journal of Neurophysiology, 83*, 2355–2373.

Hyder, F., Phelps, E.A., Wiggins, C.J., Labar, K.S., Blamire, A.M., & Shulman, R.G. (1997). Willed action: a functional MRI study of the human prefrontal cortex during a sensorimotor task. *Proceedings of the National Academy of Sciences U.S. 94*, 6989–6994.

Jacobsen, C.F. (1935). Functions of frontal association area in primates. *Archives of Neurology and Psychiatry, 33*, 558–569.

Jueptner, M., Frith, C.D., Brooks, D.J., Frackowiak, R.S.J., & Passingham, R.E. (1997). Anatomy of motor learning. II. Subcortical structures and learning by trial and error. *Journal of Neurophysiology, 77*, 1325–1337.

Koshima, S. & Goldman-Rakic, P.S. (1984). Functional analysis of spatially discriminative neurons in prefrontal cortex of rhesus monkey. *Brain Research, 291*, 229–240.

Mishkin, M. (1957). Effects of small frontal lesions on delayed alternation in monkeys. *Journal of Neurophysiology, 20*, 615–622.

Mishkin, M. & Delacour, J. (1975). An analysis of short-term visual memory in the monkey. *Journal of Experimental Psychology: Animal Behaviour and Processes, 1*, 326–334.

Niki, H. (1974). Differential activity of prefrontal units during right and left delayed response trials. *Brain Research, 70*, 346–349.

Owen, A.M., Evans, A.C., & Petrides, M. (1996). Evidence for a two-stage model of spatial working memory processing within the lateral frontal cortex: a positron emission tomography study. *Cerebral Cortex, 6*, 31–38.

Owen, A., Herrod, N.J., Menon, D.K., Clark, J.C., Downey, S.P.M.J., Carpenter, A., Minhas, P.S., Turkhemier, F.E., Williams, E.J., Robbins, T.W., Sahakian, B.J., Petrides, M., & Pichard, J.D. (1999). Redefining the functional organization of working memory processes within human lateral prefrontal cortex. *European Journal of Neuroscience, 11*, 567–574.

Paulesu, E., Frith, C.D., & Frackosizk, R.S.J. (1993). The neural correlates of the verbal component of working memory. *Nature, 362*, 342–345.

Petrides, M. (1998). Specialized systems for the processing of mnemonic information within the primate frontal cortex. In: A.C. Roberts, T.W. Robbins, & L. Weiskrantz (Eds.), *The Prefrontal Cortex* (pp. 103–116). Oxford: Oxford University Press.

Petrides, M., Alivisatos, B., Evans, A.C., & Meyer, E. (1993). Dissociation of human mid-dorsolateral from posterior dorsolateral frontal cortex in memory processing. *Proceedings of the National Academy of Sciences USA, 90*, 873–877.

Petrides, M. & Pandya, D.N. (1999). Dorsolateral prefrontal cortex: comparative cytoarchitectonic analysis in the human and the macaque brain and corticocortical connection patterns. *European Journal of Neuroscience, 11*, 1011–1036.

Pochon, J.-B., Levy, R., Poline, J.-B., Crozier, S., Lehericy, S., Pillon, B., Deweer, B., Bihan, D.L., & Dubois, B. (2001). The role of dorsolateral prefrontal cortex in the preparation of forthcoming actions: an fMRI study. *Cerebral Cortex, 11*, 260–266.

Postle, B.R. & D'Esposito, M. (1999). 'What'–Then–'Where' in visual working memory: an event-related fMRI study. *Journal of Cognitive Neuroscience, 11*, 585–597.

Postle, B.R., Berger, J.S., & D'Esposito, M. (1999). Functional neuroanatomical double dissociation of mnemonic and executive control processes contributing to working memory performance. *Proceedings of the National Academy of Sciences USA, 96*, 12959–12964.

Rowe, J. & Passingham, R.E. (2001). Working memory for location and time: activity in prefrontal area 46 relates to selection rather than to maintenance in memory. *NeuroImage, 14*, 77–86

Rowe, J., Toni, I., Josephs, O., Frackowiak, R.S.J., & Passingham, R.E. (2000). Separate fronto-parietal systems for selection versus maintenance within working memory. *Science, 288*, 1656–1660.

Rypma, B. & D'Esposito, M. (1999). The roles of prefrontal brain regions in components of working memory: effects of memory load and individual differences. *Proceedings of the National Academy of Sciences USA, 96*, 6558–6563.

Rypma, B. & D'Esposito, M. (2000). Isolating the neural mechanism of age-related changes in human working memory. *Nature Neuroscience, 2000*, 509–515.

Sakai, K., Rowe, J.B., Passingham, R.E. (2001). Active maintenance creates distractor-resistant memory: critical role of sustained activation in prefrontal area 46. *Society of Neuroscience Abstracts*, 782.10

Sawaguchi, T. & Yamane, I. (1999). Properties of delay-period activity in the monkey dorsolateral prefrontal cortex during a spatial delayed matching to sample task. *Journal of Neurophysiology, 82,* 2070–2080.

Teixeira-Ferreira, C.T., Verin, M., Pillon, B., Levy, R., Dubois, B., & Agid, Y. (1998). Spatio-temporal working memory and frontal lesions in man. *Cortex, 34,* 83–98.

Toni, I., Schluter, N.D., Josephs, O., Friston, K., & Passingham, R.E. (1999). Signal-, set- and movement-related activity in the human brain: an event-related fMRI study. *Cerebral Cortex, 9,* 35–49.

Zarahn, E., Aguirre, G.K., & D'Esposito, M. (1999). Temporal isolation of the neural correlates of spatial mnemonic processing with fMRI. *Cognitive Brain Research, 7,* 255–268.

15

Mechanisms of Conflict Resolution in Prefrontal Cortex

JOHN JONIDES, DAVID BADRE, CLAYTON CURTIS,
SHARON L. THOMPSON-SCHILL, AND EDWARD E. SMITH

Executive processes in humans are a central feature of human cognition. While there is no widespread agreement about a taxonomy of executive processes, it is generally recognized that selectively attending to one source of information to the exclusion of others is either a separate executive process or a critical feature of many executive processes (Smith & Jonides, 1999). For example, scheduling consecutive processes in complex tasks, planning a sequence of tasks, and monitoring ongoing performance all depend on control over attention, and these are generally considered examples of executive processes necessary for higher cognitive function. Consequently, an understanding of executive processing requires an understanding of the mechanisms that control the allocation of attention.

The allocation of attention is critical when there are multiple sources of information competing for processing. Of course, many everyday and laboratory tasks have this feature. In the laboratory, the Stroop task is perhaps the best-studied paradigm in which two sources of information compete for control over responses, and thus attentional allocation is demanded (Stroop, 1935). In the Stroop task, participants are presented color names that are themselves printed in ink colors. When the task is to name the color of the ink,

subjects are hindered in producing a correct response if the color name differs from the ink being named compared to a control condition in which the underlying word is not color related. For example, it takes longer to say "green" to the word "blue" printed in green ink than to say "green" to the word "bell" printed in green ink. The most frequent account of the conflict in this task is that naming words (in this case color words) is a skill better learned than naming ink colors, and so the color responses from the two sources of information (lexical and hue) conflict with one another. To resolve this conflict, there must be a mechanism that allocates attention to one response (or inhibits attention from the other). The mechanism by which this conflict resolution occurs remains an open matter, but the fact that the conflict is caused by competing sources of information vying for control is undisputed.

There are many experimental effects that depend on the resolution of interference in addition to the Stroop effect. One example is the stimulus–response compatibility effect: stimuli that are naturally and compatibly associated with some response yield faster and more accurate responses than stimuli that are arbitrarily associated with a response (Kornblum et al., 1990; Kornblum & Lee, 1995).

For example, responding with a right key press to a stimulus presented on the right of a screen and with a left key press to a stimulus on the left yields faster and more accurate responses than if the mapping is crossed. Another example is the flanker effect (Eriksen & Eriksen, 1974). When subjects are required to respond to a stimulus presented foveally, they display poorer performance if that stimulus is surrounded by stimuli that are associated with a different response. Yet other examples can be found in the large literature concerned with proactive interference on memory. In these cases, a previous association between a stimulus and a response intrudes on the encoding or retrieval of a new association. Beyond these examples, there are still other tasks, such as the go/no-go task, which can be construed as having two sources of information, one of which competes against the other (e.g., Chao & Knight, 1995; Carter et al., 1998). In a popular version of the go/no-go task, subjects are required to produce a response to a stimulus in one context, but to withhold a response to that same stimulus in another context.

What all these tasks share in common is that each features a competition between two or more sources of information that vie for control over responses. In the Stroop task, the two sources are the hue and lexical value of the stimulus. In the flanker task, they are the stimulus–response association of the central item and the stimulus–response association of the flankers. In the go/no-go task, they are the trained tendency to respond to a stimulus and the need to withhold that response when the context is inappropriate. In proactive interference situations, the two sources are the previously established association of a stimulus and a response and the current association of a stimulus with a different response.

This similarity among tasks leads naturally to the hypothesis that all these tasks share some commonality in the source of conflict resolution, a hypothesis that is largely untested. The little behavioral research that has investigated this issue has not been particularly encouraging. For example, research by Kramer et al. (1994) has revealed that correlations in performance among several tasks

that all putatively involve conflict and its resolution are quite low.

Nevertheless, there have been proposals suggesting a common theoretical tie among conflict-resolution mechanisms in tasks of this sort. Perhaps the leading such proposal comes from the work of Botvinick et al. (1999), Carter et al. (1995, 1998), and Mac-Donald et al. (2000). Consider the experiment reported by MacDonald et al. (2000). Subjects were given a Stroop task on some trials in which they had to report the hue in which a word was printed and on other trials in which they had to report the word itself. Each trial began with an instruction to either read the word or name the color. Following an 11-second delay, the target stimulus was presented, and subjects gave their response. Subjects were slower in naming the color when word and color were incongruent, consistent with the classic effect documented by Stroop (1935). Brain activations in this task were examined with event-related functional magnetic resonance imaging (fMRI) during two periods of the experiment: during five scanning sequences (each 2.5 seconds in duration) after the presentation of the task instruction and during five scanning sequences after presentation of the target stimulus. When monitoring activation after the target stimulus was presented, activation in the anterior cingulate cortex (ACC) was greater for incongruent than for congruent trials, but there was no difference in activation on these two types of trials in the dorsolateral prefrontal cortex (DLPFC). By contrast, the instruction-related fMRI activations in the ACC (Brodmann's areas 24 and 32) showed no differentiation between trials when subjects were instructed to name the hue or to read the word. But activation in the DLPFC during the instruction period (Brodmann's area 9) became increasingly larger with successive scans during the instruction period when subjects were instructed to read the hue, compared to when they read the word. Not only did activation in the DLPFC differentiate between hue-naming versus word-reading trials, individuals with more activation in the DLPFC after the color-naming instruction showed lower Stroop interference. These and other results have led these investigators to conclude that there are two fundamentally different mechanisms involved in the allocation of attention in tasks that require conflict resolution. One, lodged in the ACC, is responsible for the detection and monitoring of conflicting representations, and so this mechanism is activated once a stimulus is presented for processing. The other, lodged in DLPFC, is responsible for "representing and maintaining the attentional demands of the task" (MacDonald et al., 2000), and so it is increasingly activated when instructions indicate that the color must be named, a task that requires increased attentional resources. It is this mechanism that putatively resolves the conflict in the task.

A question that arises from this model is whether it generalizes to the larger variety of tasks that involve conflict resolution. Is there a common network of brain regions involved in resolving interference in various task contexts, and is conflict detection by ACC necessary for the enabling of prefrontal interference-resolution mechanisms? By now, there have been several imaging studies of tasks that involve conflict resolution, and so we conducted a meta-analysis of these tasks to discover whether they share a common circuitry.

META-ANALYSIS OF CONFLICT-RESOLUTION TASKS

We conducted a search of the published literature for neuroimaging experiments in which conflict-resolution tasks had been used. In these studies, the following tasks were the subject of imaging: the Stroop task, the flanker task, various stimulus–response compatibility tasks, go/no-go tasks, and the AX continuous performance task. Our criteria for including findings in the meta-analysis were the following. First, the studies had to be published in refereed venues and they had to be full archival presentations, not abstracts. Second, they had to make use of either positron emission tomography (PET) or fMRI methods tested on healthy, young participants. Third,

activations from the respective experiments had to be reported for either the subtraction of a neutral condition from an incompatible condition or a compatible condition from an incompatible condition. Fourth, the coordinates of peak activation in each region had to be reported, and these activations had to pass a relatively generous statistical criterion of $z = 2.5$ to be included in the analysis. The application of these criteria yielded the inclusion of 15 published reports in the meta-analysis, shown in Table 15–1.

The purpose of the meta-analysis was to discover whether certain common regions of the brain were activated in these studies or whether the activations were strewn throughout the brain in a haphazard manner. To discover this, we developed an iterative chi-squared technique to determine whether the foci of activation from interference-resolution tasks were distributed randomly in the brain or were clustered in certain areas greater than would be expected by chance. We describe this method only briefly here.

Activation foci were grouped by Brodmann's areas (BA), and the number of such foci represented our observed values. If there was no clustering in foci, they should be spread nonsystematically among all the areas, which became our expected values, correcting for the fact that BAs differ in volume from one to another, so the expected number of activations by chance alone would differ from one to another.

Having established expected and observed values for each BA, we computed a chi-squared statistic for the comparison of observed and expected frequencies of foci. This was reliable ($P < 0.001$). This test does not reveal the regions in which the clustering deviates from a random distribution. To locate specific regions of nonrandom clustering, we deleted each BA one at a time (by collapsing each deleted area with others) and recomputed chi-squared to determine if the significance of the model changed. Comparison of each new model with the original is possible because the difference between the chi-squared value for the original model and the chi-squared for a new model is itself distributed as chi-squared. This procedure can be

Table 15–1. Experiments included in the meta-analysis of interference-resolution tasks

Study	Experimental Condition A	Experimental Condition B	Control Condition A	Control Condition B	Imaging Modality	Num. Foci (Z > 2.5)
Bench et al., 1993	Stroop		Crosses		PET	13
Botvinick et al., 1999	°Event-related flanker				fMRI	2
Carter et al., 1995	Stroop incongruent		Congruent	Neutral	PET	10
Derbyshire et al., 1998	Stroop incongruent		Congruent		PET	2
George et al., 1997	Stroop incongruent		Color naming		PET	4
Hager et al., 1998	°Event-related CPT				fMRI	10
Humberstone et al., 1997	°Event-related go/no-go				fMRI	3
Kawashima et al., 1996	Go/no-go	Response selection	Response selection	Go/no-go	PET	46
Klingberg et al., 1997	GO/no-go		Baseline		PET	11
Konishi et al., 1998	°Event-related GO/no-go				fMRI	5
Konishi et al., 1999	°Event-related GO/no-go				fMRI	5
Paus et al., 1993	Response selection	Anti-stimulus	Baseline	Pro-stimulus	PET	30
Sweeney et al., 1996	Antisaccade		Visually guided saccade		PET	5
Taylor et al., 1994	S-R incompatible		S-R compatible		PET	2
Taylor et al., 1997	Stroop incongruent		Neutral	False fonts	PET	18

°Involved event-related comparison between incompatible and compatible trials.

repeated in an iterative fashion until it is not possible to remove any BAs without causing a significant decline in the predictability of the remaining model. The resulting BAs can then be considered the sites of nonrandom clustering in the brain.

Very few BAs contained clusters greater than would be expected by chance (Fig. 15–1 shows the areas of common activation among the various studies). The ACC was prominent among these. Brodmann's area 24 was reliably present on the left and BA 32 was reliable in both hemispheres. Brodmann's area 6, a region that mingles with anterior cingulate cortex at its most ventral extent medially, contained a cluster in the left hemisphere. There was also a cluster in right DLPFC (BA 9).

This analysis reveals a striking consistency across studies of interference-resolution tasks with respect to activation in three regions: the ACC, DLPFC, and a region of the supplementary motor area that may be continuous with the activation in the ACC. Thus, the areas of overlap among these studies are in part consistent with the prediction by Botvinick et al. (1999), Carter et al. (1998, 1995), and MacDonald et al. (2000). Tasks in which conflict is present should recruit mechanisms of ACC to detect and monitor that conflict, and they should recruit mechanisms of DLPFC in the service of controlling attention to resolve that conflict. These earlier studies are silent about activations in area 6, at least to the extent that activation in this area is separable from that in ACC.

Figure 15–1. Axial view (*top*) and sagittal view (*bottom*) of a schematic of the brain. Each of these is a "glass" view, in that all activations in the axial view, regardless of z-coordinate, are shown, and all activations in the sagittal view, regardless of x-coordinate, are shown. The plotted points represent the areas of activation that survived the iterative chi-squared analysis procedure discussed in the text, thus they show the areas of common activation across the studies included in our meta-analysis. BA, Brodmann's area.

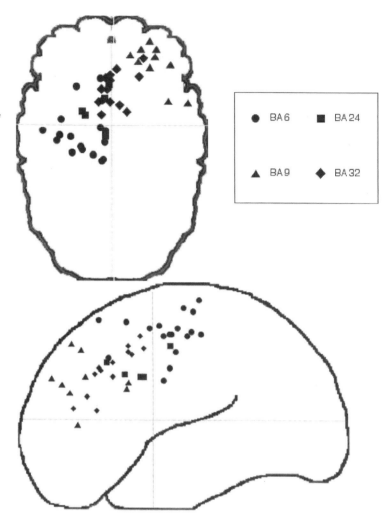

RESOLUTION OF PROACTIVE INTERFERENCE

The studies reviewed above share in common the feature that one response is prepotent— that is, one response tends to be more automatic than another. This response must be inhibited in favor of an alternative, correct response. Knowing this, it is natural to ask whether the activations that are shared in common are a direct consequence of resolving conflict in the face of a prepotent response or whether they are a result of resolving conflict in the face of possible competition somewhere earlier in the processing stream.

A striking commonality among all of the

tasks included in our meta-analysis is that the conflict that is resolved can be attributed to processes near the response end of the stream. This is certainly apt for the go/no-go and stimulus–response compatibility tasks, as these have been modeled commonly (Kornblum et al., 1990). Interference in response selection has also been implicated in the flanker task (see, e.g., Cohen et al., 1995; Cohen & Shoup, 1997). One way to show this is to compare flanker tasks in both of which the flankers differ in form from the central target item, but in one of them the flanker is associated with the same response as the target and in the other with a different response. Flankers associated with a different response yield a larger flanker effect than those associated with the same response, suggesting that interference associated with response selection is a component of the flanker effect. Similarly, the Stroop effect has also been shown to be due in part to conflict at the time of response selection. If the ensemble of colors represented in the color words is different from the ensemble of colors represented in the inks, the size of the Stroop effect is diminished, compared to a condition in which the two ensembles are identical (Klein, 1964). So, for example, if the ink colors and words are all chosen from the set "pink, green, yellow," there is a larger Stroop effect than if the inks are chosen from this set, but the color words are chosen from the set "blue, orange, red." Thus, it may be the reliance on a common stage of conflict resolution at the time of response selection that causes the activations that are revealed in our meta-analysis.

This construal of the results of the meta-analysis raises two questions: Is conflict among responses necessary to recruit processes of conflict resolution? Do processes of conflict resolution inevitably present themselves as a

network that includes the structures found in our meta-analysis regardless of whether the conflict occurs at the time of response or earlier? To address these issues, we have conducted a program of research on a conflict-resolution task that involves interference in a working memory paradigm (Jonides et al., 1998).

The paradigm is an adaptation of the classic item-recognition task devised by Sternberg (1966), and its two critical conditions are shown in Figure 15–2. The high-conflict condition is a standard item-recognition task in which a contingency is created between successive trials to create conflict that must be resolved. On each trial, subjects are presented with four randomly selected letters that serve as targets for that trial. Subjects have to store these targets during a retention interval of 3 seconds, following which a single probe-letter is presented, and subjects must decide positively or negatively whether this letter matches one of the targets. The critical feature of this high-conflict condition is that on half of the trials when the probe letter does not match any of the target items, it *does* match one of the targets from the previous trial. Thus, there

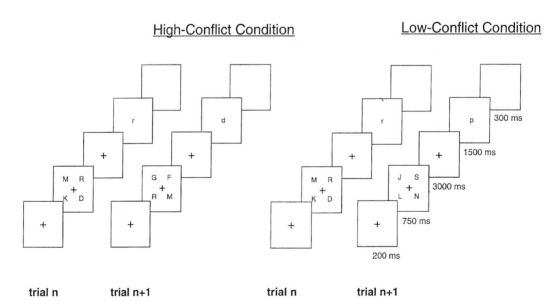

Figure 15–2. Schematic of the two critical conditions that were compared to show an effect of interference resolution. In the high-conflict condition, a probe on some trials that required a negative response because it was not a member of the target set of letters had been a member of the target set on the previous trial. In the low-conflict conditions, this sort of overlap between successive trials was not permitted. See text for further elaboration.

is a relatively high familiarity value for that probe, creating a tendency to respond positively to it; this tendency interferes with the proper response on that trial in that the probe does not match a target item. The control (low conflict) condition does not have this contingency between successive trials. In this condition, each probe that requires a negative response does not match any of the targets from the immediately preceding three trials, so little interference is created.

Behaviorally, the contrast between these conditions produced a reliable interference effect such that responses on high-conflict trials were longer in latency than responses on low-conflict trials. For example, in a practice session of this experiment, response time was 757 ms in the high-conflict condition vs. 695 ms in the low-conflict condition, and accuracies were consistent with this difference at 91% vs. 96% respectively. After these behavioral data were collected, subjects were PET scanned while they performed in the two conditions again. A subtraction of the activations of the high-conflict condition minus the low-conflict condition revealed a single region of reliable activation in left lateral prefrontal cortex (the peak voxel was at $x = -48$, $y = 21$, $z = 9$, and the region extended in superior and posterior directions; BA 45). So, this experiment showed an association between a behavioral effect and a brain activation: increased interference between the familiarity of a negative probe and its lack of membership in the current target set was associated with increased brain activation in lateral prefrontal cortex in the left hemisphere.

The fact that this outcome was realized in a PET experiment has its limitations. Of particular interest is the fact that the temporal stage of prefrontal activation in comparing the high- and low-conflict conditions cannot be surmised from the PET data. For example, if the difference in activation between these conditions is a result of brain activation during the retention interval, one might conclude that there are processes at work to heighten the trace of the current target set that is being rehearsed against the backdrop of previous target sets. This might be an effective mechanism to fight the effects of interference from

previous items. Alternatively, if the activation difference occurs at the time of encoding of each target set, then one might argue that enhanced perceptual processes were required to encode each target set in the face of competing prior alternatives. Finally, if the activation difference was due to processes at the time the probe was presented, it might be due to one of two effects. One possibility is that two responses are elicited at the time the probe is presented, and an inhibitory mechanism is activated to defeat the incorrect response. The other possibility is that at the time the probe is presented, it elicits two competing internal codes: one is a result of its familiarity from the previous trial, and the other is a result of the item's episodic code indicating that it is not a member of the present target set.

To test among these possibilities, we conducted a very similar experiment with fMRI as the imaging vehicle. This experiment had a trial structure that permitted us to examine whether the activation difference between the high- and low-conflict conditions was largely a function of encoding, retention, or retrieval differences (D'Esposito et al., 1999). The experiment included high- and low-conflict trials presented in an intermixed fashion. Each trial was stretched in length, such that target sets were presented for 1 second, following which there was a 7-second retention interval, followed by a probe presented for 2 seconds. An intertrial interval of 14 seconds permitted an examination of the activations of each trial individually. Behaviorally, the subjects in this experiment also showed a reliable difference between high-and low-Conflict trials (850ms vs. 818 ms). We then examined activation in the same left lateral prefrontal region (BA 45) that had revealed itself in a comparison of the high- and low-conflict conditions in the PET experiment. The only difference in activation between the high- and low-conflict trials in this region appeared at the time the probe letter was presented. We ruled out the possibility that this difference was somehow due to global differences between conditions by examining a different left frontal area that showed no activation differences for the two types of trials during any epoch of the experiment.

Taken together, the results of the PET and fMRI experiments using this conflict-resolution paradigm show a behavioral interference effect coupled with an activation difference in left inferior prefrontal cortex. The fMRI experiment establishes that the temporal locus of this activation is at the time of processing of the probe item. Of course, what these experiments establish is an association between brain activation and a behavioral effect; they do not establish that the brain activation is causally linked to the behavioral outcome. To examine whether there is a causal link, we undertook two further explorations.

The first involved testing normal older adults in the PET version of the task. It is by now well established that older adults have more difficulty resolving conflict between competing tasks than younger adults (e.g., Hasher & Zacks, 1988; Connelly et al., 1991; Tipper, 1991); Thus, it seemed likely that older adults would have even more difficulty than younger adults with probe items on high-conflict trials than on low-conflict trials. This failure to resolve interference on the high-conflict trials should be accompanied by a lower level of brain activation in the left lateral prefrontal site that the earlier experiments had implicated in this task, indicating that this site was causally involved in mediating conflict-resolution processes (Jonides et al., 2000).

This proved to be so. Jonides et al. (2000) compared the performance of younger and older adults on this task and found that the older adults showed a larger performance difference (combining accuracy and response time) between high-and low-conflict trials. When we compared activation between age groups in BA 45, we found that younger subjects showed reliably more activation. In fact, the older subjects themselves did not have statistically reliable activation at this site when examined individually.

The second test of causal involvement of BA 45 in conflict resolution for this task involved a patient with damage to this region (Thompson-Schill et al., 1999). The patient, R.C., was a 51-year old right-handed man who had an arteriovenous malformation resected in 1981. As a result of the procedure, he had a 53 cc lesion in the left prefrontal cortex, in-

cluding area 45. R.C.'s performance on high- and low-conflict trials was compared to that of three control groups of subjects: other patients with frontal lesions, normal age-matched older adults, and normal younger adults. The lesion locations for R.C. and the control patients are shown in Figure 15–3. Figure 15–4 shows the performance difference between high- and low-conflict trials for R.C. and the three control groups. What is stunningly obvious from the figure is that R.C. showed massively greater interference on the task than any of the control groups.

All told, then, the following picture has emerged from these investigations of conflict resolution in a working memory task. First, there is a quite reliable and robust interference effect as a result of memory codes that

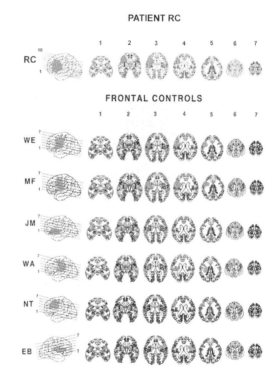

Figure 15–3. Locations of the lesions for patient R.C. and for the patients in a control group. Patient R.C., as described in the text, has a left lateral lesion that includes Brodmann's area 45. Three of the patient-controls have left frontal lesions that are centered more posteriorly; one has a left frontal lesion that is centered more inferiorly; one has a left frontal lesion that is centered more superiorly; and the final one has a right frontal lesion that includes inferior frontal gyrus.

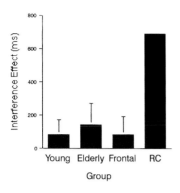 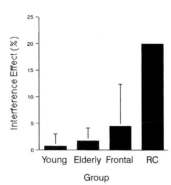

Figure 15–4. Magnitude of interference effect for patient R.C. compared to that of young and elderly normal adults and of patient-controls with frontal lesions during a working memory interference task described in the text. *Left:* Effects on response times. *Right:* Effects on error rates.

present a conflict between familiarity and episodic context. Second, there is a brain region associated with this interference effect in the inferior frontal gyrus of the left hemisphere. Third, this brain region is functionally involved in producing the resolution of conflict. This picture tightly ties the left inferior frontal gyrus to conflict resolution in this task; but how is it related to other demonstrations of conflict resolution that have emerged from the study of tasks included in our meta-analysis?

RELATIONSHIP AMONG STUDIES OF CONFLICT RESOLUTION

One might ask first whether the site of activation in our working memory task matches the sites of activation found in the meta-analysis of other tasks. It does not, in two important ways. First, the site of lateral activation in inferior left prefrontal cortex is not consistent with the sites of activation shown in Figure 15–1 for the various studies of interference-resolution tasks. The hemisphere of predominant activation differs, and beyond this, the peak of the site found in the working memory studies is inferior and posterior to the sites found in studies of the Stroop task, stimulus–response compatibility, and so on.

A second kind of mismatch concerns activations in the ACC. As we documented, this is a region that is activated commonly in tasks such as the Stroop. We did not find reliable activation in this region in our direct comparison of high- and low-conflict trials in the original report (D'Esposito et al., 1999).

We tested this further by conducting two types of region of interest (ROI) analyses. First, structural ROIs were drawn for each subject ($n = 7$) that included all of the supracallosal anterior cingulate regions. These structural ROIs included the regions that were reported reliable in the studies by Botvinick et al. (1999), Carter et al., (1998), and MacDonald et al. (2000). For each subject, activation in the ROI during the probe phase for the high-conflict trials was compared to that during low-conflict trials. Neither the average magnitude of activation (t [6] = 1.12, $P = 0.15$, one-tailed test) nor the number of active suprathreshold voxels (t [6] = 0.49, $P = 0.33$, one-tailed test) within the ROI was significantly different between the high- and low-conflict trials. Next, a functional ROI analysis was conducted by identifying all voxels within the anterior cingulate ROI that were active during the response phase for both high- and low-conflict trials combined. One subject was not included in this analysis because he showed no significant activation in the anterior cingulate ROI during the high- or low-conflict trials. Within these functionally defined ROIs, no difference in activation was found when comparing high- and low-conflict trials (t [5] = 1.59, $P = 0.09$, one-tailed test). However, it is not the case that the anterior cingulate was not active at the time of response (6/7 subjects showed many suprathreshold voxels, mean = 38.4, SD = 27.5); rather, the anterior cingulate was *equally* active during high- and low-conflict trials. Thus, within the context of the verbal item-recognition paradigm, the conflict induced by interference is unrelated to anterior cingulate activation.

Of course, a failure to find activation when

comparing high- and low-conflict conditions must be taken with caution in that it is a null result. In this case, however, there is corroboration of this null result by a report from another laboratory. Bunge et al. (submitted) conducted an fMRI experiment using the verbal item-recognition task in which they manipulated two variables. One was the very same comparison of high- and low-conflict conditions reported by Jonides et al. (1998, 2000) and D'Esposito et al. (1999). The other variable was a manipulation of the size of the memory load that subjects had to store in working memory. In this report, there was reliable activation in the ACC elicited by both variables, with the greater effect depending on the load variable. Furthermore, increased activation in the ACC due to greater memory load was associated with slowed response times, but no association was found between ACC activation and the effect that interference had on response times. The authors concluded that the activation in this region was more closely linked to working memory load than to interference resolution.

Yet another report using a different task also casts doubt on the generality of activation in the ACC as a function of conflict detection and resolution. Hazeltine and colleagues (in press) conducted an fMRI study of the flanker task. They recorded fMRI images as subjects performed congruent and incongruent trials on a flanker task involving colored stimuli, where two colors (red, green) indicated a right button-press and two other colors (blue, yellow) indicated a left button-press. When the response indicated by the central stimulus matched the response indicated by flanking stimuli, the trial was congruent (e.g., a red central target circle flanked by green distracter circles). When the flanking stimuli indicated a different response from the target, the trial was incongruent (e.g., a red central target circle flanked by blue distracter circles). They found no evidence of ACC activation when comparing the congruent and incongruent conditions.

This is an interesting contrast to the report of Botvinick et al. (1999), who did find anterior cingulate activation in this task. However, it is important to note that the activation reported by Botvinick et al. (1999) on incongruent trials appeared in a task in which there was a heavy stimulus–response compatibility component; furthermore, the activation appeared only when incompatible trials followed compatible ones. In this task, the imperative stimulus was an arrow embedded among surrounding arrows that were either compatible or incompatible. For example, the stimulus "<<<<<" would be a left-facing arrow surrounded by other left-facing arrows, whereas the stimulus "<<><<" would be a right-facing arrow surrounded by left-facing arrows. This task resulted in a flanker effect that was larger by a factor of 5 or more than that of the standard task studied by Hazeltine et al. (in press) and many others. The larger magnitude may signal that there are other factors at work in this task, such as facilitation in response due to the natural association of arrows with directions and the homogeneity of compatible stimuli on this dimension compared to incompatible stimuli. As such, the activation in the ACC may be a function in part of the jarring effect of switching from a uniform stimulus such as the former to a heterogeneous one such as the latter, an effect that would occur only on trials in which an incompatible stimulus follows a compatible one.

Overall, then, we are led to two conclusions: First, there is a noticeable similarity among activations in certain studies of conflict resolution in regions of DLPFC and ACC. Second, these similarities do not describe the activation pattern we have documented for a working memory task and that Hazeltine et al. (in press) have described for the flanker task. What might be the root of the discrepancy?

Several possibilities suggest themselves. First, consider the sheer sizes of the interference effects in question. The reports included in our meta-analysis are of phenomena that are substantial in size behaviorally. For example, the Stroop interference effect is often measured in hundreds of milliseconds. By contrast, the interference effects found for working memory and for the flanker task are substantially smaller, typically 50 ms or so in magnitude. Perhaps this difference in magnitude reveals a fundamental property of conflict-resolution mechanisms. It may be that conflict must be substantial in size to recruit a detection mechanism in the ACC and an attention-allocation mechanism in the DLPFC. Conflict that is smaller in magnitude may be handled by other mechanisms, and it may be earlier in the processing sequence as well, distinct from the later processing stages when tasks such as the Stroop have their effect. Possibly related to this is the fact that subjects performing tasks such as the Stroop are quite distinctly aware of the conflict that is present on incongruent trials, while subjects performing the working memory task and flanker tasks often have little or no awareness of the difference between high- and low-conflict trials. Awareness may be a function of the sheer size of the interference effect or whether it occurs late in the processing sequence, and it may take awareness to trigger the detection of conflict by the ACC and the allocation of attention by the DLPFC.

Another possibility is that the activation found in the ACC for some conflict tasks represents not so much detection of conflict as response to conflict after it has been detected. By this account, tasks in which the effect of conflict is sufficiently substantial to give subjects awareness of it may trigger an affective response that is a consequence of either the conflict directly or the perceived difficulty of the task in the face of conflict. This affective response may be the source of the signal in the ACC that is found in tasks such as the Stroop task or other tasks in which conflict is substantial (such as the flanker task, when it is performed under conditions of response compatibility or incompatibility, as in the report by Botvinick et al., [1999]). By this account, the activation in ACC represents not a detection of conflict for later resolution by other mechanisms, but rather a response to conflict that has elicited awareness and been detected in some other way. One piece of evidence relevant to this position comes from an event-related potential study that measured error-related negativity (ERN) in a flanker task (Gehring & Fencsik, 1999). The ERN signal is an event-related brain potential that is found when subjects produce a response in tasks that involve conflicting response possibilities. Although there is still controversy about the brain mechanisms that produce this signal, there are source-localization studies suggesting that it emanates from medial frontal structures, possibly the ACC. So, the ERN may well be a measure of the ACC signal that is measured in fMRI neuroimaging studies of conflict-resolution tasks such as those reviewed in our meta-analysis. Gehring and Fencsik (1999) found that the ERN in the flanker task began after the agonist muscle in their task showed evidence of suppressing an error in the task, and that it peaked after the onset of agonist electromyogram activity that was associated with error correction. Thus, the ERN cannot reflect a mechanism of error detection, rather, it must reflect a response to an error. If the ERN, in turn, is the temporal signal of anterior cingulate activation, this casts doubt on the view that the ACC is acting to detect errors for later correction.

There is much yet to learn about processes of conflict resolution. What we know at present is that anterior cingulate and dorsolateral prefrontal cortical regions are activated among some tasks that require processes to resolve among competing responses. We also know that these brain regions are not necessarily involved in all such tasks, but that other regions may be recruited instead. What differentiates the constellation of tasks in which these regions are recruited from those in which they are not is as yet undetermined. To make substantial progress on these issues, we will need both a better taxonomy of tasks and their psychological processes, and we will need a better corpus of brain activations that tasks may share in common.

The next several years are going to be very exciting ones for study of the role that the frontal lobe and other brain structures play in implementing executive processes of cognition. What we are discovering at this stage is that executive functioning seems best characterized in terms of a number of identifiably different processes. That this discovery is relatively new, is, of course, understandable, as there is much to learn about the range of executive processes, about the relationship of one to another, about the brain implementation of these processes, and about models that might capture the essence of how these processes work individually and in collaboration with each other. Research about all these issues is just beginning and promises to lead to rich theories of the processes that in many ways make human intelligence intelligent.

ACKNOWLEDGMENTS

Preperation of this manuscript was supported by a grant from NIMH to the University of Michigan.

REFERENCES

Bench, C.J., Frith, C.D., Grasby, P.M., Friston, K.J., Paulesu, E., Frackowiak, R.S.J., & Dolan, R.J. (1993). Investigations of the functional anatomy of attention using the Stroop task. *Neuropsychologia, 31,* 907–922.

Botvinick, M., Nystrom, L.E., Fissell, K., Carter, C., & Cohen, J.D. (1999). Conflict monitoring versus selection-for-action in anterior cingulate cortex. *Nature, 402,* 179–181.

Bunge, S.A., Ochsner, K.N., Desmond, J.E., Glover, G.H., & Gabrieli, J.D.E. (Submitted). Prefrontal regions involved in keeping information in and out of mind.

Carter, C.S., Mintun, M., & Cohen, J.D. (1995). Interference and facilitation effects during selective attention: an H2O15 PET study of stroop task performance. *Neuroimage, 2,* 264–272.

Carter, C.S., Braver, T.S., Barch, D.M., Botvinick, M.M., Noll, D., & Cohen, J.D. (1998). Anterior cingulate cortex, error detection, and the online monitoring of performance. *Science, 280,* 747–749.

Chao, L.L. & Knight, R.T. (1995). Human prefrontal lesions increase distractibility to irrelevant sensory inputs. *NeuroReport, 6,* 1605–1610.

Cohen, A. & Shoup, R. (1997). Perceptual dimensional constraints in response selection processes. *Cognitive Psychology, 32,* 128–181.

Cohen, A., Ivry, R., Rafal, R., & Kohn, C. (1995). Response code activation by stimuli in the neglected visual field. *Neuropsychology, 9,* 165–173.

Connelly, S.L., Hasher, L., & Zacks, R.T. (1991). Age and reading: the impact of distraction. *Psychology and Aging, 6,* 533–541.

Derbyshire, S.W.G., Vogt, B.A., & Jones, A.K.P. (1998). Pain and stroop interference tasks activate separate processing modules in anterior cingulate cortex. *Experimental Brain Research, 118,* 52–60.

D'Esposito, M., Postle, B.R., Jonides, J., & Smith, E.E. (1999). The neural substrate and temporal dynamics of interference effects in working memory as revealed by event-related functional MRI. *Proceedings of the National Academy of Sciences USA, 96,* 7514–7519.

Eriksen, B.A. & Eriksen, C.W. (1974). Effects of noise letters upon the identification of a target letter in a non-search task. *Perception and Psychophysics, 16,* 143–149.

Gehring, W. & Fencsik, D. (1999). Slamming on the brakes: an electrophysiological study of error response inhibition. Presented at the Annual Meeting of the Cognitive Neuroscience Society, Washington, D.C. 1999.

George, M.S., Ketter, T.A., Parekh, P.I., Rosinsky, N., Ring, H.A., Pazzaglia, P.J., Marangell, L.B., Callahan, A.M., & Post, R.M. (1997). Blunted left cingulate activitation in mood disorder subjects during a response interference task (the Stroop). *Journal of Neuropsychiatry, 9,* 55–63.

Hager, F., Volz, H.P., Gaser, C., Mentzel, H.J., Kaiser, W.A., & Sauer, H. (1998). Challenging the anterior attentional system with a continuous performance task: a functional magnetic resonance imaging approach. *European Archives of Psychiatry and Clinical Neuroscience, 248,* 161–170.

Hasher, L. & Zacks, R.T. (1988). In G.H. Bower (Ed.), *The Psychology of Learning and Motivation* (pp. 193–224). San Diego: Academic Press.

Hazeltine, E., Poldrack, R., & Gabrieli, J.D.E. (in press). Neural activation during response competition. *Journal of Cognitive Neuroscience.*

Humberstone, M., Sawle, G.V., Clare, S., Hykin, J., Coxon, R., Bowtell, R., Macdonald, I.A., & Morris, P.G. (1997). Functional magnetic resonance imaging of single motor events reveals human presupplementary motor area. *Annals of Neurology,* 632–637.

Jonides, J., Smith, E.E., Marchuetz, C., Koeppe, R.A., & Reuter-Lorenz, P.A. (1998). Inhibition in verbal working memory revealed by brain activation. *Proceedings of the National Academy of Sciences USA, 95,* 8410–8413.

Jonides, J., Marshuetz, C., Smith, E.E., Reuter-Lorenz, P.A., Koeppe, R.A., & Hartley, A. (2000). Age differences in behavior and PET activation reveal differences in interference resolution in verbal working memory. *Journal of Cognitive Neuroscience, 12,* 188–196.

Kawashima, R., Satoh, K., Itoh, H., Ono, S., Furumoto, S., Gotoh, R., Koyama, M., Yoshioka, S., Takahashi, T., Takahashi, K., Yanagisawa, T., & Fukuda, H. (1996). Functional anatomy of go/no-go discrimination and response selection—a PET study in man. *Brain Research, 728,* 79–89.

Klein, G.S. (1964). Semantic power measured through the interference of words with color-naming. *American Journal of Psychology, 77,* 576–588.

Klingberg, T. & Roland, P.E. (1997). Interference between two concurrent tasks is associated with activation of overlapping fields in cortex. *Cognitive Brain Research, 6,* 1–8.

Konishi, S., Nakajima, K., Uchida, I., Kameyama, M., Nakahara, K., Sekihara, K., & Miyashita, Y. (1998). Transient activation of inferior prefrontal cortex during set shifting. *Nature Neuroscience, 1,* 80–84.

Konishi, S., Nakajima, K., Uchida, I., Kikyo, H., Kameyama, M., & Miyashita, Y. (1999). Common inhibitory mechanism in human inferior prefrontal cortex revealed by event-related functional MRI. *Brain, 122,* 981–991.

Kornblum, S. & Lee, J.W. (1995). Stimulus–response compatibility with relevant and irrelevant stimulus dimensions that do and do not overlap with the response. *Journal of Experimental Psychology, 21,* 855–875.

Kornblum, S., Hasbroucq, T., & Osman, A. (1990). Dimensional overlap: cognitive basis for stimulus–response compatibility—a model and taxonomy. *Psychological Review, 97,* 253–270.

Kramer, A.F., Humphrey, D.G., Larish, J.F., & Logan, G.D. (1994). Aging and inhibition: beyond a unitary view of inhibitory processing in attention. *Psychology and Aging, 9,* 491–512.

MacDonald, A.W., Cohen, J.D., Stenger, V.A., & Carter, C.S., (2000). Dissociating the role of the dorsolateral prefrontal and anterior cingulate cortex in cognitive control. *Science, 288,* 1835–1838.

Paus, T., Petrides, M., Evans, A.C., & Meyer, E. (1993). Role of the human anterior cingluate in the control of oculomotor, manual, and speech responses: a positron emission tomography study. *Journal of Neurophysiology, 70,* 453–469.

Smith, E.E. & Jonides, J. (1999). Storage and executive processes in the frontal lobes. *Science, 283,* 1657–1661.

Sternberg, S. (1966). High-speed scanning in human memory. *Science, 153,* 652–654.

Stroop, J.R. (1935). Studies of interference in serial verbal reactions. *Journal of Experimental Psychology, 18,* 643–662.

Sweeney, J.A., Mintun, M.A., Kwee, S., Wiseman, M.B., Brown, D.L., Rosenberg, D.R., & Carl, J.R. (1996). Positron emission tomography study of voluntary saccadic eye movements and spatial working memory. *Journal of Neurophysiology, 75,* 454–468.

Taylor, S.F., Kornblum, S., Minoshima, S., Oliver, L.M., & Koeppe, R.A. (1994). Changes in medial cortical blood flow with a stimulus–response compatibility task. *Neuropsychologia, 32,* 249–255.

Taylor, S.F., Kornblum, S., Lauber, E.J., Minoshima, S., & Koeppe, R.A. (1997). Isolation of specific interference processing in the Stroop task: PET activation studies. *NeuroImage, 6,* 81–92.

Thompson-Schill, S.L., Jonides, J., Marshuetz, C., Smith, E.E., D'Esposito, M., Kan, I.P., Knight, R.T., & Swick, D. (1999). Impairments in the executive control of working memroy following prefrontal damage: a case study. *Abstracts of the Society for Neuroscience, 25,* 1143.

Tipper, S.P. (1991). Less attentional selectivity as a result of declining inhibition in older adults. *Bulletin of the Psychonomic Society, 29,* 45–47.

16

Fractionating the Central Executive

ALAN BADDELEY

In 1974, Graham Hitch and I proposed an alternative to the then dominant Atkinson and Shiffrin model of short-term memory. We felt that the so-called modal model had difficulty accounting for data from patients with specific short-term memory deficits (Shallice & Warrington, 1970), for the powerful impact of differential encoding on long-term memory (Craik & Lockhart, 1972), and for a range of our own results obtained using dual-task methodology. We proposed instead a system having at least three components, using the term *working memory* (Miller et al., 1960) to emphasise our concern with the functional role played by this system over and above that of simple short-term storage.

The term *working memory* is used to refer to a multicomponent system that is capable of both storing and manipulating information hence playing a central role in complex cognitive activities such as learning, comprehending, and reasoning. The temporary storage of information (short-term memory) is still assumed to be an important function of working memory, however, and two of the three subsystems proposed, namely the *phonological loop* and the *visuospatial sketch-pad*, were still primarily regarded as storage systems for verbal and visuo-spatial information respectively. However, the third component, the *central ex-*

ecutive, was postulated principally as an attentional control system, capable of integrating the two slave systems, of linking them with information from long-term memory, and of manipulating the resulting representation. In our original formulation, the executive was almost entirely underspecified, being regarded as a pool of processing capacity able to carry out the complex functions that were required to operate and combine the slave systems. It is therefore fair to say that the central executive functioned as a homunculus, the little person in the head who does all the tasks that can not currently be explained by the model.

I have to confess, however, that I am rather fond of homunculi, sharing Attneave's (1960) view that they can be very useful, if handled with care. They are, in particular, helpful in allowing one to put on one side important but currently intractable problems, while concentrating on more manageable issues. It is of course important to recognize that they do not offer a solution to a problem, merely serving a holding function.

This continued to be the role played by the central executive until Baddeley (1986), embarrassed at the lack of progress in this area, began to attempt to fill the theoretical void. The strategy employed then and since has been to attempt to specify the roles to be

246

played by the temporary homunculus, trying first to identify the tasks it needs to perform and then to explain how they are in fact achieved. By gradually splitting off and interpreting these functions, it was hoped to eventually reach a point at which the homunculus was no longer necessary, and hence could be pensioned off (Baddeley, 1996).

THE PROBLEM OF FRACTIONATION

Attempting the strategy of divide-and-rule in the analysis of executive functions is, of course, far from novel, having been used extensively in the attempt to analyze the functions of the frontal lobes (Roberts et al., 1998). The difficulty comes, however, in successfully achieving this aim.

It is a truism of neuropsychological investigation that dissociations offer a more powerful tool than associations. In the area of memory, for example, the most powerful evidence for fractionating long- and short-term memory came from single case studies of amnesic patients and patients with short-term memory deficits. When required to perform tasks that data on normal subjects suggested were dependent on short-term memory, densely amnesic patients were unimpaired (Baddeley & Warrington, 1970), while patients with grossly impaired short-term memory showed normal long-term memory (Shallice & Warrington, 1970). The section that follows describes our first steps in attempting to apply the dissociative strategy to the analysis of the central executive.

A major problem in tackling executive processes, however, is the lack of consensus as to exactly what they constitute. Much of the earlier research in this area attempted to capitalize on the probable association between frontal function and executive control, pointed out by Shallice (1982). It is certainly the case that patients with "frontal lobe syndrome" typically show both failure on a range of tasks that can plausibly be assumed to depend crucially on executive control, and damage to the frontal lobes (Shallice, 1988). However, the frontal lobes occupy a very large part of the brain, and it is by no means uncommon to find pa-

tients who clearly have lesions in this area that are apparently unaccompanied by cognitive deficit. Furthermore, examples of executive failure may occur in the absence of clear evidence of frontal lobe damage. Both of these suggest that it is unwise to conflate a cognitive deficit with its presumed anatomical underpinning, particularly given that neither of these is well understood.

Baddeley and Wilson (1988) therefore proposed that the anatomically based term *frontal syndrome* be replaced by the term *dysexecutive syndrome*. They suggested that the analysis of this wide array of cognitive symptoms should be studied in their own right, and in parallel with investigation of the neuropsychology of the frontal lobes, while accepting that it is probable that these two lines of investigation will become integrated in due course. A separation between specification at the functional and anatomical levels is, of course, very common in neuropsychology. In the case of memory, for example, our progress would be likely to have been much less had we attempted to define long-term memory in terms of the damage to a single anatomical structure such as the hippocampus. As the excellent chapter by Stuss and colleagues (Chapter 25) in this volume indicates, Baddeley and Wilson were by no means alone in proposing such a dissociation between the study of the neuroanatomy of the frontal lobes and the study of executive function.

We are, however, still left with the question of how to fractionate the central executive. One approach might be to take the tasks that have traditionally been assumed to be associated with frontal function, using them as measures of hypothetical underlying executive processes. However, as these were typically based on studies of frontal lobe lesions, such an approach seemed likely to lead us back into the structure-function conflation we were trying to escape. My colleagues and I decided therefore to step back and simply speculate on what capacities an executive would need in order to function adequately (Baddeley, 1996).

In the interests of simplicity and tractability, we assumed that the executive was purely a system for attentional control, and did not itself have any storage capacity (Baddeley & Logie, 1999). It was able to focus attention against potentially distracting irrelevant information, to switch attention between two or more stimulus sources or actions, to divide attention in order to perform two concomitant tasks, and finally to interface with long-term memory (Baddeley, 1996). We hoped to obtain measures of each of these, establishing generality by ensuring that the *same* basic executive functions could be detected by superficially different tasks using different modalities, and to investigate the separability of such functions using the classic methods of dissociation.

Our principal subject group so far, has been patients suffering from Alzheimer's disease (AD), in whom we identified a particularly marked deficit in executive control, coupled of course with their even more marked deficit in episodic memory (Spinnler et al., 1988; We selected patients in the early stages of dementia (MMSE 18–24), a point at which a clear diagnosis was possible, while cognitive capacities were still adequate for the patient to understand and follow instructions for unfamiliar experimental tasks. The exact location of any underlying anatomical deterioration was uncertain. Hence, although such patients offer the potential for studying executive function, they do not constitute an ideal group for the analysis of frontal lobe function.

EXECUTIVE CONTROL AND DUAL-TASK PERFORMANCE

Our first study occurred at a time when the central executive was almost totally unspecified, being suggested by the simple tripartite model which implied that any task that required the coordinated use of the sketchpad and the phonological loop would be likely to make demands on the central executive. We therefore combined a concurrent visuo-spatial pursuit tracking task, in which the patient was required to keep the stylus in contact with a moving spot of light, with a number of other tasks that were assumed to involve perceptual and response systems that had minimal overlap with the tracking task. Recall of span-length digit sequences is our most frequently used concurrent task. By adjusting the speed of the tracking target and the length of the digit sequences, we were able to titrate the level of difficulty to a point at which AD patients and age-matched and young control subjects were all performing at the same level of accuracy. When required to combine the two tasks, both young and normal elderly subjects showed a small but equivalent tendency for performance to decline, whereas AD patients showed a marked deficit (Baddeley et al., 1986).

A subsequent longitudinal study showed that, while the progression of the disease over a period of 12 months had minimal effect on the two tasks performed alone, it led to a clear and systematic decline in dual task performance (Baddeley et al., 1991). This result contrasted with performance on a task in which subjects attempted to classify words as belonging to one or more categories. Level of difficulty was manipulated by increasing the number of categories. The AD patients performed more slowly overall. Increasing the number of categories slowed response times for all subject groups. However, there was no interaction between subject group and category size, suggesting that an increase in difficulty does not inevitably have a disproportionate impact on the performance of AD patients. The category size effect was, however, relatively small, suggesting the need for a much closer examination of the role of level of difficulty.

Reviewing studies of the impact of AD on attentional control, Perry and Hodges (1999) suggest that dual-task performance provides the clearest evidence of a differential deficit in AD over and above that of aging. They note, however, that an alternative hypothesis in terms of lower processing speed in AD patients needs to be investigated more fully. This has recently been attempted in two separate research programms. Logie and colleagues (2000a) have independently manipulated the level of difficulty and the presence of a dual-task demand. In one study, they investigated the effect of level of difficulty when tracking and digit recall were performed as single tasks. For the digit task, span was established, after which memory was tested at two digits below span, one below span, and one and two digits above span. The results are shown in Figure 16–1, from which it is clear that simply increasing the level of difficulty does not differentially impair the performance of the AD patients. In the case of tracking, the standard pretest procedure was used to determine the target speed that resulted in 60%–70% time on target. Patients with AD and young and elderly control subjects were then tested at 50% of this speed, and at 75%, 100%, 125%, and 150%. Once again, a varying level of difficulty had the same effect on all three groups. Hence, neither task gave any support to the suggestion that AD patients are more susceptible to an increase in difficulty than control subjects.

In a further experiment, dual-task performance was studied using the easiest tracking and digit conditions. Combination of the two tasks led to an overall decrement of 12.6% in AD patients, significantly greater than that found in the elderly (2.71%) or young subjects (3.34%).

Baddeley and colleagues (2001) also chose to investigate the capacity for dual-task performance in AD patients. They attempted to tackle the difficulty hypothesis by comparing

the performance of AD patients, age-matched controls, and young controls on tasks involving focused or divided attention. One focused task involved reaction time (RT), with level of difficulty being studied by comparing simple and choice RT. Two dual-task tests were used. One was essentially a replication of earlier findings, with a visuospatial task in which subjects placed crosses in a chain of boxes, combined with a concurrent digit span task. A second experimental task was analogous to the task of a rail passenger reading a magazine in a station and waiting to hear their station name announced. The visual component involved searching an array of pictograms. Each row was preceded by a target, and the subject was required to cross out any occurrences of the target on that row, before proceeding to the next row and another target. The auditory task involved listening to a stream of town names for the name "Bristol," the city in which the testing was carried out; whenever subjects heard the target name they were required to repeat it.

Performance of the AD patients and the two control groups on simple and choice RT showed, as expected, that overall performance was better in the young subjects than the el-

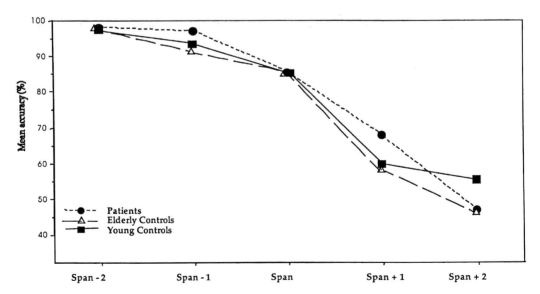

Figure 16–1. Effect of level of difficulty on the performance of patients suffering from Alzheimer's disease, and young and elderly control subjects. The difficulty of a digit span task was adjusted so that all three groups were matched under the standard condition, with performance tested at levels ranging from span − 2 to span + 2 digits.

derly controls, who responded more rapidly than the AD patients. All groups showed faster simple than choice RTs. There was a significant interaction between age and task difficulty, indicating that older subjects were more affected by increasing the number of alternatives. However, there was no evidence for a further interaction between disease and level of difficulty, as predicted by the hypothesis that more difficult tasks are simply more sensitive to AD.

When digit span was combined with the visuospatial box-crossing task, all three groups were able to maintain speed of box-crossing reasonably well under dual task conditions, although there was an interaction between condition and group, reflecting a small but significant tendency for the AD patients to work slightly more slowly. As is typically the case, however, performance on the concurrent digit span task showed a clear dual-task decrement for the AD patients, but little for either of the control groups.

Figure 16–2 shows the equivalent data for the task involving visual search and auditory detection. Rate of visual search was clearly influenced both by age and AD, and once again held up reasonably well, although there was a suggestion that the AD patients were impaired by the concurrent auditory task. However, as Figure 16–2B indicates, the dual-task requirement led to a substantial and significant increase in errors on the auditory-detection task in the case of the AD patients, but not the controls.

Thus, we again found clear evidence of a dual-task deficit in AD patients. The effect of difficulty in the absence of division of attention was shown in the simple and choice RT study. As anticipated, the older subjects responded more slowly than the young subjects, while the AD patients were yet slower. The move from simple to choice RT also increased response latency. However, there was no significant interaction between condition and group. The effect of age was at least as marked as the further effect of AD.

The combined data from the various studies of dual-task performance in AD patients strongly indicate a particular susceptibility to the requirement to perform two tasks simultaneously, a deficit that does not characterize normal elderly subjects, at least when the level of the constituent tasks is adjusted so as to equate performance across groups in the single task condition. The data from Logie et al. (2000b) and Baddeley et al. (2001) do not readily fit an interpretation in terms of an overall simple deficit in speed of processing. They suggest a qualitative distinction between the effects of increasing difficulty through requiring dual-task performance, and increasing it by increasing the level of difficulty of a single task (Baddeley et al., 1991, 2001; Logie et al., 2000a).

To what extent, however, can these findings be generalized beyond the study of AD? A similar though smaller dual-task decrement has been shown using the same paradigm in patients suffering form Parkinson's disease (Dalrymple-Alford et al., 1994), while Hartman, et al. (1992) have adapted the paradigm to study the effect of concurrent conversation by a therapist on the motor performance of brain-damaged patients. They found that conversation had no detrimental effect on control subjects, but did impair patient performance, with the effect being more marked in patients with evidence of frontal lobe damage.

The paradigm has also been applied to rehabilitation research by Alderman and colleagues (1995), who were interested in studying patients within a rehabilitation unit. The unit operated on the basis of a token economy, attempting to reduce antisocial behavior that was preventing the patients from benefiting from therapy. Most patients responded positively to the regime, but a small number did not. Such patients proved to have a particular problem in dual-task performance, suggesting the intriguing possibility that the capacity to respond appropriately in social situations might itself involve a form of dual tasking, perhaps, for example, requiring one to monitor one's own goals and aims at the same time as taking account of the needs of others.

An additional link between dual-task performance and behavioral dysfunction came

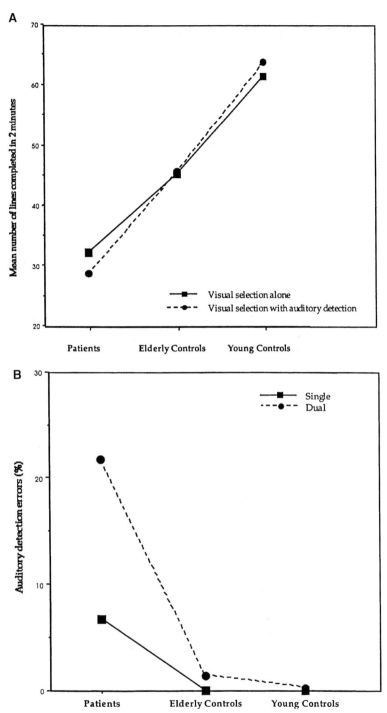

Figure 16–2. Dual-task performance in patients with Alzheimer's disease and in elderly and young control subjects. *A:* Performance on a visual-search task performed alone, and in combination with an auditory-detection task. *B:* Errors in auditory city name detection under single- and dual-task conditions.

from a study attempting to examine the relationship between dual-task performance deficit and frontal lobe damage (Baddeley, et al., 1997). Patients identified as having clear anatomical evidence of damage within the frontal lobes were tested on the Wisconsin Card Sorting Test and on a test of verbal fluency. They were also independently categorized by two judges as to whether they showed the disorganized behavior sometimes associated with frontal lobe damage. All subjects then performed two tasks, a perceptual-motor task involving crossing out a chain of boxes, in each of which a cross had to be written, and an immediate-memory task involving a series of digit sequences of span length. These tasks were performed singly and in combination. When the groups were split on the basis of the ratings of dysexecutive behavior, there was clear evidence for an association between dual-task performance and disordered behavior. There was in addition an overall impairment in performance on both the Wisconsin Card Sorting Test and verbal fluency, but no suggestion that either of these was differentially associated with dysexecutive behavior. Given that the findings of this study and of that of Alderman et al. were to some extent unexpected, this issue clearly requires further investigation before drawing any firm conclusions. If replicated, then it might still simply reflect separate cognitive and behavioral functions that happen to depend on anatomically adjacent areas. An intriguing possibility, however, is that the capacity to perform two tasks at the same time is an important and pervasive component of normal social interaction, perhaps operating through the need to combine one's own needs and aims with an appreciation of those of others.

EXECUTIVE CONTROL AND TASK SWITCHING

A third possibly separable executive function proposed was that of a capacity to switch attention from one task to another (Baddeley, 1996). Despite some highly innovative studies by Jersild in 1927, and a brief revival of interest some 50 years later (Spector & Biederman,

1976), the study of task switching has only begun to receive the attention it would appear to deserve, following an extensive series of experiments by Allport et al. (1994), which has gone on to stimulate considerable related work (e.g., Rogers & Monsell, 1995; Los, 1996; Meiran, 1996).

Following up the suggestion that task switching might depend on a specific and separable component of the central executive, Baddeley et al. (2001) decided to investigate the issue using dual-task methodology. We selected and simplified an arithmetic task initially developed by Jersild. In our version, subjects were presented with a column of single digits printed on a sheet of paper, and were required to either add 1 to each digit, or subtract 1. In the crucial switching condition, they were asked to alternate between adding and subtracting, in each case moving down the list as rapidly as possible without making errors.

We argued that if there were an important switching component to the executive, then requiring subjects to perform simultaneously another switching task should massively impair performance. Baddeley and colleagues (1998) had, in fact, developed just such a task, based on modifying the trails test. It involved the retrieval and recitation of two overlearned sequences, numbers and letters, either as single sequences, ("A, B, C, D, E, F," etc.; "1, 2, 3, 4," etc.) or in alternation ("1, A, 2, B, 3, C, 4, D," etc.). Evidence for the executive nature of the task came from combining it with a random keyboard generation task. Our verbal version of the trails task substantially disrupted random generation; indeed, degree of disruption was virtually equivalent to that resulting from performing a concurrent fluid intelligence test. As we planned to use this verbal trails task in combination with the concurrent arithmetic, we felt it necessary to avoid using numbers, opting instead for two other overlearned sequences, namely days of the week and months of the year. Hence in the blocked condition, subjects would simply recite "Monday, Tuesday," etc., or "January, February, March," etc., while in the verbal trails condition they were required to alternate ("Monday, January, Tuesday," etc.). Such a task does, of course, involve both alternation and articulatory suppression, making it necessary to include a further control condition in which subjects recited either the days of the week or the months of the year, without the requirement to alternate.

Our design, therefore, looked at the cost of switching between addition and subtraction when arithmetic was performed alone, when performed while simultaneously reciting a well-known sequence, the months of the year or days of the week, and while alternating days and months. If there is indeed a specific executive function concerned with switching of attention, then we might expect massive interference from the verbal trails task, compared to little or no effect of articulatory suppression. Finally, our study included one further small but important variable. Spector and Biederman (1976) reported that although arithmetic switching caused a substantial slowing in performance when one had to remember to alternate in the absence of plus and minus signs, accompanying each digit with the appropriate sign virtually eliminated the switch cost. We therefore ran two studies, one in which each digit was followed by the appropriate sign, and one in which the signs were omitted. The results of our two studies are shown in Figure 16–3.

Consider first Figure 16–3A, performance with signs present. Unlike Spector and Biederman, we did obtain a clear switching effect. Furthermore, performance was indeed impaired by our concurrent verbal trails task, although not dramatically so. Figure 16–3B shows performance when the plus and minus signs were omitted; first of all, there was a much more substantial switching effect, as indeed Spector and Biederman would have predicted. The concurrent verbal trails task had a major effect on performance, but note that its effect occurred for both blocked and switching conditions, suggesting that it impaired the basic arithmetic task as well as the capacity to switch. Our most unexpected finding, however, came from the articulatory suppression condition; although suppression had little effect on blocked performance, it had a marked impact when switching was required.

How should we interpret these findings? First of all, although we obtained a consistent switching cost, when the need to remember what to do next was removed by providing signs, the cost was small, despite a demanding concurrent task. Our major effects appear to come from the requirement to maintain and operate the switching program, an effect that is markedly increased by concurrent articulatory suppression. We will discuss these in turn.

Our results provide some support for a role of the central executive in task switching. However, the evidence for a specific effect on switching per se is weakened by the impact of our verbal trails task on speed of performance under the blocked condition, when switching is not required.

In contrast to our lack of success in throwing light on the proposed central executive switching process, our results do seem to have strong implications for another important issue. Whenever subjects come into a psychological laboratory to take part in an experiment, they will need a set of instructions as to how they should respond to the experimental material that will be presented. In the case of bright young students, they typically have little difficulty in absorbing quite complex instructions, going on to retain them and operate them at speed. How do they do this? In a very thoughtful article, Monsell (1996) offers this puzzle as his contribution to a book on unsolved problems of psychology. At first sight, our own study suggests that the phonological loop may play an important role in maintaining such internalized plans or programs. However, our suppression task, reciting the months of the year, while an appropriate control for the verbal trails task we used, might itself be relatively demanding. We therefore carried out a further study in which suppression simply involved repeatedly uttering the word "the". We obtained the same results, although the effects were less marked. This suggests that holding and operating the alternation program may well involve processes beyond simple articulatory rehearsal. The question of what these might comprise is discussed in the next section.

Vygotsky (1962) suggested that verbalization may be an important mechanism for the control of action, a view that was subsequently extensively supported by Luria in

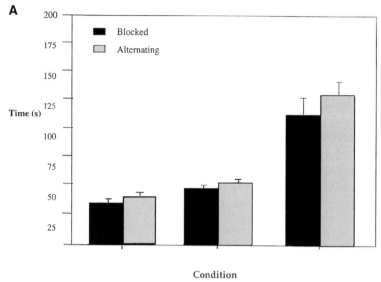

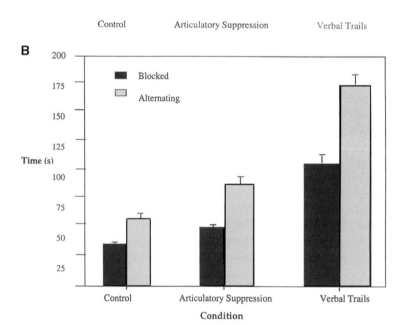

Figure 16–3. Performance on an arithmetic switching task involving alternating addition and subtraction as a function of concurrent task. The tasks involved a baseline control, an articulatory suppression condition, and a condition that itself involved alternation. *A:* Performance when plus and minus signs are present; *B:* when they are absent.

studies of both children and of patients with frontal lobe damage (Luria, 1959a, 1959b). Given that such verbal control programs need to operate over at least the duration of an experimental session, they would appear to implicate the fourth function attributed to the central executive by Baddeley (1996), namely the capacity to interface with long-term memory.

LINKING WORKING MEMORY AND LONG-TERM MEMORY: THE EPISODIC BUFFER

Over the years, although the concept of working memory has proved applicable to a very wide range of data, there has been a steady trickle of results that were not easy to accommodate within the existing framework. This was particularly so once the decision had been taken to regard the central executive purely as an attentional control system, without itself having any storage capacity (Baddeley, 1996; Baddeley & Logie, 1999). Although somewhat diverse, most apparent anomalies fall into two related categories—namely that of integrating information from the two slave systems, and interfacing with long-term memory.

The problem of integration is found even in relatively simple tasks, such as the immediate serial recall of visually presented verbal material. The presence of a powerful effect of phonological similarity indicates that such tasks typically rely heavily on phonological coding. When visual presentation is accompanied by articulatory suppression, the phonological similarity effect disappears and performance is markedly reduced. However, subjects can still remember four or five digits, and even patients with grossly defective phonological short-term memory can typically remember at least three or four digits when they are presented visually (Shallice & Warrington, 1970).

A small but consistent visual similarity effect can also be found in serial verbal recall (Logie et al., 2000b). Furthermore, digit span is greater when visually presented items comprise Arabic numerals ("7, 3, 9," etc.) than when they are presented as words ("seven, three, nine," etc.). The possibility that this is due to the greater visual complexity of the digit words is suggested by the fact that the effect was eliminated by a concurrent visuospatial task (Chincotta & Underwood, 1997a, 1997b). All of these results imply a capacity to combine information from visual and verbal sources; the working memory model as outlined by Baddeley and Logie (1999) has, however, no mechanism for achieving this combination.

The same issue occurs even more acutely in the recall of sentential material. Subjects can typically recall about 5 unrelated words, or about 16 words if they are combined into a meaningful sentence, well beyond the capacity of the phonological loop (Baddeley et al., 1987). Thus there appears to be a synergistic relationship between material held in the phonological store and that held in semantic and linguistic form, presumably in long-term memory.

A similar problem is raised by the recall of a prose passage, such as the Anna Thomson story from the Wechsler Memory Scale (Wechsler, 1945). Recall is of course measured in terms of gist rather than verbatim, and in an intelligent normal subject would comprise about 15 idea units. Performance is typically tested immediately and after a filled delay of about 20 minutes, at which point amnesic patients are likely to recall virtually nothing. On immediate recall, however, although many patients performed poorly, a few performed at a virtually normal level (Wilson & Baddeley, 1988). How could such normal performance be achieved by a densely amnesic patient? Clearly the recall of 15 idea units is well beyond the capacity of the phonological loop; indeed, the very process of recall would surely disrupt retention of later items within the phonological store, since it would introduce a filled delay of many seconds. Our suggestion (Baddeley & Wilson, in press) is that such patients were relying upon temporarily activated representations in long-term memory, a view not unlike that assumed by the concept of long-term working memory proposed by Ericsson and Kintsch (1995). Like them, we assume that the comprehension of a complex prose passage involves the activation of long-term representations at levels ranging from individual words, through phrases, to general concepts and higher-level schemata such as those proposed by Schank (1982). We assume that integrating and maintaining such novel representations is likely to place heavy demands on executive processing. In line with this view, Baddeley and Wilson found that good immediate prose recall in amnesic patients occurs only when intelligence and/or executive processes are spared. Patients suffering from AD, who typically show executive deficits, were found to perform almost uniformly poorly on immediate as well as delayed recall.

It appears to be the case, therefore, that given preserved intellect and executive control, even densely amnesic patients are able to maintain temporarily a relatively complex semantic structure. Unlike normal subjects, however, once attention is withdrawn, this structure appears to dissipate rapidly. Other similar examples have been reported in other domains. For example, Endel Tulving (personal communication) reports the case of a densely amnesic patient who retained the capacity to play bridge. Not only could he remember the contract throughout a game, but he was able to keep track of what cards had been played sufficiently well for him and his partner to win the rubber. This, like the preserved prose recall, points to some form of temporary activation, based on long-term memory but usable even in patients with gross disruption of episodic long-term retention.

The examples just described represent some but by no means all of the pieces of evidence that do not fit readily into the 1999 version of the three-component working memory model. One could, of course, abandon the model and start again, but given its success over the last 20 years in accounting for a very wide range of data, this seemed premature. Instead, a fourth component was suggested, namely the episodic buffer.

The *episodic buffer* is assumed to be a limited capacity storage system, capable of temporarily holding and manipulating information registered in terms of a multidimensional code (Baddeley, 2000a 2000b). It is termed *episodic* to reflect its capacity to hold integrated episodes that extend both spatially and temporally. It is a buffer in the sense that it offers a multidimensional code that allows information from different subsystems to be integrated with and linked to long-term memory. Such a multidimensional capacity tends to be computationally demanding, hence the limited capacity of the buffer (Hummel, 1999). The buffer is assumed to be controlled by the central executive, using conscious awareness as a major retrieval strategy (Baddeley, 1993; Baddeley & Andrade, 1998; 2000). This modified version of the working memory model is shown in Figure 16–4.

Whereas our initial approach to working memory emphasized the importance of fractionation, developing methods of establishing separate subsystems, the principal function of the episodic buffer involves integration. As

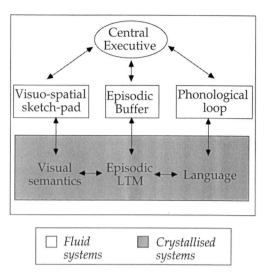

Figure 16–4. Modified version of the working memory model that includes suggested links to long-term memory (LTM), together with a new component, the episodic buffer, as proposed by Baddeley (2000a).

such, it refocuses attention on Miller's classic concept of *chunking*, whereby storage capacity is increased by integrating a number of disparate features into a single whole (Miller, 1956). Chunking can, of course, operate at a whole range of levels extending from the role of rhythmic cues in enhancing auditory digit span (Ryan, 1969) through to the use of expertise to chunk complex arrays, such as chess positions when viewed and recalled by chess masters (Saariluomi, 1995). It seems unlikely that all of these will be attentionally demanding or that all will depend on the episodic buffer. Luck and Vogel (1997), for example, present evidence to suggest that subjects are capable of encoding and retaining multiple visual dimensions when the dimensions represent the features of a single object, whereas when represented across a different range of objects, performance is much poorer. The episodic buffer is much more likely to be involved in the more complex aspects of chunking, where executive processes are likely to play an important role, creating new chunks from previously unrelated constituent features.

Postulating a new component of working memory raises a number of questions. It is important, for instance, to determine the limits of the system, in particular separating the proposed multidimensional system from the existing slave systems. This should be possible to achieve by using dual-task measures, investigating tasks that interfere with one slave system but not the other, and those that influence both (Baddeley & Andrade, 2000). The study of carefully selected single cases with specific deficits to one or another of the component systems of working memory should also be very helpful in this respect.

Another important issue concerns the relationship between the episodic buffer and long-term memory. Cowan (1999; 2001) makes similar assumptions about the utilization of long-term memory via a limited-capacity attentional control system analogous to the central executive. However, he does not postulate an additional temporary store, presumably on the assumption that the activation in long-term memory is sufficient. However, given that access to long-term memory appears to be attentionally relatively undemanding (Baddeley, et al., 1984; Craik et al., 1996), it is not clear why performance of tasks that are assumed to require the episodic buffer appear to be so dependent on executive capacity. It is also not clear how a system that simply reactivates existing material could be capable of creating and manipulating new representations. Consider, for example, the concept of a female elephant playing ice hockey. Although this is an unlikely concept, most people appear to be able to create it and, furthermore, to use it to make novel decisions. What might be the best position for such a team member? She would be capable of delivering a formidable body check, but might she be even more useful in goal?

I suggest that the episodic buffer serves as a system not only for representing the environment and making it accessible to conscious awareness, the classic binding problem, but also for utilizing past experience to model the future. Simply activating long-term memory seems unlikely to achieve this goal. A possible solution might be that such manipulation involves the maintenance of 'addresses' for representations in long-term memory. However,

it could be argued that this is not so much an alternative to a buffer as a speculation on the process underlying the operation of the episodic buffer—a necessary later step, but not one that needs to be taken at this point. This speculation does, however, lead to the important question of how the episodic buffer might conceivably be realized neurobiologically.

First of all, it seems unlikely that the episodic buffer will be represented by a single specific anatomical region or structure. Given that one of its essential functions is to link together many different codes, it must at the very least have multiple connections. Furthermore, if this system is as important as suggested, it seems likely that evolution would have built in a certain amount of anatomical redundancy to increase its robustness against potential brain damage.

There is, of course, considerable interest in mechanisms that might potentially solve the binding problem. One interesting line of research stems from the suggestion that synchronized firing might provide a way of linking multiple systems (Singer, 1999). Another possibility is through single cells that respond to the co-occurrence of two or more codes (see Chapter 6). At a more system-based level, it seems likely that areas within the frontal lobes will play a crucial part in the capacity to integrate concepts (Hummel, 1999).

A recent study using functional magnetic resonance imaging (fMRI) presents results that fit neatly into the concept of an episodic buffer. Prabakaran and colleagues (2000) required subjects to retain over a brief delay either letters or marked spatial locations. In a third condition, they were required to recall the locations, together with the letters, with the two sets of stimuli presented in parallel. In a fourth condition two sets of stimuli were combined by displaying one letter in each location. In the first three conditions, presentation of the letters activated areas associated with the phonological loop, or alternatively areas associated with the sketchpad, while the third condition involved both. However, when the letters and spatial locations were integrated, a separate frontal area became active, whereas previously active areas became less so. The authors concluded: "The present fMRI results provide evidence for another buffer, namely one that allows for temporary retention of integrated information" (Prabhakaran et al., 2000, p. 89).

One major feature of the episodic buffer concept is its emphasis on the important issue of how information is chunked. Does it represent one, two, or many different processes? How is chunking related to the more general concept of binding, and how can it best be studied? Is the capacity of the buffer set by the number of chunks it can hold (Baddeley, 2000a; Cowan, 2001), and if so, can we devise a convenient measure of episodic buffer span?

CONCLUSIONS

The concept of working memory is multifaceted and functionally defined, and as such is unlikely to map in a simple way onto an anatomical structure such as the frontal lobes. However, it is clear that the frontal lobes play an important role in integrating information from many other areas of the brain, and are crucially involved in its manipulation for purposes such as learning, comprehension, and reasoning. Given that these are precisely the roles attributed to working memory, it seems likely that the functional and anatomical approaches will continue to develop synergistically, as the complex functions assigned to working memory are tackled using an increasingly sophisticated armory of new psychological and neurobiological techniques.

ACKNOWLEDGMENTS

The support of grant G9423916 from the British Medical Research Council is gratefully acknowledged.

REFERENCES

Alderman, N., Fry, R.K., & Youngson, H.A. (1995). Improvement of self-monitoring skills, reduction of behaviour disturbance and the dysexecutive syndrome: comparisons of response cost and a new programme of self-monitoring training. *Neuropsychological Rehabilitation*, 5, 193–221.

Allport, A., Styles, E.A., & Hsieh, S. (1994). Shifting attentional set: exploring the dynamic control of tasks. In: C. Umilta & M. Moscovitch, (Eds.), *Attention and Performance XV.* (pp. 421–452) Cambridge, MA: MIT Press.

Attneave, F. (1960). In defence of humunculi. In: W. Rosenblith (Ed.), *Sensory Communication* (pp. 777–782). Cambridge, MA: Holt, MIT Press.

Baddeley, A.D. (1986). *Working Memory.* Oxford: Oxford University Press.

Baddeley, A.D. (1993). Working memory and conscious awareness. In: A.F. Collins, S.E. Gatherscole, M.A. Conway, & B.E. Morris (Eds.), *Theories of Memory* (pp. 11–28). Hove, UK: Lawrence Erlbaum Associates.

Baddeley, A.D. (1996). Exploring the central executive. *Quarterly Journal of Experimental Psychology, 49A,* 5–28.

Baddeley, A.D. (2000a). The episodic buffer: a new component of working memory? *Trends in Cognitive Sciences, 4,* 417–423.

Baddeley, A.D. (2000b). The phonological loop and the irrelevant speech effect: some comments on Neath. *Psychonomic Bulletin and Review, 7,* 544–549.

Baddeley, A.D. & Andrade, J. (1998). Working memory and consciousness: an empirical approach. In: M. Conway, S.E. Gathercole, & C. Cornoldi (Eds.), *Theories of Memory II,* (pp. 1–24). Psychology Press.

Baddeley, A.D. & Andrade, J. (2000). Working memory and the vividness of imagery. *Journal of Experimental Psychology: General, 129,* 126–145.

Baddelay, A., Chincotta, D. & Adlam, A (2001). Working memory and the control of action: Evidence from task switching. *Journal of Experimental Psychology: General, 130,* 641–657.

Baddeley, A.D. & Logie, R.H. (1999). Working memory: the multiple component model. In: A. Miyake & P. Shah (Eds.), *Models of Working Memory: Mechanisms of Active Maintenance and Executive Control* (pp. 28–61). Cambridge, UK:Cambridge University Press.

Baddeley, A.D. & Warrington, E.K. (1970). Amnesia and the distinction between long- and short-term memory. *Journal of Verbal Learning and Verbal Behavior, 9,* 176–189.

Baddeley, A.D. & Wilson, B.A. (1988). Frontal amnesia and the dysexecutive syndrome. *Brain and Cognition, 7,* 212–230.

Baddeley, A.D. & Wilson, B.A. (In press). Prose recall and amnesia: implications for the structure of working memory.

Baddeley, A.D., Lewis, V., Eldridge, M., & Thomson, N. (1984). Attention and retrieval from long-term memory. *Journal of Experimental Psychology: General, 113,* 518–540.

Baddeley, A.D., Logie, R., Bressi, S., Della Sala, S., & Spinnler, H. (1986). Dementia and working memory. *Quarterly Journal of Experimental Psychology, 38A:* 603–618.

Baddeley, A.D., Vallar, G., & Wilson, B.A. (1987). Sentence comprehension and phonological memory: some neuropsychological evidence. In: M. Coltheart (Ed.), *Attention and Performance XII: The Psychology of*

Reading (pp. 509–529). London: Lawrence Erlbaum Associates.

Baddeley, A.D., Bressi, S., Della Sala, S., Logie, R., & Spinnler, H. (1991). The decline of working memory in Alzheimer's disease: a longitudinal study. *Brain, 114,* 2521–2542.

Baddeley, A.D., Della Sala, S., Papagno, C., & Spinnler, H. (1997). Dual task performance in dysexecutive and non-dysexecutive patients with a frontal lesion. *Neuropsychology, 11,* 187–194.

Baddeley, A.D., Emslie, H., Kolodny, J., & Duncan, J. (1998). Random generation and the executive control of working memory. *Quarterly Journal of Experimental Psychology, 51A,* 818–852.

Baddeley, A.D., & Hitch, G.J. (1974) Working memory. In G.A. Bower (Ed) *Recent advances in learning and motivation.* (Vol. 8, pp. 47–90). New York: Academic Press.

Baddeley, A.D., Baddeley, H., Bucks, R., & Wilcock, G. (2001) Attentional control in Alzheimer's disease. Brain, *114,* 1492–1508.

Chincotta, D. & Underwood, G. (1997a). Bilingual memory span advantage for Arabic numerals over digit words. *British Journal of Psychology, 88,* 295–310.

Chincotta, D. & Underwood, G. (1997b). Digit span & articulatory suppression: a cross-linguistic comparison. *European Journal of Cognitive Psychology, 9,* 89–96.

Cowan, N. (1999). An embedded-processes model of working memory. In: A. Miyake & P. Shah (Eds.), *Models of Working Memory,* (pp. 67–101). Cambridge, UK: Cambridge University Press.

Cowan, N. (2001). The magical number 4 in short-term memory: a reconsideration of mental storage capacity. *Behavioral and Brain Science, 24,* 87–185.

Craik, F.I.M. & Lockhart, R.S. (1972). Levels of processing: a framework for memory research. *Journal of Verbal Learning and Verbal Behavior, 11,* 671–684.

Craik, F.I.M., Govoni, R., Naveh-Benjamin, M., & Anderson, N.D. (1996). The effects of divided attention on encoding and retrieval processes in human memory. *Journal of Experimental Psychology: General, 125,* 159–180.

Dalrymple-Alford, J.C., Kalders, A.S., Jones, R.D., & Watson, R.W. (1994). Central executive deficit in patients with Parkinson's disease. *Journal of Neurology, Neurosurgery and Psychiatry, 57,* 360–367.

Ericsson, K.A. & Kintsch, W. (1995). Long-term working memory. *Psychological Review, 102,* 211–245.

Hartman, A., Pickering, R.M., & Wilson, B.A. (1992). Is there a central executive deficit after severe head injury? *Clinical Rehabilitation, 6,* 133–140.

Hummel, J. (1999). The binding problem. In: R.A. Wilson & F.C. Keil (Eds.), *The MIT Encyclopedia of Cognitive Sciences,* (pp. 85–86). Cambridge, MA: MIT Press.

Jersild, A.T. (1927), Mental set and shift. *Archives of Psychology, 89,* 5–82.

Logie, R.H., Cocchini, C., Della Sala, S., & Baddeley, A.D. (2000a). Co-ordination of dual-task performance in working memory. Presented at the 41st Meeting of the Psychonomics Society, New Orleans, LA.,

Logie, R.H., Della Sala, S., Wynn, V., & Baddeley, A.D. (2000b). Visual similarity effects in immediate serial recall. *Quarterly Journal of Experimental Psychology, 53A,* 626–646.

Los, S.A. (1996). On the origin of mixing costs: exploring information processing in pure and mixed blocks of trials. *Acta Psychologica, 94,* 145–188.

Luck, S.J. & Vogel, E.K. (1997). The capacity of visual working memory for features and conjunctions. *Nature, 390 (6657),* 279–281.

Luria, A.R. (1959a) The directive function of speech in development and dissolution, part I. *Word, 15,* 341–352.

Luria, A.R. (1959b) The directive function of speech in development and dissolution, part II. *Word, 15,* 453–464.

Meiran, N. (1996). Reconfiguration of processing mode prior to task performance. *Journal of Experimental Psychology: Learning, Memory and Cognition, 22,* 1423–1442.

Miller, G.A. (1956). The magical number seven, plus or minus two: some limits on our capacity for processing information. *Psychological Review, 63,* 81–97.

Miller, G.A., Galanter, E., & Pribram, K.H. (1960). *Plans and the Structure of Behavior.* New York: Holt, Rinehart & Winston.

Monsell, S. (1996). Control of mental processes. In: V. Bruce (Ed.), *Unsolved Mysteries of the Mind: Tutorial Essays in Cognition* (pp. 93–148). Hove; UK: Erlbaum Associates.

Perry, R.J. & Hodges, J.R. (1999). Attention and executive deficits in Alzheimer's disease: a critical review. *Brain, 122,* 383–404.

Prabhakaran, V., Narayanan, K., Zhao, Z., & Gabrieli, J.D.E. (2000). Integration of diverse information in working memory in the frontal lobe. *Nature Neuroscience, 3,* 85–90.

Roberts, A.C., Robbins, T.W., & Weiskrantz, L. (1998). *The Prefrontal Cortex: Executive and Cognitive Functions.* Oxford: Oxford University Press.

Rogers, R.D. & Monsell, S. (1995). The cost of a predictable switch between simple cognitive tasks. *Journal of Experimental Psychology: General, 124,* 207–231.

Ryan, J. (1969). Temporal grouping, rehearsal and short-term memory. *Quarterly Journal of Experimental Psychology, 21,* 148–155.

Saariluomi, P. (1995). *Chess Players' Thinking: A Cognitive Psychological Approach.* London: Routledge.

Schank, R.C. (1982). *Dynamic Memory.* New York: Cambridge University Press.

Shallice, T. (1982). Specific impairments of planning. *Philosophical Transactions of the Royal Society of London Series D, 298,* 199–209.

Shallice, T. (1988). *From Neuropsychology to Mental Structure.* Cambridge, UK: Cambridge University Press.

Shallice, T. & Warrington, E.K. (1970). Independent functioning of verbal memory stores: a neuropsychological study. *Quarterly Journal of Experimental Psychology, 22,* 261–273.

Singer, W. (1999). Binding by neural synchrony. In: R.A. Wilson & F.C. Keil (Eds.), *The MIT Encyclopedia of Cognitive Sciences* (pp. 81–84). Cambridge, MA: MIT Press.

Spector, A. & Beiderman, I. (1976). Mental set and mental shift revisited. *American Journal of Psychology, 89,* 669–679.

Spinnler, H., Della Sala, S., Bandera, R., & Baddeley, A.D. (1988). Dementia, ageing and the structure of human memory. *Cognitive Neuropsychology, 5,* 193–211.

Vygotsky, L.S. (1962). *Thought and Language.* Cambridge, MA.: MIT Press.

Wechsler, D. (1945). A standardised memory scale for clinical use. *Journal of Psychology, 19,* 87–95.

Wilson, B.A. & Baddeley, A.D. (1988). Semantic, episodic and autobiographical memory in a post-meningitic amnesic patient. *Brain and Cognition, 8,* 31–46.

17

Fractionation of the Supervisory System

TIM SHALLICE

It is generally agreed that the lateral prefrontal cortex holds processes operating at a high level in the cognitive system (Stuss & Benson, 1986; Fuster, 1997; Miller, 2000). Theoretical accounts of how they operate are, however, remarkably few in number. One reason for this is that to understand high-level processes one must have some type of characterization of how the system (or systems) that they modulate or directly control operates. One of the few attempts to specify this and the modulation relation was that in 1980, when Norman and I argued that high-level processes modulate a system that is concerned with the *routine* control of routine motor and cognitive operations (Norman & Shallice, 1980; see also Shallice, 1982). We called this system *contention scheduling*.

We conceived of contention scheduling by analogy with a type of production system. Production systems are artificial intelligence (AI) systems that have an operation based on *productions*, which are condition–action pairs; when the conditions of a production are satisfied by perceptual representations or ones currently in working memory, then an action occurs, namely an output or a new input to working memory. Production systems differ in what happens if multiple productions have their conditions satisfied at the same time. In

our model the selection of which production (in our terminology, *schemas*) would control the special-purpose processing systems it required was based on McDermott and Forgy's (1978) approach to production system conflict resolution. In this approach, schemas each have a salience measure, activation, and there is mutually inhibitory competition as to which schema achieves an activation level that exceeds the selection threshold. This schema then operates.

From the perspective of its basic unit, the schema, our model fits with a framework used in models of lower-level actions such as reaching and grasping (e.g., Arbib, 1997). Anatomically, contention scheduling may be viewed as being based on selection processes operating in basal ganglia (Norman & Shallice, 1986) and premotor cortex (see Rumiati et al., 2001), both of which are outflow targets for dorsolateral prefrontal cortex. Moreover, neurological disorders of the carrying out of routine actions, as in action disorganization syndrome (Schwartz et al., 1991) and certain varieties of ideational apraxia, can be modelled using an implemented version of contention scheduling (see Cooper & Shallice, 2000; Rumiati et al., 2001).

In the Norman Shallice model, the key distinction between the functions of contention scheduling and the Supervisory System that is held to modulate it is between routine and nonroutine operations. The Supervisory System is thought to be located in prefrontal cortex. Evidence from a variety of methods, including animal studies (Butter, 1964), neuropsychology (e.g., Shallice & Evans, 1978; Morris et al., 1997; Daffner et al., 2000a), electrophysiology (Knight, 1984; Knight & Scabini, 1998; Daffner et al., 2000b) and functional imaging (Raichle et al., 1994; Jueptner et al., 1997), supports the idea that the prefrontal cortex is indeed much more involved in nonroutine than in routine operations. Moreover, damage to prefrontal cortex tends to lead to errors in which the patient makes the response that contention scheduling operating alone would produce, namely "capture errors," in which higher-frequency incorrect responses elicited by the task environment are produced rather than the lower-frequency correct ones (Della Malva et al., 1993). Finally, the Supervisory System–contention scheduling framework can be seen as being realized more concretely in some models of the operation of prefrontal cortex in specific tasks, e.g., those of Dehaene and colleagues (Dehaene & Changeux, 1997; Dehaene et al., 1998) on tasks such as the Wisconsin Card Sorting Task and the Tower of London Test, and somewhat less well in those of Cohen and Colleagues (1990), with tasks such as the Stroop Test. There is, however, a major problem with the Supervisory System model. The theory can explain which tasks should give difficulty if the Supervisory System is lesioned, namely those that contention scheduling alone would find difficult to undertake. However, its functions are essentially apaphatically—that is, negatively—defined; there is no specification of how it operates other than to say that it carries out all processes required for normal human cognition that are not available to contention scheduling. The issue to be addressed in this chapter is the following: Can such functions be better defined, and, in particular, can component processes of a Supervisory System be better specified?

A first attempt to specify what the component processes of the Supervisory System might be was made by Shallice and Burgess (1996) (see Fig. 17–1). That model, the Mark II Supervisory System model, was based on the assumption that a key process in coping with a nonroutine situation was to develop and apply what would be termed phenomenologically an appropriate strategy. In terms of the model, a strategy is a schema (or set of schemas) that is activated above threshold by output from the Supervisory System even though it is not sufficiently strongly activated by environmental or memory triggers. The Supervisory System was held to be able to use three different procedures to be able to activate such a schema: by direct "spontaneous schema generation," rather analogous to insight; by problem solving; or by retrieving a prespecified schema from prospective memory. Such schema selection was, however, held to be only one of a number of stages in Supervisory System operation. It was to be followed by a separate process of careful checking of its application. Moreover, a further process was held to be the setting up of intentions to be later realized as one of the three schema production processes.

THE DOMINO MODEL ANALOGY

While the set of processes hypothesized on the Mark II Supervisory System model were intuitively plausible, they appeared ad hoc. However, converging support for a related decomposition of the Supervisory System into subsystems comes from AI. A recent line of work on expert systems is specifically focused on the simulation of the key capacities required when humans confront novelty, such as reasoning about beliefs, using such reasoning to make choices, deciding in conditions of uncertainty, and acting over potentially very long periods of time to implement the actions that flow from these decisions. These are the capacities ascribed to an "intelligent agent," a term used by AI theorists to refer to artificial systems (as well as biological ones) that act on the environment and have certain of the characteristics of the human.

This degree of "humanness" is reflected in the "order" of the agent (Das et al., 1997). A *zero-order agent* responds to environmental

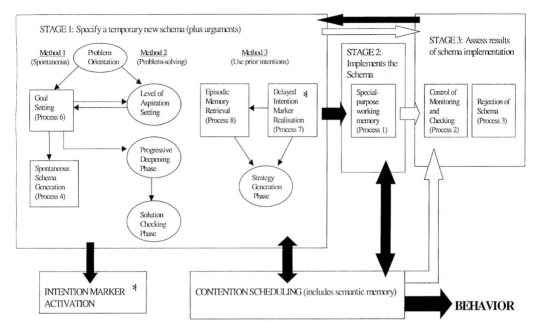

Figure 17–1. A redrawn version of the Mark II Supervisory System model developed by Shallice & Burgess (1996). All the diagram (except for the Contention Scheduling component) concerns Supervisory System processing. Within the large rectangle representing different stages of Supervisory System operation, temporally distinct phases of Supervisory System operation are represented by ellipses. Such phases of Supervisory System operation may well involve non-Supervisory processes as well as Supervisory ones. However, the numbered rectangles represent specifically Supervisory System sub-processes that are held to involve materially different subregions of prefrontal cortex in the brain. (An exception concerns processes 1 and 6, which may well involve the same structure). The individual processes are discussed in more detail in Shallice & Burgess (1996). Their correspondences with operations of the Fox and Das model (see Figure 17–2) are shown in Table 17–1. Processes 5 is not included in the diagram; it is "determination of processing mode," which is a generalization of Tulving's (1983) concept of "retrieval mode."

conditions by evaluating some function and responding on the basis of its evaluation; thus a thermostat is a zero-order agent. A *first-order agent* adds to this by containing an explicit model of the environment. A *second-order agent* contains more than one such model and so can be more adaptive than a first-order one by being able to compare alternative interpretations of the world. Finally, *third-order agents* "are second-order agents which maintain a higher-order (meta) model of their beliefs and desires, including the justifications for their beliefs and intentions and the expected consequences of their intended actions" (Das et al., 1997, p. 412). Such capacities are not available to a simple production system operating in the fashion of contention scheduling; additional systems are required (see Newell, 1990).

The recent line of work referred to above, that of Fox and Das (2000), contains both a general account of how to implement so-called third-order agents, ones that have a higher order model of their beliefs and can justify their actions, as well as the specific applications of such a model to a variety of medical decision-making situations. Their model, the so-called domino model (so named from its six sides) (see Fig. 17–2), is a collection of databases (nodes) and computational functions (arrows). It operates in the following fashion.

First it maintains a database of beliefs about a particular environment; in the medical context this includes patient data. Certain beliefs (e.g., unexplained weight loss) cause the system to raise goals (e.g., to explain the abnormal weight loss). Such goals lead to problem solving to find candidate so-

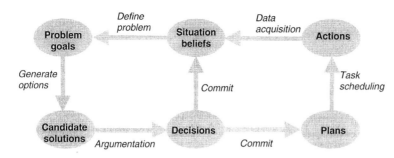

Figure 17–2. The generalized domino model of Fox and Das (2000). The ellipses refer to states of the system (representations), the arrows are processes (J. Fox, personal communication).

lutions (e.g., weight loss may be caused by cancer or peptic ulcer) and arguments are constructed for and against the candidates, by instantiating general argument schemas on the situation model (patient data) and general domain knowledge (medical knowledge). As additional data are required a point may arise where an assessment of the arguments for and against the various candidates permits the system to commit to a most probable hypothesis (e.g., cancer). This is accepted as a new belief which, while the belief is held, guides further problem solving and action. Since the new belief concerns an undesirable—indeed life-threatening—condition another goal is raised, to decide on the best therapy for the patient.

This initiates a further cycle of reasoning (Das et al., 1997), which again involves the left-hand part of Figure 17–2. "As before, candidate decision options are proposed (surgery, chemotherapy, etc.) and arguments are generated for and against the alternatives. In due course a commitment may be made to a single therapy (e.g., chemotherapy)." Das et al. (1997) then continue:

Now the process extends to the right half of the figure. Clinical therapies, such as chemotherapy, are complex procedures executed over time. Such therapies can usually be modelled as hierarchical plans that decompose into atomic actions (e.g., administer a drug) and subplans (e.g., take baseline measurements, administer several cycles of therapy, and then follow up the patient for a period). The framework acknowledges this by providing ways of representing plans and specifying the control processes required during plan execution. In particular the atomic actions of a plan must be scheduled.

A critical aspect of the system is that the different computational functions that move the system from one state (an ellipse in Fig. 17–2) to the next are implemented by programs obeying different logics. Thus the selection between candidates to produce a decision is based on a so-called logic of argument. For this stage, the system uses a variant of intuitivist logic that defines a set of inference rules for constructing arguments; the arguments do not prove their consequences, they merely indicate support or doubt (Krause, et al., 1995). They can be aggregated to produce a partial-ordering relation among the candidates specifying which are the best alternatives, which are the next best, and so on. By contrast, the stage of moving from plans to actions involves preconditions (assessing whether the basic conditions for an operation to be carried out are satisfied), the realizing of subtasks, and scheduling constraints that specify ordering relations between the subtasks and conditions under which the operation will be aborted. It also involves what Fox and Das call the "logical formalization of safety."

If one considers these two processes of decision making and of implementing a plan, then the first operates in a domain of prioritizing among alternatives, the second in terms of time and commitment of resources. The domains in which the computational functions operate have very different properties and dimensions. Now, consider by analogy posterior cortex. If the computations required involve input or output dimensions that have qualitatively very different properties, then they tend to be carried out in materially distinct systems. Take, for instance, the processes underlying movement detection compared with color identification, or the contrast within language between phonological word-form, syntactic, and semantic operations. Even within the semantic domain one has the phenomenon of category specificity whereby different types of semantic operation are separately localized (Warrington & Shallice, 1984; Gainotti et al., 1995).

This principle that qualitatively very distinct computational operations are carried out by materially distinct systems is an empirical one and *not* a theoretical a priori one. After all, a serial-processing computer can carry out highly different high-level functions on the same hardware. However, it does appear to be a rule-of-thumb principle for the nervous system and for the cortex in particular. If this simple principle were to apply to the (presumably prefrontal) processes underlying third-order agents, then suitable candidates for being naturally distinct processes could be ones implementing operations similar to those specified by Fox and Das.

On the surface, the Mark II supervisory system model and the domino model seem quite different. However, Glasspool (2000) has argued that at a deeper level they have much similarity. Although the Mark II model is the more complex in considering three alternative methods of temporary new schema generation, the two models have related central fulcra. Thus the domino model's fulcrum is the decision–plan link, while that of the Mark II model is the specification of temporary new schema–schema implementation link. Both have a common distinction between process (in Fig. 17–2 the domino model process is represented by an arrow; that of Mark II is represented by a rectangle) and state (in Fig. 17–1 the domino model state is represented by an ellipse; that of Mark II, by an arrow). Moreover, one can map between the processes and states of each (see Table 17–1). Therefore, it would appear that even though the two models were developed entirely independently, there is a good correspondance between their processes and states. On the

Table 17–1. Approximate Correspondences between the Shallice-Burgess and Fox-Das Models

Fox and Das (2000)	Shallice and Burgess (1996)
Situation beliefs	Problem orientation phase
Define problem	Goal setting (process 6)
Generate options	Spontaneous schema Generation (process 4) Progressive deepening Strategy generation phase
Argumentation	Solution checking (stage 3 and processes 2 and 3)
Commit	Implementation of temporary new schema (stage 2 and process 1) Intention Marker Activation
Task scheduling	Delayed intention marker realization (process 7)

The numbers relate to processes indicated in figure 17–1.

domino model these can be justified from an AI perspective and on the Mark II model they can be related more directly with findings of cognitive neuroscience. The correspondence between the two strengthens their plausibility.

STRATEGY SELECTION AND TOP-DOWN MODULATION OF CONTENTION SCHEDULING

The fulcrum of the domino model is the system's commitment to a course of action. This can be characterized as the adoption of an appropriate strategy on the Mark II model. Since the conceptual breakthrough of Atkinson and Shiffrin's (1968) concept of "control processes," it has been widely accepted in cognitive psychology that the performance of subjects on many tasks depends on the strategy that has been used, which they can frequently report. Patients with prefrontal damage often have a striking deficit in this respect; they do not use the strategy normal subjects standardly employ. The first published study in which patients with frontal lobe damage were reported to use relatively infrequently the standard strategy employed by normal subjects was that of Owen et al. (1990). In a complex spatial working memory task, normal subjects reduce their memory load by employing the strategy of following the same route across relevant spatial positions on a sequence of related trials. Frontal lobe–impaired patients are much less consistent in the route they follow.

Another example of this pattern occurred when Shallice and McGill (see Shallice & Burgess, 1996) used an analogue of Corsi's procedures (see Milner, 1971) for testing the ability to make recency judgments. The temporal dimension that was relevant on test trials in Corsi's procedure was replaced by that of the explicitly stated importance of the stimuli. In different conditions, words or faces were shown to the subjects, with the label "important" provided for some stimuli. On test trials one of two types of forced choice was given: one type of trial required a decision of the relative importance of the two stimuli at presentation; the other type was forced-choice recognition. Many normal subjects develop the strategy of paying less attention to stimuli not labeled important at input. This makes the relative importance judgment, which is the more difficult, much easier even though it makes the recognition judgment somewhat harder. Only 50% of patients with frontal lesions reported using this strategy, in contrast with 78% of the patients with posterior lesions.

A third relevant study was one in which we investigated the ability of subjects to inhibit a prepotent verbal response in the so-called Hayling B Task (Burgess & Shallice, 1996a). Subjects saw a sentence lacking the final word that would be strongly constrained by the rest of the sentence (e.g., "The ship sank very close to the. . . ."). Their task was to give a word that was not a completion and also had no relation to any word in the sentence. Normal subjects were again frequently found to adopt a strategy of avoiding the situation in which they would have to inhibit a prepotent response. A commonly used procedure was to generate a candidate word prior to the response and then to check to see whether it was suitable after the sentence frame was presented. To do this, two standard strategies are to give the name of an item in the room or an associate of the preceding response. When the correct responses were checked, patients with frontal lesions were found to produce responses that fitted one of these two strategies significantly less than patients with posterior lesions.

These studies do not provide any insight into whether the problem of the patients with frontal lesions in such tasks was in producing the appropriate strategy or in employing it when articulated. Indeed, in some of these patients it might be the first of these options and in others, the second. What is a strategy in information processing terms? In the language of the Supervisory System model it is required in a situation where a schema or set of schemas together with their arguments are *not* strongly activated by the current environmental, motivational, and working memory situation. When this is the case, an *indirectly triggered schema* (or set of such schemas) has to be allowed to control behavior by means other than that of being elicited by environmental triggers, and then be held in its own working memory while it is being realized.

How is a strategy produced? In the approach of Fox and Das (2000) it is the plan. There are a number of stages prior to its production. At the very least, one needs the articulation of a goal and the production of a single candidate solution. If there are more than one, then a decision must be made between them. Let us initially assume, however, that there is only one. Producing a candidate solution can involve explicit problem solving or explicit use of a prior intention. In the Mark II Supervisory System model, however, there is a third possibility. The generation of a routine run-of-the-mill strategy, such as those just discussed with respect to performing the Hayling B task, appears to arise fairly directly without conscious problem solving once the subject has the goal of producing a word in a way that is not subject to the standard difficulty that occurs in the task situation. The standard difficulty is having to inhibit the natural completion word of the sentence that would come to mind if word selection were left until after the sentence frame has been heard.

One scanning situation in which a run-of-the-mill strategy is standardly used is in the encoding of items in a categorized list when the items are presented in a random order. It has been known for many years that the optimum strategy for retaining a list containing related items is to produce an abstract structure that ties the items into a structured whole (Mandler, 1967). Subjects standardly reorder the input items for rehearsal into categories when a list that contains them is presented in random order. Our group (Fletcher et al., 1998a) presented subjects with a set of 16 words, four each drawn from four subcategories of the same broad semantic domain (e.g., for the domain *food*, there were four different meats, four fishes, four breads, and four fruits. Subjects were presented with lists constructed in three ways. Presentation order could either be *blocked* (procedure 1) or in one of two forms of *random*. In one form there were instructions prior to list presentation about what the domains and subdomains were, and these were different from those in all other lists (procedure 2). In the other form the list was presented without the subject having prior knowledge of the domain or subdomains (procedure 3). In addition, we followed the argument of Moscovitch. (1994) that a demanding secondary task would reduce frontal executive processes, which was directly supported in one of our earlier studies (Shallice et al., 1994). To do this, subjects also carried out, at the same time as list encoding, one of two secondary sensory-motor tasks, that differed in level of difficulty in anticipating the next stimulus but involved otherwise identical input and output processes, which were unrelated to those used in the memory encoding task. In one case the stimulus sequence was completely predictable, and in the other it was random. The easy or difficult secondary task conditions were combined factorially with the three methods of list presentation, to give six conditions in all.

Subjects were scanned as they encoded the lists. Later they were tested on how well they remembered the lists. The list conditions were equally well remembered except for the one condition in which the list structure was random and subjects were given no prior information as to what the subcategories were (procedure 3) and they had the demanding rather

than the easy secondary task. In this condition, subjects recalled significantly less. Moreover, their recall was less well organized into categories. Subjects were not able to use effectively the strategy of organizing the words in the list into the four subcategories and so their recall of the list was much less well structured, as well as being reduced in amount.

In only one region was the activation significantly affected by the list presentation procedure: a left dorsolateral area just above the inferior frontal sulcus. There was a large effect of difficulty of distraction on the degree of activation in this region for procedure 3 but not for the other two procedures, mirroring its effect on the ability to produce a satisfactory organization for the list (see Fig. 17–3). Thus the creation and/or use of the appropriate strategy in this situation depends upon a specific region of the left lateral prefrontal cortex.

Now, there are a number of processes involved in producing and using an appropriate strategy. In the present case, the nature of working memory demands seems a possible explanation, although there is no significant difference between procedures 1 and 2 in the activation produced in the region of the left lateral prefrontal cortex, even though the working memory requirements differ greatly. What is very specifically relevant is the production of a new organization.

Much the same region is activated when paired-associate elements have to be recoded in a re-paired form (related to the A-B A-C paradigm), compared with when new pairs have to be learned (Fletcher et al., 2000). There are two striking aspects to the regions activated in these studies. The first is that the more inferior region of Brodmann's area (BA) 45 that has been associated with simple semantic operations by Poldrack et al. (1999) is not activated; the activation is somewhat higher in lateral prefrontal cortex. The second is that the activation is limited to the left prefrontal cortex. Moreover, this seems unlikely to be just a result of lack of sensitivity, as the second study used fMRI.

The activated area is within the region of left mid-dorsolateral prefrontal cortex that Frith (2000) has associated with "sculpting the

Figure 17–3. Blood flow in left dorsolateral prefrontal cortex (coordinates: 36, 22, 28) in the three organization presentation procedures and the two distractor conditions (easy, hard). Lighter bars, no distraction; darker bars, distraction. (*Source:* From Fletcher et al., 1998a, Fig. 2 with permission)

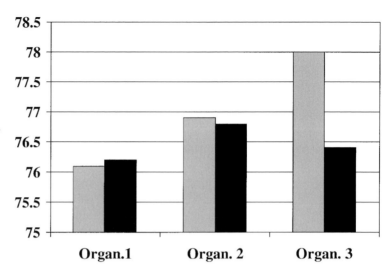

response space" (see also Thompson-Schill et al., 1997, for somewhat related ideas). Frith's idea is that when internal top-down modulation of lower-level structures occurs, as in fluency tasks, willed response tasks, and random number generation, this area needs to be activated. Frith sees the modulation occurring directly onto the representation of responses. However, in random number generation, where a very similar relation is obtained between activation and a psychological variable—in this case, degree of randomness—the left prefrontal effect seems linked to the degree of schema activation—in this case, how much ± 1 or ± 2 schemas are used (Jahanshahi et al., 2000). The "organization" experiment also does not fit well with the assumption that it is the response space that is directly controlled. However, both types of experiment are explicable under the general rubric that when structures at various levels of the output system cannot be directly triggered from stimulus representations to satisfy task requirements, then the left mid-dorsolateral prefrontal region is required to produce top-down modulation of these activation levels.

MONITORING AND CHECKING

Consider, in contrast, what in the Mark II model is a very different type of supervisory process—monitoring and checking of putative

and actual behaviors in a novel situation. The domino model uses checking in rather specific situations. In a medical application, the stage of *clinical decision making*, or *strategy production* in our terminology, is followed by that of carrying out the therapy protocol (realizing the plan) (see Fig. 17–4). A typical therapy protocol requires that monitoring be set up, which checks for the existence of certain clinical signs and for whether their triggering leads to an interruption of the existing treatment and its replacement by another. The signs that are looked for may be specific to the particular task situation and so would not be realized just by overlearned triggers.

The domino model, however, has important precursors in the AI literature. The classic AI study of a general-purpose problem-solver for coping with novel situations is that of Sussman's (1975) program HACKER, which operates in two modes. When it is posed a problem, if the answer lies in its Answer Library, then it operates in routine mode. If, however, the answer is not there, then it operates in CAREFUL mode. In CAREFUL mode it keeps both a detailed record of its solution attempts and of the changing state of the world. It must also do a lot of checking. It needs to check its behavior because the strategies it applies in a novel situation may not be effective. It keeps a detailed record so as to allow for effective fixing of any bug if a novel strategy fails. Thus a more general AI position is that

Figure 17–4. An example of a therapy protocol, for managing asthma, of the plan realization stage in a particular application of the domino model. The monitor processes operate when triggered by a check on the patient's state and lead to alteration in the therapy (personal communication, J. Fox).

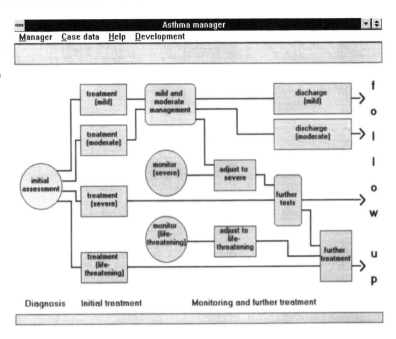

when dealing with novel situations, it is necessary to continuously check the appropriateness of the behavior to be produced.

The checking of behavior that goes on in cognition can be much more complex than merely detecting a particular state of the environment. In a protocol study of autobiographical memory retrieval, Burgess and Shallice (1996b) obtained episodes involving the detection of a memory error through the detection of an implicit contradiction between a currently retrieved memory element and the implications of a previous memory element, if the two were indeed part of the same overall episode as initially believed. Thus an event of cleaning a car (on a winter's day) was remembered as taking place at 8 P.M. Shortly thereafter, an episode within the cleaning process was recalled and it was realized that if this had taken place, it would not have been possible for the subject to have been able to see in order to clean, as the car was outside and parked in an unlighted spot. It was then realized that the prior memory of the time was incorrect and that the event in fact took place at 8 A.M. This type of process is implicit; one does not explicitly check every stage in memory retrieval. The example requires an inference depending on a number of elements: (1)

that one cannot clean without light; (2) at 8 P.M. in Britain in winter it is dark; and (3) the car was outside and in an unlighted spot. To carry out the detection of the error a complex computational process must occur.

Does one have neuropsychological evidence concerning the failure of such a process? One example of such evidence comes from the work of Stuss et al. (1994). In their study, they gave subjects three 16-word lists to remember: two contained four subcategories, one being presented blocked and the other unblocked, and one was a list of unrelated words. Subjects had to carry out both via free recall and yes/no recognition. A group with right frontal lesions and one with left frontal lesions were compared with normal control subjects. The left frontal group performed more poorly than the others on free recall. However, the group with right frontal lesions, rather than that with left lesions, produced a significantly larger number of repeated items in the free-recall protocols—more than double that of the rate of the controls. It was the right frontal group therefore that checked the output less satisfactorily.

Some of our functional imaging studies have provided a more specific localization for the key processes involved in checking in memory retrieval. Our first such study (Fletcher et al., 1998b) was the complement of the study previously discussed (Fletcher et al., 1998a) concerned with organization processes at encoding. Five minutes before scanning in the experimental, so-called internally cued, condition subjects were presented with an organized list that contained four items each from four related categories, for instance, four types of bread ("*pitta*," "ciabatta," "wholemeal," "nan"), four types of fish, four of fruit, and four of meat. During the position emission tomography (PET) scan, the subject received the "next" stimulus every 4 seconds and had to attempt to recall another word from the list. In the control, externally cued, condition there were 16 much more specific categories in each list, each with a different cue word—e.g., for "nan" the cue was "Indian bread." A different cue was presented every 4 seconds at retrieval. In addition there were two word repetition tasks as control tasks, one for each type of retrieval cue used in the two retrieval conditions. When compared with their corresponding repetition control conditions, both retrieval tasks gave rise to significantly greater activation in a large region of the right frontal cortex. In complete contrast to the organization-at-encoding task, there were no effects in left prefrontal cortex.

There was also, however, an unexpected double dissociation in the activation produced within the right prefrontal cortex. In the right dorsolateral cortex, the internally cued recall gave rise to significantly greater activation than the externally cued recall. By contrast in the posterior ventral prefrontal cortex, there was significantly greater activation in the externally cued condition, which involved paired-associate recall (see Fig. 17–5).

Why should these effects occur? As the experiment of Stuss et al. (1994) indicates, retrieval of 16 items, from a 4 × 4 structure, requires subjects to check continuously where in the structure they are and which items have and have not already been retrieved. In the externally cued condition, however, each retrieval cue is highly restricted in the items that are relevant and, indeed, only one item in the list satisfies it. If a putative response to the cue

comes to mind, it cannot have been given to a prior stimulus, so there is no need to check the relation between the retrieved item and those recalled earlier. Checking, therefore, is much less critical. Thus the significantly greater activation in the right dorsolateral region in the internally cued condition fits with this region being involved in checking processes. As free recall from a 16-item list is precisely the situation in which more item repetition errors were found in retrieval by Stuss et al., this imaging result suggests that the right dorsolateral region is critical for the process impaired in the patients studied by Stuss et al.

In three more of our studies we compared different memory retrieval conditions and found that the right dorsolateral region is more activated when more checking is required. The first of these (Henson et al., 1999b) was a PET study involving a Jacoby (1996) process dissociation framework, in which encoding and retrieval processes during memory exclusion conditions were compared with those during memory inclusion conditions. There were two parallel memory exclusion conditions. In one, subjects had to respond "yes" only when the test word had both been presented before and had been presented in the same spatial position. In a second exclusion condition the second constraint was that the test word had to be in a particular one of the two lists (list 1 or list 2), as when originally presented. There were no differences in activation between these two exclusion conditions and so they were combined. In both conditions subjects showed strong activation of dorsolateral prefrontal cortex bilaterally compared to control conditions.

Following initial recognition that a test word had previously been presented, the exclusion conditions clearly required an additional checking stage that was not required in the inclusion one. Thus the finding fits the hypothesis concerning checking developed earlier. The bilateral nature of the dorsolateral activation does differ, however, from the activation in the previous experiment, in that in this (Henson et al., 1999b) experiment there was a lateralization effect if the appro-

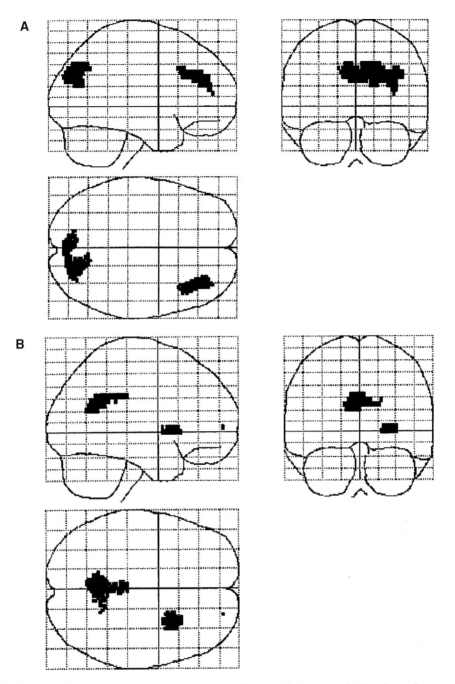

Figure 17–5. Statistical parametric mapping representation of areas that differ significantly (in each of the two directions) between recall (*A*) and paired-associate recall (*B*) (From Fletcher et al., 1998b, Fig. 2 with permission)

priate contrast was made. The activation occurring in the memory exclusion conditions was significantly weaker than that in the encoding condition in the left dorsolateral prefrontal cortex. In the right dorsolateral regions there was far stronger activation in the memory exclusion than in the encoding context. Thus, in comparing the exclusion condition with the encoding one, there was a laterality effect in dorsolateral prefrontal cortex.

In a further study (Henson et al., 1999a), in which event-related fMRI was used, we obtained surprising support for this position. The experiment involved subjects in a recognition memory experiment using a remember/know judgment in a paradigm derived from Tulving (1985) and Gardiner (1988). When results from trials on which subjects gave a "remember" judgment were compared with those from trials on which they gave a "know" judgement, significant differences in activation occurred for two regions. Surprisingly "remember" trials produced significantly greater activation in an anterior (area 8), left hemisphere region. However, more directly relevant, the "know" judgments produced a significantly greater activation of the same region of right dorsolateral prefrontal cortex, as in the previous two experiments. If one uses a familiarity/recollection framework similar to that of Mandler (1980), then following presentation of the target word and a positive familiarity impression, the subject will make an explicit check of the episodic record, if episodic retrieval has not already occurred. For "know" responses this explicit checking stage would be prolonged because it initially fails to confirm the familiarity impression by ecphory in Tulving's (1983) sense.

Another situation in which more checking is likely to occur is when the subject has low confidence. In a fourth study, also using event-related fMRI and involving recognition (Henson et al., 2000), the subject had to both decide whether the test stimulus had been presented earlier or not (yes/no) and give a confidence rating (high/low), by pressing one of four keys corresponding to "yes high," "yes low," "no low," and "no high." As one would expect from the previous studies, there was more activation in the right dorsolateral pre-

frontal regions when a subject gave a low-confidence response than with a high-confidence one. More critically, this occurred regardless of whether the subject correctly recognized that the stimulus had occurred or correctly responded that it had not. In a more anterior right prefrontal region (area 10) there was a significant difference between hits and correct rejections.

What we see in all three comparisons (Fletcher et al., 1998a, 1998b; Henson et al., 1999a, 1999b) is that when there is an equivalent encoding condition there is a significant left–right difference in dorsolateral prefrontal activation between encoding and a retrieval process that appears to be involved in increased checking of memory performance.

On the account presented for the relation between the right dorsolateral activation obtained and recognition, the effect should occur late in the retrieval process. This fits with electrophysiological findings. In a study involving both recognition judgments and cued recall, Allan and Rugg (1997) found a stronger right than left frontal potential at retrieval. However, this differential effect did not begin to occur until more than 1200 ms after the onset of the test stimulus (see also Wilding & Rugg, 1996). They argued that the right prefrontal potential was a consequence of postretrieval operations, of which checking is one. In another study on the right frontal potential, Uhl et al. (1994) found that it was greater in conditions with a higher degree of proactive interference. These are situations in which more checking has to occur, since there is a greater probability of retrieving an incorrect stimulus.

Are there not alternative explications for certain conditions producing greater right dorsolateral prefrontal activation in these experiments? One possibility is retrieval effort (Schacter et al., 1996), which presumably would be greater in the exclusion, "know" and low-confidence conditions. *Retrieval effort* has been used as an explanation of the left frontal lateralization when more shallowly studied words are retrieved (Schacter et al., 1996; Buckner et al., 1998), a situation in which checking does not seem to be a plausible alternative. Moreover, these two hypotheses have a certain degree of overlap. In their protocol study of everyday memory retrieval, Burgess and Shallice (1996b) showed that a variety of different procedures were used to check retrieval performance. An important method of checking retrieval performance is to search for further memory elements to see whether they conflict with those already obtained. Thus a checking procedure would involve further retrieval attempts and so produce greater retrieval effort.

The right dorsolateral region is also activated in other types of experimental paradigms. Lesions in the right frontal cortex affect vigilance operations (Posner & Peterson, 1990), such as a subject's ability to carry out simple monotonous tasks (e.g., Wilkins et al. 1987). In addition, Pardo et al. found (1991) that giving subjects a task that involved them being vigilant during the 1 minute of a PET scan led to activation of this region; subjects had to count the number of faint touches that had occurred when there were no more than three or four. In a study in another cognitive domain when subjects unexpectedly viewed an anomalous percept, there was strong activation in the right dorsolateral region (Fink et al., 1999). Both these paradigms would give rise to checking of performance or experience, but the checking could not be easily explained by effort.

What does checking involve? Consider the experiment of Stuss et al. (1994), in which patients with right prefrontal lesions made a significantly larger number of repeats in free recall. How do subjects prevent themselves from repeating items? In the Mandler (1980) framework for recognition it is plausible that when a repeated response comes to mind, the subject experiences increased familiarity. The familiarity needs to be detected as being greater than the threshold that must be specified by some cognitive system when recall begins. When the implicit repeat arises, an interruption must therefore occur and the subject must switch to an attempt to explicitly recognize whether the item has already been recalled or not. If a match between the implicit response and a previously retrieved item is detected, then the response must be suppressed. These series of stages involve both memory and non-memory processes, of which

only the latter could generalized to other types of study. There would seem to be three non-memory processes that may be involved: the specification of the matching criteria, the matching of the implicit familiarity response with the prespecified criteria, and the interrupt process.

CONCLUSION

In this chapter, the focus of discussion has been two supervisory processes: the top-down modulation of lower-level schemas on the one hand and checking, or monitoring, processes on the other. Both of the Burgess-Shallice and the Fox-Das models have a variety of subprocesses. Is there any evidence that any of the other subprocesses may be localized separately in prefrontal cortex?

First, consider the right ventrolateral cortex. It is activated more in retrieval tasks than in control and encoding tasks in virtually all of the memory experiments discussed in this chapter. In only one study, that of Fletcher et al. (1998b), is there differential activation of the region across different memory retrieval conditions. Why should there be more activation in the posterior ventral right prefrontal region in the externally cued condition of this study? When retrieving an organized list, subjects tended to retrieve the items in a category in succession. This means that in the internally cued recall condition, the recall specification changed only four times during retrieval, namely at the time the subject moved to the next category. In the externally cued recall condition, however, the specification of what must be searched for in memory changed with each new specific category cue; there would be sixteen different recall specifications to retrieve all items in the list. Fletcher et al. (1998b) suggested that the externally cued condition might stress the process of specifying what was being searched for in memory (see Norman & Bobrow, 1979; Burgess & Shallice, 1996b), and that this process might therefore be localized in the right ventrolateral regions (see Costello et al., 1998; Levine et al., 1998, for further supporting evidence; and Shallice, 2001, for further discussion).

This explanation would fit with the function of the use of episodic memory retrieval as providing key input to allow case-based reasoning in the problem-solving method of strategy production in the Mark II model (see Schank, 1982; Shallice, 1988).

A fourth process that is involved in the Fox and Das (2000) domino framework is the control of behavior over time, through the setting up of a task schedule to specify a series of treatment and investigation processes. In the Mark II model, this corresponds to a prefrontal process distinct from the three discussed thus far—namely the setting-up and later realization of intentions to provide the motor for the third route for strategy generation. Burgess and Shallice (1991) described three patients whose difficulties were interpreted with specific problems in the setting up and realization of intentions. While performing well on both IQ tests and many tests sensitive to frontal lobe lesions, they performed very poorly on two tests that involve carrying out a number of subtasks without any experimenter-given specification of when they should be carried out, and doing so when obeying a set of simple rules in which they had earlier been trained. Both the carrying out of a previously specified task with no signal as to when to do it and not breaking a rule in which one had earlier been trained can be thought of as involving the realization of intentions previously set up. That area 10 was a critical region for the disorder was shown in a later group study (Burgess et al., 2000). In a functional imaging study it was also shown that the area was activated when an intention to carry out a specific task at a later time had been set up (Burgess, et al. 2001).

Returning to the general theme, the overall perspective that has been outlined in this chapter is threefold. First, it is argued that there are processes that come into play specifically in nonroutine situations. This is the position initially adopted in Norman and Shallice (1980). Second, from an expert system AI perspective (the domino model), one would expect there to be a set of subprocesses that are computationally very different and have different specific roles but which also combine in coping with nonroutine situations. This is the approach taken earlier from a cognitive neuroscience perspective by the Mark II Supervisory System model. Third, from a cognitive neuroscience perspective, these subprocesses can be localized in different parts of the prefrontal cortex.

I have specifically considered four different such processes and argued that they are localized in different parts of prefrontal cortex. Two were treated in more detail; these are the top-down Supervisory System modulation of schemas in contention scheduling (left dorsolateral prefrontal cortex), and the monitoring and checking of behavior with respect to a variety of internally generated criteria (right dorsolateral prefrontal cortex). Two were considered much more briefly; these are the specification of a required memory trace (right ventrolateral prefrontal cortex) and the setting up and/or realization of intentions (area 10). All are subprocesses postulated in the Mark II Supervisory System model. Three processes also correspond well to those required by the Domino model. Indeed, these three also correspond well to three of the four temporal integration functions that Fuster postulates in Chapter 6 from a primarily neurobiological perspective as critically involving lateral prefrontal cortex. The fourth process, that of the specification of a required memory trace, relates to ideas developed by Schank (1982) that a function of episodic memory is to allow case-based reasoning in problem solving (see Shallice, 1988; Burgess & Shallice, 1996b). Most critically, however, all four processes satisfy the three general principles described in the penultimate paragraph.

First they come into play in non-routine situations. Second they are computationally very different from each other. Third they appear to be localized in different part prefrontal cortex.

REFERENCES

Allan, K. & Rugg, M.D. (1997). An event-related potential study of explicit memory on tests of word-stem cued recall and recognition memory. *Neuropsychologia, 35,* 387–397.

Arbib, M.A. (1997). Modelling visuomotor transformations. In M. Jeannerod (Ed.) *Handbook of Neuropsychology, vol II* (pp. 65–90) Amsterdam: Elsevier.

Atkinson, R.C. & Shiffrin, R.M. (1968). Human memory: a proposed system and its control processes. In K.W. Spence & J.T. Spence (Eds.), *The Psychology of Learning and Motivation: Advances in Research and Theory* 2nd ed., (pp. 90–197). New York: Academic Press.

Buckner, R.L., Koutstaal, W., Schacter, D.L., Wagner, A.D., & Rosen, B.R. (1998). Functional-anatomic study of episodic retrieval using fMRI: I. Retrieval effort versus retrieval success. *NeuroImage, 7,* 151–162.

Burgess, P. & Shallice, T. (1996a). Response suppression, initiation and strategy following frontal lobe lesions. *Neuropsychologia, 34,* 263–273.

Burgess, P. & Shallice, T. (1996b). Confabulation and the control of recollection. *Memory, 4,* 359–412.

Burgess, P., Veitch, E., Costello, A., & Shallice, T. (2000). The cognitive and neuroanatomical correlates of multitasking. *Neuropsychologia, 38,* 848–863.

Burgess, P.W., Quayle, A., & Frith, C.D. (2001). Brain regions involved in prospective memory as determined by positron emission tomography. *Neuropsychologia, 39,* 545–555.

Butter, C.M. (1964). Habituation to novel stimuli in monkeys with selective frontal lesions. *Science, 144,* 313–315.

Cohen, J.D., Dunbar, K., & McClelland, J.L. (1990). On the control of automatic processes: a parallel distributed processing account of the Stroop effect. *Psychological Review, 97,* 332–361.

Cooper, R & Shallice, T. (2000). Contention scheduling and the control of routine activities. *Cognitive Neuropsychology, 17,* 297–338.

Costello, A., Fletcher, P.C., Dolan, R.J., Frith, C.D., & Shallice, T. (1998). The origins of forgetting in a case of isolated retrograde amnesia following a haemorrhage: evidence from functional imaging. *Neurocase, 4,* 437–446.

Daffner, K.R., Mesulam, M.M., Holcomb, P.J., Calva, V., Acar, D., Chaberie, A., Kikinis, R., Jolesz, F.A., Rentz, D.M., & Scinto, L.F.M. (2000a). Disruption of attention to novel events after frontal lobe injury in humans. *Journal of Neurology, Neurosurgery and Psychiatry, 68,* 18–24.

Daffner, K.R., Mesulam, M.M., Scinto, L.F.M., Acar, D., Calvo, V., Faust, R., Chaberie, A., Kennedy, B., & Holcomb, P. (2000b). The central role of prefrontal cortex in directing attention to novel events. *Brain, 123,* 927–939.

Das, S.K., Fox, J., Hammond, P., & Elsdon, D. (1997). A flexible architecture for autonomous agents. *Journal of Experimental and Theoretical Artificial Intelligence, 9,* 407–440.

Dehaene, S. & Changeux, J.P. (1997). A hierarchical neuronal network for planning behaviour. *Proceedings of the National Acaemy of Science, USA, 94,* 13293–13298.

Dehaene, S., Kerszberg, M., & Changeux, J.P. (1998). A neuronal model of the global workspace in effortful cognitive tasks. *Proceedings of the National Academy of Sciences USA, 95,* 14529–14534.

Della Malva, C.L., Stuss, D.T., D'Alton, J., & Willmer, J. (1993). Capture errors and sequencing after frontal brain lesions. *Neuropsychologia, 31,* 363–392.

Fink, G.R., Marshall, J.C., Halligan, P.W., Frith, C.D., Driver, J., Frackowiak, R.S.J., & Dolan, R.J. (1999). The neural consequences of conflict between intention and the senses. *Brain, 122,* 497–512.

Fletcher, P.C., Shallice, T., & Dolan, R.J. (1998a). The functional roles of prefrontal cortex in episodic memory. I Encoding. *Brain, 121,* 1239–1248.

Fletcher, P.C., Shallice, T., Frith, C.D., Frackowiak, R.S.J., & Dolan, R.J. (1998b). The functional roles of prefrontal cortex in episodic memory. II Retrieval. *Brain, 121,* 1249–1256.

Fletcher, P.C., Shallice, T., & Dolan, R.J. (2000). "Sculpting the response space"—an account of left prefrontal activation at encoding. *NeuroImage, 12,* 404–417.

Fox, J. & Das, S.K. (2000). *Safe and Sound: Artificial Intelligence in Hazardous Applications.* Menlo Park, CA: AAAI Press.

Frith, C.D. (2000). The role of dorsolateral prefrontal cortex in the selection of action, as revealed by functional imaging. In: S. Monsell & J. Driver (Eds.), *Control of Cognitive Processes: Attention and Performance XVIII.* (pp. 549–565). Cambridge, MA: MIT Press.

Fuster, J. (1997). *The Prefrontal Cortex.* New York: Raven Press.

Gainotti, G., Silveri, M.C., Daniele, A., & Giustolisi, L. (1995). Neuroanatomical correlates of category-specific semantic disorder: a critical survey. *Memory, 3,* 247–264.

Gardiner, J.M. (1988). Functional aspects of recollective experience. *Memory and Cognition, 16,* 309–313.

Glasspool, D.W. (2000). The integration and control of behaviour: insights from neuroscience and AI. *Imperial Cancer Research Fund Advanced Computation Lab Tech Report No. 360.*

Henson, R.N.A., Rugg, M.D., Shallice, T., Josephs, O., & Dolan, R.J. (1999a). Recollection and familiarity in recognition memory: an event-related fMRI study. *Journal of Neuroscience, 19,* 3962–3972.

Henson, R.N.A., Shallice, T., & Dolan, R.J. (1999b). Right prefrontal cortex and episodic memory retrieval: a functional MRI test of the monitoring hypothesis. *Brain, 122,* 1367–1381.

Henson, R.N.A., Rugg, M.D., Shallice, T., & Dolan, R.J. (2000). Confidence in word recognition: dissociating right prefrontal roles in episodic retrieval. *Journal of Cognitive Neuroscience, 12,* 913–923.

Jacoby, L.L. (1996). Dissociating automatic and consciously controlled effects of study-test compatibility. *Journal of Memory and Language, 35,* 32–52.

Jahanshahi, M., Dirnberger, G., Fuller, R., & Frith, C.D. (2000). The role of dorsolateral prefrontal cortex in random number generation: a study with positron emission tomography. *NeuroImage, 12,* 713–725.

Jueptner, M., Stephan, K.M., Frith, C.D., Brooks, D.J., Frackowiak, R.S.J., & Passingham, R.E. (1997). Anatomy of motor learning. I. Frontal cortex and attention to action. *Journal of Neurophysiology, 77,* 1313–1324.

Knight, R.T. (1984). Decreased response to novel stimuli after prefrontal lesions in man. *Electroencephalography and Clinical Neurophysiology, 59,* 9–20.

Knight, R.T. & Scabini, D. (1998). Anatomic bases of event-related potentials and their relationship to novelty detection in humans. *Journal of Clinical Neurophysiology, 15,* 3–13.

Krause, P.J., Elvang-Goransson, M., & Fox, J. (1995). A logic of argumentation for uncertain reasoning. *Computational Intelligence, 11,* 113–131.

Levine, E., Black, S.E., Cabeza, R., Sinden, M., McIntosh, A.R., Toth, J.P., Tulving, E. & Sruss, D.T. (1998). Episodic memory and the self in a case of retrograde amnesia. *Brain, 121,* 1951–1973.

Mandler, G. (1967). Organization and memory. In: K. Spence & J.T. Spence (Eds.), *The Psychology of Learning and Motivation, Vol. 1* (pp. 327–372). New York: Academic Press.

Mandler, G. (1980). Recognizing: the judgment of previous occurrence. *Psychological Review, 87,* 252–271.

McDermott, J. & Forgy, C. (1978). Production system conflict resolution strategies. In: D.A. Waterman & F. Hayes-Roth (Eds.), *Pattern-Directed Inference Systems* (pp. 177–199). New York: Academic Press.

Miller, E.K. (2000). The neural basis of top-down control of visual attention in prefrontal cortex. In: S. Monsell & J. Driver (Eds.), *Control of Cognitive Processes: Attention and Performance XVIII* (pp. 511–534). Cambridge, MA: MIT Press.

Milner, B. (1971). Interhemispheric differences in the localisation of psychological processes in man. *British Medical Bulletin, 27,* 272–277.

Moscovitch, M. (1994). Cognitive resources and dual-taste interference effects at retrieval in normal people: The role of the frontal lobes and medial temporal cortex. *Neuropsychology, 8,* 524–533.

Newell, A. (1990). *Unified Theories of Cognition.* Cambridge MA: Harvard University Press.

Norman, D.A. & Bobrow, D.G. (1979). Descriptions: an intermediate stage in memory retrieval. *Cognitive Psychology, 11,* 107–123.

Norman, D.A., & Shallice, T. (1980). Attention to action: willed and automatic control of behavior. *Center for Human Information Processing, Technical Report No. 99.* Reprinted in revised form in R.J. Davidson, G.E. Schwartz, & D. Shapiro (Eds.), (1986) *Consciousness and Self-regulation, Vol 4* (pp. 1–18). New York: Plenum Press.

Owen, A.M., Downes, J.D., Sahakian, B.J., Polkey, C.E., & Robbins, T.W. (1990). Planning and spatial working memory following frontal lobe lesions in man. *Neuropsychologia, 28,* 1021–1034.

Pardo, J.V., Fox, P.T., & Raichle, M.E. (1991) Localisation of a human system for sustained attention by PET. *Nature, 349,* 61–63.

Poldrack, R.A., Wagner, A.D., Prull, M.W., Desmond, J.K., Glover, G.H., & Gabrieli, J.D.E. (1999). Func-

tional generalisation for semantic and phonological processing in the left inferior prefrontal cortex. *NeuroImage, 10,* 15–35.

Raichle, M.E., Fiez, J.A., Videen, T.O., MacLeod, A.M.K., Pardo, J.V., Fox, P.T., & Petersen, S.E. (1994). Practice related changes in human brain functional anatomy during nonmotor learning. *Cerebral Cortex, 4,* 8–26.

Rumiati, R., Zanini, S., Vorano, L., & Shallice, T. (2001). A form of ideational apraxia as a selective deficit of contention scheduling. *Cognitive Neuropsychology.*

Schacter, D.L., Reiman, E., Curran, T., Yun, L.S., Bandy, D., & McDermott, K.B. (1996). Neuroanatomical correlates of veridical and illusory recognition memory: evidence from positron emission tomography. *Neuron, 17,* 267–274.

Schank, R.C. (1982). *Dynamic Memory.* Cambridge; UK: Cambridge University Press.

Schwartz, M.F., Reed, E.S., Montgomery, M.W., Palmer, C. & Mayer, N.H. (1991). The quantitative description of action disorganization after brain damage: A case study. *Cognitive Neuropsychology, 8,* 381–414.

Shallice, T. (1982). Specific impairments of planning. *Philosophical Transactions of the Royal Society of London B: Biological Sciences, 298,* 199–209.

Shallice, T. (1988). *From Neuropsychology to Mental Structure.* Cambridge; UK: Cambridge University Press.

Shallice, T. (2001). Deconstructing 'retrieval mode'. In: M. Naveh-Benjamin, M. Moscovitch, & H.L. Roediger III (Eds.), *Perspectives on Human Memory and Cognitive Aging: Essays in Honour of Fergus Craik.* Philadelphia: Psychology Press.

Shallice, T. & Burgess, P.W. (1991). Deficits in strategy application following frontal lobe damage in man. *Brain, 114,* 727–741.

Shallice, T. & Burgess, P.W. (1996). Domains of supervisory control and the temporal organisation of behaviour. *Philosophical Transactions of the Royal Society of London B: Biological Sciences 351,* 1405–1412.

Shallice, T. & Evans, M.E. (1978). The involvement of the frontal lobes in cognitive estimation. *Cortex, 14,* 294–303.

Shallice, T., Fletcher, P.C., Frith, C.D., Grasby, P., Frackowiak, R.S.J., & Dolan, R.J. (1994). Brain regions associated with the acquisition and retrieval of verbal episodic memory. *Nature, 386,* 633–635.

Stuss, D.T. & Benson, D.F. (1986). *The Frontal Lobes.* New York: Raven Press.

Stuss, D.T., Alexander, M.P., Palumbo, C.L., Buckle, L., Sayer, L., & Pogue, J. (1994). Organizational strategies of patients with unilateral or bilateral frontal lobe injury in word list learning tasks. *Neuropsychology, 8,* 355–373.

Sussman, G.J. (1975). *A Computational Model of Skill Acquisition.* New York: Elsevier.

Thompson-Schill, S.L., D'Esposito, M., Aguirre, G.K., & Farah, M.J. (1997). Role of left inferior prefrontal cortex in retrieval of semantic knowledge: a reevaluation. *Proceedings of the National Academy of Sciences USA 94,* 14792–14797.

Tulving, E. (1983). *Elements of Episodic Memory.* New York: Oxford University Press.

Tulving, E. (1985). Memory and consciousness. *Canadian Journal of Psychology, 26,* 1–12.

Uhl, F., Podreka, I., & Deecke, L. (1994). Anterior prefrontal cortex and the effect of proactive interference in word pair learning—results of brain-SPECT. *Neuropsychologia, 32,* 241–247.

Warrington, E.K. & Shallice, T. (1984). Category-specific semantic memory impairment. *Brain, 107,* 829—854.

Wilding, E.L. & Rugg, M.D. (1996). An event-related potential study of recognition memory with and without retrieval of source. *Brain, 119,* 889–906.

Wilkins, A.J., Shallice, T., & McCarthy, R. (1987). Frontal lesions and sustained attention *Neuropsychologia, 25,* 359–365.

18

Cognitive Focus through Adaptive Neural Coding in the Primate Prefrontal Cortex

JOHN DUNCAN AND EARL K. MILLER

Many of the most conspicuous successes in systems neuroscience derive from an approach of "divide and conquer," or progressively finer and finer subdivision of the brain into local functional components. In both monkeys and humans, for example, the cortical visual system has been divided into an increasing number of subdivisions, or "visual areas," to some extent specialized for different aspects of visual function such as object recognition, perception of scene layout, visuomotor control, and so on (Desimone & Ungerleider, 1989; Tootell et al., 1998).

The success of this strategy finds its reflection in many current views of prefrontal function, with proposals that different regions of prefrontal cortex may be implicated in specific cognitive control functions such as set switching, inhibition of inappropriate behavior, strategy selection, or maintenance and organization of working memory. Many functional imaging experiments, for example, have attempted to localize specific control functions of this sort. The hope in this endeavour is to produce some road map of prefrontal functions comparable to that now available for the cortical visual system.

In this chapter we present some rather different ideas about the organization of prefrontal cortex. Rather than fixed functional spe-cialization, our view emphasizes adaptability of neural coding to fit behavioral context. In particular, we present both neuroimaging and single-unit electrophysiological evidence to suggest that, in selected regions of prefrontal cortex, neurons adapt their properties to code just that information of relevance to current behavior. This adaptation, we suggest, is a major contributor to achievement of cognitive focus and control. Although this adaptive coding model recognizes important regional specializations within prefrontal cortex, it suggests a perspective on these that is rather different from that presumed in the traditional divide-and-conquer approach. The focus of this chapter will be evidence for adaptive neural coding and its implications for prefrontal topography. For more detailed discussion of how such adaptive mechanisms can be used to orchestrate voluntary, goal-directed behavior, we refer the reader to recent papers by Miller (2000) and Miller and Cohen (2001).

IMAGING STUDIES

One important line of evidence comes from human neuroimaging studies. As we have said, a large body of imaging and other work has sought neural underpinnings for such traditional frontal functions as working memory, response inhibition, and so on. Different aspects of working memory function, for example, have been ascribed to dorsal and ventral subdivisions of the lateral frontal surface (Goldman-Rakic, 1988; Petrides, 1994). Response inhibition, traditionally associated with orbitofrontal cortex (Fuster, 1989), has more recently been linked with the anterior cingulate (Pardo et al., 1990). In a recent review (Duncan & Owen, 2000), we attempted a systematic analysis of what functional neuroimaging actually tells us about prefrontal regional specializations of this sort.

Our aim was to compare the distribution of prefrontal recruitment for different kinds of cognitive demand. In particular, we sought to combine data from published positron emission tomography (PET) and functional magnetic resonance imaging (fMRI) studies that, as carefully as possible, had manipulated only a specified demand in the context of an otherwise identical task. As it turned out, we were able to find suitable data for five aspects of cognitive demand. For each demand, we listed foci of activation within prefrontal cortex from all relevant studies we could find in the literature, allowing a comparison of overall distributions of activation for the five demand types.

As we have already mentioned, one common suggestion is that prefrontal cortex is important in suppression of strong but inappropriate response tendencies. In line with this, the first demand we analyzed was strength of response conflict. In high-conflict conditions, stimulus materials cued strong but inappropriate responses. For example, subjects might be asked to name the color of a letter string that itself spelled a conflicting color name (Stroop, 1935), or to make an eye movement in the opposite direction when a cue appeared in the peripheral visual field (Sweeney et al., 1996). In low-conflict conditions, the inappropriate response tendency was weakened or removed; for example, the letter string might now spell a neutral, non-color word, or the eye movement might now be made towards rather than away from the visual stimulus. For all six studies of this sort, we listed prefrontal activation foci for a direct comparison of high- and low-conflict conditions.

A second common theme in discussions of prefrontal function is the importance of task novelty. In particular, the suggestion is that prefrontal control is more important in the early, "attentional" phase of performance than in later, more automatic stages. To capture this we combined data from five experiments comparing early and late phases of tasks in a variety of cognitive domains (motor learning, word retrieval, etc.). We listed prefrontal activation foci for direct comparisons of early and late task phases.

In line with the recent emphasis on a prefrontal role in working memory, our next two demands concerned simple working memory tasks in which a list of one to six locations, letters, or other stimuli was to be retained for a period of a few seconds, followed by some straightforward test of either recognition or recall. We combined data from two studies manipulating the number of items to be retained, listing activation foci for direct comparisons of more and fewer items. In a separate list, we combined data from three studies manipulating delay between presentation and test, listing activation foci for direct comparisons of long and short delay.

Finally, we thought it useful to include a demand less conventionally associated with prefrontal function. For this purpose we chose perceptual difficulty, for example, object recognition under conditions of high versus low stimulus degradation. We combined data from four such experiments, listing activation foci for direct comparisons of hard and easy stimulus conditions.

The results appear in Figure 18–1. To produce this figure, all reported prefrontal activation peaks, excluding only those lying in primary motor (Brodmann's area 4) or premotor (Brodmann's area 6) cortex, have been plotted together onto a single brain. Different letters distinguish the five different types of cognitive demand. The figure shows lateral (top row) and medial (middle row) views of each hemisphere, along with views of the whole brain from above (bottom left) and below (bottom right).

A first striking result is anatomical specific-

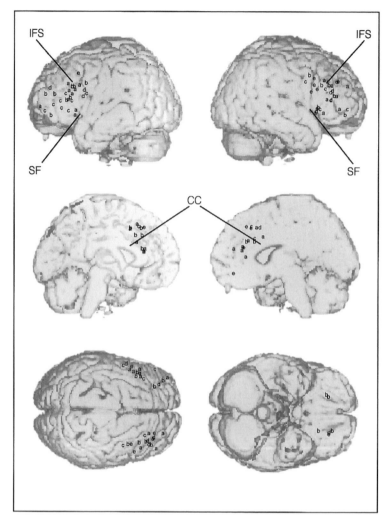

Figure 18–1. Frontal activations associated with five cognitive demands. Activations are from 20 studies addressing response conflict (a); task novelty (b); number of elements in working memory (c); working memory delay (d); and perceptual difficulty (e). Shown are lateral (*top row*) and medial (*middle row*) views of each hemisphere, along with whole brain views from above (*bottom left*) and below (*bottom right*). CC, corpus callosum; IFS, inferior frontal sulcus; SF, Sylvian fissure. (*Source:* Adapted with permission from Duncan and Owen, 2000).

ity. Although these are widely different experiments, differently conducted and analyzed and concerned with quite different cognitive demands, activations are clustered within restricted regions of prefrontal cortex. On the medial surface this clustering is particularly clear, with almost all reported activations lying in or adjacent to the dorsal part of the anterior cingulate. On the lateral surface the distribution is more diffuse, but again, there are evident clusters around the middle and posterior part of the inferior frontal sulcus (IFS), and more ventrally along the frontal operculum towards the anterior insula (appearing in Fig. 18–1 as points clustered just anterior to the Sylvian fissure). Only occasional activations appear on the orbital surface (Fig. 18–1, bottom brain view).

The second important result is essentially complete overlap of activations associated with the five different cognitive demands. Statistical comparisons between the three-dimensional distributions of activation foci associated with each possible pair of demands revealed no significant differences. Furthermore, even individual experiments often showed the full pattern of joint activation in the region surrounding the IFS, on the frontal operculum, and in the dorsal anterior cingulate. Evidently, this is a common pattern of frontal recruitment associated with increased demand or difficulty in many different cognitive domains. Indeed, once this basic pattern is recognized it is easily found in studies of perception, response selection, task switching, problem solving, language, episodic memory, and doubtless many other cognitive activities (Duncan & Owen, 2000).

On the one hand, these results offer strong evidence of regional specialization within prefrontal cortex. Certainly only restricted prefrontal regions show demand-related activation in these studies. On the other hand, this specialization takes an unexpected form—a specific set of frontal regions jointly recruited by diverse cognitive demands. Of course, there are limitations to how much we can conclude from functional imaging evidence of this sort. Limited spatial resolution, for example, leaves open the possibility that different cognitive demands are indeed associated with different recruitment patterns at a scale finer than PET or fMRI can distinguish. At the same time, the data are certainly consistent with the possibility of adaptive function in this set of frontal regions. To some extent at least, the same frontal neurons may be configured to aid in solution of many different cognitive challenges. In the following section we present more direct evidence in favor of this suggestion, coming from neurophysiological and behavioral studies in monkeys.

STUDIES IN MONKEYS

Most neurophysiological studies of monkey prefrontal cortex have focused on the lateral areas most directly connected with sensory and motor systems. This includes the dorsolateral region around and just dorsal to the principle sulcus, the ventrolateral surface just ventral to the principle sulcus, and the region around the arcuate sulcus (Fig. 18–2A). In fact, an obvious property of these neurons is their ability to adapt to behavioral context. With behavioral training, the activity of many lateral prefrontal cortex neurons comes to code information relevant to the trained task—information concerning cues, voluntary actions, and rewards that is central to cognitive control (Miller, 2000; Miller & Cohen, 2001).

An example of such adaptation to task con-

text is provided in a recent study by Freedman and colleagues (2001). A three-dimensional morphing system was used to generate stimuli spanning two categories, "cats" and "dogs". Three species of cats and three breeds of dogs served as prototypes (Fig. 18–2B); the morphed images were linear combinations of all possible prototype pairs (Fig. 18–2B, double-headed arrows). By blending different amounts of prototypes C1 and D1, for example, we were able to vary a stimulus continuously from "cat" to "dog", while by blending C1 and C2 we could continuously change from one cat to another.

In the main experiment, only the "cat–dog" categorization was relevant to the animal's task (Fig. 18–2B, two-class boundary). Specifically, animals were asked to decide whether "sample" and "choice" stimuli, each presented for 600 ms and separated by an interval of 1000 ms, came from the same or different categories. After training in this task, many prefrontal neurons gave categorical responses (Fig. 18–2C): neural activity differentiated between cats and dogs, even those close together across the category boundary, but much less between morphs within a category. Categorical "cat–dog" activity is unlikely to be a common property of prefrontal neurons outside the context of this task—in fact, monkeys had no prior experience with cats or dogs. So, already the data suggest that prefrontal neurons have been tuned to carry exactly that stimulus information of relevance to current behavior. This conclusion was directly confirmed in a follow-up study: When one animal was retrained to use new, orthogonal category boundaries (Fig. 18–B, 3-class boundaries), "cat–dog" categorization was lost from the neural response and was replaced with the new, now-relevant categorization.

Other examples of such tuning by behavioral training are easy to find. Bichot and colleagues (1996) found that neurons in the frontal eye fields (in the bow of the arcuate sulcus), which are ordinarily selective to spatial information related to voluntary eye movements and not selective to the form and color of stimuli, became selective for a color after the animal learned eye movements that were contingent on that color. In the experiments

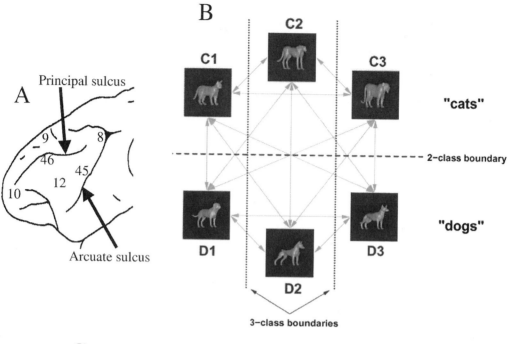

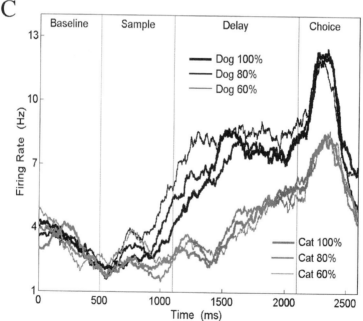

Figure 18–2. *A:* Lateral view of the macaque monkey prefrontal cortex. Cytoarchitectonic areas are numbered and shown in their approximate location. *B:* Monkeys learned to categorize randomly generated "morphs" from the vast number of possible blends of six prototypes. For neurophysiological recording, 54 sample stimuli were constructed along the 15 morph lines illustrated here. The placement of the prototypes on this figure does not reflect their similarity. *C:* Average activity of a single neuron to stimuli at the six morph blends. The vertical lines correspond (from left to right) to sample onset, offset, and choice stimulus onset. Note that this neuron responded similarly to dogs, regardless of their level of "dogness," and similarly to cats, regardless of their level of "catness." (*Source:* Adapted with permission from Freedman et al., 2001)

of Watanabe (1990, 1992), lateral prefrontal neurons (around the arcuate sulcus and posterior end of the principal sulcus) came to reflect learned associations between visual and auditory cues and whether they signaled that a reward was forthcoming or would be withheld. Fuster and colleagues (2000) recently showed that lateral prefrontal neurons reflect learned associations between visual and auditory cues.

Importantly, adaptation does not require a great deal of time or practice; changes in prefrontal neural properties can be observed after relatively little experience. As one example, Bichot and Schall (1999) found that just a few hours' experience on one day left an "impression" on the prefrontal cortex that interfered with processing on the next day when task demands had changed. They trained monkeys to search for a different visual target each day and found that neurons in the arcuate sulcus region not only discriminated the current target but also distracting stimuli that had been targets on the previous day, relative to stimuli that had been targets even earlier. This seems to have accounted for the fact that monkeys were more likely to make errors in choosing these distractors that were the previous day's targets. Asaad and colleagues (1998) reported neural correlates of stimulus–response learning in the lateral prefrontal cortex that occurred very rapidly in just 5–15 behavioral trials and over a few minutes.

Adaptability of neural response can also easily be seen following a shift of task structure or rule. Behavioral studies suggest that rule representation is a cardinal prefrontal function (Passingham, 1993; Grafman, 1994; Wise et al., 1996). Asaad and colleagues (2000) trained monkeys to switch between tasks using three different rules: matching (delayed matching to sample), associative (conditional visuomotor), or spatial (spatial delayed response). Recording from the same neurons in the three different tasks showed that, for many prefrontal neurons, activity depended on which task was currently in force. That is, a given neuron might be activated by a cue object during one task (e.g., the associative task), but be unresponsive when the same cue appeared under identical sensory conditions during another

task (e.g., the matching task). While the lateral prefrontal cortex did contain many neurons that were responsive to a given stimulus or action (saccade) across multiple tasks, the baseline activity of about half of the neurons encountered varied with the task; a given neuron might consistently show higher baseline activity whenever the monkey performed the matching task, for example. These results indicate that prefrontal neurons do not simply code stimuli or actions. Rather, they also convey their behavioral context, the pattern of associated information that is unique to a particular task or operation. White and Wise (1999) also found that the activity of up to half of lateral prefrontal neurons depended on whether the monkey was guiding behavior by a spatial rule (a cue's location indicated where the target would appear) or an associative rule (the identity of the cue indicated the target's location), and Hoshi and colleagues (1998) reported that responses to a cue in many lateral prefrontal neurons were modulated by which rule (matching shape or location) the monkey was currently using.

This flexibility may explain why different studies using different tasks to study the same prefrontal regions nonetheless all report high proportions of neurons with task-related activity. In a study by Asaad et al. (1998), for example, almost half of lateral prefrontal neurons (44%) reflected newly learned object-saccade associations. This is remarkable considering that in these and other studies from these investigators, neurons were not prescreened for responsiveness. Instead, each electrode was advanced until the activity of one or more neurons was well isolated, and then data collection began, a procedure used to ensure an unbiased estimate of prefrontal activity. Watanabe (1992) has also reported that as many as half of lateral prefrontal neurons reflect learned associations between a cue and reward, and White and Wise (1999) found that about half of lateral prefrontal neurons coded one of two rules (matching versus spatial) that the animal had learned. Plasticity in the prefrontal cortex may have resulted in neurons being co-opted for the task at hand, just as long-term training on somatosensory discrimination changes the representation of corresponding body parts in primary sensory cortex (Recanzone et al., 1992a, 1992b).

In line with the imaging studies described earlier, several general factors may influence the number of prefrontal neurons recruited for a given task. First there are the effects of long-term familiarity. Highly familiar stimuli or task conditions produce weaker activity than novel stimuli or newly learned task conditions (Asaad et al., 1998; Rainer & Miller, 2000). It may be that many neurons are recruited for the acquisition of a given task, but then as the task becomes highly familiar, neurons are winnowed from the population, leaving behind a smaller, but more robust and efficient neural representation (Li et al., 1993; Rainer & Miller, 2000). This would be consistent with the imaging studies reviewed earlier, indicating that selective prefrontal regions show diminished activity after task learning. Also in line with imaging studies, task difficulty in general is likely to be a major influence. Neurons in the extrastriate cortex (which provides a route for visual input to the lateral prefrontal cortex) have been shown to markedly increase their activity with increased task difficulty (Spitzer et al., 1988). Although there has not been a thorough, systematic study of the effects of task difficulty on lateral prefrontal neurons, there are striking differences in that a minority of neurons are engaged by tasks that, on face value, seem relatively easy, such as delayed matching-to-sample or spatial delayed response (Fuster et al., 1982; Funahashi et al., 1989), while many neurons are engaged by tasks that seem relatively difficult, such as those requiring new learning or having high attentional demands (Asaad et al., 1998; Rainer et al., 1998b).

THE ADAPTIVE CODING MODEL

A simple model sums up the above ideas. Though very much an outline, it provides an alternative perspective to the traditional emphasis on tight regional specialization. Given our emphasis on adaptability or plasticity in prefrontal function, we call this the *adaptive coding* model.

Three ideas are prominent in theoretical accounts of prefrontal function. First is the concept of *working memory,* or temporary representation of information, which is motivated by well-known deficits in delayed-response and other short-term retention tasks following prefrontal lesions in the monkey (Jacobsen, 1935). Second is the concept of *selective attention,* or focus on specific information of relevance to current behavior, which is related to distractability and processing of irrelevant input following frontal damage (Malmo, 1942; Chao & Knight, 1998). Third is the concept of *control,* or direction of mental activity in line with current task plans or goals, reflected in the general disorganization of behavior in patients with frontal lesions (Luria, 1966). The adaptive coding model has obvious similarities to other accounts based on each of these concepts (see, e.g., Norman & Shallice, 1980; Engle et al., 1999; Braver & Cohen, 2000; and in particular, Dehaene et al., 1998). Aspects of this account are extended in other recent presentations (Miller, 2000; Miller & Cohen, 2001).

The model is based on three proposals. First, we suggest that in much of frontal cortex—certainly including much of the lateral surface, and perhaps also other regions—neurons are substantially *adaptable or programmable* on the basis of current behavioral concerns. In particular, they can be configured to carry that specific information of relevance to a current task; in other words, they serve as a global working memory for currently important information. In the single-unit data, as we have seen, adaptability is directly shown by changes in the information that neurons carry in different task conditions, and indeed is strongly implied by the simple finding that, whatever (arbitrary) task a monkey has been trained to do, a high proportion of recorded frontal neurons carry information about events in that task. In imaging, adaptability is suggested by highly similar patterns of frontal recruitment for very different cognitive demands.

Second, it follows that prefrontal coding can also be seen as a *global attention system,* focusing selectively on relevant information and discarding that which is irrelevant. If a given neuron can carry different information in different task contexts, it follows that, for any given context, there is selective pruning out of all those inputs that can potentially drive the cell but currently are unwanted.

Third, we suggest that highly selective representation of task-relevant information in prefrontal cortex also serves to *control or direct* the function of other brain systems (Desimone & Duncan, 1995). In most systems, we suspect that processing is competitive, such that increased representation of one cognitive element is bought at the expense of decreased representation for others. In visual areas, for example, a strong representation of any one object in the visual input inhibits or weakens the representation of others (Reynolds et al., 1999), and we suspect that similar principles apply in other sensory modalities, in motor processing, in semantic memory activation, and so on. If strong prefrontal representation of some cognitive element strengthens or supports representation of that same element elsewhere in the brain, this will provide a basis for frontal control: multiple systems will tend to converge to represent or give dominance to just those elements or just that information required in the current task (Desimone & Duncan, 1995; Duncan, 1996). In line with the common observation that frontal lesions impair active, attentional control of behavior (Luria, 1966; Norman & Shallice, 1980; Duncan et al., 1996), we suggest that this selective convergence of mental representation on currently relevant or useful information corresponds to the subjective state of active attentional focus. We suggest that this process is fundamental in configuring a highly flexible cognitive system for coherent attack on specific current concerns.

Admittedly, this model is little more than a framework for future development. Experimental work is just beginning, for example, on interactions between frontal and posterior cortical systems (Tomita et al., 1999), and at this stage little definite is known. Neither have we addressed the question of *how* the frontal representation is able to focus on information of significance in the current behavioral context (see, e.g., Braver & Cohen, 2000). As emphasized by Shallice (1982) and others, this is the conceptual problem addressed by many planning and problem-solving systems, which must combine goals with knowledge to determine which facts and action plans are germane to goal achievement (e.g., Newell, 1990). Limited as it is, however, the adaptive coding model provides a useful context for considering a range of questions relating to prefrontal function. In the following section, we provide two illustrative examples.

APPLICATIONS

SPECIALIZATION, ADAPTATION, AND RECRUITMENT

To some extent, adaptability is the converse of specialization. In imaging data, as we have seen, different cognitive demands lead to highly similar patterns of prefrontal recruitment. In single-unit data, it certainly happens that neurons carrying many different types of task-relevant information—information about stimuli in different sensory modalities, intended actions, task rules, working memory for both location and object information, and expected or available rewards—are found mixed together over very much the same extent of the lateral frontal cortex (see, e.g., Watanabe, 1990; Quintana & Fuster, 1992; Bichot et al., 1996; Rao et al., 1997; Asaad et al., 1998; Rainer et al., 1998a; White & Wise, 1999; see Chapter 21). Different prefrontal subdivisions have partly unique, but overlapping, patterns of connections with all sensory systems, motor system structures, and brain areas processing information about motivation state and reward. Furthermore, as in much of the neocortex, most prefrontal connections are local; there are extensive interconnections between different prefrontal subregions and divisions. Thus, the prefrontal cortex seems ideally suited for intermixing of the "outputs" of other brain systems. This presumably provides a basis for their synthesis, as would be required for a system involved in the orchestration of complex behavior.

This is not to say, however, that all prefrontal neurons are equipotential for carrying all types of information. In contrast, it seems highly likely that, for any given type of information, there is some distribution across frontal cortex of neurons with potential for carrying that information. For different kinds of information, these distributions may be broad and overlapping, but quite possibly with different shapes and in particular different peaks of maximum selectivity.

This view, indeed, is supported by single-unit evidence. In one study, Ó Scalaidhe and colleagues (1999) assessed face and object selectivity in both dorsal and ventral convexities of the lateral frontal surface. Restricting analysis to a small fraction of the most selective cells (5% of the population), they found a concentration on the inferior convexity, the region directly in receipt of temporal lobe afferents. As criteria for "selectivity" were progressively relaxed, however, the distribution of object-selective cells became progressively broader.

Such results bear importantly on the form of regional specialization to be expected in imaging studies. With low statistical power, or low level of demand, two kinds of information or cognitive events might appear to recruit different prefrontal regions. This difference would indicate different regions of peak sensitivity. With greater power or demand, however, distributions of recruitment would increasingly overlap, indicating the full extent of potentially relevant tissue.

One good example concerns hemispheric specialization for stimulus materials. In working memory and other studies, there is some evidence for selective activation of the left prefrontal cortex when materials are verbal (e.g., Postle & D'Esposito, 2000). This selectivity, however, is far from absolute; homologous right hemisphere regions, strongly activated by working memory for spatial and other materials, are simply more weakly activated in the verbal case (Postle & D'Esposito, 2000). Such results are well explained by the proposal that neurons able to carry verbal information are to some extent distributed in both hemispheres, but with highest concentration on the left.

Another possible example concerns hemispheric specialization for encoding and retrieval phases of standard episodic memory tasks. Across many experiments, a strong trend has been reported for greater left frontal activation during encoding, and greater right frontal activation during retrieval. The result, however, may depend on level of demand; in a recent review, Nolde and colleagues (1998) suggest that retrieval activation becomes increasingly bilateral as retrieval difficulty is increased. This is the result we should expect if the full distribution of relevant cells is bilateral but more concentrated on the right; with increasing demand, there will be increasing recruitment of the full bilateral network.

A third possible example concerns apparent reconfiguration of frontal function following unilateral damage. As soon as 3 days after a stroke affecting the left inferior frontal gyrus, a verbal task usually activating this region can instead recruit the homologous region on the right (Thulborn et al., 1999; Rosen et al., 2000). If relevant cells are distributed in both hemispheres, but most densely on the left, then this result would not necessarily reflect any radical reconfiguration of processing after damage. In normal subjects, relatively weak recruitment would be manifest as predominant activity on the left. In patients, task demands could no longer be satisfied in this way; instead, stronger recruitment would reveal the latent, relevant cell population on the right. In line with this account, even some normal control subjects show weak right-sided activation in these tasks (Rosen et al., 2000).

Our view also bears on the form of regional specialization expected in monkey studies. For example, consider the well-known (partial) separation in the visual cortex of the processing of information about color and form used to identify an object (*what*) from that used to discern its location in space (*where*). This separation has been suggested to continue into the prefrontal cortex, with the ventrolateral region being responsible for processing *what* and the dorsolateral region being responsible for processing *where* (Wilson et al., 1993). Lesion studies in the monkey suggest some difference along these lines. Dorsolateral lesions (especially those restricted to area 46) sometimes impair spatial memory, but not object memory, tasks, while ventrolateral lesions can impair some object memory tasks (Mishkin, 1957; Gross & Weiskrantz, 1962; Mishkin & Manning, 1978). It is important to note, however, that the dissociation is not complete. Spatial-reversal tasks can show little or no impairment after dorsolateral lesions (Goldman et al., 1971; Passingham, 1975; Gaffan & Harrison, 1989); dorsolateral lesions can impair certain object tasks, such as those requiring memory for a sequence of object choices (Petrides, 1995), and ventrolateral lesions can impair some spatial tasks (Mishkin et al., 1969; Passingham, 1975). Overall, these results are more in line with a quantitative rather than qualitative distinction between dorsolateral and ventrolateral regions. Physiological data are similar, showing both *what-* and *where-*selective neurons broadly distributed across dorsal and ventral convexities (Rao et al., 1997; Rainer et al., 1998a; White & Wise, 1999), though perhaps with some differences in relative prominence from one region to another (Rainer et al., 1998a).

As we have said, the bulk of the single-unit evidence bearing on adaptive coding comes from recordings on the lateral frontal surface. On the one hand, the imaging evidence we reviewed suggests close collaboration among dorsolateral, opercular, and dorsal anterior cingulate regions, all of which are co-recruited by many forms of cognitive demand. On the other hand, this evidence suggests a definite distinction from other frontal regions, including much of the medial and orbital surfaces. In the monkey, one of the best-established functional differences between different frontal regions involves the orbitofrontal and lateral prefrontal cortices. Anatomical and behavioral studies suggest that the orbitofrontal cortex is more involved in processing "internal" information such as motivational state and reward value, whereas lateral cortex is more involved with "external" information such as stimuli and responses (see Chapter 21). At the same time, there are many interconnections between these regions, and neurons processing reward information are readily apparent in both, albeit with somewhat larger numbers in the orbitofrontal cortex (see Chapter 21). A topic for future development in the adaptive

coding approach is interaction among lateral, medial, and orbital frontal regions.

SPEARMAN'S *g*

Our second application of the adaptive coding idea concerns individual differences in cognitive activity. Perhaps surprisingly, almost any pair of tasks—whether they emphasize perception, memory, language, motor control, or any other cognitive domain—will show some positive correlation across individuals: to some extent at least, the same people tend to do well even on quite different tasks. To explain this result, Spearman (1904) originally proposed that some general, or *g* factor makes some contribution to success in diverse cognitive activities. Our proposal is that the adaptive coding function of prefrontal cortex makes a contribution to effective cognitive focus in any coherent line of activity. Could it be that this function is one major neural basis for Spearman's *g*?

At the most general level, this proposal is certainly consistent with the characteristic cognitive deficit following human frontal lobe lesions. Rather than highly focal deficits, frontal lesions are typically associated with a broad disorganization of behavior, with coherent task performance being disrupted by omission or neglect of crucial task steps, and interrupted by irrelevant, sometimes bizarre intrusions (Luria, 1966). Quantitatively, patients with frontal lesions are impaired, by comparison with controls, in performing many different tests, including those emphasizing perceptual analysis or classification (Milner, 1963), memory (Milner, 1971), simple response selections (Drewe, 1975), problem solving (Milner, 1965), and many other cognitive domains. Accepting Spearman's model, factor analysis can be used to show which tasks are the best measures of *g*; typically, these turn out to be tests of novel problem solving such as Raven's Progressive Matrices (Raven et al., 1988). Certainly patients with frontal lesions show deficits in these tests (Duncan et al., 1995), and under appropriate circumstances, normal people with poor test scores show the same, detailed neglect of crucial task requirements that is characteristic of frontal patients (Duncan et al., 1996).

In a recent study (Duncan et al., 2000) we used PET to test this hypothesis. Three tasks with high *g* correlations, measured by standard means, were compared with control tasks designed to involve some of the same basic operations but to have lower *g* involvement. The results are shown in Figure 18–3. As predicted by the adaptive coding view, the common element in comparison of the three high-*g* tasks with their corresponding low-*g* controls was activation of dorsal and (in two cases) ventral

A.

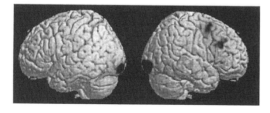

B.

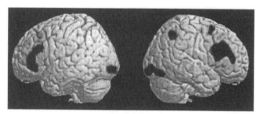

C.

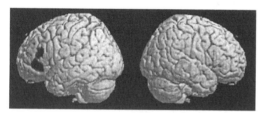

Figure 18–3. Activations for three comparisons of high- and low-*g* task pairs. *A:* Spatial problem solving minus spatial control. *B:* Verbal problem solving minus verbal control. *C:* High- minus low-*g* perceptual comparisons. (*Source:* Adapted with permission from Duncan et al., 2000)

regions of the lateral frontal cortex. Recent replications using fMRI (J. Duncan & D. Bor, unpublished data) show that this activation is commonly bilateral for both spatial and verbal tasks, although in the PET experiment only left hemisphere activity was significant in the verbal case (Fig. 18–3B). The new data also show activation of the dorsal anterior cingulate for all three high-*g* tasks. Obviously, this pattern of prefrontal recruitment is closely similar to what we have already seen in association with a broad range of perceptual, working memory, response inhibition and other cognitive demands (Fig. 18–1). These are exactly the data we should expect if *g* indeed reflects an adaptive coding function important in response to diverse cognitive challenges.

CONCLUSION

The adaptive coding model may be most useful in the direction it suggests for future work. For single-unit physiology, for example, there is perhaps little point in further experiments documenting that, once some new task is trained, many prefrontal units have properties apparently helpful for that task's control. More useful might be direct investigations of change as a task is learned and then later becomes automatized (Chen & Wise, 1995), and of short-term plasticity or reprogramming as the animal changes from one task context to another. According to the model, one key property of the prefrontal representation is its strong selectivity for task-relevant information. This suggests direct quantitative comparison of neural properties—for example, the effects of visual selective attention—in prefrontal and posterior systems (Anderson & Miller, 2000; see also Everling et al., 2000).

For imaging, similarly, there is perhaps little point in further studies documenting the co-recruitment of dorsolateral, ventral/opercular, and dorsal anterior cingulate regions in different task contexts. Instead, the key question is how these regions cooperate to respond to a general increase in task complexity or demand. In light of what we have said, one possibility is substantial flexibility of neural properties in each of these regions, making it difficult to assign them clearly different roles. Alternatively, the three regions may reflect somewhat different aspects of task difficulty or demand. For the anterior insula and adjacent frontal operculum, for example, an important function may be control of the autonomic nervous system (e.g., Mesulam & Mufson, 1982; King, et al., 1999), suggesting a possible role in the arousal/effort aspect of cognitive load (Kahneman, 1973). For the anterior cingulate, one proposal is a role in both cognitive and affective aspects of error/uncertainty detection (MacDonald et al., 2000).

In cognitive neuroscience, one major question is how cognitive and neural entities map onto one another. Although a common hope has been that a defined cognitive process will map onto one or a few defined brain regions, this, of course, is only one of many possibilities. For much of prefrontal cortex, such simple mappings may not be possible. The region may better be seen as a general computational resource, freely adapting to solve many quite different cognitive problems.

REFERENCES

Anderson, K.C. & Miller, E.K. (2000). Neural activity in the prefrontal and posterior parietal cortices during a what-then-where memory task. *Society for Neuroscience Abstracts, 30*, 975.

Asaad W.F., Rainer, G., & Miller, E.K. (1998). Neural activity in the primate prefrontal cortex during associative learning. *Neuron, 21*, 1399–1407.

Asaad, W.F., Rainer, G., & Miller, E.K. (2000). Task-specific neural activity in the primate prefrontal cortex. *Journal of Neurophysiology, 84*, 451–459.

Bichot, N.P. & Schall, J.D. (1999). Effects of similarity and history on neural mechanisms of visual selection. *Nature Neuroscience, 2*, 549–554.

Bichot, N.P. Schall, J.D., & Thompson, K.G. (1996). Visual feature selectivity in frontal eye fields induced by experience in mature macaques. *Nature, 381*, 697–699.

Braver, T.S. & Cohen, J.D. (2000). On the control of control: the role of dopamine in regulating prefrontal function and working memory. In: S. Monsell & J. Driver (Eds.), *Control of Cognitive Processes: Attention and Performance XVIII* (pp. 713–737). Cambridge, MA: MIT Press.

Chao, L.L. & Knight, R.T. (1998). Contribution of human prefrontal cortex to delay performance. *Journal of Cognitive Neuroscience, 10*, 167–177.

Chen, L.L., & Wise, S.P. (1995). Neuronal activity in the

supplementary eye field during acquisition of conditional oculomotor association. *Journal of Neurophysiology, 73*, 1101–1121.

Dehaene, S., Kerszberg, M., & Changeux, J.-P. (1998). A neuronal model of a global workspace in effortful cognitive tasks. *Proceedings of the National Academy of Sciences USA, 95*, 14529–14534.

Desimone, R. & Duncan, J. (1995). Neural mechanisms of selective visual attention. *Annual Review of Neuroscience, 18*, 193–222.

Desimone, R. & Ungerleider, L.G. (1989) Neural mechanisms of visual processing in monkeys. In: F. Boller and J. Grafman (Eds.), *Handbook of Neuropsychology, Vol. 2* (pp. 267–299). Amsterdam: Elsevier.

Drewe, E.A. (1975). Go–no go learning after frontal lobe lesions in humans. *Cortex, 11*, 8–16.

Duncan, J. (1996). Cooperating brain systems in selective perception and action. In: T. Inui & J.L. McClelland (Eds.), *Attention and performance XVI* (pp. 549–578). Cambridge, MA: MIT Press.

Duncan, J. & Owen, A.M. (2000) Common regions of the human frontal lobe recruited by diverse cognitive demands. *Trends in Neurosciences, 23*, 475–483.

Duncan, J., Burgess, P., & Emslie, H. (1995). Fluid intelligence after frontal lobe lesions. *Neuropsychologia, 33*, 261–268.

Duncan, J., Emslie, H., Williams, P., Johnson, R., & Freer, C. (1996). Intelligence and the frontal lobe: the organization of goal-directed behavior. *Cognitive Psychology, 30*, 257–303.

Duncan, J., Seitz, R.J., Kolodny, J., Bor, D., Herzog, H., Ahmed, A., Newell, F.N., & Emslie, H. (2000). A neural basis for general intelligence. *Science, 289*, 457–460.

Engle, R.W., Kane, M.J., & Tuholski, S.W. (1999). Individual differences in working memory capacity and what they tell us about controlled attention, general fluid intelligence and functions of the prefrontal cortex. In: A. Miyake & P. Shah (Eds.), *Models of Working Memory: Mechanisms of Active Maintenance and Executive Control* (pp. 102–134). Cambridge, UK: Cambridge University Press.

Everling, S., Tinsley, C.J., Gaffan, D., & Duncan, J. (2000). Neural activity in a focused attention task in monkey prefrontal cortex. *Society for Neuroscience Abstracts, 30*, 2227.

Freedman, D.J., Riesenhuber, M., Poggio, T., & Miller, E.K. (2001). Categorical representation of visual stimuli in the primate prefrontal cortex. *Science, 291*, 312–316.

Funahashi, S., Bruce, C.J., & Goldman-Rakic, P.S. (1989). Mnemonic coding of visual space in the monkey's dorsolateral prefrontal cortex. *Journal of Neurophysiology, 61*, 331–349.

Fuster, J.M. (1989). *The Prefrontal Cortex: Anatomy, Physiology, and Neuropsychology of the Frontal Lobe*, 2nd ed. New York: Raven Press.

Fuster, J.M., Bauer, R.H., & Jervey, J.P. (1982). Cellular discharge in the dorsolateral prefrontal cortex of the monkey in cognitive tasks. *Experimental Neurology, 77*, 679–694.

Fuster, J.M., Bodner, M., & Kroger, J.K. (2000). Cross-modal and cross-temporal association in neurons of frontal cortex. *Nature, 405,* 347–351.

Gaffan D. & Harrison, S. (1989). A comparison of the effects of fornix transection and sulcus principalis ablation upon spatial learning by monkeys. *Behavioural Brain Research, 31,* 207–220.

Goldman, P.S., Rosvold, H.E., Vest, B., & Galkin, T.W. (1971). Analysis of the delayed-alternation deficit produced by dorsolateral prefrontal lesions in the rhesus monkey. *Journal of Comparative and Physiological Psychology, 77,* 212–220.

Goldman-Rakic, P. (1988). Topography of cognition: parallel distributed networks in primate association cortex. *Annual Review of Neuroscience, 11,* 137–156.

Grafman, J. (1994). Alternative frameworks for the conceptualization of prefrontal functions. In: F. Boller & J. Grafman (Eds.), *Handbook of Neuropsychology* (pp. 187–202). Amsterdam: Elsevier.

Gross, C.G., & Weiskrantz, L. (1962). Evidence for dissociation of impairment on auditory discrimination and delayed response following lateral frontal lesions in monkeys. *Experimental Neurology, 5,* 453–476.

Hoshi, E., Shima, K., & Tanji, J. (1998). Task-dependent selectivity of movement-related neuronal activity in the primate prefrontal cortex. *Journal of Neurophysiology, 80,* 3392–3397.

Jacobsen, C.E. (1935). Functions of the frontal association area in primates. *Archives of Neurological Psychiatry, 33,* 558–569.

Kahneman, D. (1973). *Attention and Effort.* Englewood Cliffs, NJ: Prentice-Hall.

King, A.B., Menon, R.S., Hachinski, V., & Cechetto, D.F. (1999). Human forebrain activation by visceral stimuli. *Journal of Comparative Neurology, 413,* 572–582.

Li, L., Miller, E.K., & Desimone, R. (1993). The representation of stimulus familiarity in anterior inferior temporal cortex. *Journal of Neurophysiology, 69,* 1918–1929.

Luria, A.R. (1966). *Higher Cortical Functions in Man.* London: Tavistock.

MacDonald, A.W., Cohen, J.D., Stenger, V.A., & Carter, C.S. (2000). Dissociating the role of the dorsolateral prefrontal and anterior cingulate cortex in cognitive control. *Science, 280,* 1835–1838.

Malmo, R.R. (1942). Interference factors in delayed response in monkeys after removal of frontal lobes. *Journal of Neurophysiology, 5,* 295–308.

Mesulam, M.-M. & Mufson, E.J. (1982). Insula of the old world monkey. III: Efferent cortical output and comments on function. *Journal of Comparative Neurology, 212,* 38–52.

Miller, E.K. (2000). The prefrontal cortex and cognitive control. *Nature Reviews Neuroscience, 1,* 59–65.

Miller, E.K., & Cohen, J.D. (2001). An integrative theory of prefrontal function. *Annual Review of Neuroscience, 24,* 167–202.

Milner, B. (1963). Effects of different brain lesions on card sorting. *Archives of Neurology, 9,* 90–100.

Milner, B. (1965). Visually-guided maze learning in man: effects of bilateral hippocampal, bilateral frontal and unilateral cerebral lesions. *Neuropsychologia, 3,* 317–338.

Milner, B. (1971). Interhemispheric differences in the localization of psychological processes in man. *British Medical Bulletin, 27,* 272–277.

Mishkin, M. (1957). Effects of small frontal lesions on delayed alternation in monkeys. *Journal of Neurophysiology, 20,* 615–622.

Mishkin, M. & Manning, F.J. (1978). Nonspatial memory after selective prefrontal lesions in monkeys. *Brain Research, 143,* 313–323.

Mishkin, M., Vest, B., Waxler, M., & Rosvold, H.E. (1969). A re-examination of the effects of frontal lesions on object alternation. *Neuropsychologia, 7,* 357–364.

Newell, A. (1990). *Unified Theories of Cognition.* Cambridge, MA: Harvard University Press.

Nolde, S.F., Johnson, M.K., & Raye, C.L. (1998). The role of prefrontal cortex during tests of episodic memory. *Trends in Cognitive Sciences, 2,* 399–406.

Norman, D.A. & Shallice, T. (1980). *Attention to Action: Willed and Automatic Control of Behavior* (Report No. 8006). San Diego, CA: University of California, Center for Human Information Processing.

Ó Scalaidhe, P., Wilson, F.A.W., & Goldman-Rakic, P.S. (1999). Face-selective neurons during passive viewing and working memory performance of rhesus monkeys: evidence for intrinsic specialization of neuronal coding. *Cerebral Cortex, 9,* 459–475.

Pardo, J.V., Pardo, P.J., Janer, K.W., & Raichle, M.E. (1990). The anterior cingulate cortex mediates processing selection in the Stroop attentional conflict paradigm. *Proceedings of the National Academy of Sciences USA, 87,* 256–259.

Passingham, R. (1975). Delayed matching after selective prefrontal lesions in monkeys (*Macaca mulatta*). *Brain Research, 92,* 89–102.

Passingham, R. (1993). *The Frontal Lobes and Voluntary Action.* Oxford: Oxford University Press.

Petrides, M. (1994) Frontal lobes and working memory: evidence from investigations of the effects of cortical excisions in nonhuman primates. In: F. Boller & J. Grafman (Eds.), *Handbook of Neuropsychology, Vol. 9* (pp. 59–82). Amsterdam: Elsevier.

Petrides, M. (1995). Impairments on nonspatial self-ordered and externally ordered working memory tasks after lesions of the mid-dorsal part of the lateral frontal cortex of the monkey. *Journal of Neuroscience, 15,* 359–375.

Postle, B.R. & D'Esposito, M. (2000). Evaluating models of the topographical organization of working memory function in frontal cortex with event-related fMRI. *Psychobiology, 28,* 146–155.

Quintana, J. & Fuster, J.M. (1992). Mnemonic and predictive functions of cortical neurons in a memory task. *NeuroReport, 3,* 721–724.

Rainer, G., & Miller, E.K. (2000). Effects of visual experience on the representation of objects in the prefrontal cortex. *Neuron, 27,* 179–189.

Rainer, G., Asaad, W.F., & Miller, E.K. (1998a). Memory fields of neurons in the primate prefrontal cortex. *Pro-*

ceedings of National Academy of Sciences USA, 95, 15008–15013.

Rainer, G., Asaad, W.F., & Miller, E.K. (1998b). Selective representation of relevant information by neurons in the primate prefrontal cortex. *Nature, 393*, 577–579.

Rao, S.C., Rainer, G., & Miller, E.K. (1997). Integration of what and where in the primate prefrontal cortex. *Science, 276*, 821–824.

Raven, J.C., Court J.H., & Raven, J. (1988). *Manual for Raven's Progressive Matrices and Vocabulary Scales*. London: H.K. Lewis.

Recanzone, G.H., Merzenich, M.M., & Jenkins, W.M. (1992a). Frequency discrimination training engaging a restricted skin surface results in an emergence of a cutaneous response zone in cortical area 3a. *Journal of Neurophysiology, 67*, 1057–1070.

Recanzone, G.H., Merzenich, M.M., Jenkins, W.M., Grajski, K.A., & Dinse, H.R. (1992b). Topographic reorganization of the hand representation in cortical area 3b of owl monkeys trained in a frequency-discrimination task. *Journal of Neurophysiology, 67*, 1031–1056.

Reynolds, J.H., Chelazzi, L., & Desimone, R. (1999). Competitive mechanisms subserve attention in macaque areas V2 and V4. *Journal of Neuroscience, 19*, 1736–1743.

Rosen, H.J., Petersen, S.E., Linenweber, M., Snyder, A.Z., White, D., Chapman, L., Dromerick, A., Fiez, J.A., & Corbetta, M. (2000). Neural correlates of recovery from aphasia after damage to left inferior frontal cortex. *Neurology, 55*, 1883–1894.

Shallice, T. (1982). Specific impairments of planning. In: D.E. Broadbent & L. Weiskrantz (Eds.), *The Neuropsychology of Cognitive Function* (pp. 199–209). London: The Royal Society.

Spearman, C. (1904). General intelligence, objectively determined and measured. *American Journal of Psychology, 15*, 201–293.

Spitzer, H., Desimone, R., & Moran, J. (1988). Increased attention enhances both behavioral and neuronal performance. *Science, 240*, 338–340.

Stroop, J.R. (1935). Studies of interference in serial verbal reactions. *Journal of Experimental Psychology, 18*, 643–662.

Sweeney, J.A., Mintun, M.A., Kwee, S., Wiseman, M.B., Brown, D.L., Rosenberg, D.R., & Carl, J.R. (1996). Positron emission tomography study of voluntary saccadic eye movements and spatial working memory. *Journal of Neurophysiology, 75*, 454–468.

Thulborn, K.R., Carpenter, P.A., & Just, M.A. (1999). Plasticity of language-related brain function during recovery from stroke. *Stroke, 30*, 749–754.

Tomita, H., Ohbayashi, M., Nakahara, K., Hasegawa, I., & Miyashita, Y. (1999). Top-down signal from prefrontal cortex in executive control of memory retrieval. *Nature, 401*, 699–703.

Tootell, R.B.H., Hadjikhani, N.K., Mendola, J.D., Marrett, S., & Dale, A.M. (1998). From retinotopy to recognition: fMRI in human visual cortex. *Trends in Cognitive Sciences, 2*, 174–183.

Watanabe, M. (1990). Prefrontal unit activity during associative learning in the monkey. *Experimental Brain Research, 80*, 296–309.

Watanabe, M. (1992). Frontal units of the monkey coding the associative significance of visual and auditory stimuli. *Experimental Brain Research, 89*, 233–247.

White, I.M. & Wise, S.P. (1999). Rule-dependent neuronal activity in the prefrontal cortex. *Experimental Brain Research, 126*, 315–335.

Wilson, F.A.W., Ó Scalaidhe, S.P., & Goldman-Rakic, P.S. (1993). Dissociation of object and spatial processing domains in primate prefrontal cortex. *Science, 260*, 1955–1958.

Wise, S.P., Murray, E.A., & Gerfen, C.R. (1996). The frontal-basal ganglia system in primates. *Critical Reviews of Neurobiology, 10*, 317–356.

19

The Structured Event Complex and the Human Prefrontal Cortex

JORDAN GRAFMAN

There is no region of human cerebral cortex whose functional assignments are as puzzling to us as the human prefrontal cortex (HPFC). Over one hundred years of observation and experimentation has led to several general conclusions about its overall functions. The prefrontal cortex (PFC) is important for modulating higher cognitive processes such as social behavior, reasoning, planning, working memory, thought, concept formation, inhibition, attention, and abstraction. Yet unlike the research conducted in other cognitive domains such as object recognition or lexical/semantic storage, there has been little effort to propose and investigate in detail the underlying cognitive architecture(s) that would capture the essential features and computational properties of the higher cognitive processes presumably supported by the HPFC. Since the processes that are attributed to the HPFC appear to constitute the most complex and abstract of cognitive functions, many of which are responsible for the internal guidance of human behavior, a critical step in understanding the functions of the human brain requires us to adequately describe the cognitive topography of the HPFC. The purpose of this chapter is to argue for the validity of a representational research framework to understand PFC functioning in humans. This framework suggests that by postulating the form of the various units of representation (in essence, the elements of memory) stored in PFC, it will be much easier to derive clear and testable hypotheses that will enable rejection or validation of this and other frameworks. My colleagues and I have labeled the set of HPFC representational units alluded to above as a structured event complex (SEC). Below I will detail my hypotheses about the SEC's representational structure and features and I will attempt to distinguish the SEC framework from other cognitive models of HPFC function. Before doing so, I will briefly summarize the key elements of the biology and structure of the HPFC, the evidence of its general role in cognition based on convergent evidence from lesion and neuroimaging studies, and some key models postulating the functions of the HPFC. I will then briefly argue for a rationale that specifies why there must be representational knowledge stored in the PFC, present a short primer on the SEC framework I have adapted, and finally offer some suggestions about future directions for research of HPFC functions using the SEC framework.

INTRODUCTION

What we know about the anatomy and physiology of the HPFC is inferred almost entirely from studies in the primate and lower species (see Chapters 3–6 for a more detailed description of the anatomy and physiology of the prefrontal cortex). This research indicates that the HPFC is a proportionally large cortical region that is extensively and reciprocally interconnected with other associative, limbic, and basal ganglia brain structures. Grossly, it can be subdivided into lateral, medial, and orbital regions with Brodmann's areas providing morphological subdivisions within (and occasionally across) each of the gross regions (Barbas, 2000). It matures somewhat later than other cortex and is richly innervated with modulatory chemical systems. Finally, neurons in the PFC appear to be particularly able to fire over extended periods of time (Levy & Goldman-Rakic, 2000). If the firing of neurons in the PFC is linked to activity that "moves" the subject towards a goal rather than reacting to the appearance of a single stimulus, then potentially, those neurons could continuously fire across many stimuli or events until the goal was achieved or the behavior of the subject disrupted. This observation of sustained firing of prefrontal cortex neurons across time and events has led many investigators to suggest that the HPFC must be involved in the maintenance of a stimulus across time, i.e., working memory (Fuster et al., 2000). Besides the property of sustained firing, Elston (2000) has recently demonstrated a unique structural feature of neurons in the PFC. Elston (2000) found that pyramidal cells in the PFC of macaque monkeys are significantly more spinous than pyramidal cells in other cortical areas, suggesting that they are capable of handling a larger amount of excitatory inputs than that of pyramidal cells elsewhere. This could be one of several structural explanations for the HPFC's ability to integrate input from many sources in order to implement more abstract behaviors. These features of the HPFC map nicely onto some of the cognitive attributes of the HPFC identified in neuropsychological and neuroimaging studies as well as in the SEC framework I have adapted and described later in this chapter.

FUNCTIONAL STUDIES

The traditional approach to understanding the functions of the HPFC is to perform cognitive studies testing the ability of normal and impaired humans on tasks designed to induce the activation of processes or representational knowledge presumably stored in the HPFC (Grafman, 1999). Both animals and humans with brain lesions can be studied to determine the effects of a PFC lesion on task performance. Lesions in humans, of course, are due to an act of nature whereas lesions in animals can be more precisely and purposefully made by investigators. Likewise, "intact" animals can be studied using precise electrophysiological recordings of single neurons or neural assemblies. In humans, the powerful new neuroimaging techniques such as functional magnetic resonance imaging (fMRI) have been used to demonstrate frontal lobe activation during the performance of a range of tasks in normal subjects and patients. A potential advantage in studying humans (instead of animals) comes from the presumption that since the HPFC represents the kind of higher—order cognitive processes that distinguishes humans from other primates, an understanding of its underlying cognitive and neural architecture can only come from the study of humans.

Patients with frontal lobe lesions are generally able to understand conversation and commands, recognize and use objects, express themselves adequately enough to navigate through some social situations in the world, learn and remember routes, and even make decisions. They have documented deficits in sustaining their attention and anticipating what will happen next, in dividing their resources, in inhibiting prepotent behavior, in adjusting to some situations requiring social cognition, in processing the theme or the moral of a story, in forming concepts, abstracting, reasoning, and planning (Arnett et al., 1994; Goel & Grafman, 1995; Vendrell et al., 1995; Goel et al., 1997; Jurado et al., 1998; Dimitrov et al., 1999a; 1999b; Grafman, 1999;

Zahn et al., 1999; Carlin et al., 2000). These deficits have been observed and confirmed by investigators over the last 40 years of clinical and experimental research.

Neuroimaging investigators have published studies that show PFC activation during encoding, retrieval, decision making and response conflict, task switching, reasoning, planning, forming concepts, understanding the moral or theme of a story, inferring the motives or intentions of others, and similar high-level cognitive processing (Nichelli et al., 1994, 1995b; Goel et al., 1995; Koechlin et al., 1999; 2000; Wharton et al., 2000). The major advantage, so far, of these functional neuroimaging studies is that they have generally provided convergent evidence for the involvement of the HPFC in controlling endogenous and exogenous-sensitive cognitive processes, especially those that are engaged by the abstract characteristics of a task.

NEUROPSYCHOLOGICAL FRAMEWORKS THAT TRY TO ACCOUNT FOR HUMAN PREFRONTAL FUNCTIONS

WORKING MEMORY

Working memory has been described as the cognitive process that allows for the temporary activation of information in memory for rapid retrieval or manipulation (Ruchkin et al., 1997). It was first proposed some 30 years ago to account for a variety of human memory data that wasn't addressed by contemporary models of short-term memory (Baddeley, 1998b). Of note is that subsequent researchers have been unusually successful in describing the circumstances under which the so-called slave systems employed by working memory would be used. These slave systems allow for the maintenance of the stimuli in a number of different forms that could be manipulated by the central executive component of the working memory system (Baddeley, 1998a). Neuroscientific support for this model followed quickly. Joaquin Fuster was among the first neuroscientists to recognize that neurons in

the PFC appeared to have a special capacity to discharge over time intervals when the stimulus was not being shown prior to a memory-driven response by the animal (Fuster et al., 2000). He interpreted this neuronal activity as being concerned with the cross-temporal linkage of information processed at different points in an ongoing temporal sequence. Goldman-Rakic and colleagues later elaborated on this notion and suggested that these same PFC neurons were fulfilling the neuronal responsibility for working memory (Levy & Goldman-Rakic, 2000). In her view, PFC neurons *temporarily* hold in active memory modality-specific information *until* a response is made. This implies a restriction on the kind of memory that may be stored in prefrontal cortex. That is, this point of view suggests that there are no long-term representations in the PFC until an explicit intention to act is required and then a temporary representation is created. Miller has challenged some of Goldman-Rakic's views about the role of neurons in the PFC and argues that many neurons in the monkey PFC are modality non-specific and may serve a broader integrative function rather than a simple maintenance function (Miller, 2000). Fuster, Goldman-Rakic, and Baddeley's programs of research have had a major influence on the functional neuroimaging research programs of Courtney (Courtney et al., 1998), Smith and Jonides (Smith & Jonides, 1999), and Cohen (Nystrom et al., 2000)—all of whom have studied normal subjects to remap the HPFC in the context of working memory theory.

EXECUTIVE FUNCTION AND ATTENTIONAL/CONTROL PROCESSES

Although rather poorly described in the cognitive science literature, it is premature to simply dismiss the general notion of a central executive (Baddeley, 1998a; Grafman & Litvan, 1999b). Several investigators have described the PFC as the seat of attentional and inhibitory processes that govern the focus of our behaviors and have thus postulated the notion of a central executive operating within the confines of the HPFC. Norman and Shallice (1986) proposed a dichotomous function of the central executive in HPFC. They argued that the HPFC was primarily specialized for the supervision of attention towards unexpected occurrences. Besides this supervisory attention system, they also hypothesized the existence of a contention scheduling system that was specialized for the initiation and efficient running of automatized behaviors such as repetitive routines, procedures, and skills. Shallice, Burgess, Stuss, and others have attempted to expand this idea of the PFC as a voluntary control device and have further fractionated the supervisory attention system into a set of parallel attention processes that work together to manage complex multitask behaviors (Shallice & Burgess, 1996; Stuss et al., 1999; Burgess, 2000; Burgess et al., 2000).

SOCIAL COGNITION AND SOMATIC MARKING

The role of the HPFC in working memory and executive processes has been extensively examined, but there is also substantial evidence that the PFC is involved in controlling certain aspects of social and emotional behavior (Dimitrov et al., 1996, 1999c). Although the classic story of the nineteenth century patient Gage, who suffered a penetrating PFC lesion, has been used to exemplify the problems that patients with ventromedial PFC lesions have in obeying social rules, recognizing social cues, and making appropriate social decisions, the details of this social cognitive impairment have occasionally been inferred or even embellished to suit the enthusiasm of the storyteller—at least regarding Gage (Macmillan, 2000). Damasio and colleagues have nonetheless consistently confirmed the association of ventromedial PFC lesions and social behavior and decision-making abnormalities (Damasio, 1996; Eslinger, 1998; Anderson et al., 1999; Bechara et al., 1999, 2000; Kawasaki et al., 2001). The exact functional assignment of that area of HPFC is still subject to dispute, but convincing evidence has been presented indicating that it serves to associate somatic markers (autonomic nervous system modulators that bias activation and decision making) with social knowledge, enabling rapid social decision making—particularly for overlearned

associative knowledge. The somatic markers themselves are distributed across a large system of brain regions including limbic system structures such as the amygdala (Damasio, 1996).

ACTION MODELS

The HPFC is sometimes thought of as a cognitive extension of the functional specialization of the motor areas of the frontal lobes (Gomez Beldarrain et al., 1999), leading to the idea that it must play an essential cognitive role in determining action sequences in the real world. In keeping with that view, a number of investigators have focused their investigations on concrete action series that have proved difficult for patients with PFC lesions to adequately perform. By analyzing the pattern of errors committed by these patients, it is possible to construct cognitive models of action execution and the role of the PFC in such performance. In some patients, while the total number of errors they commit is greater than that seen in controls, the pattern of errors committed is similar to that seen in controls (Schwartz et al., 1999). Reduced arousal or effort can also contribute to a breakdown in action production in patients (Schwartz et al., 1999). However, other studies indicate that action production impairment can be due to a breakdown in access to a semantic network that represents aspects of action schema and prepotent responses (Forde & Humphreys, 2000). Action production must rely on an association between the target object or abstract goal and specific motoric actions (Humphreys & Riddoch, 2000). In addition, the magnitude of inhibition of inappropriate actions appears related to the strength in associative memory of object–goal associations (Humphreys & Riddoch, 2000). Retrieving or recognizing appropriate actions may even help subjects subsequently detect a target (Humphreys & Riddoch, 2001). It should be noted that action disorganization syndromes in patients are usually elicited with tasks that have been traditionally part of the examination of ideomotor or ideational praxis, such as brushing one's teeth, and it is not clear whether findings in patients performing such tasks apply to a breakdown in action organization at a higher level, such as planning a vacation.

COMPUTATIONAL FRAMEWORKS

A number of computational models of potential HPFC processes as well as of the general architecture of the HPFC have been developed in recent years. Some models have offered a single explanation for performance on a wide range of tasks. For example, Kimberg and Farah showed that the weakening of associations within a working memory component of their model led to impaired simulated performance on a range of tasks, such as the Wisconsin Card Sorting Test and the Stroop Test, that patients with PFC lesions are known to perform poorly on (Kimberg & Farah, 1993). In contrast, other investigators have argued for a hierarchical approach to modeling HPFC functions that incorporates a number of layers, with the lowest levels regulated by the environment and the highest levels regulated by internalized rules and plans (Changeux & Dehaene, 1998). In addition to the cognitive levels of their model, Changeux and Deahane, relying on simulations, suggest that control for transient "pre-representations" that are modulated by reward and punishment signals improved their model's ability to predict patient performance data on the Tower of London Test (Changeux & Dehaene, 1998). Norman and Shallice first ascribed two major control systems to the HPFC (Norman & Shallice, 1986). As noted earlier in this chapter, one system was concerned with rigid, procedurally based, and overlearned behaviors whereas the other system was concerned with the supervisory control over novel situations. Both systems could be simultaneously active, although one system's activation usually predominated performance. The Norman and Shallice model has been incorporated into a hybrid computational model that blends their control system idea with a detailed description of selected action sequences and their errors (Cooper & Shallice, 2000). The Cooper and Shallice (2000) model can account for sequences of response, unlike some recurrent network models, and like the Changeux and

Dehaene model is hierarchical in nature and based on interactive activation principles. It also was uncanny in predicting the kinds of errors of action disorganization described by Schwartz and Humphreys in their studies. Other authors have implemented interactive control models that use production rules with scheduling strategies for activation and execution to simulate executive control (Meyer & Kieras, 1997). Tackling the issue of how the HPFC mediates schema processing, Botvinick and Plaut have recently argued that schemas are emergent system properties rather than explicit representations (Botvinick & Plaut, 2000). They developed a multilayered recurrent connectionist network model to simulate action sequences that is somewhat similar to the Cooper and Shallice model described above. In their simulation, action errors occurred when noise in the system caused an internal representation for one scenerio to resemble a pattern usually associated with another scenerio. Their model also indicated that noise introduced in the middle of a sequence of actions was more disabling than noise presented closer to the end of the task.

Although the biological plausibility of all these models has yet to be formally compared, it is just as important to determine whether these models can simulate the behaviors and deficits of interest. The fact that models such as the ones described above are now being implemented is a major advance in the study of the functions of the HPFC.

COMMONALITIES AND WEAKNESSES OF THE FRAMEWORKS USED TO DESCRIBE HUMAN PREFRONTAL CORTEX FUNCTIONS

The cognitive and computational models briefly described above (and further explicated in Chapters 2, 5, 12, 13, 16–18, 22, 25, 27, and 34) have commonalities that point to the general role of the PFC in maintaining information across time intervals and intervening tasks, in modulating social behavior, in the integration of information across time, and in the control of behavior via temporary memory representations and thought rather than allowing behavior to depend on environmental contingencies alone. None of the major models have articulated in detail the domains and features of a representational knowledge base that would support such HPFC functions, making these models difficult to reject using error or response time analysis of patient data or functional neuroimaging.

What would one think if I described cerebral cortex in the following way. The role of cortex is to rapidly process information and encode its features, and bind these features together. This role is rather dependent on bottom-up environmental input but represents the elements of this processed information in memory. Perhaps this is not too controversial a way to describe the role of the occipital, parietal, or temporal cortex in processing objects or words. For the cognitive neuropsychologist, however, it would be critical to define the features of the word or object, the characteristics of the memory representation that led to easier encoding or retrieval of the object or word, and the psychological structure of the representational neighborhood (how different words or objects are related to each other in psychological and potentially neural space). Although there are important philosophical, psychological, and biological arguments about the best way to describe a stored unit of memory (be it an orthographic representation of a word, a visual scene, or a conceptualization), there is general agreement that memories equal representations. There is less agreement as to the difference between a representation and a cognitive process. It could be argued that processes are simply the sustained temporary activation of one or more representations.

My view is that the descriptions of the functional roles of the HPFC summarized in most of the models and frameworks already described in this chapter are inadequate to obtain a clear understanding of its role in behavior. To obtain a clear understanding of the HPFC, I believe that a theory or model must describe the cognitive nature of the representational networks that are stored in the PFC, the principles by which the representations are stored, the levels and forms of the representations, and hemispheric differences in the representational component stored that are based on the underlying computational constraints imposed by the right and left PFC. Such a model must also lead to predictions about the ease of retrieving representations stored in the PFC under normal conditions, when normal subjects divide their cognitive resources or shift between tasks, and after various forms of brain injury. None of the models noted above were intended to provide answers to any of these questions except in the most general manner.

PROCESS VERSUS REPRESENTATION: HOW TO THINK ABOUT MEMORY IN THE HUMAN PREFRONTAL CORTEX

My framework for understanding the nature of knowledge stored in HPFC depends on the idea that unique forms of knowledge are stored in the HPFC as representations. In this sense, a representation is an element of knowledge that, when activated, corresponds to a unique brain state signified by the strength and pattern of neural activity in a local brain sector. This representational element is a "permanent" unit of memory that can be strengthened by repeated exposure to the same or similar knowledge element and is a member of a local psychological and neural network composed of multiple similar representations. Defining the specific forms of the representations in HPFC so that a cognitive framework can be tested is crucial, since an inappropriate representational depiction can compromise a model or theory as a description of a targeted phenomena. It is likely that these HPFC representations are parsed at multiple grain sizes (that are shaped by behavioral, environmental, and neural constraints).

What should a representational theory claim? It should claim that a process is a representation (or set of representations) in action, essentially a representation that, when activated, stays activated over a limited or extended time domain. In order to be activated, a representation has to be primed by input from a representation located outside its region or by associated representations within its region. This can occur via bottom-up or top-down information transfer. A representation, when activated, may or may not fit within the typical time window described as working memory. When it does, we are conscious of the representation. When it doesn't, we can still process that representation but we may not have direct conscious access to all of its contents.

The idea that representations are embedded in computations performed by local neural networks and are permanently stored within those networks so that they can be easily resurrected in a similar form whenever that network is stimulated by the external world's example of that representation or via associated knowledge is not novel or free of controversy. But similar ideas of representation have dominated the scientific understanding of face, word, and object recognition and have been recognized as an acceptable way to describe how the surface and lexical features of information could be encoded and stored in the human brain. Despite the adaptation of this notion of representation to the development of cognitive architectures for various stimuli based on "lower-level" stimulus features, the application of similar representational theory to better understand the functions of the HPFC has moved much more slowly and in a more limited way.

EVOLUTION OF COGNITIVE ABILITIES

As I noted earlier in this chapter, there is both folk wisdom about, and research support for, the idea that certain cognitive abilities are uniquely captured in the human brain, with little evidence for these same sophisticated cognitive abilities having been found in other primates. Some examples of these cognitive processes include complex language abilities, social inferential abilities, and reasoning. It is not that these and other complex abilities are not present in other species, but probably, they exist only in a more rudimentary form.

The PFC, as generally viewed, is most developed in humans. Therefore, it is likely that

it has supported the transition of certain cognitive abilities from a rudimentary level to a more sophisticated one. I have already touched upon what kinds of abilities are governed by the HPFC. It is likely, however, that such abilities depend on a set of fundamental computational processes unique to humans that support distinctive representational forms in the PFC (Grafman, 1995). My goal in the remainder of this chapter is to suggest the principles by which such unique representations would be distinctively stored in the HPFC.

THE STRUCTURED EVENT COMPLEX

I define a *structured event complex* (SEC) as a set of events, structured in a particular sequence, that as a complex composes a particular kind of activity that is usually goal oriented. For example, if you had a goal to have a nice dinner at a restaurant with a friend, the structured set of events composing this activity might have the following sequence of events: leave your apartment, get in your car, pick up your friend at her apartment, drive to the restaurant, park the car, enter the restaurant, the host greets you, the host seats you, the waiter arrives with the menu, food is ordered, conversation occurs, food is served, eat the meal, receive the bill, pay the bill, leave the restaurant. The information from these events might include what constitutes their boundaries (transition between events), key features of each event (ordering, content of conversation, timing, etc.), and the abstraction of ideas across events (unstated intentions such as to get to know your friend better and to impress her). Each of these aspects of the SEC should be independently represented in the HPFC but are encoded and retrieved together as an episode, much like the features of objects are bound together to give one a complete sense of an object. On-line processing of an SEC would enable a person to predict subsequent events, but if there was damage to the HPFC that limited retrieval of part or all of an SEC, then it is likely that day-to-day behavior would be disrupted and prone to distractibility, and subjects would have a difficult time detecting behavioral and social errors in the sequence of their activities (Gehring & Knight, 2000). Below I provide more details about the nature and cognitive architecture of the SEC representation.

THE ARCHETYPE STRUCTURED EVENT COMPLEX

There must be a few fundamental principles governing evolutionary cognitive advances from other primates to humans. A key principle must be the ability of neurons to sustain their firing and code the temporal and sequential properties of ongoing events in the environment or in the mind over longer and longer periods of time. This sustained firing has enabled the human brain to code, store, and retrieve the more abstract features of behaviors whose goal or end-stage would not occur until well after the period of time that exceeds the limits of consciousness in "the present." Gradually in evolution, this period of time must have extended itself to encompass and encode all sorts of complex behaviors (Nichelli et al., 1995a; Rueckert & Grafman, 1996, 1998). Many aspects of such complex behaviors must be translated into compressed (and multiple modes of) representations (such as a verbal listing of a series of things to do and the same set of actions in visual memory), while others may have real-time representational unpacking. *Unpacking* means the amount of time and resources required to activate an entire representation and sustain it for behavioral purposes over the length of time it would take to actually perform the activity—for example, an activity composed of several linked events that take 10 minutes to perform would activate some component representations of that activity that would be active for the entire 10 minutes.

THE EVENT SEQUENCE

Neurons and assemblies firing over extended periods of time in the HPFC process *sets of input* that can be defined as *events*. Along with extended firing of neurons that allow the processing of behaviors *across time*, there must have also developed special neural pars-

ers that enabled the *editing* of these behaviors into linked sequential but individual events (much like speech can be parsed into phonological units or sentences into grammatical constituents) (Sirigu et al., 1996, 1998). In order for the event sequences, to be goal oriented and cohere, they must obey a logical sequential structure within the constraints of the physical world, the culture that the individual belongs to, and/or the individual's personal preferences. These event sequences, as a whole, can be conceptualized as units of memory within domains of knowledge (e.g., a social attitude, a script that describes cooking a dinner, or a story that has a logical plot). My colleagues and I purposely labeled the archetype event sequence the *structured event complex* (SEC), to emphasize that we believed it to be the general form of representation within the HPFC and to avoid being too closely tied to a particular description of higher-level cognitive processes contained in story, narrative processing, script, or schema frameworks.

GOAL ORIENTED

Structured event complexes are not random chains of behavior performed by normally functioning adults. They tend to have boundaries that signal their onset and offset. These boundaries can be determined by temporal cues, cognitive cues, or environmental/perceptual cues. Each SEC, however, has some kind of goal whose achievement precedes the offset of the SEC. The nature of the goal can be as different as putting a bookshelf together or determining a present to impress your child on her birthday. Some events must be more central or important to an SEC than others. Subjects can have some agreement on which ones these are when explicitly asked. Some SECs are well structured, with all the cognitive and behavioral rules available for the sequence of events to occur, and there is a clear, definable goal. Other SECs are ill structured, requiring the subject to adapt to unpredictable events using analogical reasoning or similarity judgment to determine the sequence of actions on-line (by retrieving a similar SEC from memory) as well as developing a quickly fashioned goal. Not only are SEC goals central to its execution, but the process of reaching the goal can be rewarding. Goal achievement itself is probably routinely accompanied by a reward that is mediated by the brain's neurochemical systems. Depending on the salience of this reward cue, it can become essential to the subject's subsequent competent execution of that same or similar SEC. Goal attainment is usually obvious and subjects can consciously move onto another SEC in its aftermath.

REPRESENTATIONAL FORMAT OF THE STRUCTURED EVENT COMPLEX

I hypothesize that SECs are composed of a set of differentiated representational forms that are stored in different regions of the HPFC but are activated in parallel to reproduce all the SEC elements of a typical episode (see Fig. 19–1). These distinctive memories would represent thematic knowledge, morals, abstractions, concepts, social rules, features of specific events, and grammars for the variety of SECs embodied in actions, stories and narratives, scripts, and schemas.

MEMORY CHARACTERISTICS

As just described, SECs are essentially distributed memory units with different components of the SEC, stored in various regions within the PFC. The easiest assumption to make, then, is that these memory units obey the same principles as other memory units in the brain. These principles revolve around frequency of activation based on use or exposure, association to other memory units, category specificity of the memory unit, plasticity of the representation, priming mechanisms, and binding of the memory unit and its neighborhood memory units to memory

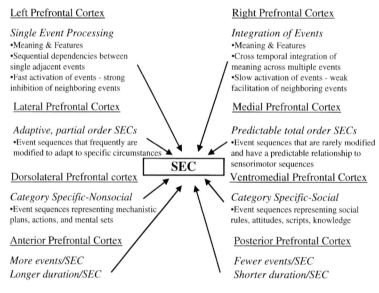

Figure 19–1. Key components of a structured event complex (SEC) mapped to prefrontal cortex topography. These SEC components are discussed in the section Representational Format of the Structured Event Complex. Note that a combination of features could be found in any SEC but that lesions might affect only certain components of the total SEC (this is based on the presumption that every SEC relies on components stored in both hemi-

spheres). For example, a patient with a left posterior ventromedial prefrontal cortex lesion would be predicted to have difficulty retrieving social rules or attitudes that are of relatively short duration and made up of a few events, especially if the task required the patient to respond to the primary meaning of the social rule/attitude or the sequential dependency between two events/stimuli composing the social rule/attitude (e.g., an object and an attitude).

units in more distant representational networks both in and remote from the territory of the PFC.

FREQUENCY OF USE AND EXPOSURE

As a characteristic that predicts a subject's ability to retrieve a memory, frequency is a powerful variable. For the SEC, the higher the frequency of the memory units composing the SEC components, the more resilient they should be in the face of PFC damage. That is, it is predicted that patients with frontal lobe damage would be most capable of performing or recognizing those SECs that they usually do as a daily routine and most impaired when asked to produce or recognize novel or rarely executed SECs. This retrieval deficit would be affected by the frequency of the specific kind of SEC component memory units stored in the damaged PFC region.

ASSOCIATIVE PROPERTIES WITHIN A HUMAN PREFRONTAL CORTEX FUNCTIONAL REGION

In order to hypothesize the associative properties of an SEC, it is necessary to adapt some general information-processing constraints imposed by each of the hemispheres (Nichelli et al., 1995b; Partiot et al., 1996; Beeman, 1998). A number of theorists have suggested that hemispheric asymmetry of information coding revolves around two distinct notions. The left hemisphere is specialized for finely tuned rapid encoding that is best at processing within-event information and coding for the boundaries between events. For example, the left PFC might be able to best process the primary meaning of an event. The right hemisphere is thought to be specialized for coarse, slower coding, allowing for the processing of information that is more distantly related (to the information currently being processed) and could be adept at integrating or synthesizing information across events in time. For example, the right PFC might be best able to process and integrate information across events to obtain the theme or moral of a story that is being processed for the first time.

When left hemisphere fine-coding mechanisms are relied on, a local memory element would be rapidly activated along with a few related neighbors with a relatively rapid deactivation. When right hemisphere coarse-coding mechanisms are relied on, there should be weaker activation of local memory elements but a greater spread of activation across a larger neighborhood of representations and for a sustained period of time—even corresponding to the true duration of the SEC currently being processed. This dual form of coding probably occurs in parallel with subjects shifting between the two, depending on task and strategic demands. Furthermore, the organization of a population of SEC components within a functionally defined region, regardless of coding mechanisms, should be based on the same principles as those argued for in other forms of associative representation, with both inhibition of unrelated memory units and facilitation of neighboring (and presumably related) memory units following activation.

ORDER OF EVENTS

The HPFC is specialized for the processing of events over time. One aspect of the SEC that is key to its representation is event order. Order is coded by the sequence of events. The stream of action must be parsed as each event begins and ends, to explicitly recognize the nature, duration, and number of events that compose the event sequence (Hanson & Hanson, 1996; Zacks & Tversky, 2001). I hypothesize that in childhood, because of the neural constraints of an immature HPFC, *individual* events are initially represented as independent memory units and only later in development are they linked together to form an SEC. Thus, in adults, there should be some redundancy of representation of the independent event (formed in childhood) and the membership of that same event within the SEC. Adult patients with PFC lesions would be expected to commit errors of order in developing or executing SECs but could wind up defaulting to retrieving the independently stored events in an attempt to slavishly carry out fragments of an activity. Subjects are aware of the sequence of events that make up an SEC and can even judge their relative importance or centrality to the overall SEC theme or goal. Each event has a typical duration and an expected onset and offset time within the time frame of the entire SEC that is coded. The order of the independent events that make up a particular SEC must be routinely adhered to by the performing subject to develop a more deeply stored SEC representation and improve the subject's ability to predict the sequence of events. The repeated performance of an SEC leads to the systematic and rigidly ordered execution of events—an observation compatible with the artificial intelligence (AI) notion of total order planning. In contrast, new SECs are constantly being encoded, given the variable and occasionally unpredictable nature of strategic thought or environmental demands. This kind of adaptive planning in AI is known as *partial order planning*, since event sequences are composed on-line, with the new SEC consisting of previously experienced events now interdigitating with novel events. Since there must be multiple SECs that are activated in a typical day, it is likely that they too (like the events within an SEC) can be activated in sequence, or additionally in a cascading or parallel manner (to manage two or more tasks at the same time).

CATEGORY SPECIFICITY

There is compelling evidence that the HPFC can be divided into regions that have predominant connectivity with specific cortical and subcortical brain sectors. This has led to the hypothesis that SECs may be stored in the HPFC on a category-specific basis. For example, it appears that patients with ventral or medial PFC lesions are especially impaired in performing social and reward-related behaviors whereas patients with lesions to the dorsolateral prefrontal cortex appear most impaired on mechanistic planning tasks (Partiot et al., 1995; Grafman et al., 1996; Dimitrov et al., 1999c; Pietrini et al., 2000; Zalla et al., 2000). Further delineation of category specificity within the HPFC awaits more precise testing, using various SEC categories as stimuli (Sirigu et al., 1998; Crozier et al., 1999).

NEUROPLASTICITY OF HUMAN PREFRONTAL CORTEX

We know relatively little about the neurobiological rules governing plasticity of the HPFC. It is probable that the same plasticity mechanisms that accompany learning and recovery of function in other cortical areas operate in the frontal lobes too (Grafman & Litvan, 1999a). For example, a change in PFC regional functional map size with learning has been noted. Shrinkage of map size is usually associated with learning of a specific element of many within a category of representation, whereas an increase in map size over time may reflect the general category of representational form being activated (but not a specific element of memory within the category). After left brain damage, right homologous HPFC assumption of at least some of the functions previously associated with Broca's area can occur. The mechanism by which the unique characteristics of PFC neurons (e.g., sustained re-entrant firing patterns or idiosyncratic neural architectures) interact with the general principles of cortical plasticity has been little explored to date. In terms of the flexibility of representations in the PFC, it appears that this area of cortex can rapidly reorganize itself to respond to new environmental contingencies or rules. Thus, although the general underlying principles of how information is represented may be similar within and across species, individual experience manifested by species or individuals within a species will be influential in what is stored in PFC and important to control for when interpreting the results of experiments trying to infer HPFC functional organization.

PRIMING

At least two kinds of priming (Schacter & Buckner, 1998) should occur when an SEC is activated. First of all, within an SEC, there should be priming of forthcoming adjacent and distant events by previously occurring events. Thus, in the case of the event that indicates that one is going into a restaurant, subsequent events such as paying the bill or ordering from the menu may be primed at that moment. This priming would activate those event representations even though they hadn't occurred yet. The activation might be too far below threshold for conscious recognition that the event has been activated, but there is a probably a relationship between the intensity of the primed activation of a subsequent event and the temporal and cognitive distance the current event is from the primed event. The closer the primed event is in sequence and time to the priming event, the more activated it should be. The second kind of priming induced by SEC activation would involve SECs in the immediate neighborhood of the one currently activated. Closely related SECs (or components of SECs) in the immediate neighborhood should be activated to a lesser degree than the targeted SEC, regardless of hemisphere. More distantly related SECs (or components of SECs) would be inhibited in the dominant hemisphere. More distantly related SECs (or components of SECs) would be weakly activated, rather than inhibited, in the nondominant hemisphere.

BINDING

Another form of priming, based on the principle of binding (Engel & Singer, 2001) of distinct representational forms *across* cortical regions, should occur with the activation of an SEC. The sort of representational forms that may be stored in the HPFC, such as thematic knowledge, should be linked to more primitive representational forms such as objects, faces, words, stereotyped phrases, scenes, and emotions. This linkage or binding enables humans to form a distributed episodic memory for later retrieval. The binding also enables priming across representational forms to occur. For example, by activating an event within an SEC that is concerned with working in the office, activation thresholds should be decreased for recognizing and thinking about objects normally found in an office, such as a telephone. In addition, the priming of forthcoming events within an SEC referred to above would also result in the priming of the objects associated with the subsequent event. Each additional representational form linked to the SEC should improve the salience of the bound con-

figuration of representations. Absence of highly SEC-salient environmental stimuli or thought processes would tend to diminish the overall activation of the SEC-bound configuration of representations and bias which specific subset of PFC representational components are activated.

HIERARCHICAL REPRESENTATION OF STRUCTURED EVENT COMPLEXES

I have previously argued for a hierarchy of SEC representations (Grafman, 1995); that is, I predicted that SECs, within a domain, would range from specific episodes to generalized events. For example, one could have an SEC representing the actions and themes of a single evening at a specific restaurant, an SEC representing the actions and themes of how to behave at restaurants in general, and an SEC representing actions and themes related to eating that are context independent. In this view, SEC episodes are formed first during development of the HPFC, followed by more general SECs, and then the context-free and abstract SECs. As the HPFC matures, it is the more general, context-free, and abstract SECs that allow for adaptive and flexible planning. Since these SECs don't represent specific episodes, they can be retrieved and applied to novel situations for which a specific SEC does not exist.

RELATIONSHIP TO OTHER FORMS OF REPRESENTATION

BASAL GANGLIA FUNCTIONS

The basal ganglia receive direct connections from different regions of the HPFC and some of these connections may carry cognitive "commands." The basal ganglia, in turn, send back to the PFC, via the thalamus, signals that reflect its own processing. Even if the basal ganglia work in concert with the PFC, their exact role in cognitive processing has yet to be defined. They appear to play a role in the storage of visuomotor sequences (Pascual-Leone et al., 1993, 1995), in reward-related behavior

(Zalla et al., 2000), and in automatic cognitive processing such as overlearned word retrieval. It is likely that the SECs in the PFC bind with the visuomotor representations stored in the basal ganglia to produce an integrated set of cognitive and visuomotor actions (Pascual-Leone et al., 1996; Koechlin et al., 2000; submitted) relevant to particular situations.

HIPPOCAMPUS AND AMYGDALA FUNCTIONS

Both the amygdala and the hippocampus have reciprocal connections with the PFC. The amygdala, in particular, has extensive connections with ventromedial PFC (Price, 1999; Zalla et al., 2000). The amygdala's signals may provide a somatic marker or cue to the stored representational ensemble in the ventromedial PFC representing social attitudes, rules, and knowledge. The more salient the input provided by the somatic cue, the more important the somatic marker becomes for biasing the activation of social knowledge and actions.

The connections between PFC and the hippocampus serve to enlist the SEC as a contextual cue that forms part of an episodic ensemble of information (Thierry et al., 2000). The more salient the context, the more important it becomes for enhancing the retrieval or recognition of episodic memories. Thus, the hippocampus also serves to help bind the activation of objects, words, faces, scenes, procedures, and other information stored in posterior cortices and basal structures to SEC-based contextual information such as themes or plans. Furthermore, the hippocampus may be involved in the linkage of sequentially occurring events. The ability to explicitly predict a subsequent event requires conscious recollection of forthcoming events, which should require the participation of a normally functioning hippocampus. Since the hippocampus is not needed for certain aspects of lexical or object priming, for example, it is likely that components of the SEC that can also be primed (see Priming, above) don't require the participation of the hippocampus. Thus a subject with amnesia might gain confidence and comfort in experiencing interactions in which they were re-exposed to the same context

(SEC) that they had experienced before. In that case, the representation of that SEC would be strengthened even without later conscious recollection of experiencing it. Thus, SEC representational priming in amnesia should be governed by the same restraints that affect word or object priming in amnesia.

TEMPORAL–PARIETAL CORTEX FUNCTIONS

The computational processes representing the major components of what we recognize as a word, object, face, or scene are stored in posterior cortex. These representations are crucial components of a context and can provide the key cue to initiate the activation of an SEC event or its inhibition. Thus, the linkage between anterior and posterior cortices is very important for providing evidence that contributes to identifying the temporal and physical boundaries delimiting the independent "events" that make up an SEC.

EVIDENCE FOR AND AGAINST THE STRUCTURED EVENT COMPLEX FRAMEWORK

The advantage of this SEC formulation of the representations stored in the HPFC is that it resembles other cognitive architecture models that are constructed in such a way as to provide testable hypotheses regarding their validity. Support for hypotheses lends confidence to the structure of the model as predicated by its architects. Rejection of hypotheses occasionally leads to rejection of the entire model, but may also lead to a revised view of a component of the model.

The other major driving forces in conceptualizing the role of the PFC have, in general, avoided the level of detail required of a cognitive or computational model and instead opted for functional attributions which can hardly be disproved. This is not entirely the fault of the investigator, as the forms of knowledge or processes stored in the PFC have perplexed and eluded investigators for more than a century. What I have tried to do by formulating the SEC framework is take the trends in cognitive capabilities observed across evolution and development, which include greater temporal and sequential processing and more capacity for abstraction, and assume what representational state(s) those trends would lead to.

The current evidence for an SEC-type representational network is supportive but still rather sparse. Structured event complexes appear to be selectively processed by anterior PFC regions (Koechlin et al., 1999; 2000). Errors in event sequencing can occur with preservation of aspects of event knowledge (Sirigu et al., 1995a). Thematic knowledge can be impaired even though event knowledge is preserved (Zalla & Cortex, in press). Frequency of the SEC can affect the ease of retrieval of SEC knowledge (Sirigu et al., 1995a; 1995b). There is evidence for category specificity in that ventromedial PFC appears specialized for social knowledge processing (Dimitrov et al., 1999c). The HPFC is a member of many extended brain circuits. There is evidence that the hippocampus and the HPFC cooperate when the sequence of events have to be anticipated (Dreher et al., submitted). The amygdala and the HPFC cooperate when SECs are goal and reward oriented or emotionally relevant (Zalla et al., 2000). The basal ganglia, cerebellum, and HPFC cooperate as well (Grafman et al., 1992; Pascual-Leone et al., 1993; Hallett and Grafman, 1997) in the transfer of performance responsibilities between cognitive and visuomotor representations. When the SEC is novel or multitasking is involved, anterior frontopolar PFC is recruited but when SECs are overlearned, slightly more posterior frontomedial PFC is recruited (Koechlin et al., 2000). When subjects rely on the visuomotor components of a task, the basal ganglia and cerebellum are more involved but when subjects have to rely on the cognitive aspects of the task, the HPFC is more involved in performance (Koechlin et al., submitted). Thus, there is positive evidence for the representation of several different SEC components within the HPFC. Although there has been little in the way of negative studies of this framework, many predictions of the SEC framework in the areas of

goal orientation, neuroplasticity, priming, associative properties, and binding have not been fully explored to date and could eventually be falsified.

FUTURE DIRECTIONS

The representational model of the structured event complex described above lends itself to the generation of testable predictions or hypotheses. To reiterate, like most representational formats hypothesized for object, face, action, and word stores, the SEC subcomponents can each be characterized by the following features: frequency of exposure/activation; imagability; association with other items/exemplars in that particular representational store; centrality of the feature to the SEC (i.e., what proportional relevance does the feature have to recognizing or executing the SEC?); length of the SEC in terms of number of events and duration of each event and the SEC as a whole; implicit or explicit activation; and association with other representational forms that are stored in other areas of the HPFC or in more posterior cortex/subcortical regions.

All these features can be characterized psychometrically by quantitative values based on normative studies using experimental methods that have obtained similar values for words, photographs, objects, and faces. Unfortunately, there have only been a few attempts to collect some of these data for SECs, such as scripts, plans, and similar stimuli. If these values for all of the features of interest of an SEC were obtained, one could then make predictions about changes in SEC performance after HPFC lesions. For example, one hypothesis from the SEC representational model described above is that the frequency of activation of a particular representation will determine its accessibility following HPFC lesions. A patient with an HPFC lesion will have had many different experiences eating dinner, including eating food with their hands as a child, later eating more properly at the dining room table, eating at fast food restaurants, eating at favorite regular restaurants, and eventually eating occasionally at special restaurants or a brand new restaurant. A patient with an HPFC lesion of moderate size should be *limited* in retrieving various subcomponents of the SEC stored in the lesioned sector of the HPFC. This patient would likely behave more predictably and reliably when eating dinner at home then when eating in a familiar restaurant, and be less predictable when eating for the first time in a new restaurant with an unusual seating or dining procedure. The kinds of errors that would characterize the inappropriate behavior would depend on which subcomponent(s) of the SEC (and thus regions within or across hemispheres) was (were) damaged. For example, if the lesion was in the right dorsolateral PFC, the patient might have difficulty integrating knowledge across dining events, so he or she would be impaired in determining the (unstated) theme of the dinner or restaurant, particularly if the restaurant procedures were unfamiliar enough that the patient could not retrieve an analogous SEC. Only one study has attempted to directly test this general idea of frequency-sensitivity, with modest success (see above; Sirigu et al., 1995a). This is just one example of many predictions that emerge from the SEC model with components that have representational features. The claim that SEC representational knowledge is stored in the HPFC in various cognitive subcomponents is compatible with claims made for models for other forms of representational knowledge stored in other areas of brain and leads to the same kind of general predictions regarding SEC component accessibility made for these other forms of knowledge following brain damage. Future studies need to test these predictions.

REPRESENTATION VERSUS PROCESS REVISITED

The kind of representational model I have proposed for the SEC balances the over-reliance on so-called process models, such as the working memory model, that dominate the field today. Process models rely on a description of performance (holding or manipulating information) without necessarily being concerned about the details of the form of

representation (i.e., memory) activated that is responsible for the performance.

Promoting a strong claim that the PFC is concerned with processes rather than permanent representations is a fundamental shift away from how we have previously tried to understand the format in which information is stored in memory. It suggests that the PFC has little neural commitment to long-term storage of knowledge, in contrast to posterior cortex. Such a shift in studying brain functions devoted to memory requires a much stronger philosophical, neuropsychological, and neuroanatomical defense for the process approach than previously offered by its proponents. The representational point of view that I offer regarding HPFC knowledge stores is more consistent with previous cognitive neuroscience approaches to understanding how other forms of knowledge, such as words or objects, are represented in the brain. It also allows for many hypotheses to be derived for further study and therefore can motivate more competing representational models of HPFC functions.

CLINICAL APPLICATIONS

There is no doubt that the impairments caused by lesions to the HPFC can be very detrimental to a person's ability to maintain their previous level of work, responsibility to their family, and social commitments (Grafman & Litvan, 1999b). There is some evidence that deficits in executive functions can have a more profound effect on daily activities and routines than sensory deficits, aphasia, or agnosia (Schwab et al., 1993). Rehabilitation specialists are aware of the seriousness of deficits in executive impairments, but there are precious few group studies detailing specific or general improvements in executive functions that are maintained in the real world and that lead to a positive functional outcome (Levine et al., 2000; Stablum et al., 2000).

The SEC representational framework proposed above may be helpful to rehabilitation specialists working on problems of executive dysfunction. One advantage that the application of SEC theory to rehabilitation method has is that an understanding of the schemas that SECs represent and the types of breakdowns in performance that may occur in carrying out SECs is easily grasped by the family members. Another advantage is in the ease of designing tasks to use to try and modify patient behavior. In keeping with the frequency characteristic of SEC components, a therapist might want to choose an SEC to work with that has a mid-range frequency of experience by the patient. This gives the patient some familiarity with the activity, but the activity is not so simple and the patient must take some care to perform it correctly. In addition to developing an error analysis of patient performance by manipulating SEC level of frequency, difficulty, and SEC event centrality, it should be much easier to see systematic differences in patient performance as patients tackle executing and understanding more difficult SECs. The SEC framework proposes that a set of stored representations that are bound together form the unified SEC. Thus, it should be possible to have several different variables measuring specific aspects of SEC performance, including accuracy of overlearned or new visuomotor procedures, acquisition or expression of integrative or event-specific thematic content, and structural knowledge of the SEC (i.e., order and timing of events). Thus, the potential richness of the SEC framework allows for fine analysis of patient breakdown and improvement in performance with training using behavioral modification methods. An additional advantage of this approach is that in the rehabilitation or research setting, SECs that patients would be trained on can be titrated to specific activities that are unique to a particular patient's experience at work, school, or home, so that behaviors can be targeted for their relevance to the patient's daily life.

CONCLUSIONS

In this chapter I have argued that an important way to understand the functions of the HPFC is to adapt the representational model that has been the predominant approach to understanding the neuropsychological aspects of, for example, language processing and object recognition. The representational approach I developed is based on the structured event complex framework, which claims that there are multiple subcomponents of higher-level knowledge that are stored throughout the HPFC as distinctive domains of memory. I have also argued that there are topographical distinctions in where these different aspects of knowledge are stored in the HPFC. Each memory domain component of the SEC can be characterized by psychological features such as frequency of exposure, category specificity, associative properties, sequential dependencies, and goal orientation, which governs the ease of retrieving an SEC. In addition, when these memory representations become activated via environmental stimuli or by automatic or reflective thought, they are activated for longer periods of time than knowledge stored in other areas of the brain, giving rise to the impression that performance dependent on SEC activation is based on a specific form of memory called *working memory*. Adapting a representational framework such as the SEC framework should lead to a richer corpus of predictions about subject performance that can be rejected or validated via experimental studies. Furthermore, the SEC framework lends itself quite easily to rehabilitation practice. Finally, there is now a substantial set of research suggesting that studying the nature of the SEC framework is a competitive and fruitful way to understand the role of the HPFC in behavior.

ACKNOWLEDGMENTS

Portions of this chapter were adapted from a chapter by J. Grafman to appear in the *Handbook of Neuropsychology*, 2nd edition, published by Elsevier Science.

REFERENCES

Anderson, S.W., Bechara, A., Damasio, H., Tranel, D., & Damasio, A.R. (1999). Impairment of social and moral behavior related to early damage in human prefrontal cortex. *Nature Neuroscience, 2,* 1032–1037.

Arnett, P.A., Rao, S.M., Bernardin, L., Grafman, J., Yetkin, F.Z., & Lobeck, L. (1994). Relationship between frontal lobe lesions and Wisconsin Card Sorting Test performance in patients with multiple sclerosis. *Neurology,* 44, 420–425.

Baddeley, A. (1998a). The central executive: a concept and some misconceptions. *Journal of the International Neuropsychological Society,* 4, 523–526.

Baddeley, A. (1998b). Recent developments in working memory. *Current Opinion in Neurobiology,* 8, 234–238.

Barbas, H. (2000). Complementary roles of prefrontal cortical regions in cognition, memory, and emotion in primates. *Advances in Neurology,* 84, 87–110.

Bechara, A., Damasio, H., Damasio, A.R., & Lee, G.P. (1999). Different contributions of the human amygdala and ventromedial prefrontal cortex to decision-making. *Journal of Neuroscience,* 19, 5473–5481.

Bechara, A., Damasio, H., & Damasio, A.R. (2000). Emotion, decision making and the orbitofrontal cortex. *Cerebral Cortex,* 10, 295–307.

Beeman, M. (1998). Coarse semantic coding and discourse comprehension. In; M. Beeman & C. Chiarello (Eds.), *Right Hemisphere Language Comprehension* (pp. 255–284). Mahwah, NJ: Lawrence Erlbaum Associates.

Botvinick, M. & Plaut, D.C. (2000). Doing without schema hierarchies: a recurrent connectionist approach to routine sequential action and its pathologies. Presented at the Annual Meeting of the Cognitive Neuroscience Society (poster presentation), San Francisco, CA, April 11, 2000.

Burgess, P.W. (2000). Strategy application disorder: the role of the frontal lobes in human multitasking. *Psychological Research,* 63, 279–288.

Burgess, P.W., Veitch, E., de Lacy Costello, A., & Shallice, T. (2000). The cognitive and neuroanatomical correlates of multitasking. *Neuropsychologia,* 38, 848–863.

Carlin, D., Bonerba, J., Phipps, M., Alexander, G., Shapiro, M., & Grafman, J. (2000). Planning impairments in frontal lobe dementia and frontal lobe lesion patients. *Neuropsychologia,* 38, 655–665.

Changeux, J.P. & Dehaene, S. (1998). Hierarchical neuronal modeling of cognitive functions: from synaptic transmission to the Tower of London. *Comptes rendus de l'Academie des sciences. Serie III, Sciences de la vie,* 321, 241–247.

Cooper, R. & Shallice, T. (2000). Contention scheduling and the control of routine activities. *Cognitive Neuropsychology,* 17, 297–338.

Courtney, S.M., Petit, L., Haxby, J.V., & Ungerleider, L.G. (1998). The role of prefrontal cortex in working memory: examining the contents of consciousness. *Philosophical Transactions of the Royal Society of London, Series B: Biological Sciences,* 353, 1819–1828.

Crozier, S., Sirigu, A., Lehericy, S., van de Moortele, P.F., Pillon, B., Grafman, J., Agid, Y., Dubois, B., & LeBihan, D. (1999). Distinct prefrontal activations in processing sequence at the sentence and script level: an fMRI study. *Neuropsychologia,* 37, 1469–1476.

Damasio, A.R. (1996). The somatic marker hypothesis and the possible functions of the prefrontal cortex. *Philo-sophical Transactions of the Royal Society of London, Series B: Biological Sciences,* 351, 1413–1420.

Dimitrov, M., Grafman, J., & Hollnagel, C. (1996). The effects of frontal lobe damage on everyday problem solving. *Cortex,* 32, 357–366.

Dimitrov, M., Grafman, J., Soares, A.H., & Clark, K. (1999a). Concept formation and concept shifting in frontal lesion and Parkinson's disease patients assessed with the California Card Sorting Test. *Neuropsychology,* 13, 135–43.

Dimitrov, M., Granetz, J., Peterson, M., Hollnagel, C., Alexander, G., & Grafman, J. (1999b). Associative learning impairments in patients with frontal lobe damage. *Brain Cognition,* 41, 213–230.

Dimitrov, M., Phipps, M., Zahn, T.P., & Grafman, J. (1999c). A thoroughly modern gage. *Neurocase,* 5, 345–354.

Dreher, J.C., Koechlin, E., Ali, O., & Grafman, J. (Submitted). Dissociation of task timing expectancy and task order anticipation during task switching.

Elston, G.N. (2000). Pyramidal cells of the frontal lobe: all the more spinous to think with. *Journal of Neuroscience,* 20, RC95 (1–4).

Engel, A.K. & Singer, W. (2001). Temporal binding and the neural correlates of sensory awareness. *Trends in Cognitive Science,* 5, 16–25.

Eslinger, P.J. (1998). Neurological and neuropsychological bases of empathy. *European Neurology,* 39, 193–199.

Forde, E.M.E. & Humphreys, G.W. (2000). The role of semantic knowledge and working memory in everyday tasks. *Brain and Cognition,* 44, 214–252.

Fuster, J.M., Bodner, M., & Kroger, J.K. (2000). Cross-modal and cross-temporal association in neurons of frontal cortex. *Nature,* 405, 347–351.

Gehring, W.J. & Knight, R.T. (2000). Prefrontal–cingulate interactions in action monitoring. *Nature Neuroscience,* 3, 516–520.

Goel, V. & Grafman, J. (1995). Are the frontal lobes implicated in "planning" functions? Interpreting data from the Tower of Hanoi. *Neuropsychologia,* 33, 623–642.

Goel, V., Grafman, J., Sadato, N., & Hallett, M. (1995). Modeling other minds. *NeuroReport,* 6, 1741–1746.

Goel, V., Grafman, J., Tajik, J., Gana, S., & Danto, D. (1997). A study of the performance of patients with frontal lobe lesions in a financial planning task. *Brain,* 120, 1805–1822.

Gomez Beldarrain, M., Grafman, J., Pascual-Leone, A., & Garcia-Monco, J.C. (1999). Procedural learning is impaired in patients with prefrontal lesions. *Neurology,* 52, 1853–1860.

Grafman, J. (1995). Similarities and distinctions among current models of prefrontal cortical functions. *Annals of the New York Academy of Sciences,* 769, 337–368.

Grafman, J. (1999). Experimental assessment of adult frontal lobe function. In: B.L. Miller & J. Cummings (Eds.), *The Human Frontal Lobes: Function and Disorder* (pp. 321–344). New York: The Guilford Press.

Grafman, J. & Litvan, I. (1999a). Evidence for four forms of neuroplasticity. In: J. Grafman & Y. Christen (Eds.), *Neuronal Plasticity: Building a Bridge from the Labo-

ratory to the Clinic (pp. 131–140). Berlin: Springer-Verlag.

Grafman, J. & Litvan, I. (1999b). Importance of deficits in executive functions. *Lancet, 354,* 1921–1923.

Grafman, J., Litvan, I., Massaquoi, S., Stewart, M., Sirigu, A., & Hallett, M. (1992). Cognitive planning deficit in patients with cerebellar atrophy. *Neurology, 42,* 1493–1496.

Grafman, J., Schwab, K., Warden, D., Pridgen, A., Brown, H.R., & Salazar, A.M. (1996). Frontal lobe injuries, violence, and aggression: a report of the Vietnam Head Injury Study. *Neurology, 46,* 1231–1238.

Hallett, M. & Grafman, J. (1997). Executive function and motor skill learning. *International Review of Neurobiology, 41,* 297–323.

Hanson, C. & Hanson, S.E. (1996). Development of schemata during event parsing: Neisser's perceptual cycle as a recurrent connectionist network. *Journal of Cognitive Neuroscience, 8,* 119–134.

Humphreys, G.W. & Riddoch, M.J. (2000). One more cup of coffee for the road: object-action assemblies, response blocking and response capture after frontal lobe damage. *Experimental Brain Research, 133,* 81–93.

Humphreys, G.W. & Riddoch, M.J. (2001). Detection by action: neuropsychological evidence for action-defined templates in search. *Nature Neuroscience, 4,* 84–88.

Jurado, M.A., Junque, C., Vendrell, P., Treserras, P., & Grafman, J. (1998). Overestimation and unreliability in "feeling-of-doing" judgements about temporal ordering performance: impaired self-awareness following frontal lobe damage. *Journal of Clinical and Experimental Neuropsychology, 20,* 353–364.

Kawasaki, H., Kaufman, O., Damasio, H., Damasio, A.R., Granner, M., Bakken, H., Hori, T., Howard, M.A., 3rd, & Adolphs, R. (2001). Single-neuron responses to emotional visual stimuli recorded in human ventral prefrontal cortex. *Nature Neuroscience, 4,* 15–6.

Kimberg, D.Y. & Farah, M.J. (1993). A unified account of cognitive impairments following frontal lobe damage: the role of working memory in complex, organized behavior. *Journal of Experimental Psychology: General, 122,* 411–428.

Koechlin, E., Basso, G., Pietrini, P., Panzer, S., & Grafman, J. (1999). The role of the anterior prefrontal cortex in human cognition. *Nature, 399,* 148–51.

Koechlin, E., Corrado, G., Pietrini, P., & Grafman, J. (2000). Dissociating the role of the medial and lateral anterior prefrontal cortex in human planning. *Proceedings of the National Academy of Sciences USA, 97,* 7651–7656.

Koechlin, E., Danek, A., Burnod, Y., & Grafman, J. (Submitted). Brain mechanisms underlying the acquisition of behavioral and cognitive sequences.

Levine, B., Robertson, I.H., Clare, L., Carter, G., Hong, J., Wilson, B.A., Duncan, J., & Stuss, D.T. (2000). Rehabilitation of executive functioning: an experimental–clinical validation of goal management training. *Journal of the International Neuropsychological Society, 6,* 299–312.

Levy, R. & Goldman-Rakic, P.S. (2000). Segregation of working memory functions within the dorsolateral pre-

frontal cortex. *Experimental Brain Research, 133,* 23–32.

Macmillan, M. (2000). *An Odd Kind of Fame: Stories of Phineas Gage.* Cambridge, MA: MIT Press.

Meyer, D.E. & Kieras, D.E. (1997). A computational theory of executive cognitive processes and multiple-task performance: Part 1. Basic mechanisms. *Psychological Review, 104,* 3–65.

Miller, E.K. (2000). The prefrontal cortex and cognitive control. *Nature Reviews: Neuroscience, 1,* 59–65.

Nichelli, P., Grafman, J., Pietrini, P., Always, D., Carton, J.C., & Miletich, R. (1994). Brain activity in chess playing. *Nature, 369,* 191.

Nichelli, P., Clark, K., Hollnagel, C., & Grafman, J. (1995a). Duration processing after frontal lobe lesions. *Annals of the New York Academy of Sciences, 769,* 183–90.

Nichelli, P., Grafman, J., Pietrini, P., Clark, K., Lee, K.Y., & Miletich, R. (1995b). Where the brain appreciates the moral of a story. *NeuroReport, 6,* 2309–2313.

Norman, D.A. & Shallice, T. (1986). Attention to action: willed and automatic control of behavior. In: R.J. Davidson, G.E. Schwartz, & D. Shapiro (Eds.), *Consciousness and Self-Regulation, Vol 4.* (pp. 1–18). New York: Plenum Press.

Nystrom, L.E., Braver, T.S., Sabb, F.W., Delgado, M.R., Noll, D.C., & Cohen, J.D. (2000). Working memory for letters, shapes, and locations: fMRI evidence against stimulus-based regional organization in human prefrontal cortex. *NeuroImage, 11,* 424–446.

Partiot, A., Grafman, J., Sadato, N., Wachs, J., & Hallett, M. (1995). Brain activation during the generation of non-emotional and emotional plans. *NeuroReport, 6,* 1397–400.

Partiot, A., Grafman, J., Sadato, N., Flitman, S., & Wild, K. (1996). Brain activation during script event processing. *NeuroReport, 7,* 761–766.

Pascual-Leone, A., Grafman, J., Clark, K., Stewart, M., Massaquoi, S., Lou, J.S., & Hallett, M. (1993). Procedural learning in Parkinson's disease and cerebellar degeneration. *Annals of Neurology, 34,* 594–602.

Pascual-Leone, A., Grafman, J., & Hallett, M. (1995). Procedural learning and prefrontal cortex. *Annals of the New York Academy of Sciences, 769,* 61–70.

Pascual-Leone, A., Wassermann, E.M., Grafman, J., & Hallett, M. (1996). The role of the dorsolateral prefrontal cortex in implicit procedural learning. *Experimental Brain Research, 107,* 479–485.

Pietrini, P., Guazzelli, M., Basso, G., Jaffe, K., & Grafman, J. (2000). Neural correlates of imaginal aggressive behavior assessed by positron emission tomography in healthy subjects. *American Journal of Psychiatry, 157,* 1772–1781.

Price, J.L. (1999). Prefrontal cortical networks related to visceral function and mood. *Annals of the New York Academy of Sciences, 877,* 383–396.

Ruchkin, D.S., Berndt, R.S., Johnson, R., Ritter, W., Grafman, J., & Canoune, H.L. (1997). Modality-specific processing streams in verbal working memory: evidence from spatio-temporal patterns of brain activity. *Brain Research: Cognitive Brain Research, 6,* 95–113.

Rueckert, L. & Grafman, J. (1996). Sustained attention deficits in patients with right frontal lesions. *Neuropsychologia, 34,* 953–963.

Rueckert, L. & Grafman, J. (1998). Sustained attention deficits in patients with lesions of posterior cortex. *Neuropsychologia, 36,* 653–660.

Schacter, D.L. & Buckner, R.L. (1998). Priming and the brain. *Neuron, 20,* 185–95.

Schwab, K., Grafman, J., Salazar, A.M., & Kraft, J. (1993). Residual impairments and work status 15 years after penetrating head injury: report from the Vietnam Head Injury Study. *Neurology, 43,* 95–103.

Schwartz, M.F., Buxbaum, L.J., Montgomery, M.W., Fitzpatrick-DeSalme, E., Hart, T., Ferraro, M., Lee, S.S., & Coslett, H.B. (1999). Naturalistic action production following right hemisphere stroke. *Neuropsychologia, 37,* 51–66.

Shallice, T. & Burgess, P.W. (1996). The domain of supervisory processes and temporal organization of behavior. *Philosophical Transactions of the Royal Society of London B, 351,* 1405–1412.

Sirigu, A., Zalla, T., Pillon, B., Grafman, J., Agid, Y., & Dubois, B. (1995a). Selective impairments in managerial knowledge following pre-frontal cortex damage. *Cortex, 31,* 301–316.

Sirigu, A., Zalla, T., Pillon, B., Grafman, J., Dubois, B., & Agid, Y. (1995b). Planning and script analysis following prefrontal lobe lesions. *Annals of the New York Academy of Sciences, 769,* 277–288.

Sirigu, A., Zalla, T., Pillon, B., Grafman, J., Agid, Y., & Dubois, B. (1996). Encoding of sequence and boundaries of scripts following prefrontal lesions. *Cortex, 32,* 297–310.

Sirigu, A., Cohen, L., Zalla, T., Pradat-Diehl, P., Van Eeckhout, P., Grafman, J., & Agid, Y. (1998). Distinct frontal regions for processing sentence syntax and story grammar. *Cortex, 34,* 771–778.

Smith, E.E. & Jonides, J. (1999). Storage and executive processes in the frontal lobes. *Science, 283,* 1657–1661.

Stablum, F., Umilta, C., Mogentale, C., Carlan, M., & Guerrini, C. (2000). Rehabilitation of executive deficits in closed head injury and anterior communicating artery aneurysm patients. *Psychological Research, 63,* 265–278.

Stuss, D.T., Toth, J.P., Franchi, D., Alexander, M.P., Tipper, S., & Craik, F.I. (1999). Dissociation of attentional processes in patients with focal frontal and posterior lesions. *Neuropsychologia, 37,* 1005–1027.

Thierry, A.M., Gioanni, Y., Degenetais, E., & Glowinski, J. (2000). Hippocampo-prefrontal cortex pathway: anatomical and electrophysiological characteristics. *Hippocampus, 10,* 411–419.

Vendrell, P., Junque, C., Pujol, J., Jurado, M.A., Molet, J., & Grafman, J. (1995). The role of prefrontal regions in the Stroop task. *Neuropsychologia, 33,* 341–352.

Wharton, C.M., Grafman, J., Flitman, S.S., Hansen, E.K., Brauner, J., Marks, A., & Honda, M. (2000). Toward neuroanatomical models of analogy: a positron emission tomography study of analogical mapping. *Cognitive Psychology, 40,* 173–97.

Zacks, J.M. & Tversky, B. (2001). Event structure in perception and conception. *Psychological Bulletin, 127,* 3–21.

Zahn, T.P., Grafman, J., & Tranel, D. (1999). Frontal lobe lesions and electrodermal activity: effects of significance. *Neuropsychologia, 37,* 1227–1241.

Zalla, T., Koechlin, E., Pietrini, P., Basso, G., Aquino, P., Sirigu, A., & Grafman, J. (2000). Differential amygdala responses to winning and losing: a functional magnetic resonance imaging study in humans. *European Journal of Neuroscience, 12,* 1764–1770.

Zalla & Cortex (in press). Story processing in patients with damage to the prefrontal cortex.

20

Chronesthesia: Conscious Awareness of Subjective Time

ENDEL TULVING

One of the most remarkable capacities that nature has seen fit to bestow on us human beings is our sense of subjective time in which we exist. We do not think much about this subjective time; we take it for granted as we take for granted the air we breathe. But we can, if we decide to do so, reflect on the fact of our protracted existence in time that extends from the present "back" into the past and "forward" into the future. We can, if we wish, close our eyes and think about what we did minutes ago, or how we celebrated our last birthday. And we can think about what we might be doing tomorrow, or next year. This kind of sense of time makes a huge difference to what we are and how we live. If we retained all our other marvelous mental capacities but lost the awareness of time in which our lives are played out, we might still be uniquely different from all other animals but we would no longer be human as we understand humanness.

This chapter is about this human sense of time. To distinguish it from other time-related and time-dependent achievements of the brain/mind, I refer to it as *chronesthesia*, which is tentatively defined as a form of consciousness that allows individuals to think about the subjective time in which they live and that makes it possible for them to "mentally travel" in such time. In this chapter, I shall attempt to explicate the concept of chronesthesia, suggest what it is (and what it is not), contrast it with other kinds of time-related mentation, discuss the origin of the concept, and, the main reason for the chapter's appearance in the present volume, speculate on chronesthesia's relation to prefrontal cortex. I shall conclude the chapter by discussing the role of chronesthesia in human evolution and human affairs.

Chronesthesia is closely related to a number of neurocognitive functions that have to do with time, and that have been studied by brain/mind scientists for a long time. These include mental activities such as remembering (or recollection of) past happenings, thinking about the past, expecting, planning, and thinking about the future. To understand the relation between chronesthesia and these other time-related cognitive activities, which may sound indistinguishable from chronesthesia as defined above, it is necessary first to draw a distinction between two aspects of organization of the brain/mind, capacity and function.

CAPACITY AND FUNCTION

A basic conceptual distinction is that between *neurocognitive (brain/mind) capacities* that individuals possess, on the one hand, and *functions (manifestations) of such general capacities* on the other hand. A (general) neurocognitive capacity (sometimes also referred to as neurocognitive or brain *system*) allows an individual to engage in mental activities and attain goals that are not possible for an individual who does not possess the capacity. Each general capacity is a property of the evolved brain that serves specific organismically useful ends. Thus, for example, the visual capacity (*vision*) allows the individual to make use of optic signals provided by the environment, that is, to see objects in space. Similarly, the auditory capacity (*audition*) allows the individual to make use of acoustic signals, that is, to hear sounds. The episodic memory capacity allows one to remember one's personal past, that is, to re-experience at time 2 happenings experienced earlier, at time 1. The biological value of these capacities and their functions is indisputable.

Examples of some of the general capacities and their functions that interest brain scientists are listed in Table 20–1. Some of them (vision, audition, and other senses) are associated with special receptors, while others (learning, memory) have no such devices for registering changes in one's external environment. Some of the latter do involve "inputs" and "outputs," whereas the operations of still others (shown in Table 20–1 as various kinds of consciousness) somehow supervene on, and

interact with, selected other processes in ways not yet completely understood.

The nature of the relation between general capacities and their specific expressions (functions) is one that is exceedingly common but has no common label. We can use the term *enabling* to designate it. Thus, a general capacity enables or allows the individual to engage in a large but circumscribed category of mental activities without specifically determining whether or how the capacity is used. A general capacity is just one of the necessary conditions of certain behavioral, cognitive, or consciousness-based achievements. The actual exercise of any capacity always depends on other factors as well.

All general capacities listed in Table 20–1 represent properties of the evolved brain, and are subserved by specific, usually widely distributed, neuronal centers and pathways. The capacities may vary among the species. Not all species have vision, and very few, perhaps only humans, have autonoetic consciousness, the kind of consciousness that allows people to be aware now of experiences of an earlier time. The capacities are also products of ontogenetic development, and usually grow, mature, and decay as an individual interacts with its physical and social environment. Being dependent on the brain, they are vulnerable to brain damage.

When a given brain/mind capacity is reasonably closely tied to known neuroanatomical structures and physiological mechanisms, we can talk about it as a neurocognitive "system": for example, the visual system, or the auditory system. When such a relation between the brain and the mind is less firmly established, as is the case for learning and memory, or as yet largely unknown, as is the case for different kinds of consciousness, we speak of the corresponding neurocognitive systems somewhat more metaphorically, simply as an expression of our faith that neural correlates of these capacities also exist even if they are not yet (or not yet completely) known.

The points just made about neurocognitive capacities, or systems, and their "expressions," or functions, are elementary, well known to and accepted by all practitioners. They are

Table 20–1. Selected Examples of General Neurocognitive Capacities and their Particular Functions

General Capacity	Function
Object vision	Seeing objects
Spatial vision	Seeing space
Color vision	Seeing colors
Motion vision	Seeing movement
Audition	Hearing sounds
Semantic memory	Knowing the world
Episodic memory	Remembering experiences
Noetic consciousness	Awareness of the world
Autonoetic consciousness	Awareness of self in time
Chronesthesia	Awareness of subjective time

mentioned here to place the concept of chronesthesia in the proper perspective.

CONSCIOUSNESS AND CHRONESTHESIA

The term *consciousness* has many different meanings. A very basic distinction can be made between the individual's general state of alertness or arousal, such as those accompanying wake–sleep cycles, or of the kind measured by the Glasgow Coma scale, on the one hand, and various cognitively and affectively experienced mental states that characterize a fully alert individual on the other.

Table 20–1 includes the reference to two particular kinds of consciousness of the latter category, noetic and autonoetic. Both have to do with experiential, or phenomenological, aspects of conscious awareness that accompany memory retrieval (recovery of stored information). Each has its own functions. *Noetic consciousness* is evolutionarily older and the more "primitive" of the two, and is the default mode of the semantic memory system. Noetic awareness accompanies an individual's memory-based interaction with aspects of its environment in the present. When individuals think about the "facts of the world," they are noetically aware of what they are thinking, as well as aware of such awareness. Noetic consciousness also provides individuals with access to their own past, but the mode of such access is one of "knowing," not "remembering" (Gardiner, 1988; Rajaram, 1993). *Autonoetic consciousness* has a more recent origin in evolution and is more advanced than noetic, because in addition to allowing people to know what happened in the past it also allows them to re-experience past experiences. Autonoetic awareness accompanies retrieval of information about one's personal past as well as projection of one's thoughts into the future. When individuals remember the past, they are autonoetically aware of what they did or thought at an earlier time, and they are also aware of such awareness. Thus, autonoetic consciousness includes but transcends noetic consciousness.

Both autonoetic and noetic consciousness are determined by the properties of the individual's brain and its general physiologic state at any given moment. A given kind of consciousness provides the individual with a potential for particular kinds of awareness; it determines what kinds of awareness or subjective experience the person *can* have. Consciousness as capacity is not directed at anything, whereas awareness is always of something. To be aware of something means to have a particular subjective experience that is determined by both the current (general) state of consciousness and the current (particular) stimulation from external and internal sources. In other words, awareness presumes consciousness, but consciousness does not imply awareness: consciousness is a necessary but not a sufficient condition of awareness. Within a given level of awareness, many particular kinds of subjective experiences may occur. We can think of (selective) attention as the primary process that determines the aspects of the stimulus situation of which the individual is aware.

Because chronesthesia is a kind of consciousness, everything that is said about consciousness in general also applies to chronesthesia. Chronesthesia is the kind of neurocognitive capability that expresses itself in individuals' awareness of the temporal dimension of their own and others' existence and that makes thinking about subjective time possible. It is a general precondition of many different kinds of *cognitive activity* that involve time. The most common and familiar expression of chronesthesia is remembering happenings from one's life, or thinking back to past events and situations. But the human time sense also extends to the future. Everybody can as readily think about the future and make plans for the future as they can think about and remember the past. I refer to the thought-about time in which one's personal experiences take place as *subjective time*. It plays a critical role in the definition of chronesthesia (on the various concepts of physical and psychological time, see Fraisse, 1963; Church, 1989; Block, 1990; Ivry, 1996; McCormack & Hoerl, 1999).

WHAT CHRONESTHESIA IS NOT

It may be useful at this point to briefly mention what chronesthesia is not, to minimize confusion and unnecessary argument. Numerous time-related concepts figure prominently in the existing literature that need to be distinguished from chronesthesia. Consider three categories of such concepts.

First, there are various behavioral and cognitive (mental) activities that clearly *depend on* chronesthesia but are not identical with it. They are the functions of chronesthesia, activities that chronesthesia makes possible. Examples are activities such as reminiscing about or recollecting past events, daydreaming, anticipation of future happenings, planning future activities (Owen, 1997; Koechlin, et al., 1999), and "prospective memory" (Mantyla & Nilsson, 1997; Einstein et al., 1999).

Second, as a special kind of consciousness, chronesthesia has properties that other forms of consciousness do not. Therefore it has to be distinguished from these other forms. For example, young children share many forms of consciousness with adults, but there is no evidence that those younger than 3 or 4 years "possess" chronesthesia (Wheeler et al., 1997).

The third category of time-related mentation that has to be differentiated from chronesthesia has to do with behavioral and cognitive activities of everyday life, and their artifactual analogues in the laboratory (*cognitive tasks*) that may appear to involve awareness of subjective time. This third category is most troublesome, because in many cases the temptation is great to think of them as dependent on chronesthesia. Examples of these include the following: *(1)* many non-episodic forms of memory whose function is to allow the organism to benefit at time 2 from what happened at time 1 (see Tulving & Markowitsch, 1998; Tulving, 1999, for further discussion); *(2)* various kinds of "serial learning" in humans (Crowder & Greene, 2000) or in nonhuman animals (Gower, 1992); *(3)* genetically programmed ("instinctive," "purposeful") evolutionary adaptations, such as rodents demonstrating temporal 'entrainment' of behavior by environmental rhythms (Moore-Ede, et al.,

1982) or crows dropping walnuts to get at the fruit (Zach, 1979), *(4)* "estimations" of temporal durations in tasks (e.g., interval reinforcement) where the duration serves as a discriminative stimulus (Church, 1989); *(5)* matching sensory-motor rhythms (e.g., finger tapping) to external sources of rhythmic stimulation (e.g., Jäncke, et al. 2000); and *(6)* the kinds of "generalized timing functions" in whose control the cerebellum plays an important role (Ivry & Fiez, 2000). Even semantic knowledge that humans possess about physical time (*chronognosia*) and expressions of such knowledge linguistically need not imply the involvement of chronesthesia.

The exclusion of these and other similar behavioral/cognitive activities as expressions of chronesthesia does not mean, of course, that they have nothing to do with chronesthesia. Indeed, it makes sense to assume that all or some of the many ways in which evolved brains deal with temporal aspects of the world represent evolutionary precursors of chronesthesia. The exclusion of these activities also does not mean that chronesthesia could not be usefully deployed in many of these activities. The hypothesis is simply that chronesthesia is not necessary for them.

CHRONESTHESIA AND RELATED CONCEPTS

If none of these other time-dependent or time-related forms of behavioral or cognitive activities are to be identified with chronesthesia, what kinds of time-related activities are? How do we know that a given bit of an individual's behavior involves or directly relies on chronesthesia?

In the first instance, of course, we can rely on individuals' telling us what they do consciously recollect of their personal happenings, that is, on their verbal reports of their past experiences and future intentions. We can also rely on their claims that they are consciously aware of the existence of subjective time, and that they understand what it means to "mentally travel" in such time.

But what do we do about nonverbal organisms, such as young children or nonhuman animals? Here we have to rely on inferential reasoning based on our extant knowledge of the world. Thus, when we observe an organism engaged in an activity that we suspect might involve chronesthesia, we ask: Would it be possible for this activity to occur without the capability of consciously thinking back to the past, or forward to the future? If the answer is positive, we act on the principle of parsimony and refrain from invoking chronesthesia; if it is negative, we postulate that the activity in question is an expression (function) of chronesthesia. Although we may not be able to achieve universal consensus on the answers to all instances of such questions, it is reasonable to expect that sufficient agreement would exist in the matter to make at least the beginning of the scientific study of chronesthesia possible. More refined approaches to chronesthesia will be worked out in the natural course of the development of cognitive neuroscience.

Although the sense of time has seen less coverage in psychology and cognitive neuroscience than has the sense of space, time-related ideas rather similar to that of chronesthesia have been proposed and discussed. These include ideas proposed by David Ingvar who, in his pioneering work on the measurement of regional cerebral blood flow, noticed chronic hyperfrontal activity and attributed it to the individual's conscious thoughts about the future (Ingvar, 1985). His prescient sentiments have been echoed in recent work in functional neuroimaging (Andreasen et al., 1995). Some time ago, Joaquin Fuster, on the basis of his findings of differential firing patterns of individual neurons (Fuster, 1973), proposed a general theory of prefrontal cortex in which temporal organization of behavior and cognition plays a central role (Fuster, 1995). Fuster's concept of "prospective set" (Fuster, 2000), one of the two major cognitive specialties of the dorsolateral prefrontal cortex in his theory (working memory is the other), designates the brain's capability of anticipating future sensory and motor acts on the basis of neurocognitive events in the present (Fuster, 2000). Prospective set can be thought of as closely related to chronesthesia. In other studies it has been observed that some patients

with brain damage can respond well to questions about the impersonal past and future, but are quite deficient on comparable questions pertaining to their own personal past and future (Dalla Barba, et al., 1997; Klein et al., 2002 [in press]). The impairment of personal temporal orientation described in these studies can be seen as possible instances of defective chronesthesia. Disturbances in consciousness of time brought about by cerebral damage have been documented by Knight and Grabowecky (1995, 2000). Finally, in developmental psychology, Haith (1997) has been engaged in a systematic research program aimed at elucidating the development of future-oriented thinking in children. Haith's concept of "future thinking" is in many ways quite similar to chronesthesia (see also Haith et al., 1994).

The concept that is most closely related to chronesthesia is *autonoetic consciousness* (or *autonoesis*), already mentioned above. It is defined as a form of consciousness that allows individuals to apprehend their subjective experiences throughout time, and to perceive the present moment as both a continuation of their past and as a prelude to their future (Nelson, 1997; Suddendorf & Corballis, 1997; Wheeler et al., 1997; Tulving, 2001; Stuss et al., 2001). Because the essence of what I attribute here to chronesthesia has previously been associated with autonoesis, one may wonder whether yet another esoteric concept such as chronesthesia is needed. I think that it is. Although both autonoesis and chronesthesia imply awareness of self in time, the emphasis on self versus time is different in the two concepts: in autonoesis the emphasis is on awareness of *self*, albeit in subjective time, whereas in chronesthesia the emphasis is on awareness of *subjective time*, albeit in relation to self. The distinction may be subtle but it is necessary, because time can be dealt with, and usually is dealt with, independently of the self, and self can be dealt with independently of time, as shown by behavioral (e.g., Gallup, 1982; Povinelli et al., 1996; Stone et al., 1998; Keenan et al., 2000) and functional neuroimaging (Craik et al., 1999; Kircher et al., 2000) research on self-recognition and self-face recognition.

CHRONESTHESIA AND THE CASE OF K.C.

The evidence supporting the postulated existence of chronesthesia is as yet scant, and what exists is largely indirect. Indeed, when relating the hypothetical ideas about chronesthesia to empirical facts, it would be pretentious to talk about evidence as such. It would be more appropriate to talk about ideas, observations, and facts that are related to the ideas concerning chronesthesia, and that can be seen as encouraging speculations about the kind of sense of time I refer to as chronesthesia.

Some relevant evidence comes from clinical cases of brain-damaged patients, such as those cases already mentioned (Dalla Barba et al., 1997, Klein et al., in press). One such case, indeed, gave rise to the concept of autonoetic consciousness, the predecessor idea of chronesthesia (Tulving, 1985). (Note: N.N. in that article is the same patient that in subsequent publications is referred to as K.C.). The case is that of a man known as K.C., now 50 years old, who at the age of 30 suffered traumatic brain injury, as a result of which he became densely amnesic. Various aspects of his case have been published previously (Tulving et al., 1988, 1991; Tulving, 1989a, 1989b, 2001; (Hayman et al., 1993; Rosenbaum et al., 2000; Westmacott et al., 2001). As shown in Figure 20–1, he has multiple cortical and white matter lesions in anterior and posterior regions, and his hippocampus and other medial–temporal lobe structures, more in the left than the right hemisphere, are also largely dysfunctional (Rosenbaum et al., 2000).

In many ways K.C.'s intellectual capabilities are comparable to those of healthy adults. His intelligence and knowledge of the world (premorbidly acquired semantic memory) is normal, language is normal, he reads and writes, his thought processes are clear, he has a good sense of self here and now, he plays the organ, can play chess and various card games (indeed, he spends a lot of time playing these games on the computer), he has no problem with immediate memory (his digit span has been measured at 8 digits), his social manners are exemplary, and he possesses a quiet sense of humour.

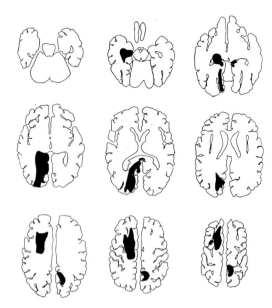

Figure 20–1. Schematic presentation of K.C.'s brain lesions, estimated from magnetic resonance imaging (MRI), rendered on axial slices of the template from Damasio and Damasio (1989). Most lesions are seen in the left hemisphere limbic, cortical, and white-matter structures, although some also appear on the right, in the medial temporal and median parietal (cuneus and precuneus) regions. (*Source:* Courtesy of Dr. Paul J Eslinger)

K.C. differs from other people primarily in two ways. First, he has no functional episodic memory: for all practical purposes he cannot remember anything that has ever happened to him. However hard he tries, and however powerfully he is prompted, he cannot mentally travel back into his past in the way that healthy people can. He has no conscious awareness of a single event, happening, or situation that he has witnessed or in which he has participated. This *global episodic amnesia* covers the period from his birth to the present day. Second, he has serious difficulties learning and retaining new information. Although he has been taught some new factual information (Tulving et al., 1991; Hayman et al., 1993); and although he has incidentally acquired some other new knowledge about the world as well as himself (Tulving, 1993; see also Klein et al., 1996), he can be classified clinically as a typical dense anterograde amnesic patient.

K.C.'s autonoesis is largely dysfunctional, or perhaps even nonexistent. He lives in a timeless world—that is, in a permanent present. When he is asked to try to "travel back in time" in his own mind, back either a few minutes or many years, he says he cannot do it. When he is asked to describe the state of his mind when he tries to turn his mind's eye towards the past, the best he can do is to say that it is "blank." Nor can he think about the future. Thus, when asked, he cannot tell the questioner what he is going to do later on that day, or the day after, or at any time in the rest of his life, any more than he can say what he did the day before or what events have happened in his life. When he is asked to describe the state of his mind when he thinks about his future, whether the next 15 minutes or the next year, he again says that it is "blank." Indeed, when asked to compare the two kinds of "blankness," one of the past and the other of the future, he says that they are "the same kind of blankness" (Tulving, 1985). Thus K.C. seems to be as incapable of imagining his future as he is of remembering his past.

It is important to note that K.C. has no greater difficulty with physical time than he has with physical space. He knows and can talk about what most other people know about physical time, its units, its structure, and its measurement by clocks and calendars. But such knowledge of time in and of itself does not allow him to remember events as having happened at a particular time. It is necessary but not sufficient. Something else is needed, and this something else—the awareness of time in which one's experiences are recorded—seems to be missing from K.C.'s neurocognitive profile. He thus exhibits a dissociation between knowing time and experiencing time, a dissociation that parallels one between knowing the facts of the world and remembering past experiences.

It was this striking pattern of K.C.'s mental life—his largely conscious thoughts about the impersonal world contrasted with his essentially nonexistent conscious thoughts about his own past and future—that first suggested the distinction between noetic and autonoetic consciousness (Tulving, 1985). K.C. possesses the former, and does not possess the latter. Because he is perfectly well aware of his timeless self—self in the present—it seems rea-

sonable to attribute his difficulties with personal past and personal future to deficient, perhaps largely lacking, chronesthesia.

CHRONESTHESIA AND PREFRONTAL CORTEX

What is the connection between chronesthesia and prefrontal cortex? What do we know in general about the neuroanatomical correlates of chronesthesia?

One reason for suspecting the involvement of prefrontal cortex in chronesthesia lies in the following general principle: If X represents a "higher"—subtle, sophisticated, intricate—form of neurocognitive capability, then chances are that frontal lobes in general and prefrontal cortex in particular figure prominently in its neural substrate. The principle was originally supported from neuropsychological studies of patients with frontal damage (Stuss & Benson, 1985), and is now further bolstered by electroencephalographic (EEG) and functional neuroimaging studies (Knight & Grabowecky, 1995, 2000).

A second reason lies in neuropsychological and functional brain imaging findings of the involvement of prefrontal cortex in many tasks that, one way or another, involve chronesthesia (e.g., Baker et al., 1996; Okuda et al., 1998; Burgess et al., 2001).

A third reason has to do with the close relation between chronesthesia and autonoesis. Autonoesis has been seen as critically dependent on prefrontal cortex, as discussed at some length by Wheeler et al. (1997). With the further refinement of the concept of autonoesis in terms of self *and* time, it would be difficult to imagine that the temporal dimension of autonoesis, that is, chronesthesia, would not critically depend on prefrontal activity.

Neuroanatomical correlates of chronesthesia, of course, are difficult to identify, for the same reason that consciousness of any kind is difficult to pin down in the brain (Moscovitch, 2000). But some suggestive evidence does exist. A relevant case is that of M.L., a patient studied at the Rotman Research Institute by Brian Levine and colleagues (Levine et al., 1998). M.L. is a young man who suffered traumatic brain injury in a traffic accident that caused a severe 'focal' retrograde amnesia (Kapur, 1993; 2000; see also Kopelman, 2000) for both episodic and semantic information. Because he had not lost his ability to acquire new semantic information, M.L. was able not only to re-acquire much of the semantic knowledge he had but also to relearn many facts about his pre-accident life. But he cannot autonoetically recollect any past happenings, possibly because of deficient chronesthesia (Levine et al., 1998). M.L.'s loss of autonoesis is accompanied by a seriously diminished affect and difficulties of self-regulation. The relevant observation is that the only magnetic resonance imaging (MRI)-detectable brain damage is a lesion in the uncinate fascicle in the right hemisphere, a fiber tract connecting prefrontal and temporal cortical regions.

Other clinical evidence suggests that patients who have suffered right anterior brain damage have difficulty in autonoetically reminiscing about their premorbid personal experiences. Thus, Calabrese and colleagues (1996) have reported the case of a post-encephalitic patient, with brain damage mainly in the right temporofrontal region, who showed a severe and enduring loss of the ability to recollect premorbid personal experiences, and less severe loss of general knowledge. Baron et al. (1994) did a position emission tomography (PET) study of a 60-year-old woman during the early recovery phase of an episode of transient global amnesia during which she exhibited severe inability for autobiographical recollection. The imaging results showed reduced cerebral blood flow and oxygen consumption over the right lateral prefrontal cortex, together with a (smaller) reduction in ipsilateral thalamic and lentiform nucleus metabolism, in the absence of any involvement of the hippocampal region. These findings suggest that the transient global amnesia in this case resulted from a metabolic dysfunction of right prefrontal cortex and consequent disturbance of retrieval, possibly because of interference with chronesthetic functions, similar to cases of lasting amnesia (Markowitsch et al., 1993; Markowitsch, 1995; Calabrese et al., 1996). A partic-

ularly revealing PET activation study was reported by Fink et al. (1996). In critical conditions of the study, subjects were scanned while they listened to two kinds of critical sentences. One kind consisted of sentences that were taken out of the subjects' own autobiographical musings that the experimenters had recorded previously. These were assumed to bring back to the subjects' minds 'affect-laden' earlier episodic experiences. The other kind consisted of comparable sentences (taken from other subjects' musings) that the subjects had been exposed to previously in the experiment. Listening to these sentences was also assumed to evoke episodic recollection, but of a type less personally relevant and less affect-laden. Fink et al. (1996) found that listening to own-life sentences was associated with largely right hemispheric activation that included temporal lobes, posterior cingulate insula, and prefrontal regions, in close proximity to M.L.'s lesion reported by Levine et al. (1998). An observation rather similar to that of Fink et al. (1996) has been described by Markowitsch and colleagues (Markowitsch et al., 1999). This was a functional imaging study with normal healthy volunteers, comparing neural networks involved in the retrieval of personal autobiographical information with those involved in retrieval of similar fictitious material. The results showed that the retrieval of autobiographical information was associated with selective activations of the right amygdala and the right ventral prefrontal cortex, again in the vicinity of the uncinate fascicle.

All these and other similar case studies suggest that damage to the frontal lobes and connected brain areas disrupts autobiographical (episodic) recollection while recall of general (semantic) knowledge of the world remains intact, or is less severely impaired. The data fit well with suggestions that frontal lobes play a critical role in self-awareness (Ingvar, 1985; Stuss & Benson, 1986). Although, typically, in these earlier discussions self-awareness was not explicitly defined in terms of time-related (autonoetic or chronesthetic) consciousness, it makes sense to do so (Wheeler et al., 1997; Wheeler, 2000). A recent case study explicitly extends these ideas into the personal past and personal future (Klein et al., in press). The data also fit well with studies that show the involvement of the frontal lobes in "theory of mind" tasks (e.g., Stone et al., 1998).

FUNCTIONAL NEUROIMAGING

Perhaps the most promising, albeit still rather indirect, evidence on chronesthesia has been provided by functional neuroimaging research concerning the similarities and differences between episodic and semantic memory. It is well established that episodic memory is like semantic memory in many ways (Tulving & Markowitsch, 1998), including the fact that both depend critically on the intact limbic system, including medial temporal lobe and diencephalic structures (Squire, 1992). For some time it was also suspected that episodic memory depends on prefrontal cortex in a way that declarative and other forms of memory do not (Schacter, 1987; Squire, 1987; Tulving, 1989b). These early ideas have received good support from more recent functional neuroimaging (PET and FMRI) studies. Most informative have been studies comparing the neuroanatomical correlates of semantic and episodic retrieval. These studies show both similarities and differences in the functional neuroanatomy of the two systems (e.g., Dalla Barba, et al., 1998; Maguire & Mummery, 1999; Wiggs, et al., 1999; Nyberg, 2002).

A remarkable empirical regularity that emerged from early studies (Shallice et al., 1994; Tulving et al., 1994) is that right prefrontal cortex is differentially more involved in retrieval of episodic than semantic information. Subsequent work reinforced this kind of hemispheric asymmetry, which has become known as one part of the hemispheric encoding/retrieval asymmetry (HERA) model (Tulving et al., 1994; Nyberg et al., 1996, 1997; Düzel et al., 1999 Cabeza & Nyberg, 2000). Under the circumstances, the question naturally arose as to the specific meaning of the right frontal activation so frequently observed in episodic retrieval but seldom in semantic retrieval.

It is known that memory retrieval is not a single process but rather consists of several subprocesses. One way of tackling the question about the theoretical meaning of right-frontal activation therefore lies in the analysis of the overall retrieval process into subprocesses, and in trying to find out to what extent these subprocesses are associated with right prefrontal cortex. A major distinction within episodic-memory retrieval process can be made between retrieval mode and recovery of stored information. *Retrieval mode* represents a mental (neurocognitive) state in which an individual attempts to remember earlier experiences, whereas *recovery* (also called *ecphory*) refers to the actual success of such an attempt. Given this distinction, it is possible to ask whether the right frontal episodic retrieval activation observed in PET and FMRI studies signifies retrieval mode or retrieval success. Although experimental evidence for both alternatives has been reported (Rugg et al., 1996, 1997; Schacter et al., 1996; Buckner et al., 1998; Nolde, et al., 1998; McDermott et al., 1999, 2000), the important fact in the present context is that right prefrontal activation has been consistently found under conditions where episodic retrieval mode is present but no recovery of previously stored information occurs (Kapur et al., 1995; Nyberg et al., 1995; Rugg et al., 1997; Buckner et al., 1998; Wagner et al., 1998). A recent multistudy analysis of PET data (Lepage et al., 2000) was undertaken to identify "retrieval mode" (REMO) sites in the brain. A *REMO site* was defined as a brain region (a cluster of voxels) that is significantly more active during episodic retrieval than during episodic encoding (or semantic retrieval), *and* that is equally so when recovery succeeds and when it fails. Semantic retrieval is usually indistinguishable from episodic encoding (Tulving et al., 1994; Cabeza & Nyberg, 2000). The data produced by this study could be regarded as especially convincing because of the large number of subjects providing the data ($n = 53$). There were six REMO sites, all of them in the frontal lobes. Five were in prefrontal cortex, three "strong" ones in the right and two "weaker" ones in the left hemisphere, and one was in the medial anterior cingulate. No similar sites were seen in any other part of the brain.

One or more, or a combination, of these prefrontal activations can be assumed to be associated with chronesthesia. The hypothesis is that they reflect the "mental time travel" (into the past) component of the recognition test. In order for subjects to be able to solve the problem posed by the task—determine whether a test item is "old" or "new"—they must be able to focus on a particular past segment of their lives, the event of studying the list. Only individuals who possess chronesthesia can "remember" such happenings from their own past. Others must solve the problem by relying on other processes, such as "knowing," or "familiarity" (or "novelty") detection (or assessment), processes whose results are expressed through noetic consciousness that does not involve chronesthesia (Mandler, 1980; Yonelinas, et al., 1998; Gardiner, 2000; Kelley & Jacoby, 2000).

CHRONESTHESIA AND EVOLUTION OF CULTURE

Living things in nature may be different from inanimate things, but they, too, exist in a physical world with its immutable laws to which everything in the world is subject. In order to come into being and to survive, all species must be able to not only fit into the world as it exists but also adapt to changes in it over time. Phylogenetic evolution tells the story of the successes and failures of such adaptation by millions of species over millions of years. The rule is simple and harsh—to live means to conform to the requirements of the world *as it exists.*

Human beings, as far as is known, are the only animals who have ever used a different, much more efficacious, solution to the problem of the fit between the species and its ecological niche: at some point in their evolutionary history, thousands of years ago, they discovered that they did not have to adapt to every feature of the world, and that one way of dealing with the physical environment was to change it to fit them. Other species exist that have used the same strategy for isolated purposes; humans learned to do it on a grand scale. The changes they have wrought on the natural world are staggering in scope and sophistication. We can use the term *culture* to collectively describe all the differences between the world—material and virtual, concrete and abstract—as it exists by virtue of human intervention and as it would have existed in the absence of such intervention, and ask the question: What kinds of events in human evolution made it possible for *Homo sapiens,* slowly but surely, to bring about the monumental achievement of culture? What prompted the initiation of cultural evolution, and what kept the momentum going?

These sorts of questions have been around for some time, and a variety of answers have been suggested. These answers have been guided by generally accepted facts about the intraspecies human evolution that occurred after the hominid species separated from the pongids some five or six million years ago. Among these facts, as revealed by available fossil evidence, one of the most telling is that for long stretches of this very long time, human culture changed exceedingly slowly. It was only in the last few tens of thousands of years (Eldredge & Tattersall, 1992) that the curve of cultural evolution began inching upward on its relentless march towards its present explosive acceleration. Thus, in addition to the questions posed earlier, we have another one: Why did this cultural evolution occur so recently?

There is good agreement that the human brain/mind has played a critical role in human evolution in general and cultural evolution in particular. Richards (1987) has noted that early evolutionists and later Darwininians alike embraced the idea that behavior and mind "drove" the evolutionary process. Thus, in addition to the gain in intricacy of neuronal organization (Tobias, 1971) and the "disproportionately large" prefrontal cortex (Deacon, 1997) that figure as candidate "drivers" of human cultural evolution, there are also obvious mental factors such as manual signaling, language, and especially speech (Donald, 1991; Lieberman, 1984; Corballis, 1998); literacy, numeracy, and abstract thought (Donald, 1991, Deacon, 1997); social learning and efficient transmission of information from one generation to the next (Boyd & Richerson, 1985); explicit instruction of others by those who had special skills and knowledge (Premack, 1984); and development of an enquiring or meditative ability exceeding simple knowledge (Santangelo, 1993).

The reason for raising the question of cultural evolution in this volume is this: I would like to propose that chronesthesia, and specifically *proscopic* (forward-looking, future-oriented) chronesthesia, was yet another "driver" of human cultural evolution, perhaps even a crucial one. The idea is simple: consciously apprehended awareness of the existence of future is a necessary, even if not a sufficient, precondition for massively changing one's environment. More specifically, the hypothesis—call it the hypothesis of chronesthetic culture—is that the development of civilization and culture was, and its continuation is, critically dependent on human beings' awareness of their own and their progeny's *continued existence* in time that includes not only the past and the present but also the future. An animal that cannot think about what might happen at a time that has not yet arrived, and that therefore does not exist, is unlikely to initiate and persist in any activity whose beneficial consequences will manifest themselves only at that physically nonexistent time. Such an animal's behavior is governed completely by the physical and biological laws of the world. These laws operate in linear time: the past can influence the present, and the present can influence the future, but there is no way in which the future, which does not yet exist, can influence anything that happens in the present—no way, except one: through a future that exists in one's conscious awareness of the world, the kind of awareness that chronesthesia makes possible. Chronesthesia is a trick that nature invented to circumvent its own most fundamental law of unidirectionality of time.

To the extent, then, that chronesthesia depends on prefrontal cortex, and to the extent that chronesthesia, once it began to evolve as a property of the human brain, became critical in the initiation and continued support of the evolution of human culture, the conclusion follows that the human prefrontal cortex, undoubtedly in collaboration with other areas of the brain, is directly responsible for the cultured world as it exists today, a world in which

not only human survival but human satisfaction and happiness are no more a matter of nature but rather depend on human beings' own wisdom, or lack of it.

PROBLEMS WITH CHRONESTHESIA

In this chapter I have outlined some ideas about a human neurocognitive capability that I have called *chronesthesia*. I have proposed that it is a kind of consciousness involving subjective time that serves many time-related behavioral and cognitive functions as a critical enabling condition. All mature humans possess chronesthesia and critically depend on it for their existence. Prefrontal cortex is probably one of the central components on the neuronal circuits that subserve chronesthesia. I assume that chronesthesia is a recent appearance in human evolution, and that it played a critical role in the evolution of culture and civilization as we know it.

There are many problems with this story (or theory) of chronesthesia. Indeed, I myself find it much easier to criticize it than find supportive ideas and evidence for it. Does it really exist as a separate neurocognitive capacity? If so, in what sense does it exist? Why classify it as a form of consciousness? Wherein lies the advantage of this assumption? In what sense is consciousness, any kind of consciousness, a neurocognitive capacity? The list of these kinds of vexing questions is long. Perhaps the most basic one of them all is this: Given that there are no easy answers to these questions, why bother to ask them? Speculation may have a legitimate role to play in science, but if it gets to be too much, does it not become counterproductive?

I am well aware of the problems that the theory of chronesthesia faces. But just because there are many problems with an idea does not necessarily mean that the we should not even try to think about it. Remember Michael Faraday and his ideas about electricity; when asked what this new thing that he called electricity was good for, he is said to have responded: "Madam, what good is a newborn baby?" Chronesthesia may not be electricity, but it does share with electricity, and all other new ideas, the feature of having a kind of future promise that nonexisting ideas do not.

REFERENCES

Andreasen, N.C., O'Leary, D.S., Cizadlo, T., Arndt, S., Rezai, K., Watkins, G.L., Ponto, L.L., & Hichwa, R.D. (1995). Remembering the past: two facets of episodic memory explored with positron emission tomography. *American Journal of Psychiatry, 152*, 1576–1585.

Baker, S.C., Rogers, R.D., Owen, A.M., Frith, C.D., Dolan, R.J., Frackowiak, R.S.J., & Robbins, T.W. (1996). Neural systems engaged by planning: A PET study of the Tower of London task. *Neuropsychologia, 34*, 515–526.

Baron, J.C., Petit-Taboue, M.C., Le Doze, F., Desgranges, B., Ravenel, N., & Marchal, G. (1994). Right frontal cortex hypometabolism in transient global amnesia. A PET study. *Brain, 117*, 545–552.

Block, R.A. (Ed.). (1990). *Cognitive Models of Psychological Time*. Hillsdale, NJ: Lawrence Erlbaum Associates.

Boyd, R. & Richerson, P.J. (1985). *Culture and the Evolutionary Process*. Chicago: University of Chicago Press.

Buckner, R.L., Koutstaal, W., Schacter, D.L., Wagner, A.D., & Rosen, B.R. (1998). Functional-anatomic study of episodic retrieval using FMRI: 1. Retrieval effort versus retrieval success. *NeuroImage, 7*, 151–162.

Burgess, P.W., Quayle, A., & Frith, C.D. (2001). Brain regions involved in prosepctive memory as determined by positrom emission tomography. *Neuropsychologia, 39*, 545–555.

Cabeza, R. & Nyberg, L. (2000). Imaging cognition II: an empirical review of 275 PET and FMRI studies. *Journal of Cognitive Neuroscience, 12*, 1–47.

Calabrese, P., Markowitsch, H.J., Durwen, H.F., Widlitzek, H., Haupts, M., Holinka, B., & Gehlen, W. (1996). Right temporofrontal cortex as critical locus for the ecphory of old episodic memories. *Journal of Neurology Neurosurgery and Psychiatry, 61*, 304–310.

Church, R.M. (1989). Theories of timing behavior. In: (S.B. Klein and R.R. Mowrer, (Eds.), *Contemporary Learning Theories: Instrumental Conditioning Theory and the Impact of Biological Constraints on Learning* (pp. 41–71). Hillsdale, NJ: Lawrence Erlbaum Associates.

Corballis, M.C. (1998). Evolution of the human mind. In M. Sabourin, F. Craik, & M. Robert (Eds.), *Advances in Psychological Science, Vol. 2: Biological and Cognitive Aspects* (pp. 31–62). Hove, UK: Psychology Press.

Craik, F.I.M., Moroz, T.M., Moscovitch, M., Stuss, D.T., Winocur, G., Tulving, E., & Kapur, S. (1999). In search of the self: a PET investigation of self-referential information. *Psychological Science, 10*, 26–34.

Crowder, R.G. & Greene, R.L. (2000). Serial learning: cognition and behavior. In: E. Tulving & F.I.M. Craik (Eds.), *The Oxford Handbook of Memory* (pp. 125–135). New York, Oxford University Press.

Dalla Barba, G., Cappelletti, J.Y., Signorini, M., & Denes, G. (1997). Confabulation: remembering 'another' past, planning 'another' future. *Neurocase, 3*, 425–436.

Dalla Barba, G., Parlato, V., Jobert, A., Samson, Y., & Pappata, S. (1998). Cortical networks implicated in semantic and episodic memory: common or unique? *Cortex, 34*, 547–561.

Damasio, H. & Damasio, A.R. (1989). *Lesion Analysis in Neuropsychology*. New York: Oxford University Press.

Deacon, T.W. (1997). *The Symbolic Species: The Co-evolution of Language and the Brain*. New York: W.W. Norton & Company.

Donald, M. (1991). *Origins of the Modern Mind*. Cambridge, MA: Harvard University Press.

Düzel, E., Cabeza, R., Picton, T.W., Yonelinas, A.P., Scheich, H., Heinze, H-J., & Tulving, E. (1999). Task-related and item-related brain processes of memory retrieval. *Proceedings of National Academy of Sciences USA, 96*, 1794–1799.

Einstein, G.O., Glisky, E.L., Rubin, S.R., Guynn, M.J., & Routhieaux, B.C. (1999), Prospective memory: a neuropsychological study. *Neuropsychology, 13*, 103–110.

Eldredge, N. & Tattersall, I. (1992). *The Myths of Human Evolution*. New York: Columbia University Press.

Fink, G.R., Markowitsch, H.J., Reinkemeier, M., Bruckbauer, T., Kessler, J., & Heiss, W.D. (1996). Cerebral representation of one's own past: neural networks involved in autobiographical memory. *Journal of Neuroscience, 16*, 4275–4282.

Fraisse, P. (1963). *The Psychology of Time*. New York: Harper & Row.

Fuster, J.M. (1973). Unit activity in prefrontal cortex during delayed-response performance: neural correlates of transient memory. *Journal of Neurophysiology, 36*, 61–78.

Fuster, J.M. (1995). *Memory in the Cerebral Cortex*. Cambridge, MA: MIT Press.

Fuster, J.M. (2000). The prefrontal cortex of the primate: a synopsis. *Psychobiology, 28*, 125–131.

Gallup, G.G. (1982). Self-awareness and the emergence of mind in primates. *American Journal of Primatology, 2*, 237–248.

Gardiner, J.M (1988). Functional aspects of recollective experience. *Memory and Cognition, 16*, 309–313.

Gardiner, J.M. (2000). On the objectivity of subjective experiences of autonoetic and noetic consciousness. In: E. Tulving (Ed.), *Memory, Consciousness, and the Brain: The Tallinn Conference* (pp. 159–172). Philadelphia: Psychology Press.

Gower, E.C. (1992). Short-term memory for the temporal order of events in monkeys. *Behavioral Brain Research, 52*, 99–103.

Haith, M.M. (1997). The development of future thinking as essential for the emergence of skill in planning. In: S.L. Friedman & E.K. Scholnick (Eds.), *The Developmental Psychology of Planning: Why, How, and When Do We Plan?* (pp. 25–42). Mahwah, NJ: Erlbaum.

Haith, M.M., Benson, J.B., Roberts, R.J., Jr, & Pennington, Bruce F. (1994). *The Development of Future-Oriented Processes*. Chicago: University of Chicago Press.

Hayman, C.A.G., Macdonald, C.A., & Tulving, E. (1993). The role of repetition and associative interference in new semantic learning in amnesia. *Journal of Cognitive Neuroscience, 5,* 375–389.

Ingvar, D.H. (1985). "Memory of the future": an essay on the temporal organization of conscious awareness. *Human Neurobiology, 4,* 127–136.

Ivry, R.B. (1996). The representation of temporal information in perception and motor control. *Current Opinion in Neurobiology, 6,* 851–857.

Ivry, R. & Fiez, J.A. (2000). Cerebellar contributions to cognition and imagery. In: M.S. Gazzaniga (Ed.), *The New Cognitive Neurosciences* (pp. 999–1011). Cambridge, MA: MIT Press.

Jäncke, L., Loose, R., Lutz, K., Specht, K., & Shah, N.J. (2000). Cortical activations during paced finger-tapping applying visual and auditory pacing stimuli. *Cognitive Brain Research, 10,* 51–66.

Kapur, N. (1993). Focal retrograde amnesia in neurological disease: a critical review. *Cortex, 29,* 217–234.

Kapur, N. (2000). Focal retrograde amnesia and the attribution of causality: an exceptionally benign commentary. *Cognitive Neuropsychology, 17,* 623–637.

Kapur, S., Craik, F.I.M., Jones, C., Brown, G.M., Houle, S., & Tulving, E. (1995). Functional role of the prefrontal cortex in retrieval of memories: a PET study. *NeuroReport, 6,* 1880–1884.

Keenan, J.P., Wheeler, M.A., Gallup, G.G., Jr., & Pascual-Leone, A. (2000). Self-recognition and the right prefrontal cortex *Trends in Cognitive Sciences, 4,* 338–344.

Kelley, C.M. & Jacoby, L.L. (2000). Recollection and familiarity: process-dissociation. In: E. Tulving and F.I.M. Craik (Eds.), *The Oxford Handbook of Memory* (pp. 215–228). New York: Oxford University Press.

Kircher, T.J., Senior, C., Phillips, M.L., Benson, P.J., Bullmore, E.T., Brammer, M., Simmons, A., Williams, S.C.R., Bartels, M., & David, A.S. (2000). Towards a functional neuroanatomy of self processing: effects of faces and words. *Cognitive Brain Research, 10,* 133–144.

Klein, S.B., Loftus, J., & Kihlstrom, J.F. (1996). Self-knowledge of an amnesic patient: toward a neuropsychology of personality and social psychology. *Journal of Experimental Psychology: General, 125,* 250–260.

Klein, S.B., Loftus, J., & Kihlstrom, J.F. 2002, in press. Memory and temporal experience: The effects of episodic memory loss on an amnesic patient's ability to remember the past and imagine the future. *Social Cognition.*

Knight, R.T. & Grabowecky, M. (1995). Escape from linear time: Prefrontal cortex and conscious experience. In: M.S. Gazzaniga (Ed.), *The Cognitive Neurosciences* (pp. 1357–1371). Cambridge, MA: MIT Press.

Knight, R.T. & Grabowecky, M. (2000). Prefrontal cortex, time and consciousness. In: M.S. Gazzaniga (Ed.), *The New Cognitive Neurosciences* (pp. 1319–1339). Cambridge, MA: MIT Press.

Koechlin, E., Basso, G., Pietrini, P., Panzer, S., & Grafman, J. (1999). The role of anterior prefrontal cortex in human cognition. *Nature, 399,* 148–151.

Kopelman, M.D. (2000). Focal retrograde amnesia and the attribution of causality: an exceptionally critical review. *Cognitive Neuropsychology, 17,* 585–621.

Lee, A.C.H., Robbins, T.W., Pickard, J.D., & Owen, A.D. (2000). Asymmetric frontal activation during episodic memory: the effects of stimulus type on encoding and retrieval. *Neuropsychologia, 38,* 677–692.

Lepage, M., Ghaffar, O., Nyberg, L., & Tulving, E. (2000). Prefrontal cortex and episodic memory retrieval mode. *Proceedings of National Academy of Sciences USA, 97,* 506–511.

Levine, B., Black, S.E., Cabeza, R., Sinden, M., McIntosh, A.R., Toth, J.P., Tulving, E., & Stuss, D.T. (1998). Episodic memory and the self in a case of isolated retrograde amnesia. *Brain, 121,* 1951–1973.

Lieberman, P. (1984). *Biology and Evolution of Language.* Cambridge, MA: Harvard University Press.

Maguire, E.A. & Mummery, C.J. (1999). Differential modulation of a common memory retrieval network revealed by positron emission tomography. *Hippocampus, 9,* 54–61.

Mandler, G. (1980). Recognizing: the judgment of previous occurrence. *Psychological Review, 87,* 252–271.

Mantyla, T. & Nilsson, L.G. (1997). Remembering to remember in adulthood: a population-based study on aging and prospective memory. *Aging, Neuropsychology, and Cognition, 4,* 81–92.

Markowitsch, H.J. (1995). Which brain regions are critically involved in the retrieval of old episodic memory? *Brain Research Review, 21,* 117–127.

Markowitsch, H.J., Calabrese, P., Liess, J., Haupts, M., Durwen, H.F., & Gehlen, W. (1993). Retrograde amnesia after traumatic injury of the fronto-temporal cortex. *Journal of Neurology, Neurosurgery, and Psychiatry, 56,* 988–992.

Markowitsch, H.J., Reinkemeier, M., Thiel, A., Kessler, J., Koyuncu, A. & Heiss, W.-D. (1999). Autobiographical memory activates the right amygdala and temporofrontal link: a PET study. *Acta Neurobiologiae Experimentalis, 59,* 219.

McCormack, T. & Hoerl, C. (1999). Memory and temporal perspective: the role of temporal frameworks in memory development. *Developmental Review, 19,* 154–182.

McDermott, K.B., Ojemannn, J.G., Petersen, S.E., Ollinger, J.M., Snyder, A.Z., Akbudak, E., Conturo, T.E., & Raichle, M.E. (1999). Direct comparison of episodic encoding and retrieval of words: an event-related FMRI study. *Memory, 7,* 661–678.

McDermott, K.B., Jones, T.C., Petersen, S.E., Lageman, S.K., & Roediger, H.L. (2000). Retrieval success is accompanied by enhanced activation in anterior prefrontal cortex during recognition memory: an event-related FMRI study. *Journal of Cognitive Neuroscience, 12,* 965–976.

Moore-Ede, M.C., Sulzman, F.M., & Fuller, C.A. (1982). *The Clocks That Time Us.* Cambridge, MA: Harvard University Press.

Moscovitch, M. (2000). Theories of memory and consciousness. In: E. Tulving and F.I.M. Craik (Eds.), *The*

Oxford Handbook of Memory (pp. 609–625). New York: Oxford University Press.

Nelson, K. (1997). Finding one's self in time. In: J.G. Snodgrass & R.L. Thompson (Eds.), *The Self Across Psychology: Self-recognition, Self-awareness and the Self-concept. Annals of the New York Academy of Sciences, 818*, (pp. 103–118). New York: New York Academy of Sciences.

Nolde, S.F., Johnson, M.K., & D'Esposito, M. (1998). Left prefrontal activation during episodic remembering: an event-related FMRI study. *NeuroReport, 9*, 3509–3514.

Nyberg, L. (2002). Where encoding and retrieval meet in the brain. In L. Squire (Ed.), *Cognitive Neuroscience of Memory and Amnesia* (pp. 193–203) New York: Guilford.

Nyberg, L., Tulving, E., Habib, R., Nilsson, L.-G., Kapur, S., Houle, S., Cabeza, R.E.L., & McIntosh, A.R. (1995). Functional brain maps of retrieval mode and recovery of episodic information. *NeuroReport, 7*, 249–252.

Nyberg, L., Cabeza, R., & Tulving, E. (1996). PET studies of encoding and retrieval: the HERA model. *Psychonomic Bulletin and Review, 3*, 135–148.

Nyberg, L., McIntosh, A.R., & Tulving, E. (1997). Functional brain imaging of episodic and semantic memory. *Journal of Molecular Medicine, 76*, 48–53.

Okuda, J., Fujii, T., Yamadori, A., Kawashima, R., Tsukiura, T., Fukatsu, R., Suzuki, K., Ito, M., Fukuda, H., (1998). Neuroscience Letters, 253, 127–130.

Owen, A.M. (1997). Cognitive planning in humans: neuropsychological, neuroanatomical and neuropharmacological perspectives. *Progress in Neurobiology, 53*, 431–450.

Plotkin, H. (1994). *Darwin Machines and the Nature of Knowledge*. Cambridge, MA: Harvard U. Press.

Povinelli, D.J., Landau, K.R., & Perilloux, H.K. (1996). Self-recognition in young children using delayed versus live feedback: evidence of a developmental asynchrony. *Child Development, 67*, 1540–1554.

Premack, D. (1984). Pedagogy and aesthetics as sources of culture. In: M.S. Gazzaniga (Ed.), *Handbook of Cognitive Neuroscience* pp. 15–35). New York: Plenum Press.

Rajaram, S. (1993). Remembering and knowing: two means of access to the personal past. *Memory and Cognition, 21*, 89–102.

Richards, R.J. (1987). *Darwin and the Emergence of Evolutionary Theories of Mind and Behavior*. Chicago: University of Chicago Press.

Rosenbaum, R.S., Priselac, S., Köhler, S., Black, S., Gao, F., Nadel, L., & Moscovitch, M. (2000) Remote spatial memory in an amnesic person with extensive hippocampal lesions. *Nature Neuroscience, 3*, 1044–1048.

Rugg, M.D., Fletcher, P.C., Frith, C.D., Frackowiak, R.S.J., & Dolan, R.J. (1996). Differential activation of the prefrontal cortex in successful and unsuccessful memory retrieval. *Brain, 119*, 2073–2083.

Rugg, M.D., Fletcher, P.C., Frith, C.D., Frackowiak, R.S.J., & Dolan, R.J. (1997). Brain regions supporting intentional and incidental memory. *NeuroReport, 8*, 1283–1287.

Santangelo, A. (1993). *The Beginning of Meaning of Culture. The Cerebral Activity Underlying It.* Milano: La Pietra.

Schacter, D.L. (1987). Memory, amnesia, and frontal lobe dysfunction. *Psychobiology, 15*, 21–36.

Schacter, D.L., Alpert, N.M., Savage, C.R., Rauch, S.L., & Albert, M.S. (1996). Conscious recollection and the human hippocampal formation: evidence from positron emission tomography. *Proceedings of National Academy of Sciences USA, 93*, 321–325.

Shallice, T., Fletcher, P. Frith, C.D., Grasby, P., Frackowiak, R.S.J., & Dolan, R.J. (1994). Brain regions associated with acquisition and retrieval of verbal episodic memory. *Nature, 368*, 633–635.

Squire, L.R. (1987). *Memory and Brain*. New York: Oxford University Press.

Squire, L.R. (1992). Memory and the hippocampus: a synthesis from findings with rats, monkeys, and humans. *Psychological Review, 99*, 195–231.

Stone, V.E., Baron-Cohen, S., & Knight, R.T. (1998). Frontal lobe contributions to theory of mind. *Journal of Cognitive Neuroscience, 10*, 640–656.

Stuss, D.T. & Benson, D.F. (1986). *The Frontal Lobes*. New York: Raven Press.

Stuss, D.T., Picton, T.W., & Alexander, M.P. (2001). Consciousness, self-awareness, and the frontal lobes. In: S.P. Salloway, P.F Malloy, & J.D Duffy (Eds.), *The Frontal Lobes and Neuropsychiatric Illness*, (pp.101–109). Washington, DC: American Psychiatric Press.

Suddendorf, T. & Corballis, M.C. (1997). Mental time travel and the evolution of the human mind. *Genetic, Social, and General Psychology Monographs, 123*, 133–167.

Tobias, P.V. (1971). *The Brain in Hominid Evolution*. New York: Columbia University Press.

Tulving, E. (1985). Memory and consciousness. *Canadian Psychology, 26*, 1–12.

Tulving, E. (1989a). Memory: performance, knowledge, and experience. *European Journal of Cognitive Psychology, 1*, 3–26.

Tulving, E. (1989b). Remembering and knowing the past. *American Scientist, 77*, 361–367.

Tulving, E. (1993). Self-knowledge of an amnesic individual is represented abstractly. In: T.K. Srull & R.S. Wyer, Jr. (Eds.), *The Mental Representation of Trait and Autobiographical Knowledge About the Self* (pp. 147–156). Hillsdale, NJ: Lawrence Erlbaum Associates.

Tulving, E. (1999). On the uniqueness of episodic memory. In: L.-G. Nilsson & H.J. Markowitsch (Eds.), *Cognitive Neuroscience of Memory* (pp. 11–42). Göttingen: Hogrefe & Huber.

Tulving, E. (2001). The origin of autonoesis in episodic memory. In: H.L. Roediger, J.S. Nairne, I. Neath, & A.M. Suprenant (Eds.), *The Nature of Remembering: Essays in Honor of Robert G. Crowder* (pp. 17–34). Washington, DC: American Psychological Association.

Tulving, E. & Markowitsch, H.J. (1998). Episodic and declarative memory: role of the hippocampus. *Hippocampus, 8*, 198–204.

Tulving, E., Schacter, D.L., McLachlan, D.R., & Moscovitch, M. (1988). Priming of semantic autobiographical knowledge: a case study of retrograde amnesia. *Brain and Cognition, 8,* 3–20.

Tulving, E., Hayman, C.A.G., & MacDonald, C.A. (1991). Long-lasting perceptual priming and semantic learning in amnesia: a case experiment. *Journal of Experimental Psychology: Learning, Memory and Cognition,* 1991, *17,* 595–617.

Tulving, E., Kapur, S., Craik, F.I.M., Moscovitsch, M., & Houle, S. (1994) Hemispheric encoding/retrieval asymmetry in episodic memory: positron emission tomography findings. *Proceedings of National Academy of Sciences USA 91,* 2016–2020.

Wagner, A.D., Desmond, J.E., Glover, G.H., & Gabrieli, J.D.E. (1998). Prefrontal cortex and recognition memory—factional-MRI evidence for context-dependent retrieval processes. *Brain, 121,* 1985–2002.

Westmacott, R., Moscovitch, M., & Leach, L. (2001). Different patterns of autobiographical memory loss in semantic dementia and medial temporal lobe amnesia: a challenge to consolidation theory. *Neurocase, 7,* 37–55.

Wheeler, M.A. (2000). Episodic memory and autonoetic awareness. In: E. Tulving & F.I.M. Craik (Eds.), *The Oxford Handbook of Memory* (pp. 597–608). New York: Oxford University Press.

Wheeler, M.A., Stuss, D.T., & Tulving, E. (1997). Toward a theory of episodic memory: the frontal lobes and autonoetic consciousness. *Psychological Bulletin, 121,* 331–354.

Wiggs, C.L., Weisberg, J., & Martin, A. (1999). Neural correlates of semantic and episodic memory retrieval. *Neuropsychologia, 37,* 103–118.

Yonelinas, A.P., Kroll, N.E.A., Dobbins, I., Lazzarra, M., & Knight, R.T. (1998). Recollection and familiarity deficits in amnesia: convergence of remember/know, process dissociation, and receiver-operating characteristics data. *Neuropsychology, 12,* 323–339.

Zach, R. (1979). Shell dropping: decision making and optimal foraging in northwestern crows. *Behaviour, 68,* 106–117.

21

Integration across Multiple Cognitive and Motivational Domains in Monkey Prefrontal Cortex

MASATAKA WATANABE

The prefrontal cortex (PFC) is considered the center of higher cognitive activity (Luria, 1980; Stuss & Benson, 1986; Fuster, 1997). The PFC plays the most important role in executive control, such as planning; decision making; estimation of value, time, and frequency; inhibition of inappropriate behavior; encoding and retrieval of episodic memory; and retention and manipulation of information in working memory (Luria, 1980; Stuss & Benson, 1986; Fuster, 1997; Roberts et al., 1998; Knight & Grabowecky, 2000). The PFC also plays important roles in motivational operations, such as emotional expression, perception of emotion, perception and control of social behavior, and estimation of reward value (Luria, 1980; Stuss & Benson, 1986; Damasio, 1994; Fuster, 1997). Neuronal mechanisms of cognitive and motivational operations in the PFC have been investigated by recording single neuronal activity from task-performing monkeys. In this chapter, I will first describe the neuronal bases of higher cognitive activity in relation to coding the stimulus' meaning across different sensory modalities. Then neuronal bases of motivational operations in primate PFC neurons will be described. Here, the focus is placed on (1) post-trial outcome–related and (2) reward expectancy-related neuronal activity observed during task perfor-

mance. To achieve a goal, several different kinds of information should be taken into consideration and integrated. The PFC appears to play the most important role in this process. Therefore, the ways in which different kinds of information interact and are integrated in the PFC for goal-directed behavior will be described, focusing on the possible roles of this brain area in the integration between motivational and cognitive information. Finally, functional segregation of the PFC in relation to motivational and cognitive operations will be discussed.

CODING THE MEANING OF THE STIMULUS ACROSS DIFFERENT SENSORY MODALITIES IN PREFRONTAL NEURONS

In the primate PFC, there are several kinds of neurons that are involved in higher cognitive activity. For example, we reported primate PFC neurons that are related to retaining information in working memory (Niki & Watanabe, 1976; Watanabe, 1981), behavioral inhibition (Watanabe, 1986b), time estimation (Niki & Watanabe, 1979), and coding the meaning of the stimulus independent of its physical properties (Watanabe, 1981, 1986a, 1990, 1992). Concerning meaning-related PFC neurons, some neurons code the *behavioral significance* of the stimulus in relation to what behavioral response the stimulus indicates to the animal while other neurons are related to coding the *associative significance* of the stimulus in relation to what specific event it is associated with. Here, I will show an example of a PFC neuron that is involved in coding the behavioral significance of the stimulus across visual and auditory modalities (Watanabe, 1996b).

In the experiment, three monkeys were trained on the visual and auditory go/no-go discrimination task with eye fixation (Fig. 21–1). In this task, the monkey was seated in a primate chair facing a panel that contained a central rectangular window above a hold lever.

The animal initiated each trial by pressing the lever. This turned on the fixation point (FP) at the center of the window, on which the animal was required to fixate. When the animal continued to fixate on the FP for 1 to 2 seconds, the discriminative visual or auditory cue was presented for 0.5 seconds (during the cue period the FP was turned off, with the eye position still being controlled). The visual cue was presented on the window, and the auditory cue was presented from a loudspeaker positioned behind the panel. When the animal further continued to fixate on the FP for 1 to 3 seconds, the FP became dim and the animal was required to perform a go or no-go response depending on the previously presented cue. On go trials, the animal had to release the lever within 0.8 seconds after dimming of the FP (immediate release) while on no-go trials, the animal had to perform a delayed release response when the dim light was turned off 1.2 seconds after it was dimmed. A juice reward was given to the animal for a correct response on both go and no-go trials. Four kinds of pattern stimuli were used as visual cues, and four kinds of sound stimuli were used as auditory cues. Two of each modality of cues were assigned to go and the other two to no-go cues. Each cue was expected to gain

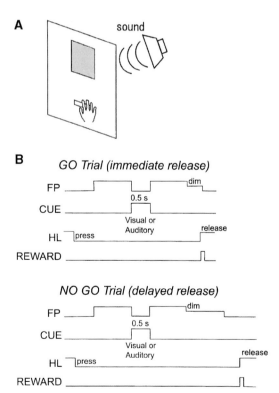

A

sound

B

GO Trial (immediate release)

FP

CUE

0.5 s

Visual or Auditory

release

HL   press

REWARD

NO GO Trial (delayed release)

FP

dim

CUE

0.5 s

Visual or Auditory

release

HL   press

REWARD

Figure 21–1. *A:* Schematic illustration of the experimental apparatus. The visual cue was presented on the window and the auditory cue was presented from behind the panel. *B:* Sequence and timing of events in the visual and auditory go/no-go discrimination task with eye fixation. FP, fixation point; HL, hold lever.

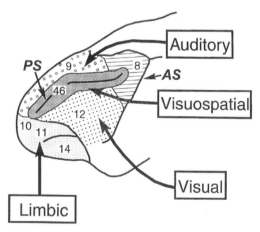

Figure 21–2. Walker's (1940) areas (areas 8, 9, 10, 11, 12, 14, and 46) in the primate prefrontal cortex (PFC) and schematic illustration of the convergence of different kinds of information in the primate PFC. Area 13 and the ventral part of area 12 do not appear in this figure. AS, arcuate sulcus; PS, principal sulcus.

behavioral significance in relation to what behavioral response (go or no-go) the cue indicated to the animal. Visual and auditory tasks
were given to the animal each in a block of
about 100 trials. Single neuronal activity was
recorded mainly from the arcuate area (area
8) and the posterior half of the principal sulcus
area (area 46) of the PFC (Fig. 21–2).

The PFC neuron shown in Figure 21–3 was
activated during the cue period when the go-

indicating cue was presented, irrespective of
differences in the cue's physical properties, on
both visual (Fig. 21–3A) and auditory (Fig.
21–3B) tasks. This neuron is thus considered
involved in coding the behavioral significance
of the stimulus across visual and auditory modalities. This consideration is strengthened by
the observation that this neuron was not activated in response to the go-indicating cue
while showing an activation to the no-go-

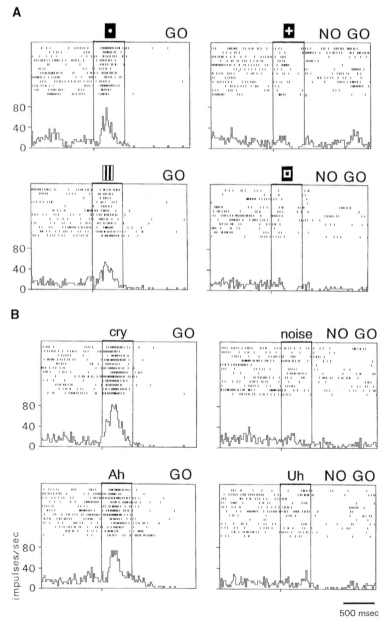

Figure 21–3. An example of the activity of a prefrontal cortex (PFC) neuron, which appeared to be involved in coding the behavioral significance of the stimulus across visual (*A*) and auditory (*B*) tasks. In the visual task, a circle and stripes were go response-indicating cues while a plus and a square were no-go–indicating cues. In the auditory task, "cry" (monkey's cry) and "Ah" (human "Ah" sound) were go-indicating cues and "noise" (loud noise) and "Uh" (human "Uh" sound) were no-go–indicating cues. Neuronal activity is shown in raster and histogram displays. For each display, the second vertical line from the left shows the time of the cue onset and the third line indicates its offset. A horizontal black bar indicates the period when a cue was being presented (0.5 seconds), and above the bar is shown the cue that was actually presented. In raster displays, each row indicates the neuronal activity of each trial for 2.56 seconds and each pulse indicates the occurrence of spike discharge(s) in a 5-ms time bin. (*Source:* From Watanabe, 1996b, with permission)

indicating cue on erroneous trials on both modalities of tasks. Among 129 PFC neurons that were examined on both visual and auditory tasks, 36 neurons responded in a similar way to both modalities of cues depending on the cue's behavioral significance, as is the case for the neuron in Figure 21–3. The remaining 93 neurons coded the behavioral significance of only the visual ($n = 85$) or auditory ($n = 8$) cue and are considered involved in modality-specific coding of the cue's behavioral significance. Neurons that coded the meaning of the stimulus across visual and auditory modalities may obtain information from these modality-specific meaning-related neurons.

Previously, I reported PFC neurons that code the associative significance of the stimulus across visual and auditory modalities (Watanabe, 1992). The PFC receives almost all kinds of highly processed sensory information from the posterior association cortices (Stuss & Benson, 1986; Barbas, 1995; Fuster, 1997). The convergence of different modalities of sensory inputs in the PFC may have functional importance for extracting the meaning of the stimulus across different sensory modalities, and cross-modal meaning-related neurons may be involved in the higher cognitive activity by integrating modality-specific information into modality-free information concerning the stimulus' meaning.

In summary, there are PFC neurons that are involved in coding the behavioral and associative significance of the stimulus across different sensory modalities. Such PFC neurons may play important roles in integrating different modalities of information to extract modality-free information concerning the stimulus' meaning, and thus to support higher cognitive activity.

POST-TRIAL PREFRONTAL NEURONAL ACTIVITY

Considerable interest in the brain mechanisms of motivational operations in the PFC has recently emerged (Damasio, 1994; Rolls, 1999; Cavada & Schultz, 2000; see Chapters 22 and 23). Here, some aspects of motivational operations in the primate PFC will first be described, with a focus on post-trial outcome-related and reward expectancy–related neuronal activity. Then, I will turn to the subject of interaction and integration of different kinds of information in this area, and describe how motivational and cognitive information interacts in primate PFC neurons.

In primate PFC neurons, four kinds of post-trial activity change are observed: (1) reward-related, (2) reinforcement-related, (3) error-related, and (4) end of trial–related. *Reward-related neurons* show activity changes whenever the food or liquid reward is delivered to the animal irrespective of whether it is given during or outside the task situation. *Reinforcement-related neurons* show activity changes only when the reward is given to the animal's correct response and do not show activity change to reward delivery outside the task situation. *Error-related neurons* show activity changes when the animal commits an error and the reward is not given to the animal. Figure 21–4 shows an example of an error-related neuron observed during a delayed go/no-go discrimination task. This neuron showed activation when the animal committed an error and could not obtain the reward. *End of trial–related neurons* show activity changes whenever the trial ends irrespective of whether the animal responds correctly, and irrespective of whether the animal obtains the reward. These neurons are considered to be involved in coding the termination of the trial.

These post-trial activity changes have been observed in the lateral PFC (LPFC) (areas 8, 46, and the lateral part of area 12 of Fig. 21–2; Niki & Watanabe, 1979; Rosenkilde et al., 1981; Watanabe, 1989, 1990), orbitofrontal cortex (OFC; areas 11, 13, 14, and ventral part of area 12; Rosenkilde et al.,1981; Aou et al., 1983 Thorpe et al., 1983; Trembley & Schultz, 1999, 2000), and anterior cingulate area (area 24; Niki & Watanabe, 1979) during the delayed response (Rosenkilde et al., 1981; Trembley & Schultz, 1999), delayed matching-to-sample (Rosenkilde et al., 1981), go/no-go discrimination (Watanabe, 1989; Trembley & Schultz, 2000), visual discrimination (Thorpe et al., 1983), bar pressing (Aou et al., 1983), delayed reaction time (Watanabe, 1990), and time estimation (Niki & Watanabe, 1979) tasks. Some neurons have combined characteristics of the second and third types, showing a different magnitude of, or reciprocal (increased versus decreased) activity changes between, reinforced and error trials.

In a study to further investigate the characteristics of reinforcement- and/or error-related PFC neurons, it was found that most of these neurons did not respond to the delivery or omission of reward during the classical conditioning situation (Niki, 1982); when a conditional stimulus (CS) of 1-second tone was associated with the unconditional stimulus (UCS) of a drop of juice, they did not respond to the delivery or omission of juice, indicating that their activity was dependent on the operant task situation.

In the go/no-go discrimination task, two other interesting aspects of the post-trial activity of LPFC neurons were found (Watan-

abe, 1989). First, there were neurons that coded the "correctness" of the response independent of the presence or absence of the reward as far as the correctness was informed to the animal. Most error-related neurons show similar activity changes when the reward is omitted after the animal's correct response as well as when the animal commits an error and no reward is given. Such neurons may be called *error- and reinforcement omission– related neurons.* However, in the task situation in which the animal was informed of the correctness of the response, some error-related neurons showed activity changes only when the animal committed an error, and did not show activity change when the reward was omitted following the animal's correct response. The neuron shown in Figure 21–4 showed clear activation when the animal recognized that it had committed an error in both

A

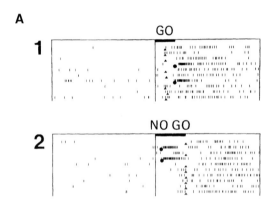
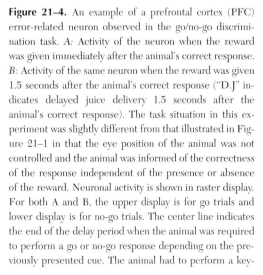

B

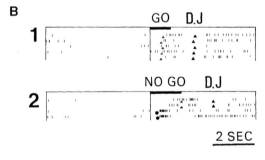

Figure 21–4. An example of a prefrontal cortex (PFC) error-related neuron observed in the go/no-go discrimination task. *A:* Activity of the neuron when the reward was given immediately after the animal's correct response. *B:* Activity of the same neuron when the reward was given 1.5 seconds after the animal's correct response ("D.J" indicates delayed juice delivery 1.5 seconds after the animal's correct response). The task situation in this experiment was slightly different from that illustrated in Figure 21–1 in that the eye position of the animal was not controlled and the animal was informed of the correctness of the response independent of the presence or absence of the reward. Neuronal activity is shown in raster display. For both A and B, the upper display is for go trials and lower display is for no-go trials. The center line indicates the end of the delay period when the animal was required to perform a go or no-go response depending on the previously presented cue. The animal had to perform a key-

release response within 1 second (go period) on go trials, but had to continue depressing the hold lever for 1.5 seconds (no-go period) on no-go trials after the end of the delay period. Horizontal black bars under headings of go and no go indicate 1 second of go period and 1.5 seconds of no-go period, respectively. Small filled triangles indicate the time of the animal's go correct response on go trials and the end of the no-go period (1.5 seconds after the end of the delay period) on no-go correct trials. Large filled triangles in B indicate the time of the delayed juiced reward delivery. Filled circles indicate the time when the animal committed an error; when the animal did not release the hold lever within 1 second of the go period and when the animal released the hold lever too early; i.e., within 1.5 seconds of the no-go period. This neuron showed activation when the animal committed an error, but did not show activation even when the reward was not given immediately after the correct response.

the immediate-reward delivery (Fig. 21–4A) and delayed-reward delivery (Fig. 21–4B) situations. However, it did not show activation when the reward delivery was delayed by 1.5 seconds and the reward was not given immediately after the animal's correct response (Fig. 21–4B), as well as when the reward was omitted following the animal's correct response (not shown in the figure). Such correctness-related neurons may play important roles in the animal's decision concerning whether the current behavioral strategies should be maintained or not. Thus, there are two kinds of reinforcement- and/or error-related neurons; one kind is related to coding the reinforcement itself or its omission, and the other kind is apparently related to coding the correctness of the response.

The second interesting findings were reward- and reinforcement-related neurons that showed differential activity to a reward delivery of the same kind and of the same magnitude after different responses (go and no-go) (Fig. 21–5). Such neurons may be involved in coding the consequence of the go and no-go responses separately and thus may be involved in facilitating learning and performance of the discrimination task.

Most post-trial activity changes in primate PFC, especially LPFC neurons, appear to be related not solely to motivational operations— i.e., not simply to coding the presence or absence of the reward, but to coding the context in which the reward is given (e.g., whether the reward is given during the operant or classical conditioning situation, or whether it is given to a go or no-go correct response) or to coding the congruence with or deviation from the expectancy; reinforcement-related neurons may be involved in coding the congruence between expectancy and the response outcome, whereas error-related neurons may be involved in coding the incongruence or mismatch between expectancy and outcome.

Human clinical studies indicate that patients with LPFC lesions are impaired in using the feedback signal to improve their performance (Luria, 1980; Milner & Petrides, 1984). Human activation studies indicate that the LPFC as well as anterior cingulate area is activated when the subject commits errors (Car-

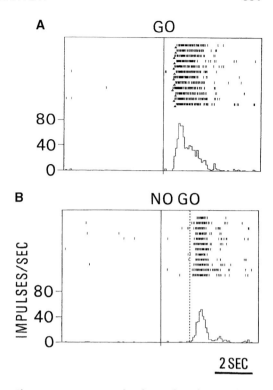

Figure 21–5. An example of a prefrontal cortex (PFC) reward-related neuron that responded differently after go and no-go correct responses despite the fact that the same amount of juice reward was given to the animal. The task situation is the same as that explained in Figure 21–4. Neuronal activity is shown in the raster and histogram displays. The upper display (*A*) shows correct go trials and lower display (*B*) shows correct no-go trials. The center line indicates the end of the delay period. The dotted line on no-go trials indicates the time of the end of the no-go period. This neuron did not show any detectable activity change when the reward was omitted after the animal's correct go response. Thus, the difference in post-trial activities after go and no-go correct responses is not considered due to the simple summation of reward-related activity and response-related activity.

ter et al., 1998; Kiehl et al., 2000). Also, in a study of error-related brain potentials in PFC patients (Gehring & Knight, 2000), it is suggested that LPFC interacts with anterior cingulate area in monitoring response outcome to adjust cognitive control based on task demands.

In summary, there are several kinds of primate neurons that show post-trial activity changes in relation to response outcome, such as reinforcement and error, in the PFC and anterior cingulate area. The PFC and anterior cingulate area of both humans and primates are considered to be involved in coding and monitoring the outcome of the response for better task performance.

REWARD EXPECTANCY AND PREFRONTAL NEURONAL ACTIVITY

Since expectancy appears to play important roles in the activity of some post-trial–related PFC neurons, it was interesting, as the next step, to look for neuronal activity in the primate cortex that might be related to reward expectancy. An expectancy wave can be recorded from the human PFC while the person anticipates the appearance of a certain event

(Walter, et al., 1964). In the primate PFC, anticipatory neuronal activity can be recorded while the animal is waiting for the presentation of the cue or triggering stimulus (Niki & Watanabe, 1979; Sakagami & Niki, 1995). As for the expectancy of the reward, reward expectancy–related neuronal activity is indeed observed in the PFC (Watanabe, 1996a; Leon & Schadlen, 1999; Trembley & Schultz, 1999; 2000; Hikosaka & Watanabe, 2000).

Behavioral experiments indicate that the monkey expects not simply a reward in general, but rather the specific reward during the task performance. In a study by Tinklepaugh (1928), the behavior of the animal in relation to reward expectancy was examined during a delayed-response task using several different kinds of rewards (Fig. 21–6). On some occa-

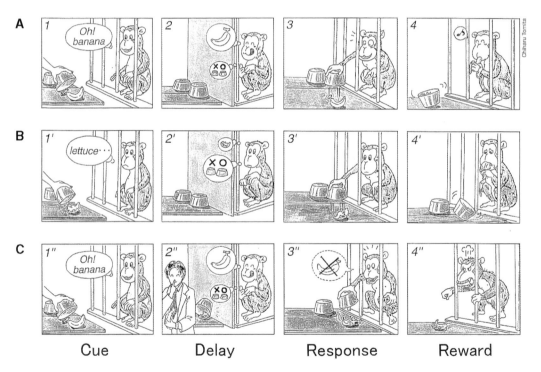

Cue   Delay   Response   Reward

Figure 21–6. Cartoon illustration of Tinklepaugh's experiment (1928). 1, cue period; 2, delay period; 3, animal's response; 4, reward delivery. A: Tinklepaugh first showed a banana (which was the animal's favorite food) in the right or left cup as a cue. During the delay period, an opaque screen was lowered in front of the animal so the animal could not see the cups. When the animal correctly responded to the cued side after the screen was raised, it was given the reward that had been shown earlier (in this case, banana). B: In this trial, the animal was shown lettuce (which was not the animal's favorite food) as a reward. The animal at least worked to obtain this non-preferred food. C: On some occasions, Tinklepaugh secretly changed the banana to lettuce during the delay period. After the correct response, when the animal found lettuce instead of the banana in the cup, it was surprised and became angry, sometimes shrieking at the experimenter.

sions (Fig. 21–6C), Tinklepaugh showed a banana (which was the animal's favorite food) in the right or left cup as a cue. During the delay period when the animal had to retain the spatial information in relation to where the food (cue) was presented, Tinklepaugh secretly exchanged the banana for lettuce (which was not the animal's favorite food, but for which the animal would, at least, work). After the correct response, when the animal found lettuce instead of banana in the cup, it was surprised and became angry, sometimes shrieking at the experimenter. It should be noted that the animal did not become angry if it was given lettuce as a reward, as long as it had been shown the lettuce during the cue period (Fig. 21–6B). It became angry only when it found a food reward that was incongruent with the expected preferred one. This experiment clearly shows that during the delay period, the monkey was expecting (although the animal was not required to do so) the delivery of the specific reward, in this case, banana, besides remembering (as a working memory) where it was presented.

To search for reward-dependent differential anticipatory activity in the primate LPFC (area 8, 46 and lateral part of area 12 of Fig. 21–2) neurons, two monkeys were trained in a modified manual delayed-response task using several kinds of food rewards (see Fig. 21–7A; Watanabe, 1996a). The animal was seated on a primate chair facing a panel that contained right and left rectangular windows, circular keys, and a hold lever below them. The animal first depressed the hold lever for 6 to 8 seconds (Pre-cue), and a red light was presented for 1 second either on the right or left key as a cue (Cue). Then there was a delay period of 5 seconds (Delay). After the delay period was over, a white light was presented on both right and left keys as a go signal (Go Signal) and the animal was required to respond to the side where the red cue had been presented (Response). Following the animal's correct response, it was given the reward that had been prepared behind the window (Reward). In this experiment, several different kinds of food rewards (such as raisin, sweet potato, apple, and cabbage) were used. In this task, the same reward was used continuously

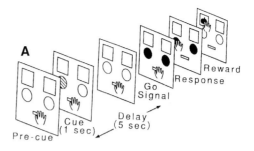

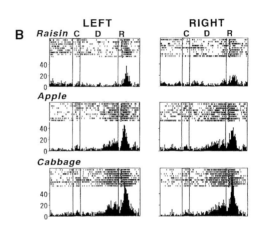

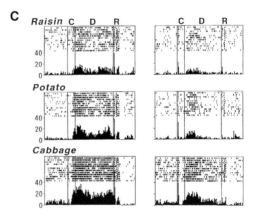

Figure 21–7. Sequence of events in the delayed-response task (*A*) and examples of reward expectancy–related prefrontal cortex neurons without (*B*) and with (*C*) spatial specificity. Neuronal activity is shown in raster and histogram displays. For each display, the second and third vertical lines indicate cue onset and offset, and the fourth vertical line indicates the end of the delay period. Each row indicates one trial, and small upward triangles in the raster indicate the time of the key-pressing responses. Only data from correct trials are shown. Left- and right-side displays are shown separately. The reward used is stated for each panel. C, cue; D, delay; R, response.

in a block of about 50 trials. Thus, the animal could know what reward was being used after experiencing a newly presented reward for two or three trials. During the delay period, the animal had to retain in working memory the spatial information concerning which side the cue was presented for correct task performance. Besides that, considering behavioral studies indicating the reward expectancy process in the monkey, it was thought that the animal was anticipating or expecting the specific reward that would be delivered.

Figure 21–7B shows an example of an LPFC delay neuron that is considered related to reward expectancy. This neuron showed differential activity during the delay period depending on differences in the reward, with the largest activity changes occurring on cabbage reward trials and almost no activity change on raisin reward trials. It should be noted that there was no external stimulus indicating a difference in the reward during the delay period. Since the same reward was used continuously in a block of about 50 trials, the animal could know what reward was being used after experiencing two or three trials and could expect the specific reward during the delay period in each trial. The differential activity observed in this neuron is considered related to the animal's expectancy for the different kind of reward. Most of these neurons showed more activity changes to the more preferred reward.

It has been well documented that there are many PFC neurons related to spatial working memory (Niki, 1974a, 1974b; Niki & Watanabe, 1976; Funahashi, et al., 1989). In my experiment on the manual delayed–response task using several kinds of reward, I also observed many delay neurons that showed spatial specificity. Interestingly, there were neurons that reflected both working memory and reward expectancy. The neuron illustrated in Figure 21–7C showed working memory–related activity by showing a higher rate of firing on left trials than on right trials during the delay period. This neuron also showed the highest rate of firing on cabbage reward trials, intermediate firing on potato reward trials, and the least firing on raisin reward trials during the delay period. Thus, in the activity of this neuron, there was an interaction between

working memory–related information and reward expectancy–related information. Such an interaction may help the animal to better prepare for obtaining a goal—i.e., to prepare for performing a certain response as well as for receiving a specific reward.

In summary, there are neurons in the primate LPFC that may be related to the reward expectancy process by showing differential anticipatory activity depending on differences in the reward to be given.

INTERACTION AND INTEGRATION OF DIFFERENT KINDS OF INFORMATION IN PRIMATE PREFRONTAL NEURONS

As I have described, the PFC receives various kinds of highly processed sensory information from the posterior association cortices. In the primate LPFC, there are neurons that are involved in retaining both space (*where*) and object (*what*) information in working memory (Watanabe, 1981; Rao, et al., 1997). Previously I reported those PFC neurons that were involved in extracting the meaning of the stimulus across different sensory modalities (Watanabe, 1992; 1996b). These "object and space working memory–related neurons" and "cross-modal meaning-related neurons" are considered to be involved in the integration of different kinds of cognitive information for executive control. Fuster (1997) has proposed that the most important role of the PFC is "temporal organization of behavior." Interestingly, Fuster and colleagues (2000) have shown, that PFC neurons represent the association of sensory items of both visual and auditory inputs and integrate these items across time. Thus, the PFC may represent both cross-modal and cross-temporal associations for executive control.

The PFC receives not only sensory and cognitive information from the posterior association cortices, but also a variety of motivational information from the limbic system (Stuss & Benson, 1986; Fuster, 1997; Figure 21–2). Thus, it is not surprising to find PFC neurons where both motivational and cognitive information interact. I have described two kinds of such LPFC neurons. One kind of neurons responded differently to the reward/no-reward delivery between operant and classical conditioning situations, or responded differently depending on differences in the behavioral response (go or no-go) of the animal (e.g., Fig. 21–5). In such neurons, there was an interaction between motivational (presence or absence of reward) and cognitive (what task situation the animal was faced with or what behavioral response the animal had performed) information. The other kind of neurons showed delay-related differential activity depending on both the difference in the reward that could be expected and the difference in the impending response (right or left—e.g., Fig. 21–7C). Also in such neurons there was an interaction between motivational (reward expectancy) and cognitive (working memory) information. A study by Leon and Shadlen (1999) has indicated that a larger reward enhances working memory–related activity in primate LPFC neurons of area 46 (principal sulcus area) during the oculomotor delayed-response task. Such enhancement of neuronal activity induced by a larger reward may facilitate learning and performance of the discrimination task. Thus, the LPFC may play important roles in the integration of motivational and cognitive information for better task performance.

In summary, cognitive and motivational information appears to interact in the activity of primate LPFC neurons. These LPFC neurons may be involved in the integration of cognitive and motivational information for better task performance.

FUNCTIONAL SEGREGATION OF PRIMATE PREFRONTAL CORTEX IN RELATION TO MOTIVATIONAL AND COGNITIVE OPERATIONS

It is generally considered that the LPFC is important for cognitive or executive function while the OFC is important for motivational function (Damasio, 1994; Fuster, 1997). Interestingly, as far as post-trial– and reward expectancy–related neuronal activities are concerned, there is no significant difference in characteristics between LPFC and OFC. Indeed, all four kinds of post-trial–related as well as reward expectancy–related neurons are observed in both LPFC and OFC, although reward-related and reinforcement-related neurons were reported to be more abundant in the LPFC than in the OFC, whereas error-related neurons were more abundant in the OFC in a study in which the neuronal activity of both LPFC and OFC was examined in the same monkey (Rosenkilde et al., 1981). Thus, it seems that the LPFC also plays important roles in motivational operations. A human activation study (Thut et al., 1997) showed that both LPFC and OFC are similarly activated in relation to the expectancy of monetary reward, indicating that the human LPFC also plays important roles in motivational operations.

Although similar post-trial– and reward expectancy– related activities are observed in both LPFC and OFC, and the LPFC appears to play as important a role in motivational operations as the OFC, there appear to be some significant differences in the properties of neuronal activity between these two PFC areas. Although there are insufficient data available, it has been indicated that working memory–related neurons are abundant in the LPFC, but quite rare in the OFC (Trembley & Schultz, 1999). The LPFC, but not the OFC neurons are reported to show both working memory–related and reward expectancy–related activity changes during the delay period of the delayed-response task (Watanabe, 1996a). The LPFC neurons appear to be more concerned than OFC neurons with coding the context in which the reward is given or omitted, such as in relation to whether the presence or absence of reward is associated with a go or no-go response (Watanabe, 1989). The LPFC, but not the OFC neurons are reported to code the correctness of the response independent of the presence or absence of the reward (Watanabe, 1989, 1998). Thus, if it is considered that (1) the LPFC receives highly processed cognitive information from the posterior association (the temporal and posterior parietal) cortices, (2) the OFC receives motivational information from the limbic system and sends the output to the LPFC (Barbas & Pandya, 1991), and (3) there is an interaction between motivational and cognitive information in the activity of LPFC neurons, it could be concluded that the LPFC, but not OFC, is involved in the integration of motivational and cognitive information for optimizing the behavior to obtain the goal.

If this is true, then the functional significance of post-trial– and reward expectancy–related neuronal activities might differ between LPFC and OFC. It appears that OFC neurons are more concerned with the hedonic aspects of reward information (Rolls, 1999), whereas LPFC neurons are more related to the integration of motivational and cognitive information (Leon & Shadlen, 1999). It may be that reward expectancy–related LPFC neurons are related more to preparing for receiving the specific outcome by integrating several different kinds of information, such as the taste, olfaction, and the visual appearance of the future reward, rather than to the expectancy of the appetitive aspects of the reward.

In summary, there appears to be functional segregation of the PFC in relation to cognitive and motivational operations, in that the OFC is predominantly involved in motivational operations while the LPFC may be involved in the integration of cognitive and motivational information.

CONCLUSIONS

For survival or for a better quality of life, an organism works to obtain a goal, such as food, liquid, a mate, and money (in the case of human beings). The goal of the behavior has motivational significance that may differ depending on the organism's motivational situation. To optimize the way to attain a goal, several different kinds of information, including both cognitive (such as current environmental situation) and motivational information (such as hunger level and attraction of the goal) should be taken into consideration and integrated. The PFC appears to play the most important role in this process. Indeed, neurons that are considered to be involved in the integration of different kinds of information have been observed in the primate PFC; some PFC neurons were related to coding behavioral or associative significance of the stimulus across different sensory modalities, and other PFC neurons appeared to be involved in integrating motivational and cognitive information (such as reward expectancy–related and working memory–related information). Compared with the OFC, which appears to be predominantly concerned with motivational operations, the LPFC appears to be more concerned with the integration of motivational and cognitive information.

To better understand the brain mechanisms of goal-directed behavior, we should further clarify how cognitive and motivational information interacts in the PFC, examining how cognition-related PFC activity is modified by motivational information as well as how motivation-related PFC activity is modulated by cognitive information. Future research along this line might facilitate a better understanding of how the PFC accommodates desire within the current situation or how the PFC works to integrate cost and benefit.

REFERENCES

Aou S., Oomura Y., & Nishino, H. (1983). Influence of acetylcholine on neuronal activity in monkey orbitofrontal cortex during bar press feeding task. *Brain Research, 275,* 178–182.

Barbas, H. (1995). Anatomic basis of cognitive-emotional interactions in the primate prefrontal cortex. *Neuroscience and Biobehavioral Reviews, 19,* 499–510.

Barbas, H. & Pandya, D.N. (1991). Patterns of connections of the prefrontal cortex in the rhesus monkey associated with cortical architecture. In: H.S. Levin, H.M. Eisenberg, & A.L. Benton (Eds.), *Frontal Lobe Function and Dysfunction* (pp. 35–58). New York: Oxford University Press.

Carter, C.S., Braver, T.S., Barch, D.M., Botvinick, M.M., Noll, D., & Cohen, J.D. (1998). Anterior cingulate cortex, error detection, and the online monitoring of performance. *Science, 280,* 747–749.

Cavada, C. & Schultz, W. (2000) The Mysterious Orbitofrontal Cortex. *Cerebral Cortex* Special Issue 10: 205–342.

Damasio, A.R. (1994). *Descartes Error: Emotion, Reason and the Human Brain.* New York: Grosset/Putnum.

Funahashi, S., Bruce, C.J., & Goldman-Rakic, P.S. (1989). Mnemonic coding of visual space in the monkey's dorsolateral prefrontal cortex. *Journal of Neurophysiology, 61,* 331–349.

Fuster, J.M. (1997). *The Prefrontal Cortex. Anatomy, Physiology and Neuropsychology of the Frontal Lobe,* 3rd ed. New York: Lippincott-Raven.

Fuster, J.M., Bodner, M., & Kroger, J.K. (2000). Cross-modal and cross-temporal association in neurons of frontal cortex. *Nature, 405,* 347–351.

Gehring, W.J. & Knight, R.T. (2000). Prefrontal-cingulate interactions in action monitoring. *Nature Neuroscience, 3,* 516–520.

Hikosaka, K. & Watanabe, M. (2000). Delay activity of orbital and lateral prefrontal neurons of the monkey varying with different rewards. *Cerebral Cortex, 10,* 263–271.

Kiehl, K.A., Liddle, P.F., & Hopfinger, J.B. (2000). Error processing and the rostral anterior cingulate: an event-related fMRI study. *Psychophysiology, 37,* 216–223.

Knight, R.T. & Grabowecky, M. (2000). Prefrontal cortex, time and consciousness. In: M.S. Gazzaniga (Ed.), *The New Cognitive Neurosciences,* 2nd ed. (pp. 1319–1339), Cambridge, MA: MIT Press.

Leon, M.I. & Shadlen, M.N. (1999). Effect of expected reward magnitude on the response of neurons in the dorsolateral prefrontal cortex of the macaque. *Neuron, 24,* 415–425.

Luria, A.R. (1980). *Higher Cortical Functions in Man.* New York: Basic Books.

Milner, B. & Petrides, M. (1984). Behavioral effects of frontal lobe lesions in man. *Trends in Neuroscience, 7,* 403–407.

Niki, H. (1974a). Prefrontal unit activity during delayed alternation in the monkey: I. Relation to direction of response. *Brain Research, 68,* 185–196.

Niki, H. (1974b). Differential activity of prefrontal units during right and left delayed response trials. *Brain Research, 70,* 346–349.

Niki, H. (1982). Reward-related and error-related neurons in the primate frontal cortex. In: S. Saito & T. Yanagita (Eds.), *Learning and Memory: Drugs as Reinforcer, Excerpta Medica, 620,* 22–34.

Niki, H. & Watanabe, M. (1976). Prefrontal unit activity and delayed response: relation to cue location versus direction of response. *Brain Research, 105,* 79–88.

Niki, H. & Watanabe, M. (1979). Prefrontal and cingulate unit activity during timing behavior in the monkey. *Brain Research, 171,* 213–224.

Rao, S.C., Rainer, G., & Miller, E.K. (1997). Integration of what and where in the primate prefrontal cortex. *Science, 276,* 821–824.

Roberts, A.C., Robbins, T.W., & Weiskranz, L. (1998). *The Prefrontal Cortex, Executive and Cognitive Functions.* Oxford: Oxford University Press.

Rolls, E.T. (1999). *The Brain and Emotion.* Oxford: Oxford University Press.

Rosenkilde, C.E., Bauer, R.H., & Fuster, J.M. (1981). Single cell activity in ventral prefrontal cortex of behaving monkeys. *Brain Research, 209,* 375–394.

Sakagami, M. & Niki, H. (1995). Encoding of behavioral significance of visual stimuli by primate prefrontal neurons: relation to relevant task conditions. *Experimental Brain Research, 97,* 423–436.

Stuss, D.T. & Benson D.F. (1986). *The Frontal Lobes.* New York: Raven Press.

Thorpe, S.J., Rolls, E.T., & Maddison, S. (1983). The orbitofrontal cortex: neuronal activity in the behaving monkey. *Experimental Brain Research, 49,* 93–115.

Thut, G., Schultz, W., Roelcke, U., Nienhusmeier, M., Missimer, J., Maguire, R.P., & Leenders, K.L. (1997). Activation of the human brain by monetary reward. *NeuroReport, 8,* 1225–1228.

Tinklepaugh, O.L. (1928). An experimental study of representation factors in monkeys. *Journal of Comparative Psychology, 8,* 197–236.

Trembley, L. & Schultz, W. (1999). Relative reward preference in primate orbitofrontal cortex. *Nature, 398,* 704–708.

Trembley, L. & Schultz, W. (2000). Reward-related neuronal activity during go–no go task performance in primate orbitofrontal cortex. *Journal of Neurophysiology, 83,* 1864–1876.

Walker, A.E. (1940). A cytoarchitectual study of the prefrontal area of the macaque monkey. *Journal of Comparative Neurology, 73,* 59–86.

Walter, W.G., Cooper, R., Aldrige, V.J., McCallum, W.C., & Winter, A.L. (1964). Contingent negative variation: an electric sign of sensori-motor association and expectancy in the human brain. *Nature, 203,* 380–384.

Watanabe, M. (1981). Prefrontal unit activity during delayed conditional discriminations in the monkey. *Brain Research, 225,* 51–65.

Watanabe, M. (1986a). Prefrontal unit activity during delayed conditional go/no-go discrimination in the monkey. I. Relation to the stimulus. *Brain Research, 382,* 1–14.

Watanabe, M. (1986b). Prefrontal unit activity during delayed conditional go/no-go discrimination in the monkey. II. Relation to go and no-go responses. *Brain Research, 382,* 15–27.

Watanabe, M. (1989). The appropriateness of behavioral responses coded in post-trial activity of primate prefrontal units. *Neuroscience Letters, 101,* 113–117.

Watanabe, M. (1990). Prefrontal unit activity during associative learning in the monkey. *Experimental Brain Research, 80,* 296–309.

Watanabe, M. (1992). Frontal units of the monkey coding the associative significance of visual and auditory stimuli. *Experimental Brain Research, 89,* 233–247.

Watanabe, M. (1996a). Reward expectancy in primate prefrontal neurons. *Nature, 382,* 629–632.

Watanabe, M. (1996b). Visual and auditory responses of the primate prefrontal neurons in relation to the significance of the stimulus. In: T. Ono, B.L. McNaughton, S. Molotchnikoff, E.T. Rolls, & H. Nishijo (Eds.), *Perception, Memory, and Emotion: Frontiers in Neuroscience* (pp. 433–444). Oxford: Pergamon Press.

Watanabe, M. (1998). Cognitive and motivational operations in primate prefrontal neurons. *Review Neuroscience 9,* 225–241.

22

Emotion, Decision Making, and the Ventromedial Prefrontal Cortex

DANIEL TRANEL

Folk wisdom has long held that making complex decisions is a task best accomplished with a "cool head," under conditions of deliberated, rational consideration of various response options, uncolored by the "heat of emotion." And one cannot question that there is some truth to this advice: take, for example, the irrational, emotion-tinged frenzy that occurs with some regularity in the stock market (Shiller, 2000), or the "crimes of passion" that are well documented in law enforcement (Tranel, in press). Against this background, it is of particular intrigue that there is new scientific evidence suggesting that *too little* emotion may be just as detrimental for good decision making as too much emotion.

This evidence derives from a series of studies that my colleagues and I have conducted in patients with damage to the ventromedial prefrontal (VMPF; see Fig. 22–1) sector of the brain (Bechara et al., 1994, 1996, 1997, 2000; Anderson et al., 1999, 2000; Tranel et al., 2000; Barrash et al. 2000). These studies have been pursued in the context of the *somatic marker hypothesis*, a theoretical framework developed to explain how emotions and feelings are used to guide decision-making processes (Damasio, 1994, 1996, 1999). This chapter focuses on three aspects of our investigations: *(1)* the development and application of a laboratory task to measure decision making and related emotional influences; *(2)* the development of a set of rating scales aimed at characterizing the personality attributes of patients with acquired VMPF dysfunction and decision-making impairments; and *(3)* studies conducted in patients who sustained damage to VMPF cortices very early in life, and who manifested lifelong social conduct and decision-making deficits. In a final section, the main features of the somatic marker framework are summarized.

MEASURING DECISION MAKING AND EMOTION IN THE LABORATORY

THE GAMBLING TASK

Many patients with VMPF damage do not evince impairments on conventional neuropsychological procedures, including quintessential "frontal lobe" tasks, even though their real-world behavior is rife with instances of poor decision making. In response to this paradox, we developed a card game (the Gambling Task), in which the goal is to maximize profit on a loan of play money, and in which response selection is guided by various schedules of immediate reward and delayed punish-

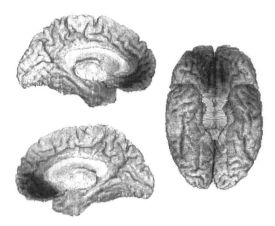

Figure 22–1. Mesial views of the left hemisphere (*upper left*) and right hemisphere (*lower left*), and ventral view of the hemispheres (*right*). The darkened area depicts lesion overlaps in the ventromedial prefrontal (VMPF) region, from more than 12 patients who have been studied in our laboratory over the past decade. The VMPF sector includes the orbital cortices, lower mesial cortices, and underlying white matter.

ment. The Gambling Task provides a valid analogue to real-world decision making, by making unpredictable rewards and punishments an explicit aspect of the situation, and by requiring delayed response gratification. Patients with VMPF lesions show a reliable pattern of disadvantageous responding on the Gambling Task, even when they are retested over various intervals of time and with various permutations on the basic theme of the task (Bechara et al., 1994; 2000). Some of the main findings are summarized below.

In the basic version of the Gambling Task, subjects are presented four decks of cards, and are given a $2000 start-up loan. Subjects are told that the game requires a long series of card selections, one card at a time, from any of the decks, until the experimenter ends the game. After each card selection, subjects receive a monetary reward; the amount is announced after the card selection, and varies from deck to deck. After some card selections, subjects are both given money and asked to pay a penalty; again, the amount is announced only after the card selection, and it varies from deck to deck and from position to position within a given deck. Subjects are told that the goal of the task is to maximize their profit; they are free to switch from any deck to another, at any time, as often as they wish. The task is discontinued after 100 card selections (subjects are not informed of this beforehand). The Gambling Task is rigged so that two of the decks (the disadvantageous decks) yield higher immediate rewards, but higher long-term penalties, such that selecting frequently from these decks will result in a net long-term loss. The other two decks (the advantageous decks) yield lower immediate rewards, but also lower long-term penalties, such that selecting frequently from these decks will result in a net long-term gain.

In an initial study (Bechara et al., 1994), three groups of subjects were compared on the Gambling Task: (*1*) six subjects with bilateral VMPF lesions; (*2*) six brain-damaged controls, who had lesions outside the VMPF region; and (*3*) 44 normal controls, who were free of neurological or psychiatric disease. To score the task, the 100 card selections were divided into five discrete blocks of 20 each, and for each block, the numbers of disadvantageous selections and advantageous selections were calculated. The results, broken down as a function of group, block, and deck type, are presented in Figure 22–2. As the task progressed, normal and brain-damaged controls gradually shifted their selections towards the advantageous decks, and by the last two blocks (trials 61–100), the subjects were choosing almost exclusively from these decks. The VMPF subjects failed to demonstrate this shift: in all but one trial block, they selected more cards from the disadvantageous decks, and on the last two trial blocks, they continued to select more frequently from the disadvantageous decks.

The same pattern of performance has been demonstrated in follow-up studies, using different permutations of the Gambling Task and larger groups of subjects (Bechara et al., 2000). For example, even when the reward–punishment contingencies of the task are completely reversed, so that the "advantageous" decks involve higher up-front punishment but higher long-term reward, and the "disadvantageous" decks involve lower up-front punishment but lower long-term reward, VMPF patients continue to opt for the disadvantageous

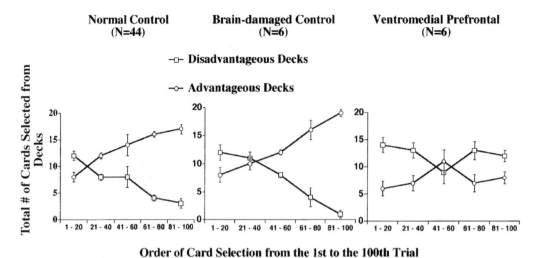

Figure 22–2. Card selections on the Gambling Task as a function of group (normal control, brain-damaged control, ventromedial prefrontal damage), deck type (disadvantageous versus advantageous), and trial block. The two control groups gradually shifted their response selections towards the advantageous decks, and this tendency became stronger as the game went on. The ventromedial prefrontal subjects did not make a reliable shift, and continued to opt for the disadvantageous decks even during the latter stages of the game, when controls had almost completely abandoned choosing from the disadvantageous decks. (*Source:* From Tranel et al., 2000, with permission)

decks. These findings suggest that patients with VMPF lesions have a fundamental insensitivity to the future consequences of their choices, whether those consequences be positive or negative, and are guided prepotently by the immediate prospects of their behavior.

ANTICIPATORY PSYCHOPHYSIOLOGICAL RESPONSES

A psychophysiological dependent variable was added to the Gambling Task, as an index of somatic state activation during the task (Bechara et al., 1996). Specifically, skin conductance responses (SCRs) during the task were measured. The format was set up to allow identification of each SCR generated in association with a specific card from a specific deck. Three types of SCRs were defined: *(1) reward* SCRs, defined as SCRs generated after the subject had selected cards for which there was a reward and no penalty; *(2) punishment* SCRs, defined as SCRs generated after the subject had selected cards for which there was a reward followed immediately by a penalty; and *(3) anticipatory* SCRs, defined as the SCRs generated immediately prior to the point at which the subject selected a card from a given deck—i.e., the time period during which the subject was deliberating their choice. Two groups of subjects were studied: *(1)* 7 subjects with bilateral VMPF lesions, and *(2)* 12 normal controls.

Both groups of subjects generated SCRs in reaction to reward and punishment, and the groups did not differ from one another in this regard. The control subjects, as they became experienced with the task, began to generate anticipatory SCRs, i.e., SCRs *prior to* the selection of some cards. The VMPF subjects failed to generate anticipatory SCRs. Also, it was found that controls generated higher-amplitude anticipatory SCRs to the disadvantageous decks than those to the advantageous decks; no such difference was evident in the VMPF subjects. The results indicated that the anticipatory SCRs generated by controls developed over time; the subjects began to respond, and responded more systematically, after selecting several cards from each deck, and thereby encountering several instances of reward and punishment. The anticipatory SCRs became more pronounced prior to the selection of cards from the disadvantageous decks.

In sum, during the Gambling Task, control subjects began to generate SCRs *prior to* their card selections, while they deliberated which deck to choose. This pattern never developed in the VMPF subjects. The findings are consistent with the idea that the absence of anticipatory SCRs in the VMPF subjects is a physiological correlate for their insensitivity to future outcomes. Within the context of the somatic marker framework (see below), the evidence indicates that these subjects fail to activate biasing signals that would serve as value markers in the distinction between choices with good or bad future outcomes. We have also proposed that these signals participate in the enhancement of attention and working memory relative to representations pertinent to the decision-making process, and that such signals hail from bioregulatory machinery that sustains somatic homeostasis and that can be expressed in emotion and feeling.

SOMATIC MARKERS CAN BE COVERT

The somatic marker hypothesis proposes that somatic markers can operate both covertly and overtly. An important prediction from this proposal is that the overt reasoning used to decide advantageously in a complex situation is actually *preceded* by a nonconscious biasing step. This prediction was tested in another study using the Gambling Task (Bechara et al., 1997). The subjects were 6 individuals with bilateral VMPF damage and 10 normal controls. Three measurements were obtained in parallel: behavioral (task performance), psychophysiological (SCRs), and self-report of the task contingencies. The self-report data were used to judge whether subjects had developed explicit knowledge of how the game worked. On the basis of these reports, we divided the task into four "knowledge periods," defined below. The reports were obtained by interrupting the Gambling Task after each subject had made 20 card selections, and asking the subject the following: *(1)* "Tell me all you know about what is going on in this game"; and *(2)* "Tell me how you feel about this game." The prompts were repeated at 10-card intervals for the remainder of the task.

After sampling from all four decks, and before encountering any punishments, subjects tended to prefer the disadvantageous decks (where there is higher immediate reward), and no anticipatory SCRs were evident. This was defined as the *pre-punishment period.* After encountering some punishments in the disadvantageous decks, the control subjects began to generate anticipatory SCRs to these decks. However, none of the subjects had yet developed any notion as to what was happening in the task, as judged from their self-reports during this phase. This was defined as the *pre-hunch period.* By about trial 50, the control subjects began to express a "hunch" that some decks were riskier and less favorable, and the subjects generated anticipatory SCRs to the disadvantageous decks. This was defined as the *hunch period.* During the remainder of the task, most of the control subjects (7/10) reported explicit knowledge regarding the task contingencies—i.e., that on balance, some decks were "bad" and some were "good." This was defined as the *conceptual period.*

The behavioral data (card selections) and anticipatory SCRs were scored as a function of the four knowledge periods (Fig. 22–3). During the pre-hunch period, the magnitude of anticipatory SCRs in the control subjects increased significantly—i.e., the subjects developed anticipatory SCRs *before* they had any notion as to what was happening in the game, and before their behavior changed clearly in favor of the advantageous decks. During the hunch and conceptual periods, the controls continued to generate anticipatory SCRs to the disadvantageous decks, and they also shifted their choices distinctly to the advantageous decks. The VMPF subjects never developed anticipatory SCRs, and they continued to select more frequently from the disadvantageous decks throughout the task. Also, the three controls who failed to reach the conceptual period still showed a shift towards the advantageous decks, and they generated anticipatory SCRs whenever they selected from the disadvantageous decks. By contrast, three of the six VMPF subjects did reach the conceptual period, but despite this, they continued to choose disadvantageously, and they failed to generate anticipatory SCRs.

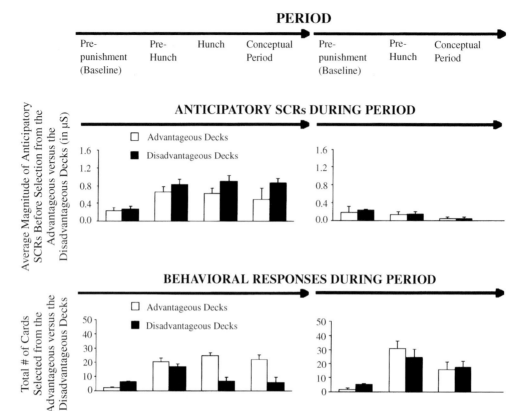

Figure 22–3. Psychophysiological (anticipatory skin conductance responses [SCRs] and behavioral (card selection) data for control subjects (*n* = 10) and subjects with ventromedial prefrontal lesions (*n* = 6), as a function of four "knowledge periods" (see text). Control subjects, even before they knew anything consciously about how the game worked (pre-hunch period), began to generate anticipatory SCRs and to shift their selections away from the bad decks. In the controls, anticipatory SCRs, especially to the bad decks, became more pronounced as the game progressed, and the subjects shifted almost exclusively to the good decks. The ventromedial prefrontal subjects never produced anticipatory SCRs, and they also continued to opt more frequently for the bad decks. This pattern occurred even in ventromedial subjects (*n* = 3) who knew at a conscious level (conceptual period) how the game worked, and that some decks were good and some were bad. (*Source:* from Tranel et al., 2000, with permission)

The autonomic responses detected in this experiment (especially those evident in the pre-hunch period) can be taken as evidence for a nonconscious signaling process, which in turn reflects access of records of previous experiences shaped by reward, punishment, and apposed emotional states. Within the somatic marker framework, these results suggest that decision-making situations lead to two nonexclusive, interacting chains of events. The first is that the sensory representation of a decision-making situation activates neural systems, including the VMPF sector, that hold dispositional knowledge related to one's previous emotional experience of similar situations. This, in turn, activates other neural regions, including autonomic and neurotransmitter nuclei. The ensuing signals (which remain nonconscious) act as covert biases on circuits that support cognitive evaluation and reasoning. In the second chain of events, the representation of a decision-making situation generates overt recall of pertinent facts, such as potential response options and probable future outcomes. Conscious reasoning strategies can then be applied to such facts. Our experiment suggests that nonconscious biases guide reasoning and decision-making behavior before conscious knowledge does; moreover, without the help of such biases, conscious knowledge may not be sufficient to ensure advantageous behavior. Other studies also support this conclusion—for example, individuals can learn and make decisions with information that is not available to conscious awareness (e.g., Lewicki et al., 1992), and they can develop "unconscious insights" (Siegler, 2000).

DEFINING AND MEASURING THE SYNDROME OF ACQUIRED SOCIOPATHY

Some of the most intriguing observations regarding patients with VMPF lesions pertain to the realm of personality. The development of certain maladaptive personality features following the onset of VMPF damage has been noted repeatedly throughout the history of neuropsychology, dating back to the description of the now-famous "crowbar" case (patient Phineas Gage), and the prescient observations of Gage's physician, John Harlow (1848, 1868; for a detailed historical review of this case, see Macmillan, 2000).

On September 13, 1848, Phineas Gage suffered a bizarre accident in which a tamping iron was propelled through the front part of his head. The bar entered his left cheek just under the eye, impaled the frontal lobes, and exited through the top front part of his head. A recent analysis of the case, based on measurements taken from Gage's skull and the tamping iron, and using modern neuroanatomical analysis techniques, established that Gage very likely sustained bilateral VMPF damage as a consequence of this accident (Fig. 22–4; Damasio et al., 1994). Despite a

remarkable recovery of intelligence, memory, speech, sensation, and movement, Gage displayed a profound change in personality and social conduct following his prefrontal injury. Before, he had been responsible, socially well adjusted, and popular with co-workers and supervisors. Afterwards, he was irresponsible, untrustworthy, irreverent, capricious, unreliable, and callous. In the words of Harlow (1868), Gage was "fitful, irreverent, indulging

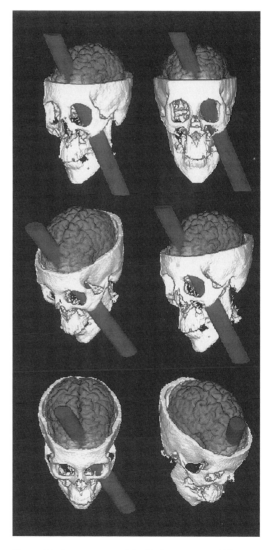

Figure 22–4. Depiction of the likely trajectory of the iron bar through the brain of Phineas Gage, as determined by a computer-assisted reconstruction based on measurements of Gage's skull and the bar. (*Source:* Modified from H. Damasio et al., 1994, with permission)

at times in the grossest profanity (which was not previously his custom), manifesting but little deference for his fellows, impatient of restraint or advice when it conflicts with his desires, at times pertinaciously obstinate, yet capricious and vacillating, devising many plans of future operation, which are no sooner arranged than they are abandoned in turn for others appearing more feasible" (pp. 339–340).

Others have called attention to the bizarre development of personality changes and abnormal social behavior following prefrontal brain injury (for review, see Damasio & Anderson, in press. The affected patients displayed a number of characteristic features: inability to organize future activity and hold gainful employment, diminished capacity to respond to punishment, a tendency to present an unrealistically favorable view of themselves, and a tendency to display inappropriate emotional reactions. Blumer and Benson (1975) noted that the personality profile of these patients (termed "pseudo-psychopathic") was characterized by puerility, a jocular attitude, sexually disinhibited humor, inappropriate and near-total self-indulgence, and complete lack of concern for others. Stuss and Benson (1986) emphasized that the patients demonstrated a remarkable lack of empathy and general lack of concern about others. The patients were described as showing boastfulness, unrestrained and tactless behavior, impulsiveness, facetiousness, and diminished anxiety and concern for the future. This personality profile bears some striking similarities to that characterized in clinical psychology and psychiatry as psychopathic (or sociopathic) (American Psychiatric Association, 1994; Sutker, 1994; Mealey, 1995). In fact, we designated this condition as "acquired sociopathy," in recognition of the fact that many prefrontal-injured patients develop personality manifestations that are reminiscent of those associated with sociopathy (Eslinger & Damasio, 1985; Damasio et al., 1990, 1991; Tranel, 1994).

The personality manifestations of VMPF patients turned out to be much like these patients' decision-making deficits, in the sense that the anomalies were blatant in the patients' everyday lives, but difficult to measure

in the laboratory. Some years ago, in an attempt to capture the syndrome of acquired sociopathy with standard personality inventories, we (Barrash et al., 1994) administered to a group of patients with VMPF damage several well-established psychometric instruments for assessing psychopathology, including the Minnesota Multiphasic Personality Inventory (MMPI and MMPI-2), the Eysenck Personality Questionnaire, the Structured Interview for DSM-III-R Personality, and the revised Hare Psychopathy Checklist. This endeavor was an unqualified failure: by and large, the VMPF patients generated normal personality profiles on these instruments, or produced profiles that were in no way faithful to the real-world personality manifestations of the patients. This outcome may be explained by the fact that many of these instruments rely on self-report, coupled with the tendency of VMPF patients to have significant anosognosia (lack of insight) for their condition; as well as the fact that the VMPF patients did, in fact, have normal personalities prior to the onset of their brain injury (Gainotti, 1993; Barrash et al., 1994; Tate, 1999).

In response to this unsuccessful effort to capture the syndrome of acquired sociopathy with standard personality instruments, we developed a set of rating scales—the *Iowa Rating Scales of Personality Change* (IRSPC)—that was designed to provide a sensitive, reliable, and valid means of characterizing acquired personality abnormalities in brain-damaged patients, especially patients with VMPF lesions. In a recent study (Barrash et al., 2000), we used the IRSPC to address two objectives: *(1)* to identify empirically the acquired personality disturbances that are most highly and specifically associated with acquired sociopathy, and *(2)* to determine the extent to which the syndrome of acquired sociopathy is specific to damage in the VMPF region.

The reader is referred to Barrash et al. (2000) for a detailed presentation of the IRSPC. Briefly, however, the IRSPC have several features that warrant emphasis. The first is that they assess functioning in the areas of emotional modulation, behavioral control, social and interpersonal behavior, and higher-order abilities such as decision-making and insight. Second, the scales are completed by an *informant*, i.e., an individual (usually a spouse or relative of the patient) who is very familiar with the patient from both before and after the onset of brain injury. The third feature is that for each characteristic, the informant rates both *level* (the extent to which that characteristic is present now) and *change* (the extent to which the current level represents a change from premorbidly). In sum, the IRSPC allow comprehensive assessment of personality changes that have occurred consequent to brain injury, while avoiding problems of self-report and clinician-based observations that are limited by restricted behavioral samples.

We studied 57 brain-damaged subjects, 7 of whom had bilateral VMPF damage. Personality characteristics that were rated as significantly more severe (higher levels) in the VMPF subjects included (in descending order of severity) lack of insight, lack of initiative, irritability, social inappropriateness, poor judgment, lack of persistence, indecisiveness, lability, blunted emotional experience, apathy, inappropriate affect, poor frustration tolerance, and inflexibility. Characteristics that were rated as significant changes in the VMPF subjects, compared to traits during the premorbid epoch, included lack of insight, lack of initiative, irritability, social inappropriateness, poor judgment, lack of persistence, lability, blunted emotional experience, inappropriate affect, poor frustration tolerance, and inflexibility. The levels and degrees of change in these characteristics were much lower in subjects with prefrontal damage outside the ventromedial region (e.g., in dorsolateral sectors) and in subjects whose damage was outside the prefrontal region entirely.

In sum, this study identified a set of personality and behavioral characteristics that comprises the core of a syndrome that we have termed *acquired sociopathy* (Table 22–1): *(1)* general dampening of emotional experience (impoverished emotional experience, low emotional expressiveness and apathy, inappropriate affect); *(2)* poorly modulated emotional reactions (poor frustration tolerance, irritability, lability); *(3)* disturbances in decision making, especially in the social realm

Table 22–1. Characteristics of Syndrome of Acquired Sociopathy

General dampening of emotional experience
Poorly modulated emotional reactions
Disturbances in decision making
Disturbances in goal-directed behavior
Disturbances in social behavior
Marked lack of insight into acquired changes

(indecisiveness, poor judgment, inflexibility, social inappropriateness, insensitivity, lack of empathy); *(4)* disturbances in goal-directed behavior (problems in planning, initiation, and persistence, and behavioral rigidity); and *(5)* marked lack of insight into these acquired changes. Moreover, this syndrome is highly and specifically associated with VMPF damage, and not with brain damage outside the ventromedial prefrontal region, or with brain damage in general. It is also important to note that the syndrome of acquired sociopathy was enduring in the VMPF patients: on average, they had manifested these characteristics for more than 10 years after the onset of brain injury. In short, VMPF damage leads to a chronic set of disturbances in emotional functioning, decision making, goal-directed behavior, social and interpersonal behavior, and insight. This set of disturbances can be empirically defined as acquired sociopathy.

The personality disturbances characteristic of patients with VMPF damage are reminiscent of many of the core features of developmental psychopathy, including shallow affect, irresponsibility, vocational instability, lack of realistic long-term goals, lack of empathy, and poor behavioral control (Hare, 1970). General dysregulation of affect has been noted in both groups (Scarpa & Raine, 1997; Zlotnick, 1999; Damasio & Anderson, in press). Similar psychophysiological abnormalities, including diminished autonomic responsiveness (especially to social stimuli), have been noted in both VMPF patients with acquired sociopathy (Damasio et al., 1990; Tranel, 1994) and developmental psychopaths (Hare et al., 1970; Schmauk, 1970; Raine et al., 2000). Finally, some developmental psychopaths manifest decision-making deficits on the Gambling Task that are reminiscent of those we have reported in VMPF patients (Schmitt et al., 1999; Mazas et al., 2000).

These parallels between developmental and acquired sociopathy raise the question as to whether the two conditions have a common pathological mechanism, namely, VMPF dysfunction. This hypothesis has received support from studies showing that developmental psychopaths may have anatomical (Raine et al., 2000), physiological (Deckel et al., 1996; Kuruoglu et al., 1996), and metabolic (Raine et al., 1998) abnormalities in prefrontal cortices. Further support comes from recent investigations demonstrating that early damage to prefrontal regions can produce a lifelong pattern of social conduct and decision-making impairments. The discussion turns now to a consideration of these investigations.

IMPAIRMENT OF SOCIAL AND MORAL BEHAVIOR FOLLOWING EARLY DAMAGE TO PREFRONTAL CORTEX

We recently had the opportunity to study two individuals who sustained damage to prefrontal cortices very early in life, specifically, prior to 16 months of age (Anderson et al., 1999; 2000). The patients were studied when they were in early adulthood, using a variety of neuropsychological, neuroanatomical, and psychophysiological techniques. Both patients were raised in stable, middle-class homes by college-educated parents, neither had any siblings with behavior problems, and neither had a family history of psychiatric disease or risk factors for behavioral disturbance other than their brain injury. Thus, direct adverse genetic or environmental contributions to the patients' behavioral problems can be largely ruled out. Against this background, both patients developed profound disturbances of social conduct and moral reasoning, which appear to be attributable to their early prefrontal injuries.

Patient 1 was normal until age 15 months, when her head was run over by the wheel of a truck. She sustained a nondepressed left parietal skull fracture, but made a rapid and apparently complete medical recovery within days of the accident. At 2 months post-injury,

she was pronounced neurologically and behaviorally normal. Around 3 years of age, however, the girl's mother noticed that she seemed largely unaffected by verbal and physical punishment. After she entered school, her teachers noted difficulty in controlling her behavior. She was able to obtain average grades, though, up until about 6th grade, when her behavior problems began to intensify. She ran away from home, shoplifted, lied, and cheated. At age 14, her school behavior became so disruptive that she was placed in the first of a series of treatment facilities. She had been placed in six different treatment facilities by age 16; typically, she was discharged for repeatedly running away, rule violations, and failure to progress toward treatment goals. She was sexually active by age 14, and became pregnant at age 18. Her maternal behavior was marked by nearly complete insensitivity to her baby's needs. She appeared to experience little empathy.

The patient continued to put herself at physical and financial risk, and eventually became entirely dependent on her parents and social agencies for financial support and oversight of her personal affairs. She did not seek employment, and did not formulate plans for the future. When employment was arranged, she could not hold the job secondary to unreliable work attendance, lack of dependability, and gross infractions of rules. Superficially, her social behavior was fairly normal, but she displayed labile affect and emotional responses that were often poorly matched to the situation. She showed complete unconcern for her behavioral transgressions, and never expressed guilt or remorse. Her conduct problems were never significantly improved by any of the various treatments to which she was exposed, including behavior management programs and pharmacological interventions.

Patient 2 was normal until age 3 months, when he was diagnosed with a right frontal tumor. The tumor was resected, and he made an excellent physical recovery; there has been no sign of tumor recurrence. When he began school, teachers noted that he had difficulty adjusting to new situations and interacting with other students, and needed frequent reminders to stay on task. By 4th grade, special education was recommended because of his poor work habits (poor attention, impulsive responses, not turning in assignments), but he did not qualify because of normal performances on standardized tests of academic achievement. He was disruptive in class and often failed to turn in assignments on time, but he managed to complete high school with only one grade repetition (12th), and he obtained average to high average scores when tested with conventional IQ and academic achievement tests.

His behavior during childhood was notable for impulsiveness and poor judgment. Personal hygiene was poor. After graduating from high school, his behavior deteriorated even further. He quit or was fired from multiple jobs. If left to his own devices, he would spend all day watching TV and listening to music. He could not manage his money; he repeatedly bought items on credit and did not make the payments, and he engaged in petty thievery. He lied frequently, had no lasting friendships, and displayed little empathy. He evinced irresponsible sexual behavior, fathering a child in a casual relationship and failing to fulfill his paternal obligations. He showed no guilt or remorse for his behavior, and could not formulate any realistic plans for the future. His parents described him as showing little worry, guilt, empathy, remorse, or fear. Failure to consider the future consequences of his actions was a prominent and constant feature of his everyday behavior.

Neither of the two patients had any neurological abnormality. The patients were studied with a magnetic resonance imaging (MRI) protocol that permitted reconstruction of their brains in three dimensions, and this revealed that both had focal damage to prefrontal regions, and no evidence of damage in other brain areas. The lesion in patient 1 was bilateral and involved the polar and ventromedial prefrontal sectors. The lesion in patient 2 was unilateral, and involved right prefrontal cortices, in mesial, polar, and lateral sectors. The lateral half of the orbital gyri and the anterior sector of the cingulate gyrus were damaged. The lesions of the two cases are depicted in Figure 22–5.

On neuropsychological testing, both pa-

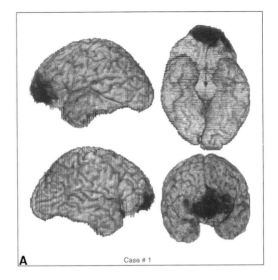

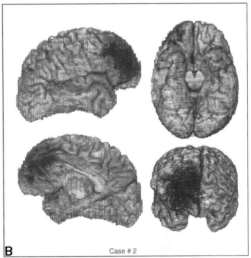

Figure 22–5. Neuroanatomical analysis of two patients with early-onset prefrontal lesions. *A:* Case 1 has a bilateral lesion in the prefrontal region, involving the anterior orbital sector, and the right mesial orbital sector and the left polar cortices. *B* Case 2 has extensive damage in the right frontal lobe, encompassing prefrontal cortices in mesial, polar, and lateral sectors. (*Source:* Modified from Anderson et al., 1999, with permission)

tients obtained average IQ scores on the Weschler Adult Intelligence Scale–Revised, and both demonstrated normal anterograde and retrograde memory, speech and language, visuoperceptual and visuospatial functioning, and visuomotor skills. On tasks of attention and working memory, both patients demonstrated mild, inconsistent deficits (which did not appear to interfere with their daily functioning). The patients showed variable performances on conventional "executive function" tests: both performed defectively on the Tower of Hanoi and Design Fluency tests, and one patient had a high number of perseverative errors on the Wisconsin Card Sorting Test (WCST). However, both patients were able to achieve all six category sorts on the WCST, and both performed normally on the Trail-making Test, the Controlled Oral Word Association Test, and the Stroop Task. Both patients had normal academic achievement performances.

The patients were administered a series of standardized procedures to assess social knowledge and moral reasoning: Standard Issue Moral Judgment (SIMJ), the Optional Thinking Test (OTT), the Awareness of Consequences Test (ACT), and the Means-Ends Problem Solving Procedure (MEPS). These procedures involve verbal presentation to the subject of moral dilemmas or social situations, and require verbal responses. In the SIMJ task, the subject is presented a conflict between two moral imperatives (a man must steal a drug in order to save his wife's life). The subject is asked to describe the protagonist's proper actions and their rationale. The OTT measures the ability to generate alternative solutions to hypothetical social dilemmas (e.g., two people disagree on what TV channel to watch). In the ACT, the subject is presented hypothetical predicaments involving temptation to transgress ordinary social conventions (e.g., receiving too much money in a business transaction), and is asked to describe how one should respond to the situation. The MEPS measures the subject's ability to conceptualize effective means of achieving social goals (e.g., how to meet people after moving to a new neighborhood).

On the SIMJ task, the two patients demonstrated moral reasoning that was conducted at a very early developmental stage—the "preconventional" stage, in Colby and Kohlberg's (1987) terms—where moral dilemmas are approached largely from the egocentric perspective of avoiding immediate punishment. This stage is characteristic of most children under the age of 9. On the other moral reasoning tasks, the patients' responses were character-

ized by limited consideration of the social and emotional implications of decisions, failure to identify the primary issues involved in social dilemmas, and very limited generation of response options for interpersonal conflicts.

The two patients also participated in the Gambling Task (as described earlier). The results were very similar to those from adult-onset VMPF patients: the two early-onset patients failed to develop a preference for the advantageous decks over the course of the Gambling Task, and continued to select more frequently from the risky decks that pay a higher reward up front but have higher long-term losses. Also similar to adult VMPF patients, the two early-onset patients failed to generate anticipatory psychophysiological responses to the risky decks. In sum, the early-onset patients demonstrated abnormal decision making and abnormal somatic marker activation during the Gambling Task.

There are two important comparisons to make in regard to these early-onset patients. The first is in relationship to adult-onset patients with VMPF lesions. There are a number of strong parallels: a shared locus of anatomical dysfunction (VMPF cortices), the development of social conduct disturbances, behavioral and emotional dysregulation, impaired decision making as indexed by defective performance on the Gambling Task, impaired psychophysiological responses in anticipation of punishment, and a lack of primary intellectual or other cognitive defects that could account for the deficits observed in the social/emotional realm. The early-onset patients, however, also show a number of distinctive features. First, their inadequate social behavior was present throughout development and into adulthood, unlike the adult-onset patients, whose behavior prior to the onset of VMPF damage was normal. Second, the social conduct disturbances in the early-onset patients seem to be more severe than those in the adult-onset patients. Adult-onset patients rarely show the sort of blatant antisocial behavior noted in the early-onset patients, e.g., stealing and violence against persons and property. Third, the early-onset patients were not able to retrieve complex social knowledge at a factual level, as shown by their failures on the moral reasoning tasks. This outcome stands in contrast with the adult-onset patients, who were remarkably competent on these verbal, off-line procedures, even though they failed to deploy such knowledge appropriately in real-world situations (Saver & Damasio, 1991; Anderson et al., 1999). These comparisons suggest that the integrity of VMPF structures is critical for the acquisition of social and moral knowledge in the first place, and that early damage to such structures blocks such acquisition. This conclusion has been hinted at in other investigations of patient populations with putative early-onset damage to VMPF structures (see Tranel & Eslinger, 2000).

The second important point of comparison is with developmental psychopaths. There are a number of striking similarities between the patients with early-onset VMPF damage and developmental psychopaths (or the conditions subsumed by the labels "Conduct Disorder" or "Antisocial Personality Disorder" in DSM-IV nosology). In the early-onset VMPF patients and in developmental psychopaths, there is a pervasive disregard for social and moral standards, consistent irresponsibility, lack of remorse and empathy, and a lack of concern for future consequences. Both types of patients evidence a lifelong pattern of social conduct disturbance. Also, it has been noted that children with antisocial tendencies have deficiencies of moral reasoning akin to those detected in our early-onset cases (Campagna & Harter, 1975; Blair, 1997). One difference we have noted is that unlike developmental psychopaths, the early-onset VMPF patients' patterns of aggression seem impulsive rather than goal directed, and have a highly transparent, almost child-like nature.

In sum, the findings from these early-onset VMPF cases suggest that antisocial behavior may depend in part on the abnormal operation of a multicomponent neural system which includes sectors of the prefrontal cortex. The causes of such abnormal operation would range from primarily biological (e.g., genetic, acting at molecular/cellular levels) to primarily environmental. In our cases, the abnormality can be traced to early damage to critical neural sectors. Moreover, the findings suggest that

defective social conduct and moral reasoning can develop independently of social and psychological factors (which did not appear to play a role in our patients). The findings also have implications in regard to issues of neural plasticity and recovery of function, suggesting that in the case of social and emotional development supported by VMPF brain sectors, it may be difficult or impossible to overcome early damage to the relevant neural structures (Eslinger et al., 1997; Taylor & Alden, 1997; Benton & Tranel, 2000).

THE SOMATIC MARKER HYPOTHESIS

The background for the somatic marker hypothesis comes from the observation that patients with VMPF damage develop profound impairments in real-life decision making, especially in situations involving ambiguity, response conflict, and social contingencies. A hallmark feature of many such situations is an inherent conflict between reward and punishment—for example, choosing a course of action that leads to an unpredictable blend of short-term reward and long-term punishment, or vice versa. Examples of such uncertainties abound in everyday life: a new acquaintance who seems wonderful at first meeting may turn out to be an ogre in the long run; going short on sleep to finish an overdue assignment may be onerous at the moment, but highly rewarding later on; having a third martini may be very appealing at 10 P.M. when one is celebrating with friends, but may have unwanted consequences the next morning; passing up the urge to cash in on an upward spike in the stock market may pay major dividends later on. It is situations like these that are especially derailing for patients with VMPF lesions—the patients repeatedly engage in courses of action that are detrimental to their best long-term interests.

This behavior is all the more puzzling when juxtaposed against the fact that these patients are usually capable of performing normally on all manner of conventional neuropsychological procedures. They do not manifest defects in conventional intellectual functions, working memory, or attention or concentration. They often perform normally on many so-called frontal lobe tests, such as the Wisconsin Card Sorting Test and Tower of Hanoi, which place demands on abstract thinking and flexible responding (see Tranel et al., 1994, for review). Moreover, as noted earlier, they even perform normally on tasks directly aimed at retrieval and application of knowledge pertaining to social conventions and moral reasoning, provided those tasks are administered in verbal format and "off-line,"—i.e., in a structured laboratory setting (Saver & Damasio, 1991; Anderson et al., 1999).

What VMPF-damaged patients do manifest is a profound inability to express emotion and to experience feeling relative to complex personal and social situations, for example, the expression and experience of embarrassment or guilt. Given that the blatant changes in social conduct and decision making that typify these patients cannot be explained by basic impairments of intellect, memory, language, attention, or working memory, we proposed that deficits in bioregulatory responses might provide a plausible explanation (Damasio et al., 1990, 1991; Damasio, 1994; 1995; 1996). In essence, the *somatic marker hypothesis* outlines the following principles:

1. Certain structures in prefrontal cortex are necessary for learning associations between various classes of complex stimuli and various internal states of the organism (such as emotions) usually experienced in connection with those classes of stimuli. The internal states are represented in the brain as transient changes in activity patterns in somatosensory maps in a large collection of structures, from the cerebral cortex to the hypothalamus and brain stem. The term *somatic* is used to denote these states, although it should be noted that *somatic* is meant to refer to all components of the soma, including the musculoskeletal and visceral, and the internal milieu.

2. When a situation from a particular class of complex stimuli recurs during one's ongoing experience, systems in the VMPF region, which previously recorded an association between that type of situation and certain types of somatic states, trigger the reactivation of the somatosensory pattern that depicts the appropriate somatic state. This can be achieved

via either of two routes: *(1)* "body" loop, in which the soma actually changes in response to the activation, with signals of those changes being relayed back to somatosensory maps; or *(2)* an "as-if-body" loop, in which reactivation signals are relayed directly to somatosensory maps, bypassing the body to prompt the appropriate pattern of activation in the somatosensory structures. Both of these mechanisms—the body loop and the as-if-body loop—can operate overtly (consciously) or covertly (nonconsciously).

3. Reactivation of the somatosensory pattern appropriate to a given situation, along with concurrent recall of factual knowledge pertinent to the situation, operates to constrain the reasoning and decision-making space, by qualifying alternatives. When the somatosensory pattern image is juxtaposed to the images that prompted the somatic state as well as to images that depict potential outcomes, the somatosensory pattern *marks* potential outcomes as good or bad. Covertly, the somatic marker provides a nonconscious biasing signal that facilitates appetitive or avoidance behavior. Overtly, the somatic marker process functions as an incentive or deterrent.

4. Somatosensory activity patterns also facilitate attention and working memory, providing an indirect influence on the decision-making process.

5. Logical reasoning is facilitated by steps 3 and 4. The VMPF cortices hold dispositional records (convergence zones; see Damasio, 1989) of temporal conjunctions of activity in various neural units (e.g., sensory cortices, limbic structures), arriving from both external and internal stimuli. The records hold signals from neural regions which were simultaneously active and which, as a set, defined certain situations. One of the key outputs of VMPF convergence zones is to autonomic effectors. When aspects of a particular exteroceptive–interoceptive conjunction are reprocessed, nonconsciously and/or consciously, activation is signaled to VMPF cortices. Those cortices then activate somatic effectors in structures such as the amygdala, hypothalamus, and brain stem. Essentially, there is an attempt to reconstruct the kind of somatic state that was part of the original conjunction.

Then, the reconstituted somatic state is signaled to cortical and subcortical somatosensory structures, triggering either a covert process that can prompt appetitive or aversive behavior, or conscious perception in the form of a *feeling*.

In this framework, emotion is considered to be a crucial component of the process of reasoning and decision making. Typically, situations involving personal and social matters are associated intimately with reward and punishment, with pleasure and pain—in short, with the regulation of homeostatic states as expressed by emotions and feelings. Assuming that the brain has a mechanism for selecting good responses from bad ones in social situations, the framework suggests that such a mechanism was co-opted for behavioral guidance. In sum, somatic markers, regardless of whether they are perceived consciously in the form of feelings, provide critical signals needed in many situations of reasoning and decision making, and especially those that occur in a social context.

It is important to note that there are other interesting views on the manner in which ventral prefrontal cortices subserve functions such as motivation and emotion. Rolls and colleagues, for example, have emphasized the idea that the orbitofrontal region contains representations of primary reinforcers from several sensory modalities (touch, taste, smell), helping to shape learning of reward and punishment contingencies (Francis et al., 1999). Specifically, Rolls (2000) has argued that the orbitofrontal cortex is crucial for learning associations between various stimuli and these primary reinforcers, and especially for controlling and modifying reward-related and punishment-related behavior in response to such associations. Many of these ideas are compatible with the somatic marker framework outlined earlier, although Rolls' position lacks the emphasis on the body-proper as a major component of emotion-related processing (Rolls, 1999). Another formulation, termed the *inhibition hypothesis*, has been advanced by Sahakian, Robbins, and colleagues (Rahman et al., 1999; Rogers et al., 1999). This hypothesis focuses on the inability of patients with VMPF dysfunction to suppress responses evoked by the immediate environment, and the reasons for the behavior of such patients being dominated by the immediate emotional impact of the stimulus at hand. Finally, there are some fascinating neurophysiology studies by Watanabe and colleagues that have shown that neurons in orbitofrontal cortex are especially concerned with motivational aspects of response outcome expectancies (Watanabe, 1998; Hikosaka & Watanabe, 2000). As Watanabe has noted, this idea is very compatible with our notion that VMPF cortices are intimately involved in the integration of cognitive and motivational information for the purposes of goal-directed behavior.

CONCLUSIONS

The investigations reviewed here suggest that too little emotion has profoundly deleterious effects on decision making; in fact, too little emotion may be just as bad for decision making as excessive emotion has long been considered to be. We have interpreted these findings as indicating that individuals utilize bioregulatory responses, including emotions and feelings, to guide decision making in many important ways, both consciously and nonconsciously. A critical component of the neural machinery subserving these processes includes the ventromedial prefrontal region.

ACKNOWLEDGMENTS

The research reported in this chapter was supported in part by Program Project Grant NINDS NS19632. I thank Drs. Donald Stuss, Robert Knight, and Natalie Denburg for helpful comments on earlier versions of the manuscript, and Dr. Ralph Adolphs for generous assistance with the figures.

REFERENCES

American Psychiatric Association (1994). *Diagnostic and Statistical Manual of Mental Disorders*, 4th ed. Washington, DC: American Psychiatric Association.

Anderson, S.W., Bechara, A., Damasio, H., Tranel, D., & Damasio, A.R. (1999). Impairment of social and moral behavior related to early damage in the human prefrontal cortex. *Nature Neuroscience*, 2, 1032–1037.

Anderson, S.W., Damasio, H., Tranel, D., & Damasio, A.R. (2000). Long-term sequelae of prefrontal cortex damage acquired in early childhood. *Developmental Neuropsychology*, 18, 281–296.

Barrash, J., Tranel, D., & Anderson, S.W. (1994). Assessment of dramatic personality changes after ventromedial frontal lesions. *Journal of Clinical and Experimental Neuropsychology, 16,* 66.

Barrash, J., Tranel, D., & Anderson, S.W. 2000. Acquired personality disturbances associated with bilateral damage to the ventromedial prefrontal region. *Developmental Neuropsychology* 18, 355–381.

Bechara, A., Damasio, A.R., Damasio, H., & Anderson, S.W. (1994). Insensitivity to future consequences following damage to human prefrontal cortex. *Cognition, 50,* 7–15.

Bechara, A., Tranel, D., Damasio, H., & Damasio, A.R. (1996). Failure to respond autonomically to anticipated future outcomes following damage to prefrontal cortex. *Cerebral Cortex, 6,* 215–225.

Bechara, A., Damasio, H., Tranel, D., & Damasio, A.R. (1997). Deciding advantageously before knowing the advantageous strategy. *Science, 275,* 1293–1295.

Bechara, A., Tranel, D., & Damasio, H. (2000). Characterization of the decision-making deficit of patients with ventromedial prefrontal cortex lesions. *Brain, 123,* 2189–2202.

Benton, A., & Tranel, D. (2000). Historical notes on reorganization of function and neuroplasticity. In: H.S. Levin & J. Grafman (Eds.), *Cerebral Reorganization of Function after Brain Damage,* (pp. 3–23). New York: Oxford University Press.

Blair, R.J.R. (1997). Moral reasoning and the child with psychopathic tendencies. *Personality and Individual Differences, 22,* 731–739.

Blumer, D. & Benson, D.F. (1975). Personality changes with frontal and temporal lobe lesions. In: D.F. Benson, & D. Blumer (Eds.), *Psychiatric Aspects of Neurologic Disease* (pp. 151–169). New York: Grune & Stratton.

Campagna, A.F. & Harter, S. (1975). Moral judgment in sociopathic and normal children. *Journal of Personality and Social Psychology, 31,* 199–205.

Colby, A. & Kohlberg, L. (1987). *The Measurement of Moral Judgment.* New York: Cambridge University Press.

Damasio, A.R. (1989). Time-locked multiregional retroactivation: a systems-level proposal for the neural substrates of recall and recognition. *Cognition, 33,* 25–62.

Damasio, A.R. (1994). *Descartes' Error: Emotion, Reason and the Human Brain.* New York: Grosset/Putnam.

Damasio, A.R. (1995). Toward a neurobiology of emotion and feeling: operational concepts and hypotheses. *Neuroscientist, 1,* 19–25.

Damasio, A.R. (1996). The somatic marker hypothesis and the possible functions of the prefrontal cortex. *Philosophical Transactions of the Royal Society of London B, 351,* 1413–1420.

Damasio, A.R. (1999). *The Feeling of What Happens.* New York: Harcourt Brace.

Damasio, A.R., & Anderson, S.W. (in press). The frontal lobes. In: K., Heilman, & E. Valenstein (Eds.), *Clinical Neuropsychology* 4th ed., (pp. –). New York: Oxford University Press.

Damasio, A.R., Tranel, D., & Damasio, H. (1990). Individuals with sociopathic behavior caused by frontal damage fail to respond autonomically to social stimuli. *Behavioural Brain Research, 41,* 81–94.

Damasio, A.R., Tranel, D., & Damasio, H. (1991). Somatic markers and the guidance of behavior: theory and preliminary testing. In: H.S. Levin, H.M., Eisenberg, & A.L. Benton, (Eds.), *Frontal Lobe Function and Dysfunction* (pp. 217–229). New York: Oxford University Press.

Damasio, H., Grabowski, T., Frank, R., Galaburda, A.M., & Damasio, A.R. (1994). The return of Phineas Gage: clues about the brain from the skull of a famous patient. *Science, 264,* 1102–1105.

Deckel, A.W., Hesselbrock, V., & Bauer, L. (1996). Antisocial personality disorder, childhood delinquency, and frontal brain functioning: EEG and neuropsychological findings. *Journal of Clinical Psychology, 52,* 639–650.

Eslinger, P.J., & Damasio, A.R. (1985). Severe disturbance of higher cognition after bilateral frontal lobe ablation: patient EVR. *Neurology, 35,* 1731–1741.

Eslinger, P.J., Biddle, K.R., & Grattan, L.M. (1997). Cognitive and social development in children with prefrontal cortex lesions. In: N.A. Krasnegor, G.R. Lyon, & P.S. Goldman-Rakic (Eds.), *Development of Prefrontal Cortex: Evolution, Neurobiology and Behavior* (pp. 295–335). Baltimore: Brookes.

Francis, S., Rolls, E.T., Bowtell, R., McGlone, F., O'Doherty, J., Browning, A., Clare, S., & Smith, E. (1999). The representation of pleasant touch in the brain and its relationship with taste and olfactory areas. *Neuroreport, 10,* 453–459.

Gainotti, G. (1993). Emotional and psychosocial problems after brain injury. *Neuropsychological Rehabilitation, 3,* 259–277.

Hare, R.D. (1970). *Psychopathy: Theory and Research.* New York: John Wiley and Sons.

Hare, R.D., Wood, K., Britain, S., & Shadman, J. (1970). Autonomic responses to affective visual stimuli. *Psychophysiology, 7,* 408–417.

Harlow, J.M. (1848). Passage of an iron rod through the head. *Boston Medical and Surgical Journal, 39,* 389–393.

Harlow, J.M. (1868). Recovery from the passage of an iron bar through the head. *Publications of the Massachusetts Medical Society, 2,* 327–347.

Hikosaka, K. & Watanabe, M. (2000). Delay activity of orbital and lateral prefrontal neurons in the monkey varying with different rewards. *Cerebral Cortex, 10,* 263–271.

Kuruoglu, A.C., Arikan, Z., Vural, G., Karatas, M., Arac, M., & Isik, E. (1996). Single photon emission computerised tomography in chronic alcoholism. *British Journal of Psychiatry, 169,* 348–354.

Lewicki, P., Hill, T., & Czyzewska, M. (1992). Nonconscious acquisition of information. *American Psychologist, 47,* 796–801.

Macmillan, M. (2000). *An Odd Kind of Fame: Stories of Phineas Gage.* Cambridge, MA: MIT Press.

Mazas, C.A., Finn, P.R., & Steinmetz, J.E. (2000).

Decision-making biases, antisocial personality, and early-onset alcoholism. *Alcohol Clinical and Experimental Research, 24*, 1036–1040.

Mealey, L. (1995). The sociobiology of sociopathy: an integrated evolutionary model. *Behavioral Brain Sciences, 18*, 523–599.

Rahman, S., Sahakian, B.J., Hodges, J.R., Rogers, R.D., & Robbins, T.W. (1999). Specific cognitive deficits in mild frontal variant frontotemporal dementia. *Brain, 122*, 1469–1493.

Raine, A., Stoddard, J., Bihrle, S., & Buchsbaum, M. (1998). Prefrontal glucose deficits in murderers lacking psychosocial deprivation. *Neuropsychiatry, Neuropsychology and Behavioral Neurology, 11*, 1–7.

Raine, A., Lencz, T., Bihrle, S., LaCasse, L., & Colletti, P. (2000). Reduced prefrontal gray matter volume and reduced autonomic activity in antisocial personality disorder. *Archives of General Psychiatry, 57*, 119–127.

Rogers, R.D., Everitt, B.J., Baldacchino, A., Blackshaw, A.J., Swainson, R., Wynne, K., Baker, N.B., Hunter, J., Carthy, T., Booker, E., London, M., Deakin, J.F.W., Sahakian, B.J., & Robbins, T.W. (1999). Dissociable deficits in the decision-making cognition of chronic amphetamine abusers, opiate abusers, patients with focal damage to prefrontal cortex, and tryptophan-depleted normal volunteers: evidence for monoaminergic mechanisms. *Neuropsychopharmacology, 20*, 322–339.

Rolls, E.T. (1999). *The Brain and Emotion*. New York: Oxford University Press.

Rolls, E.T. (2000). The orbitofrontal cortex and reward. *Cerebral Cortex, 10*, 284–294.

Saver, J. & Damasio, A.R. (1991). Preserved access and processing of social knowledge in a patient with acquired sociopathy due to ventromedial frontal damage. *Neuropsychologia, 29*, 1241–1249.

Scarpa, A. & Raine, A. (1997). Psychophysiology of anger and violent behavior. *Psychiatric Clinics of North America, 20*, 375–394.

Schmauk, F.J. (1970). Punishment, arousal and avoidance learning in sociopaths. *Journal of Abnormal Psychology, 76*, 325–335.

Schmitt, W.A., Brinkley, C.A., & Newman, J.P. (1999). Testing Damasio's somatic marker hypothesis with psychopathic individuals: risk takers or risk averse? *Journal of Abnormal Psychology, 108*, 538–543.

Shiller, R.J. (2000). *Irrational Exuberance*. Princeton, NJ: Princeton University Press.

Siegler, R.S. (2000). Unconscious insights. *Current Directions in Psychological Science, 9*, 79–83.

Stuss, D.T. & Benson, D.F. (1986). *The Frontal Lobes*. New York: Raven Press.

Sutker, P.B. (1994). Psychopathy: traditional and clinical antisocial concepts. In: D.C. Fowles, P. Sutker, & S.H. Goodman (Eds.), *Progress in Experimental Personality and Psychopathology Research*, Vol. 17 (pp. 73–120). New York: Springer-Verlag.

Tate, R.L. (1999). Executive dysfunction and characterological changes after traumatic brain injury: two sides of the same coin? *Cortex, 35*, 39–55.

Taylor, H.B. & Alden, J. (1997). Age-related differences in outcomes following childhood brain insults. *Journal of the International Neuropsychological Society, 3*, 555–567.

Tranel, D. (1994). "Acquired sociopathy": the development of sociopathic behavior following focal brain damage. In: D.C. Fowles, P. Sutker, & S.H. Goodman (Eds.), *Progress in Experimental Personality and Psychopathology Research*, Vol. 17, (pp. 285–311). New York: Springer-Verlag.

Tranel, D. (in press). Neural correlates of violent behavior. In: J. Bogousslavsky, & J. Cummings, (Eds.), *Behavior and Mood Disorders in Focal Brain Lesions*. Cambridge, UK: Cambridge University Press.

Tranel, D., Anderson, S.W., & Benton, A.L. (1994). Development of the concept of "executive function" and its relationship to the frontal lobes. In: F. Boller & J. Grafman (Eds.), *Handbook of neuropsychology*, Vol. 9 (pp. 125–148). Amsterdam: Elsevier.

Tranel, D., Bechara, A., & Damasio, A.R. (2000). Decision making and the somatic marker hypothesis. In: M.S. Gazzaniga (Ed.), *The New Cognitive Neurosciences*, (pp. 1047–1061). Cambridge, MA: MIT Press.

Tranel, D. & Eslinger, P.J. 2000. Effects of early onset brain injury on the development of cognition and behavior. *Developmental Neuropsychology, 18*, 273–280.

Watanabe, M. (1998). Cognitive and motivational operations in primate prefrontal neurons. *Reviews in the Neurosciences, 9*, 225–241.

Zlotnick, C. (1999). Antisocial personality disorder, affect dysregulation and childhood abuse among incarcerated women. *Journal of Personality Disorders, 13*, 90–95.

23

The Functions of the Orbitofrontal Cortex

EDMUND T. ROLLS

The prefrontal cortex is the cortex that receives projections from the mediodorsal nucleus of the thalamus and is situated in front of the motor and premotor cortices (areas 4 and 6) in the frontal lobe. On the basis of divisions of the mediodorsal nucleus, the prefrontal cortex may be divided into three main regions (Fuster, 1997). First, the magnocellular, medial, part of the mediodorsal nucleus projects to the orbital (ventral) surface of the prefrontal cortex (which includes areas 13 and 12). It is called the *orbitofrontal cortex*, and receives information from the ventral or object-processing visual stream, and taste, olfactory, and somatosensory inputs. Second, the parvocellular, lateral, part of the mediodorsal nucleus projects to the dorsolateral prefrontal cortex. This part of the prefrontal cortex receives inputs from the parietal cortex, and is involved in tasks such as spatial short-term memory tasks (Fuster, 1997; see Rolls & Treves, 1998). Third, the pars paralamellaris (most lateral) part of the mediodorsal nucleus projects to the frontal eye fields (area 8) in the anterior bank of the arcuate sulcus.

The functions of the orbitofrontal cortex are considered in this chapter. The cortex on the orbital surface of the frontal lobe includes area 13 caudally and area 14 medially, and the cortex on the inferior convexity includes area 12 caudally and area 11 anteriorly (see Fig. 23–1 and Carmichael & Price, 1994; Petrides & Pandya, 1994; Ongur and Price, 2000). This brain region is relatively poorly developed in rodents, but well developed in primates, including humans. Thus to understand the function of this brain region in humans, most of the studies described here were performed with macaques or with humans.

CONNECTIONS

Rolls et al. (1990) discovered a taste area in the lateral part of the orbitofrontal cortex and showed that this was the secondary taste cortex in that it receives a major projection from the primary taste cortex (Baylis et al., 1994). More medially, there is an olfactory area (Rolls & Baylis, 1994). Anatomically, there are direct connections from the primary olfactory cortex, pyriform cortex, to area 13a of the posterior orbitofrontal cortex, which in turn has onward projections to a middle part of the orbitofrontal cortex (area 11) (Price et al., 1991; Morecraft et al., 1992; Barbas, 1993; Carmichael et al., 1994; see Figs. 23–1 and

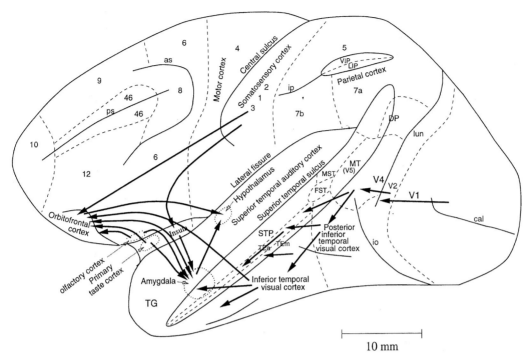

Figure 23–1. Schematic diagram showing some of the gustatory, olfactory, visual, and somatosensory pathways to the orbitofrontal cortex, and some of the outputs of the orbitofrontal cortex. The secondary taste cortex and the secondary olfactory cortex are within the orbitofrontal cortex. V1, primary visual cortex; V4, visual cortical area V4. Abbreviations: A, amygdala; as, arcuate sulcus; cc, corpus callosum; cf, calcarine fissure; cgs, cingulate sulcus; cs, central sulcus; INS, insula; io, inferior occipital sulcus; lf, lateral (or Sylvian) fissure (which has been opened to reveal the insula); lun, lunate sulcus; mos, medial orbital sulcus; os, orbital sulcus; ots, occipitotemporal sulcus; ps, principal sulcus; rhs, rhinal sulcus; sts, superior temporal sulcus; T, thalamus; TE (21), inferior temporal visual cortex; TA (22), superior temporal auditory association cortex; TF and TH, parahippocampal cortex; TG, temporal pole cortex; 12, 13, 11, orbitofrontal cortex; 35, perirhinal cortex; 51, olfactory (prepyriform and periamygdaloid) cortex.

23–2). Visual inputs reach the orbitofrontal cortex directly from the inferior temporal cortex, the cortex in the superior temporal sulcus, and the temporal pole (see Barbas, 1988, 1993; Barbas & Pandya, 1989; Seltzer & Pandya, 1989; Morecraft, et al., 1992; Barbas, 1995; Carmichael & Price, 1995). There are corresponding auditory (Barbas, 1988, 1993) and somatosensory inputs from somatosensory cortical areas 1, 2, and SII in the frontal and pericentral operculum, and from the insula (Barbas, 1988; Carmichael & Price, 1995). The caudal orbitofrontal cortex receives strong inputs from the amygdala (e.g., Price et al., 1991). The orbitofrontal cortex also receives inputs via the mediodorsal nucleus of the thalamus, pars magnocellularis,

which itself receives afferents from temporal lobe structures such as the prepyriform (olfactory) cortex, amygdala and inferior temporal cortex (see Ongur & Price, 2000). The orbitofrontal cortex projects back to temporal lobe areas such as the inferior temporal cortex and, in addition, to the entorhinal cortex (or "gateway to the hippocampus") and cingulate cortex (Insausti et al., 1987). The orbitofrontal cortex also projects to the preoptic region and lateral hypothalamus, to the ventral tegmental area (Nauta, 1964; Johnson et al., 1968), and to the head of the caudate nucleus (Kemp & Powell, 1970). Reviews of the cytoarchitecture and connections of the orbitofrontal cortex are provided by Petrides and Pandya (1994), Pandya and Yeterian

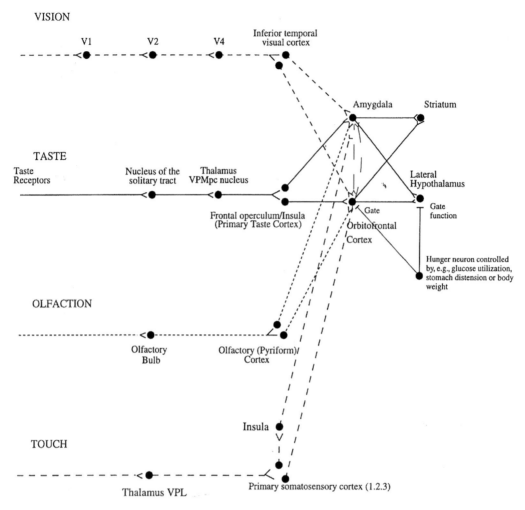

Figure 23–2. Schematic diagram showing some of the gustatory, olfactory, visual, and somatosensory pathways to the orbitofrontal cortex, and some of the outputs of the orbitofrontal cortex. The secondary taste cortex, and the secondary olfactory cortex are within the orbitofrontal cortex. V1, primary visual cortex; V2 and V4 visual cortical areas.

(1996), Carmichael and Price (1994, 1995), Barbas (1995), and Ongur and Price (2000).

EFFECTS OF LESIONS OF THE ORBITOFRONTAL CORTEX

Macaques with lesions of the orbitofrontal cortex are impaired at tasks that involve learning about which stimuli are rewarding and which ones are not, and especially in altering behavior when reinforcement contingencies change. The monkeys may respond when responses are inappropriate, e.g., are no longer

rewarded, or may respond to a non-rewarded stimulus. For example, monkeys with orbitofrontal damage are impaired on Go/No-Go task performance, in that they go on the No-Go trials (Iversen & Mishkin, 1970); in an object reversal task, as they respond to the object that was formerly rewarded with food; and in extinction as they continue to respond to an object that is no longer rewarded (Butter, 1969; Jones & Mishkin, 1972). There is some evidence for dissociation of function within the orbitofrontal cortex, in that lesions to the inferior convexity produce the Go/No-Go and object-reversal deficits, whereas damage to the caudal orbitofrontal cortex, area 13, produces the extinction deficit (Rosenkilde, 1979).

Lesions more laterally in, for example the inferior convexity, can influence performance on tasks in which objects must be remembered for short periods, e.g., delayed matching-to-sample and delayed matching-to-nonsample tasks (Passingham, 1975; Mishkin & Manning, 1978; Kowalska et al., 1991), and neurons in this region may help to implement this visual object short-term memory by holding the representation active during the delay period (Rosenkilde et al., 1981; Wilson et al., 1993; Rao et al., 1997). Whether this inferior convexity area is specifically involved in a short-term object memory (separately from a short-term spatial memory) is not yet clear (Rao et al., 1997), and a medial part of the frontal cortex may also contribute to this function (Kowalska et al., 1991). It should be noted that this short-term memory system for objects (which receives inputs from the temporal lobe visual cortical areas in which objects are represented) is different from the short-term memory system in the dorsolateral part of the prefrontal cortex, which is concerned with spatial short term memories, consistent with its inputs from the parietal cortex (see, e.g., Rolls & Treves, 1998).

Damage to the caudal orbitofrontal cortex in the monkey also produces emotional changes (e.g., decreased aggression toward humans and toward stimuli such as a snake and a doll), and a reduced tendency to reject foods such as meat (Butter et al., 1969, 1970; Butter & Snyder, 1972) or to display the normal preference ranking for different foods (Baylis & Gaffan, 1991). In humans, euphoria, irresponsibility, and lack of affect can follow frontal lobe damage (see Damasio, 1994; Kolb & Whishaw, 1996; Rolls, 1999), particularly orbitofrontal damage (Rolls et al., 1994; Hornak et al., 1996).

NEUROPHYSIOLOGY OF THE ORBITOFRONTAL CORTEX

TASTE

One of the recent discoveries that has helped us to understand the functions of the orbito-frontal cortex in behavior is that it contains a major cortical representation of taste (see Rolls, 1989, 1995b, 1997b; Rolls & Scott, 2001; Fig. 23–2). Given that taste can act as a primary reinforcer, that is, without learning as a reward or punishment, we now have the start for a fundamental understanding of the function of the orbitofrontal cortex in stimulus-reinforcement association learning. We know how one class of primary reinforcers reaches and is represented in the orbitofrontal cortex. A representation of primary reinforcers is essential for a system involved in learning associations between previously neutral stimuli and primary reinforcers, e.g., between the sight of an object and its taste.

The representation (shown by analyzing the responses of single neurons in macaques) of taste in the orbitofrontal cortex includes robust representations of the prototypical tastes sweet, salt, bitter, and sour (Rolls et al., 1990), as well as separate representations of the taste of water (Rolls et al., 1990), protein, or umami, as exemplified by monosodium glutamate (Baylis & Rolls, 1991; Rolls, 2000g) and inosine monophosphate (Rolls et al., 1996c, 1998), and of astringency, as exemplified by tannic acid (Critchley & Rolls, 1996c).

The nature of the representation of taste in the orbitofrontal cortex is that the reward value of the taste is represented. The evidence for this is that the responses of orbitofrontal taste neurons are modulated by hunger (as is the reward value or palatability of a taste). In particular, it has been shown that orbitofrontal cortex taste neurons stop responding to the taste of a food with which the monkey is fed to satiety (Rolls, et al., 1989). In contrast, the representation of taste in the primary taste cortex (Scott et al., 1986; Yaxley et al., 1990) is not modulated by hunger (Rolls et al., 1988; Yaxley, et al., 1988). Thus in the primary taste cortex, the reward value of taste is not represented, and instead the identity of the taste is represented. Additional evidence that the reward value of food is represented in the orbitofrontal cortex is that monkeys work for electrical stimulation of this brain region if they are hungry, but not if they are satiated (Mora et al., 1979; Rolls, 1994b). Furthermore, neurons in the orbitofrontal cortex are activated from many brain-stimulation reward sites (Mora et al., 1980; Rolls, et al., 1980; Rolls et al., 1980). Thus there is clear evidence that it is the reward value of taste that is represented in the orbitofrontal cortex (see Rolls, 1999a, 2000e).

The secondary taste cortex is in the caudolateral part of the orbitofrontal cortex, as defined anatomically (Baylis et al., 1994). This region projects onto other regions in the orbitofrontal cortex (Baylis et al., 1994), and neurons with taste responses (in what can be considered a tertiary gustatory cortical area) can be found in many regions of the orbitofrontal cortex (see Rolls et al., 1990; 1996; Rolls & Baylis, 1994).

In human neuroimaging experiments (e.g., with functional magnetic resonance image, [fMRI]), it has been shown (corresponding to the findings in nonhuman primate single-neuron neurophysiology) that there is an orbitofrontal cortex area activated by sweet taste (glucose) (Francis et al., 1999; Small et al., 1999), and that there are at least partly separate areas activated by the aversive taste of saline (NaCl, 0.1 M) (O'Doherty et al., 2001b), by pleasant touch (Francis et al., 1999), and by olfactory stimuli (Francis et al., 1999; O'Doherty et al., 2000).

CONVERGENCE OF TASTE AND OLFACTORY INPUTS IN THE ORBITOFRONTAL CORTEX: THE REPRESENTATION OF FLAVOR

In these further parts of the orbitofrontal cortex, not only unimodal taste neurons but also unimodal olfactory neurons are found. In addition, some single neurons respond to both gustatory and olfactory stimuli, often with correspondence between the two modalities (Rolls & Baylis, 1994; Fig. 23–2). It is probably here in the orbitofrontal cortex of primates that these two modalities converge to produce the representation of flavor (Rolls & Baylis, 1994). Forthcoming evidence will soon be described that indicates that these representations are built by olfactory–gustatory association learning, an example of stimulus-reinforcement association learning.

OLFACTORY REPRESENTATION IN THE ORBITOFRONTAL CORTEX

Takagi, and colleagues (see Takagi, 1991) described single neurons in the macaque orbitofrontal cortex that were activated by odors, and a ventral frontal region has been implicated in olfactory processing in humans (Jones-Gotman & Zatorre, 1988; Zatorre et al., 1992). Rolls and colleagues have analyzed the rules by which orbitofrontal olfactory representations are formed and operate in primates. For 65% of neurons in the orbitofrontal olfactory areas, (Critchley and Rolls, 1996a) showed that the representation of the olfactory stimulus was independent of its association with taste reward; (analyzed in an olfactory discrimination task with taste reward). For the remaining 35% of the neurons, the odors to which a neuron responded were influenced by the taste (glucose or saline) with which the odour was associated. Thus the odor representation for 35% of orbitofrontal neurons appeared to be built by olfactory-to-taste association learning. This possibility was confirmed by reversing the taste with which an odor was associated in the reversal of an olfactory discrimination task. It was found that 68% of the sample of neurons analyzed altered the way in which they responded to odor when the taste-reinforcement association of the odor was reversed (Rolls et al. 1996a). (It was also found that 25% of the neurous showed reversal, and 43% no longer discriminated after the reversal. The olfactory-to-taste reversal was quite slow, both neurophysiologically and behaviorally, often requiring 20–80 trials, which is consistent with the need for some stability of flavor representations. The relatively high proportion of neurons with modification of responsiveness by taste association in the set of neurons in this experiment was probably related to the fact that the neurons were preselected to show differential responses to the odors associated with different tastes in the olfactory discrimination task.) Thus the rule according to which the orbitofrontal olfactory representation was formed was for some neurons by association learning with taste.

To analyze the nature of the olfactory representation in the orbitofrontal cortex, Critchley and Rolls (1996b) measured the responses of olfactory neurons that responded to food while feeding the monkey to satiety. They found that most of the orbitofrontal olfactory neurons decreased their responses to the odor of the food with which the monkey was fed to satiety. Thus for these neurons, the reward value of the odor is what is represented in the orbitofrontal cortex (Rolls & Rolls, 1997). Because the neuronal responses to the food with which the monkey is fed to satiety decrease, and may even increase to a food with which the monkey has not been fed, it is the relative reward value of stimuli that is represented by these orbitofrontal cortex neurons (as confirmed by Schultz and colleagues, [2000]); and this parallels the changes in the relative pleasantness of different foods after a food is eaten to satiety (Rolls et al., 1981, 1982, 1997b; see Rolls, 1999a, 2000e). We do not yet know whether this is the first stage of processing at which reward value is represented in the olfactory system (although in rodents the influence of reward association learning appears to be present in some neurons in the pyriform cortex [Schoenbaum & Eichenbaum, 1995]).

Although individual neurons do not encode large amounts of information about which of the seven to nine odors has been presented, we have shown that the information does increase linearly with the number of neurons in the sample (Rolls et al. 1996b). This ensemble encoding results in useful amounts of information about which odour has been presented being provided by orbitofrontal olfactory neurons.

In human neuroimaging experiments, it has been shown (corresponding to the findings in nonhuman primate single-neuron neurophysiology) that there is an orbitofrontal cortex area activated by olfactory stimuli (Jones-Gotman & Zatorre, 1988; Zatorre et al., 1992, Francis et al., 1999). Moreover, the pleasantness or reward value of odor is represented in the orbitofrontal cortex, in that feeding humans to satiety decreases the activation found to the odor of that food, and this effect is relatively specific to the food eaten in the meal (O'Doherty et al., 2000).

VISUAL INPUTS TO THE ORBITOFRONTAL CORTEX

We have been able to show that there is a major visual input to many neurons in the orbitofrontal cortex, and that what is represented by these neurons is in many cases the reinforcement association of visual stimuli. The visual input is from the ventral, temporal lobe, visual stream concerned with *what* object is being seen (see Rolls, 2000a; Rolls and Deco, 2002), orbitofrontal visual neurons frequently respond differentially to objects or images depending on their reward association (Thorpe et al. 1983; Rolls, et al., 1996a). The primary reinforcer that has been used is taste. Many of these neurons show visual-taste reversal in one or a very few trials (see example in Fig. 23–3). (In a visual discrimination task, they will reverse the stimulus to which they respond, from, e.g., a triangle to a square, when the taste delivered for a behavioral response to that stimulus is reversed.) This reversal learning probably occurs in the orbitofrontal cortex, for it does not occur one synapse earlier in the visual inferior temporal cortex (Rolls, et al., 1977), and it is in the orbitofrontal cortex that there is convergence of visual and taste pathways onto the same neurons (Thorpe et al., 1983; Rolls & Baylis, 1994; Rolls et al., 1996a). The probable mechanism for this learning is Hebbian modification of synapses conveying visual input onto taste-responsive neurons, implementing a pattern association network (Rolls & Treves, 1998; Rolls, 1999a). When the reinforcement association of a visual stimulus is reversed, other orbitofrontal cortex neurons stop responding, or stop responding differentially, to the visual discriminanda (Thorpe et al., 1983). For example, one neuron in the orbitofrontal cortex responded to a blue stimulus when it was rewarded (blue S+) and not to a green stimulus when it was associated with aversive saline (green S−). However, the neuron did not respond after reversal to the blue S− or to the green S+. Similar conditional reward neurons were found for olfactory stimuli (Rolls et al., 1996a). Such conditional-reward neurons convey information about the current reinforcement status of particular stimuli, and may re-

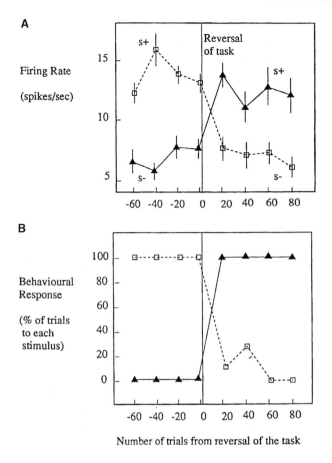

A

Firing Rate

(spikes/sec)

B

Behavioural
Response

(% of trials
to each
stimulus)

Number of trials from reversal of the task

Figure 23–3. Visual discrimination reversal of the responses of a single neuron in the macaque orbitofrontal cortex when the taste with which the two visual stimuli (triangle and square) were associated was reversed. Each point is the mean post-stimulus firing rate measured in a 0.5-second period over approximately 10 trials to each of the stimuli. Before reversal, the neuron fired most to the square when it indicated (S+) that the monkey could lick to obtain a taste of glucose. After reversal, the neuron responded most to the triangle when it indicated that the monkey could lick to obtain glucose. The response was low to the stimuli when they indicated (S−) that if the monkey licked then aversive saline would be obtained. *B:* Behavioral response to the triangle and the square, indicating that the monkey reversed rapidly. (*Source:* After Rolls et al., 1996a)

flect the fact that not every neuron that learns associations to primary reinforcers (such as taste) can sample the complete space of all possible conditioned (e.g., visual or olfactory) stimuli when acting as a pattern associator. Nevertheless, such neurons can convey very useful information, for they indicate when one of the stimuli to which they are capable of responding (given their inputs) is currently associated with reward. Similar neurons are present for punishing primary reinforcers, such as the aversive taste of salt.

In addition to these neurons that encode the reward association of visual stimuli, other neurons in the orbitofrontal cortex detect non-reward; they respond, for example, when an expected reward is not obtained when a visual discrimination task is reversed (Thorpe et al., 1983) (Table 23–1, Visual Discrimination Reversal), or when reward is no longer made available in a visual discrimination task (Table 23–1, Visual Discrimination Extinction). Dif-

ferent populations of such neurons respond to other types of non-reward, including the removal of a formerly approaching taste reward (Table 23–1, Removal) and the termination of a taste reward in the extinction of ad lib licking for juice (see Table 23–1), or the substitution of juice reward for aversive-tasting saline during ad lib licking (Thorpe et al., 1983; see Table 23–1). The presence of these neurons is fully consistent with the hypothesis that they are part of the mechanism by which the orbitofrontal cortex enables very rapid reversal of behavior by stimulus-reinforcement association relearning when the association of stimuli with reinforcers is altered or reversed (see Rolls, 1986a, 1990). The finding that different orbitofrontal cortex neurons respond to different types of non-reward (Thorpe et al., 1983) may elucidate part of the brain's mechanism that enables task or context-specific reversal to occur.

Another type of information represented in

Table 23–1. Different Types of Non-reward to Which Orbitofrontal Cortex Neurons Respond

Task	Cell Number																			
	D90	D127	D153	D154	D195	D204	D262	F466	B24	B7B	B37B	B57B	B37B	B57B	D44A	D48A	D20	D40	D61	D66
Visual discrimination																				
Reversal	1	0	1	0	0	1	1	0	—	—	—	—	—	—	0	—	—	—	—	—
Extinction	1	—	—	—	—	—	—	—	—	—	—	—	—	—	—	—	—	—	—	—
Ad lib licking																				
Reversal	1	1	—	0	0	0	—	0	1	—	—	—	—	—	—	—	—	—	—	—
Extinction	0	0	—	0	0	0	—	0	1	—	—	—	—	—	—	—	—	—	—	—
Taste of saline	0	—	0	0	0	0	0	0	1	0	0	0	0	0	0	0	0	0	0	0
Removal		0	—	0	1	1	1	0	1	0	1	1	1	1	1	1	1	1	1	1
Visual arousal	1	—	1	0	0	0	0	0	1	0	0	0	0	0	1	0	0	0	0	0

1, individual neurons responded; 0, individual neurons did not respond; —, not tested.

(*Source:* After Thorpe et al., 1983).

the orbitofrontal cortex is information about faces. A population of orbitofrontal neurons responds to such information in ways that are similar to those of neurons in the temporal cortical visual areas (see Rolls, 1984a, 1992a, 1994a, 1995a, 1996, 1997a, 2000a, Wallis & Rolls, 1997; Rolls & Deco, 2002 for a description of their properties). The orbitofrontal face-responsive neurons, first observed by Thorpe, et al. (1983), then by Rolls et al. (2002 in preparation; see Booth Rolls et al., 1998), tend to respond with longer latencies than those of temporal lobe neurons (140–200 ms typically, compared to 80–100 ms); convey information about which face is being seen, by having different responses to different faces; and are typically harder to activate strongly than temporal cortical face-selective neurons, in that many of the orbitofrontal neurons respond much better to real faces than to two-dimensional images of faces on a video monitor (Rolls & Baylis, 1986). Some of the orbitofrontal cortex face-selective neurons are responsive to facial gesture or movement. These findings are consistent with the likelihood that these neurons are activated via the inputs from the temporal cortical visual areas in which face-selective neurons are found (see Fig. 23–2). The significance of the neurons is likely to be related to the fact that faces convey information that is important in social reinforcement in at least two ways that could be implemented by these neurons. The first is

that some may encode face expression (Hasselmo et al., 1989), which can indicate reinforcement. The second way is that they encode information about which individual is present, which, by stimulus-reinforcement association learning, is important in evaluating and utilizing learned reinforcing inputs in social situations—e.g., about the current reinforcement value as decoded by stimulus reinforcement association of a particular individual.

SOMATOSENSORY INPUTS TO THE ORBITOFRONTAL CORTEX

Some neurons in the macaque orbitofrontal cortex respond to the texture of food in the mouth. Some neurons alter their responses when the texture of a food is modified by adding gelatine or methyl cellulose, or by partially liquefying a solid food such as apple (Critchley et al., 1993). Another population of orbitofrontal neurons responds when a fatty food such as cream is in the mouth. These neurons can also be activated by pure fat such as glyceryl trioleate, and by non-fat substances with a fat-like texture such as paraffin oil (hydrocarbon) and silicone oil ($Si(CH_3)_2.O)_n$). These neurons thus provide information by somatosensory pathways that a fatty food is in the mouth (Rolls et al., 1999a). These inputs are perceived as pleasant when hungry, because of the utility of ingestion of foods that are likely to contain essential fatty acids and to have a high calorific value (Rolls, 1999, 2000e). In addition to these oral somatosensory inputs to the orbitofrontal cortex, there are also somatosensory inputs from other parts of the body, and indeed, an fMRI investigation we have performed in humans indicates that pleasant and painful touch stimuli to the hand produce greater activation of the orbitofrontal cortex relative to the somatosensory cortex than do affectively neutral stimuli (Rolls et al., 1997b; in preparation; Francis et al., 1999; see below).

NEUROPHYSIOLOGICAL BASIS FOR STIMULUS-REINFORCEMENT LEARNING AND REVERSAL IN THE ORBITOFRONTAL CORTEX

The neurophysiological and lesion evidence described suggests that one function implemented by the orbitofrontal cortex is rapid stimulus-reinforcement association learning, and the correction of these associations when reinforcement contingencies in the environment change. To implement this, the orbitofrontal cortex has the necessary representation of primary reinforcers, including taste and somatosensory stimuli. It also receives information about objects, e.g., visual view-invariant information (Booth & Rolls, 1998; Rolls, 2000a), and can associate this at the neuronal level with primary reinforcers such as taste, and reverse these associations very rapidly (Thorpe et al., 1983; Rolls et al., 1996a). Another type of stimulus that can be conditioned in this way in the orbitofrontal cortex is an olfactory stimulus, although here the learning is slower. It is likely that auditory stimuli can be associated with primary reinforcers in the orbitofrontal cortex, though there is less direct evidence of this yet. The orbitofrontal cortex also has neurons that detect non-reward, which are likely to be used in behavioral extinction and reversal (Thorpe et al., 1983). They may do this not only by helping to reset the reinforcement association of neurons in the orbitofrontal cortex but also by sending a signal to the striatum, which in

turn could be routed by the striatum to produce appropriate behaviors for non-reward (Rolls & Johnstone, 1992; Williams et al., 1993; Rolls, 1994c). Indeed, it is via the striatal route that the orbitofrontal cortex may directly influence behavior when the orbitofrontal cortex is decoding reinforcement contingencies in the environment and is altering behavior in response to altering reinforcement contingencies (see Rolls, 1999). Some of the evidence for this is that neurons that reflect these orbitofrontal neuronal responses are found in the ventral part of the head of the caudate nucleus and the ventral striatum, which receive signals from the orbitofrontal cortex (Rolls et al., 1983b; Williams et al., 1993). Also, lesions of the ventral part of the head of the caudate nucleus impair visual discrimination reversal (Divac et al., 1967).

Decoding the reinforcement value of stimuli, which involves for previously neutral (e.g., visual) stimuli learning their association with a primary reinforcer, often rapidly, and which may involve not only rapid learning but also rapid relearning and alteration of responses when reinforcement contingencies change, is then a proposed function of the orbitofrontal cortex. This way of producing behavioral responses would be important in motivational and emotional behavior, such as the feeding and drinking that results when primates learn rapidly about the food reinforcement to be expected from visual stimuli (see Rolls, 1994b, 1999a). This is important, for primates frequently eat more than 100 varieties of food; vision by visual–taste association learning can be used to identify when foods are ripe; and during the course of a meal, the pleasantness of the sight of a food eaten in the meal decreases in a sensory-specific way (Rolls et al., 1983a), a function that is probably implemented by the sensory-specific satiety-related responses of orbitofrontal visual neurons (Critchley & Rolls, 1996b).

With respect to emotional behavior, decoding and rapidly readjusting the reinforcement value of visual signals is likely to be crucial, for emotions can be described as responses elicited by reinforcing signals[1] (Rolls, 1986a, 1986, 1990, 1995a, 1999, 2000d). The ability to perform this learning very rapidly is probably very important for primates in social situations, in which reinforcing stimuli are continually being exchanged and the reinforcement value of stimuli must be continually updated (relearned), based on the actual reinforcers received and given. Although the functions of the orbitofrontal cortex in implementing the operation of reinforcers such as taste, smell, tactile, and visual stimuli, including faces, are best understood, in humans the rewards processed in the orbitofrontal cortex include quite general rewards such as working for "points," as will be described shortly.

Although the amygdala is concerned with some of the same functions as the orbitofrontal cortex and receives similar inputs (see Fig. 23–2), there is evidence that it may function less effectively in the very rapid learning and reversal of stimulus-reinforcement associations, as indicated by the greater difficulty in obtaining reversal from amygdala neurons (see, e.g., Rolls, 1992b, 2000c) and by the greater effect of orbitofrontal lesions in leading to continuing choice of no longer rewarded stimuli (Jones & Mishkin, 1972). In primates, the necessity for very rapid stimulus-reinforcement re-evaluation, and the development of powerful cortical learning systems, may result in the orbitofrontal cortex effectively taking over this aspect of amygdala functions (see Rolls, 1992b, 1999a).

THE HUMAN ORBITOFRONTAL CORTEX

NEUROPSYCHOLOGY

It is of interest that a number of the symptoms of frontal lobe damage in humans appear to be related to altering behavior when stimulus-reinforcement associations alter. Humans with frontal lobe damage can show impairments in a number of tasks in which an alteration of behavioral strategy is required in response to a change in environmental reinforcement contingencies (see Goodglass & Kaplan, 1979; Jouandet & Gazzaniga, 1979; Kolb & Whishaw, 1996). For example, Milner (1963) showed that in the Wisconsin Card Sorting

Task (in which cards are to be sorted according to the color, shape, or number of items on each card depending on whether the examiner says "right" or "wrong" to each placement), patients with frontal lobe damage had difficulty in either determining the first sorting principle or in shifting to a second principle when required to. Also, in stylus mazes, these patients have difficulty in changing direction when a sound indicates that the correct path has been left (see Milner, 1982). It is of interest that, in both types of test, frontal patients may be able to verbalize the correct rules, yet may be unable to correct their behavioral sets or strategies appropriately. Some of the personality changes that can follow frontal lobe damage may be related to a similar type of dysfunction. For example, the euphoria, irresponsibility, lack of affect, and lack of concern for the present or future that can follow frontal lobe damage (see Hecaen & Albert, 1978; Damasio, 1994) may also be related to a dysfunction in altering behavior appropriately in response to a change in reinforcement contingencies. Indeed, in so far as the orbitofrontal cortex is involved in the disconnection of stimulus-reinforcer associations, and such associations are important in learned emotional responses, then it follows that the orbitofrontal cortex is involved in emotional responses by correcting stimulus-reinforcer associations when they become inappropriate.

These hypotheses, and in particular the role of the orbitofrontal cortex in human behavior, have been investigated in recent studies in humans with damage to the ventral parts of the frontal lobe. (The description *ventral* is given to indicate that there was pathology in the orbitofrontal or related parts of the frontal lobe, and not in the more dorsolateral parts of the frontal lobe.) A task directed at assessing the rapid alteration of stimulus-reinforcement associations was used, because the findings discussed above indicate that the orbitofrontal cortex is involved in this type of learning. Instead of the Wisconsin Card Sorting Task, which requires patients to shift from category (or dimension) to category, e.g., from color to shape, the task used was visual discrimination reversal, in which patients learn to obtain points by touching one stimulus when it appears on a video monitor, but to withhold a response when a different visual stimulus appears, otherwise a point is lost. After the subjects had acquired the visual discrimination, the reinforcement contingencies unexpectedly reversed. The patients with ventral frontal le-

sions made more errors on the reversal task (or on a similar extinction task in which the reward was no longer given) and completed fewer reversals than control patients with damage elsewhere in the frontal lobes or in other brain regions (Rolls et al., 1994; see Table 23–2). The

Table 23–2. Vocal and Face Expression Identification in Patients with Damage to the Ventral Parts of the Frontal Lobes and in Control Patients.

	Behavior Questionnaire	Subjective Emotional Change	Facial Expression % Corr (SD)	Vocal Expression % Corr (SD)	Reversals	Last Error	Extinction
Ventral Frontal Case							
1	6.0	–	29 (− 6.5)°°	42 (− 3.7)°°	0 (76%)	38F	—
2	4.0	2.0	84 (− 0.4)	30 (− 4.8)°°	0 (83%)	50F	30F (93%)
3	6.0	7.5	60 (− 3.1)°°	36 (− 4.9)°°	0 (75%)	20F	—
4	7.5	4.5	60 (− 3.0)°°	54 (− 2.5)°°	0 (67%)	30F	—
5	8.5	7.0	58 (− 3.2)°°	39 (− 4.0)°°	—	—	34F
6	5.0	1.5	75 (− 1.3)	67 (− 1.3)	0 (54%)	51F	53F (38%)
7	6.0	5.0	67 (− 2.3)°°	58 (− 2.1)°°	2	4	30F (86%)
8	7.0	2.5	54 (− 3.7)°°	—	0 (100%)	50F	48F (93%)
9	4.0	1.5	83 (− 0.4)	81 (+0.1)	2	5	36 (45%)
10	5.0	4.0	67 (− 2.2)°°	60 (− 1.9)°	1	23	9
11	4.5	6.5	40 (− 5.3)°°	53 (− 2.6)°°			
12	3.0		38 (− 5.6)°°	43 (− 3.5)°°			
Median	5.5	4.3	60	53	0	30	34
Nonventral							
1	0.0	0.5	79 (− 0.9)	–	2 (14%)	4	21 (43%)
2	2.5	1.0	83 (− 0.4)		2 (46%)	11	12 (36%)
3	0.5	0.0	83 (− 0.4)	61 (− 1.8)°	2 (25%)	7	4 (7%)
4	0.0	2.0	75 (− 1.4)	61 (− 1.8)°	2 (8%)	4	3 (7%)
5	0.0	1.5	71 (− 1.8)°	67 (− 1.2)	1	14	13 (21%)
6	2.0	1.0	92 (+ 0.6)	75 (− 0.5)	2 (42%)	13	100 (0%)
7	2.5	1.0	75 (− 1.4)	61 (− 1.8)°			
8	0.0	2.5	96 (+ 0.1)	78 (− 0.2)			
9	0.5	1.0	67 (− 2.3)°°				
10	1.0	1.5	79 (− 0.9)	72 (− 0.7)			
11	0.5	1.0	83 (− 0.4)	61 (− 1.8)°			
12							4 (7%)
13					2 (8%)	4	4 (7%)
Median	**0.5**	**1.0**	**79**	**64**	**2**	**7**	**4**

Also shown are the number of reversals completed in 30 trials, and the number of the last trial on which an error occurred during Reversal or Extinction.

°Scores which fall below the 5th centile of the normal distribution, i.e., SD <− 1.64 (impaired). F, failed to reach criterion in reversal or extinction.

°°Scores which fall below the 1st centile of the normal distribution, i.e., SD <− 1.96 (severely impaired).

sd, number of standard deviations above (+) or below (; ms) the means for normal subjects.

The median values for reversal and extinction are for a larger group.

The % columns refer for Reversal and Extinction to the percentage of errors of commission, that is responses made to the stimulus that was before reversal or extinction the reward−related stimulus (old S +).

⁰(*Source:* Data from Rolls et al., 1994; Hornak et al., 1996; Rolls, 1999b)

impairment correlated highly with the socially inappropriate or disinhibited behavior of the patients (assessed through a behavior questionnaire) (see Table 23–2), as well as with their subjective evaluation of the changes in their emotional state since the brain damage (see Table 23–2; Rolls et al., 1994). The patients were not impaired at performing other types of memory tasks, such as paired-associate learning. The continued choice of the no-longer rewarded stimulus in the reversal of the visual discrimination task was interpreted as a failure to reverse stimulus-reinforcer, that is, sensory-sensory, associations, and not as motor response perseveration that may follow much more dorsal damage to the frontal lobes; this is being investigated further in this type of patient. However, one of the types of evidence that bears very directly on this comes from the responses of orbitofrontal cortex neurons, which respond in relation to a sensory stimulus such as a visual stimulus when it is paired with another sensory stimulus to which the neuron responds, such as a taste stimulus. The taste stimulus is a primary reinforcer. These neurons do not respond to motor responses, and could not be involved in stimulus–to–motor response association learning. Consistent with these findings are those of Bechara and colleagues, who studied patients with frontal lobe damage performing a gambling task (Bechara et al., 1994, 1996, 1997; see also Damasio, 1994). The patients were allowed to choose cards from several decks. The patients with frontal lobe damage were more likely to choose cards from a deck that gave rewards with a reasonable probability, but also had occasional very heavy penalties resulting in lower net gains than those of choices from the other deck. In this sense, the patients were not affected by the negative consequences of their actions: they did not switch from the deck of cards providing significant rewards, even when large punishments were incurred.

It is of interest that in the reversal and extinction tasks, these patients can often verbalize the correct response, yet commit the incorrect action (Rolls et al., 1994). This pattern is consistent with the hypothesis that the orbitofrontal cortex is normally involved in executing behavior when the behavior is performed by evaluating the reinforcement associations of environmental stimuli (see below and Chapter 9 of Rolls, 1999a). The orbitofrontal cortex appears to be involved in this process in both humans and nonhuman primates, when the learning must be performed rapidly in, for example, acquisition and during reversal.

An idea of the way in which such stimulus-reinforcer learning may play an important role in normal human behavior, and may be related to the behavioral changes seen clinically in patients with ventral frontal lobe damage, can be provided by summarizing the behavioral ratings given by the caregivers of these patients. The patients were rated high on the behaviour questionnaire on at least some of the following: disinhibited or socially inappropriate behavior; misinterpretation of other people's moods; impulsiveness; unconcern or underestimation of the seriousness of their condition; and lack of initiative (Rolls et al., 1994). Such behavioral changes correlated with the stimulus-reinforcer reversal and extinction learning impairment (Rolls et al., 1994). The suggestion is, then, that the insensitivity to reinforcement changes in the learning task may be at least part of what produces the changes in behavior found in these patients with ventral frontal lobe damage. The more general impact on the behavior of these patients is that their irresponsibility tended to affect their everyday lives. For example, if such patients had received their brain damage in a road traffic accident, and compensation had been awarded, the patients often tended to spend their money without appropriate concern for the future, sometimes, for example, buying a very expensive car. Such patients often find it difficult to invest in relationships too, and are sometimes described by their family as having changed personalities, in that they care less about a wide range of factors after than before the brain damage. The suggestion that follows from this is that the orbitofrontal cortex may normally be involved in much social behavior. The ability to respond rapidly and appropriately to social reinforcers is, of course, an important aspect of primate (including human) social behavior.

Table 23–3. Facial expression identification

	Sad	Angry	Frightened	Disgusted	Surprised	Happy	Neutral
Normal subjects ($n = 11$)	68.6	94.7	77.6	81.8	92.0	100.0	93.9
Frontal patients ($n = 9$)	22.6	39.3	31.9	48.1	66.2	94.0	65.7

Group mean percent correct on each emotion in normal subjects and in patients with impaired ventral frontal lobe.
(*Source:* Data from Hornak et al., (1996; Rolls, 1999a).

To investigate the possible significance of face-related inputs to the orbitofrontal visual neurons described above, we also tested the responses of these patients to faces. We included tests of facial (and voice) expression decoding, because these are ways in which the reinforcing quality of individuals is often indicated. Impairment in the identification of facial and vocal emotional expression was demonstrated in a group of patients with ventral frontal lobe damage who had socially inappropriate behavior (Hornak et al., 1996; see Tables 23–2, 23–3, and 23–4). The expression identification impairment could occur independent of perceptual impairments in facial recognition, voice discrimination, or environmental sound recognition. The face and voice expression problems did not necessarily occur together in the same patients, providing an indication of separate processing. The impairment was found on most expressions, apart from happy (which, as the only positive facial expression, was relatively easily discriminable from the others), with sad, angry, frightened, and disgusted showing lower identification than surprised and neutral expressions (see Table 23–3). Poor performance on both expression tests was correlated with the degree of alteration of emotional experience

reported by the patients. There was also a strong positive correlation between the degree of altered emotional experience and the severity of the behavioral problems (e.g., disinhibition) found in these patients (see Hornak et al., 1996; Table 23–2). A comparison group of patients with brain damage outside the ventral frontal lobe region, without these behavioral problems, was unimpaired on the facial expression identification test, was significantly less impaired at vocal expression identification, and reported little subjective emotional change (see Hornak et al., 1996; Table 23–2). These investigations are being extended, in current studies, and it is being found that patients with facial expression decoding problems do not necessarily have impairments at visual discrimination reversal, and vice versa. This finding is consistent with some topography in the orbitofrontal cortex (see, e.g., Rolls & Baylis, 1994).

NEUROIMAGING

To further elucidate the role of the human orbitofrontal cortex in emotion, Rolls et al. (1997b; Francis et al., 1999) performed an investigation to determine where the pleasant affective component of touch is represented in the brain. Touch is a primary reinforcer that

Table 23–4. Vocal expression identification

	Sad	Angry	Frightened	Disgusted	Puzzled	Contented
Normal subjects ($n = 10$)	80.8	66.1	88.1	95.0	78.9	68.9
Frontal patients ($n = 7$)	14.7	25.0	52.8	80.9	42.8	33.3

Group mean percent correct on each emotion in normal subjects and in patients with impaired ventral frontal lobe.
(*Source:* Data from Hornak et al., 1996)

can produce pleasure. They found with fMRI that a weak but very pleasant touch of the hand with velvet produced much stronger activation of the orbitofrontal cortex than a more intense but affectively neutral touch of the hand with wood. In contrast, the affectively neutral but more intense touch produced more activation of the primary somatosensory cortex than did the pleasant stimuli. These findings indicate that part of the orbitofrontal cortex is concerned with representing the positively affective aspects of somatosensory stimuli. The significance of this finding is that a primary reinforcer that can produce affectively positive emotional responses is represented in the human orbitofrontal cortex. This provides one of the bases for the human orbitofrontal cortex to be involved in the stimulus-reinforcement association learning that provides the basis for emotional learning. In more recent studies, Rolls et al. (in preparation) have found that there is also a representation of the affectively negative aspects of touch, including pain, in the human orbitofrontal cortex. This is consistent with the reports that humans with damage to the ventral part of the frontal lobe may report that they know that a stimulus is pain producing, but that the pain does not feel very bad to them (see Freeman & Watts, 1950; Valenstein, 1974; Melzack & Wall, 1996). It will be of interest to determine whether the regions of the human orbitofrontal cortex that represent pleasant touch and pain are close topologically or overlap. Even if fMRI studies show that the areas overlap, it would nevertheless be the case that different populations of neurons would be activated, for this is what recordings from single cells in monkeys indicate about positively versus negatively affective taste, olfactory and visual stimuli (see Neurophysiology of the Orbitofrontal Cortex).

It is also of interest that nearby, but not overlapping, parts of the human orbitofrontal cortex are activated by taste stimuli (such as glucose) (Small et al., 1999; O'Doherty et al., 2001b), and it has recently been shown that the pleasantness of olfactory stimuli is represented in the human orbitofrontal cortex: orbitofrontal cortex activation decreases to an odor of food that has been eaten to satiety so that it no longer is rewarding and smells pleasant (O'Doherty et al., 2000).

In a task designed to show whether the human orbitofrontal cortex is involved in more abstract types of reward and punishment, O'Doherty et al. (2001a) found that the medial orbitofrontal cortex showed activation correlated with an amount of money just received in a probabilistic visual association task, and the lateral orbitofrontal cortex showed activation that was correlated with the amount of money just lost. This study shows that the magnitudes of quite abstract rewards and punishers are represented in the orbitofrontal cortex.

These human neuroimaging studies on the orbitofrontal cortex are thus providing confirmation that the theory of emotion and the way in which it is relevant to understanding orbitofrontal cortex function (Rolls, 1999, 2000d) also apply to humans, in that representations of many types of reward and punishment are being found in the human orbitofrontal cortex. This evidence helps us to understand behavioral changes after orbitofrontal cortex damage in humans as being related to alterations in processing and learning associations to rewards and punishments that are normally important in emotional and social behavior. The aim here is to understand the functions of the human orbitofrontal cortex in terms of the operations it performs, with the help of precise neurophysiological evidence available from studies in nonhuman primates.

NEURONAL NETWORK COMPUTATIONS IN THE PREFRONTAL CORTEX

STIMULUS-REINFORCEMENT ASSOCIATION AND REVERSAL

This reversal learning that occurs in the orbitofrontal cortex could be implemented by Hebbian modification of synapses conveying visual input onto taste-responsive neurons, implementing a pattern association network (Rolls & Treves, 1998; Rolls, 1999a, 2000b). Long-term potentiation would strengthen syn-

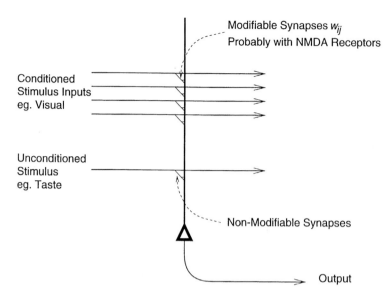

Figure 23–4. A pattern association network that could underlie the learning and reversal of stimulus-reinforcement association in the orbitofrontal cortex (see text).

apses from active conditional stimulus neurons onto neurons responding to a primary reinforcer such as a sweet taste, and homosynaptic long-term depression would weaken synapses from the same active visual inputs if the neuron was not responding because an aversive primary reinforcer (e.g., a taste of saline) was being presented (see Fig. 23–4). As noted above, the conditional-reward neurons in the orbitofrontal cortex convey information about the current reinforcement status of particular stimuli, and may reflect the fact that not every neuron that learns associations to primary reinforcers (such as taste) can sample the complete space of all possible conditioned (e.g., visual or olfactory) stimuli when acting as a pattern associator. Nevertheless, such neurons can convey very useful information, for they indicate when one of the stimuli to which they are capable of responding (given their inputs) is currently associated with reward. Similar neurons are present for punishing primary reinforcers, such as the aversive taste of salt.

The error detection neurons that respond during frustrative non-reward may be triggered by a mismatch between what was expected when the visual stimulus was shown and the primary reinforcer that was obtained, both of which are represented in the primate orbitofrontal cortex.

The dopamine projections to the prefrontal cortex and other areas are not likely to convey information about reward to the prefrontal cortex, which instead is likely to be decoded by the neurons in the orbitofrontal cortex that represent primary reinforcers, and the orbitofrontal cortex neurons that learn associations of other stimuli to the primary reinforcers. Although it has been suggested that the firing of dopamine neurons may reflect the earliest signal in a task that indicates reward and could be used as an error signal during learning (see Schultz et al., 2000), there is evidence that dopamine release is more closely related to whether active initiation of behavior is required, regardless of whether this is to obtain rewards or escape from or avoid punishments (see Rolls, 1999a, 2000d).

PREFRONTAL CORTEX NEURONAL NETWORKS FOR WORKING MEMORY

In a sense, the orbitofrontal cortex, by its rapid stimulus-reinforcer association learning, remembers the recent reward association of stimuli and implements this by synaptic plasticity, so that no ongoing neuronal firing is needed to implement stimulus-reinforcer association memory. In contrast, the inferior convexity prefrontal cortex and the dorsolateral prefrontal cortex implement a short-term memory for stimuli that is maintained by the active, continual firing of neurons. I shall now consider how this latter form of memory appears to be implemented in the prefrontal cortex.

A common way that the brain uses to implement a short-term memory is to maintain the firing of neurons during a short-memory period after the end of a stimulus (see Rolls & Treves, 1998; Rolls, 2000a). In the inferior temporal cortex of the monkey, this firing may be maintained for a few hundred ms even when the monkey is not performing a memory task (Rolls & Tovee 1994; Rolls et al., 1994, 1999b; Desimone, 1996). In more ventral temporal cortical areas such as the entorhinal cortex, the firing may be maintained for longer periods in delayed match-to-sample tasks (Suzuki et al., 1997), and in the prefrontal cortex for even tens of seconds (see Fuster, 1997). In the dorsolateral and inferior convexity prefrontal cortex, the firing of the neurons may be related to the memory of spatial responses or objects (Wilson et al., 1993; Goldman-Rakic, 1996) or both (Rao et al., 1997), and in the principal sulcus–frontal eye field–arcuate sulcus region to the memory of places for eye movements (Funahashi et al., 1989). The firing may be maintained by the operation of associatively modified recurrent collateral connections between nearby pyramidal cells producing attractor states in autoassociative networks (Amit, 1995; Rolls & Treves, 1998).

For the short-term memory to be maintained during periods when new stimuli are to be perceived, there *must* be separate networks for the perceptual and short-term memory functions, and indeed, two coupled networks—one in the inferior temporal visual cortex for perceptual functions and another in the prefrontal cortex for maintaining the short-term memory during intervening stimuli—provide a precise model of the interaction of perceptual and short-term memory systems (Renart et al., 2000, 2001; Rolls & Deco, 2002). In particular, it is shown how a prefrontal cortex attractor (autoassociation) network could be triggered by a sample visual stimulus represented in the inferior temporal visual cortex in a delayed match-to-sample task, and could keep this attractor active during a memory interval in which intervening stimuli are shown. When the sample stimulus reappeared in the task as a match stimulus, the inferior temporal cortex module showed a large response to the match stimulus, because it is activated both by the incoming match stimulus and by the consistent back-projected memory of the sample stimulus still being represented in the prefrontal cortex memory module (see Fig. 23–5).

This computational model makes it clear that in order for ongoing perception to occur

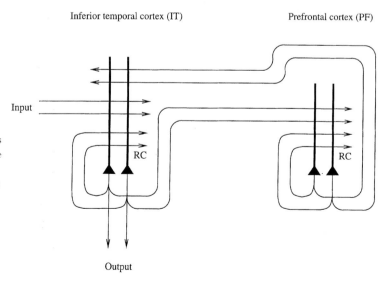

Figure 23–5. A short-term memory autoassociation network in the prefrontal cortex could hold active a working memory representation by maintaining its firing in an attractor state. The prefrontal module would be loaded with the to-be-remembered stimulus by the posterior module (in the temporal or parietal cortex) in which the incoming stimuli are represented. Back-projections from the prefrontal short-term memory module to the posterior module would enable the working memory to be unloaded to influence ongoing perception (see text). RC, recurrent collateral connections.

unhindered, implemented by posterior cortex (parietal and temporal lobe) networks, there must be a separate set of modules that is capable of maintaining a representation over intervening stimuli (Rolls and Deco, 2002). This approach emphasizes that to provide a good brain lesion test of prefrontal cortex short-term memory functions, the task set should require a short-term memory for stimuli over an interval in which other stimuli are being processed, because otherwise the posterior cortex perceptual modules could implement the short term memory function by their own recurrent collateral connections. This approach also emphasizes that there are many at least partially independent modules for short-term memory functions in the prefrontal cortex—e.g., several modules for delayed saccades in the frontal eye fields; one or more for delayed spatial (body) responses in the dorsolateral prefrontal cortex; one or more for remembering visual stimuli in the more ventral prefrontal cortex; and at least one in the left prefrontal cortex used for remembering the words produced in a verbal fluency task (Rolls & Treves, 1998; see Chapter 10). This computational approach thus provides a clear understanding of why a separate (prefrontal) mechanism is needed for working memory functions (Rolls and Deco, 2002). If a prefrontal cortex module is to control behavior in a working memory task, then it must be capable of assuming some type of executive control. There may be no need to have a single central executive in addition to the control that must be capable of being exerted by every short-term memory module.

To set up a new short-term memory attractor, synaptic modification is needed to form the new stable attractor. Once the attractor is set up, it may be used repeatedly when triggered by an appropriate cue to hold the short-term memory state active by continued neuronal firing, even without any further synaptic modification (see Kesner & Rolls, 2001). Thus agents that impair the long-term potentiation of synapses may impair the formation of new short-term memory states, but not the use of previously learned short-term memory states (see Kesner & Rolls, 2001).

CONCLUSIONS AND SUMMARY

The orbitofrontal cortex contains the secondary taste cortex, in which the reward value of taste is represented. It also contains the secondary and tertiary olfactory cortical areas, in which information about the identity and the reward value of odors is represented. The orbitofrontal cortex also receives information about the sight of objects from the temporal lobe cortical visual areas, and neurons in it learn and reverse the visual stimulus to which they respond when the association of the visual stimulus with a primary reinforcing stimulus (such as taste) is reversed. This is an example of stimulus-reinforcement association learning, and is a type of stimulus-stimulus association learning. More generally, the stimulus might be a visual or olfactory stimulus, and the primary (unlearned) positive or negative reinforcer, a taste or touch. A somatosensory input is revealed by neurons that respond to the texture of food in the mouth, including a population that responds to the mouth feel of fat. In complementary neuroimaging studies in humans, it has been found that areas of the orbitofrontal cortex are activated by pleasant touch, by painful touch, by taste, smell, and more abstract reinforcers such as winning or losing money. Damage to the orbitofrontal cortex can impair the learning and reversal of stimulus-reinforcement associations, and thus the correction of behavioral responses when these are no longer appropriate because previous reinforcement contingencies change. The information that reaches the orbitofrontal cortex for these functions includes information about faces, and damage to the orbitofrontal cortex can impair facial (and voice) expression identification. This evidence thus shows that the orbitofrontal cortex is involved in decoding and representing some primary reinforcers such as taste and touch; in learning and reversing associations of visual and other stimuli to these primary reinforcers; and in controlling and correcting reward-related and punishment-related behavior; and, thus, in emotion. The approach described here is aimed at providing a fundamental understanding of how the orbitofrontal cortex actually functions, and thus in how it is involved in motivational behavior such as feeding and drinking, in emotional behavior, and in social behavior.

ACKNOWLEDGMENTS

The author has worked on some of the experiments described here with L.L. Baylis, G.C. Baylis, R. Bowtell, A.D. Browning, H.D. Critchley, S. Francis, M.E. Hasselmo, J. Hornak, M. Kringelbach, C.M. Leonard, F. McGlone, F. Mora, J. O'Doherty, D.I. Perrett, T.R. Scott, S.J. Thorpe, E.A. Wakeman, and F.A.W. Wilson, and their collaboration is sincerely acknowledged. Some of the research described was supported by the Medical Research Council, PG8513790 and PG9826105.

NOTE

1. For the purposes of this chapter, a *positive reinforcer* or *reward* can be defined as a stimulus that the animal will work to obtain, and a *negative reinforcer* or *punishment* as a stimulus that an animal will work to avoid or escape (see Rolls, 1990, 1999).

REFERENCES

Amit, D.J. (1995). The Hebbian paradigm reintegrated: local reverberations as internal representations. *Behavioural and Brain Sciences, 18*, 617–657.

Barbas, H. (1988). Anatomic organization of basoventral and mediodorsal visual recipient prefrontal regions in the rhesus monkey. *Journal of Comparative Neurology, 276*, 313–342.

Barbas, H. (1993). Organization of cortical afferent input to the orbitofrontal area in the rhesus monkey. *Neuroscience, 56*, 841–864.

Barbas, H. (1995). Anatomic basis of cognitive–emotional interactions in the primate prefrontal cortex. *Neuroscience and Biobehavioural Reviews, 19*, 499–510.

Barbas, H. & Pandya, D.N. (1989). Architecture and intrinsic connections of the prefrontal cortex in the rhesus monkey. *Journal of Computational Neurology, 286*, 353–375.

Baylis, L.L. & Gaffan, D. (1991). Amygdalectomy and ventromedial prefrontal ablation produce similar deficits in food choice and in simple object discrimination learning for an unseen reward. *Experimental Brain Research, 86* 617–622.

Baylis, L.L. & Rolls, E.T. (1991). Responses of neurons in the primate taste cortex to glutamate. *Physiology and Behavior, 49*, 973–979.

Baylis, L.L., Rolls, E.T., & Baylis, G.C. (1994). Afferent connections of the orbitofrontal cortex taste area of the primate. *Neuroscience, 64*, 801–812.

Bechara, A., Damasio, A.R., Damasio, H., & Anderson, S.W. (1994). Insensitivity to future consequences following damage to human prefrontal cortex. *Cognition, 50*, 7–15.

Bechara, A., Tranel, D., Damasio, H., & Damasio, A.R. (1996). Failure to respond autonomically to anticipated future outcomes following damage to prefrontal cortex. *Cerebral Cortex, 6*, 215–225.

Bechara, A., Damasio, H., Tranel, D., & Damasio, A.R. (1997). Deciding advantageously before knowing the advantageous strategy. *Science, 275*, 1293–1295.

Booth, M.C.A. & Rolls, E.T. (1998). View-invariant representations of familiar objects by neurons in the inferior temporal visual cortex. *Cerebral Cortex, 8*, 510–523.

Booth, M.C.A., Rolls, E.T., Critchley, H.D., Browning, A.S., & Hernadi, I. (1998). Face-selective neurons in the primate orbitofrontal cortex. *Society for Neuroscience Abstracts, 24*, 898.

Butter, C.M. (1969). Perseveration in extinction and in discrimination reversal tasks following selective prefrontal ablations in *Macaca mulatta. Physiology and Behavior, 4*, 163–171.

Butter, C.M., & Snyder, D.R. (1972). Alterations in aversive and aggressive behaviors following orbitofrontal lesions in rhesus monkeys. *Acta Neurobiologiae Experimentalis, 32*, 525–565.

Butter, C.M., McDonald, J.A., & Snyder, D.R. (1969). Orality, preference behavior, and reinforcement value of non-food objects in monkeys with orbital frontal lesions. *Science, 164*, 1306–1307.

Butter, C.M., Snyder, D.R., & McDonald, J.A. (1970). Effects of orbitofrontal lesions on aversive and aggressive behaviors in rhesus monkeys. *Journal of Comparative and Physiological Psychology, 72*, 132–144.

Carmichael, S.T. & Price, J.L. (1994). Architectonic subdivision of the orbital and medial prefrontal cortex in the macaque monkey. *Journal of Comparative Neurology, 346*, 366–402.

Carmichael, S.T. & Price, J.L. (1995). Sensory and premotor connections of the orbital and medial prefrontal cortex of macaque monkeys. *Journal of Comparative Neurology, 363*, 642–664.

Carmichael, S.T. Clugnet, M.-C., & Price, J.L. (1994). Central olfactory connections in the macaque monkey. *Journal of Comparative Neurology, 346*, 403–434.

Critchley, H.D. & Rolls, E.T. (1996a). Olfactory neuronal responses in the primate orbitofrontal cortex: analysis in an olfactory discrimination task. *Journal of Neurophysiology, 75*, 1659–1672.

Critchley, H.D. & Rolls, E.T. (1996b). Hunger and satiety modify the responses of olfactory and visual neurons in the primate orbitofrontal cortex. *Journal of Neurophysiology, 75*, 1673–1686.

Critchley, H.D., & Rolls, E.T. (1996c). Responses of primate taste cortex neurons to the astringent tastant tannic acid. *Chemical Senses, 21*, 135–145.

Critchley, H.D., Rolls, E.T., & Wakeman, E.A. (1993). Orbitofrontal cortex responses to the texture, taste, smell and sight of food. *Appetite, 21*, 170.

Damasio, A.R. (1994). *Descartes' Error: Emotion, Reason and the Human Brain.* Putnam, New York.

Desimone, R. (1996). Neural mechanisms for visual memory and their role in attention. *Proceedings of the National Academy of Sciences USA, 93*, 13494–13499.

Divac, I., Rosvold, H.E., & Szwarcbart, M.K. (1967). Behavioral effects of selective ablation of the caudate nucleus. *Journal of Comparative Physiological Psychology, 63,* 184–190.

Francis, S., Rolls, E.T., Bowtell, R., McGlone, F., O'Doherty, J., Browning, A., Clare, S., & Smith, E. (1999). The representation of pleasant touch in the brain and its relationship with taste and olfactory areas. *NeuroReport, 10,* 453–459.

Freeman, W.J. & Watts, J.W. (1950). *Psychosurgery in the Treatment of Mental Disorders and Intractable Pain,* 2nd ed. Springfield, IL: C.C. Thomas.

Funahashi, S., Bruce, C.J., & Goldman-Rakic, P.S. (1989). Mnemonic coding of visual space in monkey dorsolateral prefrontal cortex. *Journal of Neurophysiology, 61,* 331–349.

Fuster, J.M. (1997). *The Prefrontal Cortex,* 3rd ed. New York: Raven Press.

Goldman-Rakic, P.S. (1996). The prefrontal landscape: implications of functional architecture for understanding human mentation and the central executive. *Philosophical Transactions of the Royal Society London B, 351,* 1445–1453.

Goodglass, H. & Kaplan, E. (1979). Assessment of cognitive deficit in brain-injured patient. In: M.S. Gazzaniga (Ed.), *Handbook of Behavioral Neurobiology. Vol. 2, Neuropsychology* (pp. 3–22). New York: Plenum Press.

Hasselmo, M.E., Rolls, E.T., & Baylis, G.C. (1989). The role of expression and identity in the face-selective responses of neurons in the temporal visual cortex of the monkey. *Behavioural Brain Research, 32,* 203–218.

Hecaen, H. & Albert, M.L. (1978). *Human Neuropsychology.* New York: John Wiley & Sons.

Hornak, J., Rolls, E.T., & Wade, D. (1996). Face and voice expression identification in patients with emotional and behavioural changes following ventral frontal lobe damage. *Neuropsychologia, 34,* 247–261.

Insausti, R., Amaral, D.G., & Cowan, W.M. (1987). The entorhinal cortex of the monkey. II. Cortical afferents. *Journal of Comparative Neurology, 264,* 356–395.

Iversen, S.D. & Mishkin, M. (1970). Perseverative interference in monkey following selective lesions of the inferior prefrontal convexity. *Experimental Brain Research, 11,* 376–386.

Johnson, T.N., Rosvold, H.E., & Mishkin, M. (1968). Projections from behaviorally defined sectors of the prefrontal cortex to the basal ganglia, septum and diencephalon of the monkey. *Experimental Neurology, 21,* 20–34.

Jones, B. & Mishkin, M. (1972). Limbic lesions and the problem of stimulus-reinforcement associations. *Experimental Neurology, 36,* 362–377.

Jones-Gotman, M. & Zatorre, R.J. (1988). Olfactory identification in patients with focal cerebral excision. *Neuropsychologia, 26,* 387–400.

Jouandet, M. & Gazzaniga, M.S. (1979). The frontal lobes. In: M.S. Gazzaniga (Ed.), *Handbook of Behavioral Neurobiology, Vol. 2, Neuropsychology,* (pp. 25–59). New York: Plenum Press.

Kemp, J.M. & Powell, T.P.S. (1970). The cortico-striate projections in the monkey. *Brain, 93,* 525–546.

Kesner, R.P. & Rolls, E.T. (2001). Role of long-term synaptic modification in short-term memory. *Hippocampus,* in press.

Kolb, B. & Whishaw, I.Q. (1996). *Fundamentals of Human Neuropsychology,* 4th ed. New York: Freeman Press.

Kowalska, D.-M., Bachevalier, J., & Mishkin, M. (1991). The role of the inferior prefrontal convexity in performance of delayed nonmatching-to-sample. *Neuropsychologia, 29,* 583–600.

Melzack, R. & Wall, P.D. (1996). *The Challenge of Pain.* Harmondsworth, UK: Penguin.

Milner, B. (1963). Effects of different brain lesions on card sorting. *Archives of Neurology, 9,* 90–100.

Milner, B. (1982). Some cognitive effects of frontal-lobe lesions in man. *Philosophical Transactions of the Royal Society of London B, 298,* 211–226.

Mishkin, M. & Manning, F.J. (1978). Non-spatial memory after selective prefrontal lesions in monkeys. *Brain Research, 143,* 313–324.

Mora, F., Avrith, D.B., Phillips, A.G., & Rolls, E.T. (1979). Effects of satiety on self-stimulation of the orbitofrontal cortex in the monkey. *Neuroscience Letters, 13,* 141–145.

Mora, F., Avrith, D.B., & Rolls, E.T. (1980). An electrophysiological and behavioural study of self-stimulation in the orbitofrontal cortex of the rhesus monkey. *Brain Research Bulletin, 5,* 111–115.

Morecraft, R.J., Geula, C., & Mesulam, M.-M. (1992). Cytoarchitecture and neural afferents of orbitofrontal cortex in the brain of the monkey. *Journal of Comparative Neurology, 323,* 341–358.

Nauta, W.J.H. (1964). Some efferent connections of the prefrontal cortex in the monkey. In: J.M. Warren & K. Akert (Eds.), *The Frontal Granular Cortex and Behavior* (pp. 397–407). New York: McGraw-Hill.

O'Doherty, J., Rolls, E.T., Francis, S., Bowtell, R., McGlone, F., Kobal, G., Renner, B., & Ahne, G. (2000). Sensory-specific satiety related olfactory activation of the human orbitofrontal cortex. *NeuroReport, 11,* 893–897.

O'Doherty, J., Kringelbach, M.L., Rolls, E.T., Hornak, J., & Andrews, C. (2001a). Abstract reward and punishment representations in the human orbitofrontal cortex. *Nature Neuroscience, 4,* 95–102.

O'Doherty, J., Rolls, E.T., Francis, S., McGlone, F., & Bowtell, R. (2001b). The representation of pleasant and aversive taste in the human brain. *Journal of Neurophysiology, 85,* 1315–1321.

Ongur, D., & Price J.L. (2000) The organization of network within the orbital and medial prefrontal cortex of rats, monkeys and humans. *Cerebral Cortex 10*: 206–219.

Passingham, R. (1975). Delayed matching after selective prefrontal lesions in monkeys (*Macaca mulatta*). *Brain Research, 92,* 89–102.

Pandya, D.N. & Yeterian, E.H. (1996). Comparison of prefrontal architecture and connections. *Philosophical*

Transactions of the Royal Society of London, B, 351, 1423–1431.

Petrides, M. & Pandya, D.N. (1994). Comparative architectonic analysis of the human and macaque frontal cortex. In: F. Boller & J. Grafman (Eds.), *Handbook of Neuropsychology, Vol. 9* (pp. 17–58). Amsterdam: Elsevier Science.

Price, J.L., Carmichael, S.T., Carnes, K.M., Clugnet, M.-C., Kuroda, M., & Ray, J.P. (1991). Olfactory input to the prefrontal cortex. In: J.L. Davis & H. Eichenbaum (Eds.), *Olfaction: A Model System for Computational Neuroscience* (pp. 101–20), Cambridge, MA: MIT Press.

Rao, S.C., Rainer, G., & Miller, E.K. (1997). Integration of what and where in the primate prefrontal cortex. *Science, 276,* 821–824.

Renart, A., Moreno, R., de la Rocha, J., Parga, N., & Rolls, E.T. (2001) A model of the IT-PF network in object working memory which includes balanced persistent activity and tuned inhibition. *Neurocomputing* 38–40: 1525–1531.

Renart, A., Parga, N., & Rolls, E.T. (2000). A recurrent model of the interaction between the prefrontal cortex and inferior temporal cortex in delay memory tasks. In: S.A. Solla, T.K. Leen, & K.-R. Mueller (Eds.), *Advances in Neural Information Processing Systems 12,* Cambridge MA: MIT Press.

Rolls, B.J., Rolls, E.T., Rowe, E.A., & Sweeney, K. (1981). Sensory specific satiety in man. *Physiology and Behavior, 27,* 137–142.

Rolls, B.J., Rowe, E.A., & Rolls, E.T. (1982). How sensory properties of foods affect human feeding behavior. *Physiology and Behavior, 29,* 409–417.

Rolls, E.T. (1984a). Neurons in the cortex of the temporal lobe and in the amygdala of the monkey with responses selective for faces. *Human Neurobiology, 3,* 209–222.

Rolls, E.T. (1986a). A theory of emotion, and its application to understanding the neural basis of emotion. In: Y. Oomura (Ed.), *Emotions: Neural and Chemical Control* (pp. 325–344). Tokyo: Japan Scientific Societies Press, and Basel: Karger.

Rolls, E.T. (1986b). Neural systems involved in emotion in primates. In: R. Plutchik & H. Kellerman (Eds.), *Emotion: Theory, Research, and Experience, Vol. 3, Biological Foundations of Emotion* (pp. 125–143). New York: Academic Press.

Rolls, E.T. (1989). Information processing in the taste system of primates. *Journal of Experimental Biology, 146,* 141–164.

Rolls, E.T. (1990). A theory of emotion, and its application to understanding the neural basis of emotion. *Cognition and Emotion, 4,* 161–190.

Rolls, E.T. (1992a). Neurophysiological mechanisms underlying face processing within and beyond the temporal cortical visual areas. *Philosophical Transactions of the Royal Society of London B, 335,* 11–21.

Rolls, E.T. (1992b). Neurophysiology and functions of the primate amygdala. In: J.P.Aggleton (Ed.), *The Amygdala* (pp. 143–65). New York: Wiley-Liss.

Rolls, E.T. (1994a). Brain mechanisms for invariant visual

recognition and learning. *Behavioural Processes, 33,* 113–138.

Rolls, E.T. (1994b). Neural processing related to feeding in primates. In: C.R. Legg & D.A. Booth (Eds.), *Appetite: Neural and Behavioural Bases* (pp. 11–53). Oxford: Oxford University Press.

Rolls, E.T. (1994c). Neurophysiology and cognitive functions of the striatum. *Revue Neurologique (Paris), 150,* 648–660.

Rolls, E.T. (1995a). A theory of emotion and consciousness, and its application to understanding the neural basis of emotion. In: M.S. Gazzaniga (Ed.), *The Cognitive Neurosciences* (pp. 1091–1206). Cambridge, MA: MIT Press.

Rolls, E.T. (1995b). Central taste anatomy and neurophysiology. In: R.L. Doty (Ed.), *Handbook of Olfaction and Gustation* (pp. 549–573). New York: Marcel Dekker.

Rolls, E.T. (1996). The orbitofrontal cortex. *Philosophical Transactions of the Royal Society of London B, 351,* 1433–1444.

Rolls, E.T. (1997a) A neurophysiological and computational approach to the functions of the temporal lobe cortical visual areas in invariant object recognition. In: M. Jenkin & L. Harris (Eds.), *Computational and Psychophysical Mechanisms of Visual Coding* (pp. 184–220). Cambridge, UK: Cambridge University Press.

Rolls, E.T. (1997b). Taste and olfactory processing in the brain and its relation to the control of eating. *Critical Reviews in Neurobiology, 11,* 263–287.

Rolls, E.T. (1999a). *The Brain and Emotion.* Oxford: Oxford University Press.

Rolls, E.T. (1999b). The functions of the orbitofrontal cortex. *Neurocase* 5: 301–312.

Rolls, E.T. (2000a). Functions of the primate temporal lobe cortical visual areas in invariant visual object and face recognition. *Neuron, 27,* 205–218.

Rolls, E.T. (2000b). Memory systems in the brain. *Annual Review of Psychology, 51,* 599–630.

Rolls, E.T. (2000c) Neurophysiology and functions of the primate amygdala, and the neural basis of emotion. In: J.P. Aggleton (Ed.), *The Amygdala: A Functional Analysis,* (pp. 447–478). Oxford: Oxford University Press.

Rolls, E.T. (2000d). Précis of *The Brain and Emotion. Behavioral and Brain Sciences, 23,* 177–233.

Rolls, E.T. (2000f). The orbitofrontal cortex and reward. *Cerebral Cortex, 10,* 284–294.

Rolls, E.T. (2000e). Taste, olfactory, visual and somatosensory representations of the sensory properties of foods in the brain, and their relation to the control of food intake. In H.-R. Berthoud & R.J. Seeley (Eds.), *Neural and Metabolic Control of Macronutrient Intake* (pp. 247–262). Boca-Raton, FL: CRC Press.

Rolls, E.T. (2000g). The representation of umami taste in the taste cortex. *Journal of Nutrition, 130,* S960–S965.

Rolls, E.T. & Baylis, G.C. (1986). Size and contrast have only small effects on the responses to faces of neurons in the cortex of the superior temporal sulcus of the monkey. *Experimental Brain Research, 65,* 38–48.

Rolls, E.T. & Baylis, L.L. (1994). Gustatory, olfactory and

visual convergence within the primate orbitofrontal cortex. *Journal of Neuroscience, 14,* 5437–5452.

Rolls, E.T. & Deco, G. (2002). *Computational Neuroscience of Vision.* Oxford University Press: Oxford.

Rolls, E.T. & Johnstone S. (1992). Neurophysiological analysis of striatal function. In: G. Vallar, S.F. Cappa, & C.W. Wallesch (Eds.), *Neuropsychological Disorders Associated with Subcortical Lesions* (pp. 61–97). Oxford: Oxford University Press.

Rolls, E.T. & Rolls, J.H. (1997). Olfactory sensory-specific satiety in humans. *Physiology and Behavior, 61,* 461–473.

Rolls, E.T. & Scott, T.R. (2002). Central taste anatomy and neurophysiology. In: R.L. Doty (Ed.), *Handbook of Olfaction and Gustation,* 2nd ed. New York: Marcel Dekker.

Rolls, E.T. & Tovee, M.J. (1994). Processing speed in the cerebral cortex and the neurophysiology of visual masking. *Proceedings of the Royal Society of London B, 257,* 9–15.

Rolls, E.T. & Treves, A. (1998). *Neural Networks and Brain Function.* Oxford: Oxford University Press.

Rolls, E.T., Judge, S.J., & Sanghera, M. (1977). Activity of neurones in the inferotemporal cortex of the alert monkey. *Brain Research, 130,* 229–238.

Rolls, E.T., Burton, M.J., & Mora, F. (1980). Neurophysiological analysis of brain-stimulation reward in the monkey. *Brain Research, 194,* 339–357.

Rolls, E.T., Rolls, B.J., & Rowe, E.A. (1983a). Sensory-specific and motivation-specific satiety for the sight and taste of food and water in man. *Physiology and Behavior, 30,* 185–192.

Rolls, E.T., Thorpe, S.J., & Maddison, S.P. (1983b). Responses of striatal neurons in the behaving monkey. 1. Head of the caudate nucleus. *Behavioural Brain Research, 7,* 179–210.

Rolls, E.T., Scott, T.R., Sienkiewicz, Z.J., & Yaxley, S. (1988). The responsiveness of neurones in the frontal opercular gustatory cortex of the macaque monkey is independent of hunger. *Journal of Physiology, 397,* 1–12.

Rolls, E.T., Sienkiewicz, Z.J., & Yaxley, S. (1989). Hunger modulates the responses to gustatory stimuli of single neurons in the caudolateral orbitofrontal cortex of the macaque monkey. *European Journal of Neuroscience, 1,* 53–60.

Rolls, E.T., Yaxley, S., & Sienkiewicz, Z.J. (1990). Gustatory responses of single neurons in the orbitofrontal cortex of the macaque monkey. *Journal of Neurophysiology, 64,* 1055–1066.

Rolls, E.T., Hornak, J., Wade, D., & McGrath, J. (1994). Emotion-related learning in patients with social and emotional changes associated with frontal lobe damage. *Journal of Neurology, Neurosurgery and Psychiatry, 57,* 1518–1524.

Rolls, E.T., Critchley, H., Mason, R., & Wakeman, E.A. (1996a). Orbitofrontal cortex neurons: role in olfactory and visual association learning. *Journal of Neurophysiology, 75,* 1970–1981.

Rolls, E.T., Critchley, H.D., & Treves, A. (1996b). The representation of olfactory information in the primate orbitofrontal cortex. *Journal of Neurophysiology, 75,* 1982–1996.

Rolls, E.T., Critchley, H., Wakeman, E.A., & Mason, R. (1996c). Responses of neurons in the primate taste cortex to the glutamate ion and to inosine 5'-monophosphate. *Physiology and Behavior, 59,* 991–1000.

Rolls, E.T., Francis, S., Bowtell, R., Browning, D., Clare, S., Smith, E., & McGlone, F. (1997a). Pleasant touch activates the orbitofrontal cortex. *NeuroImage, 5,* S17.

Rolls, E.T., Francis, S., Bowtell, R., Browning, D., Clare, S., Smith, E., & McGlone, F. (1997b). Taste and olfactory activation of the orbitofrontal cortex. *NeuroImage, 5,* S199.

Rolls, E.T., Critchley, H.D., Browning, A., & Hernadi, I. (1998) The neurophysiology of taste and olfaction in primates, and umami flavor. *Annals of the New York Academy of Sciences, 855,* 426–437.

Rolls, E.T., Critchley, H.D., Browning, A.S., Hernadi, I., & Lenard, L. (1999a). Responses to the sensory properties of fat of neurons in the primate orbitofrontal cortex. *Journal of Neuroscience, 19,* 1532–1540.

Rolls, E.T., Tovee, M.J., & Panzeri, S. (1999b). The neurophysiology of backward visual masking: information analysis. *Journal of Cognitive Neuroscience, 11,* 335–346.

Rolls, E.T., O'Doherty, J., Kringelbach, M.L., Francis, S., Bowtell, R., & McGlone, F. (2002). The representation of pleasant and aversive touch in the human orbitofrontal cortex.

Rolls, E.T., Critchley, H.D., & Browning, A.S. (in preparation).

Rosenkilde, C.E. (1979). Functional heterogeneity of the prefrontal cortex in the monkey: a review. *Behavioural and Neural Biology, 25,* 301–345.

Rosenkilde, C.E., Bauer, R.H., & Fuster, J.M. (1981). Single unit activity in ventral prefrontal cortex in behaving monkeys. *Brain Research, 209,* 375–394.

Schoenbaum, G. & Eichenbaum, H. (1995). Information encoding in the rodent prefrontal cortex. I. Single-neuron activity in orbitofrontal cortex compared with that in pyriform cortex. *Journal of Neurophysiology, 74,* 733–750.

Schultz, W., Tremblay, L., & Hollerman, J.R. (2000). Reward processing in primate orbitofrontal cortex and basal ganglia. *Cerebral Cortex, 10,* 272–284.

Scott, T.R., Yaxley, S., Sienkiewicz, Z.J., & Rolls, E.T. (1986). Gustatory responses in the frontal opercular cortex of the alert cynomolgus monkey. *Journal of Neurophysiology, 56,* 876–890.

Seltzer, B. & Pandya, D.N. (1989). Frontal lobe connections of the superior temporal sulcus in the rhesus monkey. *Journal of Comparative Neurology, 281,* 97–113.

Small, D.M., Zald, D.H., Jones-Gotman, M., Zatorre, R.J., Pardo, J.V., Frey, S., & Petrides, M. (1999). Human cortical gustatory areas: a review of functional neuroimaging data. *NeuroReport, 10,* 7–14.

Suzuki, W.A., Miller, E.K., & Desimone, R. (1997). Object and place memory in the macaque entorhinal cortex. *Journal of Neurophysiology, 78,* 1062–1081.

Takagi, S.F. (1991). Olfactory frontal cortex and multiple

olfactory processing in primates. *Cerebral Cortex, 9,* (133–152).

Thorpe, S.J., Rolls, E.T., & Maddison, S. (1983). Neuronal activity in the orbitofrontal cortex of the behaving monkey. *Experimental Brain Research, 49,* 93–115.

Valenstein, E.S. (1974). *Brain Control. A Critical Examination of Brain Stimulation and Psychosurgery.* New York: John Wiley & Sons.

Wallis, G. & Rolls, E.T. (1997). Invariant face and object recognition in the visual system. *Progress in Neurobiology, 51,* 167–194.

Williams, G.V., Rolls, E.T., Leonard, C.M., & Stern, C. (1993). Neuronal responses in the ventral striatum of the behaving monkey. *Behavioural Brain Research, 55,* 243–252.

Wilson, F.A.W., O'Sclaidhe, S.P., & Goldman-Rakic, P.S. (1993). Dissociation of object and spatial processing domains in primate prefrontal cortex. *Science, 260,* 1955–1958.

Yaxley, S., Rolls, E.T., & Sienkiewicz, Z.J. (1988). The responsiveness of neurones in the insular gustatory cortex of the macaque monkey is independent of hunger. *Physiology and Behavior, 42,* 223–229.

Yaxley, S., Rolls, E.T., & Sienkiewicz, Z.J. (1990). Gustatory responses of single neurons in the insula of the macaque monkey. *Journal of Neurophysiology, 63,* 689–700.

Zatorre, R.J., Jones-Gotman, M., Evans, A.C., & Meyer, E. (1992). Functional localization of human olfactory cortex. *Nature, 360,* 339–340.

24

Mapping Mood: An Evolving Emphasis on Frontal-Limbic Interactions

HELEN S. MAYBERG

Theories of human behavior have long emphasized a critical connection between emotion and cognition—a relationship now commonly attributed to neural pathways linking limbic striatal and neocortical structures, particularly the frontal lobes. While a fundamental role for limbic regions in the regulation of emotional behavior has been rigorously demonstrated in studies across many species, their links to specific frontal lobe regions are, by contrast, less well characterized. Nonetheless, empiric clinical observations of effects of transient changes in positive and negative mood on attention span, decisiveness, memory, and other cognitive abilities suggest critical interactions among these brain areas in normal emotional processing. Failure of these interactions has also been implicated as a possible mechanism for disorders of mood such as depression and anxiety, with dysregulation, dysfunction or injury to systems mediating normal emotions postulated being a likely substrate for illness. Using this model, one might further hypothesize that if healthy emotional states arise from stereotypical stimuli and produce expected responses, disease states involve the exaggeration or uncoupling of these stimulus–response events, manifesting as inappropriate initiation or persistence of an emotional state in the absence of a provoking stimulus. As such, the delineation of normal pathways mediating the various components of the emotional experience becomes critical to the understanding of emotional disorders. Alternatively, the view that disease states and normal states are fundamentally non-overlapping can also be tested by the use of parallel studies in normal and abnormal subject groups.

Functional and structural neuroimaging studies have taken on a unique role in testing these hypotheses. This chapter will focus on the use of various imaging techniques to elucidate the functional neuroanatomical substrates mediating normal and abnormal mood states. It is in this framework that a model of depression, emphasizing disruption of frontal–subcortical circuits, will be discussed.

SADNESS AND DEPRESSION: WORKING DEFINITIONS

A fundamental role for limbic structures in the regulation of mood and emotional states is now considered a virtual scientific axiom (Mesulam, 1985; Damasio, 1994; LeDoux, 1996). These regions, however, do not function in isolation, with the frontal cortex generally viewed as a critical collaborator. Early observations by Kleist (1937) demonstrating mood and emotional sensations with direct stimulation of the ventral frontal lobes (Brodmann's areas 47 and 11) focused attention on paralimbic frontal regions. Studies by Broca (1878) and, later, Papez (1937), Yakolev (1948), MaClean (1949) and Fulton (1951), elaborated many of the anatomic details of these cytoarchitecturally primitive regions of frontal cortex, as well as adjacent limbic structures, including the cingulate gyrus, amygdala, and hippocampus, and were among the first to suggest a role for these regions in emotional behaviors. Modern comparative anatomical and neurochemical studies have further delineated reciprocal pathways linking various 'limbic' structures with widely distributed brain stem, striatal, paralimbic, and frontal sites (Nauta, 1986; Vogt & Pandya, 1987; Alexander et al., 1990; Carmichael & Price, 1996. Grabiel, 1990; Mesulam & Mufson, 1992; Morecraft et al., 1992; Haber et al., 2000. Links between these regions and pathways mediating reward, motivational, and affect behaviors in animals are well documented (MacLean, 1990; Panksepp et al., 1992; Barbas, 1995; Dias et al., 1996; LeDoux, 1996; Rolls, 1996; Tremblay & Schultz, 1999).

Sadness, behaviorally defined as the sustained state of withdrawl seen in response to loss, is also observed in both animals and humans, often following the death of or separation from offspring. In this state, changes in body posture, disinterest in previously rewarding stimuli, and alterations in basic drive and circadian behaviors (i.e., feeding, reproduction, sleep, endocrine) (Harlow & Suomi, 1974, MacLean, 1990, Panksepp et al., 1991; Cowles, 1996; Levine et al., 1997; Shively et al., 1997) are all readily apparent, and in humans are commonly referred to as *grief* (Zisook & DeVaul, 1985). Despite the apparent consistency of these more chronic behavioral changes across species, there are no good transient or short term stimulus–response models to reliably study these phenomena in animals (Willner, 1991; Thiebot et al., 1992). People, on the other hand, can experience transient sadness in response to both personal internal cues and extrapersonal events. It is this capacity that has been exploited in functional imaging experiments.

SADNESS: PROVOCATION STUDIES IN HEALTHY SUBJECTS

Methods to provoke sad mood are well characterized, with recollection of past personal memories being the most commonly employed tactic (Brewer et al., 1980; Goodwin & Williams, 1982; Martin, 1990). These approaches have been used with great success to reveal brain regions mediating acute changes in emotional state. Furthermore, provocation of transient sadness can be viewed as a potential probe of putative pathways mediating chronic dysphoria in depressed patients.

Pardo et al. (1993) first described blood flow increases using position emission tomography (PET) in superior and inferior prefrontal cortex during spontaneous recollection of previous sad events. Subsequent studies by George et al. (1996), Schneider et al. (1995), Lane et al. (1997), Gemar et al. (1996), Mayberg et al. (1999), Liotti et al. (2000), and Damasio et al. (2000), using a variety of provocation methods, identified additional changes involving varying combinations of regions including the insula, hypothalamus, cerebellum, and amygdala. Across studies, increases in regional activity were most prominent. Frontal decreases reminiscent of resting-state findings in clinically depressed patients were also seen, but not consistently (Gemar et al., 1996; Mayberg et al., 1999; Damasio et al., 2000; Liotti et al., 2000). Timing of scans and the specific instructions appear to have a critical impact on both patterns and direction of regional changes. For example, Mayberg et al. (1999) and Liotti et al. (2000) employed an autobiographical memory paradigm in which scans were acquired only after the sad state was reached and sustained with subjects no longer ruminating on the specifics of the personal situation used to provoke the mood. Ventral limbic and paralimbic increases (subgenual cingulate, anterior insula, and cerebellum) and neocortical decreases (right prefrontal, inferior parietal, and posterior cingulate) were seen with this strategy, replicating some but contradicting other findings previously reported. The anterior cingulate increases closely match findings of George et al. (1996), Partiot et al. (1995), Baker et al. (1997), and Damasio et al. (2000). In contrast, the right prefrontal decreases are the reverse of previous findings, perhaps because of scanning after rather than during active recollection of the sad memory (Pardo et al., 1993; George et al., 1996). In support of this assertion, these decreases also overlap areas shown to activate with sustained attentional tasks in the absence of mood manipulations (Pardo et al., 1991; Corbetta et al., 1993)—behaviors commonly disturbed in depressed patients (Elliott, 1998).

While further corroborative studies are needed, these data suggest plausible mechanisms by which mood, motor, and cognitive states interact (Liotti & Tucker, 1992; Barbas, 1995; Tucker et al., 1995; Heilman, 1997). However, even with well-behaved provocation procedures and well-designed control states, dissociation of regions mediating subjective feelings from autonomic, somatic, and cognitive aspects of an emotional state may not be straightfoward (Lang, 1993; Damasio, 1996).

The importance of frontal, limbic, and striatal interactions in the mediation of negative emotions is further illustrated by a recent case of transient depression during deep-brain stimulation for treatment of intractable Parkinson's disease (Bejjani et al., 1999). Selective high-frequency stimulation to the left substantia nigra (2 mm below the subthalamic site, which alleviated parkinsonian symptoms) provoked a reproducible and reversible depressive syndrome in a woman with no previous psychiatric history. Stimulation-induced mood changes were associated with focal blood flow increases in the left orbital frontal cortex, amygdala, globus pallidus, anterior thalamus, and right parietal cortex. This pattern of regional activation is similar to changes seen with memory-induced sadness in healthy volunteers, although there are clear differences requiring additional further studies. Nonetheless, this remarkable case not only provides important additional clues regarding regional circuits mediating normal and abnormal mood states but also emphasizes the potential utility of carefully evaluating specific behavioral deficits in neurological disease models.

DEPRESSION: A DISEASE MODEL OF ABNORMAL MOOD REGULATION

Medical illness associated with changes in mood, particularly depression, are extremely common. Regardless of disease mechanism, the diagnosis of a major depressive episode is based on the presence of a persistent negative mood state in association with disturbances in attention, motivation, motor and mental speed, sleep, appetite, libido, as well as anhedonia, excessive or inappropriate guilt, recurrent thoughts of death with suicidal ideations, and, in some cases, suicide attempts. Unlike temporary sadness or grief, however, depressive syndromes are not necessarily precipitated by external events or personal loss (American Psychiatric Association, 1994).

Theories implicating focal lesions (Bear, 1983; Robinson et al., 1984), specific neurochemical and neuropeptide systems (Schildkraut, 1965; Fibiger, 1984; Swerdlow & Koob, 1987; Nemeroff, 1996), and selective dysfunction of known neural pathways (Drevets et al., 1992; Mayberg, 1994, 1997) have all been proposed, supported by a growing number of clinical and basic studies (Caldecott-Hazard et al., 1988; Wilner, 1991; Zacharko & Anisman, 1991; Overstreet, 1993; Sapolsky, 1994; Petty et al., 1997; Heim et al., 2000). Patient findings are complemented by parallel experiments of specific cognitive, motor, circadian, and affective behaviors mapped with functional neuroimaging techniques in healthy volunteers, which together suggest that depression is a systems-level disorder, affecting discrete but functionally linked pathways involving specific cortical, subcortical, and limbic sites and their associated neurotransmitter and peptide mediators. It is further postulated that depression is not simply dysfunction of individual regions or pathways, but is a failure of the coordinated interactions among them (Mayberg, 1997). Mechanisms mediating this "failure" are not fully characterized, although genetic vulnerability, developmental insults, and environmental stressors are considered major contributors (Fava & Kendler, 2000). Studies of specific clinical populations have provided important clues.

NEUROLOGICAL DEPRESSION MODELS

ANATOMICAL STUDIES

Neurological diseases associated with depression are common and can be grouped into three primary categories: *(1)* focal lesions such as stroke, trauma, seizure disorders, and tumor (reviewed in Starkstein & Robinson, 1993); *(2)* diseases with diffuse or random pathology such as multiple sclerosis and Alzheimer's disease (Goodstein & Ferrell, 1977; Honer et al., 1987; Zubenko & Moossy, 1988; Cummings & Victoroff, 1990); and *(3)* degenerative disorders with regionally confined pathology such as Parkinson's disease, Huntington's disease, and frontal–temporal dementia (Celesia & Wanamaker, 1972; Caine & Shoulson, 1983; Folstein et al., 1983; Mayberg & Solomon, 1995). These studies have consistently linked dysfunction of frontal cortex and less consistently temporal cortex and the striatum to the presence of mood symptoms. The role of limbic regions is less clear.

The critical role of the frontal lobes is evidenced by a number of studies of focal pathology. Reports of patients with traumatic frontal lobe injury indicate a high correlation between affective disturbances and right hemisphere pathology (Grafman et al., 1986). Studies in stroke, on the other hand, suggest that left-sided lesions of both frontal cortex and the basal ganglia are more likely to result in depressive symptoms than right lesions, where displays of euphoria or indifference predominate, although there is still considerable debate about this (Gainotti, 1972; Ross & Rush, 1981; Sinyor et al., 1986; Starkstein et al., 1987; Mendez et al., 1989; Carson et al., 2000). Further evidence supporting the lateralization of emotional behaviors is provided in studies of pathological laughing and crying. Crying is more common with left hemisphere lesions, while laughter is seen in patients with right lesions (Sackheim et al., 1982), consistent with reports of post-stroke mood changes. Lateralization of mood symptoms have also been examined in patients with temporal lobe epilepsy, although again, there is no consensus, as affective disorders have been described with left, right, and non-lateralized foci (Flor-Henry, 1969; Mendez et al., 1986ţshuler et al., 1990).

Observations of patients undergoing ablative surgery to alleviate refractory melancholia and unremitting emotional ruminations provide complementary evidence for regional localization of mood and affective behaviors (Fulton, 1951; Livingston & Escobar, 1973; Cosgrove & Rausch, 1995; Malizia, 1997). The mechanisms by which these destructive lesions improve mood are unknown, as is the precise lesion site necessary for amelioration of depressive symptoms. Improved mood, however, is seen in many severely ill patients after anterior leukotomy or subcallosal or superior cingulotomy. These seemingly paradoxical effects suggest a more complicated interaction among limbic, paralimbic, and neocortical pathways in both normal and abnormal emotional processing than the lesion-deficit literature would intimate. Also unknown is how dysphoria is related to behaviors such as apathy, executive dysfunction, mood lability, and impulsivity that often co-exist in these patients.

FUNCTIONAL IMAGING STUDIES

Functional imaging (PET, single-photon emission tomography [SPECT], and magnetic resonance spectroscopy, functional magnetic resonance imaging [fMRI]) can complement structural imaging in that the consequences of anatomic or chemical lesions on global and regional brain function (metabolism, blood flow, transmitter) can be additionally assessed. This approach has been an important tool for identifying previously unrecognized brain abnormalities and potential disease mechanisms. These methods additionally provide alternative strategies to test how similar mood symptoms occur with anatomically or neurochemically distinct disease states, or conversely, why comparable lesions do not always result in comparable behavioral phenomena. Parallel studies of primary affective disorder and patients with neurological depressions provide complementary perspectives.

Mayberg, Starkstein and colleagues, in a series of PET imaging studies (Mayberg et al.,

1990, 1991, 1992;) Starkstein et al., 1990.), focused on neurological diseases in which functional abnormalities would not be confounded by gross cortical lesions—specifically, Parkinson's disease, Huntington's disease, and lacunar infarcts involve the basal ganglia. Not only do clinical signs and symptoms in these patients mirror those seen in idiopathic depression, but specific etiological mechanisms have been postulated (Fibiger, 1984; Robinson et al., 1984; Mayeux et al., 1988; Cantello et al., 1989; Peyser & Folstein, 1990). Paralimbic (ventral prefrontal, anterior temporal) hypometabolism differentiated depressed from non-depressed patients within each group, as well as depressed from non-depressed patients, independent of disease etiology (Mayberg, 1994). These results were the first to suggest critical common pathways for the expression of depression in neurological patients, which provided important clues to possible mechanisms mediating mood symptoms in primary mood disorders. These findings have been replicated in patients with Parkinson's disease (Jagust et al., 1992; Ring et al., 1994), as well as in patients with temporal lobe epilepsy (Bromfield et al., 1992), subcortical strokes (Grasso et al., 1994), and Alzheimer's disease (Hirono et al., 1998). The regional localization of changes is similar (but not identical) to that seen in primary depression (shown in the next section) and is consistent with two known pathways: the orbital frontal–striatal–thalamic circuit (Goldman-Rakic & Selemon, 1984; Albin et al., 1989; Alexander et al., 1990), and the basotemporal limbic circuit which links orbital frontal cortex and anterior temporal cortex via the uncinate fasciculus (Papez, 1937; MacLean, 1949; Fulton, 1951; Nauta, 1971, 1986). Disease-specific disruption of converging pathways to these regions (Simon et al., 1979; Azmitia & Gannon, 1986) best explains the presence of similar depressive symptoms in patients with distinctly different disease pathologies.

Involvement of limbic regions such as the amygdala, hippocampus, and hypothalamus has not been prominent in these studies, despite the critical importance of these regions as targets of various antidepressant treatments (Hyman & Nestler, 1996; Blier & de Mon-

tigny, 1999; Duman et al., 1999). Systematic comparisons of frontal–subcortical and cortical-limbic patterns in neurological patients to those identified in patients with primary affective disorders are needed to fully characterize common functional markers of the depressive syndrome. Divergent patterns may additionally provide explanations for subtle and not-so-subtle clinical differences across different "depressed" patient groups, such as the presence of apathy or mood lability.

IDIOPATHIC DEPRESSION

ANATOMICAL STUDIES

Anatomical studies of patients with primary affective disorders have been less consistent than those of depressed patients with neurological disease (reviewed in Soars & Mann, 1997). Focal volume loss in subgenual medial orbital frontal cortex in both unipolar and bipolar depressed patients has been identified, but not consistently (Drevets et al., 1997). Cellular changes have also been reported (Ongur et al., 1998; Rajkowska et al., 1999). Reduced hippocampal and amygdala volumes have also been demonstrated in patients with recurrent major depression (Sheline et al., 1996, 1998), with a postulated mechanism of glucocorticoid neurotoxicity, consistent with both animal models (Sapolsky, 1994) and studies of patients with post-traumatic stress disorder (Bremner et al., 1995). Nonspecific changes in ventricular size and T_2-weighted MRI changes in subcortical gray and periventricular white matter have also been reported in some patient subgroups, most notably, in elderly depressed patients (Zubenko et al., 1990; Coffey et al., 1993; Dupont et al., 1995; Greenwald et al., 1996; Hickie et al., 1997). Recent reports additionally identify a more generalized orbital frontal atrophy in patients with late-life depression suggestive of early anatomical changes seen in Alzheimer's disease (Lai et al., 2000). The parallels, if any, of these observations to the regional abnormalities described in lesion and neurological patients with depression are unclear. Studies of new-onset patients, or preclinical-at-risk subjects, are needed to clarify if these changes reflect disease pathophysiology or are the consequence of chronic illness or treatment.

FUNCTIONAL IMAGING STUDIES

Resting-state PET and SPECT studies in patients with primary depression also report frontal and cingulate abnormalities, in general agreement with the pattern seen in neurological depressions. Across studies, the most robust and consistent finding is decreased frontal lobe function (Buchsbaum et al., 1986; Baxter et al., 1989; George et al., 1994; Lesser et al., 1994; Mayberg et al., 1994, 1997; Ketter et al., 1996; among others). The anatomical localization of frontal changes involves both dorsolateral prefrontal cortex (Brodmann's areas 9, 10, 46) and ventral prefrontal and orbital frontal cortices (Brodmann's areas 10, 11, 47). Findings are generally bilateral, although asymmetries have been reported. Localization of reported cingulate changes involves predominantly anterior dorsal sectors (Bench et al., 1992; Wu et al., 1992; Mayberg, 1994, 1997; Ebert & Ebmeier, 1996). Other limbic–paralimbic (amygdala anterior temporal, insula) and subcortical (basal ganglia, thalamus) abnormalities have also been identified, but the findings are more variable (Buchsbaum et al., 1986; Post et al., 1987; Drevets et al., 1992; Mayberg et al., 1994, 1997; Bonne and Krausz, 1997). Differences among patient subgroups (familial, bipolar, unipolar) and heterogeneous expression of clinical symptoms are thought to contribute to this variance, but there is not yet a consensus. Use of different analytic strategies (voxel-wise versus region of interest) likely also accounts for some of these apparent inconsistencies.

CLINICAL CORRELATES

Many studies demonstrate an inverse relationship between prefrontal activity and depression severity (reviewed by Ketter et al., 1996). Significant correlations have also been shown for psychomotor speed (negative correlations with prefrontal and angular gyrus, Bench et al., 1993a; negative correlation with ventral frontal, Mayberg et al., 1994), anxiety (positive correlation with inferior parietal lobule, Bench et al., 1993a and with parahippocampal gyrus, Osuch et al., 2000), and cognitive performance (positive correlation with medial frontal/cingulate Bench et al., 1993a; Dolan et al., 1992).

Direct mapping of these behaviors is an alternative approach, allowing head-to-head comparisons of patients and healthy controls (Dolan et al., 1993; George et al., 1997). With this type of design, one can both quantify the neural correlates of the performance decrement and identify potential disease-specific sites of task reorganization. These types of studies can be performed with any of the available functional methods, including PET, fMRI, and event-related potentials (ERP) (Whalen et al., 1998; Liotti and Mayberg, 2001).

By example, George et al. (1994, 1997) demonstrated blunting of an expected anterior cingulate increase during performance of a Stroop Task. A shift to the left dorsolateral prefrontal cortex, a region not normally recruited for this task in healthy subjects (Bench et al., 1993b; Whalen et al., 1998), was also observed. Elliot et al., (1997a), using the Tower of London test, described similar attenuation of an expected increase in dorsolateral prefrontal cortex and failure to activate anterior cingulate and caudate—regions recruited in controls. In an additional set of experiments (Elliot et al., 1997b) this group, further demonstrated that, unlike healthy subjects, depressed patients also failed to activate the caudate in response to positive or negative feedback given while they performed the task. The fact that feedback valence influenced cognitive performance in normal subjects and more dramatically in depressed individuals illustrates the highly interactive nature of mood and cognitive systems.

BRAIN CHANGES WITH ANTIDEPRESSANT TREATMENTS

An additional approach to understanding core frontal–limbic systems mediating mood states is to examine state-trait markers revealed during clinical remission. Functional changes in cortical (dorsal/ventral prefrontal, parietal), limbic–paralimbic (cingulate, insula), and subcortical (caudate, thalamus) regions have been described following various types of treatments (medication, sleep deprivation, electroconvulsive therapy [ECT], repetitive transcranial magnetic stimulation [rTMS], ablative surgery). Normalization of frontal hypometabolism is the best-replicated finding, seen mainly with medication (tricyclics, monoamine oxidase inhibitors [MAOIs], various selective serotonin reuptake inhibitors [SSRIs]), suggesting that frontal abnormalities may be state markers of the illness (Baxter et al., 1989; Martinot et al., 1990; Goodwin et al., 1993; Bench et al., 1995; Buchsbaum et al., 1997; Mayberg et al., 1999; Kennedy et al., 2001). Changes in associated limbic, paralimbic, and subcortical regions are more variable (Bonne & Krausz, 1997; Malizia, 1997; Brody et al., 1999; Mayberg et al., 1999; Smith et al., 1999; Teneback et al., 1999; Kennedy et al., 2001). Few drug-treatment studies report regional decreases; although both limbic and cortical decreases are seen in studies of (ECT) (Nobler et al., 2001). No studies have directly compared changes common to antidepressants with different modes of action, although there is a small literature on regional differences associated with response to different medications in bipolar patients (Little et al., 1996). While certain change patterns appear to occur more often than others (prefrontal, anterior cingulate increases; ventral medial frontal decreases), a consistent and reliable pattern has not been demonstrated.

RELATION TO CLINICAL RESPONSE

A critical issue in better understanding the reported variability in location and direction of regional changes with treatment is to consider that drug-induced effects may be different in patients who respond compared to those that do not, as suggested by the pretreatment resting state studies described above. In support of this hypothesis, Mayberg and colleagues (2000) examined regional metabolic changes associated with 6 weeks of fluoxetine treatment in patients with major depression. Distinct patterns of change were seen at 1 week and 6 weeks of treatment, with the time course of metabolic changes reflecting the temporal delay in clinical response. Clinical improvement was associated with limbic–paralimbic and striatal decreases (subgenual cingulate, hippocampus, pallidum, insula) and brain stem and dorsal cortical increases (prefrontal, parietal, anterior/posterior cingulate). Failed response to fluoxetine was associated with a persistent 1-week pattern (hippocampal increases; pallidal, posterior cingulate decreases) and absence of either subgenual cingulate or prefrontal changes. These findings suggest not only an interaction between limbic–paralimbic and neocortical pathways in depression, but differences among patients in adaptation of specific target regions to chronic serotonergic modulation. Failure to induce the requisite adaptive changes might be seen as a contributing cause of treatment non-response. Although specific neurochemical mechanisms for these limbic, paralimbic, and neocortical metabolic changes remain speculative, preclinical studies implicated a series of receptor second messenger and molecular events (Hyman & Nestler, 1996; Vaidya et al., 1997; Blier & de Montigny, 1999; Duman et al., 1999). As placebo responders show comparable changes in neocortex and subgenual cingulate (but not brain stem or hippocampus) to those seen with active drug, it is further hypothesized that clinical response, regardless of treatment mode, requires specific changes in critical target brain regions and pathways (Mayberg et al. 2001a). This hypothesis is the focus of ongoing research.

BASELINE PREDICTORS OF TREATMENT RESPONSE

Mechanisms mediating treatment non-response remains another important unresolved issue. While it is clear that antidepressants and, more variably, cognitive and psychotherapy are generally effective in ameliorating depressive symptoms, some patients fail or have an incomplete response. The incidence of treatment resistance can range anywhere from 20% to 40%, and at present there are no clinical, genetic, or biological markers that identify which patients are likely to respond to a given treatment, explain why one treatment modality or class of medication is effective when another is not, or predict which patients are vulnerable to relapse (Keller et al., 1983; Coryell et al., 1990; Maj et al., 1992).

Recent PET studies have demonstrated that pretreatment rostral (pregenual) cingulate metabolism may be useful in predicting response to pharmacotherapy (Mayberg et al., 1997; Brannan et al., 2000; Pizzagalli et al., 2001). Across studies, hypermetabolism was seen in eventual treatment responders, and hypometabolism in non-responders. A similar hypermetabolic pattern in a nearby region of the dorsal anterior cingulate has also been shown to predict good response to one night of sleep deprivation (Wu et al., 1992, 1999). A related observation has been made in patients with obsessive-compulsive disorder (OCD), where ventral frontal hyper- and hypometabolism preferentially respond to behavioral therapy or medication (Saxena et al., 1999). In bipolar patients, patterns predictive of response to one mood stabilizer over another have also been reported (Ketter et al., 1999). While additional studies are needed, these data suggest physiological differences among patient subgroups that may be critical to understanding brain plasticity and adaptation to illness, including propensity to respond to treatment. Evidence of persistent hypermetabolism in patients in full remission on maintenance SSRI treatment for more than a year further suggests a critical compensatory or adaptive role for rostral cingulate in facilitating and maintaining clinical response (Mayberg et al., 1998).

FRONTAL-LIMBIC DYSREGULATION: A WORKING MODEL OF DEPRESSION

Data presented in this chapter strongly support a critical role for frontal–subcortical circuits and, more specifically, frontal–limbic pathways in the mediation of clinical symptoms in patients with primary and secondary depressions. The overall pattern of cortical, subcortical, and limbic changes suggests the involvement of several well-characterized pathways, schematically organized as an interactive network model (Fig. 24–1; Mayberg, 1997; Mayberg et al., 2000).

Brain regions with known anatomical interconnections that also show consistent and synchronized changes using PET in various behavioral states—transient sadness, baseline depressed, pre- and post-treatment (as described in previous sections of this chapter)—have been grouped into two general compartments: dorsal cortical and ventral limbic. This dorsal–ventral segregation additionally defines those brain regions where an inverse relationship is seen across experiments.

The dorsal–cortical compartment includes primarily neocortical elements, and is postulated to mediate cognitive aspects of negative emotion such as apathy, psychomotor slowing, and impaired attention and executive function, on the basis of complementary structural and functional lesion-deficit correlational studies (Bench et al., 1992; Dolan et al., 1993; Mayberg et al., 1994; Devinsky et al., 1995; Maddock, 1999); symptom-specific treatment effects in depressed patients (Bench et al., 1995a; Buchsbaum et al., 1997; (Mayberg et al., 2000); activation studies designed to explicitly map these behaviors in healthy volunteers (Pardo et al., 1991; George et al., 1996; and connectivity patterns in primates Mesulam, 1985; Morecraft et al., 1993; (Petrides & Pandya, 1984; Barbas, 1995).

The ventral–limbic compartment is composed predominantly of limbic and paralimbic regions known to mediate circadian, somatic, and vegetative aspects of depression including sleep, appetite, libidinal, and endocrine disturbances, according to clinical and related animal studies (MacLean, 1990; Neafsey, 1990; Mesulam & Mufson, 1992; Augustine, 1996).

The rostral cingulate (rCg24a) is isolated from both the ventral and dorsal compartments based on its cytoarchitectural characteristics and reciprocal connections to both dorsal and ventral anterior cingulate (Vogt & Pandya, 1987; Vogt et al., 1995). Contributing to this position in the model are the observations that metabolism in this region uniquely predicts antidepressant response in acutely depressed patients (Mayberg et al., 1997) and is also the principal site of aberrant response during mood induction in remitted depressed patients (Mayberg et al., 1998). These anatomical and clinical distinctions suggest that the

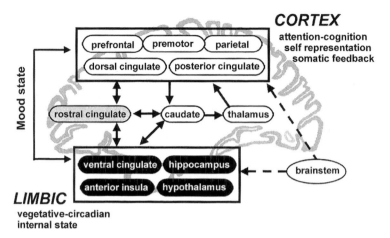

Figure 24–1. Depression model. Regions with known anatomical interconnections that also show synchronized changes using PET in three behavioral states—normal transient sadness (controls), baseline depressed (patients), and post-treatment (patients)—form the basis of this schematic. Regions are grouped into two main compartments, cortical and limbic, both with known connections to subcortical targets, as delineated. The frontal–limbic (dorsal–ventral) segregation additionally identifies those brain regions where an inverse relationship is seen across the different PET paradigms. Sadness and depressive illness are both associated with decreases in dorsal neocortical regions (mainly prefrontal) and relative increases in ventral limbic areas (subgenual cingulate). The model, in turn, proposes that illness remission occurs when there is inhibition of the overactive limbic regions and activation of the previously hypofunctioning cortical areas (solid black arrows), an effect facilitated by various forms of treatment (dotted lines). Integrity of the rostral cingulate with its direct anatomical connections to both the dorsal cortical and ventral limbic compartments is postulated to be additionally required for the occurrence of these adaptive changes, as pretreatment metabolism in this region uniquely predicts antidepressant treatment response. (*Source:* Adapted from Mayberg, 1997; Mayberg et al., 1999, 2000)

rostral anterior cingulate may serve an important regulatory role in the overall network by facilitating the interactions between the dorsal and ventral compartments Petrides & Pandya, 1984; Crino et al., 1993; Pandya & Yeterian, 1996). As such, dysfunction in this area could have significant impact on remote brain regions regulating a variety of behaviors, including the interaction between mood, cognitive, somatic, and circadian responses that characterize an emotional state.

Strategic modulation of specific subcortical (brain stem, hypothalamus, hippocampus, posterior cingulate, and striatal) "nodes" is seen as a primary mechanism for the observed widespread, reciprocal effects in ventral and dorsal cortical–limbic regions seen with various antidepressant treatments (Mayberg et al., 2000). Persistent subgenual cingulate hypometabolism in combination with rostral anterior and posterior cingulate hypermetabolism

in fully recovered, previously depressed patients on long-term maintenance SSRI treatment provides additional evidence that these may be the requisite adaptive metabolic changes needed for sustained clinical remission and mood homeostasis (Mayberg et al., 1998). While additional experimental studies are needed, it is postulated that illness remission, whether facilitated by medication, psychotherapy, ECT, or surgery, requires the reconfiguration of these reciprocally interactive pathways initiated through either top-down (cortical–limbic) or bottom-up (limbic–cortical) interventional strategies. If one assumes that both of these approaches are equally efficacious, the question shifts away from whether suppression of ventral limbic regions allows the normalization of dorsal cortical hypometabolism, or normalization of cortical activity causes a decrease in ventral limbic regions to a focus on patterns and mechanisms underlying successful and failed response to different forms of treatment. The contribution of specific frontal lobe subregions to these issues as well as more complex aspects of emotional processing and mood regulation are as yet unknown but are the focus of intense interest. Future studies examining effective functional connections among these various pathways will provide additional new insights into mechanisms mediating mood homeostasis in health and disease (McIntosh & Gonzalez-Lima, 1994; Mayberg et al., 2001b).

ACKNOWLEDGMENTS

I thank my collaborators Robert Robinson, M.D., Sergio Starkstein, M.D., Ph.D., Stephen Brannan, M.D., Mario Liotti, M.D., Ph.D., and Roderick Mahurin Ph.D., for their significant contributions to the research discussed in this chapter. This work was supported by grants from the National Institute of Mental Health (MH49553), the National Alliance for Research on Schizophrenia and Depression (NARSAD), Eli Lilly and Company, the Charles A. Dana Foundation, the Theodore and Vada Stanley Foundation and the Canadian Institute for Health Research.

REFERENCES

Albin, R.L., Young, A.B., & Penney, J.B. (1989). The functional anatomy of basal ganglia disorders. *Trends in Neuroscience, 12*, 366–375.

Alexander, G.E., Crutcher, M.D., & De Long, M.R. (1990). Basal ganglia-thalamocortical circuits: parallel substrates for motor, oculomotor, 'prefrontal' and 'limbic' functions. *Progress in Brain Research, 85*, 119–146.

Altshuler, L.L., Devinsky, O., Post, R.M., & Theodore, W. (1990). Depression, anxiety, and temporal lobe epilepsy: laterality of focus and symptoms. *Archives of Neurology, 47*, 284–288.

American Psychiatric Association (1994). *Diagnostic and Statistical Manual of Mental Disorders*, fourth edition. Washington, DC: American Psychiatric Association.

Augustine, J.R. (1996). Circuitry and functional aspects of the insular lobe in primates including humans. *Brain Research–Brain Research Reviews, 22*, 229–244.

Azmitia, E.C. & Gannon, P.J. (1986). Primate Serotonergic system: a review of human and animal studies and a report on macaca fascicularis. In S. Fahn (Ed.) *Advances in Neurology*, Vol. 43 (pp. 407–468). New York: Myoclonus, Raven Press.

Baker, S.C., Frith, C.D., & Dolan, R.J. (1997). The interaction between mood and cognitive function studied with PET. *Psychological Medicine, 27*, 565–578.

Barbas, H. (1995). Anatomical Basis of cognitive–emotional interactions in the primate prefrontal cortex. *Neuroscience and Biobehavioral Reviews, 19*, 499–510.

Baxter, L.R., Jr., Schwartz, J.M., Phelps, M.E., Mazziotta, J.C., Guze, B.H., Selin, C.E., Gerner, R.H., & Sumida, R.M. (1989). Reduction of prefrontal cortex glucose metabolism common to three types of depression. *Archives of General Psychiatry, 46*, 243–250.

Bear, D.M. (1983). Hemispheric specialization and the neurology of emotion. *Archives of Neurology, 40*, 195–202.

Bejjani, B.P., Damier, P., Arnulf I., Thivard, L., Bonnet, A.-M., Dormont, D., Cornu, P., Pidoux, B., Samson, Y., & Agid, Y. (1999). Transient acute depression induced by high-frequency deep-brain stimulation. *New England Journal of Medicine, 340*, 1476–1480.

Bench, C.J., Friston, K.J., Brown, R.G., Scott, L.C., Frackowiak, R.S., & Dolan, R.J. (1992). The anatomy of melancholia—focal abnormalities of cerebral blood flow in major depression. *Psychological Medicine, 22*, 607–615.

Bench, C.J., Friston, K.J., Brown, R.G., Franckowiak, R.S., & Dolan, R.J. (1993a). Regional cerebral blood flow in depression measured by positron emission tomography: the relationship with clinical dimensions. *Psychological Medicine, 23*, 579–590.

Bench, C.J., Frith, C.D., Grasby, P.M., Friston, K.J., Paulesu, E., Frackowiak, R.S., & Dolan, R.J. (1993b). Investigations of the functional anatomy of attention using the Stroop test. *Neuropsychologia, 31*, 907–922.

Bench, C.J., Frackowiak, R.S.J., & Dolan, R.J. (1995). Changes in regional cerebral blood flow on recovery from depression. *Psychological Medicine, 25*, 247–251.

Blier, P. & de Montigny, C. (1999). Serotonin and drug-induced therapeutic responses in major depression, obsessive compulsive and panic disorders. *Neuropsychopharmacology, 2*, 170–178.

Bonne, O. & Krausz, Y. (1997). Pathophysiological significance of cerebral perfusion abnormalities in major depression: trait or state marker? *European Neuropsychopharmacology, 7*, 225–233.

Brannan, S.K., Mayberg, H.S., McGinnis, S., Silva, J.A., Mahurin, R.K., Jerabek, P.A., & Fox, P.T. (2000). Cingulate metabolism predicts treatment response: a replication. *Biological Psychiatry, 47* (8S), 107.

Bremner, J.D., Randall, P., Scott, T.M., Bronen, R.A., Delaney, R.C., Seibyl, J.P., Southwick, S.M., McCarthy, G., Charney, D.S., & Innis R.B. (1995). MRI-based measurement of hippocampal volume in post-traumatic stress disorder. *American Journal of Psychiatry, 152*, 973–981.

Brewer, D., Doughtie, E.B., & Lubin, B. (1980). Induction of mood and mood shift. *Journal of Clinical Psychology, 36*, 215–226.

Broca, P. (1878). Anatomie comparée des circonvolutions cérébrales. Le grant lobe limbique et la scissure limbique dans la série des mammifères. *Review Anthropologia, 1*, 385–498.

Brody, A.L., Saxena, S., Silverman, D.H., Alborzian, S., Fairbanks, L.A., Phelps, M.E., Huang, S.C., Wu, H.M., Maidment, K., & Baxter, L.R. (1999). Brain metabolic changes in major depressive disorder from pre to post-treatment with paroxetine. *Psychiatry Research, 9,* 127–139.

Bromfield, E.B., Altschuler, L., Leiderman, D.B., Balish, M., Ketter, T.A., Devinsky, O., Post, R.M., & Theodore, W.H. (1992). Cerebral metabolism and depression in patients with complex partial seizures. *Archives of Neurology, 49,* 617–623.

Buchsbaum, M.S., Wu, J., DeLisi, L.E., Holcomb, H., Kessler, R., Johnson, J., King, A.C., Hazlett, E., Langston, K., & Post, R.M. (1986). Frontal cortex and basal ganglia metabolic rates assessed by positron emission tomography with 18F-2-deoxyglucose in affective illness. *Journal of Affective Disorders, 10,* 137–152.

Buchsbaum, M.S., Wu, J., Siegel, B.V., Hackett, E., Trenary, M., Abel, L., & Reynolds, C. (1997). Effect of sertraline on regional metabolic rate in patients with affective disorder. *Biological Psychiatry, 41,* 15–22.

Caine, E.D. & Shoulson, I. (1983). Psychiatric syndromes in Huntington's disease. *American Journal of Psychiatry, 140,* 728–733.

Caldecott-Hazard, S., Mazziotta, J., & Phelps, M. (1988). Cerebral correlates of depressed behavior in rats, visualized using 14C-2-deoxyglucose autoradiography. *Journal of Neuroscience, 8,* 1951–1961.

Cantello, R., Aguaggia, M., Gilli, M., Delsedime M., Chiardo Cutin I., Riccio, A., & Mutani, R. (1989). Major depression in Parkinson's disease and the mood response to intravenous methylphenidate: possible role of the "hedonic" dopamine synapse. *Journal of Neurology, Neurosurgery, and Psychiatry, 52,* 724–731.

Carmichael, S.T. & Price, J.L. (1996). Connectional networks within the orbital and medial prefrontal cortex of macaque monkeys. *Journal of Comparative Neurology, 371,* 179–207.

Carson, A.J., MacHale, S., Allen, K., Lawrie, S.M., Dennis, M., House, A., & Sharpe, M. (2000). Depression after stroke and lesion location: a sytstematic review. *Lancet, 356,* 122–126.

Celesia, G.G. & Wanamaker, W.M. (1972). Psychiatric disturbances in Parkinson's disease. *Diseases of the Nervous System, 33,* 577–583.

Coffey, C.E., Wilkinson, W.E., Weiner, R.D., Parashos, L.A., Djang, W.T., Webb, M.C., Figiel, G.S., & Spritzer, C.E. (1993). Quantitative cerebral anatomy in depression: a controlled magnetic resonance imaging study. *Archives of General Psychiatry, 50,* 7–16.

Corbetta, M., Miezin, F.M., Shulman, G.L., & Petersen, S.E. (1993). A PET study of visuospatial attention. *Journal of Neuroscience, 13,* 1020–1226.

Coryell, W., Endicott, J., & Keller, M.B. (1990). Outcome of patients with chronic affective disorders: a five-year follow-up. *American Journal of Psychiatry, 147,* 1627–1633.

Cosgrove, G.R. & Rauch, S.L. (1995). Psychosurgery. *Neurosurgery Clinic of North America, 6,* 167–176.

Cowles, K.V. (1996). Cultural perspectives of grief: an expanded concept analysis. *Journal of Advances in Nursing, 23,* 287–294.

Crino, P.B., Morrison, J.H., & Hof, P.R. (1993). Monoamine inervation of cingulate cortex. In: B.A. Vogt & M. Gabriel (Eds.), *The Neurobiology of Cingulate Cortex & Limbic Thalamus: A Comprehensive Handbook* (pp. 285–310). Boston: Birkhauser.

Cummings, J.L. & Victoroff, J.I. (1990). Noncognitive neuropsychiatric syndromes in Alzheimer's disease. *Neuropsychiatry, Neuropsychology, and Behavioral Neurology, 2,* 140–158.

Damasio, A.R. (1994). *Descartes' Error: Emotion, Reason and the Human Brain.* New York: Grosset Putnam.

Damasio, A.R. (1996). The somatic marker hypothesis and the possible functions of the prefrontal cortex. *Philosophical Transactions of the Royal Society of London Series B: Biological Sciences, 351 (1346),* 1413–1420.

Damasio, A.R., Grabowsky, T.J., Bechara, A., Damasio, H., Ponto, L.L., Parvizi, J., & Hichwa, R.D. (2000). Subcortical and cortical brain activity during the feeling of self-generated emotions. *Nature Neuroscience, 3,* 1049–1056.

Devinsky, O., Morrell, M.J., & Vogt, B.A. (1995). Contributions of anterior cingulate cortex to behavior. *Brain, 118,* 279–306.

Dias, R., Robbins, T.W., & Roberts, A.C. (1996). Dissociation in prefrontal cortex of affective and attentional shifts. *Nature, 380,* 69–72.

Dolan, R.J., Bench, C.J., Brown, R.G., Scott, L.C., Friston, K.J., & Frackowiak, R.S. (1992). Regional cerebral blood flow abnormalities in depressed patients with cognitive impairment. *Journal of Neurology, Neurosurgery and Psychiatry, 55,* 768–773.

Dolan, R.J., Bench, C.J., Liddle, P.F., Friston, K.J., Frith, C.D., Grasby, P.M., & Frackowiak, R.S. (1993). Dorsolateral prefrontal cortex dysfunction in the major psychoses; symptom or disease specificity? *Journal of Neurology, Neurosurgery and Psychiatry, 56,* 1290–1294.

Drevets, W.C., Videen, T.O., Price, J.L., Preskorn, S.H., Carmichael, S.T., & Raichle, M.E. (1992). A functional anatomical study of unipolar depression. *Journal of Neuroscience, 12,* 3628–3641.

Drevets, W.C., Price, J.L., Simpson, J.R., Jr., Todd, R.D., Reich, T., Vannier, M., & Raichle, M.E. (1997). Subgenual prefrontal cortex abnormalities in mood disorders. *Nature, 386,* 824–827.

Duman, R.S., Malberg, J., & Thome, J. (1999). Neural plasticity to stress and antidepressant treatment. *Biological Psychiatry, 46,* 1181–1191.

Dupont, R.M., Jernigan, T.L., Heindel, W., Butters, N., Shafer, K., Wilson, T., Hesselink, J., & Gillin, J.C. (1995). Magnetic resnonance imaging and mood disorders: localization of white matter and other subcortical abnormalities. *Archives of General Psychiatry, 52,* 747–755.

Ebert, D. & Ebmeier, K.P. (1996). Role of the cingulate gyrus in depression: from functional anatomy to depression. *Biological Psychiatry, 39,* 1044–1050.

Elliott, R. (1998). The neuropsycholoigcal profile in unipolar depression. *Trends in Cognitive Science, 2,* 447–454.

Elliott, R., Baker, S.C., Rogers, R.D., O'Leary, D.A., Paykel, E.S., Frith C.D., Dolan, R.J., & Sahakian, B.J. (1997a). Prefrontal dysfunction in depressed patients performing a complex planning task: a study using positron emission tomography. *Psychological Medicine, 27,* 931–942.

Elliott, R., Sahakian, B.J., Herrod, J.J., Robbins, T.W., & Paykel, E.S. (1997b). Abnormal response to negative feedback in unipolar depression: evidence for a diagnosis specific impairment. *Journal of Neurology, Neurosurgery and Psychiatry, 63,* 74–82.

Fava, M. & Kendler, K.S. (2000). Major depressive disorder. *Neuron, 28,* 335–341.

Fibiger, H.C. (1984). The neurobiological substrates of depression in Parkinson's disease: a hypothesis. *Canadian Journal Neurological Science, 11,* 105–107.

Flor-Henry, P. (1969). Psychosis and temporal lobe epilepsy. *Epilepsia, 10,* 363–395.

Folstein, S.E., Abbott, M.H., Chase, G.A., Jensen, B.A., & Folstein, M.F. (1983). The association of affective disorder with Huntington's disease in a case series and in families. *Psychological Medicine, 13,* 537–542.

Fulton, J.F. (1951). *Frontal Lobotomy and Affective Behavior: A Neurophysiological Analysis.* London: Chapman and Hall.

Gainotti, G. (1972). Emotional behavior and hemispheric side of the lesion. *Cortex, 8,* 41–55.

Gemar, M.C., Kapur, S., Segal, Z.V., Brown, G.M., & Houle, S. (1996). Effects of self-generated sad mood on regional cerebral activity: a PET study in normal subjects. *Depression, 4,* 81–88.

George, M.S., Ketter, T.A., & Post, R.M. (1994). Prefrontal cortex dysfunction in clinical depression. *Depression, 2,* 59–72.

George, M.S., Ketter, T.A., Parekh, P.I., Herscovitch, P., & Post, R.M. (1996). Gender differences in regional cerebral blood flow during transient self-induced sadness or happiness. *Biological Psychiatry, 40,* 859–871.

George, M.S., Ketter, T.A., Parekh, P.I., Rosinsky, N., Ring, H.A., Pazzaglia, P.J., Marangell, L.B., Callahan, A.M., & Post, R.M. (1997). Blunted left cingulate activation in mood disorder subjects during a response interference task (the Stroop). *Journal of Neuropsychiatry and Clinical Neurosciences, 9,* 55–63.

Goldman-Rakic, P.S. & Selemon, L.D. (1984). Topography of corticostriatal projections in nonhuman primates and implications for functional parcellation of the neostriatum. In: E.G. Jones & A. Peters (Eds.), *Cerebral Cortex* (pp. 447–466). New York: Plenum Press.

Goodstein, R.K. & Ferrel, R.B. (1977). Multiple sclerosis presenting as depressive illness. *Diseases Nervous System, 38,* 127–131.

Goodwin, A.M. & Williams, J.M.G. (1982). Mood-induction research: its implications for clinical depression. *Behavioral Research and Therapeutics, 20,* 373–382.

Goodwin, G.M., Austin, M.P., Dougall, N., Ross, M., Murray, C., O'Carroll, R.E., Moffoot, A., Prentice, N., & Ebmeier, K.P. (1993). State changes in brain activity shown by the uptake of 99mTc-exametazime with single photon emission tomography in major depression before and after treatment. *Journal of Affective Disorders, 29,* 243–253.

Grabiel, A.M. (1990). Neurotransmitters and neuromo-dulators in the basal ganglia. *Trends in Neuroscience, 13,* 244–254.

Grafman, J., Vance, S.C., Weingartner H., Salazar, A.M., & Amin, D. (1986). The effects of lateralized frontal lesions on mood regulation. *Brain, 109,* 1127–1148.

Grasso, M.G., Pantano, P., Ricci, M., Intiso, D.F., Pace, A., Padovani, A., Orzi, F., Pozzilli, C., & Lenzi, G.L. (1994). Mesial temporal cortex hypoperfusion is associated with depression in subcortical stroke. *Stroke, 25,* 980–985.

Greenwald, B.S., Kramer-Ginsberg, E., Krishnan, R.R., Ashtari, M., Aupperle, P.M., & Patel, M. (1996). MRI signal hyperintensities in geriatric depression. *American Journal of Psychiatry, 153,* 1212–1215.

Haber, S.N., Fudge, J.L. & McFarland, N.R. (2000) Striatonigrostriatal pathways in primates form an ascending spiral from the shell to the dorsolateral striatum *Journal of Neuroscience 20,* 2369–2382.

Heim, C., Newport, D.J., Heit, S., Graham, Y.P., Wilcox, M., Bonsall, R., Miller, A.H., & Nemeroff, C.B. (2000). Pituitary-adrenal and autonimic responses to stress in women after sexual and physical abuse in childhood. *Journal of the American Medical Association, 284,* 592–597.

Harlow, H.F. & Suomi, S.J. (1974). Induced depression in monkeys. *Behhavior Biology 12,* 273–296.

Heilman, K.M. (1997). The neurobiology of emotional experience. *Journal of Neuropsychiatry Clinical Neuroscience, 9,* 439–448.

Hickie, I., Scott, E., Wilhelm, K., & Brodaty, H. (1997). Subcortical hyperintensities on magnetic resonance imaging in patients with severe depression—a longitudinal evaluation. *Biological Psychiatry, 42,* 367–374.

Hirono, N., Mori, E., Ishii, K., Ikejire, Y., Imamura, T., Shimomura, T., Hashimoto, M., Yamashita, H., & Sasaki, M. (1998). Frontal lobe hypometabolism and depression in Alzheimer's disease. *Neurology, 50,* 380–383.

Honer, W.G., Hurwitz, T., Li, D.K., Palmer, M., & Paty, D.W. (1987). Temporal lobe involvement in multiple sclerosis patients with psychiatric disorders. *Archives of Neurology, 44,* 187–190.

Hyman, S.E. & Nestler, E.J. (1996). Initiation and adaptation: a paradigm for understanding psychotropic drug action. *American Journal of Psychiatry, 153,* 151–162.

Jagust, W.J., Reed, B.R., Martin, E.M., Eberling, J.L., & Nelson-Abbott, R.A. (1992). Cognitive function and regional cerebral blood flow in Parkinson's disease. *Brain, 115,* 521–537.

Keller, M.B., Lavori, P.W., & Klerman, G.L. (1983). Predictors of relapse in major depressive disorder. *Journal of the American Medical Association, 250,* 3299–3304.

Kennedy, S.H., Evans, K., Kruger, S., Mayberg, H.S., Meyer, J.H., McCann, S., Arufuzzman, A., Houle, S., & Vaccarino, F.J. (2001). Changes in regional glucose metabolism with PET following paroxetine treatment for major depression. *American Journal of Psychiatry, 158,* 899–905.

Ketter, T.A., George, M.S., Kimbrell, T.A., Benson B.E., & Post, R.M. (1996). Functional brain imaging, limbic function, and affective disorders. *Neuroscientist, 2*, 55–65.

Ketter, T.A., Kimbrell, T.A., George, M.S., Willis, M.W., Benson, B.E., Danielson, A., Frye, M.A., Herscovitch, P., & Post, R.M. (1999). Baseline cerebral hypermetabolism associated with carbamezepine response, and hypometabolism with nimodipine response in mood disorders. *Biological Psychiatry, 46*, 1364–1374.

Kleist, K. (1937). Bericht über die Gehirnpathologie in ihrer Bedeutung für Neurologie und Psychiatrie. *Zeitschrift für die Gesamte Neurologie und Psychiatrie, 158*, 159–93.

Lai, T., Payne, M.E., Byrum, C.E., Steffens, D.C., & Krishnan, K.R. (2000). Reduction of orbital frontal cortex volume in geriatric depression. *Biological Psychiatry, 14*, 971–975.

Lane, R.D., Reiman, E.M., Ahern, G.L., Schwartz, G.E., & Davidson, R.J. (1997). Neuranatomical correlates of happiness, sadness and disgust. *American Journal of Psychiatry, 154*, 926.

Lang, P.J., Greenwald, M.K., Bradley, M.M., & Hamm, A.O. (1993). Looking at pictures: affective, facial, visceral, and behavioral reactions. *Psychophysiology, 30*, 261–273.

LeDoux, J. (1996). The Emotional Brain. New York: Simon and Schuster.

Lesser, I., Mena, I., Boone, K.B., Miller, B.L., Mehringer, C.M., & Wohl, M. (1994). Reduction of cerebral blood flow in older depressed patients. *Archives of General Psychiatry, 51*, 677–686.

Levine, S., Lyons, D.M., & Schatzberg, A.F. (1997). Psychobiological consequences of social relationships. *Annals of the New York Academy of Sciences, 807*, 210–218.

Liotti, M. & Mayberg, H.S. (2001). The role of functional neuroimaging in the neuropsychology of depression. *Journal of Clinical Experimental Neuropsychology, 23*, 121–136.

Liotti, M. & Tucker, D.M. (1992). Right hemisphere sensitivity to arousal and depression. *Brain and Cognition, 18*, 138–151.

Liotti, M., Mayberg, H.S., Brannan, S.K., McGinnis, S., Jerabek, P.A., Martin, C.C., & Fox, P.T. (2000). Differential neural correlates of sadness and fear in healthy subjects: implications for affective disorders. *Biological Psychiatry, 48*, 30–42.

Little, J.T., Ketter, T.A., Kimbrell, T.A., Danielson, A., Benson, B., Willis, M.W., & Post, R.M. (1996). Venlafaxine or buproprion responders but not nonresponders show baseline prefrontal and paralimbic hypometabolism compared with controls. *Psychopharmacology Bulletin, 32*, 629–635.

Livingston, K.E. & Escobar, A. (1973). Tentative limbic system models for certain patterns of psychiatric disorders. In: V. Laitinen & K.E. Livingstone (Eds.), *Surgical Approaches in Psychiatry* (pp. 245–252). Lancaster: Medical and Technical Publishing Co.

MacLean, P.D. (1949). Psychosomatic disease and the visceral brain. Recent developments bearing on the Papez theory of emotion. *Psychosomatic Medicine, 11*, 338–353.

MacLean, P.D. (1990). *The Triune Brain in Evolution: Role in Paleocerebral Function.* New York: Plenum Press.

Maddock, R.J. (1999). The retrosplenial cortex and emotion: new insights from functional neuroimaging of the human brain. *Trends in Neuroscience, 22*, 310–316.

Maj, M., Veltro, F., Pirozzi, R., Lobrace, S., & Magliano, L. (1992). Patterns of recurrence of illness after recovery from an episode of major depression: a prospective study. *American Journal of Psychiatry, 149*, 795–800.

Malizia, A. (1997). Frontal lobes and neurosurgery for psychiatric disorders. *Journal of Psychopharmacology, 11*, 179–187.

Martin, M. (1990). On the induction of mood. *Clinical Psychology Review, 10*, 669–697.

Martinot, J.L., Hardy, P., Feline, A., Huret, J.D., Mazoyer, B., Attar-Levy, D., Pappata, S., & Syrota, A. (1990). Left prefrontal glucose hypometabolism in the depressed state: a confirmation. *American Journal of Psychiatry, 147*, 1313–1317.

Mayberg, H.S. (1994). Frontal lobe dysfunction in secondary depression. *Journal of Neuropsychiatry and Clinical Neuroscences, 6*, 428–442.

Mayberg, H.S. (1997). Limbic-cortical dysregulation: a proposed model of depression. *Journal of Neuropsychiatry and Clinical Neurosciences, 9*, 471–481.

Mayberg, H.S., Starkstein, S.E., Sadzot, B., Preziosi, T., Andrezejewski, P.L., Dannals, R.F., Wagner, H.N., Jr., & Robinson, R.G. (1990). Selective hypometabolism in the inferior frontal lobe in depressed patients with Parkinson's disease. *Annals of Neurology, 28*, 57–64.

Mayberg, H.S., Starkstein, S.E., Morris, P.L., Federoff, J.P., Price, T.R., Dannals, R.F., Wagner, H.N., & Robinson, R.G. (1991). Remote cortical hypometabolism following focal basal ganglia injury: relationship to secondary changes in mood. *Neurology, 41* (suppl), 266.

Mayberg, H.S., Starkstein, S.E., Peyser, C.E., Brandt, J., Dannals, R.F., & Folstein, S.E. (1992). Paralimbic frontal lobe hypometabolism in depression associated with Huntington's disease. *Neurology, 42*, 1791–1797.

Mayberg, H.S., Lewis, P.J., Regenold, W., & Wagner, H.N., Jr. (1994). Paralimbic hypoperfusion in unipolar depression. *Journal of Nuclear Medicine, 35*, 929–934.

Mayberg, H.S. & Solomon, D.H. (1995). Depression in PD: a biochemical and organic viewpoint. In: W.J. Weiner & A.E. Lang (Eds.), *Behavioral Neurology of Movement Disorders, Advances in Neurology Vol. 65* (pp. 49–60). New York: Raven Press.

Mayberg, H.S., Brannan, S.K., Mahurin, R.K., Jerabek, P.A., Brickman, J.S., Tekell, J.L., Silva, J.A., McGinnis, S., Glass, T.G., Martin, C.C., & Fox, P.T. (1997). Cingulate function in depression: a potential predictor of treatment response. *NeuroReport, 8*, 1057–1061.

Mayberg, H.S., Liotti, M., Brannan, S.K., McGinnis, S., Jerabek, P.A., Martin, C.C., & Fox, P.T. (1998). Disease and state-specific effects of mood challenge on rCBF. *NeuroImage, 7*, S901.

Mayberg, H.S., Liotti, M., Brannan, S.K., McGinnis, S., Mahurin, R.K., Jerabek, P.A., Silva, J.A., Tekell, J.L., Martin, C.C., Lancaster, J.L., & Fox, P.T. (1999). Reciprocal limbic-cortical function and negative mood:

converging pet findings in depression and normal sadness. *American Journal of Psychiatry, 156*: 675–682.

Mayberg, H.S., Brannan, S.K., Mahurin, R.K., McGinnis, S., Silva, J.A., Tekell, J.L., Jerabek, P.A., Martin, C.C., & Fox, P.T. (2000). Regional metabolic effects of fluoxetine in major depression: serial changes and relationship to clinical response. *Biological Psychiatry, 48*, 830–843.

Mayberg, H.S., Silva, J.A., Brannan, S.K., Tekell, J.L., Mahurin, R.K., McGinnin, S., & Jerabek, P.A. (2001a). The functional neuroanatomy of the placebo effect. *American Journal of Psychiatry*, (in press.)

Mayberg, H.S., Westmacott, R., & McIntosh, A.R. (2001b). Network analysis of trait and state abnormalities in depression. *NeuroImage, 13*, S1071.

McIntosh, A.R. & Gonzalez-Lima, F. (1994). Structural equation modeling and its application to network analysis in functional brain imaging. *Human Brain Mapping, 2*: 2–22.

Mendez, M.F., Cummings, U.L., & Benson, D.F. (1986). Depression in epilepsy. *Archives of Neurology, 43*, 766–770.

Mendez, M.F., Adams, N.L., & Lewandowski, K.S. (1989). Neurobehavioral changes associated with caudate lesions. *Neurology, 39*, 349–354.

Mesulam, M.-M. (1985). Patterns in behavioral neuroanatomy: association areas, the limbic system, and hemispheric specialization. In: M.-M. Mesulam (Ed.), *Principles of Behavioral Neurology* (pp. 1–70). Philadelphia: F.A. Davis.

Mesulam, M.-M. & Mufson, E.J. (1992). Insula of the old world monkey I, II, III. *Journal of Comparative Neurology, 212*, 1–52.

Morecraft, R.J., Geula, C., & Mesulam, M.-M. (1992). Architecture of connectivity within a cingul-fronto-parietal neurocognitive network for directed attention. *Archives of Neurology, 50*, 279–284.

Nauta, W.J.H. (1971). The problem of the frontal lobe: a reinterpretation. *Journal Psychological Research, 8*, 167–187.

Nauta, W.J.H. (1986). Circuitous connections linking cerebral cortex, limbic system, and corpus striatum. In: B.K. Doane & K.E. Livingston (Eds.), *The Limbic System: Functional Organization and Clinical Disorders* (pp. 43–54). New York: Raven Press.

Neafsey, E.J. (1990). Prefrontal cortical control of the autonomic nervous system: anatomical and physiological observations. *Progress in Brain Research, 85*, 147–66.

Nemeroff, C.B. (1996). The corticotropin-releasing factor (CRF) hypothesis of depression: new findings and new directions. *Molecular Psychiatry, 1*, 336–342.

Nobler, M.S., Oquendo, M., Kegeles, L.S., Malone, K.M., Campbell, C.C., Sackeim, H.A., & Mann, J.J. (2001). Decreased regional brain metabolism after ECT. *American Journal of Psychiatry, 158*, 305–308.

Ongur, D., Drevet, W.C., & Price, J.L. (1998). Glial reduction in the subgenual prefrontal cortex in mood disorders. *Proceedings of the National Academy of Sciences USA, 95*, 13290–13295.

Osuch, E.A., Ketter, T.A., Kimbrell, T.A., George, M.S., Benson, B.E., Willis, M.W., Hercovitch, P., & Post, R.M. (2000). Regional cerebral metabolism associated with anxiety symptoms in affective disorder patients. *Biological Psychiatry, 48*, 1020–1030.

Overstreet, D.H. (1993). The Flinders sensitive line rats: a genetic animal model of depression. *Neuroscience and Biobehavioral Review, 17*, 51–68.

Pandya, D.N. & Yeterian, E.H. (1996). Comparison of prefrontal architecture and connections. *Philosophical Transactions of the Royal Society, London, Series B: Biological Sciences, 351*, 1423–1432.

Panksepp, J., Yates, G., Ikemoto, S., & Nelson, E. (1991). Simple ethological models of depression: social-isolation induced "despair" in chicks and mice. *Animal Models in Psychopharmacology, Advances in Pharmacological Sciences* Basel: (pp. 161–181). Birkhauser Verlag.

Panksepp, J., Newman, J.D., & Insel, T.R. (1992). Critical conceptual issues in the analysis of separation-distress systems in the brain. In:K.T. Strongman (Ed.), *International Review of Studies on Emotion, Vol. 2*. (pp. 51–72). New York: John Wiley and Sons.

Papez, J.W. (1937). A proposed mechanism of emotion. *Archives of Neurology and Psychiatry, 38*, 725–743.

Pardo, J.V., Raichle, M.E., & Fox, P.T. (1991). Localization of a human system for sustained attention by positron emission tomography. *Nature, 349*, 61–63.

Pardo, J.V., Pardo, P.J., & Raichle, M.E. (1993). Neural correlates of self-induced dysphoria. *American Journal of Psychiatry, 150*, 713–719.

Partiot, A., Grafman, J., Sadato, N., Wachs, J., & Hallett, M. (1995). Brain activation during the generation of non-emotional and emotional plans. *NeuroReport, 6*, 1397–4000.

Petrides, M. & Pandya, D.N. (1984). Projections to the frontal cortex from the posterior parietal region in the rhesus monkey. *Journal of Comparative Neurology, 228*, 105–16

Petty, F., Kramer, G.L., Wu, J., & Davis, L.L. (1997). Post-traumatic stress and depression: a neurochemical anatomy of the learned helplessness animal model. *Annals of the New York Academy of Sciences, 821*, 529–532.

Peyser, C.E., & Folstein, S.E. (1990). Huntington's disease as a model for mood disorders: clues from neuropathology and neurochemistry. *Molecular and Chemical Neuropathology, 12*, 99–119.

Pizzagalli, D., Pascual-Marqui, R.D., Nitschke, J.B., Oakes, T.R., Larson, C.L., Abercrombie, H.C., Schaefer, S.M., Koger, J.V., Benca, R.M., & Davidson, R.J. (2001). Anterior cingulate activity as a predictor of degree of treatment response in major depression: evidence from brain electrical tomography analysis. *American Journal of Psychiatry, 158*, 405–415.

Post, R.M., DeLisi, L.E., Holcomb, H.H., Uhde, T.W., Cohen, R., & Buchsbaum, M.S. (1987). Glucose utilization in the temporal cortex of affectively ill patients: positron emission tomography. *Biological Psychiatry, 22*, 545–553.

Rajkowska, G., Miguel-Hidalgo, J.J., Wei, J., Dilley, G., Pittman, S.D., Meltzer, H.Y., Overholser, J.C., Roth, B.L., & Stockmeier, C.A. (1999). Morpometric evidence for neuronal and glial prefrontal cell pathology in major depression. *Biological Psychiatry, 45,* 1085–1098.

Ring, H.A., Bench, C.J., Trimble, M.R., Brooks, D.J., Frackowiak, R.S., & Dolan, R.J. (1994). Depression in Parkinson's disease. A positron emission study. *British Journal of Psychiatry, 165,* 333–339.

Robinson, R.G., Kubos, K.L., Starr, L.B., Rao, K., & Price, T.R. (1984). Mood disorders in stroke patients: importance of location of lesion. *Brain, 107,* 81–93.

Rolls, E.T. (1996). The orbitofrontal cortex. *Philosophical Transactions of the Royal Society, London, Series B: Biological Sciences, 351,* 1433–1444.

Ross, E.D. & Rush, A.J. (1981). Diagnosis and neuroanatomical correlates of depression in brain-damaged patients. *Archives of General Psychiatry, 39,* 1344–1354.

Sackeim, H., Greenberg, M.S., Weiman, A.L., Gur, R.C., Hungerbuhler, J.P., & Geschwind, N. (1982). Hemispheric asymmetry in the expression of positive and negative emotions. *Archives of Neurology, 39,* 210–218.

Sapolsky, R.M. (1994). The physiological relevance of glucocorticoid endangerment of the hippocampus. *Annals of the New York Academy of Sciences. 746,* 294–304.

Saxena, S., Brody, A.L., Maidment, K.M., Dunkin, J.J., Golgan, M., Alborzian, S., Phelps, M.E., & Baxter, L.R. (1999). Localized orbitofrontal and subcortical metabolic changes and predictors of response to paroxetine treatment in OCD. *Neuropsychopharmacology, 21,* 683–693

Schildkraut, J.J. (1965). The catecholamine hypothesis of affective disorders: a review of supporting evidence. *American Journal of Psychiatry, 122,* 509–522.

Schneider, F., Gur, R.E., Mozley, L.H., Smith, R.J., Mozley, P.D., Censits, D.M., Alavi, A., & Gur, R.C. (1995). Mood effects on limbic blood flow correlate with emotional self-rating: a PET study with O-15 labeled water. *Psychiatric Research, 61,* 265–283.

Sheline, Y.I., Wang, P.W., Gado, M.H., Csernansky, J.G., & Vannier, M.W. (1996). Hippocampal atrophy in recurrent major depression. *Proceedings of the National Academy of Sciences USA, 93,* 3908–3913.

Sheline, Y.I., Gado, M.H., & Price J.L. (1998). Amygdala core nuclei volumes are decreased in recurrent major depression. *NeuroReport, 22,* 2023–2028.

Shively, C.A., Laber-Laird, K., & Anton, R.F. (1997). Behavior and physiology of social stress and depression in female cynomolgus monkeys. *Biological Psychiatry, 41,* 871–882.

Simon, H., LeMoal, M., & Calas, A. (1979). Efferents and afferents of the ventral tegmental-A$_{10}$ region studied after local injection of [³H]-leucine and horseradish peroxidase. *Brain Research, 178,* 17–40.

Sinyor, D., Jacques, P., Kaloupek, D.G., Becker, R., Goldenberg, M., & Coopersmith, H. (1986). Post stroke depression and lesion location: an attempted replication. *Brain, 109,* 537–546.

Smith, G.S., Reynolds, C.F., Pollock, B., Derbyshire, S., Nofzinger, E., Dew, M.A., Houck, P.R., Milko, D., Melzer, C.C., & Kupfer, D.J. (1999). Cerebral glucose metabolic response to combined total sleep deprivation and antidepressant treatment in geriatric depression. *American Journal of Psychiatry, 156,* 683–689.

Soars, J.C. & Mann, J.J. (1997). The anatomy of mood disorders—review of structural neuroimaging studies. *Biological Psychiatry, 41,* 86–106.

Starkstein, S.E., Robinson, R.G., & Price, T.R. (1987). Comparison of cortical and subcortical lesions in the production of post-stroke mood disorders. *Brain, 110,* 1045–1059.

Starkstein, S.E., Mayberg, H.S., Berthier, M.L., Fedoroff, P., Price, T.R., Dannals, R.F., Wagner, H.N., Leiguarda, R., & Robinson, R.G. (1990). Mania after brain injury: neuroradiological and metabolic findings. *Annals of Neurology, 27,* 652–659.

Starkstein, S.E. & Robinson, R.G. (Eds.). (1993) *Depression in Neurologic Diseases.* Baltimore: Johns Hopkins University Press.

Swerdlow, N.R. & Koob, G.F. (1987). Dopamine, Schizophrenia, mania and depression: towards a unified hypothesis of cortico-striato-pallido-thalamic function. *Behavioral Brain Science, 10,* 197–245.

Teneback, C.C., Nahas, Z., Speer, A.M., Molloy, M., Stallings, L.E., Spicer, K.M., Risch, S.C., & George, M.S. (1999). Changes in prefrontal cortex and paralimbic activity in depression following two weeks of daily left prefrontal TMS. *Journal of Neuropsychiatry and Clinical Neuroscience, 11,* 426–435

Thiebot, M.H., Martin, P., & Puech, A.J. (1992). Animal behavioral studies in the evaluation of antidepressant drugs. *British Journal of Psychiatry, 15,* 44–50.

Tremblay, L. & Schultz, W. (1999). Relative reward preference in primate orbitofrontal cortex. *Nature, 398,* 704–708.

Tucker, P., Luu, K.H. & Pribram, K.H. (1995). Social and emotional self-regulation. *Annals of the New York Academy of Sciences, 769,* 213–239.

Vaidya, V.A., Marek, G.J., Aghajanian, G.K., & Duman, R.S. (1997). 5-HT2A receptor-mediated regulation of brain-derived neurotrophic factor mRNA in the hippocampus and the neocortex. *Journal of Neuroscience, 17,* 2785–2795.

Vogt, B.A. & Pandya, D.N. (1987). Cingulate cortex of the rhesus monkey: II. Cortical afferents. *Journal of Comparative Neurology, 262,* 271–289.

Vogt, B.A., Nimchinsky, E.A., Vogt, L.J., & Hof, P.R. (1995). Human cingulate crtex: surface features, flat maps, and cytoarchitecture. *Journal of Comparative Neurology, 359,* 490–506.

Whalen, P.J., Bush, G., McNally, R.J., Wilhelm, S., McInerney, S.C., Jenike, M.A., & Rauch, S.L. (1998). The emotional counting Stroop paradigm: a functional magnetic resonance imaging probe of the anterior cingulate affective division. *Biological Psychiatry, 44,* 1219–1228.

Willner, P. (1991). Animal models as simulations of depression. *Trends in Pharmacological Sciences, 12,* 131–136.

Wu, J.C., Gilin, J.C., Buchsbaum, M.S., Hershey, T., Johnson, J.C., & Bunney, W.E. Jr. (1992). Effect of sleep deprivation on brain metabolism of depressed patients. *American Journal of Psychiatry, 149,* 538–543.

Wu, J., Buchsbaum, M.S., Gillin, J.C., Tang, C., Cadwell,

S., Wiegand, M., Najafi, A., Klein, E., Hazen, K., Bunney, W.E., Jr., Fallon, J.H., & Keator, D. (1999). Prediction of antidepressant effects of sleep deprivation on metabolic rates in ventral anterior cingulate and medial prefrontal cortex. *American Journal of Psychiatry, 156,* 1149–1158.

Yakovlev, P.I. (1948). Motility, behavior, and the brain: stereodynamic organization and neural coordinates of behavior. *Journal of Nervous and Mental Disease, 107,* 313–335.

Zacharko, R.M. & Anisman, H. (1991). Stressor-induced anhedonia in the mesocorticaolimbic system. *Neuroscience and Biobehavioural Review, 15,* 391–405.

Zisook, S. & Devaul, R. (1985). Unresolved grief. *American Journal of Psychoanalysis, 45,* 370–379.

Zubenko, G.S., Sullivan, P., Nelson, J.P., Belle, S.H., Huff, F.J., & Wolf, G.L. (1990). Brain imaging abnormalities in mental disorders of late life. *Archives of Neurology, 47,* 1107–1111.

Zubenko, G.S. & Moossy, J. (1988). Major depression in primary dementia. *Archives of Neurology, 45,* 1182–1186.

25

Fractionation and Localization of Distinct Frontal Lobe Processes: Evidence from Focal Lesions in Humans

DONALD T. STUSS, MICHAEL P. ALEXANDER, DARLENE FLODEN, MALCOLM A. BINNS, BRIAN LEVINE, ANTHONY R. MCINTOSH, NATASHA RAJAH, AND STEPHANIE J. HEVENOR

The frontal lobes, comprising 25% to 33% of the human cortex (Stuss & Benson, 1986; Rademacher et al., 1992), most readily differentiate a primate brain from the brains of other mammals (Fuster, 1997). The functions of this region are also considered those that most strongly identify a human as human. Despite the general acceptance of the importance of frontal lobe functions, the study of these abilities has been difficult for theoretical, experimental, and clinical reasons (Stuss et al., 1995). For example, concepts such as executive control or supervisory system are difficult to make operational in experimental paradigms. In addition, even if separable processes can be defined, the relationship of these to potentially specific frontal lobe regions has been difficult to determine because of the relative infrequency of patients with limited focal frontal lobe lesions.

In this chapter, we summarize a decade or more of research on the functions of the frontal lobes through the study of patients with pathology restricted to that region (Alexander & Stuss, 2000; Stuss & Alexander, 2000). We started with one assumption: there is no unitary frontal lobe process, no central executive (Stuss & Benson, 1986; Shallice & Burgess, 1991). Rather,

the frontal lobes (in anatomical terms) or the supervisory system (in cognitive terms) do not function (in physiological terms) as a simple (inexplicable) homunculus. . . . The different regions of the frontal lobes provide multiple interacting processes. Because the level of processing allows the interaction of information from other brain regions and because of the complexity of the frontal structures, the interacting processes can provide a sophisticated control. . . . The understanding of this, however, can be completed only at the level of processes and mechanisms (Stuss et al., 1995).

In the next section, evidence will be presented from research using neuropsychological tests of frontal lobe function to demonstrate that different cognitive processes can be related to distinct regions of the frontal lobes. A very brief review of the relation of less cognitive human abilities, such as humor appreciation and theory of mind, provides some support that even higher human abilities depend on the interaction of more distinct localizable functions. We then move from the location of distinct processes to the interaction of these in networks and cognitive systems. In the final section, we will present the implications of our review.

DISTINCT PROCESSES: EVIDENCE FROM NEUROPSYCHOLOGICAL TESTS

AN APPROACH

To refine frontal lobe brain–behavior relations, we simultaneously improved our differentiation of cognitive processes, and refined the localization of regions within the frontal lobes. For cognitive processes, we tried to isolate the different components that were necessary to complete a task, or devised tests that would more directly be related to a specific cognitive function. These efforts to differentiate frontal lobe processes are exemplified below, and described in detail in the original publications.

There were several steps required to improve the identification of functionally relevant gyrus-specific frontal lobe lesions. Since lesions do not usually respect defined Brodmann's areas, we decided that it would be necessary to test as many patients as possible who might have lesions involving, and restricted to, any region of the frontal lobes. Although patients would have pathology that affected different frontal lobe areas, it was hypothesized that, if a particular region was relevant to a specific function, those individuals who had involvement in that distinct area would be impaired in that function, regardless of brain damage in other surrounding areas. In finding patients whose lesions might represent different regions of the frontal lobes, various etiologies other than single infarctions (the preferred sample) would have to be considered. Thus, patients with resected meningiomas or benign gliomas are acceptable research participants, provided that the damage from this etiology can be demonstrated to be truly focal and limited, and that such patients would be reasonably represented in all subgroups. Patients with bifrontal contusions are necessary to provide an adequate sample of subjects with inferior medial and/or polar pathology. However, such patients should not have evidence of significant diffuse axonal injury. The challenge here is that patients with restricted frontal lobe lesions fitting our inclusion and exclusion criteria are not common, and completing projects of this magnitude would take 5 to 10 years. The gamble is that the lengthy effort would be for naught, or that theoretical assumptions would no longer be relevant when the study was completed.

Over the years, we used the greater numbers of patients to evolve different approaches to localize functions within the frontal lobes. We moved from comparison of frontal versus posterior lesions to what we called the standard anatomical classification within the frontal lobes: right frontal, left frontal, and bifrontal (Della Malva et al., 1993). A somewhat more sophisticated approach can be considered "backwards engineering." That is, rather than using an a priori anatomical classification, we started from differences in performance as a means of classifying individuals. The overall goal was to reduce even further the group performance variability commonly found in patient studies by developing anatomical groupings that would be more specific than the standard anatomical classification. The grouping factor would be driven by performance itself. This is a modified case study–group approach (Shallice, 1988). As illustrated below, this method of grouping patients can be accomplished in different ways.

The success of this lesion specificity approach depends not only on the ability to separate cognitive processes but also on the precision in brain area delineation. Our anatomical classification has gradually improved with the accumulated experience of several studies. We currently use an anatomical classification based on the Petrides and Pandya (1994) architectonic divisions. The rendering of these architectonic areas onto an adult human brain is illustrated in Figure 25–1. We have also grouped these architectonic areas into more specific subgroupings, which can be further clustered into four major anatomical regions (polar, inferior medial, superior medial, and lateral). This cascade of anatomical groupings is depicted in Figure 25–2. The different levels of alignment allow flexibility in the precision of lesion identification, depending on the specificity of the available imaging data.

The identification of pathology in specific architectonic areas would be useful as an anatomical grouping method only if a very large number of patients with lesions in such areas

A

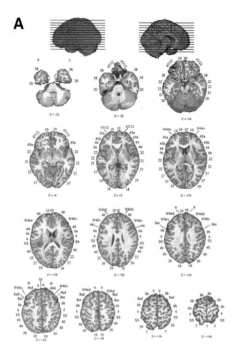

B

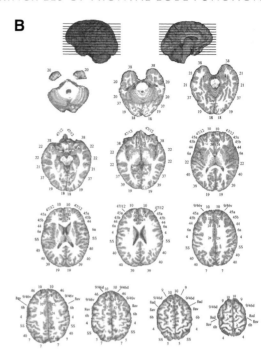

Figure 25–1. A fast T1°-weighted MRI of a young adult human brain is transformed into Talairach space (Talairach & Tournoux, 1988), enabling comparison to imaging data. On this brain, the frontal architectonic divisions of Petrides and Pandya (1994) are rendered in a manner similar to that of Damasio and Damasio (1989). For posterior areas where new architectonic divisions are not available, we continue to use Brodmann divisions on the lateral surface only. *A:* the brain is sliced in the axial plane parallel to the AC-PC line. *B:* the brain is sliced in the axial plane parallel to the orbitomedial line. Each slice is approximately 1 mm in thickness. Data from patient scans can be transferred onto the axial slices, providing a template for localizing lesions, at least in a general way, to the defined Petrides and Pandya specific architectonic areas. The subdivision of premotor area 6 is based on the Petrides and Pandya verbal descriptions of ventral and dorsal sections which we have labeled 6A and 6B, respectively.

were available. However, if a reasonable number of patients have pathology in regions of interest, then the relationship between a defined performance measure and each specific region could be calculated using various statistics, depending on the distribution of the performance measure.

Examples of these approaches are provided in the following section.

LOCALIZATION OF COGNITIVE FUNCTIONS WITHIN THE FRONTAL LOBES

An early success in discovering more precise frontal lobe–functional relationships was in a study of word list learning (Stuss et al., 1994;

see also Janowsky et al., 1989). Standard analysis of variance (ANOVA) indicated that, using the standard anatomical classification, the left frontal and bifrontal groups had a significant impairment in recognition performance. Since this was contrary to accepted wisdom at that time (see Wheeler et al., 1995, for a meta-analysis of frontal lobe memory research), we were curious about the reason for this unusual finding. All patients with frontal lobe damage were ranked in order of performance, from the best to the worst, and compared to the performance of the control group. We then used a standard criterion (2 standard deviations from the control group mean) to differentiate the good from the impaired performers. Some of the frontal pa-

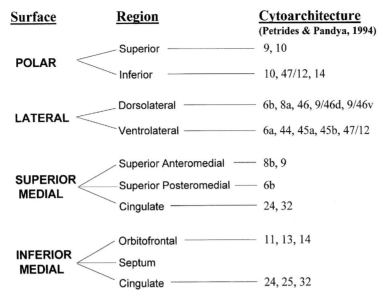

Surface	Region	Cytoarchitecture (Petrides & Pandya, 1994)
POLAR	Superior	9, 10
	Inferior	10, 47/12, 14
LATERAL	Dorsolateral	6b, 8a, 46, 9/46d, 9/46v
	Ventrolateral	6a, 44, 45a, 45b, 47/12
SUPERIOR MEDIAL	Superior Anteromedial	8b, 9
	Superior Posteromedial	6b
	Cingulate	24, 32
INFERIOR MEDIAL	Orbitofrontal	11, 13, 14
	Septum	
	Cingulate	24, 25, 32

Figure 25–2. Four major regions of the frontal lobes (which can be separated into right or left frontal areas) are depicted: polar, lateral, superior medial, and inferior medial. Each of these divisions is segmented further. The polar area can be superior polar or inferior polar, the division approximately between the 6th and 7th axial slices in Figure 25–1a. The lateral frontal lobe is divided into the dorsolateral and ventrolateral (inferior) sections at this same level with minor overlap of dorsolateral and ventrolateral cytoarchitectonic areas on the 6th and 7th slices. The superior medial division is divided into three sections: the superior medial region continuous with the polar area; the more posterior superior medial area; and the more caudal portions of the anterior cingulate gyrus. Three sections comprise the inferior medial region: the orbitofrontal gyri; the posterior inferior medial region involving the septum; and the parts of the anterior cingulate cortex somewhat inferior to the corpus callosum. All of these divisions can be further classified into the Petrides and Pandya architectonic areas as indicated, but separating these in a practical way in human pathology research is difficult. This information can be used in correlational analyses, as described in the text.

Figures 25–1 and 25–2 are used practically as follows. Information from the available scans (preferably at least 3 months post-injury) are transferred to the axial and lateral/medial views. The presence (1) or absence (0) of pathology for each architectonic area is noted on a spreadsheet. The data can then be used for each architectonic area, or collapsed in a hierarchical manner. For example, patients with discrete damage to ventrolateral 45A may exhibit a definable performance pattern. On the other hand, such a specific pattern may not be observable. That is, patients with damage to different architectonic areas of the ventrolateral area may exhibit common behavioural results indicating that the logical grouping is by the ventrolateral area in general, not by architectonic division within the area. While this is still crude, it is a considerable improvement on past localization methods for human lesion research.

tients indeed showed good recognition performance, with many performing equivalent to or better than the control group. Since many of the impaired patients had bifrontal lesions, our first hypothesis to explain the impaired recognition performance was that the frontal lobe damage in the impaired patients involved the septal–limbic memory area. This lesion location was evident in many, but not all, of the impaired patients. Further investigation revealed that the remaining individuals with impaired recognition had mild language impairment, and their pathology was in the left lateral frontal region. Thus, two separate reasons, and two distinct anatomical areas, could explain the same recognition performance deficit: left dorsolateral frontal pathology, with mild residual language impairment; and posterior inferior medial frontal damage involving the septal–limbic memory system. The implication is that the two areas are related to a verbal learning memory–encoding neural system.

This performance-based clinical approach

was completed in a more formalized manner in a study on verbal fluency (Stuss et al., 1998). For each patient, each frontal region of interest that we had defined at that time (see Stuss et al., 1995) was coded as 1 (damaged) or 0 (not damaged). Using the performance on the verbal fluency task, the Classification and Regression Tree (CART; Breiman et al., 1984) statistical procedure was used to divide patients into anatomical groups that were maximally different in terms of their performance. The standard frontal lobe anatomical classification (right, left, bifrontal) was then compared to these new anatomical groupings by fluency performance (Fig. 25–3). The original coarse anatomical classification for the frontal lobes was refined from three groups into four (left and right dorsolateral, superior medial, and inferior medial). Pathology in the right dorsolateral frontal cortical or striatal areas, or the medial inferior lobe of either hemisphere,

did not result in impaired performance in phonological fluency. Damage to the right *or* left superior medial areas, and left dorsolateral and/or striatal lesions, as well as left parietal pathology, did cause a significant deficit. These new anatomical classifications were subsequently used to assess differences in strategy performance on verbal fluency tasks (Troyer et al., 1998). In the semantic fluency task, damage to the right dorsolateral and inferior medial areas also resulted in impaired performance, suggesting that this task required other processes related to other brain regions (see Fig. 25–3).

This study exemplifies how a distinct frontal region can be demonstrated to be important for a process, regardless of the presence of brain damage in other surrounding areas. The inferior medial group who performed within the normal range on the letter fluency task tended to have pathology restricted to the inferior medial frontal area. Patients in the superior medial group, who were significantly impaired, occasionally had damage extending to the inferior medial region. The comparison of the two groups suggested that the superior medial area was most relevant for successful performance on the letter fluency task, and that the extension of pathology to the inferior medial frontal area for that group was likely not relevant to their performance.

The use of the CART to separate 35 patients with frontal lobe damage on the Wisconsin Card Sorting Test (WCST) also resulted in four different groupings: left dorsolateral, right dorsolateral, superior medial, and inferior medial (Stuss et al., 2000a). With these new groupings we were able to clarify previous results using the WCST, which tended not to emphasize the role of the medial regions. Damage to the inferior medial frontal area did not result in a deficit on the WCST (the now common finding that such patients are normal on "frontal lobe" tests), with one exception. If these patients were given the categories, they had no trouble changing categories of responses, but tended to lose set (see also Stuss et al., 1983). Patients with superior medial damage, right or left, tended to be the most impaired on all measures (categories achieved, perseverations of

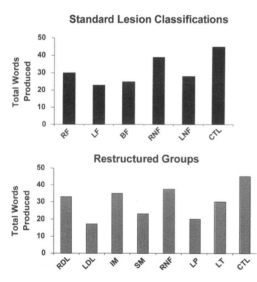

Figure 25–3. Verbal fluency results (total words produced starting with either *F, A,* or *S,* over a 1-minute period) are compared for the standard anatomical groupings (*top*) based on right frontal (RF), left frontal (LF), bifrontal (BF), right nonfrontal (RNF), and left nonfrontal (LNF) lesions to the restructured groups (*bottom*) based on Classification and Regression Tree analysis. The left nonfrontal group is now divided into left parietal (LP) and left temporal (LT) groups. The major difference for the frontal patients is the division of most of the original bifrontal group into inferior medial (IM) and superior medial (SM) groups. CTL, control.

the preceding sorting category), except for loss of set. Right and left lateral–damaged patients were also significantly impaired, although usually somewhat less than the superior medial group. There was one contrast between the right and left lateral groups: only those with right lateral damage had high set loss, even when further instructions were given to assist performance.

We noted parallel findings with an experimental concept generation task modeled after the California Card Sorting Test (Delis et al., 1989; Levine et al., 1995a), which also involves successively increasing instructions. Dorsolateral and superior medial patients were more impaired than inferior medial patients were. While all patients improved with additional instructions, the superior medial patients improved the least (Levine et al., 1995b).

The incongruent condition of the Stroop Test (Stroop, 1935) is one of the most commonly accepted measures of frontal lobe functioning, with different frontal regions considered relevant. Investigators using functional imaging have proposed a variety of frontal sites as key: left inferior lateral (Taylor et al., 1997), left superomedial (Pardo et al., 1990),

right frontal polar (Bench et al., 1993), and bilateral anterior cingulate, perhaps with right predominance (Pardo et al., 1990; Bench et al., 1993). Lesion studies have also suggested different possible frontal regions: left lateral, which is the most common region (Perret, 1974; Golden et al., 1981; Corcoran & Upton, 1993); right lateral (Vendrell et al., 1995); and superomedial (Holzt & Vilkki, 1988). The orbital frontal region is apparently not essential for successful performance on the Stroop Test (Stuss et al., 1981).

Our approach in analyzing performance on different conditions of the Stroop Test (Stuss et al., 2001b) indicated that a speed performance measure was too variable to differentiate among patients with different frontal lesions. However, the number of errors for the color-naming (name patches of colors) and incongruent (read color words printed in a different color than the word itself) conditions yielded two distinct groups (see Figure 25–4). Subjects were coded 0 for good performers or 1 for poor performers, on the basis of whether the number of errors committed fell above or below 1.5 standard deviations above the control group's mean. Only 7 of 37 frontal-

Figure 25–4. Patients with frontal lobe lesions are grouped by the number of errors they made on the Stroop test for both the color naming and incongruent conditions. The time to complete the different conditions is also presented for each group, as well as the overlaps of the lesions. In the color-naming task, the major anatomical difference was the involvement of the left dorsolateral (LDL) group. In the incongruent condition, damage in the superior medial (SM) region, particularly on the right, was the differentiating area. Since the individuals who were impaired in each condition were also slower, the difference in the errors could not be attributed to a speed–accuracy trade-off.

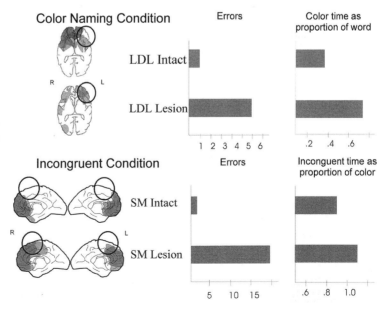

damaged patients were classified as poor performers on color naming, and their performance was highly related to their lesions in
the left lateral area. Twelve of the frontal patients made many errors in the incongruent
condition; the important pathology here was
in the superior medial areas, particularly the
right superior posteromedial region. The impaired patients in each condition were also
generally slower, but some frontal patients
who did not make errors were also slow. Time
scores alone may not be the most effective
measure of Stroop performance.

Our Stroop lesion study has several important implications. The Stroop is not just a
"frontal lobe" test. Many patients with large
frontal lobe lesions performed normally.
Grouping by performance is effective, but
sometimes the precise measure by which to
group patients by performance to maximize
information has to be sought. In addition to
the information provided by the larger anatomical divisions, the correlational methods
can yield reasonably precise gyral-specific relations. The previous lesion studies that suggested left frontal regions as being most relevant for performance of the incongruent
condition were based on straight time scores.
However, the incongruent condition also requires color naming (a condition in which the
left frontal patients *were* impaired), and a
speed measure would be confounded by the
ability to color—name. If time scores are to
be used, the incongruent time should be indexed relative to straight color-naming time.
Our Stroop results dissociate the functional
relevance of the left lateral and superior medial frontal regions.

The Trail Making Test (Army Individual
Test Battery, 1944; TMT) has been considered
by some to be a sensitive index of frontal lobe
dysfunction, in particular the switching demands of Part B, but such claims were not
based on studies assessing individuals with
documented evidence of frontal lobe dysfunction. Stuss et al. (2001a) tested this assertion
by administering the TMT to 62 patients with
focal lesions in various frontal ($n = 49$) and
nonfrontal ($n = 13$) brain regions. The time
to complete TMT Part B seemed to suggest
that this test was sensitive to frontal lobe dam-

age. This result, however, was evident only
when transformed scores were used and, if a
proportional measure that accounted for the
time taken to complete the processes required
for Part A, no frontal-posterior differences
were noted. The number of errors, however,
was discriminatory. Only subjects with frontal
lobe lesions made more than one error. Patients with right or left inferior medial frontal
and/or anterior cingulate pathology made the
fewest errors. Those who made the most errors tended to have dorsolateral pathology, although this was not significant.

We have also explored intrafrontal heterogeneity with tests that have been developed
more recently in the experimental literature.
Conditional associative learning, requiring the
acquisition of arbitrary paired associates, has
been extensively studied in both human (Petrides, 1982, 1985, 1990; Martin & Levey,
1987; Molchan et al., 1994) and animal (Halsband & Passingham, 1982; Petrides, 1982;
Rainer et al., 1998b; See Chapter 21) paradigms. In a comparison of patients with focal
frontal and posterior lesions and healthy young
and old adults, aging and focal frontal damage
produced qualitatively similar deficits (Levine
et al., 1997). These deficits, however, were not
quantitatively similar; the magnitude of impairment was much greater in the patients
with focal frontal lesions, even though they
were younger than the older adults were. Consistent with prior work, frontal patients were
not uniformly impaired. The test was sensitive
to dorsolateral prefrontal dysfunction, but not
inferior medial/orbitofrontal. This dissociation
was notable in light of the fact that the original
experimental work with this task was conducted with dorsolateral-lesioned animals and
humans.

By limiting our conditional associative
learning task to only four stimulus pairs, we
minimized the role of basic medial temporal
lobe–mediated memory processes. The specificity of the task to processes involving control
over interference was further demonstrated by
administering the stimulus pairs in a standard
paired-associate learning paradigm (in which
the examiner corrects errors rather than allowing the subject to generate their own errors
through trial-and-error learning). By enhanc-

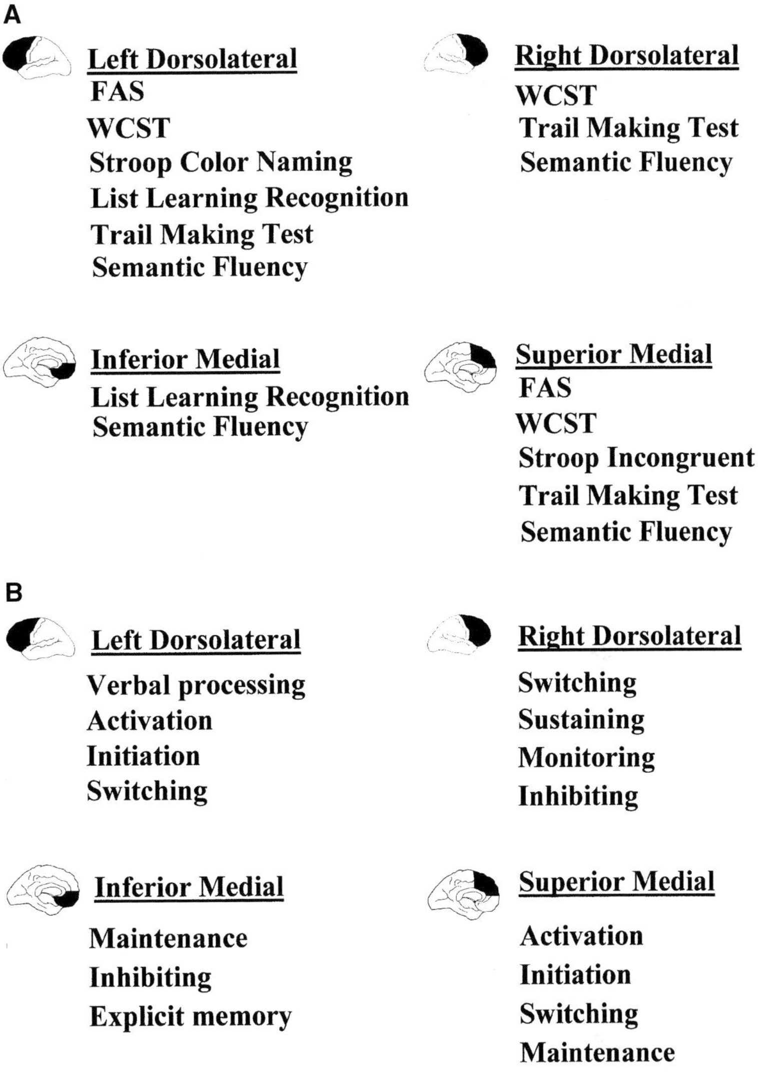

Figure 25–5. While our results have demonstrated that there are rather refined brain–behavior relationships within the frontal lobes, the major anatomical groupings that have been differentiated in our various studies are right and left dorsolateral, superior medial, and inferior medial. *A:* summarizes the relationship of the different measures from our various studies to these four groupings. *B:* Suggestions of which processes are related to those different tests. The inadequacies of our labels for the processes are evident. For example, the inhibition related to the inferior medial area is different from that to the right dorsolateral region.

A

Left Dorsolateral
FAS
WCST
Stroop Color Naming
List Learning Recognition
Trail Making Test
Semantic Fluency

Right Dorsolateral
WCST
Trail Making Test
Semantic Fluency

Inferior Medial
List Learning Recognition
Semantic Fluency

Superior Medial
FAS
WCST
Stroop Incongruent
Trail Making Test
Semantic Fluency

B

Left Dorsolateral

Verbal processing
Activation
Initiation
Switching

Right Dorsolateral

Switching
Sustaining
Monitoring
Inhibiting

Inferior Medial

Maintenance
Inhibiting
Explicit memory

Superior Medial

Activation
Initiation
Switching
Maintenance

ing structural support as in our work with the WCST, interference was reduced, and even the most impaired patients could acquire the stimulus pairs (Levine et al., 1997).

SUMMARY

The results to date suggest an anatomically and functionally discrete cognitive architecture to the frontal lobes (see Figure 25–5). At this stage, the architecture is truly an unfinished structure. Regardless, since lesion studies indicate which regions are necessary for a function, these results stand as a framework for more localized patient and imaging research in the future. In Figure 25–5a, the re-

lation of the tests to the different frontal brain areas is presented. Figure 25–5b translates these tests into likely cognitive processes.

NON-COGNITIVE CHANGES IN BEHAVIOR

The functions of the frontal lobes are far more than cognitive. A profound apathy, blunted social propriety, and a notable personality change often constitute the most striking observations in patients with frontal lobe damage, particularly bilateral orbitofrontal (ventral medial) pathology (Nauta, 1973; Stuss & Benson, 1986; Damasio et al., 1994; Stuss et al.,

2000b). The changes may be so significant that others may consider the individual not to be the same person, as in Harlow's (1868) classic description of Phineas Gage—"he was no longer Gage."

The frontal lobes also provide the individual self-awareness to use past personal knowledge to understand current behaviors, and to select and guide future responses to integrate the personal self into a social context. Stuss et al. (2001d) have proposed three interrelated hierarchical levels of self-awareness, with two of the three levels based on processes instantiated in the frontal lobes. Both of these levels appear to be related particularly to the right frontal region (Stuss, 1991; Stuss & Alexander, 1999). The highest level of self-reflectiveness has been called *autonoetic consciousness*, and is the basis for episodic memory, which is related to personal and emotionally relevant past episodes (Wheeler et al., 1997; Levine et al., 1998b). At the highest level, the self-referential abilities can be disturbed, despite normal executive or problem-solving capacities. This is a true disorder in self-reflection, a deficiency at the highest level of monitoring of behavior.

The importance of the right frontal lobe, and/or ventral medial frontal regions, in noncognitive emotional functions can be experimentally demonstrated. Patients with right frontal lobe damage, in particular the right frontal polar/medial region, could grasp slapstick humor but did not appreciate the subtleties of humor, as in jokes that depend on a "twist" at the end (Shammi & Stuss, 1999). Even when they recognized the humor, they did not show the appropriate emotional response. The right frontal lobe, certainly part of a much larger system of emotional modulation, is required for the subtle convergence of cognition and affect essential to humor.

These same types of patients, particularly if the pathology is (right) inferior medial, find it difficult to take the perspective of others to understand or guide their own behaviors (Stuss et al., 2001c). Making inferences about the actions of others requires the ability to "mentalize." Such patients may not grasp the implications of any faux pas they make (Stone et al., 1998). While such functions also require

cognitive capacity of different kinds, these deficits do not seem to be reducible to cognitive impairment.

Problems in social decisions and interactions most often occur in real-life situations, not usually in highly constrained tasks designed to isolate a limited number of cognitive operations. Progress, however, has been made in study design and new methods demanding on-line monitoring, planning, and application of strategies for behaving have been developed (e.g., Burgess et al., 1998; Levine, 1999; Levine et al., 1998a, 2000; see Chapter 33). These tests comprise multiple subgoals that have to be completed in a relatively unconstrained environment. Patients with documented frontal lobe lesions, particularly in ventral regions, who may perform normally on traditional frontal lobe tests, show strategic deficits on these measures due to impaired self-regulation (Burgess et al., 1998; Levine et al., 1998a, 1999, 2000; see also Bechara et al., 1994; and Chapter 22). The performance of these patients is striking in that they may demonstrate full awareness of the task demands even when failing to execute them (although in everyday practice this dissociation is not always observed). They incur large penalties for their real-life misconduct, yet repeat the same mistakes again, with often devastating effects on their quality of life. Accordingly, we have demonstrated that the performance of patients with traumatic brain injury (which more selectively affects ventral frontal regions; Stuss & Gow, 1992) on our strategy application task is significantly related to measures of quality-of-life outcome (Levine et al., 2000). Grafman's concept of social knowledge units provides one mechanism of explaining these real-life failures (Grafman, 1995; see Chapter 19).

FROM LOCATION AND PROCESSES TO NETWORKS AND COGNITIVE SYSTEMS

Our research on the effect of focal frontal lobe lesions on separable cognitive and noncognitive processes revealed distinct roles for different regions of the frontal lobes. Careful reading of the results leads to the conclusion that this is not a modern phrenology but a preliminary effort in the use of lesion research to understand integrated neural networks. Converging evidence from multiple methodologies compellingly argues for the regulatory role of the frontal lobes in networks involving posterior regions. The neural modeling of Cohen and Servan-Schrieber (1992) shows that the frontal lobes are capable of determining task context through excitatory connections with posterior association areas. Studies of event-related potentials (Knight, 1997), single-cell recording (Rainer et al., 1998a, 1998b), and functional neuroimaging (McIntosh et al., 1994) have each demonstrated that the frontal lobes regulate sensory cortex. The dynamic aspect of frontal lobe function within neural networks has also been captured. Event-related potential studies have demonstrated that not only are the frontal lobes involved in networks responsible for novelty detection (Halgren et al., 1998; Knight & Scabini, 1998) but frontal lobes can recruit posterior cortical areas for processing of novel events (Knight, 1996; Alain et al., 1998).

Our research focuses on how these networks can be uncovered and better understood through behavioral measures. The involvement of left dorsolateral and septal/hippocampal memory regions in recognition suggests a neural system for verbal encoding, different regions playing separate roles. In phonological fluency, for example, there were possibly several systems at work, including initiation and activation (superior medial, and possible left dorsolateral) and language-based process (left parietal and left dorsolateral frontal). Performance on the multicomponent nature of the WCST requires the functioning of a distributed neural network (superior medial and both lateral frontal regions for switching of categories; right lateral for sustained attention and monitoring; inferior medial for maintaining set under conditions of additional supervisory reflective efforts). In the Stroop Test, different regions of the frontal lobe were involved in color naming (left frontal) or maintenance of consistent activation of the intended response in the incongruent condition (bilateral superior medial frontal).

TASK COMPLEXITY AND NEURAL NETWORKS

The above studies led to considerations about how to test more actively neural networks through lesion research. We exploited the functional domain of attention, since a simple anterior–posterior dissociation of attentional abilities did not seem to encapsulate the potential complexities of the interaction between different brain regions. Patients with focal lesions in various frontal and posterior regions were compared on a location-based (select–what, respond–where) target detection task (Stuss et al., 1999). The test allowed measurement of three different attentional processes commonly linked to frontal function: *(a)* inhibiting attention to distracting information presented at the same time as the target (*interference*); *(b)* effect of previous inhibition of irrelevant information on subsequent processing (*negative priming*); *(c)* inhibition of motor responses to novel and previously processed locations (*inhibition of return*). These three attentional processes were measured under three levels of task difficulty.

Figure 25–6 summarizes our model of the regions involved in these tasks based on the

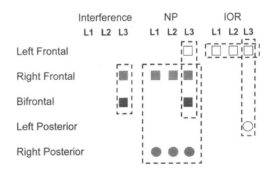

Figure 25–6. Performance of patients with right frontal, left frontal, and bifrontal lesions on a location-based (select–what, respond–where) target detection task is illustrated. There were three levels of difficulty in the task; three different attentional measures were taken (see text). The figure demonstrates that the different brain regions necessary for successful performance on the task varied depending on which attentional measure was taken, and the level of difficulty of the task. L1, lowest level of difficulty; L2, medium level of difficulty; L3, highest level of difficulty; NP, negative priming; IOR, inhibition of return.

Stuss et al. (1999) study. The presence of a symbol indicates abnormal performance for that specific attentional processes at that level of task complexity. The hypothesized neural systems are indicated by the dotted outlines grouping the task-relevant lesioned areas together.

Lesions in different brain regions affect different attentional processes. For some of the processes, impairment is found in both frontal and posterior regions, suggesting a functional neural system. Most importantly, the neural systems are dynamic and active, altering with the complexity of task demands. The functional process labeled *interference* is impaired by damage to the right frontal lobe (that is, unilateral right frontal and bifrontal damage, but not unilateral left frontal damage, results in impairment), but only at the highest level of complexity. The ability to withhold attention to irrelevant information as defined by this task appears to be a right frontal lobe function. In contrast, *inhibition of return* is affected by left frontal damage at all levels of complexity, although performance varies from abnormal facilitation to abnormal inhibition as task complexity increases. At the highest level of task difficulty there is also involvement of the left nonfrontal regions, suggesting that task difficulty or differing task demands now somehow recruit more posterior regions of left hemisphere. *Negative priming*, at the simplest level of task demands, is impaired after damage to either anterior or posterior regions of the right hemisphere, suggesting a right frontal–posterior neuronal system for inhibition of spatial selection. As difficulty increases, however, impairment is noted in all frontal groups, implying either the necessity of additional frontal lobe processes or resources.

There is no single frontal attentional deficit. A frontal supervisory attentional system is, in reality, an emergent interaction of different attentional processes, as proposed by Stuss et al. (1995). Different frontal regions support different attentional mechanisms, some in concert with posterior brain regions. These systems alter dynamically with changes in task demands or complexity. Functional neural systems are relative to the task, not absolute. The

implications for theory and clinical neuropsychological assessment are obvious.

PARTIAL LEAST SQUARES

A major stumbling block to understanding the function of neural systems is the lack of process purity, or a one-to-one mapping between tasks and processes. Traditionally, the solution to this problem has been to either develop better tasks to isolate specific processes or look at post-hoc relationships between task measures and standard neuropsychological tests in multiple domains. These methods help to clarify the role of anatomical correlates across measures. More recently, novel statistical techniques have been applied in addressing this problem (Burgess et al., 1998, 2000; see Chapter 33). Burgess and colleagues (1998) proposed several distinct processes underlying performance in their multitasking procedure. A factor analysis of the measures taken from their task, together with several neuropsychological measures, identified five theoretical constructs that contribute to multiple performance measures. Later, Burgess and colleagues (2000) employed structural equation modeling to investigate the potential relationships between underlying processes and how these might combine to produce successful (or unsuccessful) multitasking in patients with focal brain lesions. In addition, they applied a lesion analysis technique similar to that described here to identify the relevance of lesion locations to the different measures of task performance. The cognitive and lesion analyses informed each other; the lesion location analyses constrained the cognitive model, which in turn suggested the structure of neural systems supporting the contributing processes.

We have applied a different multivariate statistical method, partial least squares (PLS), to understand the relationship between our lesion findings and our behavioral measures. A full description of the matrix operations involved in the PLS procedure has been provided elsewhere (McIntosh et al., 1996). For the current analysis, we covaried a brain matrix containing binary-coded lesion location data for nine areas (septal, and left and right inferior medial, superior medial, lateral, and polar) with a behavior matrix containing age, education, and IQ-corrected scores for 24 patients with frontal lobe damage on several neuropsychological and experimental measures (see Fig. 25–7). The singular value decomposition of this covariance matrix produced sets of mutually orthogonal paired latent variables (LV). Each LV pair consists of a behavior profile across measures and a pattern of lesion locations that is optimally related to the behavior profile. The behavior profiles represent the structure of task performance most related to the pattern of lesion locations (lesion profile). The first and second LV pair accounted for 34% and 23% of the total covariance, respectively. When the analysis was subjected to a permutation test, only the first LV pair had a less than 5% probability that

these relationships could have been found by chance. However, both LV pairs showed moderate correlations between the factor scores for the lesion latent variable with the factor scores for the behavior latent variable (first LV, $r = 0.61$; second LV, $r = 0.49$), which suggests that both LV pairs reflect relatively strong relationships.

Figure 25–7 illustrates the relationship between the behavioral measures and the pattern of lesion locations that was identified by the first two LV pairs. The direction of the bars represents how the behavior and lesion profiles correlate with one another. Bars that share the same direction (upward or downward) in both the behavior and lesion profiles within an LV pair are positively related to another. Bars that point in the opposite direction for the behavior and lesion profiles within an

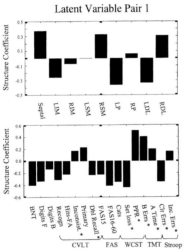
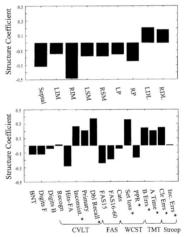

Figure 25–7. The first two orthogonal latent variable (LV) pairs identified in the partial least squares analysis. The *top* bar graphs represent the pattern of lesion locations related to each LV pair. The *bottom* bar graphs represent the profile of behavioral measures related to each LV pair. The length and direction of the bar represent the correlation of the measured variable with the LV that it contributes to. Within an LV pair, task and lesion location bars sharing the same direction (upward or downward) are positively related to one another, whereas bars that point in the opposite direction are negatively related to each other. Asterisks indicate variables for which a high score reflects poor performance. L, left; R, right; IM, inferior medial; SM, superior medial; P, polar; DL, dorsolateral; CVLT, California Verbal Learning Test; FAS, verbal fluency;

WCST, Wisconsin Card Sorting Test; TMT, Trail Making Test; BNT, Boston Naming Test; Digits F, forward digit span; Digits B, backward digit span; Recogn, recognition measure of the CVLT; Hits-FA, CVLT hits minus false alarms; Inconsist, CVLT inconsistency of recall across learning trials; Primary, CVLT primary memory estimate; Dbl Recall, CVLT within-trial recall repetition; FAS15, output over first 15 seconds; FAS16–60, output over 16–60 seconds; Cats, categories achieved in the WCST; PPR, perseveration of the preceding response in the WCST; B Errs, number of errors on the TMT; A Time, time to complete Part A of the TMT; Clr Errs, number of errors in the color-naming condition of the Stroop Test; Inc Errs, number of errors in the incongruent condition of the Stroop.

LV pair are negatively related to each other. The output of the PLS is quite complex, but the aspect of this figure that is particularly relevant to the present discussion is that the pattern of lesion correlations for the first LV pair seems to reflect a left–right contrast, whereas the pattern of lesion correlations for the second LV pair seem to reflect a dorsolateral–other areas contrast. Notice that some of the task measures are related to both lesion patterns. For example, in the first LV pair, errors on Trails B covary positively with right-sided damage. In the second LV pair, errors on Trails B covary positively with dorsolateral damage. This same relationship is also true of performance measures on the California Verbal Learning Test, verbal fluency test, and the Wisconsin Card Sorting Test. In other words, within single measures, we were able to extract unique variance related to different lesion locations. Also, in general, the patterns of behavior–lesion relationships mirror those identified in the individual analyses discussed earlier. This analysis is the first of its kind and should be regarded as a preliminary attempt to separate processes within tasks using this method. The necessary next step is to cross-validate the patterns identified here in a larger sample of patients to determine the stability of these findings. The eventual goal would be to identify unique covariance across measures that represent neuropsychological dimensions that are represented to varying degrees in their relation to lesion location.

CONCLUSIONS

The frontal lobes clearly are not homogeneous anatomical or functional monolithic structures, but are composed of morphologically distinct areas interconnected with each other and with posterior and basal brain regions to constitute complex anatomical circuitries. Such systems are an anatomical (and certainly neurochemical) infrastructure allowing for the flexible and dynamic construction of functional networks necessary for a specific task. If one considers the posterior brain regions and their functions to be more modular and hard-wired, a major

role of the processes related to the frontal lobes may be to serve the flexible and dynamic nature of such networks. Terms such as *supervisory system* or *executive control* are convenient labels to represent the sum of the processes recruited at any moment, for any task. We have identified some of the processes and marshaled evidence for their relationship to specific frontal regions.

Activation studies in neurologically intact individuals using functional magnetic resonance imaging (fMRI) and positron emission tomography (PET) also indicate that multiple regions are active during the performance of a specific task and identify how distinct frontal brain regions are related to particular elements of supervisory processes. However, such studies cannot normally differentiate all the different processes required for a complex task, since PET and fMRI are used to average results over time. Lesion research, by identifying that damage to a specific brain region impairs a relatively unique function, provides additional information related to the apparent necessity of a brain area for a specific function. In addition, functional imaging that provides temporal analysis, such as event-related potentials or magnetoencephalography, combined with source localization, would be an in vivo on-line method of dissociating processes related to brain localization. Newer methods of analysis of activation paradigms and complex networks, such as path analysis and partial least squares, may disentangle the supportive from the essential element of a brain network activated by specific supervisory processes.

ACKNOWLEDGMENTS

The research in this chapter was funded by the Canadian Institutes of Health Research, the Ontario Mental Health Foundation, and NINDS grant 26985 to the Memory Disorders Research Center of Boston University. We are indebted to the subjects for their participation, and to our colleagues involved in these studies in different ways, in particular: S. Bisschop, L. Buckle, C. Copnick, F.I.M. Craik, R. Dempster, D. Franchi, G. Gallup, L. Hamer, J. Hong, D. Izukawa, D. Katz, Wm. P. Milberg, K. Murphy, R. McDonald, P. Mathews, C. Palumbo, T. Picton, J. Pogue, A. Savas, T. Shallice, P. Shammi, E. Tulving, S. Tipper, J. Toth, and M.

Wheeler. The chapter is dedicated to the friendship and mentorship of D.F. Benson, who was so important to the careers of D.T. Stuss and M.P. Alexander, and to Edith Kaplan, who taught us to look at processes.

REFERENCES

Alain, C., Woods, D.L., & Knight, R.T. (1998). A distributed cortical network for auditory sensory memory in humans. *Brain Research, 812*, 23–37.

Alexander, M.P. & Stuss, D.T. (2000). Disorders of frontal lobe functioning. *Seminars in Neurology, 20*, 427–437.

Army Individual Test Battery. (1944). *Manual of Directions and Scoring*. Washington, DC: War Department, Adjutant General's Office.

Bechara, A., Damasio, A.R., Damasio, H., & Anderson, S.W. (1994). Insensitivity to future consequences following damage to human prefrontal cortex. *Cognition, 50*, 7–15.

Bench, C.J., Frith, C.D., Grasby, P.M., Friston, K.J., Paulesu, E., Frackowiak, R.S.J., & Dolan, R.J. (1993). Investigations of the functional anatomy of attention using the Stroop test. *Neuropsychologia, 31*, 907–922.

Breiman, L., Freidman, J.H., Olshen, R.A., & Store, C.J. (1984). *Classification and Regression Trees*. Belmont, CA: Wadsworth International Group.

Burgess, P.W., Alderman, N., Emslie, H., Evans, J., & Wilson, B.A. (1998). The ecological validity of tests of executive function. *Journal of the International Neuropsychological Society, 4*, 547–558.

Burgess, P.W., Veitch, E., Costello, A. deL., & Shallice, T. (2000). The cognitive and neuroanatomical correlates of multitasking. *Neuropsychologia, 38*, 848–863.

Cohen, J.D. & Servan-Schreiber, D. (1992). Context, cortex and dopamine: a connectionist approach to behaviour and biology in schizophrenia. *Psychology Review, 99*, 45–77.

Corcoran, R. & Upton, D. (1993). A role for the hippocampus in card sorting? *Cortex, 29*, 293–304.

Damasio, H. & Damasio, A.R. (1989). *Lesion analysis in neuropsychology*. New York: Oxford University Press.

Damasio, H., Grabowski, T., Frank, R., Galaburda, A.M., & Damasio, A.R. (1994). The return of Phineas Gage: clues about the brain from the skull of a famous patient. *Science, 264*, 1102–1105.

Delis, D., Bihrle, A., Janowsky, J., Squire, L., & Shimamura, A. (1989). Fractionation of problem-solving deficits in frontal-lobe patients [Abstract]. *Journal of Clinical and Experimental Neuropsychology, 11*, 50.

Della Malva, C.L., Stuss, D.T., D'Alton, J., & Willmer, J. (1993). Capture errors and sequencing after frontal brain lesions. *Neuropsychologia, 31*, 363–372.

Fuster, J.M. (1997). *The Prefrontal Cortex: Anatomy, Physiology, and Neuropsychology of the Frontal Lobes*. New York: Lippincott-Raven.

Golden, C.J., Osmon, D.C., Moses, J., & Berg, R.A. (1981). *Interpretation of the Halstead-Reitan Neuropsychological Test Battery: A Casebook Approach*. New York: Grune & Stratton.

Grafman, J. (1995). Similarities and distinctions among current models of prefrontal cortical functions. In: J. Grafman, K.J. Holyoak, & F. Boller (Eds.), *Structure and Functions of the Human Prefrontal Cortex* (pp. 337–368) New York: New York Academy of Sciences.

Halgren, E., Marinkovic, K., and Chauvel, P. (1998). Generators of the late cognitive potential in auditory and visual oddball tasks. *Electroencephalography and Clinical Neurophysiology, 106*, 156–164.

Halsband, U. & Passingham, R.E. (1982). The role of premotor and parietal cortex in the direction of action. *Brain Research, 240*, 368–372.

Harlow, J.M. (1868). Recovery from the passage of an iron bar through the head. *Publications of the Massachusetts Medical Society, 2*, 327–347.

Holzt, P. & Vilkki, J. (1988). Effect of frontomedial lesions on performance on the Stroop test and word fluency tests. *Journal of Clinical and Experimental Neuropsychology, 10*, 79–80.

Janowsky, J.S., Shimamura, A.P., Kritchevsky, M., & Squire, L.R. (1989). Cognitive impairment following frontal lobe damage and its relevance to human amnesia. *Behavioural Neuroscience, 103*, 548–560.

Knight, R.T. (1996). Contribution of human hippocampal region to novelty detection. *Nature, 383*, 256–259.

Knight, R.T. (1997). Distributed cortical network for visual attention. *Journal of Cognitive Neuroscience, 9*, 75–91.

Knight, R.T. & Scabini, D. (1998). Anatomic bases of event-related potentials and their relationship to novelty detection in humans. *Journal of Clinical Neurophysiology, 15*, 3–13.

Levine, B. (1999). Self-regulation and autonoetic consciousness. In: E. Tulving (Ed.), *Memory, Consciousness, and the Brain: The Tallinn Conference* (pp. 200–214). Philadelphia: Psychology Press.

Levine, B., Stuss, D.T., & Milberg, W.P. (1995a). Concept generation: validation of a test of executive functioning in a normal aging population. *Journal of Clinical and Experimental Neuropsychology, 17*, 740–758.

Levine, B., Stuss, D.T., & Milberg, W.P. (1995b). Concept generation performance in normal aging and frontal dysfunction: preliminary validation of a clinical test [Abstract]. *Journal of the International Neuropsychological Society, 1*, 208.

Levine, B., Stuss, D.T., & Milberg, & W.P. (1997). Effects of aging on conditional associative learning: process analyses and comparison with focal frontal lesions. *Neuropsychology, 11*, 367–381.

Levine, B., Stuss, D.T., Milberg, W.P., Alexander, M.P., Schwartz, M.P., & Macdonald, R. (1998a). The effects of focal and diffuse brain damage on strategy application: evidence from focal lesions, traumatic brain injury and normal aging. *Journal of the International Neuropsychological Society, 4*, 247–264.

Levine, B., Black, S.E, Cabeza, R., Sinden, M., McIntosh, A.R., Toth, J.P., Tulving, E. & Stuss, D.T. (1998b). Episodic memory and the self in a case of isolated retrograde amnesia. *Brain, 121*, 1951–1973.

Levine, B., Freedman, M., Dawson, D., Black, S., & Stuss, D.T. (1999). Ventral frontal contribution to self-regulation: convergence of episodic memory and inhibition. *Neurocase, 5,* 263–275.

Levine, B., Dawson, D., Boutet, I., Schwartz, M.L., & Stuss, D.T. (2000). Assessment of strategic self-regulation in traumatic brain injury: its relationship to injury severity and psychosocial outcome. *Neuropsychology, 14,* 491–500.

Martin, I. & Levey, A.B. (1987). Learning what will happen next: conditioning, evaluation, and cognitive processes. In: G. Davey (Ed.), *Cognitive Processes and Pavlovian Conditioning in Humans* (pp. 57–81). Toronto: John Wiley & Sons.

McIntosh, A.R., Grady, C.L., Ungerleider, L.G., Haxby, J.V., Rapoport, S.I., & Horowitz, B. (1994). Network analysis of cortical visual pathways mapped with PET. *Journal of Neuroscience, 14,* 655–666.

McIntosh, A.R., Bookstein, F.L., Haxby, J.V., & Grady, C.L. (1996). Spatial pattern analysis of functional brain images using partial least squares. *NeuroImage, 3,* 143–157.

Molchan, S.E., Sunderland, T., McIntosh, A.R., Herscovitch, P., & Schreurs, B.G. (1994). A functional anatomical study of associative learning in humans. *Proceedings of the National Academy of Science USA, 91,* 8122–8126.

Nauta, W.J.H. (1973). Connections of the frontal lobe with the limbic system. In: L.V. Laitinen & K.E. Livingston (Eds.), *Surgical Approaches in Psychiatry* (pp. 303–314). Baltimore: University Park Press.

Pardo, J.V., Pardo, P.J., Janer, K.W., & Raichle, M.E. (1990). The anterior cingulate cortex mediates processing selection in the Stroop attentional conflict paradigm. *Proceedings of the National Academy of Sciences USA, 87,* 256–259.

Perret, E. (1974). The left frontal lobe of man and the suppression of habitual responses in verbal categorical behavior. *Neuropsychology, 12,* 323–330.

Petrides, M. (1982). Motor conditional associative-learning after selective prefrontal lesions in the monkey. *Behavioral Brain Research, 5,* 407–413.

Petrides, M. (1985). Deficits on conditional associative-learning tasks after frontal- and temporal-lobe lesions in man. *Neuropsychologia, 23,* 601–614.

Petrides, M. (1990). Nonspatial conditional learning impaired in patients with unilateral frontal but not unilateral temporal lobe excisions. *Neuropsychologia, 28,* 137–149.

Petrides, M. & Pandya, D.M. (1994). Comparative architectonic analysis of the human and macaque frontal cortex. In: F. Boller & J. Grafman (Eds.), *Handbook of Neuropsychology, Vol. 9* (pp. 17–57). Amsterdam: Elsevier.

Rademacher, J., Galaburda, A.M., Kennedy, D.N., Filipek, P.A., & Caviness, V.S. (1992). Human cerebral cortex: localization, parcellation, and morphometry with magnetic resonance imaging. *Journal of Cognitive Neuroscience, 4,* 352–374.

Rainer, G., Asaad, W.F., & Miller, E.K. (1998a). Memory fields of neurons in the primate prefrontal cortex. *Proceedings of the National Academy of Sciences USA, 95,* 15008–15013.

Rainer, G., Asaad, W.F., & Miller, E.K. (1998b). Selective representation of relevant information by neurons in the primate prefrontal cortex. *Nature, 393,* 577–579.

Shallice, T. (1988). *From Neuropsychology to Mental Structure.* Cambridge, UK: Cambridge University Press.

Shallice, T. & Burgess, P.W. (1991). Deficits in strategy application following frontal lobe damage in man. *Brain, 114,* 727–741.

Shammi, P. & Stuss, D.T. (1999). Humour appreciation: a role of the right frontal lobe. *Brain, 122,* 657–666.

Stone, V.E., Baron-Cohen, S., & Knight, R.T. (1998). Frontal lobe contributions to theory of mind. *Journal of Cognitive Neuroscience, 10,* 640–656.

Stroop, J.R. (1935). Studies of interference in serial verbal reactions. *Journal of Experimental Psychology, 18,* 643–662.

Stuss, D.T. (1991). Self, awareness, and the frontal lobes: a neuropsychological perspective. In: J. Strauss & G.R. Goethals (Eds.), *The Self: Interdisciplinary Approaches* (pp. 255–278). New York: Springer-Verlag.

Stuss, D.T. & Alexander, M.P. (1999). Affectively burnt in: a proposed role of the right frontal lobe. In: E. Tulving (Ed.), *Memory, Consciousness, and the Brain: The Tallinn Conference* (pp. 215–227). Philadelphia: Psychology Press.

Stuss, D.T. & Alexander, M.P. (2000). Executive functions of the frontal lobes: a conceptual view. *Psychological Research, 63,* 289–298.

Stuss, D.T. & Benson, D.F. (1986). *The Frontal Lobes.* New York: Raven Press.

Stuss, D.T. & Gow, C.A. (1992). "Frontal dysfunction" after traumatic brain injury. *Neuropsychiatry, Neuropsychology, and Behavioral Neurology, 5,* 272–282.

Stuss, D.T., Benson, D.F., Kaplan, E.F., Weir, W.S., & Della Malva, C. (1981). Leucotomized and nonleucotomized schizophrenics: comparison on tests of attention. *Biological Psychiatry, 16,* 1085–1100.

Stuss, D.T., Benson, D.F., Kaplan, E.F., Weir, W.S., Naeser, M.A., Lieberman, I., & Ferrill, D. (1983). The involvement of orbitofrontal cerebrum in cognitive tasks. *Neuropsychologia, 21,* 235–248.

Stuss, D.T., Alexander, M.P., Palumbo, C.L., Buckle, L., Sayer, L., & Pogue, J. (1994). Organizational strategies of patients with unilateral or bilateral frontal lobe injury in word list learning tasks. *Neuropsychology, 8,* 355–373.

Stuss, D.T., Shallice, T., Alexander, M.P. & Picton, T.W. (1995). A multidisciplinary approach to anterior attentional functions. *Annals of the New York Academy of Sciences, 769,* 191–212.

Stuss, D.T., Alexander, M.P., Hamer, L., Palumbo, C., Dempster, R., Binns, M., Levine, B., & Izukawa, D. (1998). The effects of focal anterior and posterior brain lesions on verbal fluency. *Journal of the International Neuropsychological Society, 4,* 265–278.

Stuss, D.T., Toth, J.P., Franchi, D., Alexander, M.P., Tipper, S., & Craik, F.I.M. (1999). Dissociation of attentional processes in patients with focal frontal and posterior lesions. *Neuropsychologia, 37,* 1005–1027.

Stuss, D.T., Levine, B., Alexander, M.P., Hong, J., Palumbo, C., Hamer, L., Murphy, K.J., & Izukawa, D. (2000a). Card Sorting Test performance in patients with focal frontal and posterior brain damage: effects of lesion location and test structure on separable cognitive processes. *Neuropsychologia, 38,* 388–402.

Stuss, D.T., van Reekum, R., & Murphy, K.J. (2000b). Differentiation of states and causes of apathy. In: J. Borod (Ed.), *The Neuropsychology of Emotion* (pp. 340–363). New York, Oxford University Press.

Stuss, D.T., Bisschop, S.M., Alexander, M.P., Levine, B., Katz, D., & Izukawa, D. (2001a). The Trail Making Test: a study in focal lesion patients. *Psychological Assessment, 13,* 230–239.

Stuss, D.T., Floden, D., Alexander, M.P., Levine, B., & Katz, D. (2001b). Stroop performance in focal lesion patients: dissociation of processes and frontal lobe lesion location. *Neuropsychologia, 39,* 771–786.

Stuss, D.T., Gallup, G.G., & Alexander, M.P. (2001c). The frontal lobes are necessary for theory of mind. *Brain, 124,* 279–286.

Stuss, D.T., Picton, T.W., & Alexander, M.P. (2001d) Consciousness, self-awareness and the frontal lobes. In: S. Salloway, P. Malloy, & J. Duffy (Eds.), *The Frontal Lobes and Neuropsychiatric Illness* (pp. 101–112). Washington, DC: American Psychiatric Press.

Talairach, J. & Tournoux, P. (1988). *Co-Planar Stereotaxic Atlas of the Human Brain.* New York: Thieme.

Taylor, S.F., Kornblum, S., Lauber, E.J., Minoshima, S., & Koeppe, R.A. (1997). Isolation of specific interference processing in the Stroop task: PET activation studies. *NeuroImage, 6,* 81–92.

Troyer, A.K., Moscovitch, M., Winocur, G., Alexander, M.P., & Stuss, D.T. (1998). Clustering and switching on verbal fluency: the effects of focal frontal-and temporal-lobe lesions. *Neuropsychologia, 36,* 499–504.

Vendrell, P., Junque, C., Pujol, J., Jurado, M.A., Molet, J., & Grafman, J. (1995). The role of prefrontal regions in the Stroop task. *Neuropsychologia, 33,* 341–352.

Wheeler, M.A., Stuss, D.T., & Tulving, E. (1995). Frontal lobe damage produces episodic memory impairment. *Journal of the International Neuropsychological Society, 1,* 525–536.

Wheeler, M.A., Stuss, D.T., & Tulving, E. (1997). Toward a theory of episodic memory: the frontal lobes and autonoetic consciousness. *Psychological Bulletin, 121,* 331–354.

26

Neurobehavioral Consequences of Neurosurgical Treatments and Focal Lesions of Frontal–Subcortical Circuits

JEAN A. SAINT-CYR, YURI L. BRONSTEIN, AND JEFFREY L. CUMMINGS

Analyses of frontal lobe functions have typically focused on corticocortical connections. Thus, in motor control, emphasis has been placed on the relations between primary, supplementary, and premotor cortical areas (e.g., Wiesendanger & Wise, 1992), while Petrides and colleagues (Petrides & Pandya, 1999) have examined parieto-, temporo-, and retrosplenial/presubicular-frontal connections and functions. We must now integrate the evidence that a major contribution to frontal lobe function arises from the basal ganglia. These subcortical gray masses receive a full complement of cortical information, as well as brain stem and diencephalic inputs, the integrated output being largely funneled back to the frontal lobes via thalamic relays. Therefore, a thorough understanding of frontal lobe–related functions cannot ignore this crucial subcortical link. The basal ganglia contribute to the full gamut of behavioral processes from affect and motivation, through cognition, and finally into the motor domain.

Since Alexander et al. (1986) introduced the concept of parallel but segregated frontal–subcortical circuits, our understanding of the mechanism involved in their anatomy, functions, and relationship to a variety of brain–motor and brain–behavior interactions has advanced greatly. The description of five frontal–subcortical circuits has provided a basis for elucidation of how those circuits influence both behavior and movements.

Complex neurochemical interactions occur at multiple levels within the circuits and underlie the control of both behavior and movements. Multiple neurotransmitters, neuropeptides, receptor subtypes, and second messengers are intricately involved in the function of the circuitry.

Human disorders linked to dysfunction of specific frontal–subcortical circuits include personality and mood disturbances, obsessive–compulsive disorder, and Parkinson's disease (PD), among others. With improved understanding of the mechanisms and neurochemistry underlying these conditions comes a better opportunity for selective manipulation of specific frontal–subcortical circuits. This is best illustrated by current approaches to the treatment of Parkinson's disease using pallidatomy and other surgical options.

This chapter describes the neuroanatomy and neurotransmitters of frontal–subcortical circuits and the clinical behavioral syndromes associated with the specific focal lesions within the circuits. In addition, the chapter reviews the neuropsychological and behavioral consequences of posterior pallidotomy and of deep-brain stimulation in the pallidum and subthalamic nucleus in patients with Parkinson's disease. Thus, both "naturally occurring" and intentional lesions or interruption of the circuit are considered.

OVERVIEW OF FRONTAL–SUBCORTICAL CIRCUITS

Frontal–subcortical circuits can be conceptually, anatomically, and functionally grouped into as many as five subcircuits. However, some authors prefer to categorize these into only three larger families (see Parent & Hazrati, 1995a). Nevertheless, each of the circuits includes the same member structures, including the cerebral cortex, striatum, globus pallidus and substantia nigra, and thalamus, finally funneling back principally to the frontal lobe (Cummings, 1995). Within each circuit there are two pathways: a direct and an indirect one that includes the subthalamic nucleus (Alexander et al., 1990). The relative anatomic relations of the circuits are preserved as they go through the relay stations, thus the dorsolateral prefrontal cortex projects to the dorsolateral area of the caudate nucleus, the peristriate visual belt projects to the caudal body, genu, and tail of the caudate and adjacent putamen, the orbitofrontal region projects to the ventral caudate/ventral striatum, and the anterior cingulate cortex projects to the medial striatum/nucleus accumbens region (Ilinsky et al., 1985; Saint-Cyr et al., 1990; Yeterian & Pandya, 1991; Parent & Hazrati, 1995a). A similar arrangement is preserved in the globus pallidus and the thalamus. This is the principle of proximity elucidated by Kemp and Powell (1970). Yeterian and van Hoesen (1978) first demonstrated that cortical association areas, which are themselves directly interconnected, project to convergent regions of the striatum. Selemon and Goldman-Rakic (1985) then showed that those projections could terminate in interdigitating longitudinal strips which could extend throughout most of the length of the striatum. This was also shown to be the case for cortical projections arising from the anterior cingulate, interparietal sulcus, and superior temporal sulcus corticos-

triate projections (Saint-Cyr et al., 1990). Clearly, this pattern does not follow the principle of proximity.

MOTOR CIRCUIT

The motor circuit originates from neurons in the supplementary motor area, premotor cortex, primary motor cortex, and somatosensory cortex (Alexander et al., 1986, 1990). Fibers from these areas project principally to the putamen in a somatotopic distribution. While motor cortical areal somatotopic representations are proportionately maintained in the projection to putaminal matrisomes, there is only about half as large an area, proportionately, for the comparable somatosensory projection (Flaherty & Graybiel, 1995). Recently, a contribution from the anterior cingulate motor area to the putamen has also been found (Nakano, 2000). The putamen in turn projects to globus pallidus externa (GPe), ventrolateral globus pallidus interna (GPi), and caudolateral substantia nigra, pars reticulata (SNr). The indirect pathway originates in the putamen and projects to the GPe, which then acts on the subthalamic nucleus (STN) (Smith & Bolam, 1990), which in turn has excitatory projections to the GPi/SNr and all other levels of the striatum (Parent & Hazrati, 1995b). The GPe and the SNr also project to the reticular shell of the thalamus, thus exerting a modulatory control over specific thalamic relay nuclei (Kayahara et al., 1998; Paré et al., 1990; Parent & Hazrati, 1995b). The fibers from GPi connect to ventral lateral (pars oralis), ventral anterior, and centromedian nuclei of the thalamus, and from there major connections go principally to the supplementary motor area, as well as to the premotor cortex, with motor cortex completing the circuit. Thalamic nuclei have reciprocal connections with the putamen and cerebral cortex in addition to the connections within the circuit (Parent & Hazrati, 1995a; McFarland & Haber, 2000). The GPi/SNr also project caudally to the nucleus tegmentopeduncularis, pars compacta (TPC). While most of the projections of that nucleus reascend back into the basal ganglia circuitry, including the STN, connections with brain stem centers involved in locomotion and reticulospinal pathways may exist (Garcia-Rill et al., 1987).

OCULOMOTOR (FRONTAL EYE FIELDS–SUBCORTICAL) CIRCUIT

The oculomotor circuit originates in the frontal eye field (Brodmann's area 8) as well as in the prefrontal and posterior parietal cortices. Fibers from cortical regions sequentially project to the central body of caudate nucleus, dorsomedial globus pallidus and ventrolateral SNr, medial dorsal thalamic nuclei (paralamellar division), and back to frontal eye fields (Alexander et al., 1986, 1990). Recently, the frontal eye field has been further subdivided into a smooth eye movement subregion and a saccadic subregion (Tian & Lynch, 1997). These transstriatal circuits, converging on the SNr, are involved in memory-guided saccadic control, acting through the superior colliculus (Hikosaka & Wurtz, 1989).

DORSOLATERAL PREFRONTAL CIRCUIT

The dorsolateral circuit originates in Brodmann's areas 9 and 46 (prefrontal cortex) on the dorsolateral surface of the anterior frontal lobe. Contributions from the association areas of the parietal and temporal lobes are also prominent. Sequential connections are to the striosomes of the dorsolateral head of the caudate nucleus (Selemon & Goldman-Rakic, 1985; Yeterian & Pandya, 1991; Eblen & Graybiel, 1995), lateral aspect of the dorsomedial GPi, and rostrolateral SNr via the direct pathway (Parent et al., 1984; Parent & Hazrati, 1995a). The indirect pathway through the dorsal GPe and the ventromedial STN also preserves some anatomical segregation from the motor and limbic circuits. Thalamic relay stations are parvo-and magnocellular portions of the ventral anterior nucleus and the multiformis division of the mediodorsal nucleus (Ilinsky et al., 1985; Nakano, 2000). The mediodorsal thalamus closes the circuit by connecting back to areas 9 and 46 of the dorsolateral frontal lobe (Giguère & Goldman-Rakic, 1988). Projections from the ventralis anterior nucleus also terminate in the inferotemporal cortex (Middleton & Strick, 1997,

2000). Again, the GPi/SNr projection to the TPC must be considered. Studies have implicated this link to the control of arousal (Reese et al., 1995). In this context, the GPe and SNr projections to the reticular shell of thalamus may also be involved in the control of arousal Steriade et al., 1986; (Steriade & Llinás, 1988). While not identical, there is an intimate relation between attentional control and arousal, thus potentially linking the reticular thalamic and TPC connections with the prefrontal cortical executive control of attention.

The dorsolateral circuit subserves executive function (Taylor et al., 1986, 1990, Taylor & Saint-Cyr, 1995; Cummings, 1993a), which includes the ability to organize a behavioral response to solve a complex problem (i.e., working memory), activation of remote memories, maintainence and shifting of behavioral sets, generation of motor programs, environmental independence, strategy generation, and use of verbal skills and internal cues to guide behavior (Stuss & Alexander, 2000). Performance of verbal and design fluency and alternating and reciprocal sequences, performance on problem-solving tasks (e.g., the Wisconsin Card Sorting Test [WCST]) and conditional associative learning, and self-monitoring depend on executive function (Jones-Gotman & Milner, 1977; Baddeley, 1986; Cummings, 1995; Fuster, 1997). The functions of this circuit in the context of executive operations in PD have been extensively reviewed (Brown & Marsden, 1990; Dubois et al., 1991; Taylor & Saint-Cyr., 1995). In addition to these executive functions, implicit or procedural learning functions have also been attributed to this circuit (Saint-Cyr et al., 1988, 1992; Saint-Cyr & Taylor, 1992; Graybiel, 1998; see also Wise et al., 1996).

ORBITOFRONTAL CIRCUIT

The orbitofrontal circuit consists of two subcircuits originating in Brodmann's areas 10 and 11. The medial orbitofrontal circuit sends fibers to the ventral striatum and to the dorsal part of nucleus accumbens (Haber et al., 1995); the lateral orbitofrontal circuit sends projections to the ventromedial caudate. Both orbitofrontal circuits then project to the most medial portion of the caudomedial GPi and to the rostromedial SNr (Johnson & Rosvold, 1971; Parent & Hazrati, 1995a). Axons are sent from the GPi/SNr to the medial area of the magnocellular parts of the ventralis anterior thalamic nucleus (Ilinsky et al., 1985; Selemon & Goldman-Rakic, 1985). The circuit then closes with projections back to the medial or lateral orbitofrontal cortex (Ilinsky et al., 1985).

The orbitofrontal circuit mediates socially appropriate behavior; personality changes are the hallmark of orbitofrontal dysfunction (Lhermitte et al., 1986; Cummings, 1995). Animal studies have emphasized the processing of reward in the orbitofrontal areas (Rolls, 2000).

ANTERIOR CINGULATE CIRCUIT

Neurons of the anterior cingulate (Brodmann's area 24) serve as the origin of the anterior cingulate–subcortical circuit. Input travels to the ventral striatum (Selemon & Goldman-Rakic, 1985), which includes the ventromedial caudate, ventral putamen, nucleus accumbens, and olfactory tubercle, collectively named the *limbic striatum*. Fibers from the ventral striatum project to the rostromedial GPi, rostrodorsal SNr, and ventral pallidum (the region of the globus pallidus inferior to the anterior commissure, also termed the *subcommissural pallidum*) (Haber et al., 1990). There may be an indirect loop projecting from the ventral striatum to the caudal pole of GPe (Haber et al., 1990). The GPe connects to the medial STN, which returns projections to the ventral pallidum (Smith et al., 1990). The ventral pallidum connects to the magnocellular mediodorsal thalamus (Haber et al., 1993). The circuit closes with projections to the anterior cingulate (Goldman-Rakic & Porrino, 1985). The anterior cingulate circuit mediates motivated behavior, and apathy is a major consequence of the damage to the structures of this circuit.

From a functional perspective, the separation of the orbitofrontal and anterior cingulate circuits may not be possible at the striatal level, although lesions further upstream may result in different behavioral syndromes (Par-

ent & Hazrati, 1995a; Saint-Cyr et al., 1995). The ventral striatum and accumbens also receive inputs from the amygdala and, through pallidonigral relays, establish an extensive output into the basal telencephalon and limbic midbrain, including such structures as the preoptic area, lateral hypothalamus, central periaqueductal gray, mesencephalic tegmentum, and lateral habenula (Nakano, 2000). This provides a means whereby the so-called emotional circuits can directly influence autonomic and motor centers involved in the expression of motivated behaviors and emotion, without having to pass through a cortical relay.

OPEN CONNECTIONS AND INTERCONNECTIONS

As described thus far, each frontal–subcortical circuit comprises a closed loop. However, afferent and efferent open elements also contribute to each circuit (Mega & Cummings, 1994). Open elements of the circuits relate systematically to other brain regions. For example, Middleton and Strick (1997, 2000) have recently shown that striatal circuit output can act on the inferotemporal cortex, thus providing a means of contributing to memory processing. In addition to the principle of proximity, associative cortical areas, which are themselves directly interconnected, project to longitudinal, interdigitating strips in the striatum (Selemon & Goldman-Rakic, 1985). Some cortical inputs may terminate on tonically active interneurons that may cross-link striosomes and the surrounding matrix (Graybiel, 1998). Those interneurons have been shown to be active in learning (Aosaki et al., 1994a, 1994b; 1995), under dopaminergic control.

Despite the anatomical segregation of projections through the basal ganglia (recently also demonstrated with transneuronal transport of viruses) (Middleton & Strick, 1997), the extensive dendritic arbors of pallidal neurons and the proliferation of axonal terminations from the striatum and STN (see Parent & Hazrati, 1995a, 1995b, for a review) reveal the anatomical opportunity for interactions between circuits. The capacity of these circuits to function in a specific and focused manner

Table 26–1. Connections of frontal–subcortical circuits

Category	Motor	Oculomotor	Dorsolateral (Complex)
Striatal	Putamen	Caudate (body)	Caudate (head–tail)
Cortical afferents	Motor areas 9, 6, 4 Parietal areas 2, 1, 3, 7 Cingulate area 24 (mtr)	Frontal eye fields 8 Frontal 46 Parietal 7	Prefrontal areas 9, 46 Entorhinal area 28 Perirhinal area 35 Superior temporal 22
Subcortical afferents	CM VA/VLpc, VLpo VPLpo, x SNpc Dorsal raphé	CM/intralaminar SNpc Dorsal raphé	Parafascicular VA SNpc Dorsal raphé
Subcortical efferents	GPi (vl) SNr (dl) STN (dm) VLo, VApc CM, VLm, VLc TPC	GPi (dm) SNr (vl) STN (dm) MDpl CM? Superior colliculus	GPi (dm) SNr (rl) STN (rl) VAmc, pc VMp MDmf, pl Parafascicular TPC
Cortical efferent Focus	Supplementary motor area 6	Frontal eye field area 8	Prefrontal areas 9, 46 Inferotemporal cortex

Category	Orbitofrontal Circuit	Anterior Cingulate Circuit
Striatal	Caudate-putamen (ventral)	N. accumbens
Cortical afferents	Superior temporal area 22 Inferior temporal areas Orbitofrontal areas 10, 11, 12 Medial frontal area 32 Anterior cingulate areas 24, 25	Hippocampus Entorhinal area 28 Perirhinal area 35 Superior temporal area 22 Orbitofrontal area 12 Inferior temporal areas Anterior cingulate areas 24, 25
Subcortical thalamus afferents	Parafascicular (rm) STN m SN compacta (m) VTA Dorsal raphé Nucleus basalis of Meynert Amygdala	Subparafascicular Dorsal raphé VTA Nucleus basalis of Meynert Amygdala
Subcortical efferents	GPi (cm) SNr (rm) STN m VA mc, MD m VP vm, VP dl Septal region LHA, LPOA, Parav. N.	GPi (rl) (subcomm.) PAG Lateral habenula LMA TPC
Cortical efferent focus	Prefrontal area 9 Orbitofrontal areas 10, 11, 12	Anterior cingulate areas 24, 25

has been shown to be regulated by dopaminergic inputs (Filion et al., 1988, 1994). In addition, the entire concept of strict anatomical and hence functional segregation of these circuits and the validity of the current model have been criticized Percheron & Filion, 1991; Parent & Cicchetti, 1998). Table 26–1 lists the principal afferents and efferents for the frontal–subcortical circuits.

BEHAVIORAL AND NEUROPSYCHOLOGICAL MANIFESTATIONS OF CIRCUIT—RELATED LESIONS

Disruption of each of the behaviorally related circuits presents with "signature" clinical syndromes. A lesion in the orbitofrontal–subcortical circuit leads to disinhibition, a lesion of the anterior cingulate circuit causes apathy, and a lesion in the dorsolateral circuit produces a frontal dysexecutive syndrome (it has recently been suggested that we should refer to fronto striatal or frontal subcortical dysfunction to differentiate those syndromes

from impairments due to dorsolateral frontal lesions). Aside from these circuit-specific behavioral syndromes, there are circuit-related syndromes, including mood abnormalities, obsessive–compulsive spectrum disorders, and psychosis (Mega & Cummings, 1994; Cummings, 1995; Saint-Cyr et al., 1995). A variety of etiological factors have been implicated in productions of these syndromes. Behavioral abnormalities have been reported with focal lesions caused by stroke, tumors, trauma, and neurodegeneration Bhatia & Marsden, 1994; (Dubois et al., 1995).

CIRCUIT NEUROTRANSMITTERS

Each circuit involves two pathways: a direct and an indirect one. Neurons with modulatory transmitters project to these circuits and increase the complexity of neurochemical regulators. Both direct and indirect pathways begin with excitatory, glutamatergic projections from frontal cortex to specific regions of striatum. Striatal output diverges into a direct and in-

---

In this summary of some of the major anatomical relations of striatal circuits, thalamic nomenclature is taken largely from the animal literature. For correspondance with human terms, see Macchi and Jones (1997). Data are based on recent reviews by Parent and Hazrati (1995a,b), Nakano (2000), and McFarland and Haber (2000). Other references are in the text.

It should be noted that the motor circuits appear to be more focused anatomically, and include the motor area of the anterior cingulate cortex (cingulate area 24, mtr), while the complex circuits may extend their influence outside of the frontal lobes into the inferotemporal cortex. In contrast, the emotional circuitry has widespread influences extending throughout the preoptic, hypothalamic, and limbic midbrain axis, as well as the amygdala. Other summaries of these circuits have separated out a lateral orbitofrontal circuit (see Alexander et al., 1986) with cortical inputs from the anterior cingulate and temporal areas. The above scheme attributes the temporal inputs to the complex circuit and the anterior cingulate to the emotional circuits. One could also define a visual–perceptual circuit with links to both the oculomotor and complex circuits (see Saint-Cyr et al., 1990). It is also noteworthy that all of the thalamic nuclei that are in receipt of pallidonigral inputs project back into the striatum. This provides an opportunity for a wide range of inputs from spinal, brain stem, and cerebellar centers to contribute to striatal computations.

The globus pallidus interna (GPi) terminations are defined by region, rostrolateral (rl), ventrolateral (vl), dorsomedial (dm), caudal medial (cm), and subcommissural (subcomm.). Similarly, the substantia nigra pars reticulata (SNr) terminations are also defined by region, dorsolateral (dl), ventrolateral (vl), rostromedial (rm), rostrolateral (rl). The subthalamic nucleus (STN) is also compartmentalized as dorsomedial (dm), rostrolateral (rl), and medial (m). Substantia nigra pars compacta (SNpc), and the ventral tegmental area (VTA) are sources of dopamine, while the dorsal raphé contribute serotonin.

Abbreviations: *Thalamic nuclei:* CM, center median; MD, medialis dorsalis and its divisions, paralamellaris (pl), multiformis (mf), and magnocellularis (m); po, posterior group; VA, ventralis anterior and its subdivisions, parvocellularis (pc) and magnocellularis (mc); VL, ventralis lateralis and its subdivisions, oralis (o), medialis (m), and caudalis (c); VMp, posterior portion of ventralis medialis. VP, ventralis posterior and its subdivisions, ventromedial (vm), dorsolateral (dl), and lateral posterior (VPLpo); x, nucleus x.

Brain stem and hypothalamic nuclei: LHA, lateral hypothalamus; LMA, limbic midbrain area; LPOA, lateral preoptic area; PAG, periaqueductal gray; Paraven. N., paraventricular nucleus; TPC, nucleus tegmentopedunclularis, pars compacta.

direct pathway. The direct pathway sends gamma-aminobutyric acid (GABA) fibers colocalized with substance P, to neurons in the GPi and the SNr; from there, GABAergic efferents are sent to discrete regions within the thalamus that then relay information back to the striatum and frontal lobe utilizing glutamate as the thalamocortical transmitter. The indirect pathway originates from GABAergic neurons colocalized with enkephalin, which projects first to the GPe that sends GABAergic projections to the STN, which in turn sends glutamatergic fibers to the GPi/SNr, which then projects to the specific thalamic nuclei that complete the circuit by sending glutamatergic fibers back to the frontal cortical areas (and striatum).

Thus, the two principal fast-acting transmitters of the frontal–subcortical circuits are GABA and glutamate. Dopamine (DA), acetylcholine (ACh), and serotonin (5-HT) are major modulating transmitters in the circuits. Only the major transmitter systems will be reviewed here, but the reader is advised that many more neurochemical markers have been identified (Graybiel, 1990) and the histochemical compartmentation of the striatum is highly complex (Gerfen, 1992).

GABA

Within the basal ganglia, the predominant neurotransmitter is GABA. Most neurons located within the striatum are GABAergic. GABA is localized in projections neurons, interneurons, and afferent fiber terminals (Kita, 1993). Various types of GABAergic neurons have been described in the caudate-putamen (Kawaguchi et al., 1995). Other structures of circuits particularly rich in GABA are globus pallidus and substantia nigra. Inhibition of GABAergic neurons in the GPe releases (disinhibits) STN from their tonic inhibition. Similarly, striatal activation may lead to nigral inhibition and consequently to thalamic activation because of the disinhibition of the latter. It has also been shown that GPe projects directly to the reticular shell of the thalamus (also GABAergic), providing a mechanism by which the striatum can modulate thalamo-cortical attentional mechanisms (Ster-

iade & Llinás, 1988; Kayahara et al., 1998; Parent & Hazrati, 1995a).

The GABAergic system represents the output pathways of neostriatum and globus pallidus. Two distinct neuronal subpopulations are recognized by coexpression of neuropeptides in these output pathways. Striatopallidal GABAergic neurons coexpress enkephalin, whereas striatonigral GABAergic neurons coexpress substance P/dynorphin.

GABAergic neuronal terminals make contact with glutamatergic (Moratalla & Bowery, 1991), DA (Bowery, 1989), and cholinergic (DeBoer & Westerlink, 1994) neurons. It has been postulated that striatal ACh release is directly modulated by stimulation of $GABA_a$ receptors located on cholinergic neurons and indirectly modulated by stimulation of $GABA_b$ receptors located on neurons that form synapses on cholinergic neurons (Ikarashi et al., 1999).

GLUTAMATE

The striatum is driven by the massive, excitatory input from cerebral cortex and thalamostriatal connections. Both of these excitatory pathways are thought to use glutamate (Carlsson & Carlsson, 1990; Starr, 1995). Cortical glutamatergic neurons innervate the distal dentrites of medium-sized spiny striatal neurons (Kotter, 1994). Glutamatergic fibers terminate at the spine heads, where all three major glutamatergic receptor subtypes (N-methyl-D-aspartate [NMDA], AMPA, and kainate) are expressed (Kita, 1996).

Glutamate is used by input neurons from the cortex, thalamus, and brain stem to the STN, as well as by output pathways from STN to the GPI/SNr (Rouzaire-Dubois & Scarnati, 1987). The proposed mechanism of glutamate neurotransmission largely involves interactions with other neurotransmitter systems, particularly the DA system. The prevailing opinion in the literature suggests that glutamate and DA have functionally opposite effects in the striatum, however, there is still controversy as to whether glutamate stimulates or suppresses motor output from the striatum (Starr, 1995). Glutamatergic modulation of DA release in the striatum is mainly facilitatory and phasic in nature and mediated by pre- and postsynaptic NMDA and non-NMDA ionotropic receptors and probably by metabotropic glutamate receptors (mGluRs) (Morari et al., 1998). These glutamatergic–dopaminergic interactions may be highly significant in the etiopathogenesis of such disorders as PD and schizophrenia (Grace, 1992; Whitton, 1997).

ACETYLCHOLINE

Acetylcholine pathways in the frontal–subcortical circuits are divided into subsystems characterized by long cholinergic projection neurons and short intrinsic neurons in the neostriatum. The striatum contains cholinergic interneurons that receive a massive input from the thalamus but a more modest, yet potentially important, cortical input (Carpenter, 1981; Graybiel, 1998). These cholinergic interneurons express D1 and D2 DA receptors and are under dopaminergic nigrostriatal influence. They also synapse with GABAergic striatal output neurons. In this way, they may bridge the direct and indirect circuits across the striosomes and matrix, while playing a role in reinforcement learning. Dubois and colleagues (1990) have argued for a critical role of ACh in executive functions in PD, and this may involve both cortical and subcortical actions (Bédard et al., 1999).

Cholinergic afferents to the thalamus originate in the pedunculopontine nucleus and laterodorsal tegmentum and may contribute to arousal and attentional mechanisms (Reese et al., 1995). Cortical areas of frontal–subcortical circuits receive cholinergic input from nucleus basalis of Meynert via medial and lateral cholinergic pathways (Selden et al., 1998), as part of the open-loop circuit connections.

The cholinergic synapses in the striatum demonstrate specific regional distributions. The M1, M2, and M4 receptors are localized in the striatum (Levey et al., 1991); M1 and M4 receptors are particularly dense in the neostriatum and nucleus accumbens. The M2 receptor is localized in caudate-putamen and nucleus accumbens. The M3 and M4 receptors are present in the STN (Chesselet & Delfs, 1996).

Striatal ACh neurons receive three major synaptic inputs: *(1)* from intrinsic medium-sized spiny neurons; *(2)* from extrinsic DA neurons of the mesencephalic tegmentum; and *(3)* from extrinsic excitatory (glutamatergic) neurons of the intralaminar thalamus and, to a lesser degree, of the cortex (Meredith & Wouterlood, 1990). The neuronal nicotinic receptors are abundant in the striatum and SN (Perry et al., 1992). It has been shown that nicotine modulates midbrain DA neurons and cortical glutamatergic neurons (Dalack et al., 1998).

Complex interactions occur between ACh and other transmitters, particularly DA and glutamate. Acetycholine has been found to tonically facilitate striatal DA release via activation of both muscarinic and nicotonic receptors located presynaptically on DA terminals (Di Chiara & Moreli, 1993). It appears that ACh and DA exert opposite influences on striatopallidal as compared to striatonigral neurons by affecting different receptor subtypes (D1/D2; M1/M4) (Di Chiara et al., 1994).

Glutamate also modulates striatal cholinergic neurons such that blockade of NMDA receptors decreases basal ACh release (Damsma et al., 1991), whereas activation of NMDA receptors causes an increase in striatal ACh release (Scatton & Lehman, 1982).

DOPAMINE

The highest concentrations of DA receptors in the brain are in the striatum. Dopamine is involved in the regulation of a variety of functions, including locomotor activity, neuroendocrine activity, emotions, mood, and thought processes. The DA receptors are grouped into receptor subfamilies designated D1–D5. Each DA receptor subtype has a specific predilection for a specific location in the frontal–subcortical circuits. Both D1 and D2 DA receptors are present in high concentrations in the caudate and putamen. D1 receptors are found only in GPi and SNr (direct pathway), whereas D2 DA receptors are preferentially expressed by striatal projections to GPe (indirect pathway). D3 subtypes are more abundant in structures of mesolimbic system, and highest

D4 receptor expression is in the frontal lobe. Dopamine exerts complementary actions via both direct and indirect pathways to decrease tonic firing rates of intrinsic neurons in the major output nuclei of the basal ganglia. At the same time, DA projections to the frontal cortex regulate activity and excitability of the cortical neurons on which the working memory functions of the prefrontal cortex depend (Williams & Goldman-Rakic, 1995; Lewis et al., 1998).

According to Schultz and colleagues (Schultz et al., 1998; Suri & Schultz, 1998; Tremblay et al., 1998), DA appears to play two different roles in the striatum, namely a tonic nonspecific facilitation (rather neurohumoural like most monoamines) and a phasic action linked to reinforcement learning and the elimination of errors. Evidence for these functions has been gathered in single-unit recording studies in subhuman primates (Aosaki et al., 1994a, 1995b,; Bowman et al., 1996; Hollerman et al., 1998). Clinically, dopaminergic modulation of all frontal–subcortical circuits provides the anatomic basis for the complex effects of dopaminergic agents, including improvement of motor function in PD, enhanced motivation in akinetic mutism, and adverse reactions such as hallucinations and delusions (Cummings, 1991).

SEROTONIN

Serotonergic fibers project from the medial raphé to the striatum, SN, and cortex. Serotonin (5-hydroxytryptamine; 5-HT) receptors are differentially distributed in the frontal–subcortical circuits. The 5-HT1 subtype is predominantly localized in the basal ganglia; 5-HT3 receptors are more common in the ventral striatum. High densities of 5-HT2 and 5-HT1a subtypes are present in neocortex. Anatomical data indicate that the major target of serotonin axons in the prefrontal cortex is the interneuron (Smiley & Goldman-Rakic, 1996).

Serotonergic fibers modulate dopaminergic neurons, particularly when the dopaminergic neurons are activated (Palfreyman et al., 1993). Serotonin interacts with other neurotransmitters and, operating through a 5-HT2

receptor, activates GABAergic interneurons in the prefrontal cortex (Abi-Saab et al., 1999). Serotonergic dysfunction has been postulated to underlie depression in PD (Sano et al., 1990), but an interaction between biological and behavioral factors may be a more integrated perspective (Taylor & Saint-Cyr, 1990). In this view, a monoamine-based weakness in emotional control circuits results in an emotional lability, making patients more susceptible to symptom-specific and environmental stressors. Mayberg (1997) proposed a functional linkage between dorsolateral prefrontal cortex, the anterior subgenual cingulate cortex, and the ventral striatum in the control of mood.

ADENOSINE

In recent years an important role of adenosine in modulation of neurotransmitters systems in frontal–subcortical circuits has been discovered. Four different subtypes of adenosine receptors have been found in the brain: A1, A2a, A2b, and A3 (Fredholm, 1995). Striatal A1 receptors are located in intrinsic neurons and in corticostriatal afferents but not in dopaminergic afferents. Functional studies support the modulatory influences of A1 receptors on DA release (Ballarin et al., 1995). Data suggest that adenosine plays a role opposite that of DA in the striatum. Both DA antagonists and adenosine agonists produce similar effects in different behavioral tests. Adenosine receptor agonists inhibit and adenosine receptor antagonists potentiate the motor-activating effects of DA receptor agonists (Ferre, 1997). There is evidence for segregation of the DA and adenosine receptors subtypes in the two different types of striatal GABAergic efferent neurons, and data suggest that striatopallidal neurons and striatonigral neurons might be the main loci for the A2a–D2 and A1–D1 interactions, respectively (Ferre, 1997).

FUNCTIONAL NEUROIMAGING OF FRONTAL SUBCORTICAL CIRCUITS

Frontal cerebral blood flow is reduced in PD, while positron emission tomography (PET) studies have shown hypometabolism in frontal–striatal circuits (see Eidelberg, 1998; Brooks, 2000, for reviews), again demonstrating the functional unity of those interconnections. Activation paradigms (functional magnetic resonance imaging [fMRI]), which implicate the striatal circuits in cognitive operations, include visuomotor learning, visual–spatial localization, problem solving, motor sequence learning, and attentional shifting (see and Rauch & Savage, 1997: and Owen & Doyon, 1999 for reviews, and recent studies by Boeker et al., 1998, Koski et al., 1999, Poldrack et al., 1999, and Rogers et al., 2000). These studies confirm an active role of striatal circuits in executive functions with demands on attentional capacity, working memory, and new learning.

CLINICAL AND BEHAVIORAL OUTCOME OF NEUROSURGICAL TREATMENTS

Animal experiments as well as functional studies with patients have confirmed that both the GPi and STN are overly active in PD, motivating the resurgence of neurosurgical interventions (Lang & Lozano, 1998a, 1998b; Starr et al., 1998). To the extent that striatal circuits continue to play a role in motor control and cognition in PD, the interruption of pathological activity patterns via neurosurgical interventions could either impede or facilitate normal function.

This has provided a unique opportunity to study behavioral changes produced by placing focal lesions or implanting chronic deep-brain stimulation electrodes in frontal–subcortical circuits during surgical treatment of movement disorders. Surgical targets include GPi (principally to eliminate drug-induced dyskinesias and to treat primary dystonia), thalamus (to treat tremor and pain), and STN (to treat PD).

Neuropsychological outcome studies initially showed little cognitive impact, but later assessment with larger groups and more extensive testing indicated hemisphere-specific impairment and executive dysfunction after GPi posteroventral pallidotomy (Masterman et al., 1998; Trépanier et al., 1998; Green & Barnhart, 2000; Stebbins et al., 2000). Thus, after left posteroventral pallidotomy, long-standing deficits in verbal memory and verbal fluency as well as in executive functions were found. Right hemisphere lesions were more likely to be associated with transient visual–spatial dysfunction (Trépanier et al., 1998). After either left or right unilateral lesions, one in four patients may develop behavioral or personality alterations ranging from apathy and abulia to disinhibition and mania (Trépanier et al., 1998). Fortunately, these may be problematic for only a few months, but in some cases, especially in patients with antecedent psychiatric histories, the decompensation may last over 12 months. Bilateral lesions in the pallidum are unfortunately often catastrophic, resulting in marked behavioral dysfunction, characterized as a frontal behavioral syndrome (Scott et al., 1998; Trépanier et al., 1998). In the most severe cases, prolonged hospitalization and behavioral management are needed. However, some patients have been reported in whom the outcome was more benign (Ghika et al., 1999), possibly because of location or size of lesion.

Analysis of lesion location has shown that rostrodorsal placement within the GPi is associated with the greatest reduction in dyskinesia, while posteroventral lesions are associated with reduction of akinesia and tremor (Gross et al., 1999). There is also an optimal location, close to the intended posteroventral targeted location. From a neuropsychological perspective, the rostral lesions have proved to be the most toxic, being associated with reduced verbal fluency and, on the left, with impaired verbal encoding (Lombardi et al., 2000). In that same study it was also shown that the most caudal lesions are associated with a modest improvement in attentional capacity. Recently, another study has demonstrated that lesion volume, if segregated into dorsal and ventral compartments within the GPi, is associated with clinical outcome. Specifically, the volume of the posterior component was related to the reduction of drug-induced dyskinesia (Kishore et al., 2000).

The use of deep-brain stimulation of the

GPi, rather than lesions, appears to be less toxic, and permits bilateral interventions (Ardouin et al., 1999; Trépanier et al., 2000). Here also, there is a suggestion that location of stimulation within the pallidum (which may include portions of GPe) produces differential effects on parkinsonian symptoms in the on- and off-drug states (Bejjani et al., 1997).

Bilateral stimulation of the STN is now considered the treatment of choice for PD, and this fundamentally ameliorates symptoms and permits drastic reductions in medication (Krack et al., 1998; Kumar et al., 1999). The mechanism is thought to involve blocking of the action of the STN, thus reducing its widespread excitatory influence throughout the striatal circuitry (and perhaps also directly into the thalamus). In younger patients, there are few iatrogenic cognitive costs (Ardouin et al., 1999). A modest improvement in some executive functions has also been shown (Jahanshahi et al., 2000). Moreover, cessation of stimulation does not appear to alter test performance (Pillon et al., 2000). Thus, after an initial adaptation, it may be the case that a permanent reprogramming of the distribution of function has taken place, putting the striatal circuits out of the processing loop, as suggested by Marsden and Obeso (1994) with regard to motor control. However, in older patients, stimulation does lead to cognitive compromise and a more modest clinical benefit (Saint-Cyr et al., 2000). Many of these patients experience transient states of confusion lasting days to months. Otherwise, the full gamut of cognitive impairment has been seen, with those functions dependent on executive mechanisms being most at risk. Idiosyncratic behavioral and personality dysfunction is also present, sometimes requiring psychiatric management.

Mood after surgical interventions is usually improved, because of clinical benefit. However, instances of euphoria and depression/apathy (abulia) have been reported (Scott et al., 1998; Bejjani et al., 1999; Kumar et al., 1999; Trépanier et al., 2000; Pollak, personal communication).

Functional imaging studies have shown that GPi deep-brain stimulation results in activation of motor cortical areas, which were previously underactivated in PD (Davis et al., 1997). Other studies have shown that only clinically effective stimulation of the STN can normalize blood flow to the supplementary and motor association areas, whereas effective stimulation of the GPi has a less specific action (Limousin et al., 1997). These effects were only demonstrable using motor activation paradigms. Deep-brain stimulation of the STN increased activation (blood flow) of motor cortical association areas but decreased primary motor cortical activation (Ceballos-Baumann et al., 1999). These studies provide compelling evidence that the deep-brain stimulation effect is related to the recruitment of cerebellar compensatory mechanisms acting through thalamo–motor cortical pathways. Again, we are reminded of the position adopted by Mardsen and Obseo (1994) with regard to the reprogramming of motor control circuits. Comparable studies have yet to be done using cognitive paradigms.

CLINICAL SYNDROMES WITH FOCAL CIRCUIT LESIONS

ABULIA AND AKINETIC MUTISM

Akinetic mutism is a wakeful state of profound apathy, with indifference to pain, thirst, or hunger, and an absence of motor or psychic initiative, manifested by lack of spontaneous movements, absent verbalization, and failure to respond to questions or commands (Cairns et al., 1941). *Abulia* refers to a similar but less severe psychomotor syndrome.

Akinetic mutism has been described in various etiological conditions involving the ventral striatum (nucleus accumbens and ventromedial caudate), ventral globus pallidus, and medial thalamus (Mega et al., 1997). In a review of patients with discrete lesions of the basal ganglia (Bhatia & Marsden, 1994), abulia occurred with 28% of small and large caudate lesions sparing the lentiform nucleus; most lesions were unilateral. Abulia also occurs with bilateral globus pallidus lesions. Mega and Cohenour (1997) described a patient who developed a rigid akinetic mute state caused by bilateral lesions of GPi with ventral extension.

While unilateral caudate lesions are sufficient to produce abulia, akinetic mutism is most commonly accompanied by lesions involving bilateral anterior cingulate circuit structures and may be predicted by lesions that extend from the cognitive effector region posteriorly into the skeletomotor effector area of the cingulate (Mega et al., 1997).

Nemeth et al. (1986), using pathological studies, postulated that isolated damage to any of the projections of brain-stem dopaminergic nuclear groups could result in akinetic mutism. This is supported by similar findings in experimental animals in which a syndrome resembling akinetic mutism was produced by bilateral or unilateral injection of 6-hydroxydopamine into either the SN, ventral tegmentum, or nigrostriatal tract (Marshall et al., 1974).

Ross and Stewart (1981) reported a patient with akinetic mutism who responded to treatment with DA receptor agonists but not to carbidopa/levodopa or methylphenidate. This response suggests a loss of dopaminergic input to anterior cingulate cortex. Response to direct DA agonists may be poor, however, in cases where DA receptors have been damaged, e.g., in patients with lesions involving the anterior cingulate gyri.

Akinetic mutism may also be seen after bilateral lesions of the posterior midline thalamus, including the center median–parafascicular complex (Heilman et al., 1993). After successful deep-brain stimulation treatment, many patients become abulic and apathetic because of the dramatic decrease in their DA medications. This may be due to loss of compensation for the ventral tegmental area–mesolimbic loss of DA to the orbitofrontal, medial frontal–cingulate, and ventral striatal regions.

DEPRESSION

Depression has been linked to two structures of frontal–subcortical circuits, the frontal lobes and the caudate nucleus. Focal lesions of the dorsolateral prefrontal cortex and caudate may be associated with depression (Cummings, 1993b; Jorge et al., 1993). The dorsomedial prefrontal cortex was found to have reduced cerebral blood flow (CBF) in depressed but not nondepressed patients with PD (Ring et al., 1994). Hirono et al. (1998) reported decreased hypometabolism in bilateral superior frontal and left anterior cingulate cortices in depressed patients with Alzheimer's disease. Mayberg (1997) has prosed an interaction between the ventral striatum and both the prefrontal cortical areas thought to be involved in the control of compensatory strategies in depression, and the subgenual cingulate area 25, which is linked to the presence of depressive affect.

Neuroanatomical studies of idiopathic depression revealed decreased metabolism in the dorsolateral prefrontal cortex and the caudate nucleus (Baxter et al., 1989). Other functional neuroimaging studies have identified abnormalities in the orbital and medial prefrontal cortical areas and in the amygdala (Biver et al., 1994; Drevets, 1999). The posterior orbital cortex and anterior cingulate cortex ventral to genu of the corpus callosum have been shown recently in morphometric MRI and postmortem histopathological studies to have reduced gray matter volume and reduced glial cell numbers in familial major depressive disorders and bipolar disorders (Drevets, 1998, 1999). Preliminary findings suggest that patients with depression have a smaller volume of GPe on postmortem study (Baumann et al., 1999).

A substantial number of studies that examined post-stroke depression reported a significantly higher prevalence and severity of depression in patients with left hemispheric stroke, particularly in the vicinity of the frontal lobe and frontal–subcortical circuits (Robinson et al., 1987; Starkstein et al., 1987, 1988). A recent study by Beblo et al., (1999) confirmed the high prevalence of post-stroke depression after left hemispheric stroke and involvement of basal ganglia. Superimposition analysis performed by the authors revealed a maximal overlap of lesions in the caudate nucleus and posterior parts of the putamen and pallidum.

Recently, Bejjani et al. (1999) reported a remarkable case of a patient who received deep-brain stimulation to treat her intractable PD. Electrical stimulation delivered through an electrode positioned in the central region of the left SN evoked, during the course of the stimulation, unequivocal symptoms and signs of depression. Suggested mechanisms could include a de-activation of remaining SNpc DA neurons and their projections, or alteration of transthalamic circuits related to the orbitofrontal–anterior cingulate regions. Kumar and colleagues (1999) have also reported some cases.

MANIA

Mania is also a circuit-related behavior. Mania has been described with lesions or neurodegenerative disorders affecting structures of orbitofrontal–subcortical circuit, orbitofrontal cortex, caudate nucleus, and perithalamic area (Cummings & Mendez, 1984; Trautner et al., 1988; Kulisevsky et al., 1993). Cortical lesions that produce mania are rarely followed by cyclic mood disorders, whereas the subcortical lesions affecting the caudate and thalamus produce a bipolar type of mood disorder with recurrent depression and mania (Starkstein et al., 1991). Most focal lesions eliciting mania are associated with right hemisphere lesions (Cummings, 1995). Right inferior frontal lesions are recognized as the lesions most likely to produce mania (Robinson et al., 1988; Braun et al., 1999).

Transient episodes of involuntary laughter and euphoria during deep-brain stimulation of STN in a patient with PD have been reported Krack et al., 2001. Mendez et al. (1999) described a patient with involuntary laughter after bifrontal lesion following anterior cerebral artery aneurysm rupture and shunt placement for obstructive hydrocephalus. Positron emission tomography in this patient showed medial bifrontal hypometabolism. The authors postulated that the pathological neuroanatomical circuit involved in laughter includes the anterior cingulate, caudal hypothalamus, amygdala, and a pontomedullary center.

OBSESSIVE–COMPULSIVE DISORDER AND TOURETTE'S SYNDROME

Patients with idiopathic and acquired obsessive–compulsive disorder (OCD) display sim-

ilar behavioral symptoms and neuropsychological abnormalities. Etiologies of acquired OCD include pericallosal tumors compressing the posterior cingulate, left anterior cingulate contusion, subcortical lesions (particularly involving the caudate nucleus), lesions of the right posterior putamen, and post-traumatic orbitofrontal contusions (Berthier et al., 1996). Orbital, caudate, and thalamic regions have been demonstrated to be abnormal with PET in idiopathic OCD. Several authors have hypothesized that that the main pathology of OCD arises from an excessive disinhibition of the mediodorsal nucleus of thalamus (Modell et al., 1989; Baxter, 1990). Serotonin is highly implicated in the pathophysiology of OCD. The serotonergic innervation to the striatum is localized to ventromedial caudate nucleus head and ventral striatum, which receive input from the orbitofrontal and anterior cingulate cortices (Parent, 1990). Obsessive–compulsive disorder also occurs with lesions of the globus pallidus and has been reported in postencephalitic parkinsonism, anoxia, manganese intoxication, progressive supranuclear palsy (PSP), and Huntington's disease (Cummings & Cunningham, 1992).

There is substantial evidence that Tourette's syndrome involves alterations within the frontal–subcortical circuits (Singer, 1997). Neuroimaging data provide support for altered circuit acitivity in Tourette's syndrome. Singer et al. (1993) showed the putamen and lenticular region to be significantly smaller using volumetric MRI. Braun et al. (1993) used PET to demonstrate increased metabolic rates in frontal motor regions associated with hypometabolism in paralimbic prefrontal cortices and in the ventral striatum. Many patients with Tourette's syndrome exhibited OCD or OCD-like symptoms.

SUMMARY

The fractionation of corticostriatal circuits into anatomically and functionally separate families leads to the contemplation of at least three and possibly as many as five distinct sets. While recent anatomical studies have emphasized potential convergence of cortical and subcortical projections, as well as opportunities for cross-linkages between these circuits throughout their course, it is nevertheless remarkable that specific behavioral symptoms and syndromes can be seen clinically after focal lesions or specific disease processes. The secret to this functional specificity may lie in the action of transmitter systems such as DA, which appear to focus function within the circuits. Other transmitter systems also show promise as modulators of circuit functions. The final common path of these circuits was originally thought to focus exclusively on the frontal lobes. This still appears to be true for oculomotor and skeletomotor circuits, although these reach caudally to the superior colliculus and TPC nucleus, respectively. However, the influence of the complex loop, referred to as the *dorsolateral prefrontal*, has now been extended to the inferotemporal cortex. For the orbitofrontal and cingulate loops, influence clearly extends into the hypothalamic–limbic midbrain axis.

New opportunities for the study of these circuits in action are provided by single-unit studies in subhuman primates and intraoperative recordings of unit activity during surgery for movement disorders. For example, we can now study neural responses to passive and voluntary movements and sequences of movement. In addition, the use of dual microelectrodes permits us to study proximal cellular interactions and the actions of agonist and antagonist receptor–specific drugs. Functional neuroimaging may also provide a window into potential interactions between circuits and the reprogramming of function following interventional surgical or pharmacological treatments. We have been able also to study the acute effects of deep-brain stimulation on cognitive and motor activating tasks in the MRI scanner as well as with PET scanning. This may permit us to dissect the effects of the differential action of deep-brain stimulation on adjacent neuronal and fiber systems. Functional imaging, especially under conditions of activation paradigms and drug challenges, may help us select patients accordingly for surgical intervention or selective pharmacotherapy. The development of new receptor ligands for both single-photon emission computed tomography (SPECT) and PET imaging, in correlation with both clinical motor and neuropsychological status, represents another field of rapid evolution.

ACKNOWLEDGMENTS

This project was supported by a grant (AG 16570) from the National Institute on Aging Alzheimer's Disease Center, a grant from the Alzheimer's Disease Research Center of California, the Sidell-Kagan Foundation, and the Parkinson Foundation of Canada.

REFERENCES

Abi-Saab, W., Bubser, M., Roth, R., & Deutch, A. (1999). 5-HT$_2$ receptor regulation of extracellular GABA levels in the prefrontal cortex. *Neuropsychopharmacology, 20,* 92–96.

Alexander, G.E., DeLong, M.R., & Strick, P.L. (1986). Parallel organization of functionally segregated circuits linking basal ganglia and cortex. *Annual Review of Neuroscience, 9,* 357–381.

Alexander, G.E., Crutcher, M.D., & DeLong, M.R. (1990). Basal ganglia-thalamo-cortical circuits: parallel substrates for motor, oculomotor, "prefrontal" and "limbic" functions. *Progress in Brain Research, 85,* 119–146.

Aosaki, T., Graybiel, A.M., & Kimura, M. (1994a). Effect of the nigrostriatal dopamine system on acquired neural responses in the striatum of behaving monkeys. *Science, 265,* 412–415.

Aosaki, T., Tsubokawa, H., Ishida, A., Watanabe, K., Graybiel, A.M., & Kimura, M. (1994b). Responses of tonically active neurons in the primate's striatum undergo systematic changes during behavioral sensorimotor conditioning. *Journal of Neuroscience, 14,* 3969–3984.

Aosaki, T., Kimura, M., & Graybiel, A.M. (1995). Temporal and spatial characteristics of tonically active neurons of the primate's striatum. *Journal of Neurophysiology, 73,* 1234–1252.

Ardouin, C., Pillon, B., Peiffer, E., Bejjani, P., Limousin, P., Damier, P., Arnulf, I., Benabid, A.L., Agid, Y., & Pollak, P. (1999). Bilateral subthalamic or pallidal stimulation for Parkinson's disease affects neither memory nor executive functions: a consecutive series of 62 patients. *Annals of Neurology, 46,* 217–223.

Baddeley, A. (1986). *Working Memory.* Oxford: Oxford Scientific Publications.

Ballarin, M., Reiriz, J., Ambrosio, S., & Mahy, N. (1995). Effect of locally infused 2-chloradenosine, and A1 receptor agonist, on spontaneous and evoked dopamine release in rat neostriatum. *Neuroscience Letters, 6,* 29–32.

Baumann, B., Danos, P., Krell, D., Diekmann, S., Leschinger, A., Stauch, R., Wurthmann, C., Bernstein, H., & Bogerts, B. (1999). Reduced volume of limbic system–affiliated basal ganglia in mood disorders: preliminary data from a postmortem study. *Journal of Neuropsychiatry and Clinical Neuroscience 11,* 71–78.

Baxter, L.R. (1990). Brain imaging as a tool in establishing a theory of brain pathology in obsessive–compulsive disorder. *Journal of Clinical Psychiatry, 51* (Suppl), 22–26.

Baxter, L.R., Schwartz, J.M., Phelps, M.E., Mazziotta, J.C., Guze, B.H., Selin, C.E., Gerner, R.H., & Sumida, R.M. (1989). Reduction of prefrontal cortex glucose metabolism common to three types of depression. *Archives of General Psychiatry, 46,* 243–250.

Bédard, M.A., Pillon, B., Dubois, B., Duchesne, N., Masson, H., & Agid, Y. (1999). Acute and long-term administration of anticholinergics in Parkinson's disease: specific effects on the subcortico-frontal syndrome. *Brain and Cognition, 40,* 289–313.

Beblo, T., Wallesch, C.W., & Herrmann, M. (1999). The crucial role of frontostriatal circuits for depressive disorders in the postacute stage after stroke. *Neuropsychiatry, Neuropsychology, and Behavioral Neurology, 12,* 236–246.

Bejjani, B., Damier, P., Arnulf, I., Bonnet, A.M., Vidailhet, M., Dormont, D., Pidoux, B., Cornu, P., Marsault, C., & Agid, Y. (1997). Pallidal stimulation for Parkinson's disease. Two targets? *Neurology, 49,* 1564–1569.

Bejjani, B.P, Damier, P., Arnuff, I., Thivard, L., Bonnet, A.M., Dormont, D., Cornu, P., Pidoux, B., Samson, Y., & Agid, Y. (1999). Transient acute depression induced by high-frequency deep-brain stimulation. *New England Journal of Medicine, 340,* 1476–1480.

Berthier, M.L., Kulisevsky, J., Gironell, A., & Heras, J.A. (1996). Obsessive–compulsive disorder associated with brain lesions: clinical phenomenology, cognitive function, and anatomic correlates. *Neurology, 47,* 353–361.

Bhatia, K.P., & Marsden, C.D. (1994). The behavioural and motor consequences of focal lesions of the basal ganglia in man. *Brain, 117,* 859–876.

Biver, F., Goldman, S., Delvenne, V., Luxen, A., De Maertelaer, V., Hubain, P., Mendlewicz, J., & Lotstra, F. (1994). Frontal and parietal metabolic disturbances in unipolar depression. *Biological Psychiatry, 36,* 381–388.

Boecker, H., Dagher, A., Ceballos-Baumann, A.O., Passingham, R.E., Samuel, M., Friston, K.J., Poline, J.B., Dettmers, C., Conrad, B., & Brooks, D.J. (1998). Role of the human rostral supplementary motor area and the basal ganglia in motor sequence control: Investigations with O^{15}–H_2O PET. *Journal of Neurophysiology, 79,* 1070–1080.

Bowery, N. (1989). GABAb receptors and their significance in mammalian pharmacology. *Trends in Pharmacological Science, 10,* 401–407.

Bowman, E.M., Aigner, T.G., & Richmond, B.J. (1996). Neural signals in the monkey ventral striatum related to motivation for juice and cocaine rewards. *Journal of Neurophysiology, 75,* 1061–1073.

Braun, A.R., Stoetter, B., Randolph, C., Hsiao, J.K., Vladar, K., Gernet, J., Carson, R.E., Herscovitch, P., & Chase, T.N. (1993). The functional neuroanatomy of Tourette syndrome: an FDG-PET study. I. Regional changes in cerebral glucose metabolism differentiating patients and controls. *Neuropsychopharmacology, 9,* 277–291.

Braun, C.M., Larocque, C., Daigneault, S., & Montour-Proulx, I. (1999). Mania, pseudomania, depression, and pseudodepression resulting from focal unilateral cortical lesions. *Neuropsychiatry, Neuropsychology, and Behavioral Neurology, 12,* 35–51.

Brooks, D.J. (2000). Imaging basal ganglia function. *Journal of Anatomy, 196,* 543–554.

Brown, R.G. & Marsden, C.D. (1990). Cognitive function in Parkinson's disease: from description to theory. *Trends in Neuroscience, 13,* 21–29.

Cairns, H., Oldfield, R., Pennybacker, J.B., & Whitteridge, D.C. (1941). Akinetic mutism with an epidermoid cyst at the third ventricle. *Brain, 64,* 275–290.

Carlsson, M. & Carlsson, A. (1990). Interactions between glutamatergic and monoaminergic systems within the basal ganglia—implications for schizophrenia and Parkinson's disease. *Trends in Neuroscience, 13,* 272–276.

Carpenter, M.B. (1981). Anatomy of the corpus striatum and brain stem integrating system. In: V.B. Brooks (Ed.),: *Handbook of Physiology, Section 1: The Nervous System II,* (pp. 947–955). Bethesda: American Physiological Society.

Chesselet, M.F. & Delfs, J.M. (1996). Basal ganglia and movement disorders: an update. *Trends in Neuroscience, 13,* 417–422.

Ceballos-Baumann, A., Boecker, H., Bartenstein, P., von Falkenhayn, I., Riescher, H., Conrad, B., Moringlane, J., & Alesch, F. (1999). A positron emission tomography study of subthalamic nucleus stimulation in Parkinson's disease: enhanced movement-related activity of motor-association cortex and decreased motor cortex resting activity. *Archives of Neurology, 56,* 997–1003.

Cummings, J.L. (1991). Behavioral complications of drug treatment of Parkinson's disease. *Journal of the American Geriatric Society, 39,* 708–716.

Cummings, J.L. (1993a). Frontal–subcortical circuits and human behavior. *Archives of Neurology, 50,* 873–880.

Cummings, J.L. (1993b). The neuroanatomy of depression. *Journal of Clinical Psychiatry, 54* (Suppl l), 14–20.

Cummings, J.L. (1995). Anatomic and behavioral aspects of frontal–subcortical circuits. In: J. Grafman, K.J. Holyak, & F. Boller (Eds.), *Structure and Functions of the Human Prefrontal Cortex, Vol. 769* (pp. 1–13). New York: New York Academy of Sciences.

Cummings, J.L., & Cunningham, K. (1992). Obsessive–compulsive disorder in Huntington's disease. *Biological Psychiatry, 31,* 263–270.

Cummings, J.L. & Mendez, M.F. (1984). Secondary mania with focal cerebrovascular lesions. *American Journal of Psychiatry, 141,* 1084–1087.

Dalack, G., Healy, D., & Meador-Woodruff, J. (1998). Nicotine dependence in schizophrenia: clinical phenomena and laboratory findings. *American Journal of Psychiatry, 155,* 1490–1501.

Damsma, G., Robertson, G.S., Tham, C.S., & Fibiger, H.C. (1991). Dopaminergic regulation of striatal acetylcholine release: importance of D1 and *N*-methyl-D-aspartate receptors. *Journal of Pharmacology and Experimental Therapy, 259,* 1064–1072.

Davis, K.D., Taub, E., Houser, D., Lang, A.E., Dostrovsky, J.O., Tasker, R., & Lozano, A. (1997). Globus pallidus stimulation activates the cortical motor system during alleviation of parkinsonian symptoms. *Nature Medicine, 3,* 671–674.

DeBoer P. & Westerlink B. (1994). GABAergic modulation of striatal cholinergic interneurons: an in vivo microdyalisis study. *Journal of Neurochemistry, 62,* 70–75.

Di Chiara, G. & Morelli, M. (1993). Dopamine–acetylcholine–glutamate interactions in the striatum. *Advances in Neurology, 60,* 102–107.

Di Chiara, G., Morelli, M., & Consolo, S. (1994). Modulatory functions of neurotransmitters in the striatum: ACh/dopamine/NMDA interactions. *Trends in Neuroscience, 17,* 228–233.

Drevets, W.C. (1998). Functional neuroimaging studies of depression: the anatomy of melancholia. *Annual Review of Medicine, 49,* 341–361.

Drevets, W.C. (1999). Prefrontal cortical–amygdalar metabolism in major depression. *Annals of New York Academy of Sciences, 877,* 614–637.

Dubois, B., Pillon, B., Lhermitte, F., & Agid, Y. (1990). Cholinergic deficiency and frontal dysfunction in Parkinson's disease. *Annals of Neurology, 28,* 117–121.

Dubois, B., Boller, F., Pillon, B., & Agid, Y. (1991). Cognitive deficits in Parkinson's disease. In: S. Corkin, F. Boller, & J. Grafman (Eds.), *Handbook of Neuropsychology,* Vol. 5 (pp. 195–240). Amsterdam: Elsevier Science Publishers.

Dubois, B., Defontaines, B., Deweer, B., Malapani, C., & Pillon, B. (1995). Cognitive and behavioral changes in patients with focal lesions of the basal ganglia. *Advances in Neurology, 65,* 29–42.

Eblen, F. & Graybiel, A.M. (1995). Highly restricted origin of prefrontal cortical inputs to striosomes in the macaque monkey. *Journal of Neuroscience, 15,* 5999–6013.

Eidelberg, D. (1998). Functional brain networks in movement disorders [editorial]. *Current Opinion in Neurolology, 11,* 319–326.

Ferre, S. (1997). Adenosine–dopamine interactions in the ventral striatum. Implications for the treatment of schizophrenia. *Psychopharmacology, 133,* 107–120.

Filion, M., Tremblay, L., & Bédard, P.J. (1988). Abnormal influences of passive limb movement on the activity of globus pallidus neurons in parkinsonian monkeys. *Brain Research, 444,* 165–176.

Filion, M., Tremblay, L., Matsumura, M., & Richard, H. (1994). Focalisation dynamique de la convergence informationnelle dans les noyaux gris centraux. *Revue Neurologique (Paris), 150,* 627–633.

Flaherty, A.W., & Graybiel, A.M. (1995). Motor and somatosensory corticostriatal projection magnifications in the squirrel monkey. *Journal of Neurophysiology, 74,* 2638–2648.

Fredholm, B.B. (1995). Purinoreceptors in the nervous system. *Pharmacology and Toxicology, 76,* 228–239.

Fuster, J. (1997). *The Performance of Cortex: Anatomy, Physiology and Neuropsychology of the Frontal Lobe,* 3rd ed. Philadelphia: Lippencott-Raven.

Garcia-Rill, E., Houser, C.R., Skinner, R.D., Smith, W., & Woodward, D.J. (1987). Locomotion-inducing sites in the vicinity of the pedunculopontine nucleus. *Brain Research Bulletin, 18,* 731–738.

Gerfen, C.R. (1992). The neostriatal mosaic: multiple levels of compartmental organization in the basal ganglia. *Annual Reviews in Neuroscience, 15,* 285–320.

Ghika, J., Ghika-Schmid, F., Fankhauser, H., Assal, G., Vingerhoets, F., Albanese, A., Bogousslavsky, J., & Favre, J. (1999). Bilateral contemporaneous posteroventral pallidotomy for the treatment of Parkinson's disease: neuropsychological and neurological side effects. Report of four cases and review of the literature. *Journal of Neurosurgery, 91,* 313–321.

Giguère, M. & Goldman-Rakic, P.S. (1988). Mediodorsal nucleus: areal, laminar, and tangential distribution of afferents and efferents in the frontal lobe of rhesus monkey. *Journal of Comparative Neurology, 277,* 195–213.

Goldman-Rakic, P.S. & Porrino, L.J. (1985). The primate mediodorsal (MD) nucleus and projection to the frontal lobe. *Journal of Comparative Neurology, 242,* 535–560.

Grace, A.A. (1992). The depolarization block hypothesis of neuroleptic action: implications for etiology and treatment of schizophrenia. *Journal of Neural Transmission* (Suppl.) *36,* 91–131.

Graybiel, A.M. (1990). Neurotransmitters and neuromodulators in the basal ganglia. *Trends in Neurological Sciences, 13,* 244–254.

Graybiel, A.M. (1998). The basal ganglia and chunking of action repertoires. *Neurobiology of Learning and Memory, 70,* 119–136.

Green, J. & Barnhart, H. (2000). The impact of lesion laterality on neuropsychological change following posterior pallidotomy: a review of current findings. *Brain and Cognition, 42,* 379–398.

Gross, R.E., Lombardi, W.J., Lang, A.E., Duff, J., Hutchison, W.D., Saint-Cyr, J.A., Tasker, R.R., & Lozano, A.M. (1999). Relationship of lesion location to clinical outcome following microelectrode-guided pallidotomy for Parkinson's disease. *Brain, 122*(Pt 3), 405–416.

Haber, S.N., Lynd, E., Klein, C., & Groenewegen, H.J. (1990). Topographic organization of the ventral striatal efferents projections in the monkey. *Journal of Comparative Neurology, 293,* 282–298.

Haber, S.N., Lynd-Balta, E., & Mitchell, S.J. (1993). The organization of the descending ventral pallidal projections in the monkey. *Journal of Comparative Neurology, 329,* 111–128.

Haber, S.N., Kunishio, K., Mizobuchi, M., & Lynd-Balta, E. (1995). The orbital and medial prefrontal circuit through the primate basal ganglia. *Journal of Neuroscience, 15,* 4851–4867.

Heilman, K.M., Valenstein, E., & Watson, R.T. (1993). Neglect and related disorders. In: K.M. Heilman & E. Valenstein (Eds.), *Clinical Neuropsychology* (pp. 279–336). New York: Oxford University Press.

Hikosaka, O. & Wurtz, R.H. (1989). The basal ganglia. *Reviews of Oculomotor Research, 3,* 257–281.

Hollerman, J.R., Tremblay, L., & Schultz, W. (1998). Influence of reward expectation on behavior-related neuronal activity in primate striatum. *Journal of Neurophysiology, 80,* 947–963.

Hirono, N., Mori, E., Ishii, K., Ikejiri, Y., Imamura, T., Shimomura, T., Hashimoto, M., Yamahita, H., & Sasaki,

M. (1998). Frontal lobe hypometabolism and depression in Alzheimer's disease. *Neurology, 50,* 380–383.

Ikarashi, Y., Yuzurihara, M., Takahashi, A., Ishimary, H., Shiobara, T., & Maruyama, Y. (1999). Modulation of acetylcholine release via GABAa and GABAb receptors in rat striatum. *Brain Research, 816,* 238–240.

Ilinsky, L.A., Jouandet, M.L., & Goldman-Rakic, P.S. (1985). Organization of the nigrothalamocortical system in the rhesus monkey. *Journal of Comparative Neurology, 216,* 315–330.

Jahanshahi, M., Ardouin, C.M.A., Brown, R.G., Rothwell, J.C., Obeso, J., Albanese, A., Rodriguez-Oroz, M.C., Moro, E., Benabid, A.L., Pollak, P., & Limousin-Dowsey, P. (2000). The impact of deep brain stimulation on executive function in Parkinson's disease. *Brain, 123,* 1142–1154.

Johnson, T.N. & Rosvold, H.E. (1971). Topographic projections on the globus pallidus and substantia nigra of selectively placed lesions in the precommissural caudate nucleus and putamen in the monkey. *Experimental Neurology, 33,* 584–596.

Jones-Gotman, M. & Milner, B. (1977). Design fluency: the invention of nonsense drawings after focal cortical lesions. *Neuropsychologia, 15*(405), 653–674.

Jorge, R.E., Robinson, R.G., Starkstein, S.E., Arndt, S.V., Forrester, A.W., & Geisler, F.H. (1993). Secondary mania following traumatic brain injury. *American Journal of Psychiatry, 150,* 916–921.

Kawaguchi, Y., Wilson, C.J., Augood, S.A., & Emson, P.C. (1995). Striatal interneurons: chemical, physiological and morphological characterization. *Trends in Neuroscience, 18,* 527–535.

Kayahara, T. & Nakano, K. (1998). The globus pallidus sends axons to the thalamic reticular nucleus neurons projecting to the centromedian nucleus of the thalamus: a light and electron microscope study in the cat. *Brain Research Bulletin, 45,* 623–630.

Kemp, J.M., & Powell, T.P.S. (1970). The cortico-striate projection in the monkey. *Brain, 93,* 525–546.

Kishore, A., Panikar, D., Balakrishnan, S., Joseph, S., & Sarma, S. (2000) Evidence of functional somatotopy in GPi from results of pallidotomy. *Brain, 123,* 2491–2500.

Kita, H. (1993). GABAergic circuits of the striatum. *Progress in Brain Research, 99,* 51–72.

Kita H. (1996). Glutamatergic and GABAergic postsynaptic responses of striatal spiny neurons to intrastriatal and cortical stimulation recorded in slice preparations. *Neuroscience, 70,* 925–940.

Koski, L., Paus, T., Hofle, N., & Petrides, M. (1999). Increased blood flow in the basal ganglia when using cues to direct attention. *Experimental Brain Research, 129,* 241–246.

Kotter, R. (1994). Postsynaptic integration of glutamatergic and dopaminergic signals in the striatum. *Progress in Neurobiology, 44,* 163–196.

Krack, P., Pollak, P., Limousin, P., Hoffmann, D., Xie, J., Benazzouz, A., & Benabid, A.L. (1998). Subthalamic nucleus or internal pallidal stimulation in young onset Parkinson's disease. *Brain, 121,* 451–457.

Krack, P., Kumar, R., Ardouin, C., Limousin-Dowsey P.

McVicker, J.M., Benabid, A.L. & Pollak, P. (2001). Mirthful laughter induced by subthalamic nucleus stimulation. *Movement Disorders, 16,* 867–875.

Kulisevsky, J., Berthier, M.L., & Pujol, J. (1993). Hemiballismus and secondary mania following right thalamic infarction. *Neurology, 43,* 1422–1424.

Kumar, R., Krack, P., & Pollak, P. (1999). Transient acute depression induced by high frequency deep-brain stimulation. Letter to the editors. *New England Journal of Medicine, 341,* 1003–1004.

Lang, A.E. & Lozano, A.M. (1998a). Parkinson's disease—first of two parts. *New England Journal of Medicine, 339,* 1044–1053.

Lang, A.E. & Lozano, A.M. (1998b). Parkinson's disease—second of two parts. *New England Journal of Medicine, 339,* 1130–1143.

Levey, A.I., Kitt, C.A., Simonds, W.F., Price, D.L., & Brann, M.R. (1991). Identification and localization of muscarinic acetylcholine receptor proteins in brain with subtype-specific antibodies. *Journal of Neuroscience, 11,* 3218–3226.

Lewis, A.A., Sesack, S.R., Levey, A.I., & Rosenberg D.R. (1998). Dopamine axons in primate prefrontal cortex: specificity of distribution, synaptic targets, and development. *Advances in Pharmacology, 42,* 703–706.

Lhermitte, F., Pillon, B., & Serdaru, M. (1986). Human autonomy and the frontal lobes. I: Imitation and utilization behavior, a neuropsychological study of 75 patients. *Annals of Neurology, 19,* 326–334.

Limousin, P., Greene, J., Pollak, P., Rothwell, J., Benabid, A.L., & Frackowiak, R. (1997). Changes in cerebral activity pattern due to subthalamic nucleus or internal pallidum stimulation in Parkinson's disease. *Annals of Neurology, 42,* 283–291.

Lombardi, W.J., Gross, R.E., Trépanier, L.L., Lang, A.E., Lozano, A.M., & Saint-Cyr, J.A. (2000). Relationship of lesion location to cognitive outcome following microelectrode-guided pallidotomy for Parkinson's disease: support for the existence of cognitive circuits in the human pallidum. *Brain, 123,* 746–758.

Macchi, G. & Jones, E.G. (1997). Toward an agreement on terminology of nuclear and subnuclear divisions of motor thalamus. *Journal of Neurosurgery, 86,* 670–685.

Marsden, C.D. & Obeso, J.A. (1994). The functions of the basal ganglia and the paradox of stereotaxic surgery in Parkinson's disease. *Brain, 117,* 877–897.

Marshall, J.F., Richardson, J.C., & Teitelbaum, P. (1974). Nigrostriatal bundle damage and the lateral hypothalamic syndrome. *Journal of Comparative Physiology and Psychology, 87,* 808–830.

Masterman, D., DeSalles, A., Baloh, R.W., Frysinger, R., Foti, D., Behnke, E., Cabatan-Awang, C., Hoetzel, A., Intemann, P.M., Fairbanks, L., & Bronstein, J.M. (1998). Motor, cognitive, and behavioral performance following unilateral ventroposterior pallidotomy for Parkinson disease. *Archives of Neurology, 55,* 1201–1208.

Mayberg, H.S. (1997) Limbic–cortical dysregulation: a proposed model of depression. *Journal of Neuropsychiatry and Clinical Neuroscience, 9,* 471–481.

McFarland, N.R. & Haber, S.N. (2000). Convergent inputs from thalamic motor nuclei and frontal cortical areas to the dorsal striatum in the primate. *Journal of Neuroscience, 20,* 3798–3813.

Mega, M.S. & Cohenour, R.C. (1997). Akinetic mutism: disconnection of frontal–subcortical circuits. *Neuropsychiatry Neuropsychology Behavioral Neurology, 10,* 254–259.

Mega, M.S. & Cummings, J.L. (1994). Frontal–subcortical circuits and neuropsychiatric disorders. *Journal of Neuropsychiatry and Clinical Neuroscience, 6,* 358–370.

Mega, M.S., Cummings, J.L., Salloway, S., & Malloy, P. (1997). The limbic system: an anatomic, phylogenetic, and clinical perspective. *Journal of Neuropsychiatry and Clinical Neuroscience 9,* 315–330.

Mendez, M., Nakawatase, T.V., & Brown, C.V. (1999). Involuntary laughter and inappropriate hilarity. *Journal of Neuropsychiatry and Clinical Neuroscience, 11,* 253–258.

Meredith, G.E. & Wouterlood, F.G. (1990). Hippocampal and midline thalamic fibers and terminals in relation to the choline acetyltransferase-immunoreactive neurons in nucleus accumbens of the rat: a light and electron microscopic study. *Journal of Comparative Neurology, 296,* 204–221.

Middleton, F.A. & Strick, P.L. (1997). New concepts about the organization of basal ganglia output. *Advances in Neurology, 74,* 57–68.

Middleton, F.A. & Strick, P.L. (2000). Basal ganglia output and cognition: evidence from anatomical, behavioural and clinical studies. *Brain and Cognition, 42,* 183–200.

Modell, J.G., Mountz, J.M., Curtis, G.C., & Greden, J.F. (1989). Neurophysiologic dysfunction in basal ganglia/limbic striatal and thalamocortical circuits as a pathogenic mechanism of obsessive–compulsive disorder. *Journal of Neuropsychiatry and Clinical Neuroscience, 1,* 27–36.

Morari, M., Marti, M., Sbrenna, S., Fuxe, K., Bianchi, C., & Beani, L. (1998). Reciprocal dopamine–glutamate modulation of release in the basal ganglia. *Neurochemistry International, 33,* 383–397.

Moratalla, R. & Bowery, N. (1991). Chronic lesion of corticostriatal fibers reduces GABAb but not GABAa binding in rat caudate, putamen: an autoradiographic study. *Neurochemistry Research, 16,* 309–315.

Nakano, K. (2000). Neural circuits and topographic organization of the basal ganglia and related regions. *Brain and Development, 22,* S5–S16.

Nemeth, G., Hegedus, K., & Molnar, L. (1986). Akinetic mutism and locked in syndrome: the functional anatomical basis for their differentiation. *Functional Neurology, 1,* 128–139.

Owen, A.M., & Doyon, J. (1999). The cognitive neuropsychology of Parkinson's disease: a functional neuroimaging perspective. In: G.M. Stern (Ed.), *Parkinson's Disease: Advances in Neurology, Vol. 80,* (pp. 49–56). Philadelphia: Lippincott, Williams & Wilkins.

Palfreyman, M.G., Schmidt, C.J., Sorensen, S.M., Dudley, M.W., Kehne, J.H., Moser, P., Gittos, M.W., & Carr, A.A. (1993). Electrophysiological, biochemical and behavioral evidence for 5-HT2 and 5-HT3 mediated control of dopaminergic function. *Psychopharmacology, 112*(1 Suppl), S60–S67.

Paré, D., Hazrati, L.N., Parent, A., & Steriade, M. (1990). Substantia nigra pars reticulata projects to the reticular thalamic nucleus of the cat: a morphological and electrophysiological study. *Brain Research, 535,* 139–146.

Parent, A. (1990). Serotonergic innervation of the basal ganglia. *Journal of Comparative Neurolology, 299,* 1–16.

Parent, A. & Cicchetti, F. (1998). The current model of basal ganglia organization under scrutiny. *Movement Disorders, 13,* 199–202.

Parent, A. & Hazrati, L. (1995a). Functional anatomy of the basal ganglia. I. The cortico-basal ganglia-thalamo-cortical loop. *Brain Research Reviews, 20,* 91–127.

Parent, A. & Hazrati, L. (1995b). Functional anatomy of the basal ganglia. II. The place of subthalamic nucleus and external pallidum in basal ganglia circuitry. *Brain Research Reviews, 20,* 128–154.

Parent, A., Bouchard, C., & Smith, Y. (1984). The striatopallidal and striatonigral projections: two distinct fiber systems in primate. *Brain Research, 303,* 385–390.

Percheron, G. & Filion, M. (1991). Parallel processing in the basal ganglia: up to a point [letter]. *Trends in Neuroscience, 14,* 55–56.

Perry, E., Court, J., Johnson, M., Piggott, M., & Perry, R. (1992). Autoradiographic distribution of [³H] nicotine binding in human cortex: relative abundance in subicular complex. *Journal Chemical Neuroanatomy, 5,* 399–405.

Petrides, M. & Pandya, D.N. (1999) Dorsolateral prefrontal cortex: comparative cytoarchitectonic analysis in the human and the macaque brain and corticocortical connection patterns. *European Journal of Neuroscience, 11:* 1011–1136.

Pillon, B., Ardouin, C., Damier, P., Krack, P., Houeto, J., Klinger, H., Bonnet, A., Pollak, P., Benebid, A., & Agid, Y. (2000). Neuropsychological changes between "off" and "on" STN and GPi stimulation in Parkinson's disease. *Neurology, 55,* 411–418.

Poldrack, R.A. Prabhakaran, V., Seger, C.A., & Gabrieli, J.D. (1999). Striatal activation during acquisition of a cognitive skill. *Neuropsychology, 13,* 564–574.

Rauch, S.L. & Savage, C.R. (1997). Neuroimaging and neuropsychology of the striatum. Bridging basic science and clinical practice. *Psychiatric Clinics of North America, 20,* 741–768.

Reese, N.B., Garcia-Rill, E., & Skinner, R.D. (1995). The pedunculopontine nucleus—auditory input, arousal and pathophysiology. *Progress in Neurobiology, 47,* 105–133.

Ring, H.A., Bench, C.J., Trimble, M.R., Brooks, D.J., Frackowiak, R.S., & Dolan, R.J. (1994). Depression in Parkinson's disease. A positron emission study. *British Journal of Psychiatry, 165,* 333–339.

Robinson, R.G., Bolduc, P.L., & Price, T. (1987). A two-year longitudinal study of post-stroke mood disorders: diagnosis and outcome at one and two years. *Stroke, 18,* 837–843.

Robinson, R.G., Boston, J.D., Starkstein, S.E., & Price,

T.R. (1988). Comparison of mania and depression after brain injury: causal factors. *American Journal of Psychiatry, 145,* 172–178.

Rogers, R.D., Andrews, T.C., Grasby, P.M., Brooks, D.J., & Robbins, T.W. (2000). Contrasting cortical and subcortical activations produced by attention-set shifting and reversal learning in humans. *Journal of Cognitive Nueroscience, 12,* 142–162.

Rolls, E.T. (2000) The orbitofrontal cortex and reward. *Cerebral Cortex, 10:*284–294.

Ross, E.D. & Stewart, R.M. (1981). Akinetic mutism from hypothalamic damage: successful treatment with dopamine agonists. *Neurology, 31,* 1435–1439.

Rouzaire-Dubois, B. & Scarnati, E. (1987). Increase in glutamate sensitivity of subthalamic nucleus neurons following bilateral decortication: a microiontophoretic study in the rat. *Brain Research, 403,* 366–370.

Saint-Cyr, J.J. & Taylor, A.E. (1992). The mobilization of procedural learning. The "key signature" of the basal ganglia. In: N. Butters & L.R. Squire (Eds.), *Neuropsychology of Memory,* 2nd ed. (pp. 188–202). New York: Guilford Press.

Saint-Cyr, J.A., Taylor, A.E., & Lang, A.E. (1988). Procedural learning and neostriatal dysfunction in man. *Brain, 111* (Pt 4), 941–959.

Saint-Cyr, J.A., Ungerleider, L., & Desimone, R. (1990). Organization of visual cortical inputs to the striatum and subsequent outputs to the pallido-nigral complex in the monkey. *Journal of Comparative Neurology, 298,* 128–156.

Saint-Cyr, J.A., Taylor, A.E., Trépanier, L.L., & Lang, A.E. (1992). The caudate nucleus: head ganglion of the habit system. In: G. Valler, S.-F. Cappa, & C.-W. Wallesch (Eds.), *Neuropsychological Disorders Associated with Subcortical Lesions* (pp. 204–226). Oxford: Oxford Science Publications.

Saint-Cyr, J.A., Taylor, A.E., & Nicholson, K. (1995). Behavior and the basal ganglia. *Advances in Neurology, 65,* 1–28.

Saint-Cyr, J.A., Trépanier, L.L., Kumar, R., Lozano, A.M., & Lang, A.E. (2000). Neuropsychological consequences of chronic bilateral stimulation of the subthalamic nucleus in Parkinson's disease. *Brain, 123,* 2091–2108.

Sano, M., Stern, Y., Côté, L., Williams, J.B., & Mayeux, R. (1990) Depression in Parkinson's disease: a biochemical model. *Journal of Neuropsychiatry and Clinical Neuroscience, 2,* 88–92.

Schultz, W., Tremblay, L., & Hollerman, J.R. (1998). Reward prediction in primate basal ganglia and frontal cortex. *Neuropharmacology, 37,* 421–429.

Scatton, B. & Lehmann, J. (1982). N-methyl-D-aspartate type receptors mediate striatal 3H-acetylcholine release evoked by excitatory amino acids. *Nature, 297,* 422–424.

Scott, R., Gregory, R., Hines, N., Carroll, C., Hyman, N., Papanasstasiou, V., Leather, C., Rowe, J., Silburn, P., & Aziz, T. (1998). Neuropsychological, neurological and functional outcome following pallidotomy for Parkinson's disease. A consecutive series of eight simultaneous bilateral and twelve unilateral procedures. *Brain, 121*(Pt 4), 659–675.

Selden, N.R., Gitelman, D.R., Salamon-Murayma, N., Parrish, T.B., & Mesulam, M.M. (1998). Trajectories of cholinergic pathways within the cerebral hemispheres of the human brain. *Brain, 121,* 2249–2257.

Selemon, L.D. & Goldman-Rakic, P.S. (1985). Longitudinal topography and interdigitation of corticostriatal projections in the rhesus monkey. *Journal of Neuroscience, 5,* 776–794.

Singer, H.S. (1997). Neurobiology of Tourette syndrome. *Neurological Clinics, 15,* 357–379.

Singer, H.S., Reiss, A.L., Brown, J.E., Aylward, E.H., Shih, B., Chee, E., Harris, E.L., Reader, M.J., Chase, G.A., Bryan, R.N., et al. (1993). Volumetric MRI changes in basal ganglia of children with Tourette's syndrome. *Neurology, 43,* 950–956.

Smiley, J. & Goldman-Rakic, P.S. (1996). Serotonergic axons in monkey prefrontal cerebral cortex synapse predominantly on interneurons as demonstrated by serial section electron microscopy. *Journal of Comparative Neurology, 367,* 431–443.

Smith, A.D. & Bolam, J.P. (1990). The neural network of the basal ganglia as revealed by the study of synaptic connections of identified neurones. *Trends in Neuroscience, 13,* 259–265.

Smith, Y., Hazrati, L.N., & Parent, A. (1990). Efferent projections of the subthalamic nucleus in the squirrel monkey as studied by the PHA-L anterograde tracing method. *Journal of Comparative Neurology, 294,* 306–323.

Starkstein, S.E., Robinson, R.G., & Price, T. (1987). Comparison of cortical and subcortical lesions in the production of poststroke depression. *Brain, 110,* 1045–1059.

Starkstein, S.E., Robinson, R.G., Berthier, M.L., Parikh, R.M., & Price, T.R. (1988). Differential mood changes following basal ganglia vs thalamic lesions. *Archives of Neurology, 45,* 725–730.

Starkstein, S.E., Fedoroff, P., Berthier, M.L., & Robinson, R.G. (1991). Manic-depressive and pure manic states after brain lesions. *Biological Psychiatry, 29,* 149–158.

Starr, M.S. (1995). Glutamate/dopamine D1/D2 balance in the basal ganglia and its relevance to Parkinson's disease. *Synapse, 19,* 264–293.

Starr, P.A., Vitek, J.L., & Bakay, R.A. (1998). Ablative surgery and deep brain stimulation for Parkinson's disease. *Neurosurgery, 43,* 989–1013; discussion 1013–1015.

Stebbins, G.T., Gabrieli, J.D.E., Shannon, K.M., Penn, R.D., & Goetz, C.G. (2000). Impaired fronto-striatal cognitive functioning following posteroventral pallidotomy in advanced Parkinson's disease. *Brain and Cognition, 42,* 348–363.

Steriade, M. & Llinás, R.R. (1988). The functional states of the thalamus and the associated neuronal interplay. *Physiological Reviews, 68,* 649–742.

Steriade, M., Domich, L., & Oakson, G. (1986). Reticularis thalami neurons revisited: activity changes during shifts in states of vigilance. *Journal of Neuroscience, 6,* 68–81.

Stuss, D.T. & Alexander, M.P. (2000) Executive functions and the frontal lobes: a conceptual view. *Psychological Research, 63,* 289–298.

Suri, R.E. & Schultz, W. (1998). Learning of sequential movements by neural network model with dopamine-like reinforcement signal. *Experimental Brain Research, 121,* 350–354.

Taylor, A.E. & Saint-Cyr, J.A. (1990). Depression in Parkinson's disease: reconciling physiological and psychological perspectives. *Journal of Neuropsychiatry and Clinical Neuroscience, 2,* 92–98.

Taylor, A.E., Saint-Cyr, J.A. (1995). The neuropsychology of Parkinson's disease. *Brain and Cognition, 28,* 281–296.

Taylor, A.E., Saint-Cyr, J.A., & Lang, A.E. (1986). Frontal lobe dysfunction in Parkinson's disease: the cortical focus of neostriatal outflow. *Brain, 109,* 845–883.

Taylor, A., Saint-Cyr, J., & Lang, A. (1990). Memory and learning in early Parkinson's disease: evidence for a "frontal lobe syndrome". *Brain and Cognition, 13,* 211–232.

Tian, J. & Lynch, J.C. (1997). Subcortical input to the smooth saccadic eye movement subregions of the frontal eye field in cebus monkey. *Journal of Neuroscience, 17,* 9233–9247.

Trautner, R.J., Cummings, J.L., Read, S.L., & Benson, D.F. (1988). Idiopathic basal ganglia calcification and organic mood disorder. *American Journal of Psychiatry, 45,* 350–353.

Tremblay, L., Hollerman, J.R., & Schultz, W. (1998). Modifications of reward expectation–related neuronal activity during learning in primate striatum. *Journal of Neurophysiology, 80,* 964–977.

Trépanier, L.L., Saint-Cyr, J.A., Lozano, A.M., & Lang, A.E. (1998). Neuropsychological consequences of posteroventral pallidotomy for the treatment of Parkinson's disease. *Neurology, 51,* 207–215.

Trépanier, L., Kumar, R., Lozano, A., Lang, A., & Saint-Cyr, J. (2000). Neuropsychological outcome of neurosurgical therapies in Parkinson's disease: a comparison of GPi pallidotomy and deep brain stimulation of GPi or STN. *Brain and Cognition, 42,* 324–347.

Whitton, P.S. (1997). Glutamatergic control over brain dopamine release in vivo and vitro. *Neuroscience and Biobehavioral Reviews, 2,* 481–488.

Wiesendanger, M. & Wise, S.P. (1992) Current issues concerning the functional organization of motor cortical areas in nonhuman primates. *Advances in Neurology, 57,* 117–34.

Williams, G.V. & Goldman-Rakic, P.S. (1995). Modulation of memory fields by dopamine D1 receptors in prefrontal cortex. *Nature, 376,* 572–575.

Wise, S.P., Murray, E.A., & Gerfen, C.R. (1996). The frontal cortex-basal ganglia system in primates. *Critical Reviews in Neurobiology, 10,* 317–356.

Yeterian, E.H. & Pandya, D.N. (1991). Prefrontostriatal connections in relation to cortical architectonic organization in rhesus monkeys. *Journal of Comparative Neurology, 312,* 43–67.

Yeterian, E.H. & van Hoesen, G.W. (1978). Cortico-striate projections in the rhesus monkey: the organization of certain cortico-caudate connections. *Brain Research, 139,* 43–63.

27

The Role of Prefrontal Cortex in Normal and Disordered Cognitive Control: A Cognitive Neuroscience Perspective

TODD S. BRAVER, JONATHAN D. COHEN, AND
DEANNA M. BARCH

The advent of cognitive neuroscience as a discipline has accelerated research on the functions of the prefrontal cortex (PFC). The cognitive neuroscience perspective has led to greater consideration and integration of multiple different methodologies and research approaches, including basic neuroscience (neurophysiology and neuroanatomy), clinical neuroscience (neuropsychology and psychiatry), and cognitive science (experimental psychology and computer science). Moreover, researchers now have the opportunity to study the human brain "in action" through the use of functional neuroimaging methods. However, the greater focus on convergence between these different approaches and traditions has also revealed some of the conflicts between them, in terms of their traditional views of PFC function.

The first conflict concerns whether the PFC should be considered a storage buffer or an executive controller. In the neurophysiology literature, a commonly held view of PFC function is that of a short-term storage mechanism, actively holding information on-line through neural activity (Goldman-Rakic, 1995). These findings have been supported by human neuroimaging data, suggesting sustained PFC activation specifically associated with maintenance periods in tasks requiring short-term or working memory (Fiez et al., 1996; Cohen et al., 1997; Courtney, et al., 1997). In contrast, the neuropsychological literature has tended to focus on the role of the PFC in behavioral regulation and cognitive control and on the impairments in these functions following damage to the PFC (Hecaen & Albert, 1978; Damasio, 1985; Stuss & Benson, 1986). Although these differing views of PFC function are not by themselves incompatible, a prominent cognitive psychological model put forward by Baddeley and colleagues has suggested that storage and control processes should be considered architecturally distinct and strictly segregated components of a working memory system (Baddeley & Hitch, 1974; Baddeley, 1986).

A second conflict among the various literatures concerns whether the PFC functions more as a mnemonic, inhibitory, or attentional structure. Neurophysiological and neuroimaging studies have tended to focus on the role of PFC in short-term or working memory (e.g., Fuster, 1973; Funahashi et al., 1993; D'Esposito et al., 1998; Smith & Jonides, 1999). However, there is clear evidence that the PFC is critically involved in selective attention as well (Cabeza & Nyberg, 2000). The PFC is seen as playing a central role in the "anterior attentional system," in which the selection, direction, and allocation of attentional resources is endogenously controlled (Posner & Petersen, 1990). In contrast, the developmental and clinical literatures have viewed the PFC as primarily geared towards inhibitory functions, such as reducing sensory interference and overriding dominant but inappropriate response tendencies. In this literature, much has been made of findings that inhibitory control throughout the lifespan seems to parallel the time course of PFC maturation and decline (Diamond, 1990; Dempster, 1992), and that damage to the PFC often leads to a behavioral "disinhibition syndrome" in which the normal control over social and sexual behavior is released (Hecaen & Albert, 1978). In previous reviews attempting to synthesize these different literatures, some theorists have suggested that memory and inhibition should also be thought of as distinct and anatomically segregated functions of PFC (Fuster, 1989). This hypothesis has been based on neuroanatomical and neurophysiological data suggesting functional segregation of dorsolateral and ventromedial regions of PFC, with dorsolateral PFC being associated with mnemonic functions and ventromedial PFC with inhibitory function. Less focus has been placed on the anatomical locus of attention within PFC, yet the implicit view seems to be that attentional functions are one component of an anatomically based modular organizational structure within the PFC.

These functional distinctions between storage, control, and memory, inhibition, and attention present a confusing and often inconsistent picture for the theorist attempting to develop a coherent theory of PFC function. Thus, an important open question is whether and how these distinctions can be reconciled. In this chapter, we shall provide such an attempt at reconciliation, by focusing on the potential computational mechanisms associated with storage, control, inhibition, and attention. This computational approach suggests a resolution of the apparent conflicts between the different perspectives on PFC function. We suggest that a common set of computational mechanisms allow for PFC mediation of mnemonic, inhibitory, and attentional functions, where each is preferentially observable under

different task situations, and each occurs in the service of cognitive control. Specifically, we argue that the control functions of the PFC emerge as a direct consequence of two specific mechanisms: active maintenance of task-relevant context and top-down biasing of local competitive interactions that occur during processing.

We have developed our theory of PFC function using the connectionist computational modeling framework. This modeling approach involves three components: *(1)* computational analysis of the critical processing mechanisms required for cognitive control; *(2)* use of neurobiologically plausible principles of information processing; and *(3)* implementation and simulation of cognitive tasks and behavioral performance. The modeling work is complemented by a series of convergent empirical studies relying on multiple experimental methodologies. First we will describe behavioral and neuroimaging data on healthy young adults that provide validation for critical components of the model. We will then summarize our work applying the model to the clinical domain; we have tested its predictions in different population groups (older adults, schizophrenia patients) thought to suffer from PFC dysfunction. These studies highlight the power of the cognitive neuroscience approach by demonstrating how a single, integrated account of PFC function can capture a wide range of data from different methodologies and multiple populations.

A THEORY OF PREFRONTAL CORTEX FUNCTION IN COGNITIVE CONTROL

CONTEXT AND COGNITIVE CONTROL

A basic and fundamental function of cognitive control is to flexibly adapt behavior to the demands of particular tasks by facilitating processing of task-relevant information over other sources of competing information and by inhibiting habitual or otherwise prepotent responses that are inappropriate to the task. Because this control function is such a fundamental one, it occurs in even very simple task situations. As a specific example, take a situation in which a speeded response is required to a particular stimulus, but only in a particular context (e.g., respond to the letter *X* only if immediately following the letter *A*). If the context–stimulus pairing occurs frequently, the cognitive system should begin to exploit the context to prime or facilitate processing of the stimulus. In contrast, in the rare situations in which the stimulus occurs in a different context (e.g., *X* following the letter *B*), the system must rely on the information provided by the context to inhibit the tendency to respond. This example raises the question of what types of processing mechanisms could perform such a cognitive control function.

We would argue that there are at least three minimal components required of this type of cognitive control mechanism: *(1)* a representational code that conveys implications of the behavioral goal or prior context for future behavior; *(2)* a capability for actively maintaining this representation in an accessible form; and *(3)* a means of conveying an activation signal that can directly influence ongoing processing by directing attention, biasing action selection, or resolving perceptual ambiguities. In reference to the example task above, the contextual cue should be translated into a code that appropriately distinguishes between different upcoming inputs (*X* versus *not-X*) and/or their behavioral consequences (respond versus don't respond). This representation should be accessible even under conditions in which the contextual cue is temporally isolated from the relevant stimulus or response, and thus no longer externally available. Finally, the contextual cue should directly modulate processing in perceptual and/or motor pathways, such as by priming the expected response or by focusing attention towards the expected stimulus features.

Over the past 10 years we have been developing a theory which suggests that these minimal elements of cognitive control are subserved by specific neural mechanisms that are dependent on the function of the PFC (Cohen & Servan-Schreiber, 1992; Braver et al., 1995; Cohen et al., 1996; O'Reilly et al., 1999; Miller & Cohen, 2001). Moreover, we have described these neural mechanisms in terms of explicit computational principles and have implemented these principles within connectionist neural network models. Our theory is composed of three central hypotheses: *(1)* the PFC is specialized for the representation and maintenance of context information; *(2)* context information is maintained in the PFC as a stable and self-sustaining pattern of neural activity; and *(3)* context representations in the PFC mediate control through interactions that modulate the flow of information in other brain systems that more directly support task performance.

A critical aspect of our hypothesis regarding the role of the PFC in cognitive control relates to the notion of context representation. We define *context* as any task-relevant information that is internally represented in such a form that it can bias processing in the pathways responsible for task performance. Goal representations are one form of such information, which have their influence on planning and overt behavior. However, we use the more general term context to include representations that may have their effect earlier in the processing stream, on interpretive or attentional processes. For example, in the Stroop Task, the context provided by the task instructions must be actively represented and maintained to bias attentional allocation and response selection towards the ink color dimension of a visually presented word. Thus, context representations may include a specific prior stimulus or the result of processing a sequence of stimuli, as well as task instructions or a particular intended action. Representations of context are particularly important for situations in which there is strong competition for response selection. These situations may arise when the appropriate response is one that is relatively infrequent or when the inappropriate response is dominant and must be inhibited (such as the word *name* in the Stroop Task). Importantly, context representations can be maintained on-line, in an active state, such that they are continually accessible and available to influence processing. Thus, context can be thought of as a component of working memory. Specifically, context can be viewed as the subset of representations within working memory that govern how other representations are used. In this manner, context representations simultaneously subserve both storage and control functions. As described above, this aspect of the model differentiates it from Baddeley's model of working memory (Baddeley, 1986; 1993), which postulates a strict separation of representations for storage versus control.

A COMPUTATIONAL MODEL OF PREFRONTAL CORTEX FUNCTION AND CONTEXT PROCESSING

The theory of PFC involvement in context processing and cognitive control described above was developed within the connectionist, or parallel distributed processing, framework (Rumelhart & McClelland, 1986; McClelland, 1993). The connectionist framework is a natural one for concomitantly studying the neural and psychological mechanisms of cognitive control, since it provides a computational architecture that is specified in neurobiological terms and can be used to quantitatively simulate performance in cognitive tasks. In this framework, information is represented as graded patterns of activity over populations of simple units, processing takes place as the flow of activity goes from one set of units to another, and learning occurs through the modification of the connection strengths between these. From one perspective, connectionist models are highly simplified, capturing brain-style computation, without necessarily committing to the details of any particular neural

system or subsystem. However, with appropriate refinement, such models offer the opportunity to build bridges between our understanding of the low-level properties of neural systems and their participation in higher-level (system) behavior.

The theory of cognitive control put forward here can be schematized in the form of a simple canonical model in which a context module serves as an indirect pathway that modulates processing in a direct stimulus–response pathway (see Fig. 27–1). This context-processing module represents the functions of the PFC. There are two critical features of this module that provide it with the capacity for control over processing. The first is that there is strong, recurrent connectivity within the context layer, which allows for the active maintenance of information. Thus, input to the context layer can be sustained through activity recirculation along mutually excitatory connections, even when the external source of input is no longer present. The second critical feature of the context pathway is its feedback connection to the direct pathway. This provides a means for activity within the context module to provide an additional source of input, which can modulate the flow of processing within the direct pathway. In particular, feedback from the context layer serves to bias the local competition for representation that exists within each module, favoring one activation pathway or set of representations over their competitors. This biasing action of the context module can produce inhibitory effects

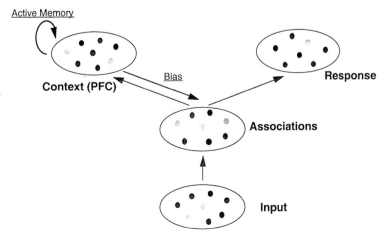

Figure 27–1. Diagram of canonical model. Key computational principles of context processing mechanism are shown: active memory through recurrent connections, and top-down bias through feedback connections. PFC, prefrontal cortex.

on processing by allowing a weak pathway to inhibit the more dominant one.

An important insight that has emerged from our work with this model is that it demonstrates how context-processing mechanisms might jointly support three cognitive functions—working memory, inhibition, and attention—that have all been suggested to be subserved by PFC, but that are often treated as independent. When a task involves a delay between a cue and a later contingent response, it is usually assumed that a working memory function is involved. However, there is no dedicated mechanism for working memory in the model. Rather, the mechanism that is used to initially represent context information can also maintain this information against the interfering and cumulative effects of noise over time. In contrast, when a task involves competing, task-irrelevant processes (as in the Stroop Task), it is often assumed that a dedicated inhibitory function is responsible for suppressing or overriding these irrelevant processes. Once again, in the model, there is no dedicated mechanism for inhibition. Rather, context representations indirectly provide an inhibitory effect by providing top-down support for task-relevant processes, allowing these to compete effectively against irrelevant ones. It is important to note that this competition is expected to occur locally, in posterior regions, rather than in the PFC itself. Finally, attention is thought to be required in tasks during which an internal or external cue signals that a specific stimulus feature or dimension has increased salience relative to others. In the model, contextual information is translated into a representational code and fed back into the system, facilitating information processing in specific stimulus–response pathways via selective support of those pathways. Yet the context mechanism is not a dedicated "attentional module," but rather just an extra source of top-down input that can be sustained over time.

Thus, the same PFC mechanism can be involved in tasks that alternatively tap working memory, inhibition, or attention; it is simply a matter of the behavioral conditions under which it operates (i.e., the source of interference) and the information it selects (task-relevant versus task-irrelevant) that lead us to label it as having a working memory, inhibitory, or attentional function. Consequently, the model suggests a clear resolution of the supposedly disparate findings of PFC involvement in working memory, attentional, and inhibitory functions by suggesting how a single mechanism might commonly subserve all three domains. Below, we discuss the computational and empirical studies we have conducted to test the model.

THE AX-CPT PARADIGM

Our investigations have focused on testing whether this model of cognitive control provides a useful account of both normal and disordered PFC function. To examine this question, we have conducted a series of studies using multiple methodologies and populations, but employing a single experimental paradigm for probing cognitive control function. Our research strategy has been to systematically examine and understand the properties and consequences of PFC activity within a single paradigm, before testing the model further in additional paradigms. The paradigm we have studied, known as the AX-CPT, was selected on the basis of a number of favorable properties. First, the AX-CPT, is derived from the well-known Continuous Performance Test (CPT; Rosvold et al., 1956), which in the clinical and neuropsychological literatures is widely used as a test of attentional control and vigilance (e.g., Nuechterlein, 1991). The more demanding versions of the CPT have been shown to strongly rely on PFC function, as evidenced by performance deficits observed in patients with frontal lesions (Glosser & Goodglass, 1990) and other syndromes thought to involve prefrontal dysfunction, such as schizophrenia (Cornblatt & Keilp, 1994) and attention-deficit disorder (ADHD) (Losier et al., 1996). Many neuroimaging studies have also used these difficult versions of the CPT to elicit PFC activity (Cohen et al., 1987; Rezai et al., 1993; Siegel et al., 1995; Seidman et al., 1998). Second, the AX-CPT appears to be sensitive to individual differences in PFC function and/or cognitive control. In previous studies, we have shown that

AX-CPT performance is correlated with performance on other widely used probes of PFC and cognitive control function, such as the N-back, Stroop, and reading span tasks (Cohen et al., 1999; Keys et al., submitted). Third, the AX-CPT probes key aspects of cognitive control, while distilling them into a task paradigm that is as simple and interpretable as possible. Because of the simplicity of the task, it can be used with many different subject populations and under a wide variety of task environments. Indeed, the task is very similar in structure to delayed-response tasks used in the neurophysiological literature on working memory (e.g., Fuster, 1973), and thus allows easy comparison with this literature. Moreover, because the task is relatively simple, it can be simulated in computational studies. Lastly, although the task is simple, it nevertheless produces multiple performance measures, which generate a rich set of data on which to base and constrain theoretical interpretations.

In the AX-CPT, subjects view sequences of letters presented one at a time as a series of cue–probe pairs in the center of a visual display. The object of the task is to make a target response to a specific probe letter (X), but only when it follows a valid cue (A), and a nontarget response in all other cases (see Fig. 27–2). Performance is dependent on the representation and maintenance of context information, insofar as the correct response to the probe depends on knowledge of the previous cue (A or not-A). In the model, the context provided by the cue is represented and maintained within the PFC. We further designed the task to selectively measure different aspects of the context processing functions subserved by PFC (working memory, attention, and inhibition).

In the task, target (AX) trials occur with high frequency (70%). This induces two types of biases in subjects. The first is a bias to make a target response to the occurrence of an X probe. On those trials in which a target response should *not* be made to the X probe (i.e., BX trials, where B refers to any non-A cue), context information must be used in an *inhibitory* fashion to override the tendency to false alarm. The second bias that occurs in the

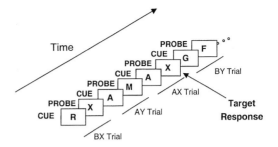

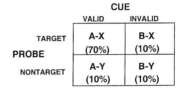

Figure 27–2. Schematic of AX-CPT paradigm. Single letters are visually displayed as a series of cue–probe pairs. A target is defined as the occurrence of an X probe immediately following an A cue. Three types of nontarget trials occur, each with equal frequency (10%): BX, AY, and BY (where B refers to any non-A cue, and Y refers to any non-X probe).

AX-CPT is an expectancy to make a target response following the occurrence of an A cue. In this case, the context provided by the cue serves a predictive function that directs *attention* to a particular response (i.e., attention-to-action; Norman & Shallice, 1986; Allport, 1989). On those trials in which the cue is an invalid predictor of the response (i.e., AY trials, where Y refers to any non-X probe), the attentional function of context creates the tendency to false alarm. This type of cue validity effect is similar to others that have been extensively studied in the attentional literature (e.g., Posner, 1980). Thus, the integrity of context processing can be examined not only through performance on AX target trials but also through an examination of performance on nontarget trials.

A key element of our theory is that both attentional and inhibitory functions in the AX-CPT should be subserved by a single underlying mechanism—the internal representation of context information within the PFC. This assumption can be tested by examining the relationship of AY to BX performance. Note that on BX trials, failure to internally represent context should impair performance, by not suppressing the inappropriate response bias. Consequently, BX false alarms can be considered *context-failure errors*. However, on AY trials, representation of context should create an inappropriate expectancy bias that leads to an increased tendency to false alarm. AY false alarms can thus be considered *context-induced errors*. Thus, if context representations are intact, more AY (context-induced) than BX (context-failure) errors should be made (with a similar pattern observable in reaction time on non-error trials). Conversely, if context representations are impaired, the opposite pattern should occur (more BX than AY errors). Performance on AX target trials should also be poorer if context processing is impaired, since determination of targets is dependent on the context provided by the cue. However, target performance may not be as impaired as BX performance, since on target trials, the response bias works in subjects' favor, by increasing the tendency to make the correct target response. Finally, a third type of nontarget trial, *BY*, provides a useful internal control, since in this condition the influence of context on performance should be relatively small (given that both the cue and the probe always map to a nontarget response).

The AX-CPT paradigm also provides a means for examining the *mnemonic* role of context information through manipulations of the cue–probe delay duration. Specifically, under conditions in which there is a long cue–probe delay (e.g., 5–10 seconds), context information must be actively maintained within working memory. Our theory suggests that context information is both represented and actively maintained within the PFC. Thus, the same context-processing mechanism that subserves inhibitory and attentional functions should also subserve active maintenance in the AX-CPT. Consequently, a strong prediction of the theory is that the effect of delay will interact with performance on AY and BX trials. If context maintenance is intact, then the strength of context representations should either hold constant or increase with delay (i.e., if it takes some period of time for context representations to reach full activation strength). Consequently, BX performance should remain constant or improve at long delays, while AY

performance should remain constant or worsen with delay. Conversely, if context maintenance is impaired, then context representations should lose strength over time. This should lead to a worsening of BX performance with a delay, but an improvement in AY performance.

As the above description of the task makes clear, our model of PFC function in cognitive control leads to a number of specific predictions for the AX-CPT that relate to normal behavioral performance, brain activation, and clinical/neuropsychological populations. A central focus of our recent work has been to systematically test these predictions through a series of studies (Braver et al., 1995, in press; Barch et al., 1997, 2001; Servan-Schreiber et al., Braver, 1997; Braver & Cohen, 1999, 2000, in press; Cohen et al., 1999). The first phase of the research was to provide initial validation of the model by examining how it can capture aspects of normal AX-CPT performance, in terms of both brain activity and behavior. The second phase of the research was to apply the model as a predictive tool for studying the consequences of impairments in PFC function and/or context processing. In this work, we have attempted to show how the model can be used to make rather specific and sometimes highly counterintuitive predictions regarding AX-CPT performance in different populations (healthy individuals performing under load, schizophrenia patients, and older adults). The remainder of the chapter discusses these two phases of our research.

MODEL VALIDATION: NORMAL COGNITIVE CONTROL

Over the past 10 years we have tested numerous healthy young adults in the AX-CPT task. From this testing it has emerged that there is a set of fairly standard characteristics of behavioral performance on the task (Braver et al., 1990b). Figure 27–3 shows error data on nontarget trials averaged from over 200 subjects performing the AX-CPT under both short (1–2 seconds) and long delay (5–10 seconds) conditions. A number of notable features can be observed. First, there are very

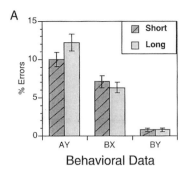

Behavioral Data   **Simulation Data**

Figure 27–3. Simulation and behavioral performance data from the AX-CPT. *A:* Behavioral data obtained from a normative sample of over 200 healthy young adults performing the AX-CPT under standard conditions. Performance on each of the three nontarget trial types is shown for short- (dark hatched bars) and long-delay (light bars) conditions. *B:* Simulation data from computational model showing performance on each the three nontarget trial types (AY, BX, and BY) under short- (dark hatched bars) and long-delay (light bars) conditions. (*Source:* Data from Braver et al, 1999b)

few errors ever made on BY trials, which serve as an internal control for baseline performance. This suggests that, overall, the task is not difficult for healthy adults to perform. Relative to the BY error rate, there are significantly more errors on BX and AY trials. This is consistent with the conflict that is present on BX and AY trials between the contextual information and the current input (Carter et al., 1998). Thus, in these conditions greater cognitive control is required. Moreover, healthy adults produce more AY (context-induced) errors than BX (context-failure) errors. As described above, this pattern indicates that context exerts a strong influence over responding—subjects are more likely to overrely on contextual information than they are to fail to utilize it. Finally, it is clear that the error pattern also interacts with delay. Specifically, at long delays AY errors are increased, BX errors are decreased, and BY errors are unchanged. This pattern indicates that context information is accurately maintained in the system over the delay period, and even appears to exert a stronger influence over performance at the longer delay interval (i.e., at the long delay there is a greater likelihood of context inducing an error and a reduced likelihood of context failing to prevent an error).

In computer simulations with our model, we found that we were able to closely capture this pattern of behavioral performance, both in qualitative and quantitative terms (see Fig. 27–3). In particular, the model exhibits all of the primary effects observed in the empirical data, including effects related to reaction time (RT) and AX target performance (not shown; see Braver et al., 1999b). However, it is important to note that a number of free parameters were adjusted in the model to optimize its fit to the data. Thus, the simulations do not provide a strong test of the theory's sufficiency or explanatory power. Nevertheless, they do serve as an initial validation of the model, suggesting that it is capable of capturing the major behavioral phenomena associated with normal AX-CPT performance. Moreover, the results increase our confidence in using the model as a starting point for generating hypotheses and predictions regarding the effects of other variables.

In a second set of studies, we directly validated the role of PFC in context processing and cognitive control postulated in our model. Specifically, brain activity was measured during AX-CPT performance through the use of functional magnetic resonance imaging (fMRI) methods. Our model suggested that in the AX-CPT task the contextual information provided by the cue should be represented in PFC and actively maintained there over an intervening delay. To test this hypothesis, we compared brain activity in the AX-CPT under short- and long-delay conditions, holding all other aspects of the task constant (such as the total trial duration). Consequently, the only thing that should have differed across conditions was the proportion of the trial period devoted to active maintenance of context information.

Our results indicated that activity within left PFC, in a dorsolateral (DL-PFC) region corresponding to Brodmann's area (BA) 46/9, was significantly increased in the long-delay condition relative to the short one (see Fig. 27–4; Barch et al., 1997). This finding has now been replicated in three subsequent studies using independent cohorts of subjects (Barch et al., 2001b; Braver & Cohen, 2001; Braver & Bongiolatti, in press). Recently, we extended our initial findings by conducting a study using newly developed event-related fMRI methods (Braver & Cohen, 2001). Event-related techniques enable measurement of the temporal dynamics and evolution of brain activity over the course of a trial (Buckner et al., 1996; Buckner & Braver, 1999). By plotting the activation time course in this left DL-PFC region across the trial, we observed a response pattern that was highly consistent with that predicted by the model. Specifically, we found that left DL-PFC activity increased immediately following cue presentation and remained high over the duration of the delay period (10 seconds), then declined following probe presentation (Fig. 27–4). Critically, we found no other brain regions outside of DL-PFC showing this characteristic activity pattern.

The neuroimaging studies of the AX-CPT provide important validation for our claims regarding the role of PFC in context processing and cognitive control. Moreover, they point to the specific region within the PFC that is activated by context processing demands during AX-CPT performance. This is critical, because the model in its current scope is rather anatomically nonspecific, in that it does not differentiate between specific PFC subregions. In one aspect, this lack of anatomical specificity is intentional, because we believe that a unifying principle of PFC function is its involvement in aspects of context processing. However, human PFC takes up nearly a third of the cerebral cortex, and there are clear anatomical subdivisions within it (ventrolateral, dorsolateral, frontopolar, medial, orbital) (Barbas & Pandya, 1989b; Fuster, 1997a). Given the structure–function relationships that exist in the brain, it is likely that these anatomic subdivisions within the PFC reflect relevant functional specialization. An important question that we shall return to at the end of the chapter is whether the model can be extended

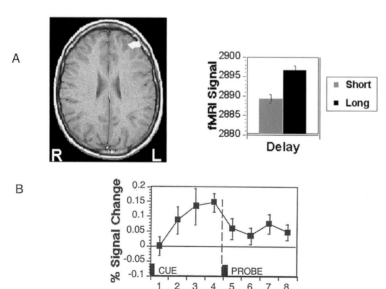

Figure 27–4. *A:* Activity in left dorsolateral (DL prefrontal cortex PFC) for short- (light bars) and long-delay (dark bars) conditions. Brain activation data are shown for a representative axial slice 24 mm superior to the AC–PC plane (centroid: -37, 42, 29). *B:* Time course of event-related activity in left DL-PFC during a long-delay trial (10 seconds). Note that there is a sustained increase in activity during the cue–probe delay period which the decays during the intertrial interval. (*Source:* From Barch et al., 1997, and Braver & Cohen, 2001)

in scope to help address and explain these functional specializations within PFC. For the current purposes, the neuroimaging studies suggest that our model of PFC context-processing functions in the AX-CPT should be considered to pertain to DL-PFC regions most directly. Moreover, the consistent observation of left DL-PFC activity during the AX-CPT in healthy young adults suggests that studies examining AX-CPT context-processing impairments in different populations and/or task conditions should focus on this region as the neural locus of dysfunction. In the next section, we will focus on a series of studies designed to test this hypothesis.

APPLYING THE MODEL: DISORDERED COGNITIVE CONTROL

Our primary research strategy has been to apply our model of cognitive control as a predictive tool for generating hypotheses regarding the relationship between PFC dysfunction and cognitive control impairments related to context processing. In particular, we adopted a cognitive neuroscience approach that sought to provide convergent evidence for the model using multiple methods. Our first step was to determine what biologically relevant parameters in the model affect context processing functions. By manipulating these parameters in computational simulations, we determined their effects on performance of the AX-CPT task, both in terms of behavior and PFC activity. The simulation results were then used to generate empirically testable predictions for populations or experimental conditions that were hypothesized to correspond to the same change in the biologically relevant parameter. Our results are from three different populations: healthy subjects performing under interference, schizophrenia patients, and older adults.

SIMULATION STUDIES

To examine the relationship between PFC dysfunction, context processing impairment,

and AX-CPT performance in the model, we simulated changing the function of the dopamine (DA) neurotransmitter projection into the PFC. A detailed description of the motivation and theory behind these simulations is beyond the scope of this chapter, and is described elsewhere (Braver & Cohen, 1999; 2000). Briefly, we hypothesized that DA provides a modulatory input into the PFC, which serves to regulate the access of incoming information. In particular, we have suggested that the connection serves as a gating mechanism. When the gate is opened, as is thought to occur following a phasic burst of DA activity, incoming information can gain access to the PFC, and thus update the current state of context representation. Conversely, when the gate is closed, access to the PFC is restricted, protecting context representations from the interfering effects of noise or other irrelevant inputs. We hypothesized that the timing of gating signals is learned through a reward prediction learning mechanism associated with the midbrain DA system (Schultz et al., 1997), which enables task-relevant information to be selected as context, because of its association with the potential for future reinforcement.

In our simulations, we found that when DA effects are reduced in the context module, the representation of context becomes less reliable (since access is partially blocked). Under conditions when DA input is noisier (i.e., more variable over time) both the representation and maintenance of context is disrupted (see Fig. 27–5; Braver, et al., 1999). The maintenance effects occur because context information is more susceptible to the interfering effects of noise and task-irrelevant inputs, and thus is more likely to decay over time. These conditions of dysfunctional context processing were also associated with clear changes in model performance on the AX-CPT (Fig. 27–5). First, we found that BX performance worsened. Recall that BX trials require inhibition of a response bias, based on context information. Thus, if the context representation is weak, then so is the ability to inhibit the response bias. In contrast, we found that AY performance was actually improved in the disturbed model. Remember that on AY trials,

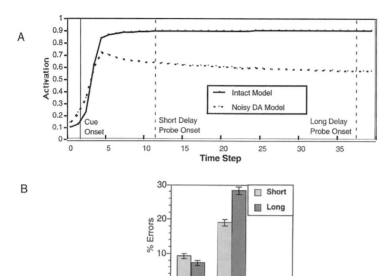

Figure 27–5. *A:* Plot of average activity level in context units during the course of an AX-CPT trial in the intact and noisy DA models. Note that context activity is attenuated in the noisy dopamine (DA) model and further declines with delay. *B:* Simulation data from computational model with noisy DA. (*Source:* Data from Braver et al., 1999b)

context sets up an expectancy that is violated by the nontarget probe letter. When context representations are weaker, so is the expectancy. The lower the expectancy, the less likely it is that a false alarm will be made.

It is important to note that this improvement of AY performance under impaired context-processing conditions represents a highly counterintuitive prediction of the model. It is typically much harder to obtain improvements in performance due to cognitive dysfunction than it is to obtain impairments. Moreover, the predicted effects on AY and BX performance suggest a crossover interaction when comparing normal and dysfunctional context-processing conditions. Predicted crossover interactions are optimal from an experimental point of view because (*1*) they are statistically powerful, and thus easier to detect (Wahlsten, 1991), and (*2*) because they obviate nonspecific interpretations of their cause, such as differential difficulty across conditions (e.g., Chapman & Chapman, 1978).

INTERFERENCE CONDITIONS

Our first test of these model predictions regarding context-processing disruption was in healthy young subjects performing the AX-CPT under interference conditions (Braver et al., 1999b). Specifically, we hypothesized that

presentation of irrelevant distractor letters during the cue–probe delay interval would disrupt context processing by increasing the probability of an inappropriate DA-mediated gating signal (causing an improper update of context). Indeed, we observed that healthy subjects under interference displayed a performance pattern similar to that predicted by the model under context disruptions. At the short delay, interference effects were minimal, with the typical effect of more AY than BX errors. However, at the long delay, the effects of interference appeared to accumulate. Specifically, BX errors increased but AY errors decreased, leaving significantly more BX than AY errors (see Fig. 27–6). We further examined the effect of interference in a neuroimaging study to determine whether performance in the interference condition was associated with changes in the activation of left DL-PFC (Braver & Cohen, 2001). We again used event-related fMRI to track DL-PFC activity dynamics over the course of a trial. Our results indicated a significant effect of interference in the left DL-PFC region that we had previously found to show delay-related activity during the task (Fig. 27–6). Under interference there is an activation response to the cue that initially increases, but then shows a rapid decay over the delay period. This finding provides fairly strong support for the idea that the

Figure 27–6. *A:* Behavioral data from young adults performing the AX-CPT under interference conditions. *B:* Time course of event-related activity in the left DLPFC under both standard and interference AX-CPT conditions. Activity declines more rapidly under the interference condition. (*Source:* Data from Braver et al., 1999, and Braver & Cohen, 2001).

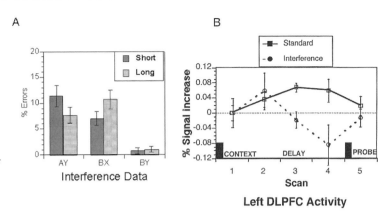

behavioral impairments related to context processing observed in AX-CPT performance under interference are linked to a change in the activity dynamics of DL-PFC.

SCHIZOPHRENIA PATIENTS

Our second set of studies examined AX-CPT performance in schizophrenia patients. Schizophrenia is a disease associated with marked cognitive disturbance. A common view is that schizophrenia patients suffer from a failure of cognitive control (Callaway & Naghdi, 1982; Nuechterlein & Dawson, 1984). There is a wealth of neuropsychological, neuroanatomical, and neuroimaging evidence suggesting that PFC dysfunction is a central component of the disease, and may be the underlying cause of the cognitive deficits (Goldman-Rakic, 1991). Additionally, the role of DA in schizophrenia is well known, and most pharmacological treatments for clinical symptoms involve agents that affect the DA system (Creese et al., 1976). More recently, investigators have suggested that some of the cognitive deficits present in schizophrenia may result from altered DA activity in PFC (Davis et al., 1991).

We have examined the performance of schizophrenia patients on the AX-CPT across a number of studies (Servan-Schreiber et al., 1996; Cohen et al., 1999; Barch et al., 2001b; Braver et al., 1999b). A consistent pattern across all of these studies is that, relative to matched controls, patients show a performance pattern that is indicative of a selective deficit in context processing and that appears

to be magnified in the long-delay condition. More recently, we have studied patients suffering their first psychotic episode and thus were not yet medicated and had never been hospitalized. This produced a very clean sample for examining schizophrenia cognitive impairments, because many of the confounding clinical variables that typically affect cognitive performance were not present (e.g., length of illness, chronic medication status, and institutionalization). We again found that this group made significantly more BX errors relative to a tightly matched control sample, but in fact made fewer AY errors, and that this effect was most pronounced at the long delay (see Fig. 27–7; Barch et al., 2001b). These findings provide support for the hypothesis that a selective context-processing deficit underlies some of the cognitive impairments observed in schizophrenia. We simulated this data in our model and found that when the DA gating mechanism was disrupted, the model produced performance patterns that were qualitatively very similar to that observed empirically (Braver et al., 1999).

We also acquired measurements of fMRI activity in this cohort of first-episode patients and matched controls during AX-CPT performance (Barch et al., 2001b). The healthy controls showed normal delay-related activation of left DL-PFC. However, the patients failed to show a delay-related increase, yielding a significant group x delay interaction in left DL-PFC (Fig. 27–7). It is noteworthy that this was the only brain region found to show such a pattern. Moreover, it was found that many other regions showed normal task-related ac-

A

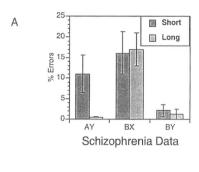
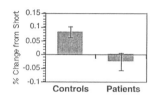

B

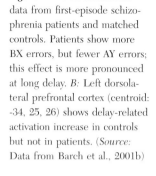

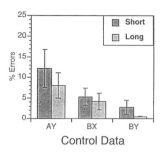

Figure 27–7. *A:* Behavioral data from first-episode schizophrenia patients and matched controls. Patients show more BX errors, but fewer AY errors; this effect is more pronounced at long delay. *B:* Left dorsolateral prefrontal cortex (centroid: -34, 25, 26) shows delay-related activation increase in controls but not in patients. (*Source:* Data from Barch et al., 2001b)

tivation in patients, including more posterior and inferior regions of PFC (e.g., Broca's area).

OLDER ADULTS

A final population that we have studied is healthy older adults. Like schizophrenia, healthy aging is associated with impairments in both PFC and DA functions, albeit at a much less severe level. Older adults perform similarly to patients with frontal lobe damage on neuropsychological batteries (West, 1996), and in some cases neuropsychological test performance has been found to correlate to the degree of age-related reductions in PFC gray matter (Raz et al., 1998). The functioning of the DA system also declines in older adults, with DA receptor concentration regularly decreasing with increasing age (de Keyser et al., 1990). Moreover, recent work has linked age-related DA receptor decreases with cognitive decline in tests sensitive to PFC function (Volkow et al., 1998). We tested whether these aging effects on DA and PFC function would be reflected in terms of selectively decreased context-processing function.

In a large sample of older adults performing the AX-CPT (in the long-delay condition only), under both baseline and interference conditions, we found the same pattern predicted by the model to be indicative of selective context-processing impairment—opposite

patterns of performance change on BX and AY trials (see Fig. 27–8; Braver et al., 2001). On BX trials, older adults made significantly more errors and showed substantial slowing of RT. However, on AY trials, older adults showed significantly fewer errors and equivalent RT. The AY RT pattern is especially striking, given that an almost ubiquitous finding in the cognitive aging literature is that older adults are slower than younger adults on any cognitive task (Cerella, 1985; Myerson & Hale, 1993). Moreover, the longer the response latency for younger adults, the greater the amount of slowing typically observed. In contrast, our results indicate that there was no age-related slowing on AY trials, even though these were the conditions that produced the longest RTs in younger adults. Without the benefit of a model, this would seem to be an anomalous and potentially difficult result to interpret. Yet it is fully consistent with our hypotheses that context-processing deficits should produce a paradoxical improvement in AY performance.

In our most recently completed work, we have followed up on the behavioral results with a fMRI study conducted in an independent sample of younger and older adults (Barch et al., 2001a). Subjects performed the long- and short-delay AX-CPT conditions in our standard design. Once again, in confirmation of our predictions, we observed a significant delay-related reduction of PFC activ-

Figure 27–8. *A:* Behavioral data from healthy older (light bars) and younger (dark bars) adults, including both errors (left) and reaction time (RT). Older adults show more BX errors, but less AY errors. The RT data show significant age-related slowing on BX trials, but no slowing on AY trials. *B:* Left dorsolateral prefrontal cortex (centroid: -43, 22, 28) shows delay-related activation increase in young but not older adults. (*Source:* Data from Barch et al., 2001a, and Braver et al., 2001)

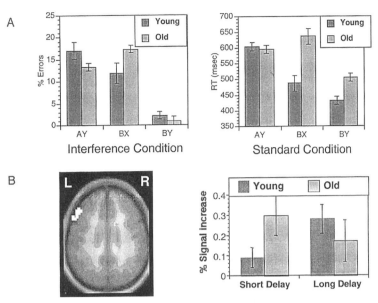

ity in older adults, located within the same left dorsolateral region identified in the previous studies (Fig. 27–8). Interestingly, this reduced DL-PFC activity contrasted with the general pattern observed across other brain regions, in which older adults actually showed greater task-related activity than younger adults. This finding is consistent with other neuroimaging studies of cognition in aging (Cabeza, 2001), and could indicate that older adults recruit additional brain regions during tasks requiring cognitive control as a means of compensating for impaired context processing functions in the PFC.

SUMMARY AND DISCUSSION

Across a series of studies, we have attempted to draw a tight link between context-processing function, AX-CPT performance, and PFC activity. In four independent samples of healthy young adults performing the AX-CPT under standard conditions, the same region of left DL-PFC (BA 46/9) was found to show increased activity when context information needed to be actively maintained over a delay period (Barch et al., 1997, 2001b; Braver & Cohen, 2001; Braver & Bongiolatti, in press). This highly replicable pattern of results suggests that the AX-CPT provides a se-

lective and focal probe of left DL-PFC function. The finding that this left DL-PFC region showed reduced activity in two different population (older adults and schizophrenia patients) thought to suffer from PFC dysfunction further supports this suggestion. Moreover, in both populations, the PFC activity pattern co-occurred with a distinctive and similar pattern of behavioral performance. This behavioral pattern included both performance impairments in some task conditions (BX trials), but also relative improvements in others (AY trials). The relationship between AX-CPT performance and left DL-PFC activity suggests that the AX-CPT paradigm has potential clinical utility as a selective neuropsychological marker. An obvious prediction of the model that is worth testing in future studies is that patients with focal left DL-PFC lesions would show a performance profile similar to that of schizophrenia patients and older adults. Another possible use of the AX-CPT worth exploring in future studies is as a diagnostic tool for suspected left DL-PFC dysfunction (i.e., when this is not immediately clear from other neuroanatomical markers). However, for this to occur, a clear amount of additional work is needed to determine whether the AX-CPT shows appropriate psychometric properties (i.e., sensitivity, specificity, and reliability) in both its behavioral and neural activity measurements to warrant such usage.

It is important to recall that not only were we able to detect differences between-groups in PFC activity associated with context-processing dysfunction, but we also observed within-subjects PFC activity differences related to experimentally induced disruptions of context processing. In particular, the findings from the interference AX-CPT studies in healthy subjects indicate that reductions in left DL-PFC activity during task performance do not necessarily indicate the presence of a neurobiological impairment. Conversely, the results also strengthen the hypothesis that the reduced left DL-PFC activity observed among older adults and schizophrenia patients was not a causally irrelevant population difference, such as being a byproduct of a more global pathophysiology. Instead, we suggest that in the AX-CPT, delay-related decreases in left DL-PFC signal the failure to appropriately represent and maintain the contextual information provided by task cues.

Although the clinical implications of our work are certainly important, our primary goal in this chapter has been to highlight the benefits of a multimethod cognitive neuroscience approach and, most importantly, the role that computational modeling can play in advancing theories of PFC function. The critical point of our studies is not that the AX-CPT activates the left DL-PFC, or that impaired activity can be observed in different populations and/or conditions, but to what these findings imply about the underlying cognitive mechanisms supporting task performance. We began with two related hypotheses: *(1)* a central function of PFC is to represent and actively maintain context or goal-relevant information; and *(2)* these context representations serve to control processing by biasing the flow of information through posterior brain pathways. These hypotheses are similar in many ways to those expressed by other investigators (Goldman-Rakic, 1987; Fuster, 1997b). In particular, the recent work of Miller and colleagues is highly consistent with our ideas. Miller suggests that representations in the PFC are not directly tied to sensory features but instead code more abstract properties such as rules or a task set

(Miller, 2000; Miller & Cohen, 2001). However, a distinguishing feature of our approach is that we have tried to make the hypotheses explicit, by implementing them within computer simulation models (c.f., Kimberg & Farah, 1993; Dehaene & Changeux, 1995). These simulation models are admittedly highly simplified and somewhat abstract in relation to many of the important neurobiological details that characterize real neural systems. Nevertheless, by developing and implementing a running simulation model, it is possible to examine how a postulated set of mechanisms interact with each other in terms of their impact on information-processing dynamics and their implications for behavioral performance within specific task contexts.

The critical insight we developed from this simulation work is that actively maintained context representations, when fed back into the rest of the system, can support multiple functions: short-term information storage (working memory), suppression of inappropriate responses (inhibition), and selection and enhancement of task-relevant input (attention). Moreover, although these functions are all subserved by the same mechanism, they are most apparent in different circumstances—storage under delay conditions, suppression under conditions involving dominant response biases, and attentional facilitation under conditions requiring robust, efficient processing (e.g., speeded conditions) or conditions with perceptually weak (or ambiguous) inputs. From this insight we designed the AX-CPT paradigm to probe each of these aspects of PFC function through different measures of performance (i.e., delay effect = working memory, BX = inhibition, AY = attention). We hypothesized that if all three functions were subserved by a common set of PFC mechanisms, then performance on the different measures should interact. Because the AX-CPT paradigm was conceptually so simple, we were able to simulate performance of the task in a quantitative manner and under multiple different conditions. The simulation results supported the hypothesis of interaction, showing that when context-processing mechanisms were disturbed (by simulating a change in DA modulation of PFC inputs), performance changed on both BX and AY trials, and the effects were modulated by delay. In addition, the behavioral effects were associated with a pattern of altered activity dynamics, such that activity was reduced in the simulated PFC units, and tended to decay over time. Thus, the primary benefit of the model was that it provided us with a means of generating explicit and highly specific predictions about the consequences of context-processing disturbances for both brain activity and behavioral performance.

The confirmation and replication of the model's predictions in different populations and with different methods suggest that it is capturing important principles related to PFC involvement in cognitive control during AX-CPT performance. It is our goal, however, to extend the model beyond the AX-CPT, to determine whether it can help explain PFC involvement in cognitive control more generally. Specifically, we have tried to show how a very simple processing mechanism of context representation and maintenance can subserve both storage and control functions, both memory and inhibition, as well as certain aspects of attentional selection. Thus, the context-processing model may provide a resolution of the various theories of PFC function that have either argued for a preferential role of PFC in one of the functions, or have suggested that the different functions are anatomically segregated and independent. Our model argues that neither of these alternatives needs to be true. A single region within PFC may be involved with multiple cognitive control functions and be critical for multiple cognitive domains, because these functions are not necessarily independent or computationally incompatible.

LIMITATIONS AND FUTURE DIRECTIONS

An important direction for future research is to determine the appropriate scope of the context-processing model. Obviously, the work presented to date is only a small first step. A clear direction for future research will be to determine if the model can be extended to examine context effects beyond the AX-CPT paradigm, in different tasks, and across different cognitive domains. Early stages of this effort have already begun (Cohen & Servan-Schreiber, 1992; Cohen et al., 1992; O'Reilly et al., in press). Another direction of future research will be to enrich our model of PFC functions. Our current model is highly simplified and, in particular, does not differentiate among PFC subregions. However, regional specializations clearly appear to be present in the PFC, in terms of both anatomy and function (Goldman-Rakic, 1987; Barbas & Pandya, 1989a; Fuster, 1997a). Thus a critical question is whether the model should only apply to DL-PFC regions (and even more specifically to left hemisphere DL-PFC), or whether it can be applied more generally.

The suggestion that the context-processing model applies only to DL-PFC regions is a plausible one and, in fact, is the only interpretation strictly supported by the results. Moreover, the dorsolateral region of PFC is most reliably implicated in cognitive control functions, in both human (Cabeza & Nyberg, 2000; Duncan & Owen, 2000; Smith & Jonides, 1999) and primate studies (Fuster, 1989; Goldman-Rakic, 1987; Smith & Jonides, 1999). We would like to speculate, however, that participation in context representation and maintenance functions may be a unifying dimension that cuts across PFC subregions. Even if this hypothesis is true, the dimensions and organizational structure that define the regional specialization of PFC remain to be discovered. The question of PFC organizational structure is being actively pursued by a number of investigators (Goldman-Rakic, 1996; Petrides, 1996; D'Esposito et al., 1998; Owen et al., 1998; Christoff & Gabrieli, 2000). One view commonly adopted is that the PFC is organized according to the information content of representations, with distinctions being drawn according to psychologically relevant categories, such as identity versus location, verbal versus nonverbal, and sensory modality (Wilson et al., 1993; Smith & Jonides, 1999; Levy & Goldman-Rakic, 2000). A second view suggests that the organizational structure is primarily based on processing rather than content specializations, such as cognitive versus emotional/motivational functions (Dias et al., 1996; Bechara et al., 1998; Rolls, 2000), and maintenance versus manipulation of information in working memory (D'Esposito et al., 1999; Postle & D'Esposito, 2000). Each of these views has met with mixed success at accounting for the full range of empirical data.

Our own view is that representational content and processing functions are likely to be tightly intertwined within the brain. Moreover, given the complexity of the computational functions performed in PFC, it is unlikely that the representational distinctions between PFC subregions will map onto easily labeled content categories. For example, the relevant dimensions of specialization within the PFC may include the temporal duration over which representations are typically activated and maintained or the number of stimulus dimensions that are simultaneously integrated. We have begun exploring models that make use of such computational specializations (O'Reilly et al., in press). Yet, regardless of which dimensions of specialization eventually prove to be the most relevant for PFC function, we feel confident that computational modeling analyses have the potential to strongly contribute to our understanding of this brain region.

REFERENCES

Allport, A. (1989). Visual attention. In: M.I. Posner (Ed.), *Foundations of Cognitive Science* (pp. 631–682). Cambridge, MA: MIT Press.

Baddeley, A.D. (1986). *Working Memory*. New York: Oxford University Press.

Baddeley, A.D. (1993). Working memory or working attention? In: A.D. Baddeley & L. Weiskrantz (Eds.), *Attention: Selection, Awareness, and Control: A Tribute to Donald Broadbent* (pp. 152–170). Oxford: Clarendon Press.

Baddeley, A.D. & Hitch, G.J. (1974). Working memory. In: G. Bower (Ed.), *The Psychology of Learning and Motivation* Vol. VIII (pp. 47–89). New York: Academic Press.

Barbas, H. & Pandya, D.N. (1989a). Architecture and intrinsic connections of the prefrontal cortex in the rhesus monkey. *Journal of Comparative Neurology, 286,* 353–375.

Barbas, H. & Pandya, D.N. (1989b). Architecture of intrinsic connections of the prefrontal cortex in the Rhesus monkey. *Journal of Comparative Neurology, 286,* 353–375.

Barch, D.M., Braver, T.S., Nystom, L.E., Forman, S.D., Noll, D.C., & Cohen, J.D. (1997). Dissociating working memory from task difficulty in human prefrontal cortex. *Neuropsychologia, 35,* 1373–1380.

Barch, D.M., Braver, T.S., Racine, C.A., & Satpute, A.B. (2001a). Cognitive control deficits in healthy aging: neuroimaging investigations. *NeuroImage, 13,* S1025.

Barch, D.M., Carter, C.S., Braver, T.S., McDonald, A., Sabb, F.W., Noll, D.C., & Cohen, J.D. (2001b). Selective deficits in prefrontal cortex regions in medication naive schizophrenia patients. *Archives of General Psychiatry, 50,* 280–288.

Bechara, A., Damasio, H., Tranel, D., & Anderson, S.W. (1998). Dissociation of working memory from decision making within the human prefrontal cortex. *Journal of Neuroscience, 18,* 428–437.

Braver, T.S. (1997). Mechanisms of Cognitive Control: A Neurocomputational Model. Ph.D. Thesis, Carnegie Mellon University, Pittsburgh, PA.

Braver, T.S., & Bongiolatti, S.R. (in press). The role of frontopolor prefrontal cortex in subgoal processing during working memory. *NeuroImage.*

Braver, T.S. & Cohen, J.D. (1999). Dopamine, cognitive control, and schizophrenia: the gating model. *Progress in Brain Research, 121,* 327–349.

Braver, T.S. & Cohen, J.D. (2000). On the control of control: The role of dopamine in regulating prefrontal function and working memory. In: S. Monsell & J. Driver (Eds.), *Attention and Performance XVIII* (pp. 713–738). Cambridge, MA: MIT Press.

Braver, T.S. & Cohen, J.D. (2001). Working memory, cognitive control, and the prefrontal cortex: Computational and empirical studies. *Cognitive Processing 2,* 25–55.

Braver, T.S. Cohen, J.D., & Servan-Schreiber, D. (1995). A computational model of prefrontal cortex function. In: D.S. Touretzky, G. Tesauro, & T.K. Leen (Eds.), *Advances in Neural Information Processing Systems,* Vol. 7 (pp. 141–148). Cambridge, MA: MIT Press.

Braver, T.S., Barch, D.M., & Cohen, J.D. (1999). Cognition and control in schizophrenia: a computational model of dopamine and prefrontal function. *Biological Psychiatry, 46,* 312–328.

Braver, T.S., Barch, D.M., Keys, B.A., Carter, C.S., Kaye, J.A., Janowsky, J.S., Taylor, S.F., Yesavage, J.A., Mumenthaler, M.S., Jagust, W.J., & Reed, B.R. (2001). Context processing in older adults: evidence for a theory relating cognitive control to neurobiology in healthy aging. *Journal of Experimental Psychology: General, 130,* 746–763.

Braver, T.S., Barch, D.M., & Cohen, J.D. (1999b). Mechanisms of cognitive control: active memory, inhibition, and the prefrontal cortex. (Technical Report PDP.CNS.99.1). Pittsburgh: Carnegie Mellon University.

Buckner, R.L., & Braver, T.S. (1999). Event-related functional MRI. In: P. Bandettini & C. Moonen (Eds.), *Functional MRI* (pp. 441–452). Berlin: Springer-Verlag.

Buckner, R.L., Bandettini, P.A., O'Craven, K.M., Savoy, R.L., Petersen, S.E., Raichles, M.E., & Rosen, B.R. (1996). Detection of cortical activation during averaged single trials of a cognitive task using functional magnetic resonance imaging. *Proceedings of the National Academy of Science USA, 93,* 14878–14883.

Cabeza, R. (2001). Functional neuroimaging of cognitive aging. In: R. Cabeza & A. Kingstone (Eds.), *Handbook of Functional Neuroimaging of Cognition* (pp. 331–337). Cambridge, MA: MIT Press.

Cabeza, R. & Nyberg, L. (2000). Imaging cognition II: an empirical review of 275 PET and fMRI studies. *Journal of Cognitive Neuroscience, 12,* 1–47.

Callaway, E. & Naghdi, S. (1982). An information processing model for schizophrenia. *Archives of General Psychiatry, 39,* 339–347.

Carter, C.S., Braver, T.S., Barch, D.M., Botvinick, M.M., Noll, D.C., & Cohen, J.D. (1998). Anterior cingulate cortex, error detection, and the online monitoring of performance. *Science, 280,* 747–749.

Cerella, J. (1985). Information processing rates in the elderly. *Psychological Bulletin, 98,* 67–83.

Chapman, L.J. & Chapman, J.P. (1978). The measurement of differential deficit. *Journal of Psychiatry, 14,* 303–311.

Christoff, K. & Gabrieli, J.D.E. (2000). The frontopolar cortex and human cognition: evidence for a rostrocaudal hierarchical organization within the human prefrontal cortex. *Psychobiology, 28,* 168–186.

Cohen, J.D. & Servan-Schreiber, D. (1992). Context, cortex and dopamine: a connectionist approach to behavior and biology in schizophrenia. *Psychological Review, 99,* 45–77.

Cohen, J.D., Servan-Schreiber, D., & McClelland, J.L. (1992). A parallel distributed processing approach to automaticity. *American Journal of Psychology, 105,* 239–269.

Cohen, J.D., Braver, T.S., & O'Reilly, R. (1996). A computational approach to prefrontal cortex, cognitive control, and schizophrenia: recent developments and current challenges. *Philosophical Transactions of the Royal Society of London Series B, 351*(1346), 1515–1527.

Cohen, J.D., Perstein, W.M., Braver, T.S., Nystrom, L.E., Noll, D.C., Jonides, J., & Smith, E.E. (1997). Temporal dynamics of brain activation during a working memory task. *Nature, 386,* 604–608.

Cohen, J.D., Barch, D.M., Carter, C., & Servan-Schreiber, D. (1999). Context-processing deficits in schizophrenia: converging evidence from three theoretically motivated cognitive tasks. *Journal of Abnormal Psychology, 108,* 120–133.

Cohen, R.M., Semple, W.E., Gross, M., Nordahl, T.E., Delisi, L.E., Holcomb, H.H., King, A.C., Morihisa, J.M., & Pickar, D. (1987). Dysfunction in a prefrontal substrate of sustained attention in schizophrenia. *Life Sciences, 40,* 2031–2039.

Cornblatt, B.A. & Keilp, J.G. (1994). Impaired attention, genetics, and the pathophysiology of schizophrenia. *Schizophrenia Bulletin, 20,* 31–62.

Courtney, S.M., Ungerleider, L.G., Keil, K., & Haxby, J.V. (1997). Transient and sustained activity in a distributed neural system for human working memory. *Nature, 386,* 608–612.

Creese, I., Burt, D.R., & Snyder, S.H. (1976). Dopamine receptor binding predicts clinical and pharmacological potencies of antischizophrenic drugs. *Science, 192,* 481–483.

Damasio, A.R. (1985). The frontal lobes. In: K.M. Heilman & E. Valenstein (Eds.), *Clinical Neuropsychology* (pp. 339–375). New York: Oxford University Press.

Davis, K.L., Kahn, R.S., Ko, G., & Davidson, M. (1991). Dopamine in schizophrenia: a review and reconceptualization. *American Journal of Psychiatry, 148,* 1474–1486.

Dehaene, S. & Changeux, J.-P. (1995). Neuronal models of prefrontal cortical function. In: J. Grafman, K. Holyoak, & F. Boller (Eds.), *Structure and Functions of the Human Prefrontal Cortex,* Vol. 769 (pp. 305–321). New York: New York Academy of Sciences.

de Keyser, J., De Backer, J.-P., Vauquelin, G., & Ebinger, G. (1990). The effect of aging on the D1 dopamine receptors in human frontal cortex. *Brain Research, 528,* 308–310.

Dempster, F.N. (1992). The rise and fall of the inhibitory mechanism: towards a unified theory of cognitive development and aging. In: G.J. Whitehurst (Ed.), *Developmental Review: Perspectives in Behavior and Cognition,* Vol. 12 (pp. 45–75). San Diego: Academic Press.

D'Esposito, M., Aguirre, G.K., Zarahn, E., Ballard, D., Shin, R.K., & Lease, J. (1998). Functional MRI studies of spatial and nonspatial working memory. *Cognitive Brain Research, 7,* 1–13.

D'Esposito, M., Postle, B.R., Ballard, D., & Lease, J. (1999). Maintenance versus manipulation of information held in working memory: an event-related fMRI study. *Brain and Cognition, 41,* 66–86.

Diamond, A. (1990). The development and neural bases of memory functions as indexed by the A-not-B and delayed response tasks in human infants and infant monkeys. In: A. Diamond (Ed.), *The Development and Neural Bases of Higher Cognitive Functions* (pp. 267–317). New York: New York Academy of Science Press.

Dias, R., Robbins, T.W., & Roberts, A.C. (1996). Dissociation in prefrontal cortex of affective and attentional shifts. *Nature, 380,* 69–72.

Duncan, J. & Owen, A.M. (2000). A similar frontal lobe network recruited by diverse cognitive demands. *Trends in Neurosciences, 23,* 475–483.

Fiez, J.A., Raife, E.A., Balota, D.A., Schwarz, J.P., Raichle, M.E., & Petersen, S.E. (1996). A positron emission tomography study of the short-term maintenance of verbal information. *Journal of Neuroscience, 16,* 808–822.

Funahashi, S. Bruce, C.J., & Goldman-Rakic, P.S. (1993). Dorsolateral prefrontal lesions and oculomotor delayed-response performance: evidence for mnemonic "scotomas". *Journal of Neuroscience, 13,* 1479–1497.

Fuster, J.M. (1973). Unit activity in prefrontal cortex during delayed-response performance: neuronal correlates of transient memory. *Journal of Neurophysiology, 36,* 61–78.

Fuster, J.M. (1989). *The Prefrontal Cortex: Anatomy, Physiology and Neuropsychology of the Frontal Lobe.* New York: Raven Press.

Fuster, J.M. (1997a). Anatomy of the prefrontal cortex. In: M. Placito, M. Bailer, & K. Bubbeo (Eds.), *The Prefrontal Cortex: Anatomy, Physiology, and Neuropsychology of the Frontal Lobe* (3rd ed. (pp. 6–42). Philadelphia: Lippincott-Raven.

Fuster, J.M. (1997b). Overview of prefrontal functions: The temporal organization of behavior. In: M. Placito, M. Bailer, & K. Bubbeo (Eds.), *The Prefrontal Cortex: Anatomy, Physiology, and Neuropsychology of the Frontal Lobe*, (3rd ed. (pp. 209–252). Philadelphia: Lippincott-Raven.

Glosser, G. & Goodglass, H. (1990). Disorders in executive control functions among aphasic and other brain-damaged patients. *Journal of Clinical and Experimental Neuropsychology, 12*, 485–501.

Goldman-Rakic, P.S. (1987). Circuitry of primate prefrontal cortex and regulation of behavior by representational memory. In: F. Plum & V. Mountcastle (Eds.), *Handbook of Physiology, The Nervous System V*, Vol. 5 (pp. 373–417). Bethesda, MD: American Physiological Society.

Goldman-Rakic, P.S. (1991). Prefrontal cortical dysfunction in schizophrenia: the relevance of working memory. In: B.J. Carroll & J.E. Barrett (Eds.), *Psychopathology and the Brain* (pp. 1–23). New York: Raven Press.

Goldman-Rakic, P.S. (1995). Cellular basis of working memory. *Neuron, 14*, 477–485.

Goldman-Rakic, P.S. (1996). The prefrontal landscape: implications of functional architecture for understanding human mentation and the central executive. In: A.C. Roberts, T.W. Robbins, & L. Weiskrantz (Eds.), *The Prefrontal Cortex: Executive and Cognitive Functions* (pp. 87–103). Oxford: Oxford University Press.

Hecaen, H. & Albert, M.L. (1978). *Human Neuropsychology*. New York: John Wiley & Sons.

Keys, B.A., Barch, D.M., Braver, T.S., & Janowsky, J.S. (submitted). Task sensitivity to age differences in working memory: relative superiority of the *N*-back paradigm.

Kimberg, D.Y. & Farah, M.J. (1993). A unified account of cognitive impairments following frontal lobe damage: the role of working memory in complex, organized behavior. *Journal of Experimental Pscyhology: General, 122*, 411–428.

Levy, R. & Goldman-Rakic, P.S. (2000). Segregation of working memory functions within the dorsolateral prefrontal cortex. *Experimental Brain Research, 233*, 23–32.

Losier, B.J., McGrath, P.J., & Klein, R.M. (1996). Error patterns on the continuous performance test in non-medicated and medicated samples of children with and without ADHD: a meta-analytic review. *Journal of Child Psychology & Psychiatry, 37*, 971–987.

McClelland, J.L. (1993). Toward a theory of information processing in graded, random, and interactive networks. In: D.E. Meyer & S. Kornblum (Eds.), *Attention and Performance XIV: Synergies in Experimental Psychology, Artificial Intelligence, and Cognitive Neuroscience* (pp. 655–688). Cambridge, MA: MIT Press.

Miller, E.K. (2000). The prefrontal cortex and cognitive control. *Nature Reviews Neuroscience, 1*, 59–65.

Miller, E.K. & Cohen, J.D. (2001). An integrative theory of prefrontal cortex function. *Annual Review of Neuroscience, 21*, 167–202.

Myerson, J. & Hale, S. (1993). General slowing and age invariance in cognitive processing: the other side of the coin. In: J. Cerella & J.M. Rybash (Eds.), *Adult Information Processing: Limits on Loss* (pp. 115–141). San Diego: Academic Press.

Norman, D.A. & Shallice, T. (1986). Attention to action: willed and automatic control of behavior. In: R.J. Davidson, G.E. Schwartz, & D. Shapiro (Eds.), *Consciousness and Self-regulation* Vol. 4, (pp. 1–18). Plenum Press.

Nuechterlein, K.H. (1991). Vigilance in schizophrenia and related disorders. In: S.R. Steinhauer, J.H. Gruzelier, & J. Zubin (Eds.), *Handbook of Schizophrenia, Vol. 5: Neuropsychology, Psychophysiology, and Information Processing* (pp. 397–433). Amsterdam: Elsevier.

Nuechterlein, K.H. & Dawson, M.E. (1984). Information processing and attentional functioning in the developmental course of schizophrenia disorders. *Schizophrenia Bulletin, 10*, 160–203.

O'Reilly, R.C., Braver, T.S., & Cohen, J.D. (1999). A biologically based computational model of working memory. In: A. Miyake & P. Shah (Eds.), *Models of Working Memory: Mechanisms of Active Maintenance and Executive Control* (pp. 102–134). Cambridge, UK: Cambridge University Press.

O'Reilly, R.C., Noelle, D.C., Braver, T.S., & Cohen, J.D. (in press). Prefrontal cortex and dynamic categorization tasks: representational organization and neuromodulatory control. *Cerebral Cortex*.

Owen, A.M., Lee, A.C.H., Williams, E.J., Kendall, I.V., Downey, S.P.M.J., Turkheimer, F.E., Menon, D.K., & Pickard, J.D. (1998). Redefining the functional organisation of working memory processes within human lateral frontal cortex. *NeuroImage, 7*, S12.

Petrides, M. (1996). Specialized systems for the processing of mnemonic information within the primate frontal cortex. *Philosophical Transactions of the Royal Society of London Series B, 351*, 1455–1462.

Posner, M.I. (1980). Orienting of attention. *Quarterly Journal of Experimental Psychology, 32*, 3–25.

Posner, M.I. & Petersen, S.E. (1990). The attention system of the human brain. *Annual Review of Neuroscience, 13*, 25–42.

Postle, B.R. & D'Esposito, M. (2000). Evaluating models of the topographical organization of working memory function in frontal cortex with event-related MRI. *Psychology, 28*, 132–145.

Raz, N., Gunning-Dixon, F.M., Head, D., Dupuis, J.H., & Acker, J.D. (1998). Neuroanatomical correlates of cognitive aging: Evidence from structural magnetic resonance imaging. *Neuropsychology, 12*, 95–114.

Rezai, K., Andreasen, N.C., Alliger, R., Cohen, G., Swayze, V., & O'Leary, D.S. (1993). The neuropsychology of the prefrontal cortex. *Archives of Neurology, 50*, 636–642.

Rolls, E.T. (2000). Orbitofrontal cortex and reward. *Cerebral Cortex, 10*, 284–294.

Rosvold, H.E., Mirsky, A.F., Sarason, I., Bransome, E.D., & Beck, L.H. (1956). A continuous performance test of brain damage. *Journal of Consulting Psychology, 20*, 343–350.

Rumelhart, D.E. & McClelland, J.L. (1986). *Parallel Distributed Processing: Explorations in the Microstructure of Cognition*, Vol. 1 and 2. Cambridge, MA: MIT Press.

Schultz, W., Dayan, P., & Montague, P.R. (1997). A neural substrate of prediction and reward. *Science, 275*, 1593–1599.

Seidman, L.J., Breiter, H.J., Goodman, J.M., Goldstein, J.M., Woodruff, P.W., O'Craven, K., Savoy, R., Tsuang, M.T., & Rosen, B.R. (1998). A functional magnetic resonance imaging study of auditory vigilance with low and high information processing demands. *Neuropsychology, 12*, 505–518.

Servan-Schreiber, D., Cohen, J.D., & Steingard, S. (1996). Schizophrenic deficits in the processing of context: a test of a theoretical model. *Archives of General Psychiatry, 53*, 1105–1113.

Siegel, B.V., Nuechterlein, K.H., Wu, J.C., & Buchsbaum, M.S. (1995). Glucose metabolic correlates of continuous performance test performance in adults with a history of infantile autism, schizophrenics, and controls. *Schizophrenia Research, 17*, 85–94.

Smith, E.E. & Jonides, J. (1999). Storage and executive processes in the frontal lobes. *Science, 283*, 1657–1661.

Stuss, D.T. & Benson, D.F. (1986). *The Frontal Lobes*. New York: Raven Press.

Volkow, N.D., Gur, R.C., Wang, G.-J., Fowler, J.S., Moberg, P.J., Ding, Y.-S., Hitzemann, R., Smith, G., & Logan, J. (1998). Association between decline in brain dopamine activity with age and cognitive and motor impairment in healthy individuals. *American Journal of Psychiatry, 155*, 344–349.

Wahlsten, D. (1991). Sample size to detect a planned contrast and a one-degree-of-freedom interaction effect. *Psychological Bulletin, 110*, 587–595.

West, R.L. (1996). An application of prefrontal cortex function theory to cognitive aging. *Psychological Bulletin, 120*, 272–292.

Wilson, F.A.W., Scalaidhe, S.P.O., & Goldman-Rakic, P.S. (1993). Dissociation of object and spatial processing domains in primate prefrontal cortex. *Science, 260*, 1955–1957.

28

Novel Approaches to the Assessment of Frontal Damage and Executive Deficits in Traumatic Brain Injury

BRIAN LEVINE, DOUGLAS I. KATZ, LAUREN DADE, AND SANDRA E. BLACK

Traumatic brain injury (TBI) is a major cause of frontal brain damage. The Centers for Disease Control estimates that 5.3 million Americans are currently living with disability as a result of TBI, with 80,000 to 90,000 people being newly disabled every year (National Center for Injury Prevention and Control, 1999). Traumatic brain injury causes 14 million restricted-activity days per year in the United States, with annual costs estimated at $48 billion annually (Lewin-ICF, 1992). While acute medical care and management of physical symptoms are undoubtedly major contributors to these costs, it is the cognitive and behavioral consequences of TBI that are truly enduring, with a greater impact being on outcome than physical symptoms (Jennett et al., 1981; Brooks et al., 1986; Dikmen et al., 1995).

The long-term cognitive and behavioral impairments in significant TBI are largely determined by damage to the frontal lobes and frontal projections. Deficits that involve capacities governed by prefrontal areas are among the most prominent and ubiquitous after TBI. Despite the well-accepted observations of prefrontal dysfunction and the particular vulnerability of the frontal lobes to traumatic damage, assessment of these impairments is challenging using standard neuropsychological

measures, and anatomical–clinical correlations are often elusive. In this chapter, we will describe interrelated streams of research aimed at improving the specificity of behavioral and brain imaging assessment of TBI. We begin with a brief review of TBI neuropathology.

DIFFUSE AND FOCAL NEUROPATHOLOGY OF TRAUMATIC BRAIN INJURY: EFFECTS ON FRONTAL SYSTEMS

The prefrontal areas are highly vulnerable to damage after TBI. Traumatic damage to prefrontal systems may result from a variety of primary and secondary brain processes. Primary processes are best conceptualized in two categories: focal injury and diffuse injury. These two injuries are important determinants of chronic-stage outcome in TBI.

Focal cortical contusions (FCC), the main form of focal injury, result from contact and acceleratory/deceleratory forces. Ventral and polar frontal and temporal regions are particularly prone to contusional damage because of excessive tissue strains in these areas against the ridges and confines of the anterior fossa and middle fossa (Courville, 1937; Ommaya &

Gennarelli, 1974; Gentry et al., 1988a). Other forms of focal damage include large deep hemorrhages from acceleratory disruption of subcortical penetrating vessels. Large deep hemorrhages may involve subcortical white and gray matter (e.g., caudate, dorsomedial, and ventral anterior thalamus), structures involved in frontal–subcortical circuits (Cummings, 1993). Secondary damage to frontal systems after focal injury may result from delayed neuronal injury (as occurs after diffuse injury), herniation syndromes (especially frontal transfalcine herniation that may compromise medial frontal lobes and anterior cerebral artery perfusion), and hypoxic–ischemic injury (including anterior cerebral artery and middle cerebral artery anterior borderzone ischemia from systemic hypotension).

Delayed complications after TBI may also disrupt frontal cortex and projections. Hydrocephalus typically compromises white matter pathways adjacent to the third and lateral ventricles, which include many prefrontal projections. Chronic subdural hematoma frequently occurs in the frontal extra-axial spaces and may cause dysfunction through compression of the underlying frontal cortex.

Diffuse axonal injury (DAI), the main form of diffuse injury, results from acceleratory/deceleratory forces leading to disruption of axonal transport progressing to axonal disconnections and distal axonal degeneration. As a consequence, there is widespread, scattered deafferentation of these axonal projections, including those involving prefrontal systems. Similarly, these forces may disrupt small blood vessels leading to scattered white matter hemorrhages. In addition to the structural damage to axons and blood vessels, DAI is accompanied by a host of other insults including disruption of small subcortical blood vessels (petechial white matter hemorrhages) and secondary neuronal damage from cascades of destructive biochemical cellular processes (e.g., excitotoxicity, membrane lipoperoxidation; see Lyeth & Hayes, 1992; Lynch & Dawson, 1994; Povlishock & Jenkins, 1995).

Elements of prefrontal dysfunction are the most common clinical effects of DAI, especially during later phases of recovery. It has been proposed that DAI may be more con-centrated in frontal areas of the brain. Although concomitant petechial hemorrhages are often more concentrated in frontal regions (Wilberger et al., 1990), microscopic DAI pathology can be found throughout the neuraxis at the gray–white matter cortical interface and in subcortical white matter and nuclei in the absence of macroscopic lesions (Povlishock, 1993). Occasionally, petechial hemorrhages involve subcortical structures with critical frontal projections, such as the ventral tegmental area of the midbrain (Goldberg et al., 1989; Adair et al., 1996) and the anterior or medial thalamus. Hypometabolism in prefrontal regions was the only correlate of executive, behavioral, and memory dysfunction in a resting positron emission tomography (PET) study of patients with DAI (Fontaine et al., 1999). It is likely that prefrontal hypometabolism and clinical signs are so prominent with DAI because of the vulnerability of prefrontal systems to any form of diffuse subcortical pathology (Goldberg & Bilder, 1987).

Despite improved understanding of pathophysiologic events after TBI and advances in structural and functional imaging techniques, the precise relationships between brain dysfunction in frontal systems and clinical consequences are not always clear. Part of the problem has been the challenge of parsing out and measuring particular prefrontal cognitive and behavioral deficits in the face of an individually unique combination of focal, diffuse, and secondary pathology associated with TBI.

The clinical effects of TBI on frontal functions are largely determined by the types, severity, and location of these combined pathophysiological events. Computation of clinical–pathological relationships is confounded by several factors: the multiplicity of pathological events; the difficulty of direct measurement of diffuse pathologies; the fact that physiological functional defects usually exceed the structural damage; difficulties in measuring executive and behavioral functions; changes in the proportional contribution of different pathologies and non-injury factors to clinical syndromes as recovery evolves. Interpretation is further compounded by non-injury factors, such as the psychosocial substrate in which the injury occurs.

Studies using structural and functional imaging have been inconsistent in demonstrating clear frontal clinical–pathological relationships. Although atrophy and depth of hemorrhagic lesions on magnetic resonance imaging (MRI) have a fairly clear relationship with overall clinical severity and outcome (Levin et al., 1988; 1990; Wilson et al., 1988), the quantity and location (mostly frontal) of petechial hemorrhages do not correlate well with severity or clinical syndrome (Wilberger et al., 1990; Kurth et al., 1994). A number of studies failed to demonstrate any robust relationship between lesion location (frontal or otherwise) and neuropsychological performance (Levin et al., 1992; Anderson et al., 1995).

Although a consistent picture has not emerged from these larger group studies, certain clinical principles can be useful in projecting natural history for individuals with TBI. Diffuse axonal injury and focal frontal injury differentially relate to outcome depending on stage of recovery. As the clinical course of DAI evolves through unconscious, confusional, and post-confusional phases, the defining cognitive impairment typically undergoes a transition from arousal, attention, and memory to executive functioning. Focal lesion effects are determined by lesion location, depth, and laterality. Delayed secondary complications such as hydrocephalus and chronic subdural hematomas commonly present as persistent or regressive frontal cognitive or behavioral problems. When executive and attentional deficits are due to DAI, they tend to evolve over a more protracted course than the similar deficits from focal injuries. When combined, a severe diffuse injury largely determines the course of recovery and masks the effects of focal pathology in the early stages (Katz & Alexander, 1994; van der Naalt et al., 1999). Focal frontal lesions may cause more persistent and prominent frontal deficits than expected from DAI alone, as recovery evolves.

Recovery depends in part on plasticity and adaptive reorganization of undamaged structures. Prefrontal functions may have more redundancy and less lateralization than some more posterior brain functions, and have a greater capacity for reorganization than other more committed brain systems (e.g., primary visual pathways, motor control of hand, and some language functions). Preservation of subcortical pathways and homologous contralateral areas may be critical factors in adaptive plasticity. For instance, patients with shallow, unilateral frontal lesions may demonstrate substantial clinical recovery and, conversely, patients with bilateral frontal lesions often recover poorly.

SUMMARY AND IMPLICATIONS

The presence of multiple and evolving injuries complicates interpretation of brain–behavior relationships in TBI, which is probably why this disease has not been a popular model for studying frontal lobe dysfunction in the cognitive neuroscience literature. Although TBI patients with focal lesions should not be regarded as equivalent to nontraumatic focal lesion patients, properly conducted TBI research can contribute to the study of frontal lobe function and to our understanding of diagnosis and treatment of TBI-related deficits. Some general guidelines for this research include the following: Large samples should be recruited to overcome the inherent variability of TBI. Smaller subgroups may be analyzed using neuropathologically based diagnosis of injury type and severity. Recovery effects should be dealt with by limiting testing to the chronic phase (e.g., 1 year or longer post-injury) or by serial testing across recovery epochs. As disability in TBI can be influenced by non-injury factors (e.g., compensation seeking), patients should be drawn from hospital admission lists rather than from clinics that attract patients with late-emerging complaints. To minimize confounds related to the psychosocial status of the TBI cohort, matched-control subjects should be drawn from friends and family members of the patients. Concurrent testing of nontraumatic focal lesion patients can be useful in teasing apart focal-lesion from diffuse-injury effects.

The remainder of this chapter describes the application of some novel research technologies designed to increase the specificity of brain–behavior relationships in TBI. For our behavioral work, we have attempted to capitalize on the location of ventral prefrontal damage in TBI by applying measures designed to be sensitive to this damage. Our imaging work seeks to quantify TBI neuropathology on chronic-phase high-resolution MRI. We will conclude with recent findings from an activation functional neuroimaging study.

ASSESSING COGNITIVE AND BEHAVIORAL CONSEQUENCES OF TRAUMATIC BRAIN INJURY

Research on the cognitive sequelea of TBI indicates a classic pattern of deficits in speeded information processing, attention (Van Zomeren et al., 1984; Stuss et al., 1989), memory (Levin & Goldstein, 1986; Crosson et al., 1989), and executive functioning (Mattson & Levin, 1990; Stuss & Gow, 1992) that corresponds with the frontal, temporal, and diffuse injury of TBI. Although this profile is widely accepted, the complexity of the clinical picture increases as emotional and psychosocial factors are considered. Patients with significant TBI can have profoundly impaired psychosocial outcome as measured by return to work, leisure activities, social and interpersonal relationships, and personality change (Jennett et al., 1981; Rappaport et al., 1989; Crépeau & Scherzer, 1993; Dikmen et al., 1996). The extent of this psychosocial disruption is not fully accounted for by the reported cognitive deficits; many patients with marked real-life disability show only mild cognitive deficits. Conversely, patients with similar cognitive deficits due to other etiologies (e.g., medial temporal lobe amnesics, Parkinson's disease patients) do not report the same degree of psychosocial disruption.

More specific behavioral and imaging measures are necessary to attain laboratory concordance with the patients' real-life disability. A generic "frontal" explanation of the real-life disability in TBI is unsatisfying as tests traditionally considered sensitive to frontal lobe lesions have been inconclusive in studies of patients with TBI (Ponsford & Kinsella, 1992; Anderson et al., 1995; Cockburn, 1995). Performance on these tests corresponds more closely with atrophy than with frontal lobe le-

sions (Vilkki et al., 1992; Duncan et al., 1997). The insensitivity of standard "frontal" tests such as the Wisconsin Card Sorting Test (WCST) may be related to the fact that these tests were developed and validated in research on the cognitive effects of dorsolateral prefrontal cortical lesions, as opposed to the ventral prefrontal regions that are specifically affected by FCC in TBI (Courville, 1937; Gentry et al., 1988a).

As discussed in detail elsewhere in this volume (see Chapters 3, 21, 22, and 23) ventral prefrontal cortex is intimately connected with limbic nuclei involved in emotional processing (Nauta, 1971; Pandya & Barnes, 1987) and is involved in the acquisition and reversal of stimulus–reward associations (Mishkin, 1964; Fuster, 1997; Rolls, 2000). The involvement of the ventral prefrontal cortex in inhibition, emotion, and reward processing suggests a role in behavioral self-regulation, as shown in numerous case studies of patients with ventral prefrontal lesions (Harlow, 1868; Ackerly, 1937; Eslinger & Damasio, 1985) whose behavior is reminiscent of that observed in patients with TBI (Stuss & Gow, 1992; Varney & Menefee, 1993).

We have used the term *self-regulatory disorder* (SRD) as shorthand for the syndrome exhibited by these patients (see Chapter 25). Self-regulatory disorder is defined as the inability to regulate behavior according to internal goals. It arises from the inability to hold a mental representation of the self on-line and to use this self-related information to inhibit inappropriate responses (Levine et al., 1998a, 1999; Levine, 1999). It therefore involves sustained attention, inhibition, and self-awareness.

This disorder is most apparent in unstructured situations (e.g., child rearing, making a major purchase, or occupational decision making), where patients fail to inhibit inappropriate responses. This is contrasted with structured situations in which environmental cues or overlearned routines determine the appropriate response, which is often the case for standard neuropsychological tests (Shallice & Burgess, 1993). As a result, many patients with SRD appear unimpaired in overlearned, structured situations, in spite of significant real-life upheaval (Mesulam, 1986; Stuss & Benson, 1986; Shallice & Burgess, 1991).

Until the last decade or so there were very few studies that quantified real-life SRD in clinical samples (as opposed to patients preselected for their highly specific lesions and clear SRD). In 1991, Shallice and Burgess attained laboratory concordance of real-life SRD in patients with ventral prefrontal damage using naturalistic multiple subgoal tasks, setting a quantitative standard for deficits that had previously been limited to qualitative description. Subsequent studies in our laboratories and elsewhere have further established the use of similar unstructured tasks in the study of patients with focal lesions (Bechara et al., 1994; Goel et al., 1997; Burgess et al., 1998, 2000; Levine et al., 1998b; Schwartz et al., 1998) and TBI (Whyte et al., 1996; Robertson et al., 1997; Levine et al., 1998b, 2000; Schwartz et al., 1999).

Our paper-and-pencil Strategy Application Test, modeled on one of the measures from the Shallice and Burgess 1991 study (the Six Element Test), requires the selection of targets with high payoff to the exclusion of readily available but lesser-valued targets. In our original study with various patient groups (Levine et al., 1998b), patients tested at 1 year post-injury were significantly impaired relative to socioeconomic- and age-matched controls.

Consistent with our hypothesis that the TBI deficit was due to ventral prefrontal damage was the finding that concurrently tested patients with nontraumatic focal ventral prefrontal lesions were uniformly impaired on this task, although they were preserved on other tests sensitive to dorsolateral prefrontal damage (Levine et al., 1995, 1997). The test was also sensitive to right hemispheric damage in both patients with TBI and those with nontraumatic focal lesions. Given similar findings in patients with right-lateralized pathology (Schwartz et al., 1999) and the right lateralization of the sustained attention system (Posner & Petersen, 1990), this finding indicated a role for sustained attention in strategy application.

We subsequently revised the test to increase its sensitivity to ventral prefrontal damage (Levine et al., 2000; see also Levine et al., 1999). This was accomplished by fostering a response pattern (completion of all items in a sequential manner) applicable early in the task but not as the task progressed, forcing a shift in strategy (selective completion of certain items to the exclusion of other items) to maintain efficiency (see Fig. 28–1). In other words, efficient performance depended on inhibition or reversal of the response pattern reinforced at the beginning of the test. Unlike the original measure, this revised Strategy Application

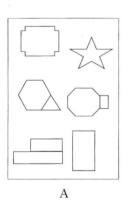 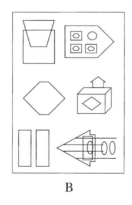 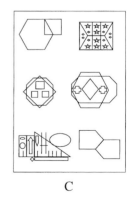

A   B   C

Figure 28–1. Sample items from the revised Strategy Application Task (R-SAT; Levine et al., 1999, 2000). On the early pages (A), all items can be traced in 5–10 seconds. As the subject progresses through the task, items increase in duration to completion but not in difficulty of completion (B, C). Given limited time and an equal amount of points per item, the best strategy is to inhibit the tendency to do all items (established on early pages) in favor of selective completion of brief items on later pages. The test is constructed such that brief items are always available. Subjects are also to complete similarly constructed sentence copying and simple counting items (not shown).

Test (R-SAT) was sensitive not only to TBI in general but also to the degree of TBI severity as measured by the 6-hour Glasgow Coma Scale (GCS) score (Levine et al., 2000). The R-SAT performance was related to patients' health-related quality of life on the Sickness Impact Profile (SIP; Bergner et al., 1976), suggesting that SRD as measured by this laboratory task is related to real-life SRD effects. This relationship held even after variance attributable to standard neuropsychological measures (including the WCST) was controlled.

The development of clinical tests of SRD has significant implications for patients whose disability is overlooked in standard exams. To date, however, the precision of lesion–behavior relationships in group studies of SRD in TBI is constrained by the use of computed tomography (CT) scanning, which is less sensitive than MRI in documenting TBI effects (Levin et al., 1987; Gentry et al., 1988b; Ogawa et al., 1992). Moreover, because of the evolving nature of TBI, scans acquired during the acute phase only partially indicate chronic-phase pathology (Wilson et al., 1988; Blatter et al., 1997). In our studies, for example, TBI patients' R-SAT performance was not related to lesion location along the anterior–posterior gradient as documented by acute CT. From these data alone, we could not tell if the lack of effect was due to insensitivity of the R-SAT or insensitivity of acute CT to chronic-phase frontal damage. The following section describes improved neuroimaging analysis technology that can be used to address such questions.

NEUROIMAGING ASSESSMENT OF TRAUMATIC BRAIN INJURY NEUROPATHOLOGY

Greater precision in brain–behavior relationships in studies of TBI patients requires, at minimum, chronic-phase MRI. A proper TBI imaging protocol should include high-resolution T1-weighted, T2-weighted, proton density, and gradient echo recalled images taken at least 70 days post-injury (Blatter et al., 1997). Even with state-of-the-art images, however, qualitative interpretation does not adequately describe TBI neuropathology, especially DAI effects. Skilled radiologists have been shown to underestimate DAI pathology on MRI (Gentry, 1990). Moreover, the small DAI lesions represent only the regions where the confluence of DAI is large enough to be visible to the naked eye (Gentry, 1990). Thus even perfect agreement among raters on DAI lesions would not truly characterize the full extent of DAI. Interpretation of focal lesions is more straightforward, but detection of focal damage due to localized atrophic changes in the absence of large lesions is subject to the same limitations as those in interpreting generalized DAI (Berryhill et al., 1995). These problems in measurement of traumatically damaged brain tissue contribute substantially to the poor precision of brain–behavior relationships in many studies of TBI.

Although axonal degeneration and cellular loss caused by DAI are microscopic, the quantification of the resultant atrophy can provide a numerical index that has greater precision than qualitative judgments and that is more amenable to research. Ventricular enlargement has been shown to reflect brain atrophy and is indicative of a disproportionately greater loss of white matter than of gray matter (Anderson & Bigler, 1994). Quantification of ventricular enlargement can be accomplished through simple linear width measures taken from CT (corrected for head size; Levin et al., 1981; Bigler et al., 1992) or by tracing of the ventricles across multiple scan slices to obtain ventricular cerebrospinal fluid (CSF) volumes (Gale et al., 1995).

More modern methods have focused on tissue compartment segmentation algorithms that capitalize on a relationship between certain properties of the MRI signal and tissue type expressed at the level of the image voxel. These quantitative analyses involving segmentation of brain volume into its constituent divisions of gray matter, white matter, and CSF have been successfully applied in the study of normal brain development (Blatter et al., 1995) as well as in the study of neurological and psychiatric disorders (Shenton et al., 1992; Reiss et al., 1993).

Several studies of TBI patients have demonstrated the utility of segmentation data in the characterization of TBI-related diffuse damage (Berryhill et al., 1995; Blatter et al., 1997; Thatcher et al., 1997). The *k*-nearest-neighbor technique used in these studies, however, is based on user sampling of the tissue compartments and does not correct for scan inhomogeneities that arise as a result of the inherent transmission and reception characteristics of radiofrequency coils used in MR scanning. Additional steps must be taken to correct for this type of error. Newly developed automated methods for MRI tissue segmentation using T1-weighted images apply local model fitting to account for inhomogeneities, and increase reliability by removing dependence on a user to identify gray matter, white matter, and CSF points (Grabowski et al., 2000). These methods are also able to accommodate variations in scan contrasts.

We have developed and validated a segmentation protocol similar to that described by Grabowski and colleagues (2000) for the purposes of rapid and reliable assessment of gray matter, white matter, and CSF compartment volumes in patients with TBI (Kovacevic et al., submitted). The following study describes preliminary data from our application of this method in our ongoing series of TBI patients.

METHODS

Imaging Parameters

Subjects were scanned on a GE Signa 1.5T MRI scanner. Sagittal T1-weighted three-dimensional (3D) volume images (TR/TE/flip angle = 35 ms/5 ms/35°, 1.0 NEX, acquisition matrix = 256 × 256; 124 slices, slice thickness = 1.3 mm; FOV = 22 cm) were acquired. Proton density/T2-weighted images were acquired using an interleaved sequence (TR/TE/flip angle = 3000 ms and 80 ms/30 ms/35°, 0.5 NEX, acquisition matrix = 256 × 256; 56 slices, slice thickness = 3 mm; FOV= 22 cm).

Image Preprocessing

Prior to segmentation of the T1 image, the skull and tissue surrounding the brain were masked out of the image, preventing the misclassification of nonbrain tissues as parenchyma. Rather than rely on fully automated software that is error-prone, we used a semi-automated process in which an automated brain–nonbrain classification on the PD/T2 weighted images was followed by manual editing, slice by slice. This was followed by a second semi-automated step in which ventricular CSF and the cerebellum were demarcated. This presegmentation procedure can be completed in less than 30 minutes per scan by a trained operator. Interrater reliability is high, as indicated by intraclass correlation coefficients of 98%–99%. The result is a mask of total brain tissue without the inclusion of skull and dura matter, and separate classifications of cerebellar tissue and ventricular CSF. This mask is then transferred onto the T1 image for tissue compartment segmentation (see Figure 28–2).

Tissue Compartment Segmentation

Four gaussian curves were fit to a two-dimensional histogram of the masked T1 image, modeling the image intensity. This information was used to find appropriate cutoff values between gray matter and CSF compartments, and between gray and white matter. To compensate for inhomogeneity of intensity values across the T1 image, segmentation was done over small regions of 50 × 50 × 30 voxels. Only the central portion of each region was segmented with overlap occurring on the outer edges of each region, so that the segmentation can occur locally yet vary smoothly across the image. All voxels were assigned gray, white, or CSF values (ventricular or sulcal as determined by the masking procedure; see Fig. 28–2). The total number of voxels in each category was then calculated as a percentage of the total intracranial capacity. Our algorithm (Kovacevic et al., submitted) is similar to that of Grabowski and colleagues (2000), but it is faster, providing the advantage of very quick computational processing time of under 1 minute for the skull-extracted T1 image.

Figure 28–2. *A:* T1-weighted image from a healthy control subject. *B:* Same slice as *A*, with skull and nonbrain tissue masked out and voxels color coded to represent gray matter, white matter, sulcal cerebraspiral fluid (CSF), and ventricular CSF on the basis of a tissue compartment segmentation algorithm.

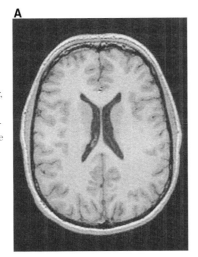
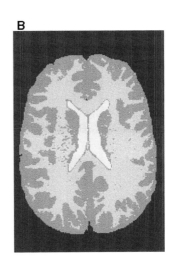

Neuropsychological Tests

We administered a small battery of standard neuropsychological tests of memory, attention, and executive functioning to 21 of the patients. These included the WCST; Trail Making, Parts A and B; phonemic word list generation; the Hopkins Verbal Learning Test, Revised (Benedict et al., 1998); and the Symbol Digit Modalities Test (Smith, 1978).

SUBJECTS

Twenty-six patients with TBI participating in our TBI research program were recruited from consecutive admissions to Sunnybrook and Women's Health Sciences Centre, Toronto, Canada's largest trauma center. According to the GCS score taken at 6 hours post-injury, six had mild TBI (GCS = 13–15), eight had moderate TBI (GCS = 9–12), and nine had severe TBI (GCS = 3–8). Clinical radiologic interpretation of these patients' MRIs taken at approximately 1 year post-injury indicated multiple tiny lesions in 70% of the patients. Thirty percent of the patients had evidence of larger focal lesions, mostly in the anterior temporal and frontal regions. Seventeen percent of the clinical reports mentioned atrophy.

Twelve healthy adults, age matched to the TBI patients, served as controls. For both groups, subjects with prior TBI, neurological

disorders, psychiatric or substance abuse disorders, and medical conditions or medications affecting brain functioning were excluded.

RESULTS

Relation to Traumatic Brain Injury Severity

The presence and degree of TBI was significantly related to tissue compartment volumes. Gray matter, white matter, and sulcal and ventricular CSF volumes were all reliably discriminated among groups, with total parenchymal volume being the most sensitive and specific. As seen in Figure 28–3, there was a significant main effect of TBI group on brain parenchyma (expressed as a percentage of total intracranial capacity; $F_{(3,36)} = 11.02$, $P < 0.0001$). By this measure, all TBI groups had significantly lower corrected parenchymal volumes than controls, and severe TBI patients had significantly lower volumes than mild TBI patients. This dose–response relationship is also apparent in the significant correlation between corrected parenchymal volume and GCS ($r_{(26)} = 0.45$, $p < 0.05$). Analysis of individual compartments revealed that ventricular CSF was more closely related to GCS than sulcal CSF (r's $_{(26)} = -0.48$, $P < 0.05$; -0.35, $P < 0.08$, respectively), and that white matter volume was more closely related to GCS than gray matter volume (r's$_{(26)} = 0.40$,

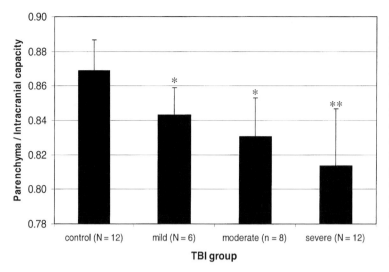

Figure 28–3. Dose–response relationship between traumatic brain injury (TBI) severity and parenchymal change. Brain parenchyma (gray + white matter, adjusted for total intracranial capacity) is plotted for controls and patients with TBI of varying levels of severity. Asterisk indicates significant atrophy relative to controls. Double asterisk indicates significant atrophy relative to controls and to mild TBI. Group differences were assessed with the Student-Newman-Keuls Test, $P < 0.05$.

$P < 0.05$; 0.25, not significant (NS), respectively).

Relation to Behavior

The tests with the strongest relation to segmentation measures were those involving speeded information processing, such as the Symbol Digit Modalities Test (speeded digit transcription, related to ventricular CSF; $r(20) = -0.63$, $P < 0.005$) and Trail Making Test, Part B (speeded alternating letter–number connection, related to parenchymal volume; $r(20) = -0.49$, $P < 0.05$). No significant relationships emerged for other tests of executive functioning and memory.

DISCUSSION

These results support the validity of our tissue compartment segmentation protocol. Although only four patients in this series were diagnosed with atrophy from standard radiologic interpretation, over half had significant atrophy as assessed by percent parenchyma > 2 standard deviations less than controls. The analysis of individual tissue compartments, while preliminary, suggests that white matter is more affected by increasing severity of TBI than gray matter. The correlation of severity with ventricular as opposed to sulcal CSF is consistent with this interpretation, as ventricular expansion would be an expected conse-

quence of white matter loss (Levin et al., 1990; Anderson & Bigler, 1994).

Parenchymal volume was moderately related to injury severity as assessed by the GCS. In using the GCS as a criterion measure in this analysis, it is important to keep in mind that it is a measure of coma depth at the time of injury. It was not designed to measure later outcome. Consciousness alteration at the time of injury can be caused by many factors, not all of which are associated with later atrophy. Figure 28–4 displays segmented images from two patients, both of whom received GCS scores of 3, but demonstrated markedly different atrophy at 1 year post-injury. Patient A had a thalamic hemorrhage at the time of injury, possibly causing altered consciousness in the absence of major DAI. Patient B, at age 58, may have been more vulnerable to DAI effects due to aging (patient A was age 19 at the time of injury). It should be noted that the degree of atrophy in this patient was far greater than that seen in age-matched controls. Whatever the explanation for the discrepancy, these patients illustrate the importance of chronic-phase brain imaging in the assessment of TBI-related brain damage as opposed to relying strictly on acute clinical signs.

Diffuse axonal injury affects the speed and efficiency of mental operations. Accordingly, DAI as indexed by tissue compartment volumes was significantly and specifically related to measures of speeded information process-

Figure 28–4. *A, B:* Two traumatic brain injury patients with severe consciousness alteration (prorated GCS = 3), but dissimilar parenchymal volumes. Tissue compartment segmentation indicated 88% parenchymal volume for patient A (in the range of controls, see Fig. 28–3), whereas patient B's percent parenchyma was 78%.

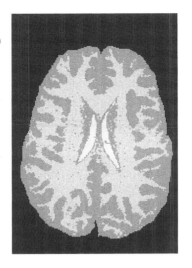

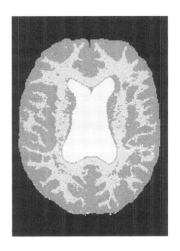

A   B

ing, but not other untimed tests. This finding suggests that these volumetric measures could be used to model the cognitive effects of general parenchymal loss.

The next step in this research program is to analyze the effects of focal damage. Chronic-phase, three-dimensional image acquisition facilitates localization and characterization of lesions. Using the Analyze software system (Biodynamic Research Unit, Mayo Foundation, Rochester, MN, USA), and comparing regions across the PD, T2, and T1 scans, areas of contusion, encephalomalacia, and hemosiderin deposits may be quantified volumetrically and localized in standard space, greatly increasing the precision of lesion classification over acute CT (e.g., Levine et al., 1998a).

A second approach to assessing focal damage in TBI is through measurement of regional atrophy, which can reveal localized effects in the absence of focal lesions (Berryhill et al., 1995). These data may be extracted from the whole-brain segmentation by co-registering a parcellated mask to the segmented image. This mask is defined by specialized algorithms that use manually and automatically identified landmarks identified on each brain to create a standard but individually customized grid (see Fig. 28–5). Segmentation data can then be derived individually for each region of interest and used to model the effects of focal tissue loss. Greater

precision in lesion identification and quantification of focal atrophy should increase brain–behavior correlations with respect to the elusive behavioral and neuropsychological deficits described above.

In summary, a properly obtained structural MRI contains a wealth of information about TBI effects that is only partially utilized in the standard radiologic examination. Quantification of atrophy can be accomplished with several different methods. Our tissue compartment segmentation algorithms provide these data rapidly and reliably, with the benefit of extension to assessment of focal atrophy. Additionally, three-dimensional acquisition in the chronic phase allows for greater precision in lesion characterization. Combining these methods with novel behavioral measures should improve the sensitivity and specificity of brain–behavior relationships in TBI.

FUNCTIONAL NEUROIMAGING

Even the most sophisticated structural imaging analysis is not informative about the functioning of brain tissue. Functional brain imaging techniques can be used to study changes in cerebral blood flow (CBF) or cerebral metabolism resulting from TBI. Most contemporary functional brain imaging studies of chronic-stage TBI effects have used single

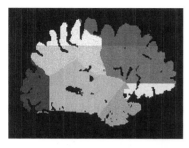

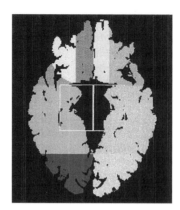

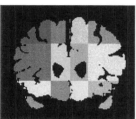

Figure 28–5. Color-coded regional parcellation mask superimposed on a healthy older adult's T1-weighted image shown in three planes. The box indicates the medial temporal region (including amygdala and hippocampus).

photon emission computed tomography (SPECT, usually with hexamethyl propyleneamine oxime [HMPAO] labeled with technetium-99m) and positron emission tomography (PET, usually with fluorodeoxyglucose [FDG]). Given the cost-effectiveness and wide availability of SPECT, it is more commonly used. It yields a greater number of cerebral abnormalities than concurrent structural imaging studies (Gray et al., 1992; Newton et al., 1992; Abdel-Dayem et al., 1998). These findings have in turn been related to neuropsychological test performance (Goldenberg et al., 1992; Ichise et al., 1994). Like SPECT, FDG PET is sensitive to functional abnormalities not appreciated by structural neuroimaging (Langfitt et al., 1986; Alavi et al., 1997), again with a meaningful relationship to neuropsychological test performance (Fontaine et al., 1999).

This functional neuroimaging research, while providing useful supplementation to structural neuroimaging findings, is still wanting with respect to elucidating brain–behavior relationships in chronic TBI. These studies are typically done with the patient in a resting state, when neural activity does not necessarily correspond to task-related neural activity (Duara et al., 1992). Cognitive testing is done separately from scanning with clinical tests of limited neuroanatomical specificity that are then compared to indices of brain function over

large brain regions. The resulting modest imaging–behavior correlations are of heuristic clinical value, but are limited in their contribution to knowledge of brain–behavior relationships in TBI. Additionally, measures of resting metabolism reflect general functional status that can be affected by factors other than brain injury (Alexander, 1995; Ricker & Zafonte, 2000)

Rather than study the relationship of these functional neuroanatomical changes at rest, when mental activity is highly variable, it makes sense to study them in response to specific tasks with reliable functional neuroanatomical properties that tap mental processes affected by TBI. $H_2^{15}O$ PET and functional MRI reflect task-related changes in regional cerebral blood flow (rCBF). There has been an explosion of cognitive functional neuroimaging research in the last decade, probing neural circuitry in response to specific tasks in all major domains of human cognition (Cabeza & Nyberg, 2000). This body of research provides useful templates against which to interpret functional imaging findings in special populations such as patients with TBI (Grady et al., 1995; Becker et al., 1996; Woodard et al., 1998). In addition to identifying focal metabolic deficits, these techniques have documented regions in patients with metabolism similar to or greater than controls, thus indicating preservation in normal task-related systems as well as reorganization in response to injury. Such functional reorganization is most explicitly seen in activation studies of patients with focal lesions following recovery from specific neuropsychological deficit, who show increased activation relative to controls in areas adjacent or homologous to damaged regions (Engelien et al., 1995; Weiller et al., 1995; Buckner et al., 1996).

Activation functional neuroimaging paradigms have been applied in a small number of cases and group studies of patients with TBI (Gross et al., 1996; Kirkby et al., 1996; Levin et al., 1996; Levine et al., 1998a; McAllister et al., 1999; Ricker et al., 2001). In a functional magnetic resonance imaging (fMRI) study of working memory in patients who sustained a mild TBI 1 month prior to scanning, McAllister and colleagues (1999) noted topographic similarity of task-related activation between patients and controls. Consistent with the findings described above, however, was the finding that the mild TBI patients showed greatly enhanced activations in task-specific regions, including the right prefrontal and right parietal cortices.

Mild TBI causes a brief alteration in consciousness, with recovery of mnemonic function occurring over days or weeks. Assessment patients with moderate to severe TBI, in which return of everyday memory is preceded by a lengthy period of post-traumatic amnesia and possibly coma, would be more informative for the study of the functional neuroanatomical correlates of mnestic recovery. Case studies in the literature have focused on focal lesion effects (Kirkby et al., 1996; Levin et al., 1996; Levine et al., 1998). In an exploratory H$_2$^{15}O PET study, a sample of five patients with severe TBI was noted to have reduced frontal activation relative during free recall, but enhanced frontal activation during recognition (Ricker et al., 2001). However, the memory activation paradigm had not been previously validated and there were only four control subjects. Additionally, structural neuroimaging data for the patients was taken from acute CT rather than chronic-phase MRI.

In a recent study with H$_2$^{15}O PET, we demonstrated reorganization of neural systems supporting memory in patients with moderate-

to-severe TBI (Levine et al., submitted). The patients, who had sustained their TBI an average of 4 years prior to the PET study, were scanned while performing a simple cued recall task that had been previously validated in studies of healthy young and older adults (Cabeza et al., 1997a; 1997b). Consistent with the functional neuroimaging findings from other populations and from studies of patients with TBI, our patients showed both reliance on normal functional systems as well as areas of increased activation (see Fig. 28–6). In particular, they showed relatively more activation of ventrolateral and dorsolateral frontal and anterior cingulate regions, including increased recruitment of left frontal regions relative to controls. We were able to relate the functional neuroimaging data to patterns of diffuse and focal injury as revealed by high-resolution structural MRI taken close in time to the PET scans. Although focal frontal lesions affected local aspects of the activation patterns, the remaining areas of increased activation were unaffected. With the exception of the anterior cingulate increase (likely associated with task difficulty in poor-performing patients; Barch et al., 1997), the overall pattern was unaffected by performance differences.

Clinical functional neuroimaging studies of chronic-stage TBI patients typically focus on hypofunctioning, interpreted within a lesion-focused framework as reduced brain activity due to focal or diffuse injury. Our findings suggest an alternative injury effect: task-related hyperactivation. Similar findings in aging and dementia have been interpreted as evidence of compensatory recruitment of additional brain areas to maintain performance (Grady et al., 1995; Cabeza et al., 1997a; Woodard et al., 1998; Bookheimer et al., 2000). Another interpretation relates to the neuropathology of DAI as described above. Widespread DAI as occurs in moderate-to-severe TBI and the resulting neuroplastic changes have functional consequences for the intact receptive fields of axotomized neurons, with functional reorganization resulting from both excitatory and inhibitory deafferentation. Neuronal function is further affected by the resulting neuroplastic changes (i.e., axonal sprouting and synaptogenesis) that may occur

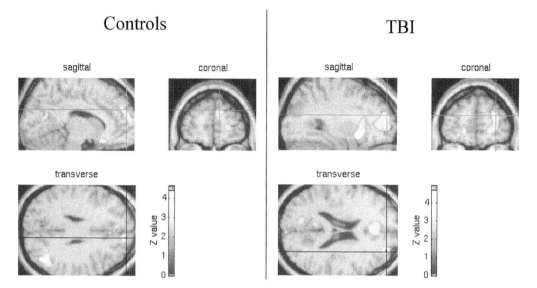

Figure 28–6. Retrieval activations (relative to an encoding baseline) in healthy controls and patients with traumatic brain injury (TBI) as displayed on a standard brain image in three planes. Activations are displayed in white in standard space on axial brain images provided with SPM96. Activations are thresholded at $P < 0.01$ for the purposes of display. Both healthy adults and patients with TBI show a right lateralized pattern of retrieval-related brain activations in frontal polar, lateral temporal, and parietal regions, and bilaterally in the anterior cingulate gyrus. Patients with TBI, however, show additional activations in anterior cingulate gyrus, cuneus, left insula, and left frontal pole. These additional activations were statistically significant in Group × Condition interaction analyses, $P < .001$.

in these fields as part of the recovery process (Povlishock et al., 1992; Christman et al., 1997). The increased spread of cortical activation observed in this study may result from such neuroplastic changes. Aging and Alzheimer's disease share with TBI both diffuse neuronal changes and, as noted above, more widespread task-related activation.

CONCLUSIONS

The advances in the acute management of TBI that have reduced mortality and morbidity have not been paralleled by diagnostic or therapeutic advances in the chronic stage, when mental and behavioral deficits predominate, including memory loss, impaired executive functioning, and personality changes. The resulting long-term disablement affects millions of North Americans, with an economic impact in the billions of dollars. While it is acknowledged that certain deficits may have a higher base rate in the cohort of individuals who sustain TBI (Dikmen et al., 1995), it is nonetheless widely accepted that the neuropsychological profile of moderate to severe TBI is related to brain damage.

The mechanisms governing these brain damage effects, including their trajectory over the recovery process, their rehabilitation, and their high variability across patients with similarly severe TBIs, however, are not well understood. While structural and functional neuroimaging measures do show correlations with behavioral and cognitive outcomes, the relationships tend to lack psychological and anatomic specificity. This state of affairs could be improved by increasing the specificity of psychological and anatomic measures.

Standard neuropsychological assessment procedures are more effective at assessing speeded information processing deficits and cognitive-executive effects of dorsolateral prefrontal cortical damage than at assessing ventral prefrontal cortical effects on emotion-related information processing (Stuss & Levine, 2002; see Chapter 25), yet in patients with

TBI, it is often the ventral prefrontal effects that determine negative outcomes. Neuropsychological assessment of these patients should include measures capable of revealing the SRD (such as our strategy application tests) that characterizes this population. It should further incorporate analysis of patients' real-life functioning, as assessed through psychosocial outcome questionnaires. These measures may reveal lesion–behavior effects not observed in laboratory assessment. A corollary point is that studies of TBI can contribute to the understanding of the human ventral prefrontal cortex, which is otherwise not a common site of frontal neuropathology.

Magnetic resonance imaging is the modality of choice for chronic-phase TBI structural neuroimaging. Not only does MRI have greater sensitivity to TBI-related focal damage, but it can also provide quantification of parenchymal loss useful in both research and clinical contexts. Such data are more appropriate to the description of chronic stage injury characterization than are acute injury data.

Functional neuroimaging studies usually involve assessment of brain metabolism at rest. Studies of task-related brain activation may show injury effects not predicted by standard clinical imaging studies. Early data have revealed task-related activation increases as an effect of DAI (and other diffuse pathologies), possibly due to deafferentation and neuroplasticity leading to reorganization in response to injury.

The future care and treatment of patients with TBI will depend on improving neuropsychological and imaging assessment with novel approaches such as those described in this chapter. Furthermore, TBI is unique for its effects on ventral frontal cortex and diffuse axonal injury. The study of the effects of these injuries provides unique insights into the function of frontal systems.

ACKNOWLEDGMENTS

Work on this chapter was supported by the Canadian Institutes of Health Research, the Canadian Neurotrauma Research Program, and The Ontario Neurotrauma Foundation. We thank Dr. Michael Schwartz for referring patients and for assistance with early clinical information, and Dr. Gordon Cheung for clinical radiological interpretation. The structural image analysis tools were developed by the Sunnybrook Cognitive Neurology neuroimaging group with the guidance of Drs. Michael Bronskill and Nancy Lobaugh and the assistance of Colleen O'Toole, Dr. Fu Chiang Gao, Peter Roy, and Conrad Rockel. Natasa Kovacevic is thanked for her invaluable contribution to the development of this software.

REFERENCES

Abdel-Dayem, H.M., Abu-Judeh, H., Kumar, M., Atay, S., Naddaf, S., El-Zeftawy, H., & Luo, J.Q. (1998). SPECT brain perfusion abnormalities in mild or moderate traumatic brain injury. *Clinical Nuclear Medicine, 23,* 309–317.

Ackerly, S. (1937). Instinctive, emotional, and mental changes following prefrontal lobe extirpation. *American Journal of Psychiatry, 92,* 717–729.

Adair, J.C., Williamson, D.J., Schwartz, R.L., & Heilman, K.M. (1996). Ventral tegmental area injury and frontal lobe disorder. *Neurology, 46,* 842–843.

Alavi, A., Mirot, A., Newberg, A., Alves, W., Gosfield, T., Berlin, J., Reivich, M., & Gennarelli, T. (1997). Fluorine-18-FDG evaluation of crossed cerebellar diaschisis in head injury. *Journal of Nuclear Medicine, 38,* 1717–1720.

Alexander, M.P. (1995). Mild traumatic brain injury: pathophysiology, natural history, and clinical management. *Neurology, 45,* 1253–1260.

Anderson, C.V. & Bigler, E.D. (1994). The role of caudate nucleus and corpus callosum atrophy in trauma-induced anterior horn dilation. *Brain Injury, 8,* 565–569.

Anderson, C.V., Bigler, E.D., & Blatter, D.D. (1995). Frontal lobe lesions, diffuse damage, and neuropsychological functioning in traumatic brain injured patients. *Journal of Clinical and Experimental Neuropsychology, 17,* 900–908.

Barch, D.M., Braver, T.S., Nystrom, L.E., Forman, S.D., Noll, D.C., & Cohen, J.D. (1997). Dissociating working memory from task difficulty in human prefrontal cortex. *Neuropsychologia, 35,* 1373–1380.

Bechara, A., Damasio, A.R., Damasio, H., & Anderson, S.W. (1994). Insensitivity to future consequences following damage to human prefrontal cortex. *Cognition, 50,* 7–15.

Becker, J.T., Mintun, M.A., Aleva, K., Wiseman, M.B., Nichols, T., & DeKosky, S.T. (1996). Compensatory reallocation of brain resources supporting verbal episodic memory in Alzheimer's disease. *Neurology, 46,* 692–700.

Benedict, R.H.B., Schretlen, D., Groninger, L., & Brandt, J. (1998). Hopkins Verbal Learning Test–Revised: normative data and analysis of inter-form and test-retest reliability. *Clinical Neuropsychologist, 12,* 43–55.

Bergner, M., Bobbitt, R.A., Pollard, W.E., Martin, D.P., & Gilson, B.S. (1976). The Sickness Impact Profile: validation of a health status measure. *Medical Care, 14,* 57–67.

Berryhill, P., Lilly, M.A., Levin, H.S., Hillman, G.R., Mendelsohn, D., Brunder, D.G., Fletcher, J.M., Kufera, J., Kent, T.A., Yeakley, J., Bruce, D., & Eisenberg, H.M. (1995). Frontal lobe changes after severe diffuse closed head injury in children: a volumetric study of magnetic resonance imaging. *Neurosurgery, 37*, 392–399; discussion 399–400.

Bigler, E.D., Kurth, S.M., Blatter, D., & Abildskov, T.J. (1992). Degenerative changes in traumatic brain injury: post-injury magnetic resonance identified ventricular expansion compared to pre-injury levels. *Brain Research Bulletin, 28*, 651–653.

Blatter, D.D., Bigler, E.D., Gale, S.D., Johnson, S.C., Anderson, C.V., Burnett, B.M., Parker, N., Kurth, S., & Horn, S.D. (1995). Quantitative volumetric analysis of brain MR: normative database spanning 5 decades of life. *American Journal of Neuroradiology, 16*, 241–251.

Blatter, D.D., Bigler, E.D., Gale, S.D., Johnson, S.C., Anderson, C.V., Burnett, B.M., Ryser, D., Macnamara, S.E., & Bailey, B.J. (1997). MR-based brain and cerebrospinal fluid measurement after traumatic brain injury: correlation with neuropsychological outcome. *American Journal of Neuroradiology, 18*, 1–10.

Bookheimer, S.Y., Strojwas, M.H., Cohen, M.S., Saunders, A.M., Pericak-Vance, M.A., Mazziotta, J.C., & Small, G.W. (2000). Patterns of brain activation in people at risk for Alzheimer's disease [see comments]. *New England Journal of Medicine, 343*, 450–456.

Brooks, N., Campsie, L., Symington, C., Beattie, A., & McKinlay, W. (1986). The five year outcome of severe blunt head injury: a relative's view. *Journal of Neurology, Neurosurgery, and Psychiatry, 49*, 764–770.

Buckner, R.L., Corbetta, M., Schatz, J., Raichle, M.E., & Petersen, S.E. (1996). Preserved speech abilities and compensation following prefrontal damage. *Proceedings of the National Academy of Sciences USA, 93*, 1249–1253.

Burgess, P.W., Alderman, N., Evans, J., Emslie, H., & Wilson, B.A. (1998). The ecological validity of tests of executive function. *Journal of the International Neuropsychological Society, 4*, 547–558.

Burgess, P.W., Veitch, E., de Lacy Costello, A., & Shallice, T. (2000). The cognitive and neuroanatomical correlates of multitasking. *Neuropsychologia, 38*, 848–863.

Cabeza, R., & Nyberg, L. (2000). Imaging cognition II: an empirical review of 275 PET and fMRI studies. *Journal of Cognitive Neuroscience, 12*, 1–47.

Cabeza, R., Grady, C.L., Nyberg, L., McIntosh, A.R., Tulving, E., Kapur, S., Jennings, J.M., Houle, S., & Craik, F.I.M. (1997a). Age-related differences in neural activity during memory encoding and retrieval: a positron emission tomography study. *Journal of Neuroscience, 17*, 391–400.

Cabeza, R., Kapur, S., Craik, F.I.M., McIntosh, A.R., Houle, S., & Tulving, E. (1997b). Functional neuroanatomy of recall and recognition: a PET study of episodic memory. *Journal of Cognitive Neuroscience, 9*, 254–265.

Christman, C.W., Salvant, J.B., Jr., Walker, S.A., & Povlishock, J.T. (1997). Characterization of a prolonged regenerative attempt by diffusely injured axons following traumatic brain injury in adult cat: a light and electron microscopic immunocytochemical study. *Acta Neuropathologica, 94*, 329–337.

Cockburn, J. (1995). Performance on the Tower of London Test after severe head injury. *Journal of the International Neuropsychological Society, 1*, 537–544.

Courville, C.B. (1937). *Pathology of the Central Nervous System, Part 4.* Mountain View, CA: Pacific Press Publishing.

Crépeau, F. & Scherzer, P. (1993). Predictors and indicators of work status after traumatic brain injury: a meta-analysis. *Neuropsychological Rehabilitation, 3*, 5–35.

Crosson, B., Novack, T.A., Trenerry, M.R., & Craig, P.L. (1989). Differentiation of verbal memory deficits in blunt head injury using the Recognition Trial of the California Verbal Learning Test: an exploratory study. *Clinical Neuropsychologist, 3*, 29–44.

Cummings, J. (1993). Frontal-subcortical circuits and human behavior. *Archives of Neurology, 50*, 873–880.

Dikmen, S.S., Ross, B.L., Machamer, J.E., & Temkin, N.R. (1995). One year psychosocial outcome in head injury. *Journal of the International Neuropsychological Society, 1*, 67–77.

Dikmen, S., Machamer, J., Savoie, T., & Temkin, N. (1996). Life quality outcome in head injury. In I. Grant & K.M. Adams (Eds.), *Neuropsychological Assessment of Neuropsychiatric Disorders*, 2nd ed. (pp. 552–576). New York: Oxford University Press.

Duara, R., Barker, W.W., Chang, J., Yoshii, F., Loewenstein, D.A., & Pascal, S. (1992). Viability of neocortical function shown in behavioral activation state PET studies in Alzheimer disease. *Journal of Cerebral Blood Flow and Metabolism, 12*, 927–934.

Duncan, J., Johnson, R., Swales, M., & Freer, C. (1997). Frontal lobe deficits after head injury: unity and diversity of function. *Cognitive Neuropsychology, 15*, 713–742.

Engelien, A., Slibersweig, D., Stern, E., Huber, W., Döring, W., Frith, C., & Frackowiak, R.S.J. (1995). The functional anatomy of recovery from auditory agnosia: a PET study of sound categorization in a neurological patient and controls. *Brain, 118*, 1395–1409.

Eslinger, P.J. & Damasio, A.R. (1985). Severe disturbance of higher cognition after bilateral frontal lobe ablation: patient EVR. *Neurology, 35*, 1731–1741.

Fontaine, A., Azouvi, P., Remy, P., Bussel, B., & Samson, Y. (1999). Functional anatomy of neuropsychological deficits after severe traumatic brain injury. *Neurology, 53*, 1963–1968.

Fuster, J.M. (1997). *The Prefrontal Cortex: Anatomy, Physiology, and Neuropsychology of the Frontal Lobe*, 3rd ed. New York: Raven Press.

Gale, S.D., Johnson, S.C., Bigler, E.D., & Blatter, D.D. (1995). Trauma-induced degenerative changes in brain injury: a morphometric analysis of three patients with preinjury and postinjury MR scans. *Journal of Neurotrauma, 12*, 151–158.

Gentry, L.R. (1990). Head trauma. In: S.W. Atlas (Ed.),

Magnetic Resonance Imaging of the Brain and Spine (pp. 439–466). New York: Raven Press.

Gentry, L.R., Godersky, J.C., & Thompson, B. (1988a). MR imaging of head trauma: review of the distribution and radiopathologic features of traumatic lesions. *American Journal of Neuroradiology, 9*, 101–110.

Gentry, L.R., Godersky, J.C., Thompson, B., & Dunn, V.D. (1988b). Prospective comparative study of intermediate-field MR and CT in the evaluation of closed head trauma. *American Journal of Neuroradiology, 9*, 101–110.

Goel, V., Grafman, J., Tajik, J., Gana, S., & Danto, D. (1997). A study of the performance of patients with frontal lobe lesions in a financial planning task. *Brain, 120*, 1805–1822.

Goldberg, E. & Bilder, R.M.J. (1987). The frontal lobes and hierarchical organization of cognitive control. In: E. Perecman (Ed.), *The Frontal Lobes Revisited* (pp. 159–187). New York: IRBN Press.

Goldberg, E. Bilder, R.M., Hughes, J.E.O., Antin, S.P., & Mattis, S. (1989). A reticulo-frontal disconnection syndrome. *Cortex, 25*, 687–695.

Goldenberg, G., Oder, W., Spatt, J., & Podreka, I. (1992). Cerebral correlates of disturbed executive function and memory in survivors of severe closed head injury: a SPECT study. *Journal of Neurology, Neurosurgery, and Psychiatry, 55*, 362–368.

Grabowski, T.J., Frank, R.J., Szumski, N.R., Brown, C.K., & Damasio, H. (2000). Validation of partial tissue segmentation of single-channel magnetic resonance images of the brain. *NeuroImage, 12*, 640–656.

Grady, C.L., McIntosh, A.R., Horwitz, B., Maisog, J.M., Ungerleider, L.G., Mentis, M.J., Pietrini, P., Schapiro, M.B., & Haxby, J.V. (1995). Age-related reductions in human recognition memory due to impaired encoding. *Science, 269*, 218–221.

Gray, B.G., Ichise, M., Chung, D.G., Kirsh, J.C., & Franks, W. (1992). Technetium-99m-HMPAO SPECT in the evaluation of patients with a remote history of traumatic brain injury: a comparison with X-ray computed tomography. *Journal of Nuclear Medicine, 33*, 52–58.

Gross, H., Kling, A., Henry, G., Herndon, C., & Lavretsky, H. (1996). Local cerebral glucose metabolism in patients with long-term behavioral and cognitive deficits following mild traumatic brain injury. *Journal of Neuropsychiatry and Clinical Neurosciences, 8*, 324–334.

Harlow, J.M. (1868). Recovery after severe injury to the head. *Publication of the Massachusetts Medical Society, 2*, 327–346.

Ichise, M., Chung, D., Wang, P., Wortzman, G., Gray, B.G., & Franks, W. (1994). Technetium-99m-HMPAO SPECT, CT, and MRI in the evaluation of patients with chronic traumatic brain injury: a correlation with neuropsychological performance. *Journal of Nuclear Medicine, 35*, 217–226.

Jennett, B., Snoek, J., Bond, M.R., & Brooks, N. (1981). Disability after severe head injury: observations on the use of the Glasgow Outcome Scale. *Journal of Neurology, Neurosurgery, and Psychiatry, 44*, 285–293.

Katz, D.I. & Alexander, M.P. (1994). Traumatic brain injury. Predicting course of recovery and outcome for patients admitted to rehabilitation. *Archives of Neurology, 51*, 661–670.

Kirkby, B.S., Van Horn, J.D., Ostrem, J.L., Weinberger, D.R., & Berman, K.F. (1996). Cognitive activation during PET: a case study of monozygotic twins discordant for closed head injury. *Neuropsychologia, 34*, 689–697.

Kovacevic, N., Lobaugh, N.J., Bronskill, M.J., Levine, B., Feinstein, A., & Black, S.E. (submitted). A robust method for extraction and automatic segmentation of brain images.

Kurth, S.M., Bigler, E.D., & Blatter, D.D. (1994). Neuropsychological outcome and quantitative image analysis of acute haemorrhage in traumatic brain injury: preliminary findings. *Brain Injury, 8*, 489–500.

Langfitt, T.W., Obrist, W.D., Alavi, A., Grossman, R.I., Zimmerman, R., Jaggi, J., Uzzell, B., Reivich, M., & Patton, D.R. (1986). Computerized tomography, magnetic resonance imaging, and positron emission tomography in the study of brain trauma. Preliminary observations. *Journal of Neurosurgery, 64*, 760–767.

Levin, H.S. & Goldstein, F.C. (1986). Organization of verbal memory after severe closed-head injury. *Journal of Clinical and Experimental Neuropsychology, 8*, 643–656.

Levin, H.S. Meyers, C.A., Grossman, R.G., & Sarwar, M. (1981). Ventricular enlargement after closed head injury. *Archives of Neurology, 38*, 623–629.

Levin, H.S., Amparo, E., Eisenberg, H.M., Williams, D.H., High, W.M., Jr., McArdle, C.B., & Weiner, R.L. (1987). Magnetic resonance imaging and computerized tomography in relation to the neurobehavioral sequelae of mild and moderate head injuries. *Journal of Neurosurgery, 66*, 706–713.

Levin, H.S., Williams, D., Crofford, M.J., High, W.M., Jr., Eisenberg, H.M., Amparo, E.G., Guinto, F.C., Jr., Kalisky, Z., Handel, S.F., & Goldman, A.M. (1988). Relationship of depth of brain lesions to consciousness and outcome after closed head injury. *Journal of Neurosurgery, 69*, 861–866.

Levin, H.S., Williams, D.H., Valastro, M., Eisenberg, H.M., Crofford, M.J., & Handel, S.F. (1990). Corpus callosal atrophy following closed head injury: detection with magnetic resonance imaging. *Journal of Neurosurgery, 73*, 77–81.

Levin, H.S., Williams, D.H., Eisenberg, H.M., High, W.M., Jr., & Guinto, F.C., Jr. (1992). Serial MRI and neurobehavioural findings after mild to moderate closed head injury. *Journal of Neurology, Neurosurgery & Psychiatry, 55*, 255–262.

Levin, H.S., Scheller, J., Rickard, T., Grafman, J., Martinkowski, K., Winslow, M., & Mirvis, S. (1996). Dyscalculia and dyslexia after right hemisphere injury in infancy. *Archives of Neurology, 53*, 88–96.

Levine, B. (1999). Self-regulation and autonoetic consciousness. In: E. Tulving (Ed.), *Memory, Consciousness, and the Brain: The Tallinn Conference* (pp. 200–214). Philadelphia: Psychology Press.

Levine, B., Stuss, D.T., & Milberg, W.P. (1995). Concept generation performance in normal aging and frontal dysfunction: preliminary validation of a clinical test. *Journal of the International Neuropsychological Society, 1,* 208.

Levine, B., Stuss, D.T., & Milberg, W.P. (1997). Effects of aging on conditional associative learning: process analyses and comparison with focal frontal lesions. *Neuropsychology, 11,* 367–381.

Levine, B., Black, S.E., Cabeza, R., Sinden, M., Mcintosh, A.R., Toth, J.P., Tulving, E., & Stuss, D.T. (1998a). Episodic memory and the self in a case of retrograde amnesia. *Brain, 121,* 1951–1973.

Levine, B., Stuss, D.T., Milberg, W.P., Alexander, M.P., Schwartz, M., & MacDonald, R. (1998b). The effects of focal and diffuse brain damage on strategy application: evidence from focal lesions, traumatic brain injury, and normal aging. *Journal of the International Neuropsychological Society, 4,* 247–264.

Levine, B., Dawson, D., Boutet, I., Schwartz, M.L., & Stuss, D.T. (2000). Assessment of strategic self-regulation in traumatic brain injury: its relationship to injury severity and psychosocial outcome. *Neuropsychology, 14,* 491–500.

Levine, B., Cabeza, R., McIntosh, A.R., Black, S.E., Grady, C.L., & Stuss, D.T. (submitted). Functional reorganization of memory systems following traumatic brain injury: a study with $H_2^{15}O$ PET.

Levine, B., Freedman, M., Dawson, D., Black, S.E., & Stuss, D.T. (1999). Ventral frontal contribution to self-regulation: convergence of episodic memory and inhibition. *Neurocase, 5,* 263–275.

Lewin-ICF. (1992). *The Cost of Disorders of the Brain.* Washington, DC: The National Foundation for the Brain.

Lyeth, B.G. & Hayes, R.L. (1992). Cholinergic and opioid mediation of traumatic brain injury. *Journal of Neurotrauma, 9,* S463–474.

Lynch, D.R. & Dawson, T.M. (1994). Secondary mechanisms in neuronal trauma. *Current Opinion in Neurology, 7,* 510–516.

Mattson, A.J. & Levin, H.S. (1990). Frontal lobe dysfunction following closed head injury. *Journal of Nervous and Mental Disease, 178,* 282–291.

McAllister, T.W. Saykin, A.J., Flashman, L.A., Sparling, M.B., Johnson, S.C., Guerin, S.J., Mamourian, A.C., Weaver, J.B., & Yanofsky, N. (1999). Brain activation during working memory 1 month after mild traumatic brain injury: a functional MRI study. *Neurology, 53,* 1300–1308.

Mesulam, M.M. (1986). Frontal cortex and behavior. *Annals of Neurology, 19,* 320–325.

Mishkin, M. (1964). Perseveration of central sets after frontal lesions in monkeys. In: J.M. Warren & K. Akert (Eds.), *The Frontal Granular Cortex and Behavior* (pp. 219–241). New York: McGraw-Hill.

National Center for Injury Prevention and Control. (1999). *Traumatic Brain Injury in the United States: A Report to Congress.* Atlanta: Centers for Disease Control and Prevention.

Nauta, W.J.H. (1971). The problem of the frontal lobe: a reinterpretation. *Journal of Psychiatric Research, 8,* 167–187.

Newton, M.R., Greenwood, R.J., Britton, K.E., Charlesworth, M., Nimmon, C.C., Carroll, M.J., & Dolke, G. (1992). A study comparing SPECT with CT and MRI after closed head injury. *Journal of Neurology, Neurosurgery and Psychiatry,* 92–94.

Ogawa, T., Sekino, H., Uzura, M., Sakamoto, T., Taguchi, Y., Yamaguchi, Y., Hayashi, T., Yamanaka, I., Oohama, N., & Imaki, S. (1992). Comparative study of magnetic resonance and CT scan imaging in cases of severe head injury. *Acta Neurochirurgica Supplementum, 55,* 8–10.

Ommaya, A.K. & Gennarelli, T.A. (1974). Cerebral concussion and traumatic unconsciousness. Correlation of experimental and clinical observations of blunt head injuries. *Brain, 97,* 633–654.

Pandya, D.N. & Barnes, C.L. (1987). Architecture and connections of the frontal lobe. In: E. Perecman (Ed.), *The Frontal Lobes Revisited* (pp. 41–72). New York: IRBN Press.

Ponsford, J. & Kinsella, G. (1992). Attentional deficits following closed-head injury. *Journal of Clinical and Experimental Neuropsychology, 14,* 822–838.

Posner, M.I. & Petersen, S.E. (1990). The attention system of the human brain. *Annual Review of Neuroscience, 13,* 25–42.

Povlishock, J.T. (1993). Pathobiology of traumatically induced axonal injury in animals and man. *Annals of Emergency Medicine, 22,* 980–986.

Povlishock, J.T. & Jenkins, L.W. (1995). Are the pathobiological changes evoked by traumatic brain injury immediate and irreversible? *Brain Pathology, 5,* 415–426.

Povlishock, J.T. Erb, D.E., & Astruc, J. (1992). Axonal response to traumatic brain injury: reactive axonal change, deafferentation, and neuroplasticity. *Journal of Neurotrauma, 9,* S189–S200.

Rappaport, M., Herrero-Backe, C., Rappaport, M.L., & Winterfield, K.M. (1989). Head injury outcome up to ten years later. *Archives of Physical and Medical Rehabilitation, 70,* 885–892.

Reiss, A.L., Faruque, F., Naidu, S., Abrams, M., Beaty, T., Bryan, R.N., & Moser, H. (1993). Neuroanatomy of Rett syndrome: a volumetric imaging study. *Annals of Neurology, 34,* 227–234.

Ricker, J.H. & Zafonte, R.D. (2000). Functional neuroimaging and quantitative electroencephalography in adult traumatic head injury: clinical applications and interpretive cautions. *Journal of Head Trauma Rehabilitation, 15,* 859–868.

Ricker, J.H., Muller, R.A., Zafonte, R.D., Black, K.M., Millis, S.R., & Chugani, H. (2001). Verbal recall and recognition following traumatic brain injury: a [0–15]-watter positron emission tomography study. *Journal of Clinical and Experimental Neuropsychology, 23,* 196–206.

Robertson, I.H., Manly, T., Andrade, J., Baddeley, B.T., & Yiend, J. (1997). 'Oops!': performance correlates of everyday attentional failures in traumatic brain injured and normal subjects. *Neuropsychologia, 35,* 747–758.

Rolls, E.T. (2000). The orbitofrontal cortex and reward. *Cerebral Cortex, 10,* 284–294.

Schwartz, M.F., Montgomery, M.W., Buxbaum, L.J., Lee, S.S., Carew, T.G., Coslett, H.B., Ferraro, M., Fitzpatrick-DeSalme, E., Hart, T., & Mayer, N. (1998). Naturalistic action impairment in closed head injury. *Neuropsychology, 12,* 13–28.

Schwartz, M.F., Buxbaum, L.J., Montgomery, M.W., Fitzpatrick-DeSalme, E., Hart, T., Ferraro, M., Lee, S.S., & Coslett, H.B. (1999). Naturalistic action production following right hemisphere stroke. *Neuropsychologia, 37,* 51–66.

Shallice, T. & Burgess, P.W. (1991). Deficits in strategy application following frontal lobe damage in man. *Brain, 114,* 727–741.

Shallice, T. & Burgess, P.W. (1993). Supervisory control of action and thought selection. In: A. Baddeley & L. Weiskrantz (Eds.), *Attention: Selection, Awareness, and Control: A Tribute to Donald Broadbent* (pp. 171–187). Oxford: Clarendon Press.

Shenton, M.E., Kikinis, R., Jolesz, F.A., Pollak, S.D., LeMay, M., Wible, C.G., Hokama, H., Martin, J., Metcalf, D., Coleman, M., et al. (1992). Abnormalities of the left temporal lobe and thought disorder in schizophrenia. A quantitative magnetic resonance imaging study. *New England Journal of Medicine, 327,* 604–612.

Smith, A. (1978). *Symbol Digit Modalities Test.* Los Angeles: Western Psychological Services.

Stuss, D.T. & Benson, D.F. (1986). *The Frontal Lobes.* New York: Raven Press.

Stuss, D.T. & Gow, C.A. (1992). "Frontal dysfunction" after traumatic brain injury. *Neuropsychiatry, Neuropsychology, and Behavioral Neurology, 5,* 272–282.

Stuss, D.T. & Levine, B. (2002). Adult clinical neuropsychology. *Annual Review of Psychology, 53,* 401–433.

Stuss, D.T., Stethem, L.L., Hugenholtz, H., Picton, T., Pivik, J., & Richard, M.T. (1989). Reaction time after traumatic brain injury: fatigue, divided and focused attention, and consistency of performance. *Journal of Neurology, Neurosurgery, and Psychiatry, 52,* 742–748.

Thatcher, R.W., Camacho, M., Salazar, A., Linden, C., Biver, C., & Clarke, L. (1997). Quantitative MRI of the gray-white matter distribution in traumatic brain injury. *Journal of Neurotrauma, 14,* 1–14.

van der Naalt, J., Hew, J.M., van Zomeren, A.H., Sluiter, W.J., & Minderhoud, J.M. (1999). Computed tomography and magnetic resonance imaging in mild to moderate head injury: early and late imaging related to outcome. *Annals of Neurology, 46,* 70–78.

Van Zomeren, A.H., Brouwer, W.H., & Deelman, B.G. (1984). Attentional deficits: the riddles of selectivity, speed and alertness. In: N. Brooks (Ed.), *Closed Head Injury: Psychological, Social, and Family Consequences* (pp. 74–107). New York: Oxford University Press.

Varney, N.R. & Menefee, L. (1993). Psychosocial and executive deficits following closed head injury: implications for the orbital frontal cortex. *Journal of Head Trauma Rehabilitation, 8,* 32–44.

Vilkki, J., Holst, P., Ohman, J., Servo, A., & Heiskanen, O. (1992). Cognitive test performances related to early and late computed tomography findings after closed-head injury. *Journal of Clinical and Experimental Neuropsychology, 14,* 518–532.

Weiller, C., Isensee, C., Rijntjes, M., Huber, W., Muller, S., Bier, D., Dutschka, K., Woods, R.P., Noth, J., & Diener, H.C. (1995). Recovery from Wernicke's aphasia: a positron emission tomographic study. *Annals of Neurology, 37,* 723–732.

Whyte, J., Polansky, M., Cavallucci, C., Fleming, M., Lhulier, J., & Coslett, H.B. (1996). Inattentive behavior after traumatic brain injury. *Journal of the International Neuropsychological Society, 2,* 274–282.

Wilberger, J.E., Jr., Harris, M., & Diamond, D.L. (1990). Acute subdural hematoma: morbidity and mortality related to timing of operative intervention. *Journal of Trauma, 30,* 733–736.

Wilson, J.T., Wiedmann, K.D., Hadley, D.M., Condon, B., Teasdale, G., & Brooks, D.N. (1988). Early and late magnetic resonance imaging and neuropsychological outcome after head injury. *Journal of Neurology, Neurosurgery, and Psychiatry, 51,* 391–396.

Woodard, J.L., Grafton, S.T., Votaw, J.R., Green, R.C., Dobraski, M.E., & Hoffman, J.M. (1998). Compensatory recruitment of neural resources during overt rehearsal of word lists in Alzheimer's disease. *Neuropsychology, 12,* 491–504.

29

Normal Development of Prefrontal Cortex from Birth to Young Adulthood: Cognitive Functions, Anatomy, and Biochemistry

ADELE DIAMOND

Dorsolateral prefrontal cortex (DL-PFC) is needed when concentration is required, as when a task is novel or complicated or when you must switch tasks. An example would be when you need to guide your actions by information that you are holding in mind, and must pay close attention so that you act according to that information and not to your natural inclination. While it is difficult to resist a natural inclination or inhibit a dominant response, after awhile such inhibition no longer requires DL-PFC action so long as you consistently do that without interruption. For example, on the classic Stroop task (Stroop, 1935; MacLeod, 1991, 1992), color words often appear in the ink of another color (for example, the word *blue* might be printed in green ink). It is difficult to report the color of the ink, ignoring the words, but it is far easier to do that over many trials than to switch back and forth between reporting the ink color and reporting the word, even though many trials in the latter condition are purportedly easy because the correct response on those trials is to make the prepotent response (that is, read the word). Task-switching paradigms (Jersild, 1927; Shaffer, 1965; Allport et al., 1994; Rogers & Monsell, 1995; Meiran, 1996; Goschke, 2000; Mayr,

2001) epitomize the twin needs of active maintenance (working memory) and inhibition, which are the hallmarks of when DL-PFC is most clearly needed. The antithesis of when DL-PFC is required is when you can go on "automatic pilot" (Reason & Mycielska, 1982; Norman & Shallice, 1986).

PFC undergoes one of the longest periods of development of any brain region, taking over two decades to reach full maturity in humans (Kostovic et al., 1988; Sowell et al., 1999a). Even during the first year of life, however, significant maturational changes occur in PFC that help to make possible important cognitive advances by 1 year of age. Other periods of life when marked changes occur in the abilities associated with prefrontal cortex are the periods from 3 to 6 years and 7 to 11 years. In this chapter I will focus on normal development, dividing it into the following epochs: 0–1 years, 1–3 years, 3–7 years, and 7 years through early adulthood. For each epoch I will try to summarize some of what is known about (*a*) the development of the working memory and inhibitory control functions that depend on PFC and (*b*) the anatomical and biochemical developmental changes in PFC during that period. First, however, I will briefly indicate where PFC is located.

LOCATING PREFRONTAL CORTEX GEOGRAPHICALLY

All of the cortex in front of the central sulcus is frontal cortex. The area just in front of the central sulcus, between it and the precentral sulcus, is primary motor cortex (Brodmann's area 4). In front of that is premotor cortex and the supplementary motor area (SMA), both subregions of Brodmann's area 6. All of the cortex in front of that is PFC (areas 8, 9, 10, 12, 44, 45, 46, 47, and 9/46). It is an extremely large area, about 25% of all the cerebral cortex in the human brain. While the brain as a whole has increased in size during evolution, the size of PFC is disproportionately large in humans (Blinkov & Glezer, 1968; Preuss, 2000). DL-PFC extends over the superior and middle frontal gyri. Areas 9, 46, and 9/46 comprise the core of DL-PFC (*mid-dorsolateral* PFC; Petrides & Pandya, 1999), with area 8 constituting the posterior portion of DL-PFC and area 10, the anterior portion. Areas 44, 45, and 47/12, all of which lie on the inferior frontal gyrus, comprise ventrolateral PFC.

DEVELOPMENT DURING THE FIRST YEAR OF LIFE

IMPROVEMENTS IN COGNITIVE FUNCTIONS THAT DEPEND ON PREFRONTAL CORTEX

The *A-not-B task* (introduced by Piaget, 1954, [1936]) has been used worldwide to study infant cognitive development (Wellman et al., 1987). Under the name *delayed response*, the almost-identical task has been widely used to study the functions of the DL-PFC subregion of PFC in rhesus monkeys since Jacobsen first introduced it for that purpose in 1935. In the A-not-B/delayed-response task, a participant watches as a desired object is hidden in one of two hiding places that differ only in left–right location. A few seconds later the participant is encouraged to find the hidden object. He or she must hold in mind over those few seconds where the object was hidden. Over trials, the participant must keep this mental record to reflect where the reward was hidden most recently. The participant is rewarded for reaching correctly by being allowed to retrieve the hidden object, thus reinforcing the behavior of reaching to that location. Hence the tendency to emit that response is strengthened. When the reward is hidden at the other location, the participant must inhibit the tendency to repeat the rewarded response and instead respond according to the representation held in mind of where the reward was hidden most recently. This task thus requires an aspect of working memory (holding information in mind), resistance to proactive interference, and inhibition of a prepotent action tendency (the tendency to repeat a positively reinforced response).

By roughly 7½ to 8 months of age, infants reach correctly at the first hiding location with delays as long as 2–3 seconds (Gratch & Landers, 1971; Diamond, 1985; see Fig. 29–1). When the reward is hidden at the other hiding location, however, infants err by reaching back to the first location (the *A-not-B error*). Infants show marked improvements in their performance on the A-not-B/delayed response task between 7½ and 12 months of age. For example, each month they can withstand delays approximately 2 seconds longer, so that by 12 months of age they can succeed with delays almost 10 seconds long (Diamond, 1985; Diamond & Doar, 1989).

In a transparent barrier detour task called "object retrieval" (Diamond, 1988, 1990, 1991), a toy is placed in a clear box, open on one side. Difficulties arise when the infant sees the toy through one of the closed sides of the box. Here, the infant must integrate seeing the toy through one side of the box with reaching through a different side. There is a strong pull to try to reach straight for the toy; that prepotent response must be inhibited when another side of the box is open. Infants progress through a well-demarcated series of five stages in performance of this task between 6 and 12 months of age (see Fig. 29–2). Infants of 6–8 months reach only at the side through which they are looking. They must look through the opening and continue to do so to reach in and retrieve the toy. As they get

A

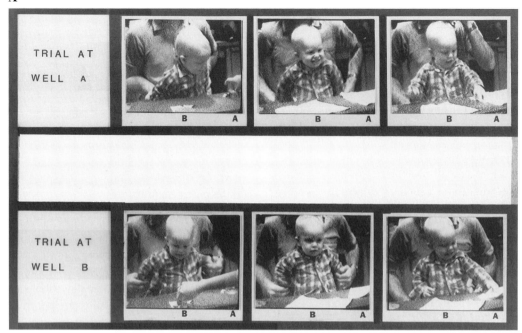

Figure 29–1. *A*: Illustration of the A-not-B task, showing an infant making the A-not-B error. The first frame (*top* and *bottom*) illustrates the experimenter hiding the desired object as the infant watches. Notice that the infant sees where the desired object is placed. The second frame of both rows illustrates the delay period. The delay begins immediately after both wells are covered. During the delay, the parent restrains the infant's arms, and the ex-perimenter calls to the infant to break the infant's visual fixation on the correct well. The third frame of both rows illustrates the infant's response. The infant uncovers a well to search for the desired object. The infant reaches correctly during the trial at the A location, but on the trial at well B the infant incorrectly searches again at well A.

(*continued*)

older, the memory of having looked through the opening is enough; infants can look through the opening, sit up, and reach in while looking through a closed side. By 11–12 months, infants do not need to look along the line of reach at all (Diamond, 1988, 1991).

Although the A-not-B/delayed response and object retrieval tasks share few surface similarities, human infants improve on these tasks during the same age period (6–12 months; Diamond, 1988, 1991) as do infant rhesus monkeys (1½–4 months; Diamond & Goldman-Rakic, 1986; Diamond, 1988, 1991). Despite marked variation among infants in the rate at which they improve on each of these tasks, the age at which a given infant reaches phase 1B on the object retrieval task is remarkably close to the age at which that same infant can first uncover a hidden object in the A-not-B/delayed response paradigm (Diamond, 1991; see Table 29–1).

There is no behavioral task more firmly linked to DL-PFC than the A-not-B/delayed response task (e.g., in ablation studies; see Butters et al., 1969; Goldman & Rosvold, 1970; Diamond & Goldman-Rakic, 1989; electrophysiology studies; see Fuster & Alexander, 1971; Fuster, 1973; Niki, 1974; localized cooling studies; see Fuster & Alexander, 1970; Bauer & Fuster, 1976; and localized injection of dopamine receptor antagonists; see Sawaguchi & Goldman-Rakic, 1991). This is one of the strongest brain–behavior relations in all of cognitive neuroscience.

Lesions of DL-PFC also disrupt performance on the object retrieval task (Diamond & Goldman-Rakic, 1985; Diamond, 1991). Injections of 1-methyl-4-phenyl-1,2,3,6-tetrahy-

B

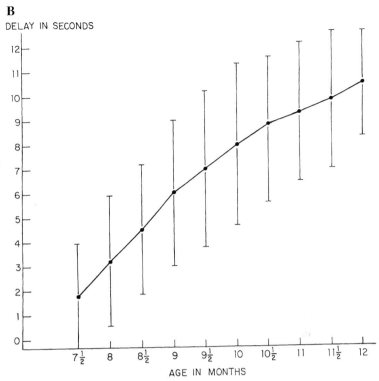

Figure 29–1 (*continued*) B: Developmental progression in the ability to withstand longer and longer delays on the A-not-B task as infants get older (based on 25 infants tested longitudinally every 2 weeks). The graph shows that as infants get older, increasingly, longer delays are required to elicit the A-not-B error. (*Source:* Reprinted with permission from Diamond, 1985)

dropyridine (MPTP), which reduce the level of dopamine in PFC, also produce deficits in object retrieval task performance (Taylor et al., 1990a,b; Schneider & Roeltgen, 1993). (MPTP also affects the level of dopamine in the striatum, but lesions of the striatum do not impair performance on the object retrieval task [Crofts et al., 1999].)

Human infants of 7½ to 9 months, infant monkeys of 1½ to 2½ months, adult monkeys in whom DL-PFC has been ablated, infant monkeys of 5 months in whom DL-PFC was ablated at 4 months, and adult monkeys who have received MPTP injections to disrupt the prefrontal dopamine system fail the A-not-B/ delayed response and object retrieval tasks under the same conditions and in the same ways (Diamond, 1988, 1991). Developmental improvements on the A-not-B/delayed response and object retrieval tasks in human infants are related to changes in the pattern of electrical activity detected by electroencephalogram (EEG) over frontal cortex and in the coherence of electrical activity detected by EEG over frontal cortex and parietal cortex (re: the

A-not-B task, see Fox & Bell, 1990; Bell & Fox, 1992, 1997; re: the object retrieval, N.A. Fox, personal communication). This does not prove that maturational changes in DL-PFC during infancy are one of the prerequisites for the age-related improvements in performance of these tasks, but it is consistent with that hypothesis.

ANATOMICAL AND BIOCHEMICAL EVIDENCE OF PREFRONTAL CORTEX MATURATION DURING THE FIRST YEAR OF LIFE

In humans the period of marked growth of the length and extent of the dendritic branches of pyramidal neurons in layer III of DL-PFC is 7½ to 12 months (Koenderink et al., 1994), coinciding exactly with the period when human infants are improving on the A-not-B/delayed response and object retrieval tasks. Pyramidal neurons in DL-PFC have a relatively short dendritic extent in 7½-month-old infants. By 12 months of age, their dendrites have reached their full mature extension.

A

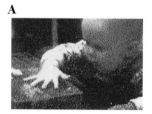 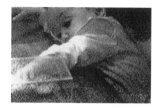 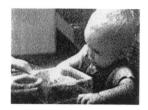

Figure 29–2. *A*: Examples of the typical performance of infants at 6–8 months, 8½ to 9 months, and 10½ to 12 months on the object retrieval task. In each frame the same transparent box is shown with a desired toy visible inside. *Frame 1* shows performance typical of Phases 1 and 1B. Here the front of the box is open, but the infant sees the toy through the closed top of the box. This 6½-month-old infant tries to retrieve the toy by reaching directly for it through the side he is looking through, as do all infants at that age. Although his hand hits the solid, impenetrable surface of the box's top, and although he may touch the top edge of the box's opening and even grasp the opening's edge, the infant tries only, though persistently, to reach through the side through which he is looking. *Frame 2* shows performance typical of Phase 2. This 8½-month-old infant still needs to look through the side she is reaching. Sitting straight up, she sees the toy through the top, and perhaps through the front of the box, but it is the right side of the box that is open. Infants at this age come up with a very creative solution to their need to match up the side through which they are looking and reaching. They lean over to look through the open side. In that position, their arm ipsilateral to the box opening is somewhat trapped under their body, so infants recruit the contralateral arm, whose movement into the box they can monitor from start to finish. This "awkward reach" may look inelegant, but it is a very creative way to get the job done, given infants' strong pull to reach through the side through which they are looking. *Frame 3* illustrates performance typical of Phase 4. This infant, now 11 months old, is the same infant pictured in Frame 1. Now the infant can sit up straight, look through the closed top of the box, and reach into the open right side of the box to retrieve the toy. No longer does the infant need to look through the box opening to retrieve the toy. Note the complex mental calculation needed to coordinate a direct line of sight to the toy through the top of the box and a circuitous detour reach through the box's right side.   (*continued*)

These dendritic branches reach a plateau—in total length, in length of uncut terminal segments, and in radial distance—at around 1 year of age, a plateau that extends at least through 27 years of age. The surface of the cell bodies of these neurons also increases between 7½ and 12 months of age (Koenderink et al., 1994). The level of glucose metabolism in DL-PFC increases during this period as well, and reaches approximately adult levels by 1 year of age (Chugani & Phelps, 1986; Chugani et al., 1987).

Dopamine is an important neurotransmitter in PFC. During the period when infant rhesus monkeys are improving on the A-not-B/delayed response and object retrieval tasks (1½–4 months), the level of dopamine increases in their brain (Brown & Goldman, 1977; Brown et al., 1979), the density of dopamine receptors increases in their PFC (Lidow & Rakic, 1992), and the distribution within their DL-PFC of axons containing the rate-limiting enzyme (tyrosine hydroxylase) for production of dopamine markedly changes (Lewis & Harris, 1991; Rosenberg & Lewis, 1995).

Indeed, even as early as the first year of life, the dopamine projection to PFC is already critical for the cognitive functions subserved by DL-PFC. Thus, if infants 6–12 months old (as well as in older children) have reduced dopamine in PFC while in other respects their central nervous systems appear to be normal, they show a selective deficit in holding information in mind and simultaneously inhibiting a prepotent response (as, for example, on the A-not-B and object retrieval tasks) while other cognitive functions appear to be spared (Diamond et al., 1997; Diamond, 2001).

Acetylcholinesterase (AChE) is an enzyme essential for metabolizing another neurotransmitter, acetylcholine. The pattern of AChE staining in various layers of DL-PFC changes dramatically during the first year of life in humans (Kostovic et al., 1988; Kostovic, 1990).

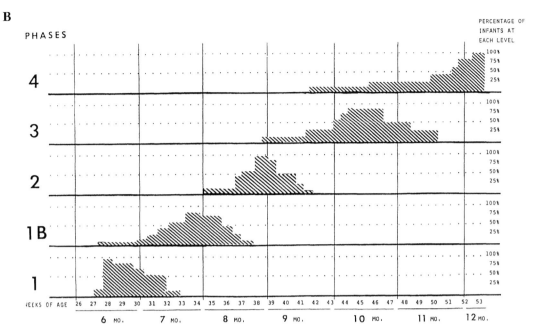

Figure 29–2 *(continued)* B: Illustration of the developmental progression on the object retrieval task. These histograms indicate the percentage, at each age, of 25 infants tested longitudinally every 2 weeks (Diamond, 1990) who were performing at each level of competence with transparent boxes on the object retrieval task. (Source: reprinted with permission from Diamond, 1988.)

DEVELOPMENT AT 1 TO 3 YEARS OF AGE

IMPROVEMENTS IN COGNITIVE FUNCTIONS THAT DEPEND ON PREFRONTAL CORTEX

Less is known about changes during this period in the cognitive functions dependent on PFC or in PFC anatomy and biochemistry than during any other period of life. It is area ripe for further investigation.

Koslowski and Bruner (1972) charted the developmental progression between the ages of 12 and 24 months in the ability to use a lazy Susan to bring a toy within reach. This task requires relating the lazy Susan and its movement to the toy and its movement. It also requires inhibition of trying to reach on a direct line of sight (as the younger children try to do) and inhibition of the tendency to push the lazy Susan in the direction one wants the toy to go (one must push left to make the toy approach on the right). Case (1985; Marini & Case, 1989) similarly reports marked improve-

ments in performance of a simple balance beam problem by children between 1½ and 2½ years of age.

Using a battery of tasks, Kochanska and colleagues (2000) found that the ability to inhibit a prepotent response in order to perform a modulated or different response improved markedly from 22 to 33 months of age and that consistency in performance across the various measures also increased from 22 to 33 months of age. In a spatial-incompatibility task appropriate for children 24 to 36 months old, Gerardi-Caulton (2000) instructed the children to press the button that matched the stimulus. For each pair of stimuli, a stimulus might appear on the same side as its associated button (spatially compatible trial) or on the side opposite its button. Thus, on roughly half the trials, children had to inhibit the prepotent tendency to respond on the same side as the stimulus. Although the location of the stimulus is irrelevant to the task, even adults perform worse on trials in which a stimulus and its associated response are on opposite sides (*the Simon effect*; e.g., Simon, 1969;

Table 29–1.   Age at which 25 infants studied longitudinally entered Phase 1B of object retrieval and could first uncover a hidden object[*]

| | Age (in weeks [and days]) of First Appearance of: | | |
Infant	Phase 1B, Object Retrieval Task	Able to Uncover a Hidden Object, One Hiding Location	A-not-B Error
Brian	28 (3) =	28 (3)	
James	28 (5)	28 (5)	30 (5)
Erin	30 (3)		32 (4)
Nina	31		29
Jennine	31 (4) =	31 (4)	33 (2)
Kate	31 (6)		33 (5)
Rachel	32 (4)		30 (6)
Isabel	32 (5) =		32 (5)
Chrissy	32 (6) =	32 (6)	34 (4)
Ryan	33 (1) =		33 (1)
Bobby	33 (2) =		33 (2)
Julia	33 (2) =		33 (2)
Lyndsey	33 (2) =		33 (2)
Jamie	34 =		34
Mariama	34		36 (3)
Michael	34		36 (4)
Emily	34 (2) =		34 (2)
Graham	34 (2) =		34 (2)
Jane	34 (5) =		34 (5)
Sarah	34 (6) =		34 (6)
Jack	35 (3) =	35 (3)	37 (5)
Blair	35 (4) =	35 (4)	37 (3)
Rusty	35 (6)		33 (5)
Tyler	36 (2)		38 (4)
Todd	39 (4) =		35 (1)

[*]Five infants were not yet ready for A-not-B testing with two wells when they could first uncover a hidden object. Note the striking similarity in age of entering object retrieval phase 1B and age of onset of the A-not-B error.

Simon et al., 1976; Lu & Proctor, 1995). By 2½ years of age, children were able to inhibit the prepotent tendency well enough to perform above chance on the spatially incompatible trials and by 3 years they were correct 90% of the time, though they (like adults) continued to be faster on the compatible than the incompatible trials.

ANATOMICAL AND BIOCHEMICAL EVIDENCE OF PREFRONTAL CORTEX MATURATION BETWEEN 1 AND 3 YEARS OF AGE

Almost nothing is known about changes in PFC during this period. One of the few things we do know is that the AChE reactivity of layer III pyramidal neurons begins to develop

during this period (Kostovic, 1990), but that is surely not the only change in PFC between 1 and 3 years of age.

DEVELOPMENT AT 3 TO 7 YEARS OF AGE

IMPROVEMENTS IN COGNITIVE FUNCTIONS THAT DEPEND ON PREFRONTAL CORTEX

The period of 3–7 years of age, and especially 3–5 years, is a time of marked improvements on a great many cognitive tasks that require holding information in mind plus inhibition (tasks such as day–night, tapping, card sorting, go/no-go, conditional discrimination, appear-

A

Abstract Designs Condition

Say "Day"   Say "Night"

Requires holding two rules in mind,
but does not require inhibiting a prepotent response.

Dog-Pig Condition

Say "Dog"   Say "Pig"

Requires holding two rules in mind, and inhibiting a
prepotent response,
BUT the response to be inhibited is not semantically
related to the response to be activated.

Standard Condition

Say "Day"   Say "Night"

Presents semantically conflicting labels.
Requires holding two rules in mind, and
inhibiting a prepotent response

Ditty Condition

Experimenter sang a little ditty:
♪ "think about the answer, don't tell me" ♪
before the child responded.

Imposes time between presentation of the stimulus and
the child's response, although that time is filled with the
experimenter's rendition of the ditty.

Ditty-between-Trials Condition

Experimenter sang a little ditty:
♪ "think about the answer, don't tell me" ♪
before displaying the stimulus the start of each trial.

Imposes additional time between trials; sessions are as
long as those in the Ditty Condition. However, the extra
time here comes *before* the stimulus is displayed.

Figure 29–3. A: Illustration of
the standard day–night task
(center) and of some variants of
it. B: Performance of 4-year-old
children on the day–night task.
Children perform at chance in
the standard condition, but succeed when the demands on inhibition are reduced (the abstract designs and dog-pig
conditions) and when forced to
allow themselves more time to
compute their answers (the
ditty condition). °°Performance
significantly better than that on
the standard condition at $P <$
0.001.

B

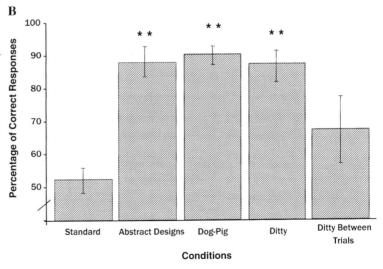

ance–reality, theory of mind, false belief, liquid conservation, and delay of gratification).
On the *day–night task* (Gerstadt et al., 1994;
Diamond et al., 2002; Fig. 29–3) a child must
hold two rules in mind, inhibit saying what the
stimuli really represent, and instead say the
opposite ("Say 'night' when shown a white

card with a picture of the sun, and say 'day'
when shown a black card with a the moon and
stars"). Children 3½ to 4½ years of age find
the task very difficult; by the age of 6–7 years
it is trivially easy. Improvement in responding
correctly is relatively continuous from 3½ to
7 years of age (see Fig. 29–4), while the im-

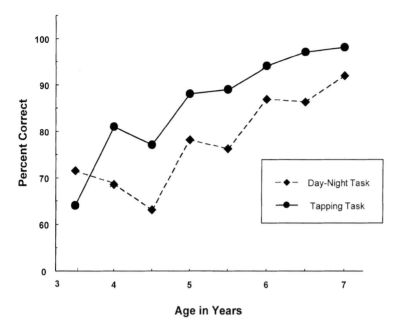

Figure 29–4. Illustration of the developmental progression of children on the day–night and tapping tasks (Source: reprinted with permission from Diamond & Taylor, 1996, Fig. 5)

provement in speed of responding occurs primarily from 3½ to 4½ years.

If abstract designs are used as the stimuli, even the youngest children have no difficulty correctly saying 'day' to one and 'night' to the other (Gerstadt et al., 1994; see Fig. 29–3). Hence, the need to learn and remember two rules is not in itself sufficient to account for the poor performance of young children. If the words to be said to the white-sun and black-moon cards are "dog" and "pig" or "dog" and "cat," even the youngest children have no difficulty (Diamond et al., 2002; see Fig. 29–3). Hence, young children can remember two rules and inhibit saying what the images on the cards represent *unless* what the children are supposed to say is semantically related to what they are not supposed to say.

Comparisons across different trials of the same child and comparisons on the same trials across different children show that when younger children take longer to respond they perform better (Gerstadt et al., 1994). Apparently, it is sufficiently difficult for them to compute the answer of saying "day" to the black-moon card or "night" to the white-sun card that it takes them quite a long time to generate the correct answer. When they rush or answer impulsively, they err. If a delay be-

tween presentation of the stimulus and when the child is able to respond is imposed by chanting a little ditty to the child ("think about the answer, don't tell me"); even young children of 4 years are able to succeed despite the potential interference from the experimenter's chanting (see Fig. 29–3). Slowing down the session by inserting the experimenter's chanting is not what helps the children because if the chanting comes before the stimulus is presented, it does not help the children (see Fig. 29–3).

Luria's *tapping test* (Luria, 1966) also requires (*a*) remembering two rules and (*b*) inhibiting a prepotent response to make the opposite response instead. Here, one needs to remember the rules, "tap once when the experimenter taps twice, and tap twice when the experimenter taps once," and inhibit the tendency to mimic what the experimenter does. Adults with large frontal lobe lesions fail this task (Luria, 1966). Performance of this task has been shown to increase activation in DL-PFC in normal adults, in comparison with mimicking the experimenter's tapping response (Brass et al., 2001). The greatest improvement in correct responding on this task occurs between 3½ and 4 years of age, and the greatest improvement in speed of responding occurs between 4½ and 5 years (Passler et al., 1985; Becker et al., 1987; Diamond & Taylor, 1996; see Fig. 29–4).

Performance on the day–night and tapping tasks is correlated, so that children whose performance on the day–night task is delayed or accelerated show a corresponding delay or acceleration in their performance of the tapping task (Diamond et al., 1997; Diamond, 2001). Indirect evidence on the neural system underlying successful performance on these tasks comes from the finding that children treated early and continuously for phenylketonuria (PKU) and who are thought to have reduced levels of dopamine in PFC are impaired in their performance of both the day–night and tapping tasks but not on an array of unrelated cognitive tasks (Diamond et al., 1997; Diamond, 2001).

Three-year-olds make an error reminiscent of infants' A-not-B error, but on a more difficult task. On this task, 3-year-olds sort cards correctly by the first criterion (regardless of whether that criterion is color or shape; see Zelazo et al., 1995, 1996; Fig. 29–5), just as infants and prefrontally-lesioned monkeys are correct at the first hiding place, and adults with PFC damage sort cards correctly according to the first criterion on the Wisconsin Card Sort Test (WCST; Milner, 1964; Drewe, 1974; Stuss et al., 2000; Fig. 29–5). Three-year-olds err when they must switch to a new sorting criterion, e.g., when cards previously sorted by color must now be sorted by shape. This error is similar to that of infants of 7½ to 9 months and prefrontally lesioned monkeys when the reward is switched to a new hiding location, and to that of adults with PFC damage when they are required to switch to a new sorting criterion. Although 3-year-old children fail to sort by the new sorting criterion, they can correctly state the new criterion (Zelazo et al., 1996), as is sometimes seen with adult patients who have sustained damage to PFC (Luria & Homskaya, 1964; Milner, 1964). Infants, too, occasionally indicate that they know the correct answer on the A-not-B task, by looking at the correct well, although they reach back incorrectly to the well that was previously correct (Diamond, 1991; Hofstadter & Reznick,

1996). By 4 years of age, most children succeed on the simple card sorting task with two dimensions, two values per dimension, and a single switch between dimensions; by 5 years of age, all succeed (Zelazo et al., 1995, 1996; Kirkham et al., 2002).

Zelazo's card sort task can be thought of as perhaps the simplest possible test of task switching. Children must first sort the cards by one dimension (e.g., color, task 1) and then switch to sorting them by the other dimension (e.g., shape, task 2). The single switch between tasks occurs between the block of trials for task 1 and the block of task 2 trials. Errors occur because of difficulty in inhibiting or overcoming what might be termed *attentional inertia*, the tendency to continue to focus on what had been initially relevant (Kirkham et al., *submitted*). For example, once a child of 3 years has focused on the "redness" of a red truck, it is difficult for the child to switch mind-sets and focus on its "truckness." The child gets stuck in thinking about a stimulus in the initially appropriate way.

That tendency never completely disappears. Traces of it can be seen in the heightened reaction times of even healthy, young adults when they are required to switch and respond on the basis of another dimension (e.g., Rogers & Monsell, 1995; Monsell & Driver, 2000; Diamond & Kirkham, 2001). No matter how much warning adults are given about which dimension will be relevant on the upcoming trial, and no matter how long the period between the forewarning and when the stimulus appears or how long the period between trials, adults are still slower to respond on trials in which the relevant dimension switches than on non-switch trials (Allport et al., 1994; Rogers & Monsell, 1995; Meiran, 1996). Remnants of attentional inertia can also be seen in the difficulty adults have in representing more than one interpretation of an ambiguous figure at a time (Chambers & Reisberg, 1985). Even when informed of the alternatives in an ambiguous figure, 3-year-old children remain stuck in their initial way of perceiving the figure; they cannot reverse (Gopnick & Rosati, 2001). By 5 years of age, most children can reverse. Seeing a stimulus in the card sort task

A

Sorting Boxes With Model Cards Affixed

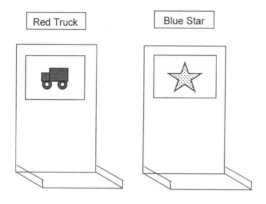

The Cards to be Sorted

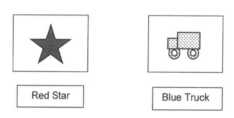

B

Model Cards

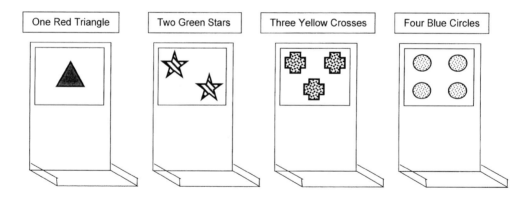

Examples of Cards to be Sorted

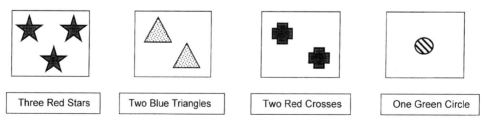

(continued)

C

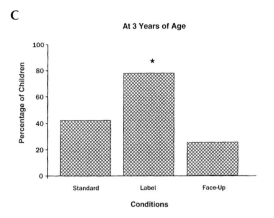

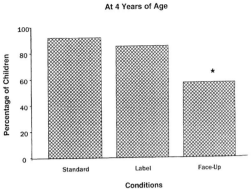

Figure 29–5. *A*: Illustration of the Kirkham et al. (submitted) version of Zelazo's card sorting task for preschoolers. When sorting by color, for example, the blue truck card should go in the bin under the blue star card. When sorting by shape, the blue truck card should go in the bin under the red truck card. *B*: Illustration of the Wisconsin Card Sorting Test (WCST), one of the classic tests for studying prefrontal cortex function in adults (Milner, 1964; Drewe, 1974; Stuss et al., 2000). Each card in this test can be sorted by color, shape, or number. The task for the participant is to deduce the correct sorting criterion on the basis of feedback and to flexibly change the manner of sorting when the experimenter changes the sorting criterion without warning. Zelazo's card sort task and the WCST are similar in that participants are to sort each of the cards in a deck under a model card, first by one dimension and then by another. There are also differences between the tasks, however, in addition to the obvious ones of two dimensions and two levels per condition in Zelazo's task and three dimensions and four levels per dimension in the WCST. For the WCST, the participant must deduce the correct sorting criterion based on feedback; in Zelazo's task, children are told what the correct criterion is and when the criterion switches. Feedback is given after each sorting response in the WCST, whereas no feedback is given after any card is sorted on Zelazo's task. Zelazo's task involves only one switch of sorting criteria; the WCST involves several. Memory load is intentionally minimized on Zelazo's card sort task by the experimenter reminding the child of the current sorting criterion on every trial; in the standard version of the WCST, no such memory aid is provided. *C*: Percentage of children who currently switched dimensions on Kirkham et al.'s (submitted) version of Zelazo's card sort task. An asterisk above a histogram indicates significantly different performance from that of children of the same age on the standard condition at *P* < 0.05.

relevant in incompatible ways to the previously relevant dimension and the newly relevant dimension (e.g., according to its color, one response would be correct, but according to its shape the other response is correct) creates a problem. There is a pull to focus on the previously relevant dimension and to respond on that basis, which must be inhibited before the correct response can be made—despite knowing full well which dimension is currently relevant and which responses are appropriate for each value along that dimension.

Similarly, children 3 years of age have difficulty with *appearance–reality tasks* (Flavell, 1986, 1993) in which they are presented, for example, with a sponge that looks like a rock. Three-year-olds typically report that it looks like a rock and really is a rock, whereas children 4–5 years of age correctly answer that it looks like a rock but really is a sponge. The problem for the younger children is in relating two conflicting identities of the same object (e.g., Rice et al., 1997) and in inhibiting the response that matches their perception. When Heberle and colleagues (1999) reduced perceptual salience in the appearance–reality task (by removing the object during questioning), they found significantly better performance by children 3–4 years of age.

Theory-of-mind and *false-belief tasks* are other tasks that require holding two things in mind about the same situation (the true state of affairs and the false belief of another person) and inhibiting the impulse to give the veridical answer. For example, the child must keep in mind where the hidden object is now and where another person saw it placed before, and must inhibit the inclination to say where the object really is, saying instead where the other person (who is mistaken) would think it is (see Fig. 29–6). Manipulations that reduce the perceptual salience of the true state of affairs aid children 3–4 years of age (e.g., telling the children where the object is really hidden but never actually showing them [Zaitchik, 1991]), as do manipulations that reduce the inhibitory demand in other ways. For example, Carlson et al. (1998) reasoned that pointing veridically is likely to be a well-practiced and reinforced response in young children, and that children of 3–4 years have trouble inhibiting that tendency when they should point to the false location on false-belief tasks. Carlson et al. (1998) found that 3- to 4-year-old children performed better

when given a novel response by which to indicate the false location.

Increasing the perceptual salience of the previous dimension impairs performance. For example, cards are normally sorted face-down in Zelazo's card sort task. If they are sorted face-up and color was the previous dimension, a red-star card would be under the red-truck model and a blue-truck card would be under the blue-star model. This emphasizes the salience of the color dimension. While almost all 4-year-olds succeed in the standard (face-down) condition, almost 50% of 4-year-olds fail the face-up condition (Kirkham et al., submitted; see Fig. 29–5C). Similarly, the cards are normally sorted face-up in the WCST. If they are sorted face down, adults perform better and adults with frontal lobe damage are especially helped. Manipu-

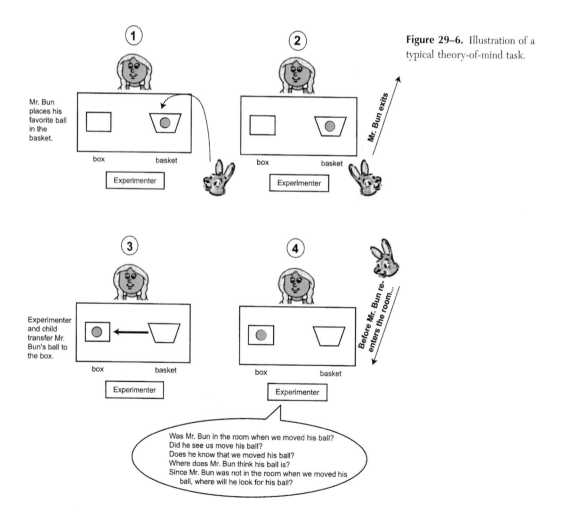

Figure 29–6. Illustration of a typical theory-of-mind task.

lations that *reduce* perceptual salience on appearance–reality tasks, by removing the object during questioning, enable children of 3–4 years to perform much better (e.g., Heberle et al., 1999).

Redirecting attention to the currently relevant dimension improves performance. At the outset of each trial in Zelazo's card sort task, the experimenter labels the new card for the child according to the relevant dimension (e.g., "Here is a truck" or "Here is a blue one"). Despite that, most 3-year-olds continue to sort by the previously correct dimension. One small change—having the child, rather than the experimenter, label the card to be sorted—enables most 3-year-olds to succeed on the switch trial. Thus, if the experimenter asks the child to label each new card (by asking on the first trial of a dimension, "What color (shape) is this?" and on the following trials, simply, "What is this?"), almost twice as many 3-year-olds are able to succeed when the sorting criterion changes (Towse et al., 2000; Kirkham et al., submitted; see Fig. 29–5C [Label Condition]). Children 3 years of age find it extremely difficult to redirect their attention to a newly relevant sorting dimension when the values of the dimension they had been using are still present; they appear to get stuck in a mind-set (a way of thinking about the stimuli) that is no longer relevant. Perhaps their own labeling of the relevant dimension gives 3-year-old children a way to use verbal mediation to help themselves (Luria, 1959; Vygotsky, 1978) inhibit the mental set that is no longer correct and refocus their attention.

Patients with frontal cortex damage are much worse at switching to sort by a different dimension and at switching tasks than are patients with damage elsewhere in the brain or normal controls. It is now fairly firmly established that being able to switch criteria on the WCST test and to resist perseverating on the previously correct dimension selectively recruits lateral prefrontal cortex, perhaps especially dorsolateral prefrontal cortex, and is particularly vulnerable to damage to DL-PFC compared with damage elsewhere in the brain, including other prefrontal regions (Milner, 1964, 1971; Stuss et al., 2000). There is also broad consensus that patients with frontal

cortex damage in the left hemisphere, in contrast with patients with damage to other areas of the brain, are impaired at switching between tasks (e.g., switching between dimensions; Shallice & Burgess, 1991; Owen et al., 1993; Rogers et al., 1998; Diedrichsen et al., 2000; Keele & Rafal, 2000). They are impaired under the same conditions as those under which children 3 years of age fail (i.e., when the stimuli are relevant to both tasks), and they fail in the same way as do 3-year-old children (by perseverating on the previously relevant dimension). Like children of 3 years, their deficit in switching to the newly relevant dimension persists over several consecutive trials (Keele & Rafal, 2000).

Neuroimaging studies of brain activity in healthy, young adults yield similar results. Activity in lateral PFC (both dorsolateral [Brodmann areas 9 & 46] and ventrolateral [areas 44 & 45]) is consistently found to be increased when people must switch between tasks, compared to when they continue doing the same task (Meyer et al., 1998; Postle & D'Esposito, 1998; Omori et al., 1999; Badre et al., 2000; Dove et al., 2000; Sohn et al., 2000; Wylie et al., 2000; Braver et al., 2001; Dreher et al., 2001; Landau et al., 2001). Similar results have been found using the WCST (for analysis with position emission tomography [PET] neuroimaging, see Berman et al., 1995; Nagahama et al., 1996; with single-photon emission computed tomograph [SPECT] neuroimaging, see Marenco et al., 1993; Rezai et al., 1993; with functional magnetic resonance imaging [fMRI] see Konishi et al., 1998, 1999a; Monchi et al., 2001). Konishi et al. (1998, 1999a) found increased activation in a posterior portion of the inferior frontal sulcus (dorsal Brodmann areas 45/44) that was time-locked to when the sorting dimension changed. This occurred even when participants were explicitly informed of the new sorting dimension (Konishi et al., 1999a; much as children are explicitly informed of the new sorting dimension on Zelazo's card sort task). Monchi et al. (2001) found that activity in area 47/12 of ventrolateral prefrontal cortex increased specifically when feedback signaled a switch in the sorting dimension on the WCST.

Zelazo's card sort task can be thought of as

a conditional discrimination task (e.g., if it is a color game, blue truck goes with blue star; if it is a shape game, blue truck goes with red truck). Indeed, the cognitive complexity and control theory espoused by Zelazo and Frye (1997) emphasizes the conditional, hierarchical rule structure implicit in the card sort task. In classic conditional discrimination paradigms participants first learn that responding to one member of a pair of stimuli is rewarded (analogous to the pre-switch block in the card sort task). Testing conditions might be as follows: Stimuli are always a circle and triangle; both are shown on every trial, always against a black background; right–left positions of the stimuli are randomly varied over trials; and choice of the circle is always rewarded. After participants reach a high level of accuracy, the stimuli are presented against a different background (say, white) and the reward contingencies are reversed (analogous to the post-switch block in the card sort task). Hence, the conditional rules for this illustration would be if the background is white, choose triangle; if the background is black, choose circle. After passing criterion on the second subtask, trials with each background are alternated or randomly intermixed (analogous to the mixed-task block in task-switching paradigms). Participants receive feedback on every trial about whether their response is correct or not (unlike the standard procedures in Zelazo's card sort task or task-switching paradigms).

When children are tested with procedures similar to those used with monkeys (minimal instruction so that the participant must deduce the rules), children cannot succeed at the task until they are 4½ to 5½ years old (Heidbreder, 1928; Jeffrey, 1961; Gollin & Liss, 1962; Gollin, 1964; 1965; Doan & Cooper, 1971). When told the rule, children younger than 4½ do much better, but perfect performance is not seen until about age 5 (Shepard, 1957; Osler & Kofsky, 1965; Gollin, 1966; Campione & Brown, 1974). Children younger than 3½ years cannot do this at all, even with explicit instruction. For example, when Gollin (1966) gave reminder trials with feedback before the mixed-task block, he found that 3½-year-olds (43–48 months) performed better, but children of 3 years still failed. Note again

the transition between the ages of 3 and 5 years.

While conditional discrimination tasks involve two relevant dimensions and participants must relate two separate things (background color and foreground shape) to one another, *only* two rules apply: if there is a black background, choose circle; if white, choose triangle. There are half as many rules as on the card sort task, yet success appears at the same age. Similarly, the day–night and tapping tasks involve only two rules (e.g., when the tester taps once, you tap twice, when the tester taps twice, you tap once), but they also require inhibition of strong stimulus–response mappings, and children of 3 years fail them miserably (Gerstadt et al., 1994; Diamond & Taylor, 1995).

Conversely, when children need to hold four rules in mind, but no inhibition or shifting of attention is required, children 3 years of age succeed. Zelazo et al. (1995) presented 3-year-old children with two manipulations of the card sort task that required memory of four rules (the same number as in the standard version) but did not require switching between two dimensions (unlike the standard version). In one condition, children were presented with four target cards of different shapes and told four rules: "If it is a plane, it goes here; if it is a car, it goes here; if it is a bus, it goes here; and if it is a boat, it goes here." Three-year-olds performed better there than on the standard version of the task, even though they were required to keep the same number of rules in mind.

Recently Brooks and colleagues (2001) and Perner and Lang (2002) independently tested children on conditional discrimination reversal tasks where the relevant dimension never changed. Their tasks contained the same number of rules (four) and the same hierarchical embedding as Zelazo's card sort task (two games, two rules each), but unlike the card sort task, the tasks of Brooks et al. and Perner and Lang contained no switch of dimensions. The same, single dimension was relevant throughout. (Indeed, being black-and-white line drawings, the stimuli contained only one dimension [shape, object identity].) In Brooks et al.'s "same" game, children were to sort airplanes with the airplane model card and dogs with the dog model card. In the "silly" game, children were to sort dogs with the airplane model card and planes with the dog model card. Similarly, in Perner and Lang's pre-switch "normal" shape game, children were to put cars with the car target card and suns with the sun target card. In the post-switch "reversed" shape game, children were to put cars with the sun target card and suns with the car target card. If the problem for children on the card sort task is its hierarchical rule structure (as the theory of Zelazo and Frye (1997) purports), 3-year-old children should fail here, for these tasks involve the same logical structure. Yet, children of 3 years succeed at these tasks. In contrast to Zelazo's card sort and conditional discrimination tasks (each of which have two relevant dimensions), 99% of 3½-year-olds succeeded in Brooks et al.'s study, as did 73% of 3-year-olds. Similarly, children of 3 and 3½ years succeeded on roughly 90% of the post-switch trials in the Perner and Lang study. When young children did not have to switch their attentional focus—i.e., did not have to shift from focusing on one dimension to another—they were able to succeed. This is true despite the fact that during the "silly" or "reversed" games, children had to sort to the opposite item, to a model card that matched the stimulus on no feature, resisting the pull to go to the model card that matched the stimulus exactly.

In these experiments, Brooks et al. and Perner and Lang used black-and-white line drawings. In a second experiment, Brooks et al. (2001) used pictures of socks and cups as the stimuli, with half of each being green and the other half yellow. Thus, a second dimension (color) was introduced, but it was irrelevant to the task throughout testing. The task was formally identical to that in Experiment 1. Under these conditions, 3-year-olds failed the task. Thus, when a second dimension was introduced, increasing the demand on attentional inhibition to avoid distraction by the irrelevant dimension, 3-year-olds failed the same task on which they succeeded in Experiment 1.

Meyer et al. (1998) found that DL-PFC activity was not increased for within-dimension switches, even though these required changing stimulus–response mappings (paralleling the success of 3-year-old children on that con-

dition [Brooks et al., 2001; Perner & Lang, 2002]). Dorsolateral prefrontal cortex activity was only required when participants needed to refocus their attention (i.e., overcome attentional inertia) and switch to a different dimension. Similarly, Pollman (2001) found that when only stimulus–response mappings needed to switch (attentional focus remained unchanged), activity did not increase in DL-PFC. (There is some suggestion from the Meyer et al. [1998] and Pollman [2001] studies that premotor cortex, in Brodmann's area 6, may be particularly important for inhibiting acting according to the previously relevant rules and switching to different stimulus–response mappings.) Conditional discriminations appear to require the frontal cortex regions which, in the monkey, border the arcuate sulcus (premotor cortex and the frontal eye fields in areas 6 and 8; see Goldman & Rosvold, 1970; Petrides, 1982, 1985, 1986; 1988; Halsband & Passingham, 1985; Lawler & Cowey, 1987; Passingham, 1988). For example, Petrides (1985) found that monkeys with lesions of the periarcuate region could learn a simple discrimination (choose the lit over the the unlit box) but they could not learn the conditional discrimination (choose the lit box in the presence of one stimulus object, and choose the unlit box in the presence of a different stimulus).

Another example of apparently knowing the correct answer but not being able to act in accord with it is provided by work with *go/no-go tasks*. Here, the child is to respond to one stimulus but do nothing when shown another. Children who are 3–4 years old can correctly restate the instructions, but they cannot get themselves to act accordingly (Tikhomirov, 1978; Bell & Livesey, 1985; Livesey & Morgan, 1991). They respond even to the no-go stimulus. Studies of go/no-go performance consistently find that children cannot succeed at the task until they are roughly 4½ years old because of inhibitory failures (errors of commission to the no-go stimulus; see Jeffrey, 1961; Luria, 1961; Birch, 1967; Beiswanger, 1968; Garber & Ross, 1968; Miller et al., 1970; Norton et al., 1971; Bronckart, 1973; Tikhomirov, 1978; Bell & Livesey, 1985; Livesey & Morgan, 1991; van der Meere & Stemerdink, 1999; Dowsett & Livesey, 2000).

Note again the transition between 3 and 5 years of age.

This is not to say that continued improvements cannot be seen with age, especially when more rapid responding is required and/or the ratio of go to no-go responses is increased. For example, Garber and Ross (1968) report that children 4¾ years of age perform significantly worse than children of 7¾ years. van der Meere and Stemerdink (1999) report more errors by 8-year-old children than by children of 10 or 12 years, and Casey et al. (1997) report more errors by 9-year-old children than by young adults of 22 years. Even adults are rarely at ceiling on the variant of the go/no-go task known as *Simon Says*. Conversely, with a slightly easier variant of the task, children of 3¾ to 4 years have been reported to perform at better than 90% correct (Jones et al., in press).

Neuroimaging studies indicate the impor-

tance of dorsolateral and ventrolateral PFC for performance of go/no-go tasks. Tsujimoto et al. (1997) report increased regional cerebral blood flow in the principal sulcus (DL-PFC) and frontal pole of macaques during performance of a go/no-go task. Konishi et al. (1998, 1999) report increased activation in the inferior frontal sulcus (ventrolateral PFC) on no-go trials compared with that on go trials. Liddle et al. (2001) report increased activity in dorsolateral and ventrolateral PFC during no-go trials. Casey et al. (1997) report increased activity in the inferior frontal gyrus (ventrolateral PFC), middle frontal gyrus (DL-PFC), and orbital frontal gyrus on no-go trials compared with that on go trials.

Many of the advances of Piaget's "concrete operational" child, who is 5–7 years old, over a "preoperational" child, who is 3–4 years of age, also reflect the development of the abilities to hold more than one thing in mind and

Step 1: Present two beakers with equal amounts of liquid.

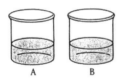

Figure 29–7. Illustration of the procedure used for testing conservation of liquid quantity. (Source: Reprinted with permission from Cole & Cole, 1989)

Step 2: Present taller, thinner beaker, and pour contents of B into it.

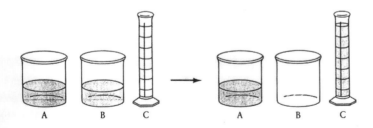

Step 3: Ask: "Which beaker has more liquid, A or C — or do they contain the same amount?"

inhibit the strongest response of the moment (Flavell, 1963). For example, children of 3 or 4 years fail tests of liquid conservation (they do not attend to both height and width, attending only to the more perceptually salient of the two dimensions; Fig. 29–7) and they fail tests of perspective-taking in which they must mentally manipulate a scene to indicate what it would look like from another perspective and must inhibit the tendency to give the most salient response (their current perspective). By 5 or 6 years of age, they can do these things. Since part of the difficulty posed by Piaget's liquid conservation task is the salience of the visual perception that the tall, thin container contains more liquid, placing an opaque screen between the child and the containers before the child answers enables younger children to perform the task better (Bruner, 1964).

In the *delay-of-gratification paradigm*, when faced with the choice of a smaller, immediate reward or a later, larger reward, many 3- to 4-year-old children are unable to inhibit going for the immediate reward, although they would prefer the larger one (Mischel & Mischel, 1983). If they cannot see the rewards or can see only pictures of the rewards, they perform much better than if the smaller reward is sitting right in front of them. On the *windows task*, in which children are rewarded for pointing to a box that is visibly empty and are not rewarded for pointing to a box in which they can see candy, many 3-year-olds fail to inhibit the tendency to point to the baited box (Russell et al., 1991). Children of 5–6 years perform well on both tasks.

ANATOMICAL AND BIOCHEMICAL EVIDENCE OF PREFRONTAL CORTEX MATURATION FROM 3 TO 7 YEARS

The density of neurons in human DL-PFC is highest at birth and declines thereafter. At 2 years of age, the density is 55% above the adult mean, but by age 7 years it is only 10% above adult levels (Huttenlocher, 1990). Thus there is a dramatic change in neuronal density in DL-PFC between 2 and 7 years of age. The synaptic density of layer III pyramidal cells in DL-PFC increases after birth and reaches its maximum at about 1 year of age; by 7 years of age the decrease in synaptic density is significant, though not yet down to adult levels (Huttenlocher, 1979). Another change during this period is a marked expansion in the dendritic trees of layer III pyramidal cells in human DL-PFC between 2 and 5 years of age (Mrzlijak et al., 1990). In addition, the density of neuropeptide Y–immunoreactive neurons in human DL-PFC increases between the ages of 2–4 years and 6–7 years (DeLalle et al., 1997). (Neuropeptide Y–immunoreactive neurons are a class of local circuit intrinsic neurons [Hendry et al., 1984; Hendry, 1993].)

DEVELOPMENT FROM 7 YEARS OF AGE THROUGH EARLY ADULTHOOD

IMPROVEMENTS IN THE COGNITIVE FUNCTIONS THAT DEPEND ON PREFRONTAL CORTEX

Aspects of memory that do not depend on PFC, such as the ability to recognize or recall what one has previously seen, even after a long delay, or the ability to hold information in mind (without an added requirement of manipulating that information or exercising inhibition), develop very early, are robust by the preschool years, and show little improvement with age (Brown, 1975; Dempster, 1985; Diamond, 1995). Where improvements with age, even after 7 years, and in most cases even until early adulthood, are seen are in (1) speed of processing, (2) the ability to use strategies, (3) the ability to hold information in mind *and* work with it (manipulating, monitoring, or transforming it), and (4) the ability to hold information in mind and exercise inhibition (resisting interference, resisting attentional inertia, or resisting a prepotent response tendency). Interestingly, each of these four classes of abilities appears to be tied to the PFC, especially DL-PFC.

Speed of Processing

Speed of processing increases markedly until early adolescence and continues improving, though more gradually, until early adulthood (Kail, 1988, 1991a,b; Hale, 1990; Kail & Park, 1992; Fry & Hale, 1996; Miller & Vernon, 1997). There is a strong, well-replicated relation between speed of processing and performance on tasks either known or hypothesized to tap DL-PFC functions (Case et al., 1982; Fry & Hale, 1986; Salthouse, 1992; Kail & Salthouse, 1994; Duncan et al., 1995), although the reason for this association is not yet fully understood.

Improvements in speed of processing with age account for a good deal of what has been taken to be age-related improvements in the ability to hold information in mind. For example, Case et al. (1982) found that the faster people were able to repeat back the word they had just heard, the more words they could hold in mind, and as the speed of word repetition improved with age so too did word span. When Case et al. equated the speed at which adults and 6-year-olds could repeat back words (by presenting adults with unfamiliar words), they found equivalent word spans in adults and children. Similarly, when they equated adults and children in the speed at which they could count (by requiring adults to count in a foreign language), they found equivalent counting spans in adults and 6-year-olds.

Speed of encoding is another aspect of speed of processing. Item recognition time decreases with age (e.g., Samuels, et al., 1975–1976; Chi, 1977) and speed of item identification is related to the number of items (span) that can be held in mind and retrieved (Dempster, 1981). Individuals who have shorter naming times (within and between ages) have larger memory spans. For example, people generally have larger spans for digits than for words and people can generally name a digit faster than a word; people generally have larger spans for words than pictures, and words are identified faster than pictures (Mackworth, 1963). Chi (1977) found that when adults were only allowed to view picture stimuli for half as long as 5-year-olds (to offset the faster encoding speed of adults), the age difference in the number of pictures that could be held in mind was dramatically reduced. Similarly, Zald and Iacono (1998)

found that, given the same amount of time for encoding, 20-year-olds were significantly more accurate than 14-year-olds at indicating, from memory, the location of an object in space, even after a brief delay of only 500 ms. Although they found little difference among age-groups in the rate of degradation of the internal representation, they did find a developmental improvement in how accurately the information could be encoded in a given amount of time.

Use of Strategies

As children get older they are more likely to use strategies and to improve in their use of strategies. Rehearsal strategies as a memory aid generally emerge around the age of 7 years and are rarely seen in younger children, even when overt attempts are made to try to encourage their use (Flavell, et al., 1966; Johnston, et al., 1987; Gathercole & Hitch, 1993; Gathercole, 1998). Patients with DL-PFC damage are notorious for being unsystematic and for failing to avail themselves of strategies to aid their performance (e.g., Owen et al., 1996; Mangels, 1997; Baldo & Shimamura, 1998). When the material does not lend itself to use of any particular strategy, age differences in memory span are greatly reduced (Ross, 1969; Dempster, 1978; Hess & Radke, 1981), as are performance differences between frontal patients and controls and as is the difference in degree of PFC activation (Bor et al., 2001).

The Ability to Hold Information in Mind and Work with it (Manipulating, Monitoring, or Transforming it)

Piaget (1958) proposed that beginning at about 7 years of age, children begin to be able to simultaneously take into account more than one perspective and to simultaneously think about two aspects of something. Beginning at this age, according to Piaget, children become able to mentally combine, separate, order, and reorder. They become more flexible in their thinking, and can think about alternatives when solving problems.

Baddeley, who coined the term *working*

memory, defined it as involving both temporarily maintaining information in mind and manipulating that information (Baddeley, 1992). This definition of working memory—"temporary storage + manipulation of information"—has received widespread acceptance. Neuroimaging studies have repeatedly demonstrated that activation of DL-PFC is far greater when information must be both held in mind and manipulated than when it must only be held in mind (e.g., D'Esposito et al., 1995, 1998; Petrides, 1995; Cohen et al., 1997; Owen, 1997; Smith et al., 1998; Smith & Jonides, 1999).

Thus, for example, the forward digit span task (recalling numbers in the order in which they are heard) requires less DL-PFC involvement, and performance of this task is less impaired in patients with PFC damage than that of backward digit span (repeating back numbers in the order opposite that in which they were presented), which requires not only holding the information in mind but also manipulating it (Hoshi et al., 2000). Similarly, there is much less improvement with age in performing forward digit span than there is with backward digit span. From ages 7 to 13 years, the number of digits that can be held in mind for forward digit span increases by little more than 1.5 digits (Dempster, 1981). Over the same age period, it increases by twice that for backward digit span (3 digits). Indeed, from ages 6 to 13 years there is a fivefold increase in backward digit span.

Moreover, involvement of DL-PFC and marked improvements in performance of a variety of tasks over the school-age years appear to be found regardless of how the information held in mind is to be manipulated—e.g., ordering randomly presented information (in alphabetical or numerical order) or mentally adding or multiplying numbers. This is true whether monitoring a list of randomly presented numbers to determine which one was omitted, generating all the numbers from 1 to 10 in random order without repeating any (Petrides et al., 1993; Jahanshahi et al., 2000), trying to remember which stimuli were already chosen so that each one is choosen once and none more than once (Petrides, 1995; 2000), or keeping in mind a main goal while performing concurrent subgoals (Koechlin et al.,

1999). Developmental differences are consistently greatest on those tasks that require some (or any) kind of transformation of information held in mind (Dempster, 1985). These findings may describe the limited capacity system independently hypothesized by Daneman and Carpenter (1980, coming from a cognitive science perspective) and by Case et al. (1982, coming from a developmental psychology perspective) that subserves both processing (i.e., manipulation) and storage such that the more information that must be held in mind the fewer resources there are for acting on that information, and the more extensive the processing needed the fewer items of information that can be maintained in mind.

Ability to Hold Information in Mind While Exercising Inhibition (Resisting Interference, Resisting Attentional Inertia, or Resisting a Prepotent Response Tendency)

Engle and Kane have defined working memory slightly differently from Baddeley. They define it as the ability to (*a*) maintain selected information in an active, easily retrievable form while (*b*) blocking or inhibiting other information from entering that active state (Conway & Engle, 1994; Kane & Engle, 2000; 2002; see Hasher and Zacks [1988] for a somewhat similar perspective on the role of inhibition in working memory).

Task-switching paradigms epitomize the twin needs of activate maintenance and inhibition captured by this perspective on working memory, as such paradigms require that one activate the information and rules relevant for the current task and inhibit the mind-set relevant to the other task. Children 4 years of age can begin to perform such switching paradigms, but only poorly. Improvement on task-switching paradigms occurs throughout childhood and into adulthood. On one simple paradigm devised by Meiran (1996; see Fig. 29–8), by age age 11 years children are correct on virtually all non-switch trials but on only 80% of the switch trials, and by age 11 years children are still not performing at adult levels (Cohen et al., 2001). As noted in the section Development at 3 to 7 Years of Age (above), switching tasks elicits increased activation of

A

Task A: Is target in TOP or BOTTOM half?

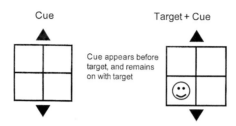

B

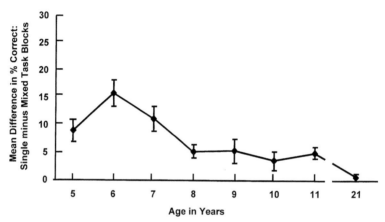

Figure 29–8. *A:* Illustration of Meiran's task-switching paradigm. Participants are to press the "3" key on the keyboard number pad to indicate a response of "down" or "right" and are to press the "7" key to indicate a response of "up" or "left." *B:* Difference in percentage of correct responses on mixed-task blocks versus single-task blocks. Children were significantly less accurate on switch than on nonswitch trials at every age, and on both kinds of trials in mixed-task blocks than on trials in single-task blocks.

Indeed, children were correct on significantly fewer non-switch trials in mixed-task blocks than on exactly the same type of trials (non-switch trials) in single-task blocks. Just knowing that sometimes they would have to switch tasks impaired their performance on all trials in the block. Although the difference in accuracy decreased continuously with age, even 11-year-old children showed a significantly larger difference in accuracy (a significantly larger "switch cost") than did adults.

PFC, and task switching is impaired in patients with PFC damage.

Several bodies of work indicate that the ability to exercise inhibitory control continues to improve until early adulthood. In the *directed-forgetting paradigm*, participants are

directed to forget some of the words they are shown and to remember others. Even children 11 years of age show more intrusions of the to-be-forgotten words than do adults (e.g., Harnishfeger & Pope, 1996; Lehman et al., submitted). The *anti-saccade task* requires participants to suppress the tendency to reflexively look at (saccade to) a visual stimulus in the periphery, and instead look away in the opposite direction. Performance of this task depends especially on the frontal eye fields (Brodmann's area 8; Guitton et al., 1985; O'Driscoll et al., 1995) as well as on the supplementary eye fields and DL-PFC (Luna et al., 2001). Performance of the task improves continuously from 8 through 20–25 years of age (Fischer et al., 1997; Munoz et al., 1998; Luna et al., 2001). Luna et al. (2001) report that while activation in the frontal eye fields, supplementary eye fields, and DL-PFC increased during anti-saccade performance in participants of all ages, increased activation of the thalamus, striatum, and cerebellum was seen only in adults, suggesting perhaps late maturation of the circuit connecting PFC with subcortical regions.

Further evidence of the very protracted de-velopmental progression of the ability to exercise inhibitory control comes from testing with the *directional Stroop task* (Diamond et al., 1998; Davidson et al., 1999; see Fig. 29–9), in which participants are given a response box with two buttons (one for the left thumb and one for the right). When stimulus A appears to the left or right, the participant is to press the button on the same side as the stimulus. When stimulus B appears, the participant is to press the button on the side opposite the stimulus, which requires inhibition of the tendency to respond on the same side as the stimulus. (The tendency to respond on the same side as a stimulus is well documented. People are slower and less accurate to respond on the side opposite a stimulus than they are to respond on the same side. This type of response is called "spatial incompatibility" or the "Simon effect" [Simon, 1969; Craft & Simon, 1970; Simon & Berbaum, 1990; Hommel,

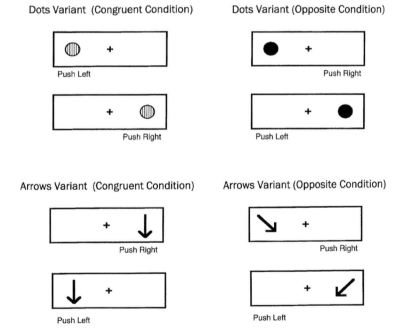

Figure 29–9. Illustration of two of the conditions in the directional Stroop task. In the *dots variant*, when a striped dot appears, the participant is to press the response button on the same side as the stimulus. When a gray dot appears, the participant is to press the button on the side opposite the stimulus. Similarly, in the *arrows variant*, when the arrow points straight down, the participant is to press the button on that side, and when the arrow points diagonally to the opposite side, the participant is to press the button on the side opposite the arrow. The dots-variant requires holding two rules in mind and, when the dot is gray, inhibiting the tendency to respond on the same side as the stimulus. The arrows-variant also requires inhibiting that tendency (when the arrow is diagonal), but it requires little memory because the stimulus itself points to where the participant should respond.

1995; Lu & Proctor, 1995].) The two kinds of stimuli are randomly intermixed over trials. In a comparison of the percentage of correct answers, or reaction time, on trials in which participants are to respond on the same side as the stimulus versus on the opposite side, one finds that the cost (in accuracy and speed) of inhibiting the natural tendency to respond on the same side as the stimulus shows a protracted developmental course, improving linearly from 4 to 26 years of age (Davidson et al., 1999; see Fig. 29–10).

Most tests of working memory require both (*a*) manipulation of information held in mind and (*b*) inhibition of potentially competing information from intruding and potentially competing responses from being made. Indeed,

one perspective on the reason for speed of item identification being so highly correlated with memory span is that both are usually tested under high-interference conditions requiring inhibition (Dempster, 1981), as, for example, in the counting span and spatial span tasks (see Fig. 29–11). On each trial of the counting span task (Case et al., 1982), the participant is asked to count a set of blue dots embedded in a field of yellow dots, touching each blue dot and enumerating it. Immediately thereafter, the participant is to give the answer for that display and the answers for all preceding displays in correct serial order. Thus, this task requires (*1*) selective attention (inhibiting attention to the yellow dots), (*2*) holding of information in mind while execut-

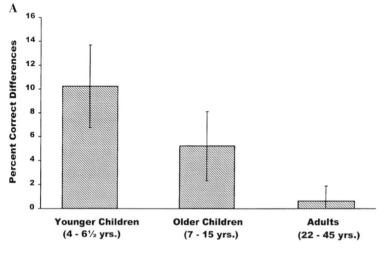

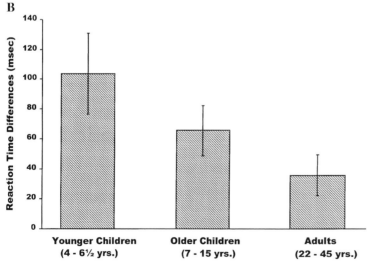

Figure 29–10. *A:* Accuracy when inhibitory control was not required (congruent trials [spatial conflict absent]) minus accuracy when inhibitory control was required (opposite or incongruent trials [spatial conflict present]) on both the dots and arrows variants. *B:* Reaction time when inhibitory control was required (opposite or incongruent trials [spatial conflict present]) minus when inhibitory control was *not* required (congruent trials [spatial conflict absent]) on both the dots and arrows variants. It was sufficiently difficult for children to inhibit responding on the same side as the stimulus that their performance on trials requiring such inhibition was significantly worse (as indexed by either accuracy or speed) at every age (4 through 15 years) than their performance on congruent trials. Even 15-year-olds did not perform at adult levels, although the difference in performance on these two trial types decreased continuously with age.

A

Figure 29–11. *A*: Sample of the kinds of trials presented on the counting span task. *(continued)*

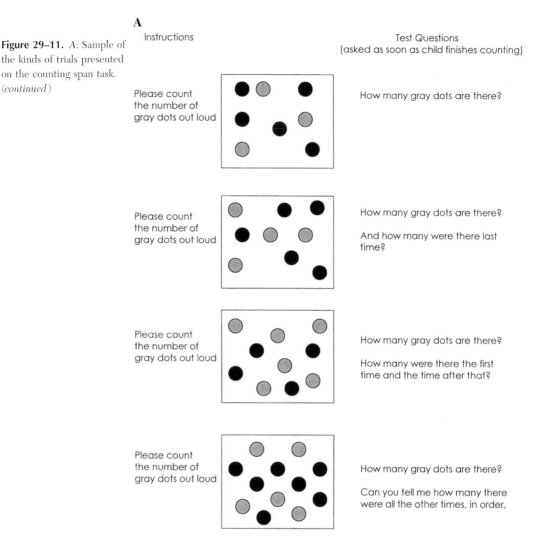

Instructions

Test Questions
(asked as soon as child finishes counting)

Please count the number of gray dots out loud

How many gray dots are there?

Please count the number of gray dots out loud

How many gray dots are there?

And how many were there last time?

Please count the number of gray dots out loud

How many gray dots are there?

How many were there the first time and the time after that?

Please count the number of gray dots out loud

How many gray dots are there?

Can you tell me how many there were all the other times, in order,

ing another mental operation (counting), *(3)* updating of the information held in mind on each trial, and *(4)* temporal order memory (keeping track of the order of the totals computed across trials).

In the spatial span task (Case, 1992a; b) the participant inspects a 4 × 4 matrix on each trial, noting which cell is shaded in. A filler pattern is then shown, and then a second 4 × 4 grid. The second grid is empty; the participant is to point to the cell that had been shaded in on that trial. Several blocks of trials are presented. The number of shaded cells increases by 1 for each subsequent block. Interference from prior trials and from the filler pattern is very high.

A meta-analysis by Case (1992a; b) of 12 cross-sectional studies showed remarkably similar developmental progressions on both of these tasks (see Fig. 29–11). Continuous and marked improvements are seen on both tasks from 4½ to 8 years of age, and continued, more gradual improvement is seen until performance asymptotes on both tasks at around 10–11 years of age.

Quite parallel developmental progressions have also been seen on the compound stimulus visual information (CSVI) task, the pattern span task, and the WCST. In the *CSVI task* (Pascual-Leone, 1970), the participant is taught a different novel response (e.g., raise your hand, clap your hands) for each of several

B
Level 1

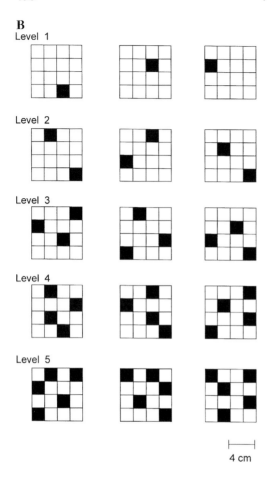

different visual cues (e.g., a square shape or red color). After learning these to criteria, compound stimuli (e.g., red square) are presented, each for 5 seconds, and the participant is to "decode the message" by producing every response called for by the stimuli. The number of correct responses increases until about age 11 (Case, 1972, 1995).

The *pattern span task* is similar to the spatial span task except that several cells are filled in. First, the participant gets a quick look at the pattern. At test, one of the cells that had been filled-in is now unfilled and the participant must point to that cell. The number of filled-in cells increases until the participant's accuracy falls below criterion. Performance on this task also improves greatly between 5 and 11 years of age, when it reaches roughly adult levels (Wilson et al., 1987; Miles et al., 1996).

On the WCST, one of the classic tests of PFC function in adults, the participant must deduce the rule for sorting cards, which can be sorted by color, shape, or number, and must flexibly switch sorting rules, without warning, on the basis of feedback of whether each response is correct or not. Children begin to reach adult levels of performance on this task at about 10–11 years old (Chelune & Baer, 1986; Welsh et al., 1991).

4 cm

C

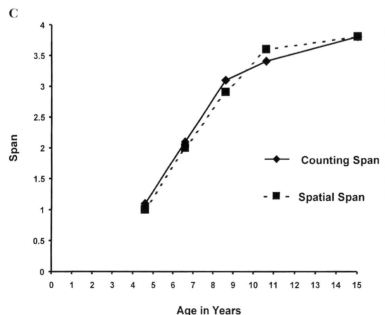

Figure 29-11 (*continued*) *B*: Sample of the kinds of trials presented on the spatial span task. *C*: Developmental progression in the number of items that could be held in mind (span) on the counting span and spatial span tasks. The data for the counting span task are from Crammond (1992), and for the spatial span task, are from Menna (1989).

On the *listening span task* (Daneman & Carpenter, 1980) the participant needs to process incoming information (auditorially presented sentences) while retaining, in correct temporal sequence, the final words of each of the preceding sentences he or she heard. Performance on this task improves from 6 years until at least 15 years of age (Siegel, 1994).

ANATOMICAL AND BIOCHEMICAL EVIDENCE OF PREFRONTAL CORTEX MATURATION FROM AGE 7 UNTIL EARLY ADULTHOOD

Myelination of PFC is protracted and does not reach adult levels until adolescence (Yakovlev & LeCours, 1967; Huttenlocher, 1970; Giedd et al., 1999). For example, using MRI and following the same children longitudinally, Giedd et al. (1999) were able to show that the amount of white matter (i.e., myelinated axons) increased linearly in frontal cortex from 4 to 13 years of age.

Portions of the neuron that are unmyelinated, such as the cell body, have a gray appearance. In their longitudinal study, Giedd et al. (1999) found that gray matter in frontal cortex increased until adolescence, reaching its maximum size at age 12 for males and age 11 for females. However, in cross-sectional volumetric studies, Jernigan et al. (1991) and Sowell et al. (1999a) report *reductions* in gray matter volume between childhood and adolescence, with the most dramatic changes occurring in dorsal frontal and parietal cortex. Sowell et al. (2001) related these gray matter changes to cognitive performance and found that, between 7 and 16 years of age, gray matter in frontal cortex (which included in their analyses not only PFC but also motor cortex, the supplementary motor area, and premotor cortex) decreased in size and the ability to accurately remember which words had and had not been presented earlier (i.e., the ability to remember which words had been seen in the present context and to discriminate them from other familiar words) improved. More impressively, gray matter thinning in frontal cortex was significantly correlated with this source memory, independent of chronological age. Indeed, whereas the relation between frontal cortex gray matter thinning and this ability remained significant even while controlling for age, the relation between age and source memory was no longer significant when controlling for frontal gray matter changes.

Synaptogenesis occurs concurrently with myelination. Huttenlocher (1979) reported that the synaptic density of layer III pyramidal cells in DL-PFC increases until about the age of 1 year, and then decreases, finally reaching adult levels at about 16 years of age. Huttenlocher and Dabholkar (1997) reported that the formation of synaptic contacts in DL-PFC reaches its maximum after 15 months of age, and synapse elimination occurs late in childhood, extending to mid-adolescence for DL-PFC.

Developmental changes in PFC continue on into adulthood. Sowell et al. (1999b) reported a reduction in the density of gray matter in frontal cortex between adolescence (12–16 years) and adulthood (23–30 years). They also reported a reduction in the striatum (primarily in the putamen and globus pallidus) over five times greater in size during this period. Kostovic et al. (1988) reported that AChE reactivity of layer III pyramidal cells in DL-PFC, which begins to develop after the first postnatal year, finally reaches its peak intensity in young adults.

CONCLUSIONS AND UNANSWERED QUESTIONS

Clearly, the ability to exercise inhibitory control over one's thoughts, attention, and action and the ability to interrelate, reorder, and play with information held in mind both show a protracted developmental progression that is matched by the protracted maturation of DL-PFC into early adulthood. Yet, advances in these abilities, as well as maturational changes in DL-PFC, are evident even during the first year of life. While this chapter has generally focused on memory and inhibition rather than on attention, clearly the abilities discussed here are critical for focused, selective, divided, and sustained attention. Indeed, can attention and working memory really be distinguished from one another? The difference is, in part, merely semantic—one can say that information is held in working memory for several seconds or that focused attention on the information was sustained for several seconds; they mean the same thing. The same PFC system that enables us to selectively keep our mind focused on the information we want to hold in mind also helps us to selectively attend to stimuli in our environment (tuning out irrelevant stimuli; e.g., Awh et al., 2000; Awh & Jonides, 2001; Casey et al., 2001). Awh and colleagues (Awh et al., 1998; Awh & Jonides, 2001) have shown, for example, that people are quicker to see, and respond to, stimuli in a location they are holding in working memory; if forced to orient their attention away from a memorized location, their memory accuracy declines. Individual differences in working memory capacity (using the Engle and Kane definition of working memory, see Ability to Hold Information in Mind While Exercising Inhibition, above) correspond to individual differences in selective attention (Conway et al., 1999).

What is the relation between the ability to hold information in mind and inhibition? Is inhibition necessary to keep the relevant information, and only the relevant information, on the stage of one's mind? How can one know what to inhibit unless one is holding the information on what is relevant in mind? Are the abilities to hold information in mind and to exercise inhibitory control, then, fundamentally intertwined? Certainly individuals who perform better on tests of working memory are better at blocking out, or inhibiting, distracting information (Hasher & Zacks, 1988; Gernsbacher, 1993; Conway & Engle, 1994; Rosen & Engle, 1997; Conway et al., 1999). Individuals with better working memory perform better on tasks that tax inhibition, but have minimal memory demands, such as the anti-saccade task (Kane et al., 2001). Vulnerability to proactive interference may determine working memory span scores (May et al., 1999). Conversely, taxing working memory can impair one's ability to resist distractors (de Fockert et al., 2001) and to perform tasks that demand inhibition of prepotent response ten-

dencies, such as the anti-saccade task (Roberts et al., 1994). One view is that working memory and inhibition depend on the same limited capacity system so that increasing the demand on either affects one's ability to do the other (e.g., Kane & Engle, 2002). Another view is that working memory is primary and inhibition is derivative (Goldman-Rakic, 1987; Kimberg & Farah, 1993; Munakata, 2000).

Are inhibition and working memory separable, and if so, under what circumstances? Evidence has been presented in this chapter that these abilities can be dissociated during development (e.g., Davidson et al., 1999). There is also evidence that they can be dissociated neurally (e.g., Bunge et al., 2001). If they are separable, are holding information in mind + manipulating it and holding information in mind + exercising inhibition separable? What are the relations between self-control (or its inverse, compulsions or addictions) and working memory or attention? For example, impairments in the executive functions discussed in this chapter, especially inhibition, are prominent problems in obsessive–compulsive disorder (OCD; see, e.g., Cox, 1997; Hartston & Swerdlow, 1999; Rosenberg, et. al., 1997). What is the role of PFC in compulsive behavior and do all addictions share a common neural substrate? There is a burgeoning literature on this (see, e.g., Lyvers, 2000; Goldstein et al. 2001; Schroeder et al. 2001).

Are the different aspects of inhibitory control dissociable from one another? For example, is the same neural system required to resist internal and external distractions? Is the neural system that subserves inhibition in attention (selective attention [inhibiting attention to distractors], switching the focus of one's attention) the same neural system that subserves inhibition in action (inhibiting a prepotent response tendency, switching stimulus–response mappings)? There is some evidence that inhibition in attention, memory, or cognition may require anterior portions of dorsolateral and ventrolateral PFC, whereas switching stimulus–response mappings may require posterior DL-PFC and the premotor cortex immediately behind it (e.g., Goldman & Rosvold, 1970; Petrides, 1982; Halsband &

Passingham, 1985; Meyer et al., 1998; Wylie et al., 2000; Pollman, 2001). Might developments in inhibition and in working memory appear earlier at the behavioral level and then later at the cognitive level? If so, would behavioral inhibition appear before cognitive inhibition, and might the ability to hold information in mind + exercise inhibitory control appear earlier than the ability to hold information in mind + mentally manipulate it?

Is the neural system required to inhibit an action and not act at all (e.g., on no-go trials) the same as the system required to inhibit one action to do another? The work of Petrides (1986) and de Jong and colleagues (1995) suggests it is not. Is the neural system that underlies the ability to inhibit an unwanted action the same system as that which underlies the ability to check a desired action (e.g., as in not swinging at a poorly pitched ball or as on the stop-signal task [Logan, 1994])? Do all of these forms of inhibition develop concurrently and are they equally susceptible to disruption because of a particular genetic abnormality or environmental insult during development? If they are separable, how are we to divide them into components (see, e.g., Nigg, 2000; Casey, 2001)?

In this chapter I have discussed the ability to simultaneously hold information in mind plus manipulate it in a host of different ways, monitor it, or inhibit prepotent thoughts, stimuli, or action tendencies. This ability requires DL-PFC and develops during the course of the first two decades of life as DL-PFC develops. Is DL-PFC to be understood as some sort of general, all-purpose central executive? If so, how is that possible at the neural level? The most consistent finding across all neuroimaging studies is that activity in DL-PFC is greater when a task—any task—is more difficult (e.g., D'Esposito et al., 1998; Diamond et al., 1998; Duncan & Owen, 2000)—when the task demands greater concentration, for example, when it is new and unfamiliar, and when small changes in the neural or mental signal-to-noise ratio are most likely to result in significant consequences for performance. How are we to understand the seemingly pervasive involvement of DL-PFC in so many different functions and behavioral tasks? Can dif-

ferential developmental profiles in these functions and/or in performance on these tasks provide a clue? Are the developmental profiles of these dissociable?

Is the close relation between developmental improvements in speed of processing and developmental improvements in holding information in mind + manipulating it or + inhibiting intruding perceptions, thoughts, or actions just a coincidence? Is the close relation between the degradation of each of these abilities with advancing old age (e.g., Hasher & Zacks, 1988; Salthouse, 1990, 1993; Salthouse & Meinz, 1995) also a coincidence? Is it simply that faster, more efficient processing is helpful to the development of any cognitive functions, including those dependent on DL-PFC but by no means limited to them? Might the functions dependent on DL-PFC be particularly sensitive to system-wide improvements (and impairments) in the tuning of signal-to-noise ratios, and is speed an index of that? Or, could it be that speed measures are also sensitive to distraction and interference, and so the relation between measures of speed and those of working memory consists in their both requiring the exercise of inhibition? Might it be that a more mature, better functioning DL-PFC is able to reduce signal-to-noise ratios in diverse neural regions, permitting faster and more efficient cognitive functioning?

This chapter has been concerned with the development of working memory and inhibitory functions, and the focus has been on how maturation of DL-PFC may be one of the factors contributing to the development of those cognitive functions. However, the anterior cingulate cortex has also been linked to many of these same cognitive functions (e.g., Posner & Rothbart, 1998; Carter et al., 1999; Bush et al., 2000; Cohen et al., 2000). How are the differences between the functions of DL-PFC and those of the anterior cingulate, or the interdependence between DL-PFC and the anterior cingulate in subserving common functions, to be understood? Similarly, the cerebellum is consistently activated during any cognitive task in which DL-PFC is activated (independent of any motor requirements of the task), and cerebellar and DL-PFC activation is remarkably closely linked, such that when activation of one increases (or decreases) so does activation of the other (for review, see Diamond, 2000). Moreover, the cerebellum shows the same protracted developmental progression as does DL-PFC and it has undergone the same explosion in size during primate evolution (Leiner et al., 1987; 1994–95). How is the interrelation between DL-PFC and the cerebellum in subserving cognitive functions to be understood? Does the cerebellum (traditionally thought of as being important for motor functions) play a role in the working memory and inhibitory functions linked to DL-PFC?

Certainly, PFC does not subserve any of its functions in isolation from other neural regions. We are only beginning to understand the components of the neural systems through which the functions associated with DL-PFC are realized. DL-PFC sends a heavy projection to the caudate nucleus. What roles do the basal ganglia play in the cognitive functions discussed in this chapter? The caudate matures much earlier than DL-PFC. Might maturational changes involving the caudate be responsible for any of the developmental changes during the first years of life that I have attributed to maturational changes in DL-PFC? DL-PFC, posterior parietal cortex, and the superior temporal cortex send reciprocal projections to one another, and send intricately interdigitated projections *throughout* the brain, providing multiple opportunities for these neural regions to communicate with, and influence, one another (Goldman-Rakic & Schwartz, 1982; Schwartz & Goldman-Rakic, 1984; Selemon & Goldman-Rakic, 1985, 1988; Johnson et al., 1989). What roles do those neural regions play in the cognitive functions discussed here? Since DL-PFC, posterior parietal cortex, and superior temporal cortex communicate directly with one another, why has the brain evolved in such a way that these neural regions are also able to communicate with one another at so many different levels throughout the brain and to *simultaneously* influence those diverse neural regions?

What are the developmental changes in the prefrontal neural system that underlie improvements in the cognitive functions it subserves? We still know little about that. What is the developmental timetable in the functional connectivity between PFC and the other neural regions with which it is interconnected? What is the relation between that timetable and the age-related cognitive advances discussed in this chapter? If DL-PFC subserves inhibitory control functions, what is the wiring diagram and neurochemical basis by which it does that? What roles do pruning and increased arborization in PFC play in cognitive advances discussed here? What roles do hormones play in PFC development? What role does exposure to stress play in PFC development? What roles do changes in various neurotransmitter systems in the PFC play in prefrontal maturation and in the development of the cognitive functions dependent on DL-PFC? Little is known about the roles of neurotransmitters other than dopamine and norepinephrine in DL-PFC, although we know that serotonin, acetylcholine, and other neurotransmitters are present there (Goldman-Rakic et al., 1990; Kritzer & Kohama, 1999; Lambe et al., 2000; Passetti et al., 2000). Indeed, the region that is source of the dopamine projection to PFC (the ventral tegmental area) sends a much heavier projection of GABA to PFC than of dopamine (Carr & Sesack, 2000). What roles do changes in these neurotransmitter systems play in developmental changes in the cognitive functions subserved by PFC? The neurotransmitters in PFC interact. What are the mechanisms and consequences of those interactions in adults and during development?

We share with even simple creatures such as worms and sea slugs the ability to be conditioned (to be affected by our experience) and, like them, we come into the world with certain biological predispositions. Even in humans, these are by far the two strongest influences on behavior. However, because having PFC enables us to hold in mind things we cannot see and to inhibit our predispositions and conditioned responses—however fragile and incomplete those abilities may be—we have the possibility to exercise choice and control over what we do. This is important not just for cognitive development but for social and emotional development as well. Now is an exciting time in front lobe research because finally we have the tools to begin to answer many of the still unanswered questions about the development of PFC and the abilities it subserves. Finding the answers to these questions is particularly pressing because PFC is important for so many diverse cognitive functions and for so much of what makes us proud to be human.

REFERENCES

Allport, A., Styles, E.A., & Hsieh, S. (1994). Shifting intentional set: exploring the dynamic control of tasks. In C. Umilta & M. Moscovitch (Eds.), *Attention and Performance XV* (pp. 421–452). Cambridge, MA: MIT Press.

Awh, E. & Jonides, J. (2001). Overlapping mechanisms of attention and spatial working memory. *Trends in Cognitive Science, 5,* 119–126.

Awh, E., Jonides, J., & Reuter-Lorenz, P.A. (1998). Rehearsal in spatial working memory. *Journal of Experimental Psychology: Human Perception and Performance, 24,* 780–790.

Awh, E., Anllo-Vento, L., & Hillyard, S.A. (2000). The role of spatial selective attention in working memory for locations: evidence from event-related potentials. *Journal of Cognitive Neuroscience, 12,* 840–847.

Baddeley, A. (1992). Working memory. *Science, 255,* 556–559.

Badre, D.T., Jonides, J., Hernandez, L., Noll, D.C., Smith, E.E., & Chenevert, T.L. (2000). Behavioral and neuroimaging evidence of dissociable switching mechanisms in executive functioning. *Cognitive Neuroscience Society Annual Meeting Abstracts, 1,* 108.

Baldo, J.V. & Shimamura, A.P. (1998). Letter and category fluency in patients with frontal lobe lesions. *Neuropsychology, 12,* 259–267.

Bauer, R.H. & Fuster, J.M. (1976) Delayed-matching and delayed-response deficit from cooling dorsolateral prefrontal cortex in monkeys. *Journal of Comparative and Physiological Psychology, 90,* 293–302.

Becker, M.G., Isaac, W., & Hynd, G.W. (1987). Neuropsychological development of nonverbal behaviors attributed to "frontal lobe" functioning. *Developmental Neuropsychology, 3,* 275–298.

Beiswenger, H. (1968). Luria's model of the verbal control of behavior. *Merrill-Palmer Quarterly, 14,* 267–284.

Bell, J.A., & Livesey, P.J. (1985). Cue significance and response regulation in 3- to 6- year old children's learning of multiple choice discrimination tasks. *Developmental Psychobiology, 18,* 229–245.

Bell, M.A. & Fox, N.A. (1992). The relations between frontal brain electrical activity and cognitive development during infancy. *Child Development, 63,* 1142–1163.

Bell, M.A. & Fox, N.A. (1997). Individual difference in object permanence performance at 8 months: locomotor experience and brain electrical activity. *Developmental Psychobiology, 31,* 287–297.

Berman, K.F., Ostrem, J.L., Randoulph, C., Gold, J., Goldberg, T.E., Coppola, R., Carson, R.E., Herscov-

itch, P., & Weinberger, D.R. (1995). Physiological activation of a cortical network during performance of the Wisconsin Card Sorting Test: a positron emission tomography study. *Neuropsychologia, 33,* 1027–1046.

Birch, D. (1967). Verbal control of nonverbal behavior. *Journal of Experimental Child Psychology, 4,* 266–275.

Blinkov, S. & Glezer, I. (1968). *The Human Brain in Figures and Tables*. New York: Basic Books.

Bor, D., Owen, A.M., & Duncan, J. (2001). Prefrontal cortex activation increases in association with an easier variant of the spatial span task. *NeuroImage, 13,* S301.

Brass, M., Zysset, S., & von Cramon, D.Y. (2001). *The inhibition of imitative response tendencies: A functional MRI study.* Poster presented at the Annual Meeting of the Cognitive Neuroscience Society, March 2001, New York, NY.

Braver, T., Sikka, S., Satpute, A., & Ollinger, J. (2001). Dissociating prefrontal cortex involvement in sustained vs. transient components of task-switching. *NeuroImage, 13,* S302.

Bronckart, J.P. (1973). The regulating role of speech. *Human Development, 16,* 417–439.

Brooks, P.J., Hanauer, J.B., & Rosman, H. (2001). Examining the effect of stimulus complexity on preschoolers' rule use using a novel dimensional card sort. Paper presented at the Biennial Meeting of the Society for Research in Child Development, Minneapolis, MD, April, 2001.

Brown, A.L. (1975) The development of memory: knowing, knowing about knowing, and knowing how to know. In H.W. Reese (Ed.), *Advances in Child Development and Behavior,* Vol. 10 (pp. 103–152). New York: Academic Press.

Brown, R.M. & Goldman, P.S. (1977). Catecholamines in neocortex of rhesus monkeys: regional distribution and ontogenetic development. *Brain Research, 127,* 576–580.

Brown, R.M., Crane, A.M., & Goldman, P.S. (1979). Regional distribution of monoamines in the cerebral cortex and subcortical structures of the rhesus monkey: concentrations and in vivo synthesis rates. *Brain Research, 168,* 133–150.

Bruner, J.S. (1964). The course of cognitive growth. *American Psychologist, 19,* 1–15.

Bunge, S.A., Ochsner, K.N., Desmond, J.E., Glover, G.H., & Gabrieli, J.D. (2001). Prefrontal regions involved in keeping information in and out of mind. *Brain, 124,* 2074–2086.

Bush, G., Luu, P., & Posner, M.I. (2000). Cognitive and emotional influences in anterior cingulate cortex. *Trends in Cognitive Sciences, 4,* 215–222.

Butters, N., Pandya, D., Sanders, K., & Dye, P. (1969). Behavioral deficits in monkeys after selective lesions within the middle third of sulcus principalis. *Journal of Comparative and Physiological Psychology, 76,* 8–14.

Campione, J.C. & Brown, A.L. (1974). The effects of contextual changes and degree of component mastery on transfer of training. *Advances in Child Development and Behavior, 9,* 69–114.

Carlson, S.M., Moses, L.J., & Hix, H.R. (1998). The role of inhibitory processes in young children's difficulties with deception and false belief. *Child Development, 69,* 672–691.

Carr, D.B. & Sesack, S.R. (2000). GABA-containing neurons in the rat ventral tegmental area project to the prefrontal cortex. *Synapse, 38,* 114–123.

Carter, C.S., Botvinick, M.M., & Cohen, J.D. (1999). The contribution of the anterior cingulate cortex to executive processes in cognition. *Reviews in the Neurosciences, 10,* 49–57.

Case, R. (1972). Validation of a neo-Piagetian capacity construct. *Journal of Experimental Child Psychology, 14,* 287–302.

Case, R. (1985). *Intellectual Development: Birth to Adulthood.* New York: Academic Press.

Case, R. (1992a). *The Mind's Staircase: Exploring the Conceptual Underpinnings of Children's Thought and Knowledge.* Hillsdale, NJ: Lawrence Erlbaum Associates.

Case, R. (1992b). The role of the frontal lobes in the regulation of cognitive development. *Brain and Cognition, 20,* 51–73.

Case, R. (1995) Capacity-based explanations of working memory growth: a brief history and reevaluation. In: F.E. Weinert & W. Schneider (Eds.), *Memory Performance and Competencies: Issues in Growth and Development* (pp. 23–44). Mahwah, NJ: Lawrence Erlbaum Associates.

Case, R., Kurland, D.M., & Goldberg, J. (1982). Operational efficiency and short-term memory span. *Journal of Experimental Child Psychology, 33,* 386–404.

Casey, B.J. (2001). *Development and Disruption of Inhibitory Mechanisms of Attention*, Vol. 28. Hillsdale, NJ: Lawrence Erlbaum Associates.

Casey, B.J., Trainor, R.J., Orendi, J.L., Schubert, A.B., Nystrom, L.E., Cohen, J.D., Noll, D.C., Giedd, J., Castellanos, X., Haxby, J., Forman, S.D., Dahl, R.E., & Rapoport, J.L. (1997). A pediatric functional MRI study of prefrontal activation during performance of a go-no-go task. *Journal of Cognitive Neuroscience, 9,* 835–847.

Casey, B.J., Martinez, A., Thomas, K., Worden, M., & Durston, S. (2001). A developmental fMRI study of attentional conflict. *NeuroImage, 13,* S306.

Chambers., D. & Reisberg, D. (1992). What an image depicts depends on what an image means. *Cognitive Psychology, 24,* 145–74.

Chelune, G.J., & Baer, R.A. (1986). Developmental norms for the Wisconsin Card Sorting Test. *Journal of Clinical and Experimental Neuropsychology, 8,* 219–228.

Chi, M.T.H. (1977). Age differences in memory span. *Journal of Experimental Child Psychology, 23,* 266–281.

Chugani, H.T. & Phelps, M.E. (1986). Maturational changes in cerebral function in infants determined by 18FDG positron emission tomography. *Science, 231,* 840–843.

Chugani, H.T., Phelps, M.E., & Mazziotta, J.C. (1987). Positron emission tomography study of human brain functional development. *Annals of Neurology, 22,* 487–497.

Cohen, J.D., Perlstein, W.M., Braver, T.S., Nystrom, L.E., Noll, D.C., Jonides, J., & Smith, E.E. (1997). Temporal dynamics of brain activation during a working memory task. *Nature, 386,* 604–607.

Cohen, J.D., Botvinick, M., & Carter, C.S. (2000). Anterior cingulate and prefrontal cortex: who's in control? *Nature Neuroscience, 3,* 421–423.

Cohen, S., Bixenman, M., Meiran, N., & Diamond, A. (2001). Task switching in children. Presented at the South Carolina Bicentennial Symposium on Attention, University of South Carolina, Columbia, SC, May, 2001.

Cole, M., & Cole, S.R. (1989). *The Development of Children,* 2nd ed. New York: Scientific American Books.

Conway, A.R.A. & Engle, R.W. (1994). Working memory and retrieval: a resource-dependent inhibition model. *Journal of Experimental Psychology: General, 123,* 354–373.

Conway, A.R.A., Tuholski, S.W., Shisler, R.J., & Engle, R. (1999). The effect of memory load on negative priming: an individual differences investigation. *Memory and Cognition, 27*(6), 1042–1050.

Cox, C.S. (1997). Neuropsychological abnormalities in obsessive-compulsive disorder and their assessments. *International Review of Psychiatry, 9,* 45–60.

Craft, J.L. & Simon, J.R. (1970). Processing symbolic information from a visual display: interference from an irrelevant directional cue. *Journal of Experimental Psychology, 83,* 415–420.

Crammond, J. (1992). Analyzing the basic cognitive developmental processes of children with specific types of learning disability. In: R. Case (ed.), *The Mind's Staircase: Exploring the Conceptual Underpinnings of Human Thought and Knowledge* (pp. 285–303). Hillsdale, NJ: Lawrence Erlbaum Associates.

Crofts, H.S., Herrero, M.T., Del Vecchio, A., Wallis, J.D., Collins, P., Everitt, B.J., Robbins, T.W., & Roberts, A.C. (1999). Excitotoxic lesions of the caudate nucleus in the marmoset: comparison with prefrontal lesions on discrimination learning, object retrieval and spatial delayed response. *Society for Neuroscience Abstracts, 25,* 891.

Daneman, M. & Carpenter, P. (1980). Individual differences in working memory and reading. *Journal of Verbal Learning and Verbal Behavior, 19,* 450–466.

Davidson, M., Cruess, L., Diamond, A., O'Craven, K.M., & Savoy, R.L. (1999). Comparison of executive functions in children and adults using directional Stroop tasks. Presented at the Biennial Meeting of the Society for Research in Child Development, Albuquerque, NM, April, 1999.

de Fockert, J., Rees, G., Frith, C., & Lavie, N. (2001). The role of working memory in visual selective attention. *Science, 291,* 1803–1806.

de Jong, R., Coles, M.G.H., & Logan, G.D. (1995). Strategies and mechanisms in nonselective and selective inhibitory motor control. *Journal of Experiemental Psychology: Human Perception and Performance, 21,* 498–511.

DeLalle, I., Evers, P., Kostovic, I., & Uylings, H.B.M. (1997). Laminar distribution of neuropeptide Y–immunoreactive neurons in human prefrontal cortex during development. *Journal of Comparative Neurology, 379,* 515–522.

Dempster, F.N. (1978). Memory span and short-term memory capacity: a developmental study. *Journal of Experimental Child Psychology, 26,* 419–431.

Dempster, F.N. (1981). Memory span: sources of individual and developmental differences. *Psychological Bulletin, 89,* 63–100.

Dempster, F.N. (1985). Short-term memory development in childhood and adolescence. In: C.J. Brainerd & M. Pressley (Eds.), *Basic Processes in Memory Development: Progress in Cognitive Development Research.* New York: Springer-Verlag.

D'Esposito, M., Detre, J.A., Aslop, D.C., Shin, R.K., Atlas, S., & Grossman, M. (1995). The neural basis of the central executive system of working memory. *Nature, 378,* 279–281.

D'Esposito, M., Ballard, D., Aguirre, G.K., & Zarahn, E. (1998). Human prefrontal cortex is not specific for working memory: a functional MRI study. *NeuroImage, 8,* 274–282.

Diamond, A. (1985). Development of the ability to use recall to guide action, as indicated by infants' performance on A-not-B. *Child Development, 56,* 868–883.

Diamond, A. (1988). Differences between adult and infant cognition: is the crucial variable presence or absence of language? In: L. Weiskrantz (Ed.), *Thought without Language* (pp. 337–370). Oxford: Oxford University Press.

Diamond, A. (1990). Developmental time course in human infants and infant monkeys, and the neural bases, of inhibitory control in reaching. *Annals of the New York Academy of Sciences, 608,* 637–676.

Diamond, A. (1991). Neuropsychological insights into the meaning of object concept development. In: S. Carey & R. Gelman (Eds.), *The Epigenisis of Mind: Essays on Biology and Cognition* (pp. 67–110). Hillsdale, NJ: Lawrence Erlbaum Associates.

Diamond, A. (1995). Evidence of robust recognition memory early in life even when assessed by reaching behavior. *Journal of Experimental Child Psychology, 59* (special issue), 419–456.

Diamond, A. (2000). Close interrelation of motor development and cognitive development and of the cerebellum and prefrontal cortex. *Child Development, 71* (special issue: *New Directions for Child Development in the 21st Century*), 44–56.

Diamond, A. (2001). A model system for studying the role of dopamine in prefrontal cortex during early development in humans. In: C. Nelsen and M. Luciana (Eds.), *Handbook of Developmental Cognitive Neuroscience* (pp. 433–472). Cambridge, MA: MIT Press.

Diamond, A. & Doar, B. (1989). The performance of human infants on a measure of frontal cortex function, the delayed response task. *Developmental Psychobiology, 22* (3), 271–294.

Diamond, A. & Goldman-Rakic, P.S. (1985). Evidence for involvement of prefrontal cortex in cognitive changes during the first year of life: comparison of performance of human infant and rhesus monkeys on a detour task with transparent barrier. *Society for Neuroscience Abstracts, 11,* 832.

Diamond, A. & Goldman-Rakic, P.S. (1986). Comparative development in human infants and infant rhesus monkeys of cognitive functions that depend on prefrontal cortex. *Society for Neuroscience Abstracts, 12,* 742.

Diamond, A. & Goldman-Rakic, P.S. (1989). Comparison of human infants and rhesus monkeys on Piaget's A-not-B task: evidence for dependence on dorsolateral prefrontal cortex. *Experimental Brain Research, 74,* 24–40.

Diamond, A. & Kirkham, N. (2001). Card sorting by children of 3 & 4 years and task switching by older children: Inhibition needed to overcome "attentional inertia." Presented at the Cognitive Development Society Annual Meeting, Virginia Beach, VA, October.

Diamond, A. & Taylor, C. (1996). Development of an aspect of executive control: development of the abilities to remember what I said and to "do as I say, not as I do". *Developmental Psychobiology, 29,* 315–334.

Diamond, A., Prevor, M., Callender, G., & Druin, D.P. (1997). Prefrontal cortex cognitive deficits in children treated early and continuously for PKU. *Monographs of the Society for Research in Child Development, 62(4),* Monograph #252, 1–207.

Diamond, A., O'Craven, K.M., & Savoy, R.L. (1998). Dorsolateral prefrontal cortex contributions to working memory and inhibition as revealed by fMRI. *Society for Neuroscience Abstracts, 24,* 1251.

Diamond, A., Kirkham, N., & Amso, D. (2002). Conditions under which young children CAN hold two rules in mind and inhibit a prepotent response. *Developmental Psychology, 38,*

Diedrichsen, J., Mayr, U., Dhaliwal, H., Keele, S., & Ivry, R.B. (2000). Task-switching deficits in patients with prefrontal lesions or Parkinson's disease. Presented at Cognitive Neuroscience Society Annual Meeting, San Francisco, CA, April, 2000.

Doan, H.M. & Cooper, D.L. (1971). Conditional discrimination in children: two relevant factors. *Child Development, 42,* 209–220.

Dove, A., Pollmann, S., Schubert, T., Wiggins, C.J., & von Cramon, Y.D. (2000). Prefrontal cortex activation in task switching: an event-related fMRI study. *Cognitive Brain Research, 9,* 103–109.

Dowsett, S.M. & Livesey, D.J. (2000). The development of inhibitory control in preschool children: effects of "executive skills" training. *Developmental Psychobiology, 36,* 161–174.

Dreher, J.C., Kohn, P.D., & Berman, K. (2001). The neural basis of backward inhibition during task switching. *NeuroImage, 13,* S311.

Drewe, E.A. (1974). The effect of type and area of brain lesion on Wisconsin Card Sorting Test performance. *Cortex, 10,* 159–170.

Duncan, J. & Owen, A.M. (2000). Common regions of the human frontal lobe recruited by diverse cognitive demands. *Trends in Neurosciences, 23,* 475–483.

Duncan, J., Burgess, P., & Emslie, H. (1995). Fluid intelligence after frontal lobe lesions. *Neuropsychologia, 33,* 261–268.

Fischer, B., Biscaldi, M., & Gezeck, S. (1997). On the development of voluntary and reflexive components in human saccade generation. *Brain Research, 754,* 285–297.

Flavell, J.H. (1963). *The Developmental Psychology of Jean Piaget.* Princeton, NJ: Van Nostrand.

Flavell, J.H. (1986). The development of children's knowledge about the appearance-reality distinction. *American Psychologist, 41,* 418–425.

Flavell, J.H. (1993). The development of children's understanding of false belief and the appearance–reality distinction. *International Journal of Psychology, 28,* 595–604.

Flavell, J.H., Beach, D.R., & Chinsky, J.M. (1966). Spontaneous verbal rehearsal in a memory task as a function of age. *Child Development, 37,* 283–299.

Fox, N.A. & Bell, M.A. (1990). Electrophysiological indices of frontal lobe development: relations to cognitive and affective behavior in human infants over the first year of life. *Annals of the New York Academy of Sciences, 608,* 677–704.

Fry, A.F. & Hale, S. (1996). Processing speed, working memory, and fluid intelligence: evidence for a developmental cascade. *Psychological Science, 7*, 237–241.

Fuster, J.M. (1973). Unit activity in prefrontal cortex during delayed-response performance: neuronal correlates of transient memory. *Journal of Neurophysiology, 36*, 61–78.

Fuster, J.M. & Alexander, G.E. (1970). Delayed response deficit by cryogenic depression of frontal cortex. *Brain Research, 61*, 79–91.

Fuster, J.M. & Alexander, G.E. (1971). Neuron activity related to short-term memory. *Science, 173*, 652–654.

Garber, H.L., & Ross, L.E. (1968). Intradimensional and extradimensional shift performance of children in a differential conditioning task. *Psychonomic Science, 10*, 69–70.

Gathercole, S. (1998). The development of memory. *Journal of Child Psychology and Psychiatry, 39*, 3–27.

Gathercole, S.E. & Hitch, G.J. (1993). Developmental changes in short-term memory: a revised working memory perspective. In: A. Collins, S.E. Gathercole, M.A. Conway, & P.E. Morris (Eds.), *Theories of Memory* (pp. 189–210). Hove, UK: Lawrence Erlbaum Associates.

Gerardi-Caulton, G. (2000). Sensitivity to spatial conflict and the development of self-regulation in children 24–36 months of age. *Developmental Science, 3*, 397–404.

Gernsbacher, M.A. (1993). Less skilled readers have less efficient suppression mechanisms. *Psychological Science, 4*, 294–298.

Gerstadt, C., Hong, Y., & Diamond, A. (1994). The relationship between cognition and action: performance of 3.5–7 year old children on a Stroop-like day-night test. *Cognition, 53*, 129–153.

Giedd, J.N., Blumenthal, J., Jeffries, N.O., Castellanos, F.X., Liu, H., Zijdenbos, A., Paus, T., Evans, A.C., & Rapoport, J.L. (1999). Brain-development during childhood and adolescence: a longitudinal MRI study. *Nature Neuroscience, 2*, 861–863.

Goldman, P.S. & Rosvold, H.E. (1970). Localization of function within the dorsolateral prefrontal cortex of the rhesus monkey. *Experimental Neurology, 29*, 291–304.

Goldman-Rakic, P.S. (1987). Development of cortical circuitry and cognitive function. *Child Development, 58*, 601–622.

Goldman-Rakic, P.S., & Schwartz, M.L. (1982). Interdigitation of contralateral and ipsilateral columnar projections to frontal association cortex in primates. *Science, 216*, 755–757.

Goldman-Rakic, P.S., Lidow, M.S., & Gallagher, D.W. (1990). Overlap of the dopaminergic, adrenergic, and serotoninergic receptors and complementarity of their subtypes in primate prefrontal cortex. *Journal of Neuroscience, 10*, 2125–2138.

Goldstein, R.Z., Volkow, N.D., Wang, G., Fowler, J.S., & Rajaram, S. (2001). Addiction changes orbitofrontal gyrus function: involvement in response inhibition. *NeuroReport: For Rapid Communication of Neuroscience Research, 12*, 2595–2599.

Gollin, E.S. (1964). Reversal learning and conditional discrimination in children. *Journal of Comparative and Physiological Psychology, 58*, 441–445.

Gollin, E.S. (1965). Factors affecting conditional discrim-ination in children. *Journal of Comparative and Physiological Psychology, 60*, 422–427.

Gollin, E.S. (1966). Solution of conditional discrimination problems by young children. *Journal of Comparative and Physiological Psychology, 62*, 454–456.

Gollin, E.S. & Liss, P. (1962). Conditional discrimination in children. *Journal of Comparative and Physiological Psychology, 55*, 850–855.

Gopnick, A. & Rosati, A. (2001). Duck or rabbit? Reversing ambiguous figures and understanding ambiguous representations. *Developmental Science, 4*, 175–183.

Goschke, T. (2000). Intentional reconfiguration and involuntary persistence in task set switching. In: S. Monsell & J. Driver (Eds.), *Control of Cognitive Processes: Attention and Performance XVIII* (pp. 331–355). Cambridge, MA: MIT Press.

Gratch, G. & Landers, W.F. (1971). Stage IV of Piaget's theory of infant's object concepts: a longitudinal study. *Child Development, 42*, 359–372.

Guitton, D., Buchtel, H.A., & Douglas, R.M. (1985). Frontal lobe lesions in man cause difficulties in suppressing reflexive glances and in generating goal-directed saccades. *Experimental Brain Research, 58*, 455–472.

Hale, S. (1990). A global development trend in cognitive processing speed. *Child Development, 61*, 653–663.

Hale, S., Bronik, M.D., & Fry, A.F. (1997). Verbal and spatial working memory in school-age children: developmental differences in susceptibility to interference. *Developmental Psychology, 33*, 364–371.

Halsband, U. & Passingham, R.E. (1985). Premotor cortex and the conditions for movement in monkeys (*Macaca mulatta*). *Behavioural Brain Research, 18*, 269–277.

Harnishfeger, K.K. & Pope, R.S. (1996). Intending to forget: the development of cognitive inhibition in directed forgetting. *Journal of Experimental Child Psychology, 62*, 292–315.

Hartston, H.J. & Swerdlow, N.R. (1999). Visuospatial priming and Stroop performance in patients with obsessive compulsive disorder. *Neuropsychology, 13*, 447–457.

Hasher, L. & Zacks, R.T. (1988). Working memory, comprehension, and aging: a review and a new view. In: G.H. Bower (Ed.), *The Psychology of Learning and Motivation: Advances in Research and Theory*, Vol. 22 (pp. 193–225). San Diego, CA: Academic Press.

Heberle, J.F., Clune, M., & Kelly, K. (1999). Development of young children's understanding of the appearance–reality distinction. Presented at the Biennial Meeting of the Society for Research in Child Development, Albuquerque, NM, April, 1999.

Heidbreder, E.F. (1928). Problem solving in children and adults. *Journal of Genetic Psychology, 35*, 522–545.

Hendry, S.H.C. (1993). Organization of neuropeptide Y neurons in the mammalian central nervous system. In: W.F. Colmers and C. Wahlestedt (Eds.), *The Biology of Neuropeptide Y and Related Peptides* (pp. 65–156). Totowa, NJ: Human Press.

Hendry, S.H., Jones, E.G., & Emson, P.C. (1984). Morphology, distribution, and synaptic relations of somatostatin- and neuropeptide Y–immunoreactive neurons in rat and monkey neocortex. *Journal of Neuroscience, 4*, 2497–2517.

Hess, T.M. & Radtke, R.C. (1981). Processing and memory factors in children's reading comprehension skill. *Child Development, 52,* 479–488.

Hofstadter, M. & Reznick, J.S. (1996). Response modality affects human infant delayed-response performance. *Child Development, 67,* 646–658.

Hommel, B. (1995). Stimulus–response compatibility and the Simon effect: toward an empirical clarification. *Journal of Experimental Psychology: Human Perception and Performance, 21,* 764–775.

Hoshi, Y., Oda, I., Wada, Y., Ito, Y., Yamashita, Y., Oda, M., Ohta, K., Yamada, Y., & Tamura, M. (2000). Visuospatial imagery is a fruitful strategy for the digit span backward task: a study with near-infrared optical tomography. *Cognitive Brain Research, 9,* 339–342.

Huttenlocher, P.R. (1970). Myelination and the development of function in immature pyramidal tract. *Neurology, 29,* 405–415.

Huttenlocher, P.R. (1979). Synaptic density in human frontal cortex—developmental changes and effects of aging. *Brain Research, 163,* 195–205.

Huttenlocher, P.R. (1990). Morphometric study of human cerebral cortex development. *Neuropsychologia, 28,* 517–527.

Huttenlocher, P.R. & Dabholkar, A.S. (1997). Regional differences in synaptogenesis in human cerebral cortex. *Journal of Comparative Neurology, 387,* 167–178.

Jacobsen, C.F. (1935). Functions of the frontal association areas in primates. *Archives of Neurology and Psychiatry, 33,* 558–560.

Jahanshahi, M., Dirnberger, G., Fuller, R., & Frith, C.D. (2000). The role of the dorsolateral prefrontal cortex in random number generation: a study with positron emission tomography. *NeuroImage, 12,* 713–725.

Jeffrey, W.E. (1961). Variables in early discrimination learning: III. Simultaneous vs. successive stimulus presentation. *Child Development, 32,* 305–310.

Jensen, A.R. & Figueroa, R.A. (1975). Forward and backward digit span interaction with race and I.Q.: Predictions from Jensen's theory. *Journal of Educational Psychology, 67,* 882–893.

Jernigan T.L., Trauner D.A., Hesselink J.R., & Tallal P.A. (1991). Maturation of human cerebrum observed in vivo during adolescence. *Brain, 114,* 2037–2049.

Jersild, A.T. (1927). Mental set and shift. *Archives of Psychology, 89.*

Johnson, P.B., Angelucci, A., Ziparo, R.M., Minciacchi, D., Bentivoglio, M., & Caminiti, R. (1989). Segregation and overlap of callosal and association neurons in frontal and parietal cortices of primates: a spectral and coherency analysis. *Journal of Neuroscience, 9,* 2313–2326.

Johnston, R.S., Johnson, C., & Gray, C. (1987). The emergence of the word length effect in young children: the effects of overt and covert rehearsal. *British Journal of Developmental Psychology, 5,* 243–248.

Jones, L.B., Rothbart, M.K., & Posner, M.I. (submitted). Development of inhibitory control in preschool children.

Kail, R. (1988). Developmental functions for speeds of cognitive processes. *Journal of Experimental Child Psychology, 45,* 339–364.

Kail, R. (1991a). Development of processing speed in childhood and adolescence. In: H.W. Reese (Ed.), *Ad-*

vances in Child Development and Behavior, 23, (pp. 151–185). New York: Academic Press.

Kail, R. (1991b). Developmental change in speed of processing during childhood and adolescence. *Psychological Bulletin, 109,* 490–501.

Kail, R. & Park, Y. (1992). Global developmental change in processing time. *Merrill-Palmer Quarterly, 38,* 525–541.

Kail, R. & Salthouse, T.A. (1994). Processing speed as a mental capacity. *Acta Psychologica, 86,* 199–225.

Kane, M.J. & Engle, R.W. (2000). Working-memory capacity, proactive interference, and divided attention: limits on long-term memory retrieval. *Journal of Experimental Psychology: Learning, Memory, & Cognition, 26,* 336–358.

Kane, M.J., Bleckley, M., Conway, A.R., & Engle, R.W. (2001). A controlled-attention view of working-memory capacity. *Journal of Experimental Psychology: General, 130,* 169–183.

Kane, M.J. & Engle, R.W. (2002). Full frontal fluidity: Working memory capacity, attention, intelligence, and the prefrontal cortex. *Psychonomic Bulletin and Review* (in press).

Keele, S. & Rafal, R. (2000). Deficits of task set in patients with left prefrontal cortex lesions. In: S. Monsell & J. Driver (Eds.), *Control of Cognitive Processes, Attention and Performance XVIII* (pp. 627–652). Cambridge, MA: MIT Press.

Kimberg, D.Y., & Farah, M.J. (1993). A unified account of cognitive impairments following frontal lobe damage: the role of working memory in complex, organized behavior. *Journal of Experimental Psychology, 122,* 411–428.

Kirkham, N., Cruess, L., & Diamond, A. (submitted). Helping children apply their knowledge to their behavior on a dimension-switching task. *Cognition.*

Kochanska, G., Murray, K.T., & Harlan, E.T. (2000). Effortful control in early childhood: continuity and change, antecedents, and implications for social development. *Developmental Psychology, 36,* 220–232.

Koechlin, E., Basso, G., Pietrini, P., Panzer, S., & Grafman, J. (1999). The role of the anterior prefrontal cortex in human cognition. *Nature, 399,* 148–151.

Koenderink, M.J.Th., Ulyings, H.B.M., & Mrzljiak, L. (1994). Postnatal maturation of the layer III pyramidal neurons in the human prefrontal cortex: a quantitative Golgi analysis. *Brain Research, 653,* 173–182.

Konishi, S., Nakajima, K., Uchida, I., Kameyama, M., Nakahara, K., Sekihara, K., & Miyashita, Y. (1998). An fMRI study of Wisconsin Card Sorting Test: transient activation in inferior prefrontal cortex time-locked to dimensional shift, and its load-dependent increase. *NeuroImage, 1,* S891.

Konishi, S., Kawazu, M., Uchida, I., Kikyo, H., Asakura, I., & Miyashita, Y. (1999a). Contribution of working memory to transient activation in human inferior prefrontal cortex during performance of the Wisconsin Card Sorting Test. *Cerebral Cortex, 9,* 745–753.

Konishi, S., Nakajima, K., Uchida, I., Kikyo, H., Kameyama, M., & Miyashita, Y. (1999b). Common inhibitory mechanism in human inferior prefrontal cortex revealed by event-related functional MRI. *Brain, 122,* 981–999.

Koslowski, B. & Bruner, J.S. (1972). Learning to use a lever. *Child Development, 43,* 790–799.

Kostovic, I. (1990). Structural and histochemical reorganization of the human prefrontal cortex during perinatal and postnatal life. *Progress in Brain Research, 85,* 223–240.

Kostovic, I., Skavic J., & Strinovic D. (1988). Acetylcholinesterase in the human frontal associative cortex during the period of cognitive development: early laminar shifts and late innervation of pyramidal neurons. *Neuroscience Letters, 90,* 107–112.

Kritzer, M.F. & Kohama, S.G. (1999). Ovarian hormones differentially influence immunoreactivity for dopamine beta-hydroxylase, choline acetyltransferase, and serotonin in the dorsolateral prefrontal cortex of adult rhesus monkeys. *Journal of Comparative Neurology, 409,* 438–451.

Lambe, E.K., Krimer, L.S., & Goldman-Rakic, P.S. (2000). Differential postnatal development of catecholamine and serotonin inputs to identified neurons in prefrontal cortex of rhesus monkey. *Journal of Neuroscience, 20,* 8780–8787.

Landau, S.M., Schumacher, E.H., Hazeltine, E., Ivry, R., & D'Esposito, M. (2001). Frontal contributions to response competition and response selection during task switching. Presented at Cognitive Neuroscience Society Annual Meeting, New York, NY, April, 2001.

Lawler, K.A. & Cowey, A. (1987). On the role of posterior parietal and prefrontal cortex in visuo-spatial perception and attention. *Experimental Brain Research, 65,* 695–698.

Lehman, E., Srokowski, S.A., Hall, L.C., & Renkey, M.E. (submitted). Directed forgetting of related words: evidence for the inefficient inhibition hypothesis.

Leiner, H.C., Leiner, A.L., & Dow, R.S. (1987). Cerebrocerebellar learning loops in apes and humans. *Italian Journal of Neurological Sciences, 8,* 425–436.

Leiner, H.C., Leiner, A.L., & Dow, R.S. (1994–1995). The underestimated cerebellum. *Human Brain Mapping, 2,* 244–254

Lewis, D.A. & Harris, H.W. (1991). Differential laminar distribution of tyrosine hydroxylase-immunoreactive axons in infant and adult monkey prefrontal cortex. *Neuroscience Letters, 125,* 151–154.

Liddle, P.F., Kiehl, K.A., & Smith, A.M. (2001). Event-related fMRI study of response inhibition. *Human Brain Mapping, 12,* 100–109.

Lidow, M.S. & Rakic, P. (1992) Scheduling of monoaminergic neurotransmitter receptor expression in the primate neocortex during postnatal development. *Cerebral Cortex, 2,* 401–416.

Livesey, D.J., & Morgan, G.A. (1991). The development of response inhibition in 4- and 5-year-old children. *Australian Journal of Psychology, 43,* 133–137.

Logan, G.D. (1994). On the ability to inhibit thought and action: a users' guide to the stop signal paradigm. In: D. Dagenbach & T.H. Carr (Eds.), *Inhibitory Processes in Attention, Memory, and Language* (pp. 189–239). New York: Academic Press.

Lu, C.H. & Proctor, R.W. (1995). The influence of irrelevant location information on performance: a review of the Simon and spatial Stroop effects. *Psychonomic Bulletin and Review, 2,* 174–207.

Luna, B., Thulborn, K.R., Munoz, D.P., Merriam, E.P., Garver, K.E., Minshew, N.J., Keshavan, M.S., Genovese, C.R., Eddy, W.F., & Sweeney, J.A. (2001). Maturation of widely distributed brain function subserves cognitive development. *NeuroImage, 13,* 786–793.

Luria, A.R. (1959). The directive function of speech in development and dissolution. *Word, 15,* 341–352.

Luria, A.R. (1961). The development of the regulatory role of speech. In: J. Tizard (Ed.), *The Role of Speech in the Regulation of Normal and Abnormal Behavior* (pp. 50–96). New York: Liveright Publishing.

Luria, A.R. (1966). *The Higher Cortical Functions in Man.* New York: Basic Books.

Luria, A.R. & Homskaya, E.D. (1964). Disturbance in the regulative role of speech with frontal lobe lesions. In: J.M. Warren & K. Akert (Eds.), *The Frontal Granular Cortex and Behavior* (pp. 353–371). New York: McGraw Hill.

Lyvers, M. (2000). "Loss of control" in alcoholism and drug addiction: a neuroscientific interpretation. *Journal of Experimental Clinical Psychopharmacology, 8,* 225–249.

Mackworth, J.F. (1963). The relation between the visual image and post-perceptual immediate memory. *Journal of Verbal Learning and Verbal Behavior, 2,* 75–85.

MacLeod, C.M. (1991). Half a century of research on the Stroop effect: An integrative review. *Psychological Bulletin, 109,* 163–203.

MacLeod, C.M. (1992). The stroop task: the "gold standard" of attentional measures. *Journal of Experimental Psychology: General, 121,* 12–14.

Mangels, J.A. (1997). Strategic processing and memory for temporal order in patients with frontal lobe lesions. *Neuropsychology, 11,* 207–221.

Marenco, S., Coppola, R., Daniel, D.G., Zigun, J.R., & Weinberger, D.R. (1993). Regional cerebral blood flow during the Wisconsin Card Sorting Test in normal subjects studied by xenon-133 dynamic SPECT: comparison of absolute values, percent distribution values, and covariance analysis. *Psychiatry Research, 50,* 177–192.

Marini, Z. & Case, R. (1989). Parallels in the development of preschoolers' knowledge about their physical and social worlds. *Merrill-Palmer Quarterly, 35,* 63–88.

May, C.P., Hasher, L., & Kane, M.J. (1999). The role of interference in memory span. *Memory and Cognition, 27,* 759–767.

Mayr, U. (2001). Age differences in the selection of mental sets: the role of inhibition, stimulus ambiguity, and response-set overlap. *Psychology and Aging, 16,* 96–109.

Meiran, N. (1996). Reconfiguration of processing mode prior to task performance. *Journal of Experimental Psychology: Learning, Memory, and Cognition, 22,* 1423–1442.

Menna, R. (1989). Working Memory and Development: An EEG Investigation. Master's thesis, University of Toronto.

Meyer, D.E., Evans, J.E., Lauber, E.J., & Gmeindl, L. (1998). The role of dorsolateral prefrontal cortex for executive processes in task switching. Paper presented at the Cognitive Neuroscience Society Annual Meeting, San Francisco, CA, April, 1998.

Miles, C., Morgan, M.J., Milne, A.B., & Morris, E.D.M. (1996). Developmental and individual differences in visual memory span. *Current Psychology, 15,* 53–67.

Miller, L.T. & Vernon, P.A. (1997). Developmental

changes in speed of information processing in young children. *Developmental Psychology, 33,* 549–554.

Miller, S.A., Shelton, J., & Flavell, J.H. (1970). A test of Luria's hypotheses concerning the development of verbal self-regulation. *Child Development, 41,* 651–665.

Milner, B. (1964). Some effects of frontal lobectomy in man. In: J.M. Warren & K. Akert (Eds.), *The Frontal Granular Cortex and Behavior* (pp. 313–334). New York: McGraw Hill.

Milner, B. (1971). Interhemispheric differences in the localization of psychological processes in man. *British Medical Bulletin, 27,* 272–277.

Mischel, H.N. & Mischel, W. (1983). The development of children's knowledge of self-control strategies. *Child Development, 54,* 603–619.

Monchi, O., Petrides, M., Petre, V., Worsley, K., & Dagher, A. (2001). Wisconsin Card Sorting revisited: distinct neural circuits participating in different stages of the task identified by event-related functional magnetic resonance imaging. *Journal of Neuroscience, 21,* 7733–7741.

Monsell, S. & Driver, J. (Eds.) (2000). *Control of Cognitive processes: Attention and Performance XVIII.* Cambridge, MA: MIT Press.

Mrzljak, L., Uylings, H.B.M., van Eden, C.G., & Judas, M., (1990). Neuronal development in human prefrontal cortex in prenatal and postnatal states. In: H.B.M. Uylings, C.G. van Eden, J.P.C. de Bruin, M.A. Corner, and M.G.P. Feenstra (Eds.), *The Prefrontal Cortex: Its Structure, Function, and Pathology. Progress in Brain Research,* Vol. 85 (pp. 185–222). Amsterdam: Elsevier.

Munakata, Y. (2000). Challenges to the violation of expectation paradigm: throwing the conceptual baby out with the perceptual processing bathwater? *Infancy,* 471–477.

Munoz, D., Broughton, J., Goldring, J., & Armstrong, I. (1998). Age-related performance of human subjects on saccadic eye movement tasks. *Experimental Brain Research, 217,* 1–10.

Nagahama, Y., Fukuyama, H., Yamauchi, H., Matsuzaki, S., Konishi, J., Shibasaki, H., & Kimura, J. (1996). Cerebral activation during performance of a card sorting test. *Brain, 119,* 1667–1675.

Nigg, J.T. (2000). On inhibition/disinhibition in developmental psychopathology: views from cognitive and personality psychology and a working inhibition taxonomy. *Psychological Bulletin, 126,* 220–246.

Niki, H. (1974). Differential activity of prefrontal units during right and left delayed response trials. *Brain Research, 70,* 346–349.

Norman, D.A., & Shallice, T. (1986). Attention to action. In: R.J. Davidson, G.E. Schwartz, & D. Shapiro (Eds.), *Consciousness and Self-regulation* (pp. 1–18). New York: Plenum Press.

Norton, G.R., Muldrew, D., & Strub, H. (1971). Feature-positive effect in children. *Psychonomic Science, 23,* 317–318.

O'Driscoll, G.A., Alpert, N.M., Matthysse, S.W., Levy, D.L., Rauch, S.L., & Holzman, P.S. (1995). Functional neuroanatomy of antisaccade eye movements investigated with positron emission tomography. *Proceedings of the National Academy of Sciences USA, 92,* 925–929.

Omori, M., Yamada, H., Murata, T., Sadato, N., Tanaka, M., Ishii, Y., Isaki, K., & Yonekira, Y. (1999). Neuronal substrates participating in attentional set-shifting of rules for visual guided motor selection: a functional magnetic resonance imaging investigation. *Neuroscience Research, 33,* 317–323.

Osler, S.F. & Kofsky, E. (1965). Stimulus uncertainty as a variable in the development of conceptual ability. *Journal of Experimental Child Psychology, 2,* 264–279.

Owen, A.M. (1997). The functional organization of working memory processes within human lateral frontal cortex: the contribution of functional neuroimaging. *European Journal of Neuroscience, 9,* 1329–1339.

Owen, A.M., Roberts, A.C., Hodges, J.R., Summers, B.A., Polkey, C.E., & Robbins, T.W. (1993). Contrasting mechanisms of impaired attentional set shifting in patients with frontal lobe damage or Parkinson's disease. *Brain, 116,* 1159–1175.

Owen, A.M., Morris, R.G., Sahakian, B.J., Polkey, C.E., & Robbins, T.W. (1996). Double dissociations of memory and executive functions in a self-ordered working memory task following frontal lobe excision, temporal lobe excisions or amygdalahippocampectomy in man. *Brain, 119,* 1597–1615.

Pascual-Leone, J.A. (1970). A mathematical model for transition in Piaget's developmental stages. *Acta Psychologia, 32,* 301–345.

Passetti, F., Dalley, J.W., O'Connell, M.T., Everitt, B.J., & Robbins, T.W. (2000). Increased acetylcholine release in the rat medial prefrontal cortex during performance of a visual attentional task. *European Journal of Neuroscience, 12,* 3051–3058.

Passingham, R.E. (1988). Premotor cortex and preparation for movement. *Experimental Brain Research, 70,* 590–596.

Passler, P.A., Isaac, W., & Hynd, G.W. (1985). Neuropsychological development of behavior attributed to frontal lobe functioning in children. *Developmental Neuropsychology, 4,* 349–370.

Perner, J., & Lang, B. (2002). What causes 3-year olds' difficulty on the dimensional change card sorting task? *Infant and Child Development* (in press).

Petrides, M. (1982). Motor conditional associative-learning after selective prefrontal lesions in the monkey. *Behavioral Brain Research, 5,* 407–413.

Petrides, M. (1985). Deficits in non-spatial conditional associative learning after periarcuate lesions in the monkey. *Behavioural Brain Research, 16,* 95–101.

Petrides, M. (1986). The effect of periarcuate lesions in the monkey on the performance of symmetrically and asymmetrically reinforced visual and auditory go, no-go tasks. *Journal of Neuroscience, 6,* 2054–2063.

Petrides, M. (1988). Performance on a nonspatial self-ordered task after selective lesions of the primate frontal cortex. *Society for Neuroscience Abstracts, 14,* 2.

Petrides, M. (1995). Impairments on nonspatial self-ordered and externally ordered working memory tasks after lesions of the mid-dorsal part of the lateral frontal cortex in the monkey. *Journal of Neuroscience, 15,* 359–375.

Petrides, M. (2000). Mid-dorsolateral and mid-ventrolateral prefrontal cortex: two levels of executive control for the processing of mnemonic information. In: S. Monsell & J. Driver (Eds.), *Control of Cognitive Processes: Attention and Performance XVIII.* Cambridge, MA: MIT Press.

Petrides, M. & Pandya, D.N. (1999). Dorsolateral prefrontal cortex: comparative cytoarchitectonic analysis in the human and the macaque brain and corticocortical connection patterns. *European Journal of Neuroscience, 11,* 1011–1036.

Petrides, M., Alivisatos, B., Meyer, E., & Evans, A.C. (1993). Functional activation of the human frontal cortex during performance of verbal working memory tasks. *Proceedings of the National Academy of Sciences USA, 90,* 878–882.

Piaget, J. (1954 [1936]). *The Construction of Reality in the Child.* (M. Cook, trans.). New York: Basic Books.

Piaget, J. (1958). Principal factors determining intellectual evolution from childhood to adult life. In: E.L. Hartley & R.E. Hartley (Eds.), *Outside Readings in Psychology,* 2nd ed. (pp. 43–55). New York: Crowell.

Pollman, S. (2001). Switching between dimensions, locations, and responses: the role of the left frontopolar cortex. *NeuroImage, 14,* 118–124.

Posner, M.I. & Rothbart, M.K. (1998). Attention, self-regulation and consciousness. *Philosophical Transactions of the Royal Society of London. Series B: Biological Sciences, 353,* 1915–1927.

Postle, B.R. & D'Esposito, M. (1998). Homologous cognitive mechanisms and neural substrates underlie dissociable components of set-shifting and task-switching phenomena. Society for Neuroscience Abstracts, 24, 506.

Preuss, T.M. (2000). What's human about the human brain? In: M.S. Gazzaniga (Ed.), *The New Cognitive Neurosciences,* 2nd ed. (pp. 1219–1234). Cambridge, MA: MIT Press.

Reason, J. & Mycielska, K. (1982). *Absent-Minded? The Psychology of Mental Lapses and Everyday Errors.* Englewood Cliffs, NJ: Prentice-Hall.

Rezai, K., Andreasen, N.C., Alliger, R., Cohen, G., Swayze, V.N., & O'Leary, D.S. (1993). The neuropsychology of the prefrontal cortex. *Archives of Neurology, 50,* 636–642.

Rice, C., Koinis, D., Sullivan, K., Tager-Flusberg, H., & Winner, E. (1997). When 3-year-olds pass the appearance-reality test. *Developmental Psychology, 33,* 54–61.

Roberts, R.J., Hager, L.D., & Heron, C. (1994). Prefrontal cognitive processes: working memory and inhibition in the antisaccade task. *Journal of Experimental Psychology: General, 123,* 374–393.

Rogers, R.D. & Monsell, S. (1995). Costs of a predictable switch between simple cognitive tasks. *Journal of Experimental Psychology, 124,* 207–231.

Rogers, R.D., Sahakian, B.J., Hodges, J.R., Polkey, C.E., Kennard, C., & Robbins, T.W. (1998). Dissociating executive mechanisms of task control following frontal lobe damage and Parkinson's disease. *Brain, 121,* 815–842.

Rosen, V.M., & Engle, R.W. (1997). The role of working memory capacity in retrieval. *Journal of Experimental Psychology, 126,* 211–227.

Rosenberg, D. & Lewis, D. (1995). Postnatal maturation of the dopaminergic innervation of monkey prefrontal and motor cortices: a tyrosine hydroxylase immunohistochemical analysis. *Journal of Comparative Neurology, 358,* 383–400.

Rosenberg, D.R., Dick, E.L., O'Hearn, K.M., & Sweeney, J.A. (1997). Response-inhibition deficits in obsessive-compulsive disorder: an indicator of dysfunction in frontostriatal circuits. *Journal of Psychiatry and Neuroscience, 22,* 29–38.

Ross, B.M. (1969). Sequential visual memory and the limited magic of the number seven. *Journal of Experimental Psychology, 80,* 339–347.

Russell, J., Mauthner, N., Sharpe, S., & Tidswell, T. (1991). The "windows task" as a measure of strategic deception in preschoolers and autistic subjects. *British Journal of Developmental Psychology, 9,* 101–119.

Salthouse, T.A. (1990). Working memory as a processing resource in cognitive aging. *Developmental Review, 10,* 101–124.

Salthouse, T.A. (1992). Influence of processing speed on adult age differences in working memory. *Acta Psychologica, 79,* 155–170.

Salthouse, T.A. (1993). Speed mediation of adult age differences in cognition. *Developmental Psychology, 29,* 722–738.

Salthouse, T.A. & Meinz, E.J. (1995). Aging, inhibition, working memory, and speed. *Journal of Gerontology Series B, Psychological Sciences and Social Sciences, 50,* 297–306.

Samuels, S.J., Begy, G., & Chen, C.C. (1975–1976). Comparison of word recognition speed and strategies of less skilled and more highly skilled readers. *Reading Research Quarterly, 11,* 72–86.

Sawaguchi, T. & Goldman-Rakic, P.S. (1991). D1 dopamine receptors in prefrontal cortex: involvement in working memory. *Science, 251,* 947–950.

Schneider, J.S. & Roeltgen, D.P. (1993). Delayed matching-to-sample, object retrieval, and discrimination reversal deficits in chronic low dose MPTP-treated monkeys. *Brain Research, 615,* 351–354.

Schroeder, B.E., Binzak, J.M., & Kelley, A.E. (2001). A common profile of prefrontal cortical activation following exposure to nicotine- or chocolate-associated contextual cues. *Neuroscience, 105,* 535–545.

Schwartz, M.L. & Goldman-Rakic, P.S. (1984). Callosal and intrahemispheric connectivity of the prefrontal association cortex in rhesus monkey: relation between intraparietal and principal sulcal cortex. *Journal of Comparative Neurology, 226,* 403–420.

Selemon, L.D. & Goldman-Rakic, P.S. (1985). Longitudinal topography and interdigitation of corticostriatal projections in the rhesus monkey. *Journal of Neuroscience, 5,* 776–794.

Selemon, L.D. & Goldman-Rakic, P.S. (1988). Common cortical and subcortical target areas of the dorsolateral prefrontal and posterior parietal cortices in the rhesus monkey: evidence for a distributed neural network subserving spatially guided behavior. *Journal of Neuroscience, 8,* 4049–4068.

Shaffer, L.H. (1965). Choice reaction with variable S-R mapping. *Journal of Experimental Psychology, 70,* 284–288.

Shallice, T. & Burgess, P.W. (1991). Higher-order cognitive impairments and frontal lobe lesions in man. In: H.S. Levin, H.M. Eisenberg, & A.L. Benton (eds.), *Frontal Lobe Function and Dysfunction* (pp. 125–138). Oxford: Oxford University Press.

Shepard, W.O. (1957). Learning set in preschool children. *Journal of Comparative & Physiological Psychology, 50,* 15–17.

Siegel, L. (1994). Working memory and reading: a lifespan perspective. *International Journal of Behavioural Development, 17*, 109–124.

Simon, J.R. (1969). Reactions toward the source of stimulation. *Journal of Experimental Psychology, 81*, 174–176.

Simon, J.R., Acosta, E., Mewaldt, S.P., & Speidel, C.R. (1976). The effect of an irrelevant directional cue on choice reaction time: duration of the phenomenon and its relation to stages of processing. *Perception and Psychophysics, 19*, 16–22.

Simon, R.J. & Berbaum, K. (1990). Effect of conflicting cues on information processing: the 'Stroop effect' vs. the 'Simon effect'. *Acta Psychologia, 73*, 159–170.

Smith, E.E. & Jonides, J. (1999). Storage and executive processes in the frontal lobes. *Science, 283*, 1657–1661.

Smith, E.E., Jonides, J., Marshuetz, C., & Koeppe, R.A. (1998). Components of verbal working memory: evidence from neuroimaging. *Proceedings of the National Academy of Sciences USA, 95*, 876–882.

Sohn, M.H., Ursu, S., Anderson, J.R., Stenger, V.A., Carter, C.S. (2000). Inaugural article: the role of prefrontal cortex and posterior parietal cortex in task switching. *Proceedings of the National Academy of Sciences USA 97*, 13448–13453.

Sowell, E.R., Thompson, P.M., Holmes, C.J., Batth, R., Jernigan, T.L., & Toga, A.W. (1999a). Localizing age-related changes in brain structure between childhood and adolescence using statistical parametric mapping. *NeuroImage, 9*, 587–597.

Sowell, E.R., Thompson, P.M., Holmes, C.J., Jernigan, T.L., & Toga, A.W. (1999b). In vivo evidence for post-adolescent brain maturation in frontal and striatal regions. *Nature Neuroscience, 2*, 859–861.

Sowell, E.R., Delis, D., Stiles, J., & Jernigan, T.L. (2001). Improved memory functioning and frontal lobe maturation between childhood and adolescence: a structural MRI study. *Journal of the International Neuropsychological Society, 7*, 312–322.

Stroop, J.R. (1935). Studies of interference in serial verbal reactions. *Journal of Experimental Psychology, 18*, 643–662.

Stuss, D.T., Levine, B., Alexander, M.P., Hong, J., Palumbo, C., Hamer, L., Murphy, K.J., & Izukawa, D. (2000). Wisconsin Card Sorting Test performance in patients with focal frontal and posterior brain damage: effects of lesion location and test structure on separable cognitive processes. *Neuropsychologia, 38*, 388–402.

Taylor, J.R., Elsworth, J.D., Roth, R.H., Sladek, J.R., Jr., & Redmond, D.E., Jr. (1990a). Cognitive and motor deficits in the acquisition of an object retrieval detour task in MPTP-treated monkeys. *Brain, 113*, 617–637.

Taylor, J.R., Roth, R.H., Sladek, J.R., Jr., & Redmond, D.E., Jr. (1990b). Cognitive and motor deficits in the performance of the object retrieval detour task in monkeys (*Cercopithecus Aethiops sabaeus*) treated with MPTP: long-term performance and effect of transparency of the barrier. *Behavioral Neuroscience, 104*, 564–576.

Tikhomirov, O.K. (1978). The formation of voluntary movements in children of preschool age. In: M. Cole (Ed.), *The Selected Writings of A.R. Luria* (pp. 229–269). New York: M.E. Sharpe.

Towse, J.N., Redbond, J., Houston-Price, C.M.T., & Cook, S. (2000). Understanding the dimensional change card sort: Perspectives from task success and failure. *Cognitive Development, 15*, 347–365.

Tsujimoto, T., Ogawa, M., Nishikawa, S., Tsukada, H., Kakiuchi, T., & Sasaki, K. (1997). Activation of the prefrontal, occipital and parietal cortices during go/no-go discrimination tasks in the monkey as revealed by positron emission tomography. *Neuroscience Letters, 224*, 111–114.

van der Meere, J. & Stemerdink, N. (1999). The development of state regulation in normal children: an indirect comparison with children with ADHD. *Developmental Neuropsychology, 16*, 213–225.

Vygotsky, L.S. (1978). *Mind in Society: The Development of Higher Psychological Processes*. Cambridge, MA: Harvard University Press.

Wellman, H.M., Cross, D., & Bartsch, K. (1987). Infant search and object permanence: a meta-analysis of the A-not-B error. *Monographs of the Society for Research in Child Development, 51*, 1–67.

Welsh, M.C., Pennington, B.F., & Groisser, D.B. (1991). A normative-developmental study of executive function: a window on prefrontal function in children. *Developmental Neuropsychology, 7*, 131–149.

Wilson, J.T.L., Scott, J.H., & Power, K.G. (1987). Developmental differences in the span of visual memory for pattern. *British Journal of Developmental Psychology, 5*, 249–255.

Wylie, G.R., Frith, C.D., & Allport, D.A. (2000). An fMRI study of task-switching: control in preparation and action. *Cognitive Neuroscience Society Annual Meeting Abstracts, 1*, 115.

Yakovlev, P.I. & LeCours, A.R. (1967). The myelogenetic cycles of regional maturation of the brain. In: A. Minkowski (Ed.), *Regional Development of the Brain in Early Life* (pp. 3–70). Oxford: Blackwell.

Zaitchik, D. (1991). Is only seeing really believing?: sources of the true belief in the false belief task. *Cognitive Development, 6*, 91–103.

Zald, D.H., & Iacono, W.G. (1998). The development of spatial working memory abilities. *Developmental Neuropsychology, 14*, 563–578.

Zelazo, P.D., & Frye, D. (1997). Cognitive complexity and control: a theory of the development of deliberate reasoning and intentional action. In: M. Stamenov (Ed.), *Language Structure, Discourse, and the Access to Consciousness* (pp. 113–153). Philadelphia: John Benjamins.

Zelazo, P.D., Reznick, J.S., & Piñon, D.E. (1995). Response control and the execution of verbal rules. *Developmental Psychology, 31*, 508–517.

Zelazo, P.D., Frye, D., & Rapus, T. (1996). An age-related dissociation between knowing rules and using them. *Cognitive Development, 11*, 37–63.

30

Executive Functions after Frontal Lobe Injury: A Developmental Perspective

VICKI ANDERSON, HARVEY S. LEVIN, AND RANI JACOBS

The frontal lobes are critical for normal development because of their rich connections with other cerebral regions and their central role in efficient executive function. These structures develop rapidly through childhood and early adolescence. This development is paralleled by increases in executive abilities such as planning, reasoning, and flexibility. Current research suggests that damage to frontal regions during childhood may interrupt normal maturational processes, leading to irreversible changes in brain structure and organization and associated impairments in neurobehavioral development. Such impairments may hinder the child's capacity to function in day-to-day life, to acquire new skills, and to make use of teaching and instruction. To fully appreciate the implications of such insults, it is necessary to consider the developmental context of the child. In particular, an understanding of normal maturational processes occurring within the central nervous system (CNS) and the associated development of cognitive abilities provides a backdrop for interpreting the possible impairments of children who have sustained frontal injuries.

This chapter examines these issues and contrasts normal cerebral and cognitive development with that of children who have sustained frontal pathology. The consequences of frontal pathology may be quite global in the young child, having an impact on a wide range of cognitive domains. We have chosen to focus specifically on the domain of executive function, with the assumption that frontal regions are essential to the development and implementation of efficient executive skills. We will discuss two studies from our research teams that illustrate the impact of frontal lobe pathology during childhood and the problems of assessing these skills accurately with current methodologies. The first study describes an ongoing program of research that examines the range of executive deficits exhibited by children who have sustained traumatic brain injury involving the frontal regions. The second study investigates the impact of focal frontal lesions during childhood, with an emphasis on approaches to the measurement of executive function.

EXECUTIVE FUNCTIONS

Historically, the frontal structures of the brain have been closely linked to the implementation of executive abilities. These executive functions may be conceptualized as the *central executive* of the information-processing system, which directs attention, monitors activity, and coordinates and integrates information and activity. Lezak (1995) states that executive functions are "capacities that enable a person to engage successfully in independent, purposeful, self-serving behaviors" (p. 42). Stuss (1992) has proposed an integrated model of executive function, including a set of associated skills that allow the individual to develop goals, hold them in active memory, monitor performance, and control for interference to achieve those goals. Other authors have included processes such as focused and sustained attention, generation and implementation of strategies, and monitoring and utilization of feedback under the umbrella term *executive functions* (Stuss & Benson, 1986; Glosser & Goodglass, 1990; Mateer & Williams, 1991). Shallice (1990) and Walsh (1978) have fine-tuned the concept further, suggesting that executive functions may not be activated during the execution of well-learned, routine behaviors, but are enlisted in novel or unfamiliar circumstances, in which no previously established routines for responding exist.

Such definitions may be operationalized to include three separable but integrated components: *(1) attentional control*, which includes selective attention, sustained attention, and response inhibition; *(2) goal setting*, incorporating initiating, planning, problem solving, and strategic behavior; and *(3) cognitive flexibility*, which entails working memory, attentional shift, self-monitoring, conceptual transfer, and self-regulation (Neisser, 1967; Luria, 1973; Duncan, 1986; Shallice, 1990; Lezak, 1995; Anderson, et al., in press). Thus *executive dysfunction* may be reflected by poor planning and organization, difficulties generating and implementing strategies for problem solving, perseveration, inability to correct errors or use feedback, and rigid or concrete thought processes (Walsh, 1978; Stuss & Benson, 1986). Qualitative features of executive dysfunction may include poor initiation inflexibility, reduced self-control, impulsivity, erratic or careless response behaviors, and deficient high-level communication skills (Lezak, 1995). While these behaviors are commonly considered deviant in adults following frontal injury, a similar interpretation may not be warranted for children. Before determining whether such behaviors are indicative of executive dysfunction in children, developmental expectations need to be considered.

There is a growing body of developmental research that describes sequential progression of executive functions throughout childhood that coincides with growth spurts in frontal lobe development (Welsh & Pennington, 1988; Levin et al., 1991; Thatcher, 1991, 1992; Bell & Fox, 1992; Luciana & Nelson, 1998; Anderson et al., in press). Such findings provide support for the mediation of executive functions via anterior cerebral regions, and the prefrontal cortex specifically. While this may be the case, these cerebral regions are dependent on input from other brain areas, making it difficult to isolate frontal functions from those of other developing cerebral structures. It may be that the gradual emergence of executive function demonstrated throughout childhood reflects the integrity of development throughout the brain. Furthermore, the development of executive functions may be inextricably linked with the gradual progression of other cognitive capacities, as there is ample evidence for associated increments in skills such as language (Gaddes & Crockett, 1975; Halperin et al., 1989), attention (Miller & Weiss, 1962; McKay et al., 1994), speed of processing (Howard & Polich, 1985), and memory capacity (Simon, 1975; Case, 1985; Baddeley, 1986; Hale et al., 1997).

PHYSIOLOGICAL DEVELOPMENT UNDERPINNING EXECUTIVE FUNCTIONS

Knowledge of CNS maturation is steadily advancing because of increased sophistication of technical methodologies. It is now well established that cerebral development continues throughout childhood and into adolescence. Brain weight increases from around 400 grams at birth to 1500 grams at maturity in early adulthood, although most maturation is thought to occur during the first decade of life (Caeser, 1993). Prenatal development is primarily concerned with structural formation, while postnatal development is associated with elaboration of the CNS (Yakovlev, 1962; Orzhekhovskaya, 1981). Processes such as dendritic aborization, myelination, and synaptogenesis have all been reported to progress during early childhood in a primarily hierarchical manner, with anterior regions being the last to reach maturity (Kolb & Fantie, 1989; Jernigan & Tallal, 1990; Fuster, 1993). Initially, progress in child neuropsychology was hindered by a view that the frontal lobes were "functionally silent" in infancy and early childhood, with executive skills not being measurable until the second decade of life (Golden, 1981). A number of neurophysiological studies now refute this view, documenting frontal lobe activity even in infancy. For example, Chugani and colleagues (1987) measured local cerebral metabolic rates of glucose in infants and young children, and found evidence of frontal activation in infants as young as 6 months of age. Similarly, Bell and Fox (1992) have documented changes in scalp-recorded electroencephalograms (EEGs) in frontal regions during the first year of life and related these to improvements in behavioral performances. Many investigators now support the notion that these biological growth markers account for age-related variation in nonbiological development during childhood, such as cognition (Thatcher, 1991; 1992; Caeser, 1993).

The basic neural structures subsuming executive function may be the same regardless of developmental stage. However, important differences exist with respect to their maturity. Results from a variety of methodological approaches (EEG studies, functional and structural imaging, metabolic analyses) have demonstrated major growth periods within the frontal regions, the first being between birth to 2 years, another documented from 7 to 9 years, and a final spurt occurring in late adolescence (16 to 19 years) (Hudspeth & Pribram, 1990; Jernigan & Tallal, 1990; Fuster, 1993; Huttenlocher & Dabholkar, 1997; Klinberg et al., 1999; see Chapter 29). Progressive myelination of frontal structures, prefrontal RNA development, and changes in patterns of metabolic activity and levels of various enzymes during childhood and adolescence have each been described (Yakelov & Lecours, 1967; Thatcher, R.W. (1997). Uemura & Hartmann, 1978; Kennedy et al., 1982; Hudspeth & Pribram, 1990; Jernigan & Tallal, 1990;

Staudt et al., 1993; Giedd et al., 1996; Hale et al., 1997; Huttenlocher & Dabholkar, 1997; Klinberg et al., 1999). With ongoing maturation, children and adolescents may gradually acquire the capacity for more efficient information processing, because transmission of nerve impulses is more rapid with increasing myelination of nerve tracts (Halford & Wilson, 1980; Klinberg et al., 1999; Sowell et al., 2001). The incomplete development of frontal lobes during childhood and adolescence implies a limited ability to apply effective executive skills. This suggestion has been supported by a range of developmental researchers who have plotted increments in executive function throughout childhood (Simon, 1975; Todd, et al., 1996; Bjorklund, 1989; Levin et al., 1991; Welsh et al., 1991; V. Anderson et al., 1995; Luciana & Nelson, 1998).

Together, these findings support the view of hierarchical organization within the frontal lobes, with all areas receiving input from posterior and subcortical cerebral regions. In particular, the prefrontal cortex, thought to be the primary mediator of executive functions, has rich bidirectional connections with all areas of the frontal and posterior neocortex (Barbas, 1992; Fuster, 1993). Thus sensory and perceptual data are processed by the frontal lobes where actions are organized and executed. This pattern of connectivity suggests that, while prefrontal regions may "orchestrate" behavior, they are also dependent on all other cerebral areas for input, with efficient functioning being reliant on the quality of information received from other cerebral regions.

Synaptogenesis appears to be simultaneous in multiple areas and layers of the cortex in infrahuman primates (Rakic et al., 1986), with neurotransmitter receptors throughout the brain being reported to mature at the same time (Lidow & Goldman-Rakic, 1991). Such findings suggest concurrent development, in which posterior and anterior structures develop along approximately the same timetable. However, synaptogenesis and later pruning in human frontal cortex is delayed relative to auditory cortex (Huttenlocher & Dabholkar, 1997). Consequently, it appears that hierarchical development with relative delay in frontal cortical development may be specific to humans.

To summarize, these various lines of inquiry suggest that cerebral development is likely to be primarily hierarchical, both within and across cerebral regions, with frontal areas reaching maturity relatively late, possibly in late puberty. Furthermore, there is substantial support for a step-wise model of development, rather than a gradual progression, with convergent evidence that growth spurts occur in early infancy, and again around 7 to 10 years of age, with a final spurt described during adolescence.

PSYCHOLOGICAL DEVELOPMENT

A number of links may be made between patterns of neuroanatomic change and cognitive development. Numerous studies have reported that executive functions emerge in a stage-like manner, consistent with growth spurts identified within anterior brain regions. Historically, cognitive models have strongly supported such a hierarchical view of development. In particular, Piaget's theory of cognitive development (Piaget, 1963), while providing no reference to possible neural substrates, is compatible with current understandings of cerebral development. Piaget described four sequential cognitive stages: sensorimotor (birth to 2 years), preoperational (2 to 7 years), concrete operational (7 to 9 years), and formal operational (early adolescence). While contemporary developmental psychology disputes many of the principles of Piagetian theory (e.g., Flavell, 1992), it is noteworthy that Piaget's hypothesized timing of transitions between his cognitive stages parallels growth spurts documented within the CNS.

Some researchers have used Piagetian techniques to investigate the relationship of cerebral development to early cognitive development (Diamond & Goldman-Rakic, 1985; 1989; Goldman-Rakic, 1987; Diamond, 1988), finding evidence that frontally mediated, goal-directed, planful behavior is present as early as 12 months of age in human infants. Others have attempted to map developmental trajec-

tories for aspects of executive function in older children (Chelune & Baer, 1986; Passler et al, 1985; Becker, et al, 1987; Welsh et al., 1991), documenting a stage-like progression of executive skills, with mastery still not being achieved in many areas by age 12 years.

More recently, a number of researchers have examined the possibility that the various components of executive function may emerge at different stages during childhood. To do this, most researchers have employed a *battery model*, incorporating into their study protocols a variety of tests purported to measure executive function. Such an approach, while providing developmental trajectories for each of these tasks, also enables investigation of possible relationships among measures, thus addressing the crucial issue of test validity. One informative study was conducted by Levin and colleagues (1991), who evaluated 52 normal children and adolescents across three age groups: 7–8 years, 9–12 years, and 13–15 years. They administered a range of executive ability measures and identified developmental gains across all tasks, reflecting progress in concept formation, mental flexibility, and goal-setting skills throughout childhood. They identified three factors associated with specific aspects of executive function, as well as unique developmental patterns. Factor 1 tapped semantic association/concept formation and factor 3 was primarily concerned with problem solving; proficiency in each of these abilities showed a gradual progression over the three age ranges. Factor 2 was related to impulse control and mental flexibility and these behaviors were noted to reach adult levels by age 12.

With the central aim of establishing normative data for a number of commonly used clinical executive function tests, Anderson and colleagues (P. Anderson, et al., 1995; V. Anderson, et al., 1995, V. Anderson et al, (in press); have also examined age trends in the executive domain. Their sample included 430 children, aged 7 to 17 years, selected as representative of the general population with respect to social factors and gender. The test battery included the following measures: the Complex Figure of Rey (CFR; Rey, 1964),

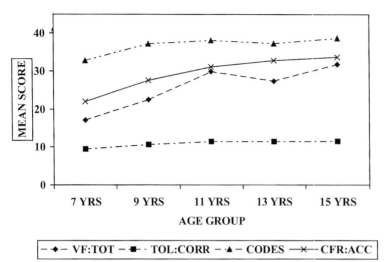

Figure 30–1. Mastery scores for children and adolescents on executive function tasks. CFR: ACC, accuracy score of Complex Figure of Rey; CODES, number correct on Code Test; TOL:CORR, number of items correct on Tower of London; VF:TOT, total words generated on Verbal Fluency Test.

Verbal Fluency Test (VF: Gaddes & Crockett, 1975), Tower of London (Shallice, 1982; P. Anderson, et al., 1995), Contingency Naming Test (CNT: P. Anderson et al., 2001), and Codes (Test of Everyday Attention for Children: Manly et al., 1999). In line with the work of Levin et al. (1991) and Welsh et al. (1991), data indicated significant improvements in executive skills through middle to late childhood (7 to 11 years), with stabilization being evident by mid-adolescence.

Figures 30–1 and 30–2 illustrate that age-related improvements are present for both test mastery scores and strategic measures specific to executive function (e.g., impulsive errors, planning ability). Such developmental progression can also be depicted qualitatively, as shown by the improved reproductions of the CFR displayed in Figure 30–3. These three copies of the CFR were produced by normal, healthy children, aged 6, 8 and 12 years old, with comparable intellectual abilities falling within the high-average range. The relative lack of planning evident in the 6-year-old child's copy is consistent with findings from Chelune and Baer (1986), who argued that younger children perform similarly to adults with frontal lesions on tests tapping executive function, suggesting that these skills are relatively immature at this stage of childhood. In contrast, by 14 years of age, performance is equivalent to adult levels.

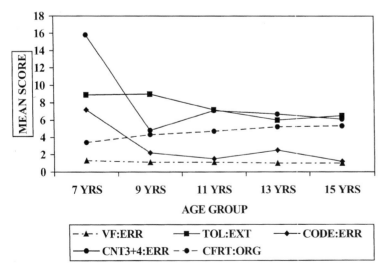

Figure 30–2. Strategy scores for children and adolescents on executive function tasks. CFRT: ORG, organization score of Complex Figure of Rey; CODE: ERR, number of errors on Code Test; CNT3+4:ERR, number of errors on subtests 3 and 4 of Contingency Naming Test; TOL:EXT, number of extra attempts on Tower of London; VF:ERR, number of errors on Verbal Fluency Test.

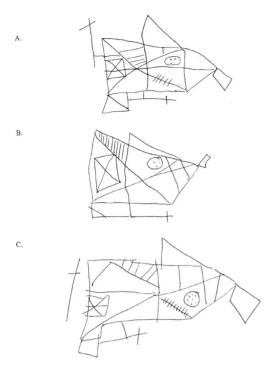

Figure 30–3. Complex Figure of Rey productions from three healthy children. A: Twelve-year-old boy, superior intelligence. B: Eight-year-old boy, high-average intelligence. C: Six-year-old boy, high average intelligence. All productions fall within age expectations, based on normative data for accuracy and organizational level.

The parallels between the patterns of emergence of executive functions described in these studies and the stages reported in neurophysiological research are difficult to ignore. Furthermore, the data suggest that executive functions, rather than being a unitary concept, may be divided into a number of subcomponents possessing different developmental trajectories and possibly maturing at different rates. These varying patterns may reflect mediation by specific areas within the frontal lobes, which also mature at different rates. The likely impact of similar maturational processes occurring in other cerebral areas must also be considered. For example, the quality of neural transmission from posterior and subcortical regions may have an impact on the functioning of the frontal and prefrontal cortices, which have rich connections with all cerebral areas. Maturation of these posterior regions may then enhance the functioning of anterior cerebral areas. From a cognitive viewpoint, similar processes are important. The gradual increase in memory capacity, advances in language skills, and faster speed of processing may all enhance the child's capacity to function on the multidimensional measures of executive functioning employed in the studies described above. While tentative links have been established, further investigation is needed to define relationships between development of executive skills and frontal structures, or to isolate cognitive gains specific to executive functions, divorced from lower-order cognitive capacities. Advancing functional brain imaging technology may provide the necessary tools for such investigations. Regardless, this convergence of evidence emphasizes the importance of close communication among disciplines involved in improving our understanding of brain–behavior relationships in the developing child.

FRONTAL LOBE PATHOLOGY: DISRUPTION TO DEVELOPMENT?

In the neuropsychology literature, the terms *frontal lobe function* and *executive function* have developed in parallel. They are often used interchangeably, most likely because of early observations of executive dysfunction in individuals with frontal lobe damage (Benton, 1968; Luria, 1973; Walsh, 1978; 1985; Welsh & Pennington, 1988; Parker & Crawford, 1992). Despite this common co-occurrence, the practice of localizing executive functions to the frontal lobes has been questioned, with similar patterns of behavioral disturbance being identified in patients whose pathology is not restricted to frontal regions (Albert & Kaplan, 1980; Walsh, 1985; Glosser & Goodglass, 1990). While frontal regions play a central role in the mediation of executive function, the integrity of the entire brain is likely to be necessary for intact performance in this domain. Alternatively, executive function may be interpreted purely as a psychological concept, relating to a set of observable behaviors, without any reference to possible anatomical underpinnings (Stuss, 1992).

The impact of frontal lobe injury and related executive deficits on long-term development is as yet unknown. In one of the earliest studies in the area, Mateer (1990) examined a small group of children who had sustained an early cerebral insult, documenting perseveration, reduced attention, rigidity, lability, and social difficulties in her sample. Her findings suggest intact or mildly depressed intellectual ability, despite presence of frontal pathology, which is consistent with adult patterns of impairment. A handful of case studies of adults sustaining damage in childhood has revealed the expected pattern of poor problem solving, reduced planning, and inappropriate social skills (Ackerly & Benton, 1948; Anderson, 1988; Eslinger et al., 1992, 1997, 1999). In keeping with the model of emerging deficits originally outlined by Dennis (1989), Eslinger and colleagues (1992) reported a pattern of delayed onset of impairments in their patients, with difficulties being identified only as executive skills failed to "come on-line" and mature at critical stages throughout development. Several group studies have recently reported on the effects of specific frontal pathology in children (Levin et al., 1994; 1997b; 2000, 2001; Anderson & Moore, 1995; Garth, et al., 1997; Pentland, et al., 1998; Todd et al., 1996). While each of these authors note the expected deficits in aspects of executive function in their sample, such as planning and reasoning, there is also a suggestion of relative deterioration or lack of normal development in children with frontal pathology. Such ongoing difficulties may reflect the inadequacy of the damaged brain to acquire skills in a normal manner, and have major implications for the needs of these children throughout their lifetime.

This hypothesized lack of normal development, or *emergence of deficits*, may be best illustrated on an individual case basis. The following case description plots the progress of a young child who suffered a severe head injury and later demonstrated a lack of expected development and a gradual fall-off in performance relative to peers her age.

Katy was aged 3 years, 11 months, when she was hit by a truck, sustaining severe head injuries. Prior to her accident, Katy had been a healthy, active toddler. She had no previous medical history and had exhibited normal to advanced developmental milestones. Katy was unconscious at the scene of the accident and was taken to a local hospital by ambulance. On admission to hospital Katy was diagnosed as suffering from a severe head injury. Radiological investigations detected frontal lobe contusions and hemorrhage.

Katy remained unconscious for 4 weeks. She received intensive rehabilitation, but remained functionally impaired. On discharge, 9 weeks post-injury, Katy displayed continued impairments in language, attention, and gross and fine motor skills. Even many years post-injury, Katy's speech was slow and labored, restricting her capacity for normal communication. Difficulties with mobility and coordination persisted, and she was unable to participate in sporting activities.

Katy was first comprehensively assessed almost 7 months post-injury, and then on a number of subsequent occasions until the age of 12. On each occasion, qualitative features of presentation included high levels of distractibility and impulsivity. Figure 30–4 plots her performance at each assessment on standardized measures of IQ, receptive language, memory, and visuomotor coordination. The scores are presented as age equivalents to enable direct comparison across tests. As these results suggest, Katy exhibited age-expected progress in the first 18 months to 2 years post-injury, probably reflecting some recovery of function plus slightly slowed developmental progression. After this time her progress reduced, showing little improvement in the following years. By 8 years post-injury, Katy's best results on neuropsychological test measures were at the level expected for a 7-and-a-half year-old child.

This lack of developmental progress is consistent with her school history. Katy commenced school at age 6 years. She attended a mainstream school, with full-time support and a modified educational curriculum. After several years, Katy's reduced abilities became difficult to manage within the classroom, and

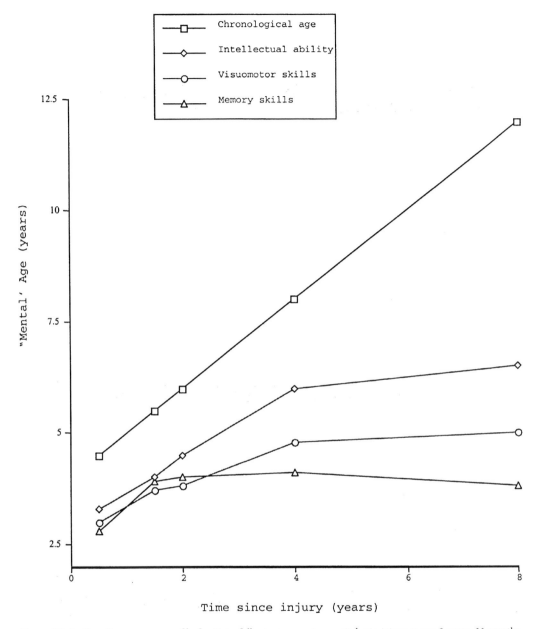

Figure 30–4. Cognitive recovery profile for Katy, following severe traumatic brain injury at age 3 years, 11 months.

she was transferred to a special school for children with intellectual impairment. Even in this environment, Katy experienced ongoing difficulties, both social and academic. In a recent review aimed at looking at her future vocational options, it was evident that Katy is unlikely to live independently or to attain employment. While she is able to manage basic daily living skills, including bathing, washing, dressing, and feeding, she is unable to perform more complex activities without supervision, for example, cooking or shopping. Katy displays limited insight regarding her problems. She progressed through her early school years quite happily. As she moves through adolescence, she has developed some degree of insight, inventing a special friend who had also had a brain injury. Through her friend she has been able to express some of her feelings of sadness and anger about being different from her peers.

Such cases emphasize the impact of disruption to frontal regions during early development. In contrast to the specific deficits often reported in adults, it appears that children may experience more global deficits, with increasing cerebral pathology and associated failure to develop in a normal manner. Furthermore, systematic research is required to fully understand the impact of such insults. To date, the findings in this area are limited. Samples are often heterogeneous with respect to brain pathology and timing of insult. Studies are cross-sectional and unable to demonstrate patterns of development. Measures are multidimensional, leading to difficulties isolating executive impairments from other lower-order impairments in language, visual skills, and motor function. Further studies are needed that incorporate accurate indicators of location and extent of cerebral pathology as well as appropriate and reliable measures of cognitive outcome. In the following discussion of two research programs, we aim to highlight the importance of these factors in the search for a clearer understanding of outcome following frontal injury during childhood.

STRUCTURAL LESIONS IN THE FRONTAL LOBES ASSOCIATED WITH TRAUMATIC BRAIN INJURY

In the following sections we will characterize the relationship of frontal lesions to neurobehavioral sequelae of traumatic brain injury (TBI) in children sustaining closed head injury (CHI) in which the injury mechanism is sudden acceleration or deceleration of the freely moving brain. Detection of structural lesions in the frontal lobes depends on the post-injury interval and imaging protocol, in addition to the severity and biomechanics of injury. Acute frontal lesions (e.g., contusions) seen on computed tomography (CT) within 24 hours after injury might resolve prior to follow-up assessment, whereas late magnetic resonance imaging (MRI) can detect areas of gliosis or hemosiderin that were not detected by early CT. Specific MRI sequences (e.g., FLAIR) are especially sensitive to gliosis and hemosiderin, whereas other sequences (e.g., T1 volume sequence) provide greater anatomic detail. In general, MRI performed at about 3 months after injury is appropriate for detecting chronic lesions and sufficiently delayed for resolution of acute, reversible lesions. Consequently, the following sections are based on late MRI findings obtained in research protocols in which radiologists interpreted the images independently of the neuropsychological findings. Although the studies described below indicate that frontal lesion volume contributes to cognitive impairment, caution is advised in interpreting these findings, because frontal and nonfrontal regions of dysfunction have been documented by magnetic resonance spectroscopy (Ashwal et al., 2000; Garnett et al., 2000) even in the absence of structural lesions. In a recent functional MRI (fMRI) study of adults recovering from mild TBI, McAllister et al. (1999) showed that the pattern of frontal activation in relation to memory load was altered as compared to uninjured controls. Consequently, the absence of structural lesions in the frontal region does not imply normal function, and the extent of frontal dysfunction is not necessarily confined to the boundaries of a structural lesion. Finally, the circuitry associated with the frontal cortex could be disrupted by diffuse axonal injury and thereby contribute to executive dysfunction in the absence of lesions involving the frontal cortex.

FREQUENCY AND SITES OF FOCAL BRAIN LESIONS

In a project on executive functions after nonmissile TBI in children, Levin et al. (1997a) performed MRI in a prospective sample of 169 children who sustained TBI at least 3 months earlier and in a retrospective sample of 82 children who had a TBI 3 years post-injury. Both cohorts included the spectrum of acute severity of TBI as reflected by the

Glasgow Coma Scale (GCS) of Teasdale and Jennett (1974) and were recruited from consecutive hospital admissions to mitigate selection bias. The neuroradiologist coded each area of abnormal signal using templates developed by Damasio (1989). The frontal lobe white matter was the most common site of lesion, including 54 left frontal and 51 right frontal lesions. Of the frontal lobe cortical subregions, the orbital gyri were most frequently involved (22 left and 21 right), with approximately equal frequencies of lesions occurring for the inferior, middle, and superior frontal gyri.

CONTRIBUTION OF FRONTAL LESIONS TO COGNITIVE SEQUELAE OF TRAUMATIC BRAIN INJURY

Analysis of the contribution of frontal lesions to the neurobehavioral outcome of TBI is complicated by frequent cases of multifocal lesions, which are not confined to a single lobe. Limiting analysis to children with focal lesions restricted to the frontal region would constrain the sample size and the findings would not be representative of children with TBI. Focal brain lesions are also associated with TBI severity, a potential confound in the interpretation of lesion effects. To mitigate this problem, Levin et al. (1993) performed multiple hierarchical regression in which the lesion size was entered into the equation after entering the lowest post-resuscitation GCS score for 76 children and adolescents who were studied at least 3 months post-injury. This approach determined the relationship of lesion volume to cognitive performance after taking account of overall TBI severity. Children with lesions in the region of interest for each analysis (e.g., frontal) were included despite extension of their lesion(s) to other (e.g., extrafrontal) regions. The outcome measures emphasized executive functions as described earlier in this chapter. As shown in Figure 30–5, left frontal lesion volume was related to performance on the Wisconsin Card Sorting Test (number of categories) and go/no-go task (trials to criterion), and approached significance for total words produced on Controlled Oral Word Association. Right frontal lesion size was also re-

lated to word association, semantic organization of items on the California Verbal Learning Test as reflected by percent of words from the same category clustered in recall, and a marginal finding on the go/no-go task (P = 0.09). Volume of extrafrontal lesions was not related to performance on any of the executive function measures (Fig. 30–5). A similar analysis of the Tower of London Test in a similar study (Levin et al., 1997b) also showed that left frontal lesion volume was related to the percent of problems solved on trial 1 and on the initial planning time, whereas left extrafrontal lesion volume was related to the number of broken rules. Inclusion of a small number of cognitive measures that were not considered to assess executive functions (e.g., receptive vocabulary, matching faces) has generally supported the specificity of the relationship of frontal lesion volume to executive function performance.

RELATIONSHIP OF FRONTAL LESIONS TO EPISODIC MEMORY AFTER TRAUMATIC BRAIN INJURY

The relationship of frontal lesions to episodic memory in head-injured children has been studied using the California Verbal Learning Test–Children's Version (CVLT-C) of Delis et al. (1994). As noted in the preceding section, Levin et al. (1993) found that frontal lesion size was related to semantic clustering on the CVLT-C. In a recent study (Levin et al., 2000) the performance of groups of children who sustained frontal (n = 13) or extrafrontal (n = 7) lesions was compared after determining that their severity of TBI and demographic features did not differ. The frontal lesion group recalled fewer words from the Monday list after a short or long delay relative to the performance of children who had extrafrontal lesions. In contrast, the frontal and extrafrontal groups did not differ in their estimation of the frequency and recency of presentation of words and nonverbal stimuli. In a related study by this group, Di Stefano et al. (2000) measured hippocampal formation volume in addition to focal lesion volume for children who had undergone MRI at least 3 months after sustaining a TBI. In view of earlier neu-

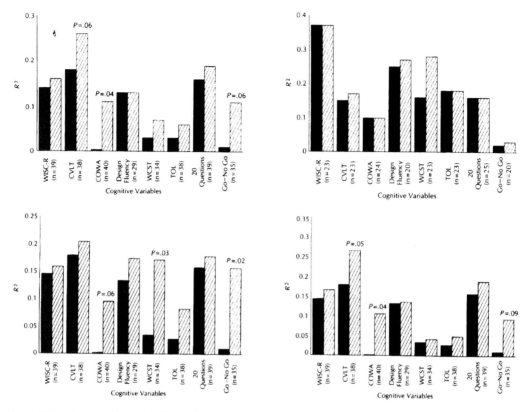

Figure 30–5. Summary of results of hierarchical multiple regression analysis that evaluated the contributions of frontal (*top left*) and extrafrontal (*top right*) lesions to making the variance in cognitive test scores incremental, as explained by the lowest post-resuscitation Glasgow Coma Scale score. The regressions were repeated to evaluate specifically the contributions of left frontal (*bottom left*) and right frontal (*bottom right*) lesions. Closed bars indicate R^2; hatched bars, incremental R^2. COWA, Con-trolled Oral Word Association; CVLT, California Verbal Learning Test; TOL, Tower of London Test; WCST, Wisconsin Card Sorting Test; WISC-R, Wechsler Intelligence Scale for Children–Revised. (*Source* From Levin, H.S., Culhane, K.A., Mendelsohn, D., Lilly, M.A., Bruce, D., Fletcher, J.H.M., Chapman, S.B., Harward, H., & Eisenberg, H.M. [1993]. Cognition in relation to MRI in head injured children and adolescents. *Archives of Neurology*, 50, 897–905, reprinted with permission)

ropathological studies (Kotapka et al., 1993) demonstrating hippocampal damage in fatal pediatric TBI, Di Stefano et al. postulated that morphometric analysis of MRI would reveal reduced hippocampal volume in children who were at least 3 months post-injury. Frontal lesion volume, but not hippocampal volume, was predictive of recall on various measures of immediate and delayed recall on the CVLT-C (Fig. 30–6). Di Stefano et al. also found that hippocampal formation volume was only marginally reduced after severe TBI. The positive findings for frontal lesion volume are in agreement with studies of adults showing that frontal lesions are associated with impaired word

list recall (Jetter et al., 1986; Janowsky et al., 1989).

METACOGNITION

The term *metacognition* has been used in the developmental literature to describe two different processes. The first meaning refers to awareness of one's cognitive abilities (Flavell, 1971), a skill that is thought to emerge in middle childhood. In contrast, *metacognition* also denotes the self-regulatory aspect of cognitive processes (Brown, 1978), which is thought to develop in early childhood. Metacognitive abilities are engaged in tasks such as self-

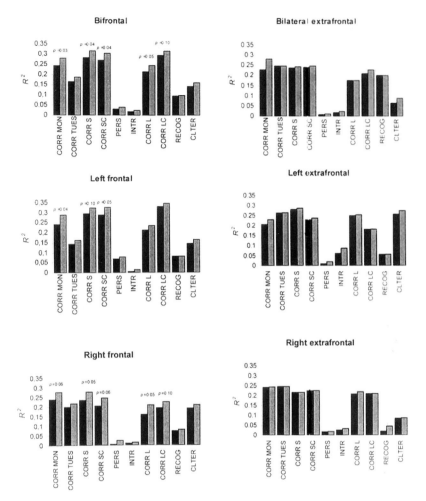

Figure 30–6. Summary of results of hierarchical multiple regression analysis that evaluated the incremental contributions of bilateral frontal (*top left*), bilateral extrafrontal (*top right*), left frontal (*middle left*), left extrafrontal (*middle right*), right frontal (*bottom left*), and right extrafrontal (*bottom right*) lesions to predicting the verbal learning and memory test scores after entering the severity of injury and age at testing alone. Closed bars indicate R^2 when entering Glasgow Coma Score and age at testing into the regression equation; hatched bars indicate incremental R^2 when additionally entering lesion size into the regression equation. CLTER, clusters on Monday list recall; CORR L, correct word on long-delay free recall; CORR LC, correct word on long-delay cued recall; CORR MON, correct words on Monday list; CORR TUES, correct words on Tuesday list; CORR S, correct words on short-delay free recall; CORR SC, correct words on short-delay cued recall; INTR, intrusions on Monday list recall; PERS, perseverations on Monday list recall; RECOG, correct recognitions. (*Source:* From Di Stefano, G., Bachevalier, J., Levin, H.S., Song, J.X., Scheibel, R.S., & Fletcher, J.M. (2000). Volume of focal brain lesions and hippocampal formation in relation to memory function after closed head injury in children. *Journal of Neurology, Neurosurgery, and Psychiatry, 69, 210–216,* reprinted with permission from the BMJ Publishing Group)

checking arithmetic, altering strategy in response to changes in reward contingencies, and determining when the amount of studying is sufficient to pass an examination. Metamemory, as reflected by using rehearsal as a mnemonic strategy, appears in children by 6 to 7 years and is thought to be dependent on frontal lobe functioning (Shimamura et al., 1991). Both self-awareness and self-regulation are considered to be dependent on the maturation and integrity of the prefrontal region. In children who have focal lesions in the prefrontal area following TBI, it is plausible that metacognition is impaired.

Dennis et al. (1996) administered a sentence anomaly task in which the child was asked to determine whether the sentence was correct or not, and then to repair the sentence if it had an anomaly. These investigators found that TBI complicated by a frontal lesion and TBI occurring before age 7 years were associated with more severe metacognitive deficit. To extend this finding, Hanten, and colleagues (1999) studied detection and repair of sentence anomalies, including a working memory manipulation in 12 children who had sustained a severe TBI at least 10 months previously. The child was asked to decide if the sentence presented auditorily was acceptable or not, to identify the problem if it was unacceptable, and to repair the sentence. Placing the anomaly after the verb reduced the working memory load (e.g., "Near the boat swam the boy, the dog, and the bicycle together with the fish") because the patient could detect an unacceptable sentence based on retaining the verb "swam." An interaction between memory load and group reflected the TBI children's disproportionate difficulty in detecting sentence anomalies under a high memory load condition (i.e., when the anomaly preceded the verb; Fig. 30–7). In contrast to the Dennis et al. study, Hanten and co-workers found that children had difficulty identifying the anomaly (i.e., explaining what was not correct), even if they could detect that the sentence did not sound correct.

Moreover, brain-injured children frequently were unable to repair an anomaly despite correctly detecting it. With a small sample size, Hanten et al. were unable to show an effect of prefrontal lesions on comprehension of sentence anomalies. Implications of this study include the possibility that training in metacognitive skills could enhance pediatric rehabilitation and special education for children following TBI.

In a preliminary metacognitive study, Hanten and colleagues (2000) investigated judgment of learning by children aged 7 to 13 years who had sustained a TBI. All but one child was at least 1 year post-injury and 7 of the 9 children had frontal lesions on CT or MRI performed within a year of testing. The metacognitive judgment task was embedded in a multitrial learning and recall procedure. The child was asked first to read each word aloud and to judge the ease or difficulty of learning each of the 15 words on a scale ranging from very easy to learn to very hard to learn. Following four study and recall trials, the child was then given a printed list of the words and asked to judge how sure they were of remembering each word (four-point scale) over a 2-hour interval. A delayed-recall trial was given 2 hours later. As shown in Figure 30–8, the distributions of ratings for TBI children were skewed toward the "easy" end of the continuum for both ease of learning and judgment of learning. Overall recall performance of the two groups did not significantly differ. Ease-of-learning judgments were analyzed for

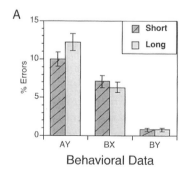

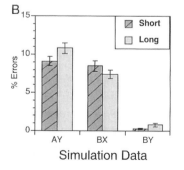

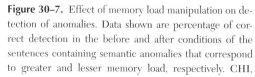

Figure 30–7. Effect of memory load manipulation on detection of anomalies. Data shown are percentage of correct detection in the before and after conditions of the sentences containing semantic anomalies that correspond to greater and lesser memory load, respectively. CHI, closed head injury. (*Source:* From Hanten, G., Levin, H.S., & Song, J. (1999). Working memory and metacognition in sentence comprehension by severely head-injured children: a preliminary study. *Developmental Neuropsychology, 16,* 393–414, reprinted with permission.)

Figure 30–8. Average number of words rated by children with traumatic brain injury (TBI) and control children for ease of learning (A) and judgment of learning (B). Standard deviations are shown as error bars. (*Source:* From Hanten, G., Bartha, M., & Levin, H.S. (2000). Metamemory following pediatric traumatic brain injury: a preliminary study. *Developmental Neuropsychology, 18,* 383–398, reprinted with permission)

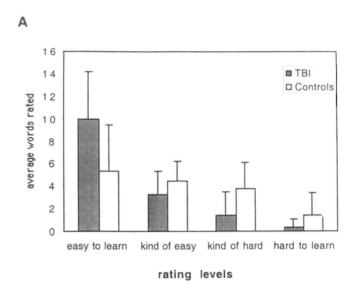

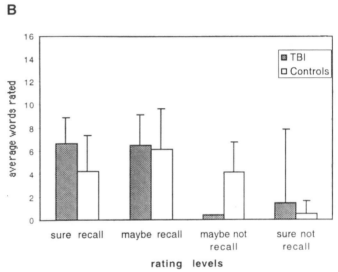

words rated 1 or 2 (easy to learn), with the TBI group exhibiting a lower proportion of correct recall (0.49), compared to that of 0.65 for the typically developing children. Corresponding proportions of correct delayed recall for the words rated as being easy to remember (1 or 2) were 0.55 for the TBI group and 0.73 for the controls. These differences in proportions of correct recall of words judged to be easy to learn (trials 1–4) and recall (2-hour delayed recall) were significant. Hanten et al. considered alternative explanations of this pattern, including immature development of self-knowledge of one's learning capacity. Deficient monitoring of learning could also be invoked to explain the

tendency of brain-injured children to overestimate their retention of words. Pending replication, these preliminary findings raise the question of whether remediation techniques could improve the accuracy of metacognitive judgments about learning.

EXPRESSIVE LANGUAGE AND EXECUTIVE FUNCTIONS

Expressive language impairments, including reduced spontaneous speech and word fluency, deficient writing to dictation, and discourse formulation, are frequent sequelae of severe TBI. Levin et al. (2000) studied word fluency, an ability that has been viewed as sensitive to executive functions, in addition to linguistic competence. Compromised spontaneity, initiative, attention, and productivity under restricted search and retrieval conditions are factors potentially contributing to impaired word fluency after TBI. Working memory to monitor words already mentioned, inhibition of words that do not conform to the rules of the task (e.g., proper nouns), and cognitive flexibility in shifting from one word to the next are also thought to contribute to word fluency performance. Consistent with this conceptualization of word fluency, Levin et al. (2000) postulated that the left frontal region mediates the linguistic component of the task, whereas the executive function aspects are subserved by both left and right prefrontal areas. Levin et al. (2000) posited that severe diffuse TBI at a young age would disrupt development of the prefrontal circuitry involved in age-related improvement of word fluency, whereas the adverse effects of a focal left frontal lesion would increase with age of the child, reflecting cortical specialization for this function. The longitudinal study included 78 children who sustained a severe

TBI (mean age at injury = 9.6 years) and 44 children who had a mild TBI (mean age at injury was 9.8 years). Both groups returned for at least three follow-up examinations over a 3-year period. As seen in Figure 30–9, severely injured children had impaired word fluency relative to that of patients with mild TBI, despite a general trend of age-related improvement in performance. However, a triple interaction of TBI severity, age at injury, and occasion reflected an increasing gap in development of word fluency between severe and mild TBI groups in the youngest age range, whereas older, severely injured patients exhibited recovery relative to similarly aged children who sustained a mild TBI.

To analyze the effect of left frontal lesions, we selected 39 patients with severe TBI in the longitudinal study who completed both the 3- and 36-month fluency tests and categorized them according to presence (23 children) or absence (16 patients) of a left frontal lesion. The two groups did not differ in demographic features or severity of TBI. However, children in both groups frequently had lesions in other sites, such as a contralateral homologous area. Regression analysis, which fitted age at injury, lesion group, and their interaction, showed a

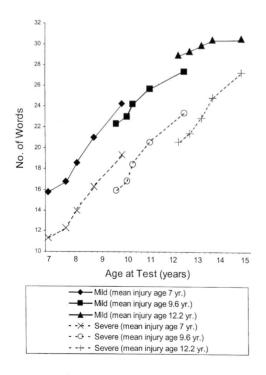

Figure 30–9. Mean total number of words recalled by mild and severe closed head–injured (CHI) children from three age-at-injury groups in longitudinal study. Growth curves show that younger children exhibit less improvement in word fluency after severe CHI than do younger children who sustained mild CHI and older children following severe CHI. (Source: From Levin, H.S., Song, J., Ewing-Cobbs, L., Chapman, S.B., & Mendelsohn, D. (2001). Word fluency in relation to severity of closed head injury, associated frontal brain lesions, and age at injury in children. *Neuropsychologia, 39,* 122–131, reprinted with permission from Elsevier Science)

significant interaction between age at injury and lesion group. Figure 30–10 shows that the difference in the total number of words generated across the three trials increased with age (i.e., the relative impairment associated with left frontal lesions was greater in the older children and adolescents). The main effects of age at injury and occasion were significant. A parallel analysis of the right frontal lesion effect disclosed no effect on word fluency. The left frontal lesion effect in older children and adolescents could reflect the more established functional commitment of this region to expressive language and word fluency in particular than that in young children with a similar lesion. This interpretation is compatible with the finding of synaptic elimination in the middle frontal gyrus, which continues into mid-adolescence (Huttenlocher & Dabholkar, 1997) and beyond the period of pruning in other cortical regions, and with a recent fMRI study (Gaillard et al., 2000), which found an age-related increase in a left frontal localization of activation. It is plausible that young children sustaining a left frontal le-

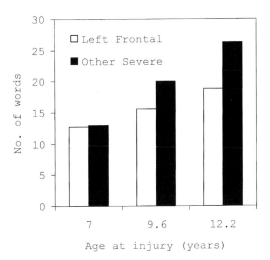

Figure 30-10. Histogram showing left frontal effect on mean total number of words recalled in longitudinal study, reflecting a greater lesion effect on word fluency in older children than in younger children. Reprinted from *Neuropsychologia, 39,* Levin, Song, Ewing-Cobbs, Chapman, & Mendelsohn, Word fluency in relation to severity of closed head injury, associated frontal brain lesions, and age at injury in children, 122–131, 2001, with permission from Elsevier Science.

sion were able to recruit a right frontal homologous area to subserve expressive language. Positron emission tomography (PET) has shown that a peak of cortical glucose metabolism occurs between ages 4 and 9 years, a finding viewed as evidence for a window of cerebral plasticity that enhances interhemispheric transfer of function (Chugani et al., 1987).

Studies of narrative discourse following severe TBI in children have also identified impairments that reflect both linguistic and executive function deficits (Chapman et al., 1992; Brookshire et al., 2000). In these studies, narrative discourse was assessed at least 1 year (Chapman et al., 1992) or more than 3 years (Brookshire et al., 2000) post-injury. When asked to retell stories immediately after they were read by the examiner, severely injured, but not mildly injured children tended to lose the gist or central point of the stories and their productions were disorganized. Other features of the story-retelling by children who had sustained severe TBI included less complex sentences, fewer words, and reduced content. Although the discourse-processing deficits were related to measures of executive function, the findings were not specific to children with prefrontal lesions.

Limitations in this area of research include the characterization of frontal pathology, which can be detected with functional brain imaging in the absence of structural lesions. Analysis of lesion volume is also problematic because many children have lesions overlapping frontal and extrafrontal regions. Consequently, structural MRI provides an incomplete assessment of frontal injury effects in children who have sustained TBI. Future studies could mitigate this limitation by incorporating functional brain imaging, such as fMRI or magnetic resonance spectroscopy.

FOCAL FRONTAL LESIONS IN CHILDREN

Focal lesions to frontal regions (in particular, prefrontal cortex) in adults have demonstrated that these regions can be subdivided according to specific behavioral characteristics and executive functions. It is unclear whether the immature frontal regions in young children, are similarly structured, or even if there is any lateralization of frontal function. To understand the role of the frontal lobes in early development, we investigated the effects of interruption to these cerebral regions. The aims of the study were to examine the neuropsychological abilities of children who had sustained focal frontal brain injuries during childhood and, in particular, to document presence and laterality of executive impairments. To do this, the study employed a number of clinical measures purported to assess specific components of executive function–attentional control, goal setting, and cognitive flexibility, were used, with an emphasis on identifying tasks relevant and interesting to children.

Traditionally, tests of executive ability have been scored on the basis of a summary or "endpoint" score, incorporating a range of cognitive skills and thereby not facilitating the isolation and quantification of specific features of those skills such as planning, problem solving, reasoning, and attention (Anderson, 1998). One of the novel aspects of this study was the implementation of a scoring method that included typical summary scores but also acknowledged that such scores represent the contribution of a range of lower-level cognitive abilities in addition to executive skills. It was predicted that, while summary scores would detect general levels of cognitive impairment, more process-oriented scores would enable discrimination within groups with frontal lobe damage. This approach has been previously described by Garth et al. (1997), who divided task performance as follows: (1) *mastery* is a summary score that provides a general indicator of performance reflecting a range of cognitive skills, such as speed, accuracy, perception, and language; (2) *rate* is the time taken to complete a task; and (3) *strategy* refers to measures of adaptive or "high-level" aspects of performance that are predicted to be specifically impaired in frontal injuries. Typically, these aspects are not analyzed on traditional measures of executive

function. The validity of this measurement approach has been described in a number of child-based studies conducted by our research team (V. Anderson et al., 1995, Anderson et al., 1998 Garth et al., 1997; P. Anderson, et al., 2001; Matthews et al., 2001).

In contrast to the study of structural lesions in the frontal lobe associated with TBI (discussed above) in this research we excluded TBI patients in an attempt to focus on skills specific to the frontal lobes. We examined 27 children with focal brain lesions involving the prefrontal cortex as documented on MRI scan. Children with additional pathology were excluded from the study. Etiology of frontal pathology was diverse and included stroke, penetrating head injury, tumor, and dysplasia. The timing of lesion varied, with some lesions resulting from developmental abnormalities ($n = 7$) and others being related to acquired disorders ($n = 20$). A healthy control group ($n = 20$) was also included in the study to match the demographic characteristics of the frontal group (gender, age, socioeconomic status) as closely as possible. Demographic, intellectual, and neurological characteristics of the sample are presented in Tables 30–1 and 30–2.

The study aimed to evaluate the three components of executive function previously described: (1) attentional control, by means of the Digit Span Task (Wechsler, 1991) and the Sky Search Dual Task (SSDT; Manly et al., 1999); (2) goal setting, by means of the Tower of London Test (TOL; Shallice, 1982; P. Anderson et al., 1995) and the Complex Figure

Table 30–1. Demographics of clinical and control samples

Factor	Frontal Lesions ($n = 27$)	Control Sample ($n = 20$)
Number of males	18	14
Age in years, mean (SD)	11.1 (2.9)	10.1 (2.2)
Socioeconomic status, mean (SD)	4.8 (1.4)	3.7 (0.9)
Full-scale IQ, m (SD)	88.9 (9.1)	106.2 (13.6)

SD, Standard deviation.

Socioeconomic status derived using scale developed by Daniel (1983).

Table 30–2. Characteristics of frontal lesion group

Factor	Left-sided Lesions ($n = 11$)	Right-sided Lesions ($n = 9$)
Age in years, mean (SD)	11.6 (2.5)	10.7 (3.5)
Intellectual ability		
Full-scale IQ, mean (SD)	91.9 (9.0)	89.7 (8.0)
Verbal IQ mean (SD)	89.6 (11.3)	95.6 (12.6)
Performance IQ, mean (SD)	96.4 (11.6)	88.4 (8.5)
Neurological characteristics		
Acquired lesions (n)	7	7
Seizures (n)	7	3
Seizure onset (years) mean (SD)	7.7 (4.2)	6.3 (4.5)

SD, standard deviation. No statistically significant differences between left & right sided lesion groups.

Table 30–3. Mastery scores for neuropsychological function following frontal lesions

Measure	Frontal Group Mean (SD)	Controls Mean (SD)
Digit span (SS)°	8.3 (2.5)	10.1 (3.2)
SSDT (targets correct)	16.7 (3.4)	18.1 (1.5)
SSDT (counts correct)°	4.8 (2.7)	7.5 (3.6)
TOL (no. correct)	10.8 (1.2)	10.8 (1.0)
CFR (copy accuracy)	28.2 (9.1)	23.2 (10.5)
COWAT (total words)°	16.5 (7.5)	24.8 (7.9)
20QT (% constraint)	40.8 (27.2)	41.8 (19.4)

CFR, Complex Figure of Rey; COWAT, Controlled Oral Word Association Test; SSDT, Sky Search Dual Task; TOL, Tower of London Test, 20QT, 20 Questions Test.

°$P < 0.05$, by Analysis of Covariance (ANCOVA) covarying for age.

of Rey (CFR; Rey, 1964; P. Anderson et al., 2001); and (3) cognitive flexibility, by means of the Controlled Oral Word Association Test (COWAT; Gaddes & Crocket, 1975 and the 20 Questions Test (20Q; Denny & Denny, 1973). In addition, the variables derived from these measures were designed to focus on three components of executive function, in line with our previous research (Garth et al., 1997; Anderson, 1998), incorporating indices of rate and strategy as well as mastery scores.

COMPARISONS BETWEEN FRONTAL LESIONS AND CONTROLS

Initial analyses of children with focal frontal lesions ($n = 27$) and control children were conducted, with all analyses including age as a covariate. Intellectual quotient (IQ) was not used as a covariate, as the development of IQ is likely to be intimately linked to deficient executive functions in children. The results of these comparisons are shown in Tables 30–3 and 30–4.

While trends for poorer performance were evident for children with frontal lesions, group differences across mastery, rate, and strategy measures were surprisingly small. For mastery scores, children with frontal lesions exhibited poorer attentional control (Digit Span, SSDT)

Table 30–4. Rate and strategy scores for neuropsychological function following frontal lesions

Measure	Frontal Group Mean (SD)	Controls Mean (SD)
Rate		
SSDT (completion time)	113.3 (36.2)	135.3 (48.1)
TOL (% planning time)	19.5 (5.7)	21.2 (11.9)
TOL (total time)	272.9 (68.4)	279.8 (78.9)
CFR (copy time)	214.7 (84.0)	247.9 (101.4)
20QT (solution time)°	63.3 (20.8)	85.4 (37.1)
Strategy scores		
SSDT (decrement score)	4.8 (9.1)	3.1 (4.4)
TOL (failed attempts)	9.2 (3.6)	7.7 (3.3)
TOL (perseverative errors)†	2.2 (1.6)	1.2 (1.8)
TOL (rule breaks)	0.9 (1.5)	0.7 (1.3)
CFR (organization)	3.9 (1.2)	4.3 (1.0)
COWAT (errors)	2.6 (2.4)	2.1 (2.2)
20QT (% pseudo-constraint)°	9.8 (10.9)	21.7 (17.2)
20QT (% hypothesis)	49.4 (37.3)	37.3 (27.6)

CFR, Complex Figure of Rey; COWAT, Controlled Oral Word Association Test; SSDT, Sky Search Dual Task; TOL, Tower of London Test; 20QT, 20 Questions Test.

°$P < 0.05$; †$P < 0.1$, by Analysis of Covariance (ANCOVA) covarying for age.

and generated fewer words on fluency tasks (COWAT). Mastery-level scores on tasks tapping goal setting and planning abilities (i.e., TOL, CFR) were unimpaired relative to controls.

In the domain of strategy, results were in the predicted direction, although group differences were often not substantial. Children with focal frontal lesions made more perseverative errors on the TOL, and asked more "pseudo-constraint" questions on the 20Q; this finding suggests a lower capacity for strategic behavior and evidence of cognitive inflexibility. There was also a trend toward poorer attentional control, higher error levels, and less planful behavior.

Interestingly, healthy control children tended to take longer to complete all executive function tasks. This finding is not consistent with adult findings, which suggest slowing of processing speed following brain insult (Ponsford & Kinsella, 1992). Similar findings have been documented, however, in other studies of childhood brain disease (V. Anderson et al., in press; Catroppa & Anderson, submitted). In both the current study and these previous studies, faster response speeds were not related to better overall performances. One interpretation for the slow performance of normal children is that the quicker responses of the frontal group are abnormal, possibly reflecting impulsive responses or a lack of attention to detail. This explanation is supported by the higher mean levels of errors and self-corrections recorded in the frontal group, which suggest that in the trade-off between speed and accuracy, children with frontal lesions are more likely to choose speed, which may indicate impulsivity. Thus such quick performances are not necessarily advantageous, because overall efficiency may be compromised, as shown on the Contigency Narning Test (CNT): efficiency measure.

WITHIN GROUP COMPARISONS LEFT AND RIGHT FRONTAL LESIONS

It is often argued within the adult literature that simple comparisons of clinical and control groups may mask subtle deficits demonstrated by subsets of the clinical sample. In an at-

tempt to address this issue, we further divided our clinical sample according to laterality of frontal pathology. We expected that children with left-sided lesions would perform more poorly on tasks requiring primarily verbal skills, including verbal generation and fluency skills (e.g., COWAT, 20Q), while those with right frontal pathology would achieve poorest results for nonverbal tasks, including attentional control (e.g., on the SSDT, TOL, and CFR).

Results pertinent to these comparisons are presented in Tables 30–5 and 30–6. Overall laterality effects appeared to be test specific and as predicted. The left frontal group appeared to perform most similarly to controls overall, and this group performed better than the right lesion group on all measures.

Right frontal lesions were associated with the poorest performances on measures of attentional control, goal setting, and cognitive flexibility, regardless of the primary modality of the task, as has been described in relevant literature on adults (Knight et al., 1981). Children with right frontal lesions appeared to have greater difficulties on the executive aspects of these tasks. These results cannot be explained in terms of severity, timing, or size of lesion. On the basis of this pattern of findings, it may be postulated that, in early childhood, executive functions are primarily subsumed by the right frontal lobe, or damage to

Table 30–5. Mastery scores of laterality effects following frontal lobe lesions

Measure	Left ($n = 11$) Mean (SD)	Right ($n = 9$) Mean (SD)
Digit Span (SS)	8.4 (2.5)	8.1 (2.6)
SSDT (targets correct)	17.2 (2.4)	16.1 (4.5)
SSSDT (counts correct)	5.0 (2.6)	4.4 (3.2)
TOL (no. correct)	11.0 (0.9)	10.7 (1.4)
CFR (copy accuracy)	28.2 (9.1)	23.2 (10.5)
COWAT (total words)	15.5 (7.6)	17.8 (7.6)
20QT (% constraint)°	54.5 (10.5)	28.6 (32.0)

CFR, Complex Figure of Rey; COWAT, Controlled Oral Word Association Test; SSDT; Sky Search Dual Task; SSSDT, Score Dual Task; TOL, Tower of London Test; 20QT, 20 Questions Test.

°$P < 0.05$; by t-tests.

Table 30–6. Rate and strategy scores of laterality effects following frontal lobe lesions

Measure	Left (n = 11) Mean (SD)	Right (n = 9) Mean (SD)
Rate		
SSDT (completion time)	113.4 (50.4)	113.1 (48.2)
TOL (% planning time)	19.7 (6.2)	19.2 (5.5)
TOL (total time)	264.5 (71.2)	282.2 (68.1)
CFR (copy time)	210.9 (87.8)	219.6 (85.6)
20QT (solution time)	67.0 (24.1)	60.5 (18.9)
Strategy scores		
SSDT (decrement score)	3.7 (5.5)	6.2 (12.7)
TOL (failed attempts)†	7.8 (2.9)	10.7 (3.9)
TOL (perseverative errors)	1.9 (1.1)	2.6 (1.9)
TOL (rule breaks)	0.7 (1.4)	1.1 (1.7)
CFR (organization)	4.3 (0.9)	3.4 (1.4)
COWAT (errors)	2.4 (2.4)	2.9 (2.6)
20QT (% pseudo-constr)	12.2 (11.5)	7.9 (10.7)
20QT (% hypothesis)°	31.3 (15.3)	63.5 (35.3)

CFR, Complex Figure of Rey; COWAT, Controlled Oral Word Association Test; SSDT, Sky Search Dual Task; TOL, Tower of London Test; 20QT, 20 Questions Test.

°$P < 0.05$; †$P < 0.1$ by t-tests.

right frontal regions has a global impact on the development of executive skills. As the brain matures, executive skills may become progressively lateralized, leading to the verbal–nonverbal distinction described in adults with such injury. This suggestion is not inconsistent with the theory of nonverbal learning disability (Rourke, 1987), a developmental syndrome, which describes the right hemisphere as being particularly vulnerable to early insult. When such insult occurs, development is disrupted, with symptoms including motor impairments, nonverbal processing deficits, as well as problems with higher-order functions, such as planning, reasoning, cognitive flexibility, and attention.

In summary, mastery, rate, and strategy measures may all provide valuable information on executive function in children. Results from the present study suggest less clear laterality-specific function within the brain than has been described in adults, perhaps with the exception of verbal production, a skill argued to be clearly lateralized from infancy (Johnson, 1997). Rather, it appears that the right

frontal lobe may have a critical role in the early development of executive skills, a finding consistent with the work of Rourke (1987). It remains unclear whether these skills may be gradually lateralized in children with frontal damage or remain within the damaged lobe.

Alternatively, it may be that executive functions develop primarily in right frontal regions, then gradually transfer and become lateralized with age. Thus, when right frontal damage occurs in childhood, the efficient maturation and transfer of these skills is disrupted. However, when early left frontal damage occurs, development can continue unaffected in the right hemisphere. Transfer of function may then not occur at all, with all functions being maintained within the healthy right hemisphere, or transfer may occur after some recovery to the damaged left frontal regions. A final possibility that the tests we have chosen in this study, while supposedly tapping a variety of executive components, may have failed to tap those subsumed by left frontal regions.

CONCLUSIONS

Damage to frontal brain regions has wide-ranging implications for ongoing development in children. Deficits in many aspects of neurobehavioral function have been observed, including attention, impulse control, language, and memory. In contrast to the often focal consequences observed in adults, children who sustain frontal lobe pathology are likely to present with more globally depressed cognitive profiles, with the likelihood of developing emerging deficits over time. The possible explanations for these generalized impairments may relate to the impact of such injuries on the child's capacity to acquire new skills. Alternatively, there may be a biological basis reflecting the timing of injury and the capacity for functional reorganization and recruitment within the developing brain.

Current research limitations restrict our ability to come to any firm conclusions about prefrontal functions in children. In particular, research has been flawed because of problems in the accurate detection and characterization of frontal pathology, the confounding effects of extrafrontal injury, and the lack of consensus regarding the essential features of executive functions, their most appropriate indicators in children, and their developmental trajectories. Many widely used measures of executive function are complex and underpinned by a range of skills, thus complicating efforts to specify or manipulate hypothesized processes such as inhibition or working memory. Hypothesis-driven studies in which tasks designed to measure specific cognitive processes are used could contribute to advancements in assessment and cognitive intervention. Moreover, neuroscientific research concerning the pharmacologic modulation of executive functioning and effects on prefrontal cortex (see Chapter 4) provide an opportunity to develop treatment strategies for children with post-traumatic frontal dysfunction.

ACKNOWLEDGMENTS

Research presented in this chapter was supported by grants NS21889, H133B990014 and from the Australian National Health & Medical Research Council. The authors are indebted to Angela D. Williams for editorial assistance.

REFERENCES

Ackerly, S.S. & Benton, A.L. (1948). Report of a case of bilateral frontal lobe defect. *Association for Research on Nervous and Mental Disorders, 27,* 479–504.

Albert, M.S. & Kaplan, E.F. (1980). Organic implications of neuropsychological deficits in the elderly. In: L.W. Poon, J. Fozard, L. Cermak, D. Arenberg, & L.W. Thompson (Eds.), *New Directions in Memory and Aging: Proceedings of the George A. Talland Memorial Conference* (pp. 403–432). Hillsdale, NJ: Lawrence Erlbaum Associates.

Anderson, P., Anderson, V., & Lajoie, G. (1995). The Tower of London Test: validation and standardization for pediatric populations. *Clincal Neuropsychologist, 10,* 54–65.

Anderson, P., Anderson, V., & Garth, J. (2001 [a]). A process-oriented approach to scoring the Complex Figure of Rey. *Clinical Neuropsychologist, 15,* 81–94.

Anderson, P., Anderson, V., & Northam, E., & Taylor, H.G. (2001 [b]). Standardization of the Contingency Naming Test (CNT) for school-aged children: a measure of reactive flexibility. *Clinical Neuropsychological Assessment,* (1), 247–273.

Anderson, V. (1998). Assessing executive functions in children: biological, psychological, and developmental considerations. *Neuropsychological Rehabilitation, 8,* 319–349.

Anderson, V. (1988). Recovery of function in children: the myth of cerebral plasticity. In: M. Matheson & H. Newman (Eds.), *Brain Impairment: Proceedings from the Thirteenth Annual Brain Impairment Conference, ASSBI, Sydney.* (pp. 223–247).

Anderson, V. & Moore, C. (1995). Age at injury as a predictor of outcome following pediatric head injury. *Child Neuropsychology, 1,* 187–202.

Anderson, V., Lajoie, G., & Bell, R. (1995). Neuropsychological assessment of the school-aged child. Department of Psychology, University of Melbourne, Australia.

Anderson, V., Fenwick, T., Robertson, I., & Manly, T. (1998). Attentional skills following traumatic brain injury in children: a componential analysis. *Brain Injury, 12,* 937–949.

Anderson, V., Anderson, P., Northam, E., Jacobs, R., Catroppa, C. (in press). Development of executive function through late childhood and adolescence in an Australian sample. *Developmental Neuropsychology.*

Ashwal, S., Holshouser, B.A., Shu, S.K., Simmons, P.L., Perking, R.M., Tomasi, L.G., Knierim, D.S., Sheridan, C., Craig, K., Andrews, G.H., & Hinshaw, D.B., Jr. (2000). Predictive value of proton magnetic resonance spectroscopy in pediatric closed head injury. *Pediatric Neurology, 23,* 114–125.

Baddeley, A. (1986). *Working Memory.* Oxford: Oxford University Press.

Barbas, H. (1992). Architecture and cortical connections of the prefrontal cortex in the rhesus monkey. In: P. Chauvel & A. Delgado-Esceuta (Eds.), *Advances in Neurology* (pp. 91–115). New York: Raven Press.

Becker, M.G., Isaac, W., & Hynd, G. (1987). Neuropsychological development of non-verbal behaviors attributed to the frontal lobes. *Developmental Neuropsychology, 3,* 275–298.

Bell, M.A. & Fox, N.A. (1992). The relations between frontal brain electrical activity and cognitive development during infancy. *Child Development, 63,* 1142–1163.

Benton, A.L. (1968). Differential behavioral effects of frontal lobe disease. *Neuropsychologia, 6,* 53–60.

Bjorklund, D.F. (1989). *Children's Thinking: Developmental Function and Individual Differences.* Pacific Grove, CA.: Brooks/Cole.

Brookshire, B.L., Chapman, S.B., Song, J., & Levin, H.S. (2000). Cognitive and linguistic correlates of children's discourse after closed head injury: a three-year follow-up. *Journal of the International Neuropsychology Society, 6,* 741–751.

Brown, A.L. (1978). Knowing when, where, and how to remember: a problem of metacognition. In R. Glaser (ed.), *Advances in Instructional Psychology,* Vol. 1, (pp. 77–165). Hillsdale, NJ: Lawrence Erlbaum Associates.

Caeser, P. (1993). Old and new facts about perinatal brain development. *Journal of Child Psychology and Psychiatry, 34,* 101–109.

Case, R. (1985). *Intellectual development: Birth to Adulthood*. Orlando, FL: Academic Press.

Catroppa, C. & Anderson, V. (submitted). Children's sustained attention skills two years post-TBI: An experimental analysis.

Chapman, S.B., Culhane, K.A., Levin, H.S., Harward, H., Mendelsohn, D., Ewing-Cobbs, L., Fletcher, J.M., & Bruce, D. (1992). Narrative discourse after closed head injury in children and adolescents. *Brain and Language, 43*, 42–65.

Chelune, G.J. & Baer, R.A. (1986). Developmental norms for the Wisconsin Card Sorting Test. *Journal of Clinical and Experimental Neuropsychology, 8*, 219–228.

Chugani, H.T., Phelps, M.E., & Mazziotta, J.C. (1987). Positron emission tomography study of human brain functional development. *Annals of Neurology, 22*, 287–297.

Damasio, H. (1989). Neuroanatomy of frontal lobe in vivo: a comment on methodology. In: H.S. Levin, H.M. Eisenberg, & A.L. Benton (Eds.), *Frontal Lobe Function and Dysfunction* (pp. 92–124). New York: Oxford University Press.

Daniel, A. (1983). *Power, Privilege and Prestige: Occupations in Australia*. Melbourne: Longman-Cheshire.

Delis, D.C., Kramer, J.H., Kaplan, E., Ober, B.H. (1986). *The California Verbal Learning Test: Research Edition*. New York: Psychological Corporation.

Dennis, M. (1989). Language and the young damaged brain. In: T. Boll & B.K. Bryant (Eds.), *Clinical Neuropsychology and Brain Function: Research, Measurement and Practice* (pp. 89–123). Washington: American Psychological Association.

Dennis, M., Barnes, M.A., Donnelly, R.E., Wilknson, M., & Humphreys, R. (1996). Appraising and managing knowledge: metacognitive skills after childhood head injury. *Developmental Neuropsychology, 12*, 77–103.

Denny, D.R. & Denny, N.W. (1973). The use of classification for problem solving: a comparison of middle and old age. *Developmental Psychology, 9*, 275–278.

Diamond, A. (1988). Differences between adult and infant cognition: is the crucial variable presence or absence of language? In: L. Weiskrantz (Ed.), *Thought Without Language* (pp. 337–370). New York: Oxford University Press.

Diamond, A. & Goldman-Rakic, P.S. (1985). Evidence for involvement of prefrontal cortex in cognitive changes during the first year of life: comparison of human infants and rhesus monkeys on a detour task with transparent barrier. *Neurosciences Abstracts (Pt. II), 11*, 832.

Diamond, A. & Goldman-Rakic, P.S. (1989). Comparison of human infants and rhesus monkeys on Piaget's AB task: evidence for dependence on dorsolateral prefrontal cortex. *Experimental Brain Research, 74*, 24–40.

Di Stefano, G., Bachevalier, J., Levin, H.S., Song, J.X., Scheibel, R.S., & Fletcher, J.M. (2000). Volume of focal brain lesions and hippocampal formation in relation to memory function after closed head injury in children. *Journal of Neurology, Neurosurgery, and Psychiatry, 69*, 210–216.

Duncan, J. (1986). Disorganization of behavior after frontal lobe damage. *Cognitive Neuropsychology, 3*, 271–290.

Eslinger, P., Grattan, L., Damasio, H., & Damasio, A. (1992). Development consequences of childhood frontal lobe damage. *Archives of Neurology, 49*, 764–769.

Eslinger, P., Biddle, K., & Grattan, L. (1997). Cognitive and social development in children with prefrontal cortex lesions. In: N. Krasnegor, G. Lyon, & P.S. Goldman-Rakic (Eds.), *Development of the Prefrontal Cortex: Evolution, Neurology, and Behaviour* (pp. 295–336). Baltimore: Brookes.

Eslinger, P., Biddle, K., Pennington, B., & Page, R. (1999). Cognitive and behavioral development up to 4 years after early right frontal lobe lesion. *Developmental Neuropsychology, 15*, 157–191.

Flavell, J.H. (1971). First discussant's comments: what is memory development the development of? *Human Development, 14*, 272–278.

Flavell, J.H. (1992). Cognitive development: past, present, and future. *Developmental Psychology, 28*, 998–1005.

Fuster, J. (1993). Frontal lobes. *Current Opinion in Neurobiology, 3*, 160–165.

Gaddes, W.H. & Crockett, D.J. (1975). The Spreen Benton Aphasia Tests: normative data as a measure of normal language development. *Brain and Language, 2*, 257–279.

Gaillard, W.E., Hertz-Pannier, L., Mott, S.H., Barnett, A.S., LeBihan, D., & Theodore, W.H. (2000). Functional anatomy of cognitive development: fMRI of verbal fluency in children and adults. *Neurology, 54*, 180–185.

Garnett, M.R., Blamire, A.M., Rajagopalan, B., Styles, P., & Cadoux-Hudson, T.A.D. (2000). Evidence for cellular damage in normal-appearing white matter correlates with injury severity in patients following traumatic brain injury. A magnetic resonance spectroscopy study. *Brain, 123*, 1403–1409.

Garth, J., Anderson, V., & Wrennall, J. (1997). Executive functions following moderate-to-severe frontal lobe injuries: impact of injury and age at injury. *Pediatric Rehabilitation, 1*, 99–108.

Giedd, J., Snell, J., Lange, N., Rajapaske, J., Casey, B., Kozuch, P., Vaitus, A., Vauss, Y., Hamburger, S., Kaysen, D., & Rapoport, J. (1996). Quantitative magnetic resonance imaging of human brain development: ages 4–18. *Cerebral Cortex, 6*, 551–560.

Glosser, G. & Goodglass, H. (1990). Disorders in executive control functions among aphasic and other brain damaged patients. *Journal of Clinical and Experimental Neuropsychology, 12*, 485–501.

Golden, C.J. (1981). The Luria-Nebraska Children's Battery: theory and formulation. In: G.W. Hynd & J.E. Obrzut (Eds.), *Neuropsychological Assessment of the School-Aged Child* (pp. 277–302). New York: Grune & Stratton.

Goldman-Rakic, P.S. (1987). Development of cortical circuitry and cognitive function. *Child Development, 58*, 601–622.

Hale, S., Bronik, M., & Fry, A. (1997) Verbal and spatial working memory in school-aged children: developmental differences in susceptibility to interference. *Developmental Psychology, 33*, 364–371.

Halford, G.S. & Wilson, W.H. (1980). A category theory approach to cognitive development. *Cognitive Psychology, 12,* 356–411.

Halperin, J.M., Healey, J.M., Zeitchik, E., Ludman, W.L., & Weinstein, L. (1989). Developmental aspects of linguistic and mnestic abilities in normal children. *Journal of Clinical and Experimental Neuropsychology, 11,* 518–528.

Hanten, G., Levin, H.S., & Song, J. (1999). Working memory and metacognition in sentence comprehension by severely head-injured children: a preliminary study. *Developmental Neuropsychology, 16,* 393–414.

Hanten, G., Bartha, M., & Levin, H.S. (2000) Meta-memory following pediatric traumatic brain injury: a preliminary study. *Developmental Neuropsychology, 18,* 383–398.

Howard, L. & Polich, J. (1985). P300 latency and memory span development. *Developmental Psychology, 21,* 283–289.

Hudspeth, W. & Pribram, K. (1990). Stages of brain and cognitive maturation. *Journal of Educational Psychology, 82,* 881–884.

Huttenlocher, P. & Dabholkar, A. (1997). Developmental anatomy of prefronatl cortex. In: N. Krasnegor, G. Reid Lyon, & P. Goldman-Rakic (Eds.), *Development of the Prefrontal Cortex: Evolution, Neurobiology, and Behavior.* (pp. 69–84). Baltimore: Brookes.

Janowsky, J.S., Shimamura, A.P., Kritchevsky, M., & Squire, L.R. (1989). Cognitive impairment following frontal lobe damage and its relevance to human amnesia. *Behavioral Neuroscience, 103,* 548–560.

Jernigan, T.L. & Tallal, P. (1990). Late childhood changes in brain morphology observable with MRI. *Developmental Medicine and Child Neurology, 32,* 379–385.

Jetter, W., Poser, U., Freeman, R.B., Markowitsch, H.J. (1986). A verbal long term memory deficit in frontal lobe damaged patients. *Cortex, 22,* 229–242.

Johnson, M. (1997). *Developmental Cognitive Neuroscience.* Oxford: Blackwell.

Kennedy, C., Sakurada, O., Shinohara, M., & Miyaoka, M. (1982). Local cerebral glucose utilization in the newborn macaque monkey. *Annals of Neurology, 12,* 333–340.

Klinberg, T., Vaidya, C., Gabrieli, J., Moseley, M., & Hedehus, M. (1999). Myelination and organization of the frontal white matter in children: a diffusion tensor study. *NeuroReport, 10,* 2817–2821.

Knight, R., Hillyard, S., Woods, D., & Neville, H. (1981). The effects of frontal cortex lesions on event-related potentials during auditory selective attention. *Electroencephalography and Clinical Neurophysiology, 52,* 571–582.

Kolb, B. & Fantie, B. (1989). Development of the child's brain and behavior. In: C. Reynolds & E. Fletcher-Janzen (Eds.), *Handbook of Clinical Child Neuropsychology* (pp. 17–39). New York: Plenum Press.

Kotapka, M.J., Graham, D.I., Adams, J.H., Doyle D., & Gennarelli, T.A. (1993). Hippocampal damage in fatal pediatric head injury. *Neuropathology and Applied Neurobiology, 19,* 128–133.

Levin, H.S., Culhane, K.A., Hartmann, J., Evankovich, K., Mattson, A.J., Harward, H., Ringholz, G., Ewing-Cobbs, L., & Fletcher, J.M. (1991). Developmental changes in performance on tests of purported frontal lobe functioning. *Developmental Neuropsychology, 7,* 377–395.

Levin, H.S., Culhane, K.A., Mendelsohn, D., Lilly, M.A., Bruce, D., Fletcher, J.H.M., Chapman, S.B., Harward, H., & Eisenberg, H.M. (1993). Cognition in relation to MRI in head injured children and adolescents. *Archives of Neurology, 50,* 897–905.

Levin, H.S., Mendelsohn, D., Lilly, M.A., Fletcher, J.M., Culhane, K.A., Chapman, S.B., Howard, H., Kusnerik, L., Bruce, D., & Eisenberg, H.M. (1994). Tower of London performance in relation to magnetic resonance imaging following closed head injury in children. *Neuropsychology, 8,* 171–179.

Levin, H.S., Mendelsohn, D., Lilly, M.A., Yeakley, J., Song, J., Scheibel, R.S., Harward, H., Fletcher, J.M., Kufera, J.A., Davidson, K.C., & Bruce, D. (1997a). Magnetic resonance imaging in relation to functional outcome of pediatric closed head injury: a test of the Ommaya-Gennarelli model. *Neurosurgery, 40,* 432–440.

Levin, H.S., Song, J., Scheibel, R.S., Fletcher, J.M., Harward, H., Lilly, M., & Goldstein, F. (1997b). Concept formation and problem-solving following closed head injury in children. *Journal of the Internationl Neuropsychological Society, 3,* 598–607.

Levin, H.S., Song, J., Scheibel, R.S., Fletcher, J.M., Harward, H.N., & Chapman, S.B. (2000). Dissociation of frequency and recency processing from list recall after severe closed head injury in children and adolescents. *Journal of Clinical and Experimental Neuropsychology, 22,* 1–15.

Levin, H.S., Song, J., Ewing-Cobbs, L., Chapman, S.B., & Mendelsohn, D. (2001). Word fluency in relation to severity of closed head injury, associated frontal brain lesions, and age at injury in children. *Neuropsychologia, 39,* 122–131.

Lezak, M. (1995). *Neuropsychological Assessment.* New York: Oxford University Press.

Lidow, M. & Goldman-Rakic, P.S. (1991). Synchronized overproduction of neurotransmitter receptors in diverse regions of the primate cerebral cortex. *Proceedings of the National Academy of Science USA, 88,* 10218–10221.

Luciana, M. & Nelson, S. (1998). The functional emergence of frontally guided working memory systems in four- to eight-year old children. *Neuropsychologia, 36,* 273–293.

Luria, A.R. (1973). *The Working Brain.* New York: Basic Books.

Manly, T., Robertson, I., Anderson, V., & Nimmo-Smith, I. (1999). *The Test of Everyday Attention for Children.* Cambridge, UK: Thames Valley Test Copmpany.

Mateer, C.A. (1990). Cognitive and behavioral sequalae of face and forehead injury in childhood. *Journal of Clinical and Experimental Neuropsychology, 12,* 95.

Mateer, C.A. & Williams, D. (1991). Effects of frontal lobe injury in childhood. *Developmental Neuropsychology, 7,* 69–86.

Matthews, L., Anderson, P., & Anderson, V. (2001). Assessing the validity of the Rey Complex Figure as a diagnostic tool: process and accuracy scores in children with brain insult. *Clinical Neuropsychological Assessment, 2*, 85–99.

McAllister, T.W., Saykin, A.J., Flashman, L.A., Sparling, M.B., Johnson, S.C., Guerin, S.J., Mamourian, A.C., Weaver, J.B., & Yanofsky, N. (1999). Brain activation during working memory 1 month after mild traumatic brain injury: a functional MRI study. *Neurology, 153*, 1300–1308.

McKay, K.E., Halperin, J.M., Schwartz, S.T., & Sharma, V. (1994). Developmental analysis of three aspects of information processing: sustained attention, selective attention, and response organization. *Developmental Neuropsychology, 10*, 121–132.

Miller, P.H. & Weiss, M.G. (1962). Children's attentional allocation, understanding of attention, and performance on the incidental learning task. *Child Development, 52*, 1183–1190.

Neisser, U. (1967). *Cognitive Psychology.* New York: Appleton-Century-Crofts.

Orzhekhiovskaya, N.S. (1981). Fronto-striatal relationships in primate ontogeny. *Neuroscience and Behavioral Physiology, 11*, 379–385.

Parker, D.M. & Crawford, J.R. (1992). Assessment of frontal lobe dysfunction. In: J.R. Crawford, D.M. Parker, & W.W. McKinlay (Eds.), *A Handbook of Neuropsychological Assessment* (pp. 267–294). London: Lawrence Erlbaum Associates.

Passler, M.A., Isaac, W., & Hynd, G.W. (1985). Neuropsychological development of behavior attributed to frontal lobe functioning in children. *Developmental Neuropsychology, 1*, 349–370.

Pentland, L., Todd, J.A., & Anderson, V. (1998). The impact of head injury severity on planning ability in adolescence: a functional analysis. *Neuropsychological Rehabilitation. 8*, 301–317.

Piaget, J. (1963). *The Origins of Intelligence in Children.* New York: W.W. Norton.

Ponsford, J. & Kinsella, G. (1992). Attentional deficits following closed-head injury. *Journal of Clinical and Experimental Neuropsychology, 14*, 822–838.

Rakic, P., Bourgeois, J.P., Eckenhoff, M., Zecevic, N., & Goldman-Rakic, P. (1986). Concurrent overproduction of synapses in diverse regions of the primate cerebral cortex. *Science, 232*, 232–235.

Rey, A. (1964). *L'examen Clinique en Psychologie.* Paris: Presses Universitaires de France.

Rourke, B.P. (1987). Syndrome of nonverbal learning disabilities: the final common pathway of white-matter disease/dysfunction. *Clinical Neuropsychologist, 1*, 209–234.

Shallice, T. (1990). *From Neuropsychology to Mental Structure.* New York: Cambridge University Press.

Shimamura, A.P., Janowsky, J.S., & Squire, L.R. (1991). What is the role of frontal lobe damage in amnesic disorders? In: H.S. Levin, H.M. Eisenberg, & A.L. Benton (Eds.), *Frontal Lobe Function and Dysfunction* (pp. 173–195). New York: Oxford University Press.

Simon, H.A. (1975). The functional equivalence of problem solving skills. *Cognitive Psychology, 7*, 268–288.

Sowell, E., Delis, D., Stiles, J., & Jernigan, T. (2001). Improved memory functioning and frontal lobe maturation between childhood and adolescence: a structural MRI study. *Journal of the International Neuropsychological Society, 7*, 312–322.

Staudt, M., Schropp, C., Staudt, F., Obletter, N., Bise, K., & Breit, A. (1993). Myelination of the brain in MRI: a staging system. *Pediatric Radiology, 23*, 169–176.

Stuss, D.T. (1992). Biological and psychological development of executive functions. *Brain and Cognition, 20*, 8–23.

Stuss, D.T. & Benson, D.F. (1986). *The Frontal Lobes.* New York: Raven Press.

Teasdale, G, & Jennett, B. (1974). Assessment of coma and impaired consciousness. *Lancet, 2*, 81–84.

Thatcher, R.W. (1991). Maturation of the human frontal lobes. Physiological evidence for staging. *Developmental Neuropsychology, 7*, 397–419.

Thatcher, R.W. (1992). Cyclical cortical reorganization during early childhood. *Brain and Cognition, 20*, 24–50.

Thatcher, R.W. (1997). Human frontal lobe development: a theory of cyclical cortical reorganization. In: N. Krasnegor, G. Reid Lyon, & P. Goldman-Rakic (Eds.). *Development of the Prefrontal Cortex: Evolution, Neurobiology, and Behavior* (pp. 85–116). Baltimore: Brookes.

Todd, J.A., Anderson, V.A., & Lawrence, J. (1996). Planning skills in head injured adolescents and their peers. *Neuropsychological Rehabilitation, 6*, 81–99.

Uemura, E. & Hartmann, H.A. (1978). RNA content and volume of nerve cell bodies in human brain: I. Prefrontal cortex in aging normal and demented patients. *Journal of Neuropathology and Experimental Neurology, 37*, 487–496.

Walsh, K.W. (1978). *Neuropsychology: A Clinical Approach.* New York: Churchill Livingston.

Walsh, K.W. (1985). *Understanding Brain Damage: a Primer of Neuropsychological Evaluation.* New York: Churchill Livingston.

Wechsler, D. (1991). *Manual for the Wechsler Scale of Children's Intelligence-III.* New York: Psychological Corporation.

Welsh, M.C. & Pennington, B.F. (1988). Assessing frontal lobe functioning in children: views from developmental psychology. *Developmental Neuropsychology, 4*, 199–230.

Welsh, M.C., Pennington, B.F., & Groisser, D.B. (1991). A normative-developmental study of executive function: a window on prefrontal function in children. *Developmental Neuropsychology, 7*, 131–149.

Yakovlev, P.I. (1962). Morphological criteria of growth and maturation of the nervous system in man. *Research Publications Association for Research in Nervous and Mental Disease, 39*, 3–46.

Yakovlev, P.I. & Lecours, A.R. (1967). The myelogenetic cycles of regional maturation of the brain. In: A. Minkiniwski (Ed.), *Regional Development of the Brain in Early Life* (pp. 3–70). Oxford: Blackwell.

31

Aging, Memory, and Frontal Lobe Functioning

FERGUS I.M. CRAIK AND CHERYL L. GRADY

Older adults often complain that their memory performance is not as good as it was when they were younger, and this observation is generally borne out by the results of laboratory studies (Craik & Jennings, 1992; Balota et al., 2000; Zacks et al., 2000). However, these studies are also consistent in showing that age-related memory losses are very task-dependent; performance on some tasks drops substantially with increasing age, whereas performance on other tasks shows essentially no change across the adult years. This differential pattern of strengths and weaknesses can presumably give researchers some clues, about both the cognitive organization of memory systems and the underlying neural correlates of these different systems. The purpose of this chapter is first to provide an account of age-related memory losses at the behavioral level and then to assess the compatibility between this account and current findings and ideas from neuroimaging. In particular, we address the question of how far the pattern of memory losses associated with normal aging can be understood as a consequence of an age-related decline in the efficiency of frontal lobe functioning—the so-called frontal lobe hypothesis of cognitive aging (Albert & Kaplan, 1980; Dempster, 1992; West, 1996).

The idea that the frontal lobes are particularly vulnerable to the effects of aging comes from both the behavioral literature and the literature on structural changes in the brain with age. For example, behavioral studies have shown that older adults have particular difficulty with memory tasks that make heavy demands on the frontal lobes, such as working memory and free recall (West, 1996). Most of the data on changes in brain structure with age come from magnetic resonance imaging (MRI) studies that have examined age-related differences in the volume of various brain regions. A recent review by Raz (2000) indicates that the volume of frontal cortex is somewhat more strongly correlated with age than other cortical areas, such as the temporal or parietal lobes, although it should be noted that some subcortical areas (such as the caudate nucleus) show a correlation with age similar to that seen in the frontal lobes. These two bodies of work together have been taken as evidence that declines in frontal lobe function underlie many of the age-related changes seen in cognitive abilities. However, a recent review of the evidence for the frontal lobe aging hypothesis (Greenwood, 2000) concluded that too little attention has been paid to evidence for changes seen elsewhere in the brain and advocates a network approach to this issue, rather than a localization one. As we shall see below, the neuroimaging evidence indicates a critical role not only for the frontal lobes in cognitive aging but also for other areas as well.

AGING AND MEMORY: BEHAVIORAL EVIDENCE

It is abundantly clear that human memory cannot be thought of as a monolithic entity that performs either poorly or well. Rather, it is a set of loosely related cognitive abilities whose various functions have been attributed to either different memory systems (e.g., Tulving, 1983; Tulving & Schacter, 1990) or different cognitive processes (e.g., Craik, 1983; Jacoby, 1983; Kolers & Roediger, 1984). The experimental literature on cognitive aging typically deals with adults aged between 20 and 90, and there is general agreement that performance on some memory tasks holds up well across this age range whereas performance on other tasks declines substantially from young to old adulthood (see Craik & Jennings, 1992; Balota et al., 2000; Zacks et al., 2000, for recent reviews). It is assumed that this differential pattern of task performance reflects the fact that different memory tasks tap the different systems or processes to various degrees; also, some systems or processes are more vulnerable than others to the effects of aging.

Tasks that show little change as a function of aging include procedural memory tasks, priming and other "implicit memory" tasks, episodic recognition memory, and semantic memory tasks. *Procedural memory tasks* are those reflecting learned skills—either motor skills such as typing or cognitive skills such as reading. *Implicit memory tasks* show benefits from a previous event in the absence of conscious recollection of that event. For example, recent experience of a word primes later perception of that same word, even if the subject does not remember seeing the word in the previous phase of the experiment. *Semantic memory* is the person's general knowledge of facts, vocabulary, etc., and the ability to access and use this knowledge changes only slightly with increasing age. Finally, although *episodic memory* for specific events is generally vul-

nerable to the effects of aging, if the test is recognition (as opposed to recall), the effects are typically small (Craik & McDowd, 1987). Large age-related decrements, however, are usually seen in the free recall of previously experienced episodes, in recollection of context and source, in working memory, and in prospective memory. Thus, for example, older adults can recollect facts that they have acquired, but be unable to remember the *source* of that fact—whether it was heard on the radio, seen on TV, or read in a newspaper. *Working memory tasks* are those that involve the active manipulation of material held in mind—mental arithmetic, for example, or repeating back a string of words in the reverse order. *Prospective memory* involves remembering to carry out a planned action at some future time, as in mailing a letter, buying a birthday gift, or even collecting a specific book from another room; older people are often less efficient at carrying out such tasks.

The crucial scientific problem is therefore to find common factors that underlie these strengths and weaknesses, first at the level of psychological description and then at the level of brain functions. One possible basis of organization is the memory systems viewpoint proposed by Endel Tulving and colleagues (Tulving, 1983; Tulving & Schacter, 1990). Tulving has suggested that there are five major memory systems: procedural memory, the perceptual representational system, working memory, semantic memory, and episodic memory. Is it possible that aging affects some of these systems but not others, thereby giving rise to the previously described pattern of strengths and weaknesses? Age-related differences are slight in both procedural memory and various perceptual memory systems (Craik & Jennings, 1992), so this observation fits the systems viewpoint. For the other systems the fit is not so good, however, as there are strengths and weaknesses *within* each system. For example, working memory tasks show substantial age-related declines (see Balota et al., 2000; Zacks et al., 2000, for reviews), but other closely related short-term memory tasks (e.g., span measures and primary memory tasks) show little change (Craik & Jennings, 1992). Semantic memory holds up well with age, yet the tendency to forget proper *names* (clearly semantic memory information) is universally reported by older people. Older adults' performance on episodic memory tasks is generally poor, yet their performance on episodic *recognition* tasks, as opposed to recall tasks, is comparatively good (Craik & McDowd, 1987). All in all, then, the systems viewpoint does not provide a very satisfactory account of the pattern of memory deficits seen in older people.

An alternative approach in terms of different *processes* was suggested by Craik (1983, 1986), who theorized that encoding processes are driven partly by internal mental states, primarily by those associated with the perception, comprehension, and elaboration of the original event (Craik & Lockhart, 1972; Craik & Tulving, 1975), and partly by the external context. All of these variables are incorporated into the encoded representation of the event. Successful retrieval is largely a question of re-creating the same pattern of mental activities that occurred at the time of encoding, and the reestablishment of this pattern is helped greatly if the external environment is similar to the encoding context and thus induces the same mental operations. To the extent that such environmental support is lacking, the person must recruit self-initiated processing in an attempt to re-create the original pattern; Craik's (1983) suggestion was that such self-initiated processing depends substantially on the integrity of the frontal lobes. Also, some tasks require more self-initiated processing than others. Recognition memory involves the re-presentation of the items (along with new lures or distractor items) and so is moderately high in environmental support. Free recall, by contrast, is typically carried out in the complete absence of cues and often in a different environment from the original encoding context, so this task is low in environmental support and must therefore rely heavily on self-initiated activities. The general scheme, showing the complementary relations between environmental support and self-initiated processing, is shown in Figure 31–1. If normal aging is associated with a reduction in the efficiency of frontal lobe functioning, then older people should be especially penalized on tasks

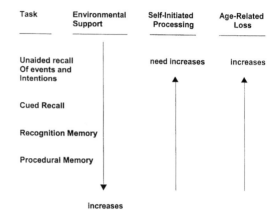

Figure 31–1. Scheme illustrating the relations among environmental support, self-initiated processing, and age-related memory loss.

that require a lot of self-initiated processing. That is, they should be poor on recall tasks but perform comparatively well on recognition and procedural memory tasks, and this is what the data show.

Before examining the plausibility of Craik's suggestion further, we will consider the evidence on aging and frontal lobe functioning, with an emphasis on recent findings from functional neuroimaging.

NEUROIMAGING STUDIES OF AGING, MEMORY, AND THE FRONTAL LOBES

There are two aspects of brain activity changes with age during cognitive tasks that have been addressed with functional neuroimaging: brain areas where older adults have reduced activity compared to that of young adults, and areas where older adults have increased activity. Reduced activity can reasonably be assumed to reflect a reduced level of functioning, particularly when accompanied by poorer performance on the task. Therefore, if the frontal lobes are vulnerable to the effects of aging, older adults should show reduced frontal activity during memory tasks, particularly those memory tasks that older adults find especially difficult. Unfortunately, no neuroimaging experiments to date have examined free recall, the memory task on which older adults show the greatest deficit. However, a number of experiments have used recognition tasks, to examine both encoding and retrieval in elderly adults, and a few have used cued recall. These experiments have found support for the idea that older individuals are particularly disadvantaged during encoding (Craik & Byrd, 1982). During encoding of unfamiliar faces, young adults show increased activity in left inferior prefrontal cortex, as well as in temporal regions, both medially and laterally (Haxby et al., 1996; Bernstein et al., 2002). Older adults show less activation of left prefrontal and temporal regions during face encoding than that in younger adults (Grady et al., 1995, in press). Similar results were found in a verbal memory study in which young and old adults were scanned during encoding of paired associates (Cabeza et al., 1997). As in the face memory study, the old adults showed less activation during encoding in the areas that were active in young adults—i.e., left prefrontal and temporal regions. This finding was replicated by Anderson et al. (2000), who showed further that divided attention during encoding and aging both reduced encoding-related activity in left prefrontal cortex. This result suggests that the reductions in memory accuracy due to aging and divided attention may have a common mechanism in that both reduce the ability to engage in elaborative encoding that is mediated, at least in part, by left prefrontal cortex.

During retrieval the picture is somewhat different. During recognition of faces, both young and old adults show activation of right prefrontal and parietal cortices with little or no difference in the magnitudes of this activation (Grady et al., 1995, in press). Right prefrontal activity is also seen during verbal retrieval in both young and old adults, during both cued recall (Cabeza et al., 1997) and recognition (Cabeza et al., 1997; Madden et al., 1999b). Sometimes, however, right prefrontal activity is reduced in the older group during cued recall (Anderson et al., 2000) or is in a different location than that of young adults (Schacter et al., 1996). Other areas of reduced activity in the elderly during retrieval include the thalamus (Madden et al., 1999b; Anderson et al., 2000), temporal regions (Bäckman et al., 1997; Cabeza et al., 1997), and visual cortex (Grady et al., 1995; Anderson et al., 2000). Thus, in terms of prefrontal regions, older adults consistently show reduced levels of activity in prefrontal areas that mediate encoding—mainly left inferior prefrontal cortex. In contrast, older adults often can engage the right prefrontal regions involved in retrieval relatively normally, particularly if memory is tested via recognition; this finding is consistent with the behavioral evidence of less age-related reduction during recognition than during recall. Thus, if one examines the results in terms of reduced frontal activity in the elderly, the findings are consistent with the idea that older individuals have difficulty with both stages of memory, particularly the encoding stage and when memory is assessed with more effortful forms of retrieval. In addition, these difficulties are mediated by not only reductions in the frontal lobes but also reduced activity in posterior cortical regions.

In contrast to these *reductions* in brain activation, which imply a reduction in processing resources, a number of investigators have now reported *increased* utilization of some brain regions by older adults during memory tasks, primarily in prefrontal regions during memory retrieval. The study of paired-associate memory mentioned above (Cabeza et al., 1997) and one of face memory experiments (Grady et al., in press) found that both young and old adults had right prefrontal activity during retrieval, but the old adults also had left prefrontal activity during this task. Similar findings were reported in experiments by Cabeza et al. (2000) and by Madden and colleagues (1999b), who examined recognition of single words and found that young adults had right prefrontal activation during word recognition, whereas the old adults had bilateral prefrontal activation. Bäckman and colleagues (1997) also reported bilateral prefrontal activation in older adults during cued recall of learned words; in young adults activation was in the right hemisphere. These experiments, together with those examining encoding (discussed above), indicate that older adults do not engage left prefrontal cortex during encoding, but often do so during retrieval and to a greater extent than young adults. This suggests that the cognitive processes mediated by left prefrontal cortex during memory tasks are not necessarily unavailable to the elderly, but are used differently. These age-related differences are summarized in Figure 31–2.

Differential use of prefrontal and other regions of cortex also has been found in short-term or working memory experiments. Two recent experiments of working memory for letters in which similar paradigms were used, found decreased activity in left prefrontal cortex (Jonides et al., 2000; see Fig. 31–2) and bilateral dorsolateral prefrontal cortex in older adults, than that in younger adults (Rypma D'Esposito, 2000). Interestingly, the study by Rypma and D'Esposito (2000) showed that this age-related difference was seen only when participants made their responses to the memory probe and not during encoding or the 10-second retention period. Other working memory studies have shown increases as well as decreases in activation in older adults. One such experiment involved short-term recognition of unfamiliar faces using a delayed match-to-sample (DMS) paradigm (Grady et al., 1998). When the delayed recognition condi-

tions were compared to a baseline condition, both young and old adults had activation of occipitotemporal and prefrontal cortices bilaterally. However, young adults had greater activation of right ventral prefrontal cortex, and old individuals showed greater activation in left dorsolateral prefrontal cortex (see Fig. 31–2). In addition, the older adults also had greater activity during the working memory tasks in occipital cortex. This study is therefore an interesting example of both reduced use of resources (in right frontal) and increased use of resources (left frontal and occipital) in the elderly. Reuter-Lorenz and colleagues (2000) examined working memory for verbal and spatial information and found that young adults had lateralized prefrontal activity during these tasks—in the left hemisphere during the verbal task and in the right hemisphere during the spatial task. Older adults, by contrast, had bilateral prefrontal activity during both tasks, a finding similar to the reports of bilateral prefrontal activity in the elderly during episodic retrieval, discussed above.

The obvious question raised by these data is how one should interpret this recruitment of brain activity in the elderly. In some cases, this additional activity occurs during a task that the older adults are able to perform as well as young adults, leading to the suggestion that recruitment of additional areas is com-

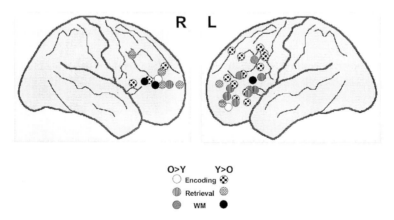

Figure 31–2. Schematic right and left hemispheres showing areas where functional neuroimaging studies have found differences between older (o) and younger (y) adults in brain activation during the encoding and retrieval phases of episodic memory experiments and during working memory (WM) experiments. Data were extracted from the following studies: Grady et al., (1995, 1998, 1999, in press); Schacter et al. (1996); Madden et al., 1996, 1999; Bäckman et al. (1997); Cabeza et al. (1997, 2000); Anderson et al. (2000); Jonides et al. (2000).

pensatory (Grady et al., 1994; Cabeza et al., 1997). Another way of looking at this issue is to examine correlations between brain activity and task performance. In an experiment examining brain activity during working memory for simple visual stimuli (McIntosh et al., 1999), both young and old adults showed regions of cortex where activity was correlated with better memory performance, but the specific regions were different in the two groups. This result suggests that memory performance depends on the function of different sets of brain regions as we age. A similar result was reported for face memory, in that younger adults showed positive correlations between activity in medial temporal regions and accuracy of face recognition, whereas older adults showed correlations between activity in dorsolateral prefrontal regions and face memory (Grady et al., in press). In addition, Rypma and D'Esposito (2000) found that faster reaction times were related to increased dorsolateral prefrontal activity in older but not younger adults. This evidence of differential correlations between brain activity and memory performance suggests that older adults might be able to recruit brain areas, particularly dorsolateral prefrontal cortex, during certain tasks to compensate for reduced activity elsewhere in the brain. As a consequence of this compensation, task performance would be maintained. Dorsolateral prefrontal cortex increases its activity, however, when tasks emphasize executive functions (e.g. D'Esposito et al., 1995, 1999) or become more difficult (e.g., Grady et al., 1996; Braver et al., 1997). It is possible, then, that increased prefrontal activity in the elderly reflects greater need or use of executive functions at lower levels of task demand than would be necessary for activation of this area in young adults. This might

be the most likely explanation in those situations where older adults have increased prefrontal activation yet show reduced performance levels compared to those of younger adults (e.g., Madden et al., 1999a).

BEHAVIORAL EVIDENCE RE-EXAMINED

Much of the evidence from the behavioral experiments and neuroimaging studies reviewed above points to inefficient encoding processes in the elderly as being the major source of age-related memory problems. The similarity between the effects of aging and the effects of divided attention on memory (Craik, 1982) suggests further that the encoding problems may be a consequence of reduced attentional processing resources in the older brain (Craik & Byrd, 1982). This account has its problems, however. If encoding processes are impaired in older people, then manipulations that boost encoding should benefit older people differentially, yet typically they do not. Rather, such manipulations benefit younger and older adults to the same extent. One example of this pattern comes from an experiment carried out by Rabinowitz and colleagues, reported by Craik and Byrd (1982). Younger and older adults were given either lists of words or lists of pictures of objects to recall or recognize. It is well known that pictures boost encoding processes and are associated with higher levels of subsequent recall. This was true in the present case also (Table 31–1), but the picture superiority effect was the same for younger and older groups. Interestingly, the age-related decrement was eliminated when picture presentation was coupled with a *recognition* test at the time of retrieval. An imaging study using this design of comparing picture and word

Table 31–1. Mean proportions recalled and recognized as a function of age and type of material (Craik & Byrd, 1982)

| Age Group | Recall | | Recognition | |
	Words	Pictures	Words	Pictures
Young	0.33	0.52	0.73	0.84
Old	0.17	0.36	0.63	0.83

recognition showed results consistent with these behavioral findings. Both younger and older adults had brain activity patterns that differentiated picture and word encoding, with visual cortex and medial temporal areas being more active during picture encoding, indicating that the mechanisms used to provide the picture superiority effect were similar regardless of age (Grady et al., 1999).

A second example of equal benefits to younger and older subjects comes from a recent Swedish study using subject-performed tasks (SPTs) Rönnlund et al., submitted). It is known that lists of simple verbal commands such as "point to the book" and "pick up the orange" are recalled better if the actions are actually performed, rather than if they are read. In the study by Rönnlund et al. (Submitted), participants ranging in age from 35 to 80 years were given lists of verbal commands or SPTs to recall. The results, shown in Figure 31–3, demonstrate that SPTs boosted recall (presumably by enhancing the effectiveness of encoding processes) but did so equivalently for subjects of all ages.

Good episodic memory performance reflects the depth and elaboration of encoding accomplished at the time the event was originally encountered (Craik & Lockhart, 1972; Craik & Tulving, 1975). In these terms it seems possible that one consequence of a re-

duction in processing resources, associated speculatively with both normal aging and division of attention in young adults, is a reduction in the depth and elaboration of processing achieved during encoding (Eysenck, 1974; Craik & Byrd, 1982; Naveh-Benjamin et al., 2000). A reduction in depth of processing implies an impairment in semantic processing, yet some recent studies cast doubt on whether older adults are impaired, at least in the *amount* of semantic processing carried out during encoding. Experiments on "false memories" show that older people make at least as many such errors as do younger adults (Balota et al., 1999; Kensinger & Schacter, 1999; Benjamin, in press). A typical experiment in this vein involves the presentation of a series of words that are highly related to a nonpresented target word. For example, the nonpresented target word might be *needle*, and the presented words would be *pin, sharp, sew*, etc. The finding is that subjects falsely recall and recognize the target word with high probability, and that older subjects make such errors at least as frequently as young adults do (Balota et al., 1999; Kensinger & Schacter, 1999; Benjamin, 2001). It seems, then, that the *amount* of semantic processing is not impaired in older people, but it may well be the case that the specificity and distinctiveness of encoding is impaired by aging and by division of attention, and that this impairment leads both to a decrease in the retrieval of presented events and an increase in the liability to make false-positive errors. Again, imaging studies can shed some light on this issue. When older adults are required to learn new stimuli using semantic strategies, they can recruit the brain areas necessary for semantic encoding as readily as young adults, at least when the stimuli are pictures of objects, but not when the stimuli are words (Grady et al., 1999). This suggests that the "amount" of semantic processing is similar in young and old for at least some types of stimuli, but perhaps not all. An intriguing idea raised by the imaging data reviewed above is that the additional left prefrontal activity seen in older adults during retrieval is an attempt to overcome the deficit in specificity of semantic processing during encoding by increased semantic processing during retrieval.

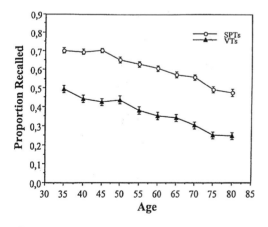

Figure 31–3. Proportions of phrases recalled by adults of different ages as a function of whether the phrases were presented as subject-performed tasks (SPTs) or verbal tasks (VTs). (*Source:* Data from Rönnlund et al., submitted)

Some recent evidence from Craik's laboratory suggests that division of attention in young people may impair encoding in a rather different way. Experiments reported by Craik and Kester (2000) showed that memory performance was lower following divided attention than that after full attention at encoding, even when the amount of semantic elaboration achieved during the encoding process was equated between the two conditions. This result implies that division of attention has some further detrimental effect beyond the encoding stage, and Craik and Kester (2000) speculated that this further effect may be connected with the consolidation or binding process. Speculatively, the positive relationship between depth and elaboration of processing on the one hand and memory performance on the other may be modulated by division of attention such that the level of memory performance associated with a particular amount of semantic processing at encoding is reduced as attentional resources are withdrawn. By extension, the same mechanism may be a factor in normal aging. It is certainly the case that amnesic patients process information deeply and semantically, yet remember very little. The present speculative suggestion is that a similar phenomenon occurs in dual-task situations and with older adults, and that in these cases the modulating variable is withdrawal of attentional resources.

If encoding difficulties in the elderly do not account for all instances of memory failure, what other types of impairment may play a part? The obvious candidate is the set of processes that underlie retrieval; is there evidence for an age-related increase in retrieval difficulties? Clearly the answer is yes. First, older adults very often report problems in retrieving names, even names that they know well and were clearly well encoded. A second indication of age-related retrieval difficulties is the effectiveness of environmental support (Craik, 1983) in reducing the size of memory decrements in older people. The observation here is that older adults typically benefit differentially as more cues and context are supplied at the time of retrieval. For example, age-related memory decrements are less in recognition than in free recall (Craik & McDowd, 1987).

A third example comes from dual-task experiments in which subjects encode and retrieve information either under full-attention conditions or while carrying out a demanding secondary task. The results of such studies have shown that memory performance is reduced by the presence of the secondary task to about the same extent in younger and older adults, but that performance on the secondary task itself is more impaired in older people, especially when the secondary task is performed at the time of retrieval (Nyberg et al., 1997; Anderson et al., 1998). Again, this example shows that retrieval processes are less efficient, or require more processing resources, in older than in younger adults. Finally, recent work by Jacoby and colleagues has shown that older people have specific problems with the conscious recollection of events and their contexts, as opposed to situations in which a simple judgment of familiarity is sufficient (Jacoby, 1991; Jennings & Jacoby, 1993; Hay & Jacoby, 1999). All of these examples make it clear that some substantial part of older people's memory problems is attributable to an age-related reduction in the efficiency of retrieval processes. It also should be noted that although older adults consistently have reductions in a number of critical brain areas during encoding, there is evidence for reduced activity in retrieval-related areas under some conditions. Thus, the neuroimaging data are consistent with the idea that older adults have deficits at both encoding and retrieval.

One way of characterizing such a reduction in efficiency is the suggestion that specific detail becomes harder to retrieve, whereas relatively general global information remains accessible to retrieval. Examples showing that older people have particular difficulties with specific detail include their problems in remembering names and retrieving words in response to their definitions or pictorial representations (see Light, 1992, for a review). A second example comes from the recall of text material; Byrd (1981) showed that the age-related decrement in recall was greater for detailed information than for general gist information. The poorer performance of older people in the recollection of contextual detail, as opposed to central item information (Spencer & Raz, 1995), is a further case in point. Finally, the very fact that older people perform less well than their younger counterparts on episodic memory tasks—in which specific events must be recalled—again points to a particular difficulty with the recollection of specific detail.

Two further comments may be made at this point. First, given that older adults show difficulties both in the recollection of names from the semantic memory system and of events from the episodic memory system, it is suggested that the primary age-related difficulty is associated with the specificity of information to be recalled, rather than with a particular memory system. Second, one congenial way of describing the difficulty associated with the recollection of detail is to say that the resolving power of retrieval processing is impaired. Interestingly, Fuster (see Chapter 6) suggested that one consequence of frontal lobe damage is a failure of discrimination or of analytic power.

Figure 31–4 illustrates the general idea that the cognitive system is organized hierarchically, or more likely that the system is organized along a number of different dimensions, each of which may be depicted in hierarchical terms. Figure 31–4 shows two of these dimensions, one running from representations of specific episodic instances to generalized, context-free representations of the features common to those instances. As an example, the specific instances could be the various occasions on which one met a person, encoded along with details of time and place, and the higher-level representations would encode one's general knowledge of that person. The

higher levels may be designated "semantic memory" and the lower levels "episodic memory," but in the present scheme these different levels are graded levels in an overall hierarchy rather than different memory systems. Recent work in which experimental participants judge that they either "remember" some event along with its contextual details or merely "know" that an event occurred (Gardiner & Richardson-Klavehn, 2000) may be represented as tapping different levels of the hierarchy.

A second cut through the same cognitive system represents a more taxonomic hierarchy within general knowledge, running from specific names of people, plants, animals, etc. to global concepts of these people and objects. The relevance of these ideas in the present context is that older adults appear to have greater difficulty retrieving information from the lower levels of hierarchical representations than from higher levels.

Lesion studies provide another source of evidence linking age-related memory impairments to frontal lobe function and dysfunction. Stuss and colleagues (1996) compared groups of younger and older individuals' performance on a verbal learning task to three groups of patients who had lesions in left frontal, right frontal, and bilateral frontal regions, respectively. The qualitative nature of recall performance was similar between the older normal group and the group of patients with right frontal lesions, especially on measures of organization and in the types of error shown at retrieval. The overall pattern of performance exhibited by the older adults resembled that shown by frontal patients much

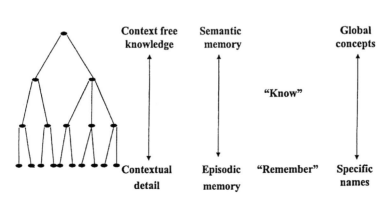

Figure 31–4. Hierarchical representation of knowledge and memory.

more than it resembled the pattern usually found in patients with temporal lobe pathology. In particular it seemed that a deficiency in executive processes was the most important factor underlying the relatively poor performance of the older participants.

CONCLUSION

The behavioral evidence makes it clear that age-related declines in memory do occur, but that these declines are much greater in the performance of some tasks (e.g., recall and working memory tasks) than that of others (e.g., recognition memory and implicit memory tasks). Age-related declines in brain volume are also differential, with the greatest amounts of atrophy being seen in the prefrontal cortex and neostriatum (Raz, 2000). It is now clear that age-related changes in prefrontal cortical structure and function are related to the changes observed in memory performance, although the research is still in its early days.

Some findings are already clear, however. During memory encoding, areas in the left inferior frontal cortex are less activated in older than in younger adults (Grady et al., 1995; Cabeza et al., 1997). Interestingly, analogous reductions in left prefrontal activation were observed in young adults encoding under divided attention conditions (Anderson et al., 2000), a finding that lends support to the notion that division of attention mimics aging in many respects (Craik, 1982). One possibility is that both conditions involve reductions in attentional processing resources (Craik & Byrd, 1982). Such reductions can be compensated for by increases in environmental support (Fig. 31–1, Craik, 1983). As one example, presenting stimuli as pictures instead of words raises the level of memory performance in older adults, and also changes the pattern of frontal activation (Grady et al., 1999).

Older people also show retrieval difficulties—in both episodic and semantic memory. These difficulties tend to be greatest in tasks requiring a great deal of self-initiated activity; thus age-related decrements are greater in recall than in recognition (Craik & McDowd,

1987). This difference is also found in neuroimaging studies; for example, age-related reductions in prefrontal activity occur in cued recall (Schacter et al., 1996) but not in recognition (Grady et al., 1995). Young adults show a marked asymmetry during retrieval, in that the right prefrontal cortex is more active than the left, but interestingly, older adults show much less asymmetry; specifically older adults show greater amounts of left prefrontal activity during retrieval than young adults do (Cabeza et al., 1997; Grady et al., in press). This age-related reduction in prefrontal asymmetry may reflect compensatory activity in the older brain or may reflect the process of "de-differentiation"—that is, older adults may recruit frontal and other cortical areas in a less selective manner (see Buckner & Logan, 2001; Cabeza, 2001, for recent reviews).

Thus some progress has been made in specifying the roles of the frontal lobes in memory encoding and retrieval, and how these functions change as a function of normal aging. Two interesting problems for future explorations are first, the notion of a breakdown with age in appropriate control processes, which is perhaps associated with the age-related failures of inhibitory processes documented by Hasher and colleagues (e.g., Zacks et al., 2000), and second, the role of the frontal lobes in the resolution and reactivation of specific detail during episodic and semantic retrieval.

Finally, how does the frontal hypothesis of aging fare in light of the evidence presented here? Although it seems likely that age-related inefficiencies of many different areas of the brain play a role in the decline of many memory functions with age, the present evidence suggests that the frontal lobes play a crucial role, perhaps in conjunction with other areas. First, aging is associated with a decline in activation levels of the left prefrontal cortex during encoding—an area that appears to be important for semantic processing and thus for subsequent memory performance. Second, this same area shows a decline in activation when participants encode under conditions of divided attention. This is an interesting finding given the behavioral similarities observed between older adults and young adults working in divided-attention situations in memory studies. Third, patients with right frontal lesions show a pattern of memory performance similar to that shown by normal older adults, especially in organizational processes and in the types of error made. Fourth, several neuroimaging studies have now found that older adults exhibit compensatory activation of areas of the left prefrontal cortex during retrieval; again the age-related difference lies in the frontal regions. Finally, deficiencies in working memory performance are typical of older adults, and the executive control of such tasks has been located in dorsolateral prefrontal regions.

Despite these many reasons to link aging with a decline in frontal lobe functioning, it seems certain that other areas also contribute to age-related memory losses. In particular, age-related declines in the function of both lateral medial temporal regions are likely to be involved, as mentioned above. An exciting new approach to neuroimaging data involves the use of analyses that examine the functional connections between brain regions during cognitive tasks, or so-called network approaches (McIntosh & Gonzalez-Lima, 1994). The use of these methods is based on the assumption that cognition is the result of the integrated activity of dynamic brain networks rather than the action of any one region acting independently. The few studies to apply this approach to data from older adults have shown that the brain networks supporting cognitive processes can be quite different from those seen in younger adults. For example, Della-Maggiore et al. (2000) found that the hippocampus was functionally connected to different regions in young and old participants during a visual memory task, with the older adults showing stronger influences from occipital and temporal regions into the hippocampus. Differential functional connections between hippocampus and frontal regions also were found. Thus, although the frontal cortex plays a major role in age-related changes in memory function, an understanding of the way in which the frontal lobes communicate with other brain areas is likely to be equally if not more important in ultimately determining the brain mechanisms underlying these changes.

REFERENCES

Albert, M.S. & Kaplan, E. (1980). Organic implications of neuropsychological deficits in the elderly. In: L.W. Poon, J.L. Fozard, L.S. Cermak, D. Arenberg & L.W. Thompson (Eds.), *New directions in memory and aging* (pp. 403–432). Hillsdale, NJ: Lawrence Erlbaum Associates.

Anderson, N.D., Craik, F.I.M., & Naveh-Benjamin, M. (1998). The attentional demands of encoding and retrieval in younger and older adults: I. Evidence from divided attention costs. *Psychology and Aging, 13,* 405–423.

Anderson, N.D., Iidaka, T., Cabeza, R., Kapur, S., McIntosh, A.R. & Craik, F.I.M. (2000). The effects of divided attention on encoding- and retrieval-related brain activity: a PET study of younger and older adults. *Journal of Cognitive Neuroscience, 12,* 775–792.

Bäckman, L., Almkvist, O., Andersson, J., Nordberg, A., Winblad, B., Reineck, R., & Langstrom, B. (1997). Brain activation in young and older adults during implicit and explicit retrieval. *Journal of Cognitive Neuroscience, 9,* 378–391.

Balota, D.W., Cortese, M.J., Duchek, J.M., Adams, D., Roediger, H.L., III, McDermott, K.B., & Yenys, B.E. (1999). Veridical and false memories in healthy older adults and dementia of the Alzheimer's type. *Cognitive Neuropsychology, 16,* 361–384.

Balota, D.A., Dolan, P.O., & Duchek, J.M. (2000). Memory changes in healthy older adults. In: E. Tulving & F.I.M. Craik (Eds.), *The Oxford Handbook of Memory* (pp. 395–409). New York: Oxford University Press.

Benjamin, A.S. (2001). On the dual effects of repetition on false recognition. *Journal of Experimental Psychology: Learning, Memory, and Cognition 27,* 941–947.

Bernstein, L.J., Beig, S., Siegenthaler, A., & Grady, C.L. (2002). The effect of encoding strategy on the neural correlates of memory for faces. *Neuropsychologia 40,* 86–98.

Braver, T.S., Cohen, J.D., Nystrom, L.E., Jonides, J., Smith, E.E., & Noll, D.C. (1997). A parametric study of prefrontal cortex involvement in human working memory. *NeuroImage, 5,* 49–62.

Buckner, R.L. & Logan, J.M. (2001). Frontal contributions to episodic memory encoding in the young and elderly. In: A.E. Parker, E.L., Wilding, & T. Bussey (Eds.). *The Cognitive Neuroscience of Memory Encoding and Retrieval.* Philadelphia: Psychology Press.

Burke, D.M. & Light, L.L. (1981). Memory and aging: the role of retrieval processes. *Psychological Bulletin, 90,* 513–546.

Byrd, M. (1981). *Age differences in memory for prose passages.* Unpublished Ph.D. thesis, University of Toronto, Toronto.

Cabeza, R. (2001). Functional neuroimaging of cognitive aging. In: R. Cabeza & A. Kingstone (Eds.), *Handbook of Functional Neuroimaging of Cognition.* Cambridge, MA: MIT Press.

Cabeza, R., Grady, C.L., Nyberg, L., McIntosh, A.R., Tulving, E., Kapur, S., Jennings, J.M., Houle, S., & Craik, F.I.M. (1997). Age-related differences in neural activity during memory encoding and retrieval: a positron emission tomography study. *Journal of Neuroscience, 17*, 391–400.

Cabeza, R., Anderson, N.D., Houle, S., Mangels, J.A., & Nyberg, L. (2000). Age-related differences in neural activity during item and temporal-order memory retrieval: a positron emission tomography study. *Journal of Cognitive Neuroscience, 12*, 197–206.

Craik, F.I.M. (1982). Selective changes in encoding as a function of reduced processing capacity. In: F. Klix, J. Hoffmann, & E. van der Meer (Eds.), *Cognitive Research in Psychology* (pp. 152–161). Berlin: Deutscher Verlag der Wissenschaften.

Craik, F.I.M. (1983). On the transfer of information from temporary to permanent memory. *Philosophical Transactions of the Royal Society Series B 302*, 351–359.

Craik, F.I.M. (1986). A functional account of age differences in memory. In: F. Klix & H. Hagendorf (Eds.), *Human Memory and Cognitive Capabilities, Mechanisms and Performances* (pp. 409–422). Amsterdam: Elsevier.

Craik, F.I.M. & Byrd, M. (1982). Aging and cognitive deficits: The role of attentional resources. In: F.I.M. Craik & S. Trehub (Eds.), *Aging and Cognitive Processes* (pp. 191–211). New York: Plenum Press.

Craik, F.I.M. & Jennings, J.J. (1992). Human memory. In F.I.M. Craik & T.A. Salthouse (Eds.), *The Handbook of Aging and Cognition* (pp. 51–110). Hillsdale, NJ: Lawrence Erlbaum Associates.

Craik, F.I.M. & Kester, J.D. (2000). Divided attention and memory: impairment of processing or consolidation? In: E. Tulving (Ed.), *Memory, Consciousness, and the Brain: The Tallinn Conference* (pp. 38–51). Philadelphia: Psychology Press.

Craik, F.I.M. & Lockhart, R.S. (1972). Levels of processing: a framework for memory research. *Journal of Verbal Learning and Verbal Behavior, 11*, 671–684.

Craik, F.I.M. & McDowd, J.D. (1987). Age differences in recall and recognition. *Journal of Experimental Psychology: Learning, Memory, and Cognition, 13*, 474–479.

Craik, F.I.M. & Tulving, E. (1975). Depth of processing and the retention of words in episodic memory. *Journal of Experimental Psychology: General, 104*, 268–294.

Della-Maggiore, V., Sekuler, A.B., Grady, C.L., Bennett, P.J., Sekuler, R. & McIntosh, A.R. (2000). Corticolimbic interactions associated with performance on a short-term memory task are modified by age. *Journal of Neuroscience, 20*, 8410–8416.

Dempster, F.N. (1992). The rise and fall of the inhibitory mechanisms: toward a unified theory of cognitive development and aging. *Developmental Review, 12*, 45–75.

D'Esposito, M., Detre, J.A., Alsop, D.C., Shin, R.K., Atlas, S., & Grossman, M. (1995). The neural basis of the central executive system of working memory. *Nature, 378*, 279–281.

D'Esposito, M., Postle, B.R., Ballard, D., & Lease, J. (1999). Maintenance versus manipulation of information held in working memory: an event-related fMRI study. *Brain and Cognition, 41*, 66–86.

Eysenck, M.W. (1974). Age differences in incidental learning. *Developmental Psychology, 19*, 936–941.

Gardiner, J.M. Richardson-Klavehn, A. (2000). Remembering and knowing. In F.I.M. Craik E. Tulving (Eds.), *The Oxford Handbook of Memory* (pp. 229–244). New York. N.Y. Oxford University Press.

Grady, C.L., Maisog, J.M., Horwitz, B., Ungerleider, L.G., Mentis, M.J., Salerno, J.A., Pietrini, P., Wagner, E., & Haxby, J.V. (1994). Age-related changes in cortical blood flow activation during visual processing of faces and location. *Journal of Neuroscience, 14*, 1450–1462.

Grady, C.L., McIntosh, A.R., Horwitz, B., Maisog, J.M., Ungerleider, L.G., Mentis, M.J., Pietrini, P., Schapiro, M.B., & Haxby, J.V. (1995). Age-related reductions in human recognition memory due to impaired encoding. *Science, 269*, 218–221.

Grady, C.L., Horwitz, B., Pietrini, P., Mentis, M.J., Ungerleider, L.G., Rapoport, S.I., & Haxby, J.V. (1996). The effect of task difficulty on cerebral blood flow during perceptual matching of faces. *Human Brain Mapping, 4*, 227–239.

Grady, C.L., McIntosh, A.R., Bookstein, F., Horwitz, B., Rapoport, S.I., & Haxby, J.V. (1998). Age-related changes in regional cerebral blood flow during working memory for faces. *NeuroImage, 8*, 409–425.

Grady, C.L., McIntosh, A.R., Rajah, M.N., Beig, S., & Craik, F.I.M. (1999). The effects of age on the neural correlates of episodic encoding. *Cerebral Cortex, 9*, 805–814.

Grady, C.L., Bernstein, L., Siegenthaler, A., & Beig, S. (in press). The effects of encoding strategy on age-related differences in the functional neuroanatomy of face memory. *Psychology and Aging.*

Greenwood, P.M. (2000). The frontal aging hypothesis evaluated. *Journal of the International Neuropsychological Society, 6*, 705–726.

Haxby, J.V., Ungerleider, L.G., Horwitz, B., Maisog, J.M., Rapoport, S.I., & Grady, C.L. (1996). Storage and retrieval of new memories for faces in the intact human brain. *Proceedings of the National Academy of Science USA, 93*, 922–927.

Hay, J.F. & Jacoby, L.L. (1999). Separating habit and recollection in young and older adults: effects of elaborative processing and distinctiveness. *Psychology and Aging, 14*, 122–134.

Jacoby, L.L. (1983). Remembering the data: analyzing interactive processes in reading. *Journal of Verbal Learning and Verbal Behavior, 22*, 485–508.

Jacoby, L.L. (1991). A process dissociation framework: separating automatic from intentional uses of memory. *Journal of Memory and Language, 30*, 513–541.

Jennings, J.M. & Jacoby, L.L. (1993). Automatic versus intentional uses of memory: aging, attention, and control. *Psychology and Aging, 8*, 283–293.

Jonides, J., Marsheutz, C., Smith, E.E., Reuter-Lorenz, P.A., Koeppe, R.A., & Hartley, A. (2000). Age differences in behavior and PET activation reveal differences in interference resolution in verbal working memory. *Journal of Cognitive Neuroscience, 12*, 188–196.

Kensinger, E.A. & Schacter, D.L. (1999). When true

memories suppress false memories: effects of aging. *Cognitive Neuropsychology, 16*, 399–415.

Kolers, P.A. & Roediger, H.L., III (1984). Procedures of mind. *Journal of Verbal Learning and Verbal Behavior, 23*, 425–449.

Light, L.L. (1992). The organization of memory in old age. In: F.I.M. Craik & T.A. Salthouse (Eds.), *The Handbook of Aging and Cognition* (pp. 111–165). Hillsdale, NJ: Lawrence Erlbaum Associates.

Madden, D.J., Gottlob, L.R., Denny, L.L., Turkington, T.G., Provenzale, J.M., Hawk, T.C., & Coleman, R.E. (1999a). Aging and recognition memory: changes in regional cerebral blood flow associated with components of reaction time distributions. *Journal of Cognitive Neuroscience, 11*, 511–520.

Madden, D.J., Turkington, T.G., Provenzale, J.M., Denny, L.L., Hawk, T.C., Gottlob, L.R., & Coleman, R.E. (1999b). Adult age differences in the functional neuroanatomy of verbal recognition memory. *Human Brain Mapping, 7*, 115–135.

McIntosh, A.R. & Gonzalez-Lima, F. (1994). Structural equation modeling and its application to network analysis in functional brain imaging. *Human Brain Mapping, 2*, 2–22.

McIntosh, A.R., Sekuler, A.B., Penpeci, C., Rajah, M.N., Grady, C.L., Sekuler, R., & Bennett, P.J. (1999). Recruitment of unique neural systems to support visual memory in normal aging. *Current Biology, 9*, 1275–1278.

Naveh-Benjamin, M., Craik, F.I.M., Gavrilescu, D., & Anderson, N.D. (2000). Asymmetry between encoding and retrieval: evidence from divided attention and a calibration analysis. *Memory & Cognition, 28*, 965–976.

Nyberg, L., Nilsson, L.G., Olofsson, U., & Bäckman, L. (1997). Effects of division of attention during encoding and retrieval on age differences in episodic memory. *Experimental Aging Research, 23*, 137–143.

Raz, N. (2000). Aging of the brain and its impact on cognitive performance: integration of structural and functional findings. In: F.I.M. Craik & T.A. Salthouse (Eds.), *The Handbook of Aging and Cognition, 2nd. ed.* (pp. 1–90). Mahwah, NJ: Lawrence Erlbaum Associates.

Reuter-Lorenz, P.A., Jonides, J., Smith, E.E., Hartley, A., Miller, A., Marshuetz, C., & Koeppe, R.A. (2000). Age differences in the frontal lateralization of verbal and spatial working memory revealed by PET. *Journal of Cognitive Neuroscience, 12*, 174–187.

Rönnlund, M., Nyberg, L., Bäckman, L., & Nilsson, L.G. (Submitted). Recall of subject-performed tasks, verbal tasks, and cognitive activities across the adult life span: parallel age-related deficits. Submitted for publication.

Rypma, B. & D'Esposito, M. (2000). Isolating the neural mechanisms of age-related changes in human working memory. *Nature Neuroscience, 3*, 509–515.

Schacter, D.L., Savage, C.R., Alpert, N.M., Rauch, S.L., & Albert, M.S. (1996). The role of hippocampus and frontal cortex in age-related memory changes: a PET study. *NeuroReport, 7*, 1165–1169.

Spencer, W.D. & Raz, N. (1995). Differential effects of aging on memory for content and context: a meta-analysis. *Psychology and Aging, 10*, 527–539.

Stuss, D.T., Craik, F.I.M., Sayer, L., Franchi, D., & Alexander, M.P. (1996). Comparison of older people with patients with frontal lesions: evidence from word list learning. *Psychology and Aging, 11*, 387–395.

Tulving, E. (1983). *Elements of Episodic Memory*. New York: Oxford University Press.

Tulving, E. & Schacter, D.L. (1990). Priming and human memory systems. *Science, 247*, 301–306.

West, R.L. (1996). An application of prefrontal cortex function theory to cognitive aging. *Psychological Bulletin, 120*, 272–292.

Zacks, R.T., Hasher, L., & Li, K.Z.H. (2000). Human memory. In: F.I.M. Craik & T.A. Salthouse (Eds.), *The Handbook of Aging and Cognition, 2nd ed.* (pp. 293–357). Mahwah, NJ: Lawrence Erlbaum Associates.

32

Frontal Lobe Plasticity and Behavior

BRYAN KOLB AND ROBBIN GIBB

The goal of this chapter is to consider how the structure of the frontal lobe changes over time, how this relates to behavior, and how the rest of the brain changes when the frontal lobe is injured. In thinking about the relationship between the frontal lobe and behavior, there is a tendency to presume constancy in frontal lobe function, rather than change and variability. Thus, as we try to understand frontal lobe function, there is a tendency to focus on the similarities in the functional data across individuals. Indeed, it could be argued that one of the reasons that we know so much about frontal lobe function is because there is so much constancy in brain organization, not only across subjects within a species but across species as well. But the burgeoning literature on plastic changes in the brain is making it clear that change and variability are as basic to brain function as uniformity. The first goal of this chapter is to summarize some of the work on the nature of the plastic changes in frontal lobe structure and function in the normal brain. The second goal is to consider how the rest of the brain changes in response to perturbations of the frontal lobe and how this in turn contributes to behavioral change.

This review will focus on studies that have analyzed both structure and function and, in particular, those that have estimated the change in synaptic space after some treatment. The simplest way to do this is to use some type of technique that allows one to visualize an entire neuron. The most common technique is the Golgi technique, which has the advantage that a small percentage of neurons (1%–5%) are stained and these neurons are stained completely. It is thus possible to draw the individual neurons and to quantify the amount of dendritic space available, as well as the location and density of dendritic spines. These measures are used because they can be taken as estimates of the total space for synapses (i.e., dendritic length) and of the density of excitatory synapses (i.e., spine density). It is estimated that about 95% of excitatory synapses are located on dendrites and most of those are found on spines (e.g., Buell & Coleman, 1985).

FRONTAL LOBE PLASTICITY IN THE NORMAL BRAIN

EXPERIENCE-DEPENDENT CHANGES

It has been known since the early 1960s that experience can alter cortical structure, and there is now an extensive literature showing that the structure of cortical neurons is influenced by various types of sensory and motor experience (for a review see Kolb & Whishaw, 1998). For example, if laboratory animals, ranging from rats to cats and monkeys, are placed in complex environments instead of standard lab cages, there are large changes in dendritic length and synapse number throughout the primary visual and somatosensory cortex (e.g., Greenough et al., 1985; Beaulieu & Colonnier, 1987). Similarly, if rats are trained on neuropsychological learning tasks such as a visual maze or a skilled motor learning task, then there are changes in cells in occipital cortex and motor cortex, respectively (Greenough & Chang, 1989). These changes are specific, however, as visual training does not influence motor cortex neurons and visa versa. Curiously, few studies have looked at frontal regions outside of the motor cortex. With this in mind, we examined the changes in the medial prefrontal region (Zilles' area Cg3), occipital cortex (Oc1), and somatosensory cortex (Zilles' Par1) in animals that were placed either in complex environments or standard lab cages for 4 months. The results were intriguing because they showed that although cells in both the occipital and parietal cortex showed large changes in dendritic length (about 10%), there was no change in cells in Cg3 (Kolb et al., in submitted 2002). The simplest conclusion from this result is that placing animals in complex environments does not engage the prefrontal cortex and thus the cells do not change. In contrast, the complex environments do engage the sensory and motor regions and, as a result, they do change. These conclusions suggest that the presence of the prefrontal cortex is not necessary for cortical neurons to show experience-dependent change in complex housing studies (Kolb & Gibb, 1991a).

The key question that we might ask at this point is just what types of experience are likely to engage prefrontal neurons and lead to structural changes. One prediction would be that training animals in tasks that have high demands on the temporal organization of behavior (e.g., Fuster, 1989) would change neurons in the prefrontal cortex. We are unaware of any such study, but the prediction is that if the prefrontal cortex really does function in

such tasks, then training animals on this type of task should lead to changes in the structure of neurons in the prefrontal region. (Of course, it is possible that the reason that we did not see experience-dependent changes in frontal neurons is that frontal neurons are relatively unchanged by experience, but we shall see below that this is not the case.)

One hypothesis that comes from thinking in this way about the relation between structure and functions is that if specific tasks do activate specific regions of the frontal lobe, then it ought to be possible to infer functional differences in different frontal subregions from an analysis of the anatomical changes. This is, of course, the intent of positron emission tomography (PET) and functional magnetic resonance imaging (fMRI) studies, but there is a fundamental difference. The imaging studies identify those regions that are actively engaged in behaviors. The anatomical changes reflect a chronic change in the processing by frontal lobe areas as a result of having been engaged in behaviors. In other words, anatomical changes would reflect how the frontal lobe has been altered by its activation in problem solving and this, in turn, is expected to alter how the frontal lobe works in the future. The effect of psychoactive drugs (see next section) provides an example of this type of phenomenon.

There is, however, another explanation for why we failed to find increased dendritic length in prefrontal cortex of rats placed in the complex environments. Specifically, it is possible that experience changes the prefrontal cortex in a different manner, compared to other cortical areas. With this possibility in mind, we measured the density of spines on distal regions of the dendrites of pyramidal cells in prefrontal, parietal, and occipital cortex of the rats housed in the complex environments. To our surprise, we found that although the prefrontal cells did not grow longer dendrites, they did have increased spine density (Fig. 32–1), which means that there was an increase in synapses per cell but they were distributed differently than in control animals. All previous reports of experience-dependent spine changes in adult animals have shown that when there is an in-

Figure 32–1. The prefrontal cortex responds differently to experience than other cortical areas. For example, when animals are placed in complex environments, most cortical areas show an increase in dendritic length and an increase in spine density. In contrast, the prefrontal cortex shows only an increase in spine density. □, cage-housed; ■, housed in complex environment. (*Source:* After Kolb, et al., in submitted)

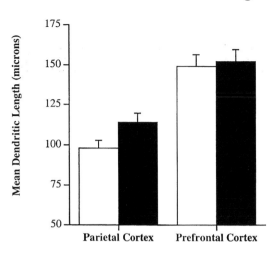

Basilar Dendritic Length

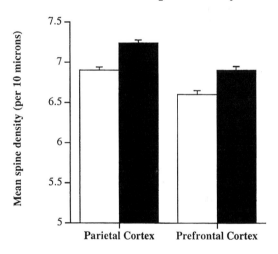

Basilar Spine Density

crease in spine density, it is always associated with increased dendritic length (e.g., Globus et al., 1973; Kolb et al., 2002). There is, however, a precedent for spine changes independent of dendritic length: two studies have shown that stimulation in infant animals leads to a decrease in spine density independent of changes in dendritic length (Bock & Braun, 1998; Kolb et al., 2002). These findings have been interpreted to show that experience during development produces changes in the brain that are different from those as a result of similar experience in adulthood. Using the same logic, we can conclude that experience in adulthood may change the prefrontal cortex in a different manner than experience changes other cortical areas. This possibility is intriguing and certainly worth pursuing. It also suggests that if we are to look for synaptic changes related to the performance of cognitive tests that engage the prefrontal cortex, these changes may not be the same as those that are found in motor or visual cortex when animals learn motor or visual tasks, respectively.

To summarize, neurons in the prefrontal cortex change in response to experience but do so differently than cells in other forebrain

Table 32–1. Summary of effects of factors on frontal cortical plasticity

Factor	Result	Reference
Complex housing	Increased spine density	Kolb et al., submitted
Psychoactive drugs	Increased dendritic length Increased spine density	Robinson & Kolb, 1999a
Cocaine self-administratation	Pathological structure of pre-frontal neurons	Robinson et al., 2001
Nerve growth factor	Increased dendritic length Increased spine density	Kolb et al., 1997
Gonadal hormones	Alter neuronal structure during development	Kolb & Stewart, 1991
	Removal of estrogen stimulates dendritic growth	Forgie & Kolb, submission
Hippocampal injury	Infant hippocampal lesions reduce synapse number	Lipska et al., 2000

areas. Specifically, many studies have shown that cortical neurons in motor and sensory cortex show experience-dependent increases in dendritic length, whereas those in prefrontal cortex show increases in spine density (Table 32–1). Past studies of experience-dependent change in prefrontal cortex that have not examined changes in spine density may thus have missed effects that were actually present.

PSYCHOACTIVE DRUGS

The repeated intermittent administration of many drugs of abuse results in a progressive increase in their psychomotor activating and rewarding effects, a phenomenon known as *behavioral sensitization* (e.g., Robinson & Berridge, 1993). Behavioral sensitization is interesting in the current context for several reasons. First, it is a compelling example of experience-dependent behavioral change. Sensitized animals remain hypersensitive to the psychomotor activating and rewarding effects of drugs for months to years. Second, the neuroadaptations that underlie behavioral sensitization may contribute to drug-induced psychopathology in humans (e.g., Segal & Schuckit, 1983). Third, the rewarding effects of psychomotor stimulant drugs are mediated by the mesolimbic dopamine system and, in particular, the projections from the dopamine-

containing cells in the ventral tegmental area to the glutamate-containing cells of the prefrontal cortex (e.g., Wise & Bozarth, 1987; Wise, 1996). Finally, it has been proposed that drugs of abuse may act on prefrontal neurons, leading to various behavioral disorders including paranoid psychosis and addiction (e.g., Berridge & Robinson, 1995). The question, therefore, is whether psychoactive drugs actually do change the structure of neurons in the frontal cortex, and if so, what does this mean about frontal lobe function.

Rats were given intermittent doses of one of several different drugs, including amphetamine, cocaine, and nicotine. Neurons in the medial frontal region (Cg 3) and parietal and occipital cortex were later analyzed using Golgi methods (e.g., Robinson & Kolb, 1997; 1999a; 1999b; Brown & Kolb, 2001; Robinson et al., 2001). The results were unequivocal: all of these drugs increased dendritic length and spine density in Cg 3 but there were no effects of the drugs on dendritic measures in the neurons in parietal or occipital cortex (Fig. 32–2). These results are remarkable because this pattern of dendritic change was exactly the opposite of what we observed in animals placed in complex housing instead of lab caging (see above). Thus, the absence of plastic changes in response to experience in the prefrontal neurons was not simply a reflection of reduced plasticity in prefrontal neurons but rather

Saline   **Amphetamine**

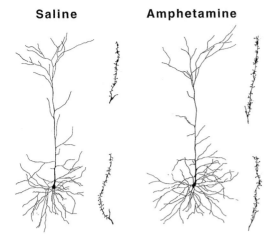

Figure 32–2. Examples of representative drawings of neurons of rats that received repeated administration of either amphetamine or saline. (*Source:* After Robinson & Kolb, 1997)

more likely indicated the engagement of the frontal neurons in response to the drugs. We should note here that the dendritic growth was not simply an artifact of increased activity in the drug-treated rats, because animals forced to run in running wheels or to bar press for food showed no dendritic changes in the neurons in Cg 3 (or Par 1).

One additional question that we addressed was whether self administration of the drugs would produce similar changes to those seen when the drugs were experimenter administered. Rats were therefore trained to self-administer cocaine for a period about as long as the rats in the initial studies had been given experiment-administered drugs. The result was clear, as there were even larger increases in the Cg 3 neurons in response to the cocaine self-administration. In addition, we found that the Cg 3 showed pathology in the form of bead-like protuberances along the distal portions of the apical dendrites (Robinson et al., 2001). It is unclear what this pathology might reflect, but one can speculate that it would lead to abnormalities in frontal lobe functioning. This is an intriguing notion, because there is accumulating evidence suggesting that cocaine addicts show neurobiological and neuropsychological signs of frontal lobe dysfunction (e.g., Bolla et al., 1998).

In sum, it appears that neurons in the frontal cortex are altered by psychomotor stimulants and that these neuronal changes may be related to changes in frontal lobe functioning. The reason for the action of the drugs is presumably because of alterations in the dopaminergic inputs to the frontal lobe. It has been hypothesized that the dopaminergic input to the frontal lobe is related to the frontal lobe's role in affect and possibly in reward, and there is little doubt that psychomotor stimulants act to alter affective experience (e.g., Tzschentke, 2000). What is still puzzling, however, is what the nature of the change in affective behavior might be after repeated exposure to psychomotor stimulants, and especially to nicotine.

NEUROTROPHIC FACTORS

Proteins known as *neurotrophic factors* are manufactured in the brain and act to influence development and maintenance of neurons. Nerve growth factor (NGF) was the first neurotrophic factor to be described and it is still the best characterized. Intraventricular infusions of NGF stimulate dendritic growth and increased spine density in cortical pyramidal cells, including those in the medial frontal region (Kolb et al., 1997). Indeed, the effect of NGF on neurons in Cg 3 is even larger than the effect of psychomotor stimulants. It is not known whether other neurotrophic factors might also influence cortical organization, but it does seem likely, and there is reason to think that at least some actions might be specific to prefrontal cortex. For example, Flores and Stewart (2000) have found that rats given sensitizing doses of amphetamine show an increase in basic fibroblast growth factor (bFGF) expression in medial frontal cortex but not in more posterior cortex. They note that bFGF may thus participate in the development of structural changes brought about by amphetamine. Importantly, although the structural changes in neurons are long-lasting and possibly permanent, the changes in bFGF are not maintained. This makes sense if the bFGF activity is involved in stimulating the dendritic changes because once changed, the bFGF would no longer be needed. It is not known whether administration of bFGF might selectively change the structure of neurons in the frontal lobe, but it seems likely. The interesting question is how this might be manifested behaviorally.

GONADAL HORMONES

In the course of studying the effects of frontal lesions in male and female rats, it became clear to us that there were sex-related differences in the behavioral outcome (e.g., Kolb & Cioe, 1996), a result that is similar to observations in both humans (e.g., Kimura, 1999) and rhesus monkeys (Clark & Goldman-Rakic, 1989). This led us to investigate whether there might be sex-related differences in the structure of cells in the prefrontal regions—namely differences between the medial frontal (Cg 1, Cg 3) and the ventral frontal regions—and, indeed, we found this to be the case (Kolb & Stewart, 1991). In general, males showed more extensive dendritic fields in the midline regions whereas females showed more extensive dendritic fields in the ventral frontal regions. These differences were hormone-dependent, as neonatal castration or ovariectomy eliminated the differences in adulthood. The presence of sexually dimorphic cell structure in different regions of the frontal cortex of rats implies that there must be some type of hormone-dependent difference in function of the different frontal cortical regions. The nature of this difference is, at present, unknown.

The presence of hormone-dependent differences in the organization of the frontal cortex of rats led us to wonder if there might be sex-related differences in the actions of gonadal hormones on neurons in the frontal cortex of adult rats. To test this possibility, we removed the ovaries or testes of adult rats, waited 3 months, and then examined the structure of cortical neurons. The results were surprising: ovariectomy resulted in an extensive increase in both dendritic length and spine density of pyramidal cells in both the medial frontal and parietal cortex (Stewart & Kolb, 1994; Forgie & Kolb, in submitted). Furthermore, this dendritic growth could be blocked by the administration of estrogen. In contrast, castration had no effect on dendritic

length, but did increase spine density. These results suggest that the circuitry of the frontal cortex is somehow influenced by gonadal hormones in the adult brain. One intriguing question is whether the slow loss of gonadal hormones has the same effect on the cortex as a sudden loss. To test this idea, we have looked at the cortical pyramidal neurons in 3-year old female rats, with and without estrogen supplements, over the last year of their life. The results were unexpected: the untreated females showed a significant atrophy and reduction in spine density, which was significantly reduced in the estrogen-treated animals. It appears that there is a difference between the sudden loss of estrogen after ovariectomy and the slow decline in estrogen levels in old age.

The results of gonadal manipulations in female rats led us to wonder whether the presence or absence of gonadal hormones influences the cortical response to experience or to injury. This question becomes especially important when we consider the effect that menopause might have on cortical organization and function. We have begun to investigate this question by examining the effects of estrogen on recovery from medial frontal injury in postmenopausal female rats (Forgie & Kolb, in submitted). The behavioral data show that the absence of estrogen actually produced a small enhancement in recovery, relative to estrogen-treated rats with lesions. This result has important implications for the treatment of stroke in human females and certainly warrants further study.

In sum, it is clear that gonadal hormones (especially estrogen) have both organizational (developmental) and activational (adult) influences on the intrinsic circuitry of the frontal lobe. It also appears that at least estrogen may influence outcome after frontal injury. What is not known yet is how gonadal hormones might influence experience-dependent changes in the frontal lobe. Given that gonadal hormones do affect hippocampal plasticity (e.g., Juraska, 1990), it seems reasonable to expect that there may be some influence on frontal lobe plasticity as well. Furthermore, Janowsky, and colleagues (2000) have shown that testosterone can modulate working memory in older men, suggesting that testosterone is able to alter the structure (or at least function) of neurons in the prefrontal cortex.

FRONTAL LOBE PLASTICITY IN THE INJURED BRAIN

When the brain is injured, there are two obvious routes to repair: *(1)* reorganization of existing circuits; and *(2)* the creation of new circuits, either by forming new connections among remaining neurons or by generating new neurons. Studies over the past decade have shown that both routes to repair are used by the brain but, curiously, there is little known about the nature of changes in the frontal lobe after injury elsewhere. Two obvious outcomes are possible. First, it is reasonable to expect that if regions of the brain that have extensive connections with the frontal cortex are damaged, then the absence of such connections could produce dendritic atrophy. At least one study shows this: when rats are given strokes that involve the motor and somatosensory regions, there is an atrophy of the neurons in Cg 3 (Kolb et al., 1997), presumably reflecting the loss of afferents from the damaged regions. Second, we could predict that if there were some form of adaptation to the injury, which could take the form of partial recovery or perhaps even the emergence of new behavioral symptoms, and if this adaptation involves frontal lobe activity, then there might be changes in frontal lobe organization. Although there are virtually no studies investigating this possibility after injuries in adult animals, a recent study in young animals is instructive. Weinberger and colleagues developed an animal model of schizophrenia in which infant rats receive lesions of the ventral hippocampus (e.g., Raedler. et al., 1998). In adulthood, these animals show various symptoms characteristic of rats with frontal lobe injuries, such as hyperactivity and deficits in social behavior and working memory (e.g, Sams-Dodd et al., 1997). These functional deficits are ameliorated by antipsychotic drugs and are associated with a decrease in the metabolites of dopamine in the medial frontal region, which has led the authors to propose that schizophrenia might result from

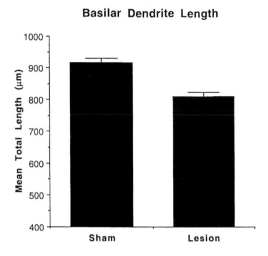

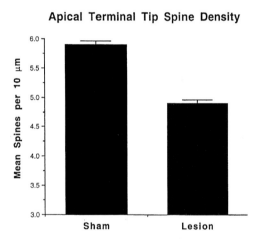

Figure 32–3. Summary of the effects of ventral hippocampal lesions in infant rats on spine density and dendritic length in neurons in the prefrontal cortex in adulthood. (*Source:* After Lipska et al., 2000)

developmental abnormalities in the hippocampal formation. (Lipska et al., 1992). Given that psychomotor stimulants enhance dopaminergic-mediated activity in the frontal lobe and produce an expansion of dendritic fields in medial frontal cortex in rats, it is reasonable to predict that decreased prefrontal dopaminergic activity after infant hippocampal lesions might decrease dendritic arborization and spine density in prefrontal cortex. This is indeed the case, as there is a reduction in dendritic arborization and a drop in spine density in prefrontal, but not parietal cortex, in rats with early hippocampal lesions (Fig. 32–3);

Lipska et al., 2000). This is an exciting result, because it suggests that injury elsewhere in the brain may alter connectivity in the frontal lobe, and that, in turn, may alter behavior.

CORTICAL PLASTICITY AFTER FRONTAL LOBE INJURY

We are aware of only two studies that examined changes in cortical neurons after frontal lesions in adulthood (Kolb & Gibb, 1991a; Kolb, 1995). These studies showed that there is a gradual improvement in maze performance, but not skilled motor behavior, after frontal injury in rats. Subsequent Golgi-Cox analyses revealed that there is an initial atrophy of dendritic fields in remaining frontal regions but this reverses over a 1 to 3 month period, resulting in an expansion of the dendritic fields in the same cells. (A parallel result is seen after lesions in the hippocampal system as well [Steward, 1991]). It seems likely that the observed recovery is supported, at least in part, by the reorganization of intrinsic cortical circuits. We hasten to point out, however, that this reorganization is insufficient to influence recovery of skilled motor sequences or of species' typical behaviors (e.g., food hoarding, nest building, social behavior). This rather limited functional recovery after frontal lobe lesions is not only observed in rats but is also typical of humans with frontal cortical excisions (Kolb, 1995). There is, however, a circumstance under which there is much better functional recovery after frontal injury and that is during development. The privileged status of the infant brain has been known since the time of Broca as he noted that children with lesions of the left frontal operculum are virtually never chronically aphasic, the only exception being if there are bilateral lesions. There is now an extensive literature on the effects of early frontal injury in rats, cats, and monkeys, which we shall consider in some detail.

BEHAVIORAL SEQUELAE OF EARLY FRONTAL LESIONS

Perhaps the best-known studies on the effects of early brain injury on behavior were those performed by Margaret Kennard in the late 1930s (e.g., Kennard, 1942). She made unilateral motor cortex lesions in infant and adult monkeys. The behavioral impairments in the infant monkeys were milder than those in the adults, which led Kennard to hypothesize that there had been a change in cortical organization in the infants and these changes supported the behavioral recovery. In particular, she hypothesized that if some synapses were removed as a consequence of brain injury, "others would be formed in less usual combinations" and that "it is possible that factors which facilitate cortical organization in the normal young are the same by which reorganization is accomplished in the imperfect cortex after injury" (Kennard, 1942, p. 239). Although Kennard had much to say regarding the limitations of functional recovery after early brain injury (see review by Finger & Almli, 1988), it was her demonstration that the consequences of motor cortex lesions in infancy were less severe than similar injury in adulthood that is usually associated with her name, and is commonly referred to as the *Kennard principle*.

Kennard was aware that early brain damage might actually produce more severe deficits than expected, but it was Hebb (1947; 1949) who emphasized this possibility. On the basis of his studies of children with frontal lobe injuries, Hebb concluded that an early injury may prevent the development of some intellectual capacities that an equally extensive injury, at maturity, would not have destroyed. Hebb believed that this outcome resulted from a failure of initial organization of the brain, thus making it difficult for the child to develop many behaviors, especially socioaffective behaviors. During the 1960s and 1970s several groups examined the effects of frontal lobe lesions in infant monkeys (e.g., Harlow et al., 1964; Goldman, 1974). Although the initial studies appeared to support Kennard's earlier conclusions, it became clear by the mid-1970s that there was far less functional recovery in the infant operates than had been claimed, unless the injuries were induced prenatally (e.g., Goldman & Galkin, 1978). The Goldman studies were important because they pointed to the need for a thorough analysis of the precise age at injury during development. This type of study is impractical in monkeys, but because rats are born early in gestation, it is possible to manipulate age at injury ex utero in rats and there is indeed a very tight relationship between functional recovery and age at injury. Consider the following example.

We have removed the frontal cortex of different groups of rats at various ages ranging from embryonic day 18 (the gestation period of a rat is about 22 days) through infancy and adolescence (e.g., Kolb, 1995). The behavioral results can be illustrated by the spatial navigation performance of rats with removal of the frontal cortex on embryonic day 18 (E18), postnatal day 1 (P1), 5, 10, or 90 (i.e., adult). Rats are trained to find a hidden platform in a swimming pool. Figure 32–4 shows that rats with lesions in adulthood or on day 1 show severe deficits relative to control animals whereas rats with lesions on day 5 show intermediate deficits and those with E18 or P10 lesions show very little or no deficit at all. Parallel results can be seen on other behavioral tests as well. Functional outcome thus clearly varies with precise age at injury. On the basis of our studies we can reach the following conclusion: damage during the period of neurogenesis, which in the rat cortex is from about

E12 to E20, appears to be associated with a good functional outcome (see also Hicks & D'Amato, 1961); damage in the first week of life, which is a time of neural migration and the initiation of synaptic formation, is associated with a dismal outcome; damage in the second week of life, which is a time of maximal astrocyte generation and synapse development, results in an excellent functional outcome; and damage after 2 weeks leads to progressively more severe chronic behavioral loss. A similar pattern of results can be seen in parallel studies of the effects of cortical lesions in kittens by Villablanca and colleagues (e.g., Villablanca et al., 1993). A key point here is that birth date is irrelevant. It is the developmental stage of the brain at injury that is critical. Thus, because rats and kittens are born at an embryologically younger age than primates, including humans, the time scale for functional outcome must be adjusted to match the neural events that are underway at the time of injury. Because neural generation is most intense during the second trimester in humans and is largely complete by the third trimester, the second trimester is probably most similar to the last week of gestation in the rat. Similarly, because the third trimester in humans is a time of active cell migration and the beginning of differentiation, the third trimester of humans parallels the first week of life in the infant rat. From these observations we would predict that the worst time for injury during development in the human frontal lobe would likely be the third trimester whereas there should be relatively good compensation for injuries during the second trimester (see Chapter 30).

In sum, there is a clear relationship between age at prefrontal injury and functional recovery. Rats or cats with lesions during the time of neuronal migration show a very poor functional outcome whereas similar lesions during the time of peak synaptogenesis lead to a very good functional outcome. Similar results can be seen in human infants as well (see Chapter 30). Given that there are qualitative changes in the growth of the prefrontal cortex of infants and children (e.g., Thompson et al., 2000), it is reasonable to wonder if there might be additional age-related variations in functional outcome during the more pro-

Morris Water Task Latency

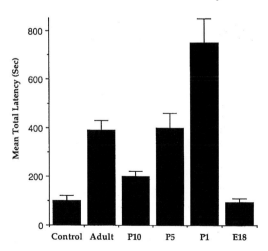

Figure 32–4. Summary of the effects of large frontal cortex lesions at different ages on water task performance. Animals with lesions at embryonic day 18 (E18) do not differ from control animals. Animals with lesions on postnatal day (P10) have a slight impairment in contrast to the animals with lesions at P1, P5, or in adulthood.

longed development of the prefrontal cortex in children.

BRAIN PLASTICITY AFTER EARLY FRONTAL INJURY

One of the most obvious, and consistent, changes in the brain after early frontal injury is that brain size in adulthood is directly related to the postnatal age at injury: the earlier the injury, the smaller the brain and the thinner the cortical mantle. Thus, rats with perinatal lesions have very small brains whereas those with lesions at day 10 have larger brains. Curiously, however, the day 10 brains still are markedly smaller than the brains of rats with lesions later in life, such as at day 25, even though the behavioral outcome is far better (Kolb & Whishaw, 1981; Kolb et al., 1996). Therefore, it must be the organization of the brain rather than its size that predicts recovery in the day 10 animal. Changes in organization can be inferred from an analysis of dendritic organization, cortical connectivity, and evidence of neurogenesis. (We note here that it is not just age at injury that determines the adult brain size. Thus, although rats with prenatal frontal lesions do have small brains, they are larger than those of animals with lesions in the first postnatal week. This, of course, correlates with the observed functional outcome.)

DENDRITIC ORGANIZATION

Golgi analyses of cortical neurons of rats with perinatal lesions consistently show a general stunting of dendritic arborization and a drop in spine density across the cortical mantle (e.g., Kolb & Gibb, 1991b; 1993; Kolb et al., 1994). In contrast, rats with cortical lesions around 10 days of age show an increase in dendritic arbor and an increase in spine density relative to normal control littermates. Thus, animals with the best functional outcome show the largest dendritic fields whereas animals with the worst functional outcome have the smallest dendritic arbor relative to control animals. Furthermore, factors that act

to increase dendritic space also enhance functional outcome whereas those that act to decrease dendritic space act to retard functional outcome (see below).

CHANGES IN CORTICAL CONNECTIVITY

There is a tendency to presume that animals with nearly complete functional recovery after early injury will show extensive reorganization of connections throughout the brain. We noted earlier, however, that most connections of pyramidal cells are with neighboring cells and that in most instances plastic changes reflect reorganization of intrinsic circuitry, which is reflected in the dendritic changes. To examine the possibility that there might also be changes in cortical connectivity with other structures, we used retrograde tracing techniques to map the cortical–cortical, cortical–thalamic, and cortical–fugal pathways after frontal lesions on days 1 or 10. The results were surprising, as animals with frontal lesions on day 1 showed massive changes in cortical connectivity but these animals had the worst behavioral outcome (Kolb et al., 1994). Furthermore, we showed that the abnormal pathways did not reflect the creation of new connections so much as they reflected a failure of pruning of connections that are normally discarded during development. This was demonstrated by our finding that newborn animals have extensive aberrant pathways that die off during the first week of life. If the cortex is damaged during this time, however, some of these pathways fail to die off, leaving the animal with apparently novel circuitry that is not seen in normally developing animals. Some of this unusual circuitry could prove helpful after an injury, but given that normal animals shed such circuitry it seems likely that it could prove equally disadvantageous to maintain such circuitry. Indeed, both hypotheses are confirmed. Rats with infant motor cortex lesions do show sparing of some motor skills (Whishaw & Kolb, 1988), but apparently at the price of impairments in other cognitive functions (e.g. Kolb et al., 2000). It therefore seems likely that the presence of abnormal corticofugal pathways after early cortical injury may be as disruptive as it is helpful. This possibility has been termed *crowding* to reflect the idea that the normal functions of a cortical region can be crowded out by the development of abnormal connections (e.g., Teuber, 1975).

CHANGES IN NEUROGENESIS

In the course of studies of the effect of restricted lesions of the medial frontal cortex or olfactory bulb, we discovered that, in contrast to lesions elsewhere in the cerebrum, midline telencephalic lesions on postnatal days 7–12 led to spontaneous regeneration of the lost regions, or at least partial regeneration of the lost regions (Fig. 32–5). Similar injuries either before or after this temporal window did not produce such a result. Analysis of the medial frontal region showed that the area contained newly generated neurons that formed at least some of the normal connections of this region (Kolb et al., 1998c). Furthermore, animals

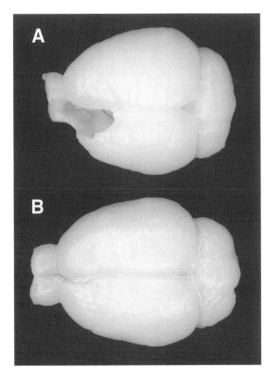

Figure 32–5. Photographs illustrating the regeneration of unilateral midline frontal cortex after a lesion on postnatal day 10 (A) but not after a similar lesion on postnatal day 1 (B).

with this regrown cortex appeared virtually normal on many, although not all, behavioral measures (e.g., Kolb et al., 1996). Additional studies showed that if we blocked regeneration of the tissue with prenatal injections of the mitotic marker bromodeoxyuridine (BrdU), the lost frontal tissue failed to regrow and there was no recovery of function (Kolb et al., submitted), a result that implies that the regrown tissue was supporting recovery. Parallel studies in which we removed the regrown tissue found complementary results: removal of the tissue eliminated the functional recovery (Dallison & Kolb, submitted). Thus, in the absence of the regrown tissue, whether we blocked the growth or removed the tissue, function was lost.

One question that arises is whether the regeneration of lost brain during infancy influences later plastic events in the brain. For example, does the generation of so many new cells during infancy compromise the brain's ability to generate cells for the olfactory bulb or hippocampus in adulthood? To test this possibility we made frontal lesions in mice at P7, and later in adulthood we removed the stem cells from the subventricular zone and placed them in vitro with neurotrophic factors (Kolb et al., 1999). When stem cells are placed in such a medium they normally divide rapidly, producing large numbers of new stem cells and progenitor cells (e.g., Weiss et al., 1996). In contrast to the cells from control mice, which produced thousands of new cells in vitro, the cells from the brains of the animals with previous P7 lesions produced few new cells. The early brain damage followed by regeneration of the lost tissue appears to have used up the proliferative potential of the subventricular stem cells, leading to an abnormal response in adulthood. We do not yet know what implications this result has for the normal endogenous production of new neurons in adulthood, but it seems likely that it will not be normal. Once again, there appears to be a price to be paid for plastic changes in the infant brain.

In sum, it appears that neurogenesis can be reinitiated after frontal lesions on postnatal days 7–12. The reason for the particularity of this time and place for neurogenesis is unclear, but these results show that regeneration of lost tissue is possible. This regeneration may not be without cost to later plastic changes in the brain, however.

In conclusion, studies of laboratory rats with cortical lesions at different developmental ages have shown that there are a variety of morphological changes that follow early cortical injury (see Table 32–2). These changes include either increases or decreases in synaptic space, alterations in corticofugal connectivity, and the regeneration of cortical tissue. Functional recovery correlates with increases in cortical synaptic space and the generation of new neurons, but changes in corticofugal connections may be as disruptive as helpful in stimulating functional recovery.

THE FUTURE: STIMULATING PLASTICITY

We have examined the changes produced in the structure of neurons in the frontal lobe in response to both experience, including drug experience and injury elsewhere in the brain, and to the changes in the brain after frontal lobe injury. There are two obvious directions for the future: *(1)* correlating anatomical change with behaviors that engage the frontal lobe; and, *(2)* using information on brain plasticity to stimulate functional recovery after injury to both the frontal lobe and beyond.

ANATOMICAL CHANGE AND FRONTAL LOBE FUNCTION

We noted earlier that imaging studies function in part to identify cortical regions that are *actively engaged* in particular behaviors. The literature and other chapters in this volume have now shown many such examples. We noted too that, in contrast, anatomical changes reflect a *chronic change* in the processing by frontal lobe areas as a result of having been engaged in behaviors. Thus, anatomical changes can be seen to reflect how the synaptic organization of the frontal lobe has been altered by its activation in problem solving. Such changes in frontal lobe organization can be expected to alter how the frontal lobe works in the future. To date, there are few studies of this sort; this is an area of research that is ripe for new investigations. A good example in the normal brain would be to study the nature of the changes in frontal lobe structure during development. We know, for example, that the frontal lobe of children is very late in functional development (e.g., Kolb et al., 1992). We would predict, therefore, that there should be prolonged change in the synaptic organization of the frontal cortex and we can speculate that these changes are likely to be heavily influenced by experiences of various sorts. One could expect that many experiences, including social, sexual, and cognitive experiences, as well as hormones, drugs, and neurotrophic factors would influence the development of the synaptic organization of the frontal lobe of laboratory animals and, by ex-

Table 32–2. Summary of effects of frontal cortical injury at different ages

Age at Injury	Result	Reference
E18	Cortex regrows with odd structure Functional recovery	Kolb et al., 1998a
P1–P6	Small brain, dendritic atrophy Dismal functional outcome	Kolb & Gibb, 1990 Kolb, 1987
P7–P12	Dendrite and spine growth Cortical regrowth Functional recovery	Kolb & Gibb, 1991b Kolb et al., 1998c
P120	Dendritic atrophy, then growth Partial return of function	Kolb, 19957

E18, embryonic day 18; P*x*, postnatal day *x*.

tension, children. Consider, for example, that Donald Hebb (1949) believed that the frontal lobe's activity was essential for the development of normal intellectual capacities. He noted that frontal lobe injuries in children often produced larger functional deficits than similar injury in adulthood and he concluded that early injury may prevent the development of some intellectual capacities that, once developed, would not have been influenced by injury in adulthood. We noted too, that damage to the hippocampus in infancy results in abnormal morphology of cells in the frontal lobe, a condition that may be a model of schizophrenia. One question that immediately comes to mind is whether treatments for schizophrenia, such as antipyschotic drugs, might act to normalize the structure of these cells. Such studies could have important implications for our understanding of both the etiology and treatment of schizophrenia, and presumably other disorders as well.

STIMULATING FUNCTIONAL RECOVERY

Although it is generally assumed that behavioral therapies will improve recovery from cerebral injury in humans, there have been few direct studies of how this might work, when the optimal time for therapy might be, or even whether it is actually effective (e.g., Kwakkel et al., 1997). Furthermore, as we try to develop animal models of cognitive or motor therapies, we are left with the problem of determining what an appropriate therapy might be. One approach to this challenge has been to focus on manipulations that we know are capable of changing the brain of intact animals and then expose brain-injured animals, especially those with poor functional outcomes, to the same experiences. We know, for example, that sensory and motor experience, psychomotor stimulants, gonadal hormones, and neurotrophic factors all change the normal brain. The question, therefore, is whether these factors might also facilitate recovery in the injured brain, and especially in the brain with frontal lobe injury (for reviews see Kolb et al., 1998a; 2000). For example, given that nicotine can stimulate synaptic change in the cortex, one would predict that the injured brain could

be treated by use of nicotine as a postinjury treatment. Furthermore, given that we know that behavioral experience, such as complex housing or motor or cognitive training, can stimulate synaptic change as well, we might predict that a combination of nicotine and behavioral therapy might be expected to stimulate considerable synaptic change, and presumably functional recovery. This is likely to be an active area of research over the next decade, both in laboratory studies and in the clinic.

In sum, although the history of the neuropsychological study of frontal lobe function and organization has been devoted largely to constancy in frontal lobe function, it is clear that an understanding of its change and variability provides a complementary broth of information that should attract more researchers over the coming decades.

CONCLUSIONS

1. Experience-dependent changes in the synaptic organization of the cortex (i.e., cortical plasticity) can tell us a great deal about what the functions of the prefrontal cortex are. Because synaptic organization can be inferred from changes in the dendritic morphology of prefrontal neurons, it is possible to do postmortem studies on neurons in the frontal lobe of both humans and laboratory animals with different types of experiential histories.

2. The prefrontal cortex is plastic, but its plasticity is different from that of other forebrain areas. For example, housing animals in complex environments increases dendritic length of cells in all sensory and motor areas as well as in the striatum and hippocampus, but does not alter medial prefrontal neurons. Surprisingly, placing animals in complex environments increases spine density in prefrontal neurons even though the dendritic length is unaffected. In contrast, exposure to psychomotor stimulants, certain neurotrophic factors, and gonadal hormones increases dendritic length in prefrontal neurons but not those in sensory or motor regions.

3. The organization of prefrontal cortex is

affected by injury, and especially perinatal injury, in other parts of the brain.

4. Other parts of the brain change when the prefrontal cortex is damaged.

5. Various factors modulate the injury-related changes observed after frontal lobe injury. These include experience, psychomotor stimulants, gonadal hormones, neurotrophic factors, and neuromodulators.

REFERENCES

Beaulieu, C. & Colonnier, M. (1987). Effect of the richness of the environment on the cat visual cortex. *Journal of Comparative Neurology, 266,* 478–494.

Berridge, K.C. & Robinson, T.E. (1995). The mind of an addicted brain: neural sensitization of wanting versus liking. *Current Directions in Psychological Science, 4,* 71–76.

Bock, J. & Braun, K. (1998). Differential emotional experience leads to pruning of dendritic spines in the forebrain of domestic chicks. *Neural Plasticity, 6,* 17–27.

Bolla, K.I., Cadet, J.L., & London, E.D. (1998). The neuropsychiatry of chronic cocaine abuse. *Journal of Neuropsychiatry and Clinical Neuroscience, 10,* 280–289.

Brown, R.W. & Kolb, B. (2001). Nicotine sensitization increases dendritic length and spine density in the nucleus accumbens and cingulate cortex. *Brain Research, 899,* 94–100.

Buell, S.J. & Coleman, P.D. (1985). Regulation of dendritic extent in developing and aging brain. In C.W. Cotman (Ed.), *Synaptic Plasticity,* (pp. 311–333). New York: Raven Press.

Clark, A.S. & Goldman-Rakic, P.S. (1989). Gonadal hormones influence the emergence of cortical function in nonhuman primates. *Behavioral Neuroscience, 103,* 1287–1295.

Dallison, A. & Kolb, B. (submitted). Recovery from infant frontal cortical lesions in rats can be reversed by cortical lesions in adulthood.

Finger, S. & Almli, C.R. (1988). Margaret Kennard and her "principle" in historical perspective. In S. Finger, T.E. Le Vere, C.R. Almli, & D.G. Stein (Eds.), *Brain Injury and Recovery: Theoretical and Controversial Issues* (pp. 117–132). New York: Plenum Press.

Flores, C. & Stewart, J. (2000). Changes in astrocytic basic fibroblast growth factor expression during and after prolonged exposure to escalating doses of amphetamine. *Neuroscience, 98,* 287–293.

Forgie, M. & Kolb, B. (Submitted) Ovariectomy and senescence in female rats alters cortical neuronal morphology in different ways.

Fuster, J. (1989). *The Prefrontal Cortex.* New York: Plenum Press.

Globus, A., Rosenzweig, M.R., Bennett, E.L., & Diamond, M.C. (1973). Effects of differential experience on dendritic spine counts in rat cerebral cortex. *Journal of Comparative and Physiological Psychology, 82,* 175–181.

Goldman, P.S. (1974). An alternative to developmental plasticity: Heterology of CNS structures in infants and adults. In: D.G. Stein J.J., Rosen & N. Bulters (Eds.) *Plasticity and Recovery of Function in the Central Nervous System.* New York: Academic Press (pp. 149–174).

Goldman, P.S. & Galkin, T.W. (1978). Prenatal removal of frontal association cortex in the fetal rhesus monkey: Anatomical and functional consequences in postnatal life. *Brain Research, 152,* 451–485.

Greenough, W.T. & Chang, F.F. (1989). Plasticity of synapse structure and pattern in the cerebral cortex. In A. Peters & E.G. Jones (Eds.), *Cerebral Cortex, Vol. 7,* 391–440. New York: Plenum Press.

Greenough, W.T., Larson, J.R., & Withers, G.S. (1985). Effects of unilateral and bilateral training in a reaching task on dendritic branching of neurons in the rat motor-sensory forelimb cortex. *Behavioral and Neural Biology, 44,* 301–314.

Harlow, H.F., Akert, K., & Schlitz, K.A. (1964). The effects of bilateral lesions on learned behavior of neonatal, infant, and preadolescent monkeys. In: J.M. Warren & K. Akert (Eds.), *The Frontal Granular Cortex and Behavior* (pp. 126–148). New York: McGraw-Hill.

Hebb, D.O. (1947). The effects of early experience on problem solving at maturity. *American Psychologist, 2,* 737–745.

Hebb, D.O. (1949). *The Organization of Behavior.* New York: McGraw-Hill.

Hicks, S. & D'Amato, C.J. (1961). How to design and build abnormal brains using radiation during development. In: W.S. Fields & M.M. Desmond (Eds.), *Disorders of the Developing Nervous System* (pp. 60–79). Springfield, IL: C.C. Thomas.

Janowsky, J.S., Chavez, B., & Orwoll, E. (2000). Sex steroids modify working memory. *Journal of Cognitive Neuroscience, 12,* 407–414.

Juraska J.M. (1990). The structure of the cerebral cortex: effects of gender and the environment. In B. Kolb & R. Tees (Eds.), *The Cerebral Cortex of the Rat,* (pp. 483–506). Cambridge, MA: MIT Press.

Kennard, M. (1942). Cortical reorganization of motor function. *Archives of Neurology, 48,* 227–240.

Kimura, D. (1999). *Sex and Cognition.* Cambridge, MA: MIT Press.

Kolb, B. (1987). Recovery from early cortical damage in rats. I. Differential behavioral and anatomical effects of frontal lesions at different ages of neural maturation. *Behavioural Brain Research, 25,* 205–220.

Kolb, B. (1995). *Brain Plasticity and Behavior.* Mahwah, NJ: Lawrence Erlbaum Associates.

Kolb, B. & Cioe, J. (1996). Sex-related differences in cortical function after medial frontal lesions in rats. *Behavioral Neuroscience, 110,* 1271–1281.

Kolb, B. & Gibb, R. (1991a). Environmental enrichment and cortical injury: behavioral and anatomical consequences of frontal cortex lesions. *Cerebral Cortex, 1,* 189–198.

Kolb, B. & Gibb, R. (1991b). Sparing of function after neonatal frontal lesions correlates with increased cortical dendritic branching: a possible mechanism for the Kennard effect. *Behavioural Brain Research, 43,* 51–56.

Kolb, B. & Gibb, R. (1993). Possible anatomical basis of recovery of spatial learning after neonatal prefrontal lesions in rats. *Behavioral Neuroscience, 107,* 799–811.

Kolb, B. & Stewart, J. (1991). Sex-related differences in dendritic branching of cells in the prefrontal cortex of rats. *Journal of Neuroendocrinology, 3,* 95–99.

Kolb, B. & Whishaw, I.Q. (1981). Neonatal frontal lesions in the rat: Sparing of learned but not species-typical behavior in the presence of reduced brain weight and cortical thickness. *Journal of Comparative and Physiological Psychology, 95,* 863–879.

Kolb, B. & Whishaw, I.Q. (1998). Brain plasticity and behavior. *Annual Review of Psychology, 49,* 43–64.

Kolb, B., Wilson, B., & Taylor, L. (1992). Development of face emotion recognition in children. *Brain and Cognition, 20,* 74–84.

Kolb, B., Gibb, R., & van der Kooy, D. (1994). Neonatal frontal cortical lesions in rats alter cortical structure and connectivity. *Brain Research, 645,* 85–97.

Kolb, B., Petrie, B., & Cioe, J. (1996). Recovery from early cortical damage in rats. VII. Comparison of the behavioural and anatomical effects of medial prefrontal lesions at different ages of neural maturation. *Behavioural Brain Research, 79,* 1–13.

Kolb, B., Cote, S., Ribeiro-da-Silva, R., & Cuello, A.C. (1997). NGF stimulates recovery of function and dendritic growth after unilateral motor cortex lesions in rats. *Neuroscience, 76,* 1139–1151.

Kolb, B., Cioe, J., & Muirhead, D. (1998a) Cerebral morphology and functional sparing after prenatal frontal cortex lesions in rats. *Behavioural Brain Research, 91,* 143–155.

Kolb, B., Gibb, R., Gorny, G., & Whishaw, I.Q. (1998c). Possible brain regrowth after cortical lesions in rats. *Behavioural Brain Research, 91,* 127–141.

Kolb, B., Gibb, R., Martens, D.J., Coles, B., & van der Kooy, D. (1999). Proliferation of neural stem cells in vitro and in vivo is reduced by infant frontal cortex lesions or prenatal BrdU. *Society for Neuroscience Abstracts, 25.*

Kolb, B., Cioe, J., & Whishaw, I.Q. (2000). Is there an optimal age for recovery from motor cortex lesions? Behavioural and anatomical sequelae of bilateral motor cortex lesions in rats on postnatal days 1, 10, and in adulthood. *Brain Research, 882,* 62–74.

Kolb, B., Gibb., R., & Gorny, G. (2002) Experience-dependent changes in dendritic arbor and spine density in neocortex vary qualitatively with age and sex. *Neurobiology of Learning and Memory.*

Kolb, B., Pedersen, B., & Gibb, R. (submitted). Recovery from frontal cortex lesions in infancy is blocked by embryonic pretreatment with bromodeoxyuridine.

Kolb, B., Gorny, G., & Robinson, T. (submitted). Complex housing increases dendritic arborization and spine density in sensory cortex and striatum but not in prefrontal cortex.

Kwakkel, G., Wagenaar, R.C., Koelman, T.W., Lankhorst,

G.J., & Koetsier, J.C. (1997). Effects of intensity of rehabilitation after stroke. A research synthesis *Stroke 28,* 1550–1556.

Lipska, B.K., Jaskiw, G.E., Chrapusta, S., Karoum, F., & Weinberger, D.R. (1992). Ibotenic acid lesion of the ventral hippocampus differentially affects dopamine and its metabolites in the nucleus accumbens and prefrontal cortex in the rat. *Brain Research, 585,* 1–6.

Lipska, B.K., Weinberger, D.R., & Kolb, B. (2000). Synaptic pathology in prefrontal cortex and nucleus accumbens of adult rats with neonatal hippocampal damage. Presented at the American College of Neuropsychopharmacology Annual Meeting, San Juan, Puerto Rico, 2000.

Raedler, T.J., Knable, M.B., & Weinberger, D.R. (1998). Schizophrenia as a developmental disorder of the cerebral cortex. *Current Opinion in Neurobiology, 8,* 157–161.

Robinson, T.E. & Berridge, K.C. (1993). The neural basis of drug craving: an incentive–sensitization theory of addiction. *Brain Research Reviews, 18,* 247–291.

Robinson, T.E. & Kolb, B. (1997). Persistent structural adaptations in nucleus accumbens and prefrontal cortex neurons produced by prior experience with amphetamine. *Journal of Neuroscience, 17,* 8491–8498.

Robinson, T.E. & Kolb, B. (1999a). Alterations in the morphology of dendrites and dendritic spines in the nucleus accumbens and prefrontal cortex following repeated treatment with amphetamine or cocaine. *European Journal of Neuroscience, 11,* 1598–1604.

Robinson, T.E. & Kolb, B. (1999b). Morphine alters the structure of neurons in nucleus accumbens and neocortex. *Synapse, 33,* 160–162.

Robinson, T., Mitton, E., Gorny, G., & Kolb, B. (2001). Self administration of cocaine modifies neuronal morphology in nucleus accumbens and prefrontal cortex. *Synapse, 39,* 257–266.

Sams-Dodd, F., Lipska, B.K., & Weinberger, D.R. (1997). Neonatal lesions of the rat ventral hippocampus result in hyper locomotion and deficits in social behaviour in adulthood. *Psychopharmacology, 132,* 303–310.

Segal, D.S. & Schuckit, M.A. (1983). Animal models of stimulant-induced psychosis. In I. Creese (Ed.), *Stimulants: Neurochemical, Behavioral and Clinical Perspectives,* (pp. 131–167. New York: Raven Press.

Steward, O. (1991). Synapse replacement on cortical neurons following denervation. In A. Peters, & E.G. Jones (Eds.) *Cerebral cortex, 9,* 81–132. New York: Plenum.

Stewart, J. & Kolb, B. (1994). Dendritic branching in cortical pyramidal cells in response to ovariectomy in adult female rats: suppression by neonatal exposure to testosterone. *Brain Research, 654,* 149–154.

Thompson, P.M., Giedd, J.N., Woods, R.P., MacDonald, D., Evans, A.C., & Toga, A.W. (2000). Growth patterns in the developing brain detected by using continuum mechanical sensory maps. *Nature, 404,* 190–193.

Teuber, H.L. (1975). Recovery of function after brain injury in man. In: *Outcome of Severe Damage to the Ner-*

vous System, Ciba Foundation Symposium 34. Amsterdam: Elsevier North-Holland.

Tzschentke, T.M. (2000). The medial prefrontal cortex as a part of the brain reward system. *Amino Acids, 19,* 211–219.

Villablanca, J.R., Hovda, D.A., Jackson, G.F., & Infante, C. (1993). Neurological and behavioral effects of a unilateral frontal cortical lesion in fetal kittens: II. Visual system tests, and proposing a 'critical period' for lesion effects. *Behavioural Brain Research, 57,* 79–92.

Weiss, S., Reynolds, B.A., Vescovi, A.L., Morshead, C., Craig, C.G., & van der Kooy, D. (1996). Is there a neu-

ral stem cell in the mammalian forebrain? *Trends Neuroscience, 19,* 387–393.

Whishaw, I.Q. & Kolb, B. (1988). Sparing of skilled forelimb reaching and corticospinal projections after neonatal motor cortex removal or hemidecortication in the rat: support for the Kennard doctrine. *Brain Research, 451,* 97–114.

Wise, R.A. (1996). Neurobiology of addiction. *Current Opinion in Neurobiology, 6,* 243–51.

Wise, R.A. & Bozarth, M.A. (1987). A psychomotor stimulant theory of addiction. *Psychological Review, 94,* 469–492.

33

Principles of the Rehabilitation of Frontal Lobe Function

PAUL W. BURGESS AND IAN H. ROBERTSON

The aim of this chapter is to outline the practical rehabilitation implications of current theories and models of executive deficits following frontal lobe damage. We do not intend to review comprehensively the literature concerning the rehabilitation of executive functions, nor to provide clinical guidelines (see Mateer, 1999; Robertson, 1999). Moreover, we do not aim to address the treatment of the motor and language functions of the frontal lobes, but concentrate instead on the executive functions of the frontal lobes. Within this area, we shall attempt to outline the practical rehabilitation implications of current theories and models of frontal lobe function, with the aim of providing some provisional principles for the rehabilitation of the dysexecutive patient.

INTRODUCTION

Many of the symptoms that rehabilitation practitioners find particularly difficult to treat are those associated with frontal lobe abnormalities (e.g., apathy; Okada et al., 1997). Moreover, frontal executive dysfunction can affect a patient's ability to benefit from therapy aimed at ameliorating other forms of deficit (e.g., physical therapy) and is often asso-

ciated with a generally poor response to treatment (e.g., Alderman, 1996; Tamamoto et al., 2000). Additionally, dysexecutive problems are common in neurological patients, as we shall see below. For these reasons, it is vital that a theory of how the workings of rehabilitation might work is developed as quickly as possible. There are two main obstacles at present. The first is the myriad of symptoms of frontal lobe dysfunction, and the second is the theoretical complexity involved in investigating (and therefore understanding) them. As regards the theoretical complexity, although very significant gaps in our knowledge still exist (see Burgess, 1997), the current volume is a testament to the very rapid progress now being made in this area, which gives us every reason to be optimistic. However, as we shall see, it is still not always easy to bridge the gap between experimental work and the treatment of real-life symptoms. Nevertheless, we firmly believe that it is possible to do so (within limits).

As regards the range of symptoms of executive dysfunction, consider Table 33–1. This lists the twenty most commonly reported symptoms of frontal lobe dysfunction that were described in the seminal works of Stuss and Benson (1984, 1986). There are also many other symptoms that are less common but

Table 33–1. Frequencies of reporting dysexecutive symptoms°

Symptom	Patients Reporting Problem (%)	Caregivers Reporting Problem (%)	Rank of Disagreement†	Scaled Disagreement in Ranks‡
Poor abstract thinking	17	21	16.5	−9
Impulsivity	22	22	19.5	−10
Confabulation	5	5	19.5	+3
Planning	16	48	1	+8
Euphoria	14	28	5	+7
Poor temporal sequencing	18	25	15	−8
Lack of insight	17	39	3	+5
Apathy	20	27	13	−5
Disinhibition (social)	15	23	13	−3
Variable motivation	13	15	18	−7
Shallow affect	14	23	10.5	+1
Aggression	12	25	6	+6
Lack of concern	9	26	4	+9
Perseveration	17	26	10.5	−1
Restlessness	25	28	16.5	−6
Can't inhibit responses	11	21	9	+4
Know–do dissociation	13	21	13	−2
Distractibility	32	42	8	+1
Poor decision making	26	38	7	−3
Unconcern for social rules	13	38	2	+10

°Only ratings of 3 or 4 (out of a maximum of 4) for each item on the dysexecutive (DEX) questionnaire (Burgess et al., 1996a) were considered as indicating a problem. These correspond to classification of the symptom as "often" or "very often" observed. These results are based on data gathered as part of the study by Wilson et al., (1996).

†This number represents the rank size of the disagreements (in proportions reporting the symptom) between patients and controls, where 1 = largest disagreement. In other words, 1 means that caregivers reported this symptom much more often than patients.

‡This number reflects the relative disagreement in rank frequency of reporting between patients and controls, scaled from −10 to +10, with 0 being absolute agreement in rank position of that symptom. This scale takes into account the tendency for patients to report fewer symptoms overall. On this scale, −10 means that this was a relatively commonly reported symptom by patients, but not by caregivers, and +10 means that caregivers reported this symptom frequently, but it was relatively uncommon for patients to report it.

which might also have been included (e.g., utilization behavior, [Shallice et al., 1989], bizarre behavior [Burgess & Shallice, 1996a], multitasking problems [Shallice & Burgess, 1991a; Burgess et al., 2000], and attentional difficulties [Stuss et al., 1999]. In addition, one might also include the difficulties with spoken language, visual perception, and motor control that occur following frontal lobe damage (for review, see Passingham, 1993; Fuster, 1997) but are traditionally considered under other topic headings in cognitive neuroscience and so are not considered here. To include all of these symptoms under one topic heading (e.g., "frontal lobe [dys] function") is a pragmatic solution. But there is a danger that it implies the possibility of finding a single, uni-

fying explanation for them, and thus a single rehabilitative method. We will show that the present evidence suggests that this will not be possible.

GOING FROM THEORY TO PRACTICE

There are a number of obstacles that have to be overcome in making practical suggestions for rehabilitation based on evidence from experimental (theoretical) research. However, acknowledgment of them is a precondition for resolution, and we hope that the following brief exposition will encourage rehabilitation practitioners and theoreticians alike to consider whether these obstacles are actually helpful to either party. It is our contention that the best practice of either would actually look more similar than is (largely) the case at present.

OBSTACLE 1: FUNCTION VERSUS CONSTRUCT

The first obstacle is that while rehabilitation is necessarily concerned with specific functions (i.e., the patient cannot do X (e.g., remember to switch off the oven), experimental study tends to focus on constructs (i.e., hypothetical abilities or sets of processes, e.g., prospective memory). This has quite practical consequences: ideally, we would be able to discuss individually the specific impairments or disabilities given in Table 33–1. But our (theoretical, experimental) knowledge of the executive demands made by much real-world behavior is so basic that this is not currently possible. In this way, the study of executive frontal lobe function differs from other areas of cognitive neuroscience: there is often a far less obvious correspondence between the experimental paradigms used in research and the situations normally encountered by people in everyday life (Burgess, 1997).

Let us consider an example. When cognitive neuroscientists study planning, the most commonly used task is the Tower of London and its variants (e.g., Shallice, 1982; Morris, 1988; Owen et al., 1990, 1995). However the situation that this task presents for a participant is almost completely unlike say, where they are planning a weekend trip away, or a holiday, or a meal for friends; in other words, what most people would give as examples of the activity "planning." Contrast this situation with the study of motor control: in typical studies of reaching and grasping, for instance, the situation being presented to the subject is extremely similar to those they will often encounter in everyday life.

In the study of executive functions, It can be argued, of course, that there is some similarity at the process level between the experimental task (e.g., Tower of London) and real-life demands (e.g., planning a vacation), for instance, in the involvement of some imaginary construct such as "lookahead" (e.g., McCarthy & Warrington, 1990). The evidence for such constructs is extremely weak, however. There are many different types of performance failure on the Tower of London Test, and it may even be that a given type of failure may have more than one reason (see, e.g., Goel & Grafman, 1995; Welsh et al., 1999; Carlin et al., 2000; Miyake et al., 2000). Additionally, there is almost certainly a complex network of brain systems whose operation is required for task success (e.g., Baker et al., 1996; Dagher et al., 1999). Moreover, prima facie small differences in task structure or administration may have profound performance (and psychometric) effects (see Welsh et al., 2000; and Stuss et al., 2000 for an example with an alternative paradigm). We have used the Tower of London Test as an example here. But similar arguments could be made for most experimentally derived executive tasks.

OBSTACLE 2: ARE EXPERIMENTAL PARADIGMS SIMPLIFIED MODELS OF THE WORLD?

Of course, the principal reason for studying experimental paradigms that are quite unlike "real" situations is that the real situation is so complex or difficult to study that one needs to create a simplified model situation. This model will permit observation of systematic change in response to a given manipulation that will permit the discovery of basic principles of cognition.

Recent evidence shows, however, that many experimental tasks (e.g., the Tower of London) do not appear to be significantly less complex than the real situation. For instance, it may be the case that understanding the entire dynamics of performance on the Tower of London Test (and the brain systems involved) is much easier than understanding the dynamics of how someone plans a short vacation. But it is certainly not obvious that this is the case.

OBSTACLE 3: WHAT DO EXPERIMENTAL PARADIGMS AND REAL-WORLD ACTIVITIES HAVE IN COMMON?

Unless we understand the cognitive demands of everyday activities, we will never know how the results of experimental studies (or indeed, any emergent principles of cognition) might relate to them. Unfortunately, the research that is necessary to show these relations has only recently begun (e.g., Burgess et al., 1998). Of course, this requirement would be considerably reduced if at least some experimental paradigms were more like real-world situations. Fortunately, there is a recent move in this direction (e.g., Robertson et al., 1996; Wilson et al., 1996; Burgess et al., 2000). Some investigators are even studying real-life behavior in situ. For instance, Alderman et al. (submitted) and Shallice and Burgess (1991a) have studied real-world shopping behavior. Robertson et al. (1996) used a range of tasks, such as map reading, telephone directory searching and listening to a simulated broadcast of winning lottery numbers, to try to sample distinct types of attention, based on hypothesized anatomically differentiated supramodal attentional systems (Robertson et al., 1996). In this way, it is thus likely that the results of future experimental studies will have more obvious relevance for the rehabilitation of executive dysfunction. And knowing more about the dynamics of the real situations in which patients experience problems should help in the design of rehabilitative methods.

WHAT CAN WE LEARN FROM THEORIES OF FRONTAL LOBE FUNCTION?

We have described some of the obstacles that currently prevent the straightforward translation of experimental theoretical research to rehabilitation. While these obstacles preclude making straightforward recommendations for rehabilitation on the basis of experimental evidence, it is our view that experimental theorizing still provides the most promising source of provisional hypotheses concerning which techniques might be worth trying. After all, every putative rehabilitation method first requires a theory of how it might work. Thus we take theories of frontal lobe function that have been based on (largely) experimental evidence, and attempt to translate these into their practical implications for rehabilitation.

Most of these current theories of frontal

lobe function are (in the terms of Morton & Bekerian, 1986) more accurately characterized as frameworks than falsifiable theories. For this reason, they can seem of rather distant help when faced with a specific symptom. However, some general principles emerge. The greatest level of distinction that has implications for rehabilitation method concerns the way in which the theory was developed. The main differences are those between single-account theories, construct-led theories, multiple-account theories, and single-symptom theories. We cannot cover all of the theories in this chapter, so we have chosen a few illustrative ideas that have been developed by other authors appearing in this volume. In this way, interested readers can refer to the relevant chapters should they want more detailed exposition.

SINGLE-PROCESS THEORIES

COHEN'S CONTEXT INFORMATION THEORY

Single-process theories are those that hold that damage to a single process or system is responsible for a number of different dysexecutive symptoms. A good example is the theory of Cohen and colleagues (e.g., Cohen et al., 1990, 1998; Cohen & Servan-Schreiber, 1992), which is derived from connectionist modeling of simple tasks such as the Stroop paradigm. Cohen et al.'s theory is that prefrontal cortex (PFC) is used to represent "context information," which they define as the "information necessary to mediate an appropriate behavioural response" (Cohen et al., 1998, p. 196). This information may be a "set of task instructions, a specific prior stimulus or the result of processing a sequence of prior stimuli (e.g., the interpretation resulting from processing a sequence of words in a sentence)" (Cohen et al., 1998, p. 196). It is argued that at least two functions of PFC may be effected by this system: active memory and behavioral inhibition. They argue that both these functions reflect the operation of the context layer under different task conditions. Under the conditions of response competition, when a strong response tendency must be overcome for appropriate behavior, the context module plays an inhibitory role by supporting the processing of task-relevant information. When there is a delay between information relevant to a response and the execution of that response, the context module plays a role in memory by maintaining that information over time.

Interestingly, Cohen et al. (1998) criticize their own theory as incomplete. They maintain that for a more general account of cognitive control (as opposed to one that is constrained chiefly to explaining patterns of Stroop and Continous Performance Test [CPT] performance), they need mechanisms that deal with management of interference, identification of task-relevant information, and representation of many different information types. A strength of this theory, however, is that various aspects of it can be tested. For instance, Cohen et al. (1998) make the prediction from the model that memory deficits should emerge earlier than inhibitory deficits in schizophrenia (p. 199).

IMPLICATIONS FOR REHABILITATION

These accounts have the advantage of parsimony. And Cohen et al.'s account in particular holds the promise that apparently quite different symptoms might share a common cause. In this respect, careful consideration of the precise demands of the situations in which patients demonstrate their impairment is encouraged. It also holds the promise that rehabilitation of the critical function might result in improvement over a wide range of symptoms, although it may be difficult to predict the exact form that this improvement would take in any one case. In practical terms, perhaps a suggestion of this theory is that dysexecutive patients might be helped by a system of reminding patients what they are supposed to be doing, and how far they have yet to go in achieving their goal—in other words, moment-by-moment feedback system. This implication for rehabilitation leads us to *provisional principle 1:* Consider the use of feedback systems to modify dysexecutive behavior,

especially for symptoms of disinhibition and distractibility.

DUNCAN'S THEORY OF GOAL NEGLECT

Duncan (1986; 1995; Duncan et al., 1995, 1996, 2000) has pointed out that much of human behavior is controlled by goal lists, or lists of goals and subgoals constructed in response to environmental or internal demands (e.g., get ready for guests to arrive). When the current state of affairs does not match the goal state, a store of actions is consulted, and actions are then activated to resolve the discrepancy in an iterative process. However, actions can also be activated in response to competing and sometimes irrelevant input (e.g., the letter on the desk). A function of the goal list is to impose coherence on behavior by controlling the activation or inhibition of actions that promote or oppose task completion. An important aspect of goal-directed behavior is the selection of new actions when previously selected actions fail to achieve the goal. According to Duncan et al. (1996), much of the disorganized behavior seen in patients with frontal systems dysfunction can be attributed to impaired construction and use of such goal lists. One fundamental feature of such impairment is a restricted capacity for maintaining goals in working memory such that particular goals will be extinguished or neglected, leading to behavioral disorganization.

IMPLICATIONS FOR REHABILITATION

In contrast to Cohen's theory, the implications of Duncan's theory have been put to rehabilitation test. Robertson (1996) developed a rehabilitation method based on Duncan's theory of frontal lobe function. This goal management training, given over two 1-hour sessions in a randomized trial to executively impaired subjects with traumatic brain injury, taught the steps of stopping current activity and orienting towards the task, defining the main goal and component subgoals, rehearsing the steps necessary to tackle the problem, and monitoring the outcome. After such training significant reductions in errors rates in naturalistic and varied cooking tasks, were found, and patients reported fewer everyday difficulties (Levine et al., 2000).

A further study examined whether the provision of brief auditory stimuli could act in a bottom-up fashion to interrupt current activity and cue patients to consider their overall goal, thus reducing goal neglect (Manly et al., in press a). Ten brain-injured patients completed a modification of Shallice and Burgess' six elements Test (Shallice & Burgess, 1991a; Burgess et al., 1996b) under two conditions. In the 'hotel' test, the patients were asked to try and do some of five subtasks within 15 minutes. As the total time to complete all of the tasks would exceed an hour, the measure emphasizes patients' ability to monitor the time, switch between the tasks, and keep track of their intentions. Without the external auditory cues, the patients performed significantly more poorly than age- and IQ-matched control volunteers, a common error being continuing to perform one task to the detriment of beginning others or allowing sufficient time for them. When exposed to the interrupting tones, however, their performance was both significantly improved and no longer significantly different from that of the control group. The results have assessment value in helping to attribute poor performance to goal neglect, rather than, for example, poor memory or comprehension. They also suggest that providing environmental support to one aspect of executive function may facilitate monitoring and behavioral flexibility, and thus the useful expression of other skills that may be relatively intact. The implications of Duncan's theory for rehabilitation lead us to *provisional principle 2:* Some dysexecutive patients fail to carry out intended tasks, despite being able to recall (when prompted) what it is they have to do. Consider the use of simple interrupts in their treatment.

WORKING MEMORY THEORIES

Two of the most commonly encountered working memory theories are those by Petrides and colleagues (e.g., Petrides, 1994) and Goldman-Rakic and colleagues (e.g.,

Goldman-Rakic, 1995). Petrides's position concerns the roles of the mid-dorsolateral and mid-ventrolateral aspects of the frontal lobes. He believes that the mid-dorsolateral region (areas 9 and 46) supports a brain system "in which information can be held on-line for monitoring and manipulation of stimuli" (Petrides, 1998, p. 106). By "monitoring" he refers to the process of considering a number of possible alternative choices. This system enables people to maintain and monitor their self-generated choices and thus the occurrence of events. By contrast, the mid-ventrolateral region "subserves the expression within memory of various first-order executive processes, such as [the] active selection, comparison and judgement of stimuli" (p. 107). It is used for the explicit encoding and retrieval of information (see Chapter 3 for a detailed discussion).

Goldman-Rakic's position is rather different. She maintains that the various different frontal lobe regions all perform a similar role in working memory, but that each processes a different type of information (Goldman-Rakic, 1995). *Working memory* is defined as the ability to "hold an item of information 'in mind' for a short period of time and to update information from moment to moment" (Goldman-Rakic, 1998, p. 90). She argues that dysfunction of this system can cause a variety of deficits. Problems on the verbal fluency and Stroop tasks are explained as a failure to suppress a prepotent response due to an inability to use working memory to initiate the correct response. Perseveration and disinhibition may result from the "loss of the neural substrate necessary to generate the correct response" (Goldman-Rakic, 1998, p. 93). There is less disagreement between Petrides and Goldman-Rakic about which brain areas subserve working memory, as Goldman-Rakic also places emphasis on the lateral aspects of the frontal lobes (see Chapter 5 for further discussion).

An interesting aspect of these theories is that they make the strongest connection between function and neurochemistry. Links are consistently made between working memory, dorsolateral PFC, and dopaminergic systems (See Diamond, 1998 for review, and Chapter

11, this volume, for more detailed discussion on the working memory role of lateral PFC). Indeed, there is a link here with Cohen's theory, in which dopaminergic neuromodulation plays a critical role (e.g., Cohen et al., 1998, pp. 207–208).

IMPLICATIONS FOR REHABILITATION

Two possible avenues for rehabilitation emerge from the working memory accounts of dysexecutive symptoms. The first is drug therapy, as suggested by the link between working memory deficits and dopaminergic system dysfunction. The uses of drugs that alter the action of dopamine in the brain are, of course, well developed for treating schizophrenia. They are less well developed for the treatment of brain injury, although evidence of the potential of such treatment is now beginning to emerge (e.g., Powell et al., 1996; Karli et al., 1999; see Chapter 32). Thus working memory theories may suggest a role for neurochemistry in the treatment of patients whose pattern of deficits is consistent with working memory problems (see also Chapter 4).

The second possibility arising from these theories is the use of simple and varied instruction as well as use of quite basic methods of reinforcement. This possibility stems from both Petrides' and Goldman-Rakic's theories Petrides' claims that the root of many dysexecutive patients' problems is that they cannot (1) hold in mind a number of things at one time and (2) select, compare, and make judgements on incoming stimuli. Goldman-Rakic holds that working memory systems might be information or modality-specific (e.g., verbal, visual, tactile etc.). These characterizations have quite straightforward implications for the way that rehabilitation should be conducted (see also Baddeley and Della Sala, 1998), and lead us to *provisional principle 3:* Keep instructions simple and unambiguous.

Reasoning with someone about their behavior requires that the person track the various arguments as they are being said and compare the various aspects of the argument. This may well be beyond the capabilities of the patient with working memory problems.

Rehabilitation implications from the working memory theories also include *provisional principle 4:* Use simple reinforcement and reward techniques, if possible Petrides maintains that the ventrolateral working memory system is implicated in the encoding and recall of complex material. If this system is damaged, patients may have trouble with encoding for themselves the salient aspects of the learning situation. So it may be better if verbal reinforcement alone is not relied on; actual acts of reward may be more effective. Moreover, for treatment to be effective, it may be unwise to rely on the patient's ability to encode and actively later remember the the content of previous sessions. Gradual behavioral shaping may be a better option. Above all, one might expect a statement to a patient such as, "it would be better to do X because . . ." or general talking therapies to be relatively ineffective for treating dysexecutive symptoms that may be secondary to working memory impairment. According to Goldman-Rakic, this might include disinhibition, which, as Table 33–1 shows, is a quite common dysexecutive symptom.

PROBLEMS OF SINGLE-FACTOR AND WORKING MEMORY THEORIES

A number of problems emerge for any executive function theory that rests on a single, unitary process:

1. In group studies of either neurological patients or healthy subjects, correlations between performance on different executive tasks are typically very low (see, e.g., Burgess & Shallice, 1994; Robbins, 1998; Miyake et al., 2000).

2. Group studies also show a number of clusters of behavioral symptoms of the dysexecutive syndrome rather than just one factor (Burgess et al., 1998).

3. At the single case level, symptoms such as confabulation or multitasking deficits may be seen independently of virtually any other signs (e.g., Shallice & Burgess, 1991a; Burgess & McNeil, 1999; Burgess, 2000b; Burgess et al., 2000).

4. Also at the single case level, deficits such as response suppression and initiation problems can doubly dissociate (Shallice, 1988) on executive tests (e.g., Burgess & Shallice, 1996c).

5. Different behavioral symptoms are associated with performance decrements on different clinical executive tasks (Burgess et al., 1998).

6. As a group, frontal lobe patients can show a range of different forms of error on the same executive test (e.g. Burgess & Shallice, 1996c; Stuss et al., 2000).

7. Brain lesions in different parts of the frontal lobes can be associated with decrements on different executive tasks and with different types of failure (e.g., Stuss, et al., 1994, 1999; Troyer et al., 1998; Burgess et al., 2000; Stuss & Alexander, 2000.)

8. Functional imaging and electrophysiological studies of the frontal lobes suggest potential fractionation of the executive system (Knight & Nakada, 1998; Gehring & Knight, 2000; see also Chapters 7 and 11).

Together, these results suggest that although there may well be cognitive control/executive processes that are used in many different situations as the single-process and construct-led accounts claim, it is doubtful that they can be complete accounts of the entire frontal cognitive system (as the authors themselves generally admit). As a consequence, some theorists have presented more complex models that attempt to take these potential fractionations into account: the multiple-process theories.

MULTIPLE-PROCESS THEORIES

These theories propose that the frontal lobe executive system consists of a number of components that typically work together in everyday actions, but can be examined relatively independently in experimental studies.

FUSTER'S TEMPORAL INTEGRATION FRAMEWORK

Fuster (1997; see also chapter 6) provides one of the most concisely articulated examples of this type of theory. He states, "the prefrontal cortex is essential for the formulation and execution of novel plans or structures of behaviour. These gestalts of action, with their goals, are represented in neuronal networks of this cortex in the form of abstract *schemas*. The simpler components of those structures of action are represented in frontal or subcortical networks at lower levels of the motor hierarchies" (Fuster, 1997 p. 251). The frontal cortex exerts its influence through connective and reciprocal links with posterior cortical regions, and the overall frontal system performs three functions:

1. *Working memory:* the provisional retention of information for prospective action. This function is mainly supported by dorsolateral prefrontal cortical (DLPFC) areas.

2. *Set:* the selection and preparation of particular (established) motor acts. The DLPFC and the anterior medial cortex also support this function.

3. *Inhibitory control:* serves to suppress interference, either from external distractors, or from internal inappropriate sensory and motor memories. This function is supported primarily by the orbitomedial PFC.

STUSS'S ANTERIOR ATTENTIONAL FUNCTIONS

The idea in Fuster's model that the frontal lobes serve control functions over more basic schemas is one of the enduring ideas in modern frontal lobe theorizing (e.g., Luria & Homskaya, 1964; Norman & Shallice, 1986). Recently, Stuss et al., (1995) have expanded upon how they see the relationship between the schema and the executive system might operate (see also Chapter 25).

Stuss et al. (1995) describe a *schema* as being a network of connected neurons that can be activated by sensory input, by other schemata, or by the executive control (i.e., frontal lobe) system. In turn, it can recruit other schemata to cognitive control processing so as to produce its required response(s). In addition, they suggest that schemata provide feedback to the executive system concerning its level of activity. Different schemata compete for the control of thought and behavior by means of a process called "contention scheduling" (a concept described originally by Norman & Shallice, [1986]), which is mediated by lateral inhibition. They suggest that each schema contains multiple internal connections, some of which provide internal feedback. Once activated, a schema remains active for a period of time, depending on its goals and processing characteristics. This might be only a few seconds in situations such as reaction-time tasks. But over longer periods that require activity without triggering input, activation has to be maintained by repeated input from the executive control system.

The focus of Stuss et al.'s theory is attention. They propose seven different attentional functions, each of which has its own neuronal correlates: sustaining (right frontal); concentrating (cingulate); sharing (cingulate plus orbitofrontal); suppressing (DL-PFC); switching (DL-PFC plus medial frontal); preparing (DL-PFC); and setting (left DL-PFC).

SHALLICE'S SUPERVISORY ATTENTIONAL SYSTEM

The notion that the frontal lobes are crucially involved in attention is also reflected in one of the most influential modern theories of frontal lobe function. This theory was developed by Shallice and colleagues over the last 20 years (e.g., Norman & Shallice, 1986 [initially published as a technical report in 1980]; Shallice, 1988; Shallice et al., 1989; Shallice & Burgess, 1991a, 1991b, 1993, 1996; Burgess & Shallice, 1997; Burgess et al., 2000; see Chapter 17). The use of the term *attention* in this theory is broad, and refers in a general sense to the allocation of processing resources (Shallice, 1988).

The first version of this theory (Norman & Shallice, 1986) is principally concerned with outlining in broad terms the organization of the executive control system over well-rehearsed behavioral (and thought) routines. There are four levels of increasing organization. The first level consists merely of "cognitive or action units," which are the basic abilities one has (e.g., reaching for an object, reading a word). Schemata exist at the second level. These are nests of first-level units that

had come to be closely associated through repetition, as described above. The third level, was a process called "contention scheduling," is the basic triggering interface between incoming stimuli (including thoughts) and the schemata. Its purpose is to effect the quick selection of routine behaviors in well-known situations. Of course, many situations (or aspects of them) that we encounter are not well rehearsed. In this situation one has to consciously decide what to do. The cognitive system that effects this conscious deliberation is called the "supervisory attentional system" (SAS).

In the early versions of the theory, the SAS was merely represented as a single entity. This was not because it was thought that the system comprised only one process or construct, but merely that there was little empirical evidence at that time concerning potential fractionation (see points 1–8 in Problems of Single-Factor and Working Memory Theories, above). More recently, the putative organization of the SAS has been articulated in more detail (Shallice & Burgess, 1996; see also Chapter 17). In this model, the SAS plays a part in at least eight different processes: working memory; monitoring; rejection of schema; spontaneous schema generation; adoption of processing mode; goal setting; delayed intention marker realization; and episodic memory retrieval. (A more detailed description of this theory, together with a figure of the model, can be found in Chapter 17).

IMPLICATIONS FOR REHABILITATION

The strength of the multiple-process theories is that they encapsulate the results from many different types of studies, and they attempt to explain behavior in many different kinds of situations. As such, they stand a better chance of explaining a variety of dysexecutive symptoms (see Table 33–1). Their disadvantage is that they are difficult to disprove. If a new dissociation between tasks or symptoms is found, it is easy to either "bolt-on" another process to the theory, or explain it as a refinement of one of the existing concepts. It is difficult to see at what stage such a theory could ever be completely rejected.

For rehabilitation, the suggestions of these models is more complex than for the single-process or construct-led theories. These theories suggest that one first needs to isolate the locus of the impairment(s). In practical terms, this would require administration of the sets of procedures on which the model was based (or as close as is practically possible). This is likely to be a much more time-consuming procedure than for the other types of theory. However, it is less likely that an important impairment would be missed. Moreover, a number of the hypothesized processes are only tapped in certain situations; one needs to assess a patient in a wide range of them. Thus we come to *provisional principle 5:* Pre- and post-treatment evaluation of dysexecutive problems requires assessment of competence in a wide range of situations.

If this principle is followed, rehabilitation efforts can then be targeted to the specific situations in which the patient has problems. In this way, the implications for rehabilitation of the multiple-process models are quite different from those of the previous theories, which suggested that rehabilitation could be performed out of the everyday situations in which the patient has problems. The question then becomes, are there any grounds for establishing a basic minimum set of investigations that should be performed as a first-stage assessment of the dysexecutive patient?

The results of a study by Burgess et al. (1998) may give some answers to this question. In this study, the caregivers or relatives of 92 mixed-etiology neurological patients were given a questionnaire (the DEX; Burgess et al., 1996a) which asked them to rate the frequency of occurrence of the 20 most common dysexecutive symptoms in the patients they knew well. These symptoms are listed in Table 33–1. When the results were subjected to factor analysis (orthogonal rotation), five factors were selected: inhibition (principally problems with response suppression and disinhibition); intentionality (everyday deficits in planning and decision making); executive memory (e.g., confabulation, perseveration); and two purely affective factors—positive (e.g., euphoria) and negative (e.g., apathy) affective changes. A range of neuropsychological

tests was also administered to the patients, which allowed examination of the relationships between the scores for these behavioral symptom factors and individual psychometric test performances. Burgess et al. found a distinct pattern of relationships between test performances and the behavioral symptoms. Performance on none of the psychometric tests was associated with either of the affective symptom factor scores. However, performance on many executive tests (Cognitive Estimates, Verbal Fluency, Trail-Making, and the Six Element Test of the Behavioural Assessment of the Dysexecutive Syndrome (BADS) battery (Wilson et al., 1996) was significantly associated with inhibition factor scores, as were Wechsler Adult Intelligence Scale (WAIS) Full-Scale IQ scores. Modified Wisconsin Card Sorting Test (MWCST) performance and verbal fluency was associated with the executive memory factor scores. And only 1 test (out of a total of 22) was significantly associated with the intentionality factor scores: the Six Element Test (Shallice & Burgess, 1991a; Burgess et al., 1996b). From these results, Burgess et al. (1998) recommended that, at the very least, an assessment of a dysexecutive patient should include tests that measure each of these symptom clusters (the affective aspects will be dealt with below). Broadly, these would include the following:

1. A general measure of inhibitory abilities (impairments of which are detected by a wide range of tasks, including those of intellectual function)
2. Measures of executive memory abilities, both short-term (i.e., working memory) and long-term (i.e., accuracy of episodic recollection)
3. A measure of multitasking ability (the subcomponents of which include planning, prospective memory, and task switching; see Burgess, 2000a, for more detail).

The degree of concordance of these empirical results with the multiple-process theories outlined above is striking. Two of Fuster's three temporal integration functions are closely replicated, and if one takes a broad view of preparatory set, then there is further agreement. Stuss's inhibition, switching, preparation, and attention maintenance aspects are also all reflected in these empirical findings. Shallice's model fares particularly well; it explicitly mentions as separate processes inhibition (in the form of both schema rejection and adoption of processing mode); working memory and episodic retrieval; and both components of multitasking (prospective memory as "delayed intention marker realization" and planning as the set of processes in method 2 of new schema formation). Thus the multiple-process theories explain quite well the multitude of symptoms that can follow frontal lobe damage.

These theories also suggest a general approach to investigating the root causes of everyday dysexecutive impairments. Following formal assessment of function as outlined above, one would examine how the particular impairments contribute to disability in everyday life. This requires componential analysis of the situations that present the greatest problem (as identified, for instance, by ABC analysis). It is most unfortunate that experimental paradigms are so often unlike real-world situations (see Obstacle 3: What Do Experimental Paradigms and Real-World Activities Have in Common), since if this were not the case, much of the work would already have been done for the rehabilitation specialist and this stage would be largely redundant. The final stage would of course be intervention, the exact method of which would depend on the nature of the impairment, the situation in which it manifests itself, the intact abilities the patient shows, and other relevant clinical variables.

This argument raises two important and interconnected matters for the rehabilitation of executive function. The first concerns the relative importance of the various symptoms, and the second concerns patients' awareness of them.

THE PROBLEM OF AWARENESS

From Table 33–1 it is quite apparent that some symptoms are reported more frequently than others by caregivers of dysexecutive patients. Indeed, some (e.g., planning problems) were reported as a problem by relatives in almost half of the cases that formed the sample in the study from which these data were taken (Burgess et al., 1998).

Table 33–1 also shows that patients are often unaware of the extent of their problems. This problem is not confined to executive dysfunction: many amnesics or people with neglect may also be unaware of their problems, at least in the early stages of their disability. The problem of unawareness is nonetheless both prevalent and persistent for dysexecutive patients (see also Prigatano, 1991a, 1991b) and should at least in part guide the agenda for their rehabilitation. All other matters being equal, treatment of a problem that the patients does not notice or acknowledge will always be more problematic than for one of which the patient complains. Table 33–1 shows that two of the symptoms where there is typically greatest disagreement between patients and caregivers both involve a lack of concern. This presents an interesting conundrum: how does one make a patient concerned that they are unconcerned? Perhaps consideration of the item of greatest disagreement between patients and caregivers provides an answer: planning problems. One might suggest, in a simple-minded fashion, that a consequence of not considering the future or the consequences of ones actions is likely to be a lack of concern. So if one can first facilitate this planning function, the problem with concern is likely to show concomitant improvement. In this example it would make most sense to target one's rehabilitation efforts first towards the deficits in planning. This argument suggests a further dysexecutive rehabilitation principle, *provisional principle 6:* When deciding which dysexecutive behavior to treat first, do not necessarily start with the most troublesome. Also consider the order in which the symptoms should be treated (see also Chapter 32).

To continue this example into the domain of more practical treatment delivery, the first stage in facilitating planning is to demonstrate the consequences of failures at the most basic level—in other words, to provide a feedback mechanism. Alderman and colleagues (1995) have described a form of this feedback training, which they call "self-monitoring training." This consists of five stages. The first is a baseline stage (of target behavior frequency). The second stage is "spontaneous self-monitoring," in which the patient is given a counting device (e.g., mechanical clicker) and is asked to keep a record of how many times they show the target behavior while performing an attention-demanding ongoing task. In the third stage, the second stage is repeated with one modification: on each occasion the subject engages in the target behavior but does not record it; the therapist gives a verbal prompt for them to do so. The purpose of this stage of the training is to encourage subjects to monitor their own behavior more accurately and get into the habit of routinely recording their behavior. The aim of the fourth stage is to withdraw external structure and facilitate self-monitoring. This is done by rewarding subjects if their recording is within a given range of the same recording made independently by the therapist (verbal prompts are not given during this stage). The subject's accuracy may be steadily "shaped" using ever-stricter criteria for reward. The aim of the final stage of training is to encourage inhibition of the target behavior. This typically involves rewarding the participant if they have not engaged in the target behavior more than a given number of times over a set period. With success, the reward criterion number is gradually reduced until the target behavior is within acceptable limits. This method has been used successfully with a range of behavioral problems, when patients showed little awareness of them (e.g., Alderman et al., 1995; Alderman & Burgess, 2001).

SINGLE-SYMPTOM THEORIES

The final category of theories of frontal lobe dysfunction is those that seek to explain specific dysexecutive symptoms (see Table 33–1). Often these theories quite directly suggest treatment interventions. An example is the treatment of a confabulating patient reported by Burgess and McNeil (1999). Based on the

Burgess and Shallice (1996b) model of the processes damaged in confabulation, Burgess and McNeil successfully implemented a simple diary-keeping method for the treatment of a patient with a persistant confabulatory problem. Single-symptom theories of this type are likely to hold great rehabilitation potential. However, since it is likely that some executive impairments might be the root cause of more than one behavioral symptom, it is unlikely that it will be possible to develop explanatory theories of individual symptoms in isolation from larger-scale theories. A full review of the rehabilitation implications of all possible theories of all possible dysexecutive symptoms is beyond the scope of this chapter, as the focus of this chapter is general treatment principles, which are less likely to emerge from symptom-specific theories. We believe, however, that single-symptom theories set in the context of larger-scale theories will prove to be a particularly powerful tool for progress in rehabilitation technique.

MECHANISMS OF RECOVERY

We have discussed some of the leading theories on the means by how the frontal lobes exert their control over behavior. And we have outlined in broad terms some of the implications for the rehabilitation of patients with executive control deficits. In some cases, the form of rehabilitation might be termed *cognitive prosthetics*—in other words, the aim is to improve function rather than ameliorate the cognitive impairment by the use of external aids (e.g., the Neuropage system [Wilson et al., 1997; Evans et al., 1998]). In other cases, rehabilitation may reduce the need for the impaired ability by changing the environment. A third type of rehabilitation aims to establish behavior patterns that rely on intact systems—in other words, to alter the construct demands of the old function (a rather simple example might be when a patient with severe speech production problems is encouraged to write messages to communicate). A fourth type aims to improve the actual cognitive impairment itself. How might such an improvement occur in the damaged brain?

One possibility is that at least part of the impairment in a given executive function may be attributable to insufficient input from a malfunctioning system that normally provides input to it. Arousal is a case in point. Even circadian fluctuations in basic arousal within the intact brain alter executive control over behavior, including slips of action (Manly et al., in press b). Many pathologies that contribute to frontal damage—particularly traumatic brain injury—also damage the white matter and other structures responsible for the regulation of arousal in the brain, resulting in significant and rather general problems of arousal regulation. The effects of periodic auditory alerts on complex executive function described above (Manly et al., in press a) may well have exerted effects through bottom-up modulation of arousal as well as activating top-down monitoring of current goals. Modulation of arousal through both behavioral (Robertson et al., 1995) and pharmacological means is possible, and it is entirely plausible that these relatively simple manipulations may produce effects in complex, multifactorial systems in a way that sophisticated interventions that tackle the systems themselves may have more difficulty achieving.

CONCLUSION

There must be a theory of the cause of an impairment before a treatment can be designed. However, currently there is a gap between pure experimental work from which such theories might evolve and potential treatment applications. As we have seen, there are two reasons for this discrepancy. First, the kinds of situations and techniques studied in pure experimental work are often unlike those in everyday rehabilitation. Second, rehabilitation is necessarily concerned with function, but experimental work in this area has historically been more concerned with constructs. It is our opinion that there is actually more potential cross-talk between these concerns than might at first appear. To demonstrate this viewpoint, we have explored the practical implications for rehabilitation of some current leading theories of executive frontal lobe function, and developed six provisional principles for treatment (see Table 33–2). These should be regarded as hypotheses for the moment; they are untested predictions from theoretical studies made with no regard for the myriad of clinical considerations that actually bear upon treatment. Nevertheless, the extent to which they conform to the kinds of approaches already being developed is encouraging. It is our contention that if rehabilitation of frontal lobe executive functions is to develop equivalence to other forms of therapy in this area (e.g., speech and language therapy), such principles must be formally developed and tested. The quite astonishing advance in our understanding of the frontal lobes over the last 20 years suggests that this might not be unnecessarily optimistic, given the right circumstances. However, this will require extensive collaboration between experimental researchers, who may be in a position to suggest new avenues to explore, and clinicians, who can determine how these suggestions might be implemented. To this end, we hope that both sides will make

Table 33–2. Provisional rehabilitation principles emerging from frontal lobe theories

1. Consider the use of feedback systems to modify dysexecutive behavior, especially symptoms of disinhibition and distractibility (i.e., loss of goal).
2. Some dysexecutive patients fail to carry out intended tasks despite being able to recall (when prompted) what it is they have to do. Consider the use of simple interrupts in their treatment.
3. Keep instructions and advice simple and unambiguous.
4. Use simple reinforcement and reward techniques, if possible.
5. Pre- and post-treatment evaluation of dysexecutive problems requires assessment of competence in a wide range of situations.
6. When deciding which dysexecutive problem to treat first, do not necessarily start with the most troublesome. Also consider the order in which the symptoms should be treated, since treatment of certain problems may benefit greatly by initial groundwork elsewhere.

sound efforts to make their work accessible to each other.

ACKNOWLEDGMENTS

Paul W. Burgess is supported by Wellcome Trust grant ref. 049241/Z/96/Z/WRE/HA/JAT. We are grateful to Barbara A. Wilson, Nick Alderman, Jon J. Evans, and Hazel Emslie for letting us describe in Table 33–1 data collected as part of their study.

REFERENCES

Alderman, N. (1996). Central executive deficit and response to operant conditioning methods. *Neuropsychological Rehabilitation, 6,* 161–186.

Alderman, N. & Burgess, P.W. (2001). Assessment and rehabilitation of the dysexecutive syndrome. In: R. Greenwood, T.M. McMillan, M.P. Barnes, & C.D. Ward (Eds.), *Handbook of Neurological Rehabilitation,* 2nd Ed. Hove, UK: Psychology Press.

Alderman, N., Fry, R.K., & Youngson, H.A. (1995). Improvement of self-monitoring skills, reduction of behaviour disturbance and the dysexecutive syndrome: comparison of response cost and a new programme of self-monitoring training. *Neuropsychological Rehabilitation, 5,* 193–221.

Alderman, N., Burgess, P.W., Knight, C., & Henman, C. (submitted). Ecological validity of a simplified version of the multiple errands shopping test.

Baddeley, A.D. & Della Sala, S. (1998). Working memory and executive control. In: A.C. Roberts, T.W. Robbins, & L. Weiskrantz (Eds.), *The Prefrontal Cortex: Executive and Cognitive Functions* (pp. 9–21). Oxford: Oxford University Press.

Baker, S.C., Rogers, R.D., Owen, A.M., Frith, C.D., Dolan, R.J., Frackowiak, R.S., & Robbins, T.W. (1996). Neural systems engaged by planning: a PET study of the Tower of London task. *Neuropsychologia, 34,* 515–526.

Burgess, P.W. (1997). Theory and methodology in executive function research. In: P. Rabbitt (Ed.), *Methodology of Frontal and Executive Function* (pp. 81–116). Hove, UK: Psychology Press.

Burgess, P.W. (2000a). Real-world multitasking from a cognitive neuroscience perspective. In: S. Monsell & J. Driver (Eds.), *Control of Cognitive Processes: Attention and Performance XVIII* (pp. 465–472). Cambridge, MA: MIT Press.

Burgess, P.W. (2000b). Strategy application disorder: the role of the frontal lobes in human multitasking. *Psychological Research, 63,* 279–288.

Burgess, P.W. & McNeil, J.E. (1999). Content-specific confabulation. *Cortex, 35,* 163–182.

Burgess, P.W. & Shallice, T. (1994). Fractionnement du syndrome frontal. *Revue de Neuropsychologie, 4,* 345–370.

Burgess, P.W. & Shallice, T. (1996a). Bizarre responses, rule detection and frontal lobe lesions. *Cortex, 32,* 241–260.

Burgess, P.W. & Shallice, T. (1996b). Confabulation and the control of recollection. *Memory, 4,* 359–411.

Burgess, P.W. & Shallice, T. (1996c). Response suppression, initiation and strategy use following frontal lobe lesions. *Neuropsychologia, 34,* 263–276.

Burgess, P.W. & Shallice, T. (1997). The relationship between prospective and retrospective memory: neuropsychological evidence. In: M.A. Conway (Ed.), *Cognitive Models of Memory.* Hove, UK: Psychology Press.

Burgess, P.W., Alderman, N., Emslie, H., Evans, J.J., & Wilson, B.A. (1996a). The dysexecutive questionnaire. In: B.A. Wilson, N. Alderman, P.W. Burgess, H. Emslie, & J.J. Evans (Eds.), *Behavioural Assessment of the Dysexecutive Syndrome* Bury St. Edmunds, UK: Thames Valley Test Company.

Burgess, P.W., Alderman, N., Emslie, H., Evans, J.J., Wilson, B.A., & Shallice, T. (1996b). The simplified Six Element Test. In: B.A. Wilson, N. Alderman, P.W. Burgess, H. Emslie, & J.J. Evans (Eds.), *Behavioural Assessment of the Dysexecutive Syndrome* Bury St. Edmunds, UK: Thames Valley Test Company.

Burgess, P.W., Alderman, N., Evans, J., Emslie, H., & Wilson, B.A. (1998). The ecological validity of tests of executive function. *Journal of the International Neuropsychological Society, 4,* 547–558.

Burgess, P.W., Veitch, E., Costello, A., & Shallice, T. (2000). The cognitive and neuroanatomical correlates of multitasking. *Neuropsychologia, 38,* 848–863.

Carlin, D., Bonerba, J., Phipps, M., Alexander, G., Shapiro, M., & Grafman, J. (2000). Planning impairments in frontal lobe dementia and frontal lobe lesions. *Neuropsychologia, 38,* 655–665.

Cohen, J.D., Braver, T.S., & O'Reilly, R.C. (1998). A computational approach to prefrontal cortex, cognitive control, and schizophrenia: recent developments and current challenges. In: A.C. Roberts, T.W. Robbins, & L. Weiskrantz (Eds.), *The Prefrontal Cortex: Executive and Cognitive Functions* (pp. 195–220). Oxford: Oxford University Press.

Cohen, J.D. & Servan-Schreiber, D. (1992). Context, cortex and dopamine: a connectionist approach to behaviour and biology in schizophrenia. *Psychological Review, 99,* 45–77.

Cohen, J.D., Dunbar, K., & McClelland, J.L. (1990). On the control of automatic processes: a parallel distributed processing account of the Stroop effect. *Psychological Review, 97,* 332–61.

Dagher, A., Owen, A.M., Boecker, H., & Brooks, D.J. (1999). Mapping the network for planning: a correlational PET activation study with the Tower of London task. *Brain, 122,* 1973–1987.

Diamond, A. (1998). Evidence for the importance of dopamine for prefrontal cortex functions early in life. In A.C. Roberts, T.W. Robbins, & L. Weiskrantz (Eds.), *The Prefrontal Cortex: Executive and Cognitive Functions* (pp. 117–130). Oxford: Oxford University Press.

Duncan, J. (1986) Disorganisation of behaviour after frontal lobe damage. *Cognitive Neuropsychology 3*, 271–290.

Duncan, J. (1995). Attention, intelligence and the frontal lobes. In M.S. Gazzaniga (Eds.), *The Cognitive Neurosciences* (pp. 721–733). Cambridge, MA: MIT Press.

Duncan, J., Burgess, P.W., & Emslie, H. (1995). Fluid intelligence after frontal lobe lesions. *Neuropsychologia, 33*, 261–268.

Duncan, J., Emslie, H., Williams, P., Johnson, R., & Freer, C. (1996). Intelligence and the frontal lobe: the organisation of goal-directed behaviour. *Cognitive Psychology, 30*, 257–303.

Duncan, J., Seitz, R.J., Kolodny, J., Bor, D., Herzog, H., Ahmed, A., Newell, F.N., & Emslie, H. (2000). A neural basis for intelligence. *Science, 289 (5478)*, 457–460.

Evans, J.J., Emslie, H., & Wilson, B.A. (1998). External cueing systems in the rehabilitation of executive impairments of action. *Journal of the International Neuropsychological Society, 4*, 399–408.

Fuster, J.M. (1997). *The Prefrontal Cortex: Anatomy, Physiology and Neuropsychology of the Frontal Lobe 3rd Ed.* Philadelphia: Lippincott-Raven.

Gehring, W.J. & Knight, R.T. (2000). Prefrontal–cingulate interactions in action monitoring. *Nature Neuroscience, 3*, 516–520.

Goel, V. & Grafman, J. (1995). Are the frontal lobes implicated in "planning" functions? Interpreting data from the Tower of Hanoi. *Neuropsychologia, 33*, 623–642.

Goldman-Rakic, P.S. (1995). Architecture of the prefrontal cortex and the central executive. *Annals of the New York Academy of Science, 769*, 212–220.

Goldman-Rakic, P.S. (1998). The prefrontal landscape: implications of functional architecture for understanding human mentation and the central executive. In: A.C. Roberts, T.W. Robbins, & L. Weiskrantz (Eds.), *The Prefrontal Cortex: Executive and Cognitive Functions* (pp. 87–102). Oxford: Oxford University Press.

Karli, D.C., Burke, D.T., Kim, H.J., Calvanio, R., Fitzpatrick, M., Temple, D., MacNeil, M., Pesez, K., & Lepak, P. (1999). Effects of dopaminergic combination therapy for frontal lobe dysfunction in traumatic brain injury rehabilitation. *Brain Injury, 13*, 63–68.

Knight, R.T. & Nakada, T. (1998). Cortico-limbic circuits and novelty: a review of EEG and blood flow data. *Review of Neuroscience, 9*, 57–70.

Levine, B., Robertson, I.H., Clare, L., Hong, J., Wilson, B.A., Duncan, J., & Stuss, D.T. (2000). Rehabilitation of executive functioning: an experimental–clinical validation of goal management training. *Journal of the International Neuropsychological Society, 6*, 299–312.

Luria, A.R. & Homskaya, E.D. (1964). Disturbance in the regulative role of speech with frontal lobe lesions. In: J.M. Warren & K. Akert (Eds.), *The Frontal Granular Cortex and Behavior* (pp. 353–371). New York: McGraw-Hill.

Manly, T., Hawkins, K., Evans, J., Woldt, K., & Robertson, I.H. (In press a). Rehabilitation of executive function: facilitation of effective goal management on complex tasks using periodic auditory alerts. *Neuropsychologia.*

Manly, T., Lewis, G.H., Robertson, I.H., Watson, P.C., &

Datta, A. (In press b). "Coffee in the cornflakes": time of day, routine response control and subjective sleepiness. *Neuropsychologia.*

Mateer, C.A. (1999). The rehabilitation of executive disorders. In: D.T. Stuss, G. Winocur, & I.H. Robertson (Eds.), *Cognitive Neurorehabilitation* (pp. 314–332). Cambridge, UK: Cambridge University Press.

McCarthy, R.A. & Warrington, E.K. (1990). *Cognitive Neuropsychology: A Clinical Introduction.* London: Academic Press.

Miyake, A., Friedman, N.P., Emerson, M.J., Witzki, A.H., Howerter, A., & Wager, T.D. (2000). The unity and diversity of executive functions and their contributions to complex "frontal lobe" tasks: a latent variable analysis. *Cognitive Psychology, 41*, 49–100.

Morris, R.G., Downes, J.J., Sahakian, B.J., Polkey, C.E., & Robbins, T.W. (1988). Planning and spatial working memory in Parkinson's disease. *Journal of Neurology, Neurosurgery and Psychiatry, 51*, 757–766.

Morton, J. & Bekerian, D.A. (1986). Three ways of looking at memory. In: N.E. Sharkey (ed.), *Advances in Cognitive Sciences I* (pp. 43–71). Chichester: Ellis Horwood Ltd.

Norman, D. & Shallice, T. (1986). Attention to action. In: R.J. Davidson, G.E. Schwartz, & D. Shapiro (Eds.), *Consciousness and Self-Regulation* (pp. 1–18). New York: Plenum Press.

Okada, K., Kobayashi, S., Yamagata, S., Takahashi, K., & Yamaguchi, S. (1997). Poststroke apathy and regional cerebral blood flow. *Stroke, 28*, 2437–2441.

Owen, A.M., Downes, J.J., Sahakian, B.J., Polkey, C.E., & Robbins, T.W. (1990). Planning and spatial working memory following frontal lobe lesions in man. *Neuropsychologia, 28*, 757–766.

Owen, A.M., Sahakian, B.J., Hodges, J.R., Summers, B.A., Polkey, C.E., & Robbins, T.W. (1995). Dopamine-dependent fronto-striatal planning deficits in early Parkinson's disease. *Neuropsychology, 9*, 126–140.

Passingham, R. (1993). *The Frontal Lobes and Voluntary Action.* Oxford: Oxford University Press.

Petrides, M. (1994). Frontal lobes and working memory: evidence from investigations of the effects of cortical excisions in nonhuman primates. In: F. Boller & J. Grafman (Eds.), *Handbook of Neuropsychology*, Vol. 9 (pp. 59–82). Amsterdam: Elsevier.

Petrides, M. (1998). Specialized systems for the processing of mnemonic information within the primate frontal cortex. In: A.C. Roberts, T.W. Robbins, & L. Weiskrantz (Eds.), *The Prefrontal Cortex: Executive and Cognitive Functions* (pp. 103–116). Oxford: Oxford University Press.

Powell, J.H., al-Adawi, S., Morgan, J., & Greenwood, R.J. (1996). Motivational deficits after brain injury: effects of bromocriptine in 11 patients. *Journal of Neurology, Neurosurgery and Psychiatry, 60*, 416–421.

Prigatano, G.P. (1991a). Disturbances of self-awareness of deficit after traumatic brain injury. In: G.P. Prigatano & D.L. Schacter (Eds.), *Awareness of Deficit after Brain Injury: Clinical and Theoretical Issues.* New York: Oxford University Press.

Prigatano, G.P. (1991b). The relationship of frontal lobe

damage to diminished awareness: studies in rehabilitation. In: H.S. Levin, H.M. Eisenberg, & A.L. Benton (Eds.), *Frontal Lobe Function and Dysfunction* (pp. 381–397). New York: Oxford University Press.

Robbins, T.W. (1998). Dissociating executive functions of the prefrontal cortex. In: A.C. Roberts, T.W. Robbins, & L. Weiskrantz (Eds.), *The Prefrontal Cortex: Executive and Cognitive Functions* (pp. 117–130). Oxford: Oxford University Press.

Robertson, I.H. (1996). *Goal Management Training: A Clinical Manual.* Cambridge, UK: PsyConsult.

Robertson, I.H. (1999). The rehabilitation of attention. In D.T. Stuss, G. Winocur, & I.H. Robertson (Eds.), *Cognitive Neurorehabilitation* (pp. 302–313). Cambridge, UK: Cambridge University Press.

Robertson, I.H., Tegner, R., Tham, K., Lo, A., & Nimmo-Smith, I. (1995). Sustained attention training for unilateral neglect: theoretical and rehabilitation implications. *Journal of Clinical and Experimental Neuropsychology, 17,* 416–430.

Robertson, I.H., Ward, T., Ridgeway, V., & Nimmo-Smith, I. (1996). The structure of normal human attention: the Test of Everyday Attention. *Journal of the International Neuropsychological Society, 2,* 525–534.

Shallice, T. (1982). Specific impairments of planning. *Philosophical Transactions of the Royal Society of London B, 298,* 199–209.

Shallice, T. (1988). *From Neuropsychology to Mental Structure.* New York: Cambridge University Press.

Shallice, P.W. & Burgess, P.W. (1991a). Deficits in strategy application following frontal lobe damage in man. *Brain, 114,* 727–741.

Shallice, T. & Burgess, P.W. (1991b). Higher-order cognitive impairments and frontal lobe lesions in man. In: H.S. Levin, H.M. Eisenberg, & A.L. Benton (Eds.), *Frontal Lobe Function and Dysfunction* (pp. 125–138). New York: Oxford University Press.

Shallice, T. & Burgess, P.W. (1993). Supervisory control of action and thought selection. In: A.D. Baddeley & L. Weiskrantz (Eds.), *Attention: Selection, Awareness and Control.* Oxford: Oxford University Press.

Shallice, T. & Burgess, P.W. (1996). The domain of supervisory processes and the temporal organisation of behaviour. *Philosophical Transactions of the Royal Society of London B, 351,* 1405–1412. [Reprinted in: A.C. Roberts, T.W. Robbins, & L. Weiskrantz (Eds.), *The Prefrontal Cortex: Executive and Cognitive Functions* (pp. 22–35). Oxford: Oxford University Press, 1998.]

Shallice, T., Burgess, P.W., Schon, F., & Baxter, D.M. (1989). The origins of utilisation behaviour. *Brain, 112,* 1587–1598.

Stuss, D.T. & Alexander, M.P. (2000). Executive functions and the frontal lobes: a conceptual view. *Psychological Research, 63,* 289–298.

Stuss, D.T. & Benson, D.F. (1984). Neuropsychological studies of the frontal lobes. *Psychological Bulletin, 95,* 3–29.

Stuss, D.T. & Benson, D.F. (1986). *The Frontal Lobes.* New York: Raven Press.

Stuss, D.T., Eskes, G.A., & Foster, J.K. (1994). Experimental neuropsychological studies of frontal lobe functions. In: F. Boller & J. Grafman (Eds.), *Handbook of Neuropsychology,* Vol. 9. Amsterdam: Elsevier Science B.V.

Stuss, D.T., Shallice, T., Alexander, M.P., & Picton, T.W. (1995). A mulitidisciplinary approach to anterior attentional functions. *Annals of the New York Academy of Sciences, 769,* 191–211.

Stuss, D.T., Toth, J.P., Franchi, D., Alexander, M.P., Tipper, S., & Craik, F.I.M. (1999). Dissociation of attentional processes in patients with focal frontal and posterior lesions. *Neuropsychologia, 37,* 1005–1027.

Stuss, D.T., Levine, B., Alexander, M.P., Hong, J., Palumbo, C., Hamer, L., Murphy, K.J., & Izukawa, D. (2000). Wisconsin Card Sorting Test performance in patients with focal frontal and posterior brain damage: effects of lesion location and test structure on separable cognitive processes. *Neuropsychologia, 38,* 388–402.

Tamamoto, F., Sumi, Y., Nakanishi, A., Okayasu, K., Maehara, T., & Katayama, H. (2000). Usefulness of cerebral blood flow (CBF) measurements to predict the functional outcome for rehabilitation in patients with cerebrovascular disease (CVD). *Annals of Nuclear Medicine, 14,* 47–52.

Toyer, A.K., Moscovitch, M., Winucur, G., Alexander, M.P., & Stuss, D. (1998). Dissociation of attentional processes in patients with focal frontal and posterior lesions. *Neuropsychologia, 37,* 1005–1027.

Welsh, M.C., Saterlee-Cartmell, T., & Stine, M. (1999). Towers of Hanoi and London: contribution of working memory and inhibition to performance. *Brain and Cognition, 41,* 231–242.

Welsh, M.C., Revilla, V., Strongin, D., & Kepler, M. (2000). Towers of Hanoi and London: is the nonshared variance due to differences in task administration? *Perceptual and Motor Skills, 90,* 562–572.

Wilson, B.A., Alderman, N., Burgess, P.W., Emslie, H., & Evans, J.J. (1996). *Behavioural Assessment of the Dysexecutive Syndrome (BADS).* Bury St. Edmunds, UK: Thames Valley Test Company.

Wilson, B.A., Evans, J.J., Emslie, H., & Malinek, V. (1997). Evaluation of NeuroPage: a new memory aid. *Journal of Neurology, Neurosurgery and Psychiatry, 6,* 113–115.

34

Prefrontal Cortex: The Present and the Future

ROBERT T. KNIGHT AND DONALD T. STUSS

The frontal lobes have provided the tools to now study how tools are actually devised in the human mind.
R.T. Knight and D.T. Stuss 2001

In this chapter the current neuropsychological and physiological evidence linking lateral and orbital prefrontal cortex (PFC) to human cognition and social interchange will be reviewed in an attempt to provide a summary of much of the work presented in this book and elsewhere. We will begin with our view of the contributions of lateral PFC to executive control. This book provides evidence of a remarkable convergence of lesion, electrophysiological, and functional magnetic resonance imaging (fMRI) and data on the role of lateral PFC in inhibitory control, excitatory modulation, working memory, and novelty processing. The electrophysiological data accrued from humans and animals provide important information on the timing of PFC modulation of cognitive processing. These data are complemented by fMRI findings defining the spatial characteristics of PFC involvement in a variety of cognitive tasks, with evidence mounting for engagement of interleaved inhibitory and excitatory processes during a host of cognitive processes. Finally, the neuropsychological data provide the crucial behavioral confirmation of

electrophysiological and fMRI findings obtained in normal populations. In our view the most complete picture will emerge from the fusion of classic neuropsychological approaches informed by cognitive theory with powerful new techniques to measure human brain physiology. We will first review the findings concerning the role of lateral PFC in executive control of cognition and then discuss the relevant literature on the contributions of orbital PFC to social and emotional control. This chapter will not address the role of medial PFC cortex in various aspects of motor planning, nor will we discuss language and PFC, which is reviewed by Alexander in Chapter 10. A possible separate role for the polar regions may exist, but the evidence is currently inadequate to introduce in this review.

LATERAL PREFRONTAL CORTEX

INTRODUCTION

Evidence from neuropsychological, electrophysiological, and neuroimaging research supports a critical role of PFC in executive control of goal-directed behavior. Lateral PFC, including portions of the inferior, middle, and superior frontal gyri, is involved in multiple domains, including language, attention, and memory (Stuss & Benson, 1984, 1986; D'Esposito et al., 1995, 1999a, 1999b, Chao & Knight, 1998; Corbetta, 1998; Knight et al., 1998; D'Esposito and Postle, 1999; Dronkers et al., 2000; Fuster et al., 2000; McDonald et al., 2000). Functional MRI and event-related potential (ERP) research have defined the spatial and temporal contributions of lateral PFC in working memory, attention, response conflict, and novelty processing (Jonides et al., 1993, 1998; Knight et al., 1998; Owen et al., 1998; Botvinick et al., 1999; Barch et al., 2000; Prabhakaran et al., 2000). A meta-analysis of neuroimaging studies (Duncan & Owen, 2000) reveals activation of common regions of lateral PFC in diverse cognitive tasks. The PFC activations in these seemingly diverse cognitive domains center in the posterior portions of the lateral PFC at the junction of the middle and inferior frontal gyri, including portions of dorsal and ventral PFC (Brodmann's areas 9, 44, 45, and 46; Rajkowska & Goldman-Rakic, 1995a, 1995b). This suggests that common regions of the human PFC are able to control many aspects of human cognition. Furthermore, fMRI research has revealed that extensive areas of dorsal and ventral PFC are crucial for sustaining neural activations during cognitive performance and more dorsal portions of PFC appear to be crucial for manipulating neural activity during cognitive performance. Thus, a more complete behavioral and physiological picture of the functions of subregions of human lateral PFC is emerging.

The extensive reciprocal PFC connections to virtually all cortical and subcortical structures place PFC in a unique neuroanatomical position to monitor and manipulate diverse cognitive processes. Lateral prefrontal damage in humans results in behavioral deficits in attention, working memory, planning, response selection, temporal coding, metamemory, judgment, and insight. In advanced bilateral lateral PFC damage, the patient has a flattened affect, manifests perseverative behavior, and is unable to properly manage everyday affairs. The patient may be incorrectly diagnosed as being depressed, although careful evaluation actually reveals indifference and an amotivational state rather than true feelings of depression. This amotivational state can be differentiated from the amotivation seen in patients with pure superior medial or orbitofrontal pathology (Stuss, et al., 2000). The amotivational state extends to both the cognitive and emotional domain. For instance, cognitive flexibility and creativity as well as sexual drive are frequently reduced. Frontal release signs (primitive reflexes including snout, rooting, suck, grasp, and palmomental) are often observed (Knight & Grabowecky, 2000). Performance of the Luria handsequencing task, in which the patient is required to repetitively produce the sequence fist–palm of hand–edge of hand, is often abnormal because of perseverative and random errors.

It should be emphasized that the severe lateral prefrontal syndrome is typically observed in bilateral PFC damage, as might be observed in degenerative disease, infiltrating tumors, or multiple cortical or subcortical infarctions. This clinical observation emphasizes the inherent redundancy in the capacity of lateral PFC function to control cognitive processing. This is not to say that clear behavioral and physiological deficits are not apparent after unilateral damage. Rather, these deficits are not as obvious as one might expect. One intact PFC is able to control bilateral hemispheric processing to some degree. The way in which this redundancy of function is accomplished is not clear, although recent animal work suggests that processing may be accomplished by callosal transfer of information to the intact PFC (Rossi et al., 1999; Tomita et al, 1999). The use of the intact processes in the undamaged frontal lobe to overcome or compensate for the deficit in the damaged region of the prefrontal lobe has also been hypothesized (Stuss, et al., 1987).

NEUROPSYCHOLOGY

Human behavior is paralleled by a massive expansion of the PFC, which occupies up to 35% of the neocortical mantle in humans. In contrast, the PFC occupies about 10%–12% of the cortical mantle in high-level nonhuman primates such as gorillas (Fuster, 1989). Since lateral PFC is involved in so many aspects of behavior, characterization of a mild prefrontal syndrome can be elusive. Prefrontal damage from strokes, tumors, trauma, or degenerative disorders is notoriously difficult to diagnose, since deficits in creativity and mental flexibility may be the only salient findings (Knight, 1991). Patients may complain that they are not able to pay attention as well and that their memory is not quite as sharp. An early lateral PFC syndrome may become clinically obvious only if the patient has a job requiring some degree of mental flexibility and decision making. However, if the patient has a routinized job or lifestyle, prefrontal damage can be quite advanced before a diagnosis is made. Indeed, many prefrontal tumors are extensive at initial diagnosis. As unilateral prefrontal disease progresses or becomes bilateral pronounced, abnormalities invariably become evident. Deficits in attention, planning, response selection, temporal coding, metamemory, judgment, and insight predominate. In advanced bilateral lateral PFC damage, perseveration, manifesting behaviorally as being fixed in the present and unable to effectively go forward or backward in time, becomes evident. In association with these deficits, confidence about many aspects of behavior deteriorates. Indeed, patients with prefrontal damage may be uncertain about the appropriateness of their behavior even when it is correct.

The behavioral changes that arise from damage to the PFC are notoriously difficult to capture with many standardized neuropsychological tests. Patients with large prefrontal lesions can perform within the normal range on tests of memory, intelligence, and other cognitive functions, one observation that has led to the often-cited "paradox" or "riddle" of the frontal lobes. Even supposedly frontal lobe–sensitive tests such as the Wisconsin Card Sorting Test (WCST) sometimes fail to discriminate patients with frontal lesions from people with normal function or those with lesions in other regions (Eslinger & Damasio, 1985; Grafman et al., 1990). This is due in part to a mixing of lesion location. Clinicians and researchers often do not differentiate regions within the frontal lobes. However, when one segregates subregions of PFC damage, a clearer pattern of regional specificity emerges. For instance, tests such as the WCST appear to be more sensitive to dorsolateral than orbitofrontal PFC damage (see chapter 25). In addition, there is often a lack of specificity as to the precise process that is impaired. For example, the notion that only perseverative errors are made by PFC lesioned patients in the WCST may contribute to some of the confusion in the literature. Recent findings in patients with lateral PFC damage indicate that these patients make as many random errors as perseverative errors (Barcelo & Knight, in press). Perseverative errors are traditionally viewed as a failure in inhibition of previous response patterns. A perseverative error on the WCST is due to failure to shift set to a new sorting criterion. Random errors that are as frequent as perseverative errors reflect a different problem in these patients. A random error occurs when a patient is sorting correctly and switches to a new incorrect sorting category without any prompt from the examiner. Random errors can be viewed as a transient failure in maintaining the goal at hand and may represent a problem with maintenance of neural activity during the sorting task. As will be discussed later, excitation-dependent maintenance of distributed neural circuits appears to be a key aspect of PFC function (for reviews see Knight et al., 1998; D'Esposito and Postle, 1999). Other tasks often employed by clinical neuropsychologists to capture lateral PFC deficits include variations of the Stroop Test, which is particularly sensitive to failures in inhibitory control, and tests of divided attention. However, tests of divided attention are also failed by patients with inferior parietal lobe damage and do not provide a specific assay of PFC function. It should be emphasized that patients with lesions in different parts of the brain may fail the same task, but for different reasons.

While conventional neuropsychological tests such as the Wecshler Adult Intelligence Scale (WAIS) may be normal or only show minimal deficits, patients with lateral PFC cortex damage may be quite impaired in their daily lives. How can this paradox of relatively good performance on standardized tests be reconciled with impaired functioning in daily life? We will first review the current experimental neuro-psychological literature on lateral PFC dysfunction and then we will present some new concepts drawn from the cognitive psychology literature that may provide additional insight into understanding the human lateral PFC syndrome. After reviewing the neuropsychological literature, we will then discuss the physiological data, including ERPs and fMRI, which delineate of the role of lateral PFC in human cognition.

Temporal Processing

Patients with frontal lobe lesions are impaired in tasks involving temporal ordering, such as the sequencing of recent or remote events Milner, et al., 1985; Moscovitch, 1989; Shimamura, et al., 1990; McAndrews & Milner, 1991). These patients are also impaired in making recency judgments (Milner, 1971; Janowsky et al., 1989a; 1989b; Milner, et al., 1985), a process that also relies on the correct temporal coding of events. Performance of self-ordered pointing, a task in which the patient must remember the order in which objects have been indicated, is also impaired in patients with frontal lesions (Petrides & Milner, 1982). Patients with extensive frontal lesions also have little concern for either the past or the future (Goldstein, 1944; Ackerly & Benton, 1947). These patients are "stuck" in the present world, with severe perseveration representing the penultimate example of failure to move across the time dimension. To fluidly move from the present to either the past or the future, one must be able to both inhibit the current mental context and find or construct a new mental image, requiring excitation-dependent activation of neural ensembles. This PFC dependent interplay between inhibitory and excitatory activity will become apparent when physiological data relevant to PFC function are reviewed.

Explicit Memory, Source Memory, and Metamemory

While some sources suggest that explicit memory is normal in patients with lateral PFC damage, a meta-analysis of the published data shows significant deficits in explicit memory in patients with lateral PFC damage (Wheeler et al., 1995). These deficits are typically not as severe in patients with medial temporal amnesia, but this distinction is compromised by the fact that most studies have compared unilateral PFC lesions to bilateral medial temporal amnestics such as that occurring from CA1 hypoxic damage or herpes simplex. In other studies, patients with Korsakoff's syndrome or ruptured anterior communicating aneurysms have been compared to unilateral PFC patients. Thus, the true degree of explicit memory dysfunction in patients with bilateral PFC damage has probably been underestimated. If the pathology is in the left PFC or involves septal/basal-forebrain areas, an encoding deficit is revealed (Stuss et al., 1994). Patients with damage to PFC show a disproportionate impairment in the memory for source of information (Schacter et al., 1984; Shimamura & Squire, 1987; Janowsky, et al., 1989b). Factual information is correctly recalled, but the spatiotemporal context in which the information was acquired is forgotten. These patients also have a diminished ability to make metamemory judgments (Janowsky et al., 1989b). *Metamemory* includes an ability to judge whether or not the answer to a factual question has been or will be correctly retrieved. Patients with frontal lesions are impaired at making these judgments even though their memory for the facts is intact. In contrast, patients with medial temporal amnesia have explicit memory impairments but are quite confident about the limited number of items they recall.

Inhibitory Control

There is long-standing evidence that distraction due to a failure in inhibitory control is a key element of the deficit observed in monkeys on delayed-response tasks (Malmo, 1942; Brutkowski, 1965; Bartus & Levere, 1977). For example, simple maneuvers such as turning off the lights in the laboratory or mildly sedating the animal, which would typically impair performance in intact animals, improved delay performance in animals with PFC lesions. Despite this evidence, remarkably few data have been obtained on humans with PFC damage. The extant data center on failures in inhibition of early sensory input as well as problems in inhibition of higher-level cognitive processes.

In the sensory domain, it has been shown that inability to suppress irrelevant information is associated with difficulties in sustained attention, target detection, and match-to-sample paradigms in both monkeys and humans (Woods & Knight, 1986; Richer et al., 1993; Chao & Knight, 1995, 1998). Delivery of task-irrelevant sensory information disproportionately reduces performance in patients with lateral PFC lesions. For example, presentation of brief, high-frequency tone pips during a tone-matching delay task markedly reduces performance in PFC patients. In essence, the patient with a lateral PFC lesion functions in a noisy environment because of a failure to gate out extraneous sensory information.

In the cognitive domain, inhibitory deficits in cognitive tasks requiring suppression of prior learned material are also observed in patients with lateral PFC lesions (Shimamura et al., 1995; Mangels et al., 1996). Prior learned information now irrelevant to the task intrudes on performance. For example, words from a prior list of stimuli employed in a memory task may be inappropriately recalled during recall of a subsequent list of words. In essence, the PFC patient is unable to sweep the internal mental slate clean, thus previously learned material maintains an active neural representation. Inability to suppress previous incorrect responses may underlie the poor performance of PFC subjects on a wide range of neuropsychological tasks, such as the Wisconsin Card Sorting Task, and Stroop Task (Shimamura et al., 1992). Interestingly, there is some evidence that inhibitory failure extends to some aspects of motoric control. For instance, lateral PFC damage results in a deficit in suppressing reflexive eye movements to task-irrelevant spatial locations (Guitton et al., 1985).

Working Memory and Attention

Working memory and attention are core concepts necessary to understand lateral PFC function. *Working memory* refers to the ability to maintain information over a delay and to manipulate the contents of this short-term memory storage system. Working memory is ubiquitous to many cognitive tasks. A trivial example of working memory would be remembering a phone number just obtained from the operator. This task would only require maintenance of the numbers over a few-second period and would typically not be impaired in unilateral disease. However, if one were asked to remember the same number over the same few-second delay but now also respond at the end of the delay as to whether this number matched a number given a few minutes previously, deficits would be apparent in patients with lateral PFC disease. In the second situation, both maintenance and manipulation of the contents of working memory are required, and both of these are dependent on lateral PFC. Experimental findings provide a critical link between the animal and human working memory literature. Monkeys with bilateral frontal lesions involving the sulcus principalis, proposed to be equivalent to human lateral PFC (Brodmanns areas 9 and 46; Rajkowska & Goldman-Rakic, 1995a, 1995b), are severely impaired at delayed-response tasks (Jacobsen, 1935). In delayed-response tasks, information critical to perform a certain task is initially presented. The experimenter then interposes a delay period before the animal or human is allowed to perform the task. For successful performance, the information must be reliably held in a short-term working memory buffer during the delay period. Ablation, cryogenic depression, or dopamine depletion in the sulcus principalis area results in an inability of the monkey to retain the critical information at intervals as short as 1 second (Funahashi et al., 1993).

Subsequent animal research showed that problems with inhibition of extraneous inputs contributed to the delayed-response deficit. Simple maneuvers such as turning off the lights in the laboratory or mildly sedating the animal, which would typically impair performance in intact animals, improved delay performance in prefrontal-lesioned animals. These observations led to the formulation of the *distractibility hypothesis* (Malmo, 1942; Bartus & Levere, 1977), which postulates that prefrontal patients are unable to suppress responses to irrelevant stimuli during delay tasks. Impairments in inhibitory control in prefrontal patients and fMRI evidence linking lateral PFC to inhibitory control provides further support for the prefrontal–distractibility hypothesis. Successful performance on the delayed-response task, of course, requires more than inhibitory control. Subjects must select and activate distributed brain regions, depending on task-specific parameters. Data from neurological patients has revealed that lateral PFC modulates excitatory pathways projecting into subregions of visual and auditory association cortices during attention and working memory tasks. In accord with these physiological deficits in inhibition and excitation, prefrontal patients are distractible and unable to maintain the focus of attention.

Working memory tasks in humans, widely viewed as dependent on lateral PFC, share a core task structure with the monkey delayed-response task. Single-unit, lesion, ERP, blood flow, and neural models (Funahashi et al., 1993; Jonides et al., 1993: Cohen et al., 1996; Chao & Knight, 1998; Rainer et al., 1998a, 1998b) have shown that lateral PFC is required to perform any task requiring a delay. Thus, delayed-response tasks and working memory share some common neural mechanisms in animals and humans. Despite the clear link between working memory, delayed-response performance, and PFC, there have been a limited number of experimental studies on working memory capacity in humans with PFC lesions. Moreover, working memory tasks are infrequently employed in clinical neuropsychological work. However, all studies examining working memory in patients with lateral PFC lesions have reported deficits (Chao & Knight, 1995, 1998; Harrington et al., 1998; Stone et al., 1998).

Patients with prefrontal lesions are also impaired in their ability to focus attention on task-relevant stimuli (Knight et al., 1981; Damasio, 1985; Woods & Knight, 1986). It should be noted that attention deficits are often more severe after right PFC damage. Patients with right prefrontal damage show electrophysiological and behavioral evidence of a dense hemi-inattention to left ear stimuli (Woods & Knight 1986), as in the human hemi-neglect syndrome, which is more common after right prefrontal or temporal–parietal lesions (Kertesz & Dobrolowski, 1981; Mesulam, 1981, 1998). Increased size of the right frontal lobe in humans may provide the anatomical basis for the hemi-inattention syndrome in humans. The left hemi-neglect syndrome subsequent to right temporal–parietal damage may be due to remote effects of disconnection from asymmetrically organized prefrontal regions.

Novelty Processing

The capacity to detect novelty in the stream of external sensory events or internal thoughts and the ability to produce novel behaviors are crucial for new learning, creativity, and flexible adjustments to perturbations in the environment. Indeed, creative behavior in fields extending from science to the arts is commonly defined in direct relation to the degree of novelty. Prefrontal patients have problems with the solving of novel problems (Goldberg et al., 1994; Godfrey & Rousseaux, 1997) and the generation of novel behaviors (Daffner et al., 2000a, 2000b). In advanced disease indifference, loss of creativity, and deficits in orienting to novel stimuli emerge. In accord with these clinical observations, prefrontal damage markedly reduces the scalp electrophysiological response to unexpected novel stimuli in the auditory (Knight, 1984; Knight & Scabini, 1998), visual (Knight, 1997), and somatosensory modalities (Yamaguchi & Knight, 1991, 1992). The physiological link between PFC and novelty processing will be expanded in the Physiology section (below).

Behavioral Monitoring

Behavioral output is constantly monitored so that incorrect responses can be detected and corrected. One notices this system in operation in everyday behavior, such as reaching for the wrong object on a table and attempting to on-line correct the incorrect movement. Another example might be attempting to stop a swing at a baseball pitch that is not in the strike zone. One might extend this notion to the monitoring of complex cognitive and social exchange. For instance, two linked classes of higher-level cognitive operations, simulation behavior and reality checking, are proposed to be impaired after lateral PFC damage (Knight & Grabowecky, 2000). *Simulation* refers to the process of generating internal models of external reality. These models may represent an accurate past or an alternative past, present, or future and include models of the environment, of other people, and of the self. *Reality checking* refers to processes that monitor information accrued from interactions with the external world in an effort to accurately represent their spatiotemporal context (Kahneman & Miller, 1986). These monitoring processes are critical for discriminating between simulations of alternate possibilities and veridical models of the world. Simulation and reality checking are considered "supervisory" (Shallice, 1988) or "executive" (Milner & Petrides, 1984; Stuss & Benson, 1986; (Baddeley & Wilson, 1988) and are essential for behavior to be integrated, coherent, and contextually appropriate. Simulation behavior and reality checking are necessary for permitting actions to be dissociated from current environmental constraints. They permit humans to create mental representations of the world that may either draw on prior experience or be entirely innovative. A patient who cannot simulate alternatives to a situation becomes "stimulus bound" (Luria, 1966; Lhermitte, 1986; Lhermitte et al., 1986) and is incapable of responding flexibly. Without reality checking, a patient cannot discriminate between internally generated possibilities and the model of the external world as it currently exists. Simulation and reality checking work in concert, allowing humans to simulate manipulations of the external environment, evaluate the consequences of those manipulations, and act on the results of those simulations.

Stimulus bound behavior is typical in patients with PFC damage (Luria, 1966; Lhermitte, 1986). The patients studied by Lhermitte and colleagues included those with large lateral PFC lesions that extended into the orbital and basal ganglia regions in some subjects. Thus, precise behavioral–anatomical conclusions must be tempered. Objects placed in front of prefrontal patients in the Lhermitte studies were picked up and used (utilization behavior) without the patient being asked to do so (Lhermitte, 1986). Behavior of the experimenter may be imitated, even when this behavior is bizarre and socially inappropriate. Thus, patients with frontal lesions appear excessively bound by environmental cues. Patients with PFC lesions have also been described as lacking insight and foresight, as being incapable of planning either for the near or distant future, and as being deficient in creativity (Hebb & Penfield, 1940; Ackerly & Benton, 1948; Damasio, 1985; Eslinger & Damasio, 1985). This set of abnormal behaviors may be a consequence of a deficit in the ability to simulate alternative scenarios of the current situation. Once again, precise behavioral–anatomical conclusions cannot be obtained, since clear lesion definition is only provided in the Damasio cohort as predominantly orbital damage.

The term *reality checking* refers to those aspects of monitoring the external world that have been called "reality testing" when they concern the present, and "reality monitoring" when they concern the past. Reality checking includes both an awareness of the difference between an internally generated alternate reality and a current reality, and the maintenance of a true past in the presence of counterfactual alternatives that one might construct (Kahneman & Varey, 1990). Reality checking is essential for simulation processes to be carried out without compromising the ability to respond to the objective environment. Simulation processes generate an alternate reality that must be evaluated in relation to its divergence from the current reality. Memories are created for both events experienced in the world and events experienced through internally constructed simulations. These two sources of memories must be treated differently for them to be used effectively. Given that both internal and external events create memory representations, what cues differentiate our internal models of reality from our internal simulations of reality? Johnson and Raye (1981) studied normal subjects' abilities to discriminate between memories of external events and those of internally generated events. Rich memory traces with many sensory features were ascribed to external experience. Memories of external events tend to be more detailed and have more spatial and temporal contextual information. Internally generated memories tend to be abstract and schematic, lacking in detail. These two memory representations form overlapping populations, and similar internal and external events may become confused. Reality checking involves a continual assessment of the relationship between behavior and the environment. As an individual acts on the environment, the consequences of the action must be incorporated into existing plans. If the environment deviates from expectations, one needs to detect this change and plans must be reassessed. It is proposed that these processes of continual reality checking and simulation are impaired in patients with frontal lobe lesions (Knight & Grabowecky, 2000). There is a paucity of neuropsychological literature linking simulation and reality monitoring to PFC, although some data indicate that monitoring in memory is related to dorsolateral areas, more on the right (Stuss et al., 1994). Reality monitoring has also been proposed as a major mechanism underlying different disturbances of self-awareness (Stuss, 1991; Stuss et al., 2001b).

PHYSIOLOGY

Physiological research strongly supports and extends the results demonstrated in the neuropsychological literature. The physiological literature demonstrates the temporal unfolding of frontal lobe processes. In this section, we will emphasize that basic concepts such as inhibitory and excitatory control, a bias to novelty, and response monitoring can provide useful physiological constructs for beginning to understand PFC function.

Inhibitory Control

The PFC inhibitory control of subcortical (Edinger et al., 1975) and cortical regions has been documented in a variety of mammalian preparations (Alexander et al., 1976; Skinner & Yingling, 1977; Yingling & Skinner, 1977). Galambos (1956) provided the first physiological evidence of an inhibitory auditory pathway

in mammals with the description of the brain stem olivocochlear bundle. The olivocochlear bundle projects from the olivary nucleus in the brain stem to the cochleus in the inner ear. Stimulation of this bundle results in inhibition of transmission from the cochlea to the brain stem cochlear nucleus as measured by reductions in evoked responses in the auditory nerve. This pathway provides a system for early sensory suppression in the auditory system. The evidence for sensory filtering at the cochlear or brain stem level in humans is controversial, with most laboratories finding no evidence of attention-related manipulation of the brain stem auditory-evoked response (Woods & Hillyard, 1978; Woldorff & Hillyard, 1991).

Subsequent research in the 1970s reported evidence of a multimodal prefrontal–thalamic inhibitory system in cats that regulates sensory flow to primary cortical regions. Reversible suppression of the cat PFC by cooling (cryogenic blockade) increased the amplitudes of evoked responses recorded in primary cortex in all sensory modalities (Skinner & Yingling, 1977; Yingling & Skinner, 1977). Conversely, stimulation of the thalamic region (nucleus reticularis thalami) surrounding the sensory relay nuclei resulted in modality-specific suppression of activity in primary sensory cortex. This effect is also observed in all sensory modalities. These data provided the first physiological evidence of a prefrontal inhibitory pathway regulating sensory transmission through thalamic relay nuclei. This prefrontal–thalamic inhibitory system provides a mechanism for modality-specific suppression of irrelevant inputs at an early stage of sensory processing. As noted, this system is modulated by an excitatory lateral PFC projection to the nucleus reticularis thalami, although the precise course of anatomical projections between these structures is not well understood. The nucleus reticularis thalami, in turn, sends inhibitory GABA-ergic projections to sensory relay nuclei, providing a neural substrate for selective sensory suppression (Guillery et al., 1998).

There is also evidence in humans that the PFC exhibits control on other cortical and subcortical regions. For example, ERP studies in patients with focal PFC damage have shown that primary auditory and somatosensory evoked responses are enhanced (Knight et al., 1989a; Yamaguchi & Knight, 1990; Chao & Knight, 1998), suggesting disinhibition of sensory flow to primary cortical regions. In a series of experiments, task-irrelevant auditory and somatosensory stimuli (monaural clicks or brief electric shocks to the median nerve) were presented to patients with comparably sized lesions in lateral PFC, the temporal–parietal junction, or lateral parietal cortex. Evoked responses from primary auditory (Kraus et al., 1982) and somatosensory (Leuders et al., 1983; Sutherling et al., 1988; Wood et al., 1988) cortices were recorded from these patients and age-matched controls. Damage to primary auditory or somatosensory cortex in the temporal–parietal lesion group reduced the early latency (20–40 ms) evoked responses generated in these primary cortical regions. Posterior association cortex lesions in the lateral parietal lobe sparing primary sensory regions had no effect on early sensory potentials and served as a brain-lesioned control group. Lateral PFC damage resulted in enhanced amplitudes of both the primary auditory and somatosensory evoked responses (Knight et al., 1989a; Yamaguchi & Knight, 1990; Chao & Knight, 1998). Spinal cord and brain stem potentials were not affected by lateral PFC damage, suggesting that the amplitude enhancements were due to abnormalities in either a prefrontal–thalamic or a prefrontal–sensory cortex mechanism. These results are in accord with the findings reported in the 1970s by Yingling and Skinner in their cat model of PFC dependent sensory gating.

Behavioral and imaging evidence of the involvement of lateral PFC in inhibitory control (Konishi et al., 1998) does not provide direct support for the hypothesis that there are inhibitory signals from the PFC directed either toward early sensory cortices or excitatory PFC inputs to the GABAergic nucleus reticularis thalami, resulting in a net inhibitory control of sensory flow. In contrast, the combined ERP/patient studies described above are able to measure the temporal dynamics of inhibitory control and provide powerful evidence in humans that the PFC provides a net inhibitory regulation of early sensory transmission.

Excitatory Control

Attention allows us to select from the myriad of closely spaced and timed environmental events. Attention is crucial for virtually all cognitive abilities. Indeed, recent cognitive theorists have begun to refer to attention/working memory, highlighting that these two constructs are inextricably linked. In addition to suppressing responses to irrelevant stimuli, subjects must excite and sustain neural activity in distributed brain regions to perform attention/working memory tasks. Computational modeling employing prefrontal excitatory modulation of distributed brain regions has successfully modeled prefrontally medicated behaviors in people with normal function and prefrontal dysfunction (e.g., patients with schizophrenia) (Cohen & Servan-Scrieber, 1992; Cohen et al., 1996). These authors postulate that dorsal PFC controls task context by regulating posterior association cortex through excitatory connections. Desimone (1998) has proposed a competition-based model of visual attention in which visual neurons involved in the processing of different aspects of the visual world are mutually inhibitory. In this view, an excitatory signal to selective visual neurons would result in inhibition of nearby non–task-relevant visual neurons, resulting in a sharpening of the attentional focus. Patients with focal prefrontal damage fail to maintain excitatory control of posterior association cortex, resulting in failures in attention/working memory.

Selective attention to an ear, a region of the visual field, or a digit increases the amplitude of sensory evoked potentials to all stimuli delivered to that sensory channel (Hillyard et al., 1973). There is evidence that attention reliably modulates neural activity at early sensory cortices, including secondary and perhaps primary sensory cortex (Woldorff et al., 1993; Grady et al., 1997; Somers et al., 1999; Steinmetz et al., 2000). Visual attention involves modulation in the excitability of extrastriate neurons through descending projections from hierarchically ordered brain structures (Hillyard & Anllo-Vento, 1998). Single-cell recordings in monkeys (Funahashi et al., 1993; Rainer et al., 1998a, 1998b; Fuster et al., 2000), lesion studies in humans (Knight, 1997; Knight et al., 1998; Nielsen-Bohlman & Knight, 1999; Barcelo et al., 2000) and monkeys (Rossi et al., 1999), and blood flow data (McIntosh et al., 1994; Büchel & Friston, 1997; Rees et al., 1997; Corbetta, 1998; Chawla et al., 1999; Kastner et al., 1999; Hopfinger et al., 2000) have linked PFC to control of extrastriate cortex during visual attention.

Modulation of visual pathway activity has been extensively investigated in humans through the use of ERPs. Attended visual stimuli evoke distinct ERP signatures. Attention enhances extrastriate ERP amplitudes for all stimuli in an attended channel with changes apparent in the initial 100–200 ms after delivery of a to-be-attended visual stimulus (Heinze et al., 1994; Mangun, 1995; Woldorff et al., 1997; Martinez et al., 1999). These early human ERP components have been linked to increased firing of extrastriate neurons in monkeys (Luck et al., 1997), providing a powerful parallel between the human and animal literature.

From ERP studies in patients with lateral PFC damage, evidence has accumulated that human lateral PFC regulates attention-dependent extrastriate neural activity through three distinct mechanisms. These mechanisms include (1) an attention dependent enhancement of extrastriate cortex; (2) a tonic excitatory influence on ipsilateral posterior areas for all sensory information, including attended and nonattended sensory inputs; and (3) a phasic excitatory influence of ipsilateral posterior areas to correctly perceived task-relevant stimuli. In these ERP studies, patients with unilateral PFC lesions (centered in Brodmann's areas 9 and 46) performed a series of visual attention experiments. In the task, non-target stimuli consisted of upright triangles, which were presented rapidly to both visual fields (4° from the fovea). Targets were rarely presented (10% of all stimuli) and consisted of inverted triangles presented randomly in each visual field. In one experiment,

patients and age-matched controls were asked to press a button whenever a target appeared in either visual field (Barcelo et al., 2000). In another experiment, subjects were required to allocate attention to only one visual field (Yago & Knight, 2000).

An interesting pattern of results emerged from these two experiments. First, both experiments revealed that lateral PFC provides a tonic excitatory influence to ipsilateral extrastriate cortex. Specifically, the P1 component of the visual ERP is markedly reduced in amplitude for all stimuli presented to the contralesional field. Importantly, this tonic influence is attention independent, since a reduced P1 potential in extrastriate cortex was found ipsilateral to PFC damage for all visual stimuli (attended and nonattended targets and nontargets) presented to the contralesional field. This tonic component may be viewed as a modulatory influence on extrastriate activity.

As noted previously, it is well known that attention increases the amplitude of extrastriate ERPs in normals with effects onsetting by about 50–100 ms post-stimulus delivery. The second experiment (allocating attention to only one visual field) provided evidence of the temporal kinetics of prefrontal–extrastriate interactions. In essence, attention effects on extrastriate cortex were normal in the first 200 ms of processing in PFC patients and severely disrupted after 200 ms (Yago & Knight, 2000). This finding suggests that other cortical areas are responsible for attention-dependent regulation of extrastriate cortex in the first 200 ms. A candidate structure for this influence based on the neuroimaging and clinical literature would be inferior parietal cortex. It is conceivable that inferior parietal cortex is responsible for the early reflexive component of attention, whereas PFC is responsible for more controlled and sustained aspects of visual attention onsetting after the parietal signal to extrastriate cortices.

The third observation from these experiments is the finding that lateral PFC has been shown to send a top-down signal to extrastriate cortex when a task-relevant event is detected during an attention task. There are two types of stimuli typically presented in an attended channel—one that is task-irrelevant and one requiring detection and a behavioral response. The amplitude of both the irrelevant and relevant stimuli is enhanced in an attended channel. As discussed previously, PFC is responsible for regulating this channel-specific attention enhancement. When a relevant target event is detected in an attended channel, another distinct electrophysiological event is generated in addition to the channel-specific enhancement. This top-down signal onsets at about 200 ms after a correct detection, extends throughout the ensuing 500 ms, and is superimposed on the channel-specific ERP attention enhancement (Suwazono et al., 2000). Damage to lateral PFC results in marked decrements in the top-down signal, accompanied by behavioral evidence of impaired detection ability (Barcleo et al., 2000).

The temporal parameters of this human PFC–extrastriate attention modulation are in accord with single-unit recordings in monkeys that show enhanced prefrontal stimulus detection–related activity 140 ms post-stimulus onset (Rainer et al., 1998a, 1998b) and other studies showing top-down activation of inferior temporal neurons 180–300 ms post-target detection (Tomita et al., 1999). Finally, there is a vigorous debate in the single-unit and fMRI research domains on whether lateral PFC is organized by modality (Wilson et al., 1993; Courtney et al., 1998; Romanski et al., 1999) or whether lateral PFC, and, more particularly, dorsolateral PFC, functions in a modality-independent executive manner during working memory and object and spatial integration (Rao et al., 1997; Assad et al., 1998; D'Esposito et al., 1999a; Miller, 1999; Fuster et al., 2000). Evidence from PFCx lesioned patients (Muller et al., in press) supports the notion that the lateral portion of PFC may function in a task-independent manner to control and integrate distributed neural activity in some cognitive tasks.

Projections from prefrontal areas 45 and 8 to inferior temporal (IT) areas TE and TEO have been demonstrated in monkeys (Webster et al., 1994), providing a possible glutamatergic pathway by which lateral prefrontal cortex could facilitate visual processing. A similar failure of prefrontal excitatory modulation is observed in the auditory modality. Prefrontal lesions markedly reduce the attention-sensitive N100 component throughout the hemisphere ipsilateral to damage (Chao & Knight, 1998). There are well-described prefrontal projections to the superior temporal plane, which may subserve this excitatory PFC–auditory cortex input (Alexander et al., 1976). The auditory and visual data provide clear evidence that lateral PFC cortex is crucial for maintaining distributed intrahemispheric neural activity during auditory and visual attention/working memory tasks.

Novelty Processing

The neural mechanisms of novelty detection and the production of novel behavior have been receiving increasing attention. Multiple experimental approaches have focussed on the biological mechanisms of novelty processing. Behavioral and electrophysiological data have shown that novel events are better remembered (Von Restorff, 1933; Karis et al., 1984). On a molecular basis, genetic studies of novelty seeking behavior in humans have provided a link to the short arm of chromosome 11 and the dopamine D4 receptor gene (Benjamin et al., 1996; Ebstein et al., 1996). Integrative neuroscience approaches including neuropsychological, electrophysiological, and cerebral blood flow techniques have revealed that a distributed neural network, including lateral PFC, temporal–parietal junction, hippocampus, and cingulate cortex is engaged both by novelty detection and during the production of novel behaviors.

Studies in normals have shown that novel items generate a late-positive ERP peaking in amplitude at about 300–500 ms that is maximal over the anterior scalp. This novelty ERP is proposed to be a central marker of the orienting response (Sokolov, 1963; Courchesne et al., 1975; Knight, 1984; Yamaguchi & Knight, 1991; Bahramali et al., 1997; Escera et al., 1998). The ERP evidence derived from neurological patients with lateral PFC damage (Knight et al., 1989b; Yamaguchi & Knight, 1991, 1992; Verleger et al., 1994; Knight, 1996; 1997) and intracranial ERP recordings in presurgical epileptics (Halgren et al., 1998) has revealed that a distributed neural network including lateral and orbital PFC, hippocampal formation, anterior cingulate and temporal–perietal cortex is involved in detecting and encoding novel information (Halgren et al., 1998). Neuroimaging results have confirmed the lesion and intracranial evidence on the neuroanatomy of the novelty-processing system (Tulving et al., 1994, 1996; Stern et al., 1996; McCarthy et al., 1997; Menon et al., 1997; Linden et al., 1999; Opitz et al., 1999a, 1999b; Yoshiura et al., 1999; Clark et al., 2000; Downar et al., 2000; Kiehl et al., in press). The lateral PFC contribution is a key component of this novelty network. For instance, unlike posterior cortical and hippocampal activity, PFC novelty activation recorded with ERPs or neuroimaging habituates to repeated exposures to novel events and is modality independent (Knight, 1984; Yamaguchi & Knight, 1991; Raichle et al., 1994; Knight & Scabini, 1998; Peterson et al., 1999). Importantly, lateral PFC also appears to initiate the novelty detection cascade prior to activation of other brain regions, as revealed by lesion-ERP studies. If the novel event is sufficiently engaging, posterior cortical and medial temporal regions are recruited for further processing (Ahlo et al., 1994; Knight, 1996; Alain et al., 1998).

Novelty, of course, is an elusive concept dependent on both the sensory parameters of an event and the context in which it occurs. As an example, the unexpected occurrence of a visual fractal would typically engage the novelty system. Conversely, if one were presented with a stream of visual fractals and suddenly a picture of an apple occurred, this would also drive the novelty system. In the first case, the visual complexity of the fractal drives the novelty response. In the second situation, the local context of repeated fractals would be violated by the insertion of a picture of an apple and this would also engage the novelty network. Sensory parameters and local context have powerful effects on electrophysiological and behavioral response to novelty (Comerchero & Polich, 1998, 1999; Katayama & Polich, 1998), and this effect is also dependent on lateral PFC (Barcelo & Knight, in press; Suwazono et al., 2000).

Neuroimaging findings in people with normal function also support a critical role for PFC in responding to novel events and solving new problems (see Duncan & Owen, 2000, for a review). These neuropsychological, ERP, and neuroimaging findings support a central role of lateral prefrontal cortex in the processing of novelty (Kimble et al., 1965; Godfrey & Rousseaux, 1997). Single-unit data from monkeys also support a prefrontal bias towards novelty (Rainer & Miller, 2000).

Response Monitoring

Major advances have developed in our understanding of the neural basis of implementing neural control of behavioral output. First, the discovery of an ERP response referred to as the *error-related negativity* (ERN) has provided an on-line measure of a subject's performance monitoring (Gehring et al., 1993). Second, neuroimaging data have implicated a prefrontal–cingulate network in error response monitoring and correction (Kiehl et al., 2000; McDonald et al., 2000). Finally, lesion–ERP evidence obtained from patients with lateral PFC damage supports the notion that PFC controls cingulate-related error activity (Gehring & Knight, 2000). Cohen and colleagues have suggested that the role of PFC in response monitoring is to provide a stable representation of the task at hand (Carter et al., 1999; Cohen et al., 2000). This permits better suppression of distracting information, lessening the chance of an error. These authors suggest that the cingulate ERN and fMRI blood flow response to errors is a manifestation of conflict detection by the anterior cingulate (areas 24 and 32). Thus, if the representation of the task is weakened by PFC damage, conflict increases on all trials and an ERN is generated to all stimuli. This view places the PFC in an executive position regarding anterior cingulate function. An alternative model consistent with the accrued data posits that the activity reflected in the ERN represents an affective or motivational signal. In this view, the cingulate signal as measured by the ERN would serve an alerting function that mobilizes affective systems, rather than immediate corrective action, perhaps via cingulate connections with the amygdala and brainstem autonomic nuclei. This conception of the ERN would be consistent with dissociations between ERN activity and compensatory behavior and with reports of medial frontal ERN-like activity in response to stimuli with negative hedonic significance (Falkenstein et al., 2000; Vidal et al., 2000; Luu et al., 2000).

CASE REPORT, THE LATERAL PREFRONTAL SYNDROME: PATIENT W.R.

A case study exemplifies the effects of lateral prefrontal lesions. W.R., a 31-year-old lawyer, presented to the neurology clinic with family concern over his lack of interest in important life events. When queried as to why he was in the clinic, the patient stated that he had "lost his ego." His difficulties began 4 years previously, in 1978, when he had a tonic–clonic seizure after staying up all night and drinking large amounts of coffee while studying for midterm exams in his final year of law school. An extensive neurological evaluation conducted at that time at the National Institutes of Health (NIH) including electroencephalogram (EEG), computed tomography (CT) scan, and positron emission tomography (PET) scan were all unremarkable. The diagnosis of generalized seizure disorder exacerbated by sleep deprivation was given and he was placed on dilantin. W.R. graduated from law school but did not enter a practice because he couldn't decide where to take the bar exam. Over the next year he worked as a tennis instructor in Florida. He then broke off a 2-year relationship with a woman and moved to California to live near his brother, who was also a lawyer. His brother reported that he was indecisive, procrastinated in carrying out planned activities, and was becoming progressively isolated from family and friends. The family attributed these problems to a "mid-life crisis." Four months prior to neurological consultation, W.R.'s mother died. At the funeral and during the time surrounding his mother's death the family noted that he expressed no grief regarding his mother's death. The family decided to have the patient re-evaluated. W.R. was pleasant but somewhat indifferent to the situation. General neurological exam was unremarkable. A mild snout reflex was present.

W.R. made both perseverative and random errors on the Luria hand-sequencing task and was easily distracted during the examination. His free recall was two out of three words at a 5-minute delay. He was able to recall the third word with a semantic cue. On questioning about his mother's death, W.R. confirmed that he did not feel any strong emotions, either about his mother's death or about his current problem. The patient's brother mentioned that W.R. "had never lost it" emotionally during the week after his mother's death, at which point W.R. immediately interjected "and I'm not trying not to lose it." Regarding his mother's death, he stated "I don't feel grief, I don't know if that's bad or good." These statements were emphatic, but expressed in a somewhat jocular fashion (witzelsucht). W.R. was asked about changes in his personality. He struggled for some minutes to describe changes he had noticed, but did not manage to identify any. He stated, "being inside, I can't see it as clear." He was distractible and perseverative, frequently reverting to a prior discussion of tennis, and repeating phrases such as "yellow comes to mind" in response to queries of his memory. When asked about either the past or the future, his responses were schematic and stereotyped. He lacked any plans for the future, initiated no future-oriented actions, and stated, "It didn't matter that much, it never bothered me," that he never began to practice law. A CT scan revealed a left lateral prefrontal glioblastoma, which had grown through the corpus callosum into the lateral right frontal lobe. After discussion of the serious nature of the diagnosis, W.R. remained indifferent. The family were distressed by the gravity of the situation and showed appropriate anxiety and sadness. Interestingly, they noted that their sadness was alleviated when in the presence of W.R.

Discussion of Patient W.R.

W.R. remained a pleasant and articulate individual despite his advanced frontal tumor. However, he was unable to carry out the activities to make him a fully functioning member of society. His behavior was completely constrained by his current circumstances. His jocularity was a reaction to the social situation of the moment, and was not influenced by the larger context of his recent diagnosis. He appeared to have difficulty with explicit memory and source monitoring, with little confidence in his answers to memory queries, complicated by frequent intrusions from internal mental representations. Thus, metamemory was impaired, and he was unable to sustain working memory processes. He was distractible and was unable to sustain normal working memory. Perseverative errors were common in both the motor and cognitive domain. A prominent aspect of his behavior was a complete absence of counterfactual expressions. In particular, W.R. expressed no counterfactual emotions, being completely unable to construe any explanation for his current behavioral state. He seemed unable to feel grief or regret, nor was he bothered by their absence, even though he was aware of his brother's concern over his absence of emotion. These observations suggest that damage in lateral PFC leads to deficits in reality monitoring, a process that is essential for the normal planning and decision-making functions necessary for normal human behavior. Behavioral analysis of this case highlights the role of lateral PFC in virtually all aspects of human cognition.

ORBITOFRONTAL CORTEX

INTRODUCTION

In the simplest formulation, lateral PFC may be viewed as the central executive for cognitive control, with orbitofrontal cortex serving as the central executive for emotional and social control. In contrast to lateral prefrontal damage, orbitofrontal damage spares many cognitive skills but dramatically affects all spheres of social behavior (Bechera et al., 1998; Stone et al., 1998). The patient with orbitofrontal damage is frequently impulsive, hyperactive, and lacking in proper social skills, despite showing intact cognitive processing on a range of tasks typically impaired in the lateral PFC–lesioned patient. In some cases, the behavioral syndrome is so severe that the term

acquired sociopathy has been used to describe the resultant personality profile of the orbitofrontal patient. However, unlike true sociopaths, orbitofrontal patients typically feel remorse for their inappropriate behavior. Primitive reflexes such as snout, suck, rooting, and grasp are not often observed. Severe social and emotional dysfunction is typically observed only in bilateral orbital disease, as might be observed after head trauma, orbital meningioma, or certain degenerative disorders such as frontal–temporal dementia. Thus, there appears to be redundancy in both lateral and orbital human PFC, with one intact PFC being able to sustain many aspects of cognitive and social function. Similar to recent advances in segregating function of lateral PFC into dorsal and ventral divisions, progress has been made in parcellation of orbital PFC function. The ventromedial portion of the orbital PFC has been associated with the use of internal autonomic states in the guidance of goal-directed behavior. The ventromedial portion of human orbital PFC has also been proposed to be involved in inhibitory processing of emotional stimuli. The lateral portions of orbital PFC have been implicated in the rapid establishment of reward–punishment associations (Shimamura, 2000; see Chapter 23). Tests of social and cognitive skills reveal a double dissociation between lateral and orbital PFC damage. Lateral PFC damage impairs working memory and attention capacity but spares theory of mind. Conversely, orbital PFC damage leaves working memory intact but impairs theory of mind. There is some suggestion of an important role of the polar region, but this has not yet been conclusively determined.

Disorders of emotional control and social regulation are frequent accompaniments of acquired neurological disease and are receiving increasing attention in the clinical and research arena (Stuss & Alexander, 2000; Stuss et al, 2001a). In the 1930s, Kluver & Bucy (1939) described prominent affective and visual processing changes in monkeys with bilateral anterior temporal ablations. During this same period, Papez (1937) described the classic "circle of Papez" or limbic brain in humans encompassing the anterior cingulate, hippocampus, septum, and hypothalamus. However, the two most critical components of the human emotional control network, orbitofrontal cortex and amygdala, were not included in the original concept proposed by Papez. A seminal observation linking brain damage and personality alteration can be traced to 1848 in Cavendish, Vermont. A well-respected train company employee, Phineas Gage, was working at clearing rocks for the laying down of a new rail line. An unfortunate accident propelled an iron tamping rod through his skull. Remarkably, given that the rod weighed 13 pounds, was over 3 feet long, and antibiotics were not yet discovered, Gage survived. However, marked changes in his previous calm and organized personality ensued. Gage became more labile and disinhibited in his behavior and was noted to use profanity and make irreverent statements. His acquaintances noted that "Gage was no longer Gage." His problems continued unabated until he died of uncontrolled seizures 12 years later in San Francisco. Inspection of his skull indicates that the tract of the bar injured bilateral orbitofrontal cortex and the anterior portion of the left temporal lobe. The role of orbitofrontal cortex in social behavior was largely neglected, however, until the 1960s.

The most common cause of orbitofrontal and amygdala damage is closed head injury, with about 100,000 people per year in the U.S. alone experiencing a closed head injury severe enough to damage these critical brain injuries. Orbitofrontal and amygdala damage is not limited to head trauma and can also be observed in dementing disorders such as Pick's disease or frontotemporal dementia, which has been linked to abnormalities in chromosome 17 in some cases. In addition, tumors including meningiomas and gliomas can affect these areas and infections such as herpes simplex have a particular predilection for the limbic brain. Patients with an acquired nonprogressive lesion such as that due to head trauma may return to a high level of pre-injury cognitive function. However, as predicted by the Gage case, patients with orbitofrontal or amygdala damage are impaired to varying degrees in emotional control, social interaction, and decision making involving interpersonal choices

and behaviors. Many patients are initially diagnosed incorrectly with a personality disorder when, in fact, they have damaged their emotional brain. Neurological examination, other than for frequent anosmia, is invariably normal if damage is restricted to orbital PFC and there was no significant axonal shear at the initial time of injury. Frontal release signs including snout, suck, grasp, and rooting are absent. Remarkably little is known about the neural underpinnings of this severely compromised social self.

NEUROPSYCHOLOGY

Several investigators have provided neuropsychological data implicating orbital/ventral–medial PFC in emotional and social regulation (Grafman et al., 1993; Bechera et al., 1994; 1997; 2000; Rolls et al., 1994; Tranel & Damasio, 1994; Stone et al., 1998; Shammi & Stuss, 1999; Hartikainen et al., 2000). Disorders of emotional control and social regulation due to orbital PFC dysfunction are frequent accompaniments of psychiatric disease such as obsessive–compulsive disorder and drug abuse (London et al., 2000; Volkow & Fowler, 2000), as well as acquired neurological disease, including head trauma, dementia, and tumors. Thus, the societal costs of orbital PFC dysfunction are immense. Developmental aspects of acquired orbital PFC damage in children and adolescents are even less well understood than adult dysfunction (Price et al., 1990). Patients with adult acquired orbital PFC are aware of their problems and know the actual rules of proper social behavior despite failures to properly implement them. Childhood-acquired orbital PFC damage may result in a failure to both implement and learn the rules of proper social discourse (Anderson et al., 1999). Changes in emotional disposition are routinely observed in patients who have suffered damage to the orbitofrontal cortex. Damage to this brain region has been associated with a variety of social–emotional dysfunctions, including personality change, risk taking, impulsivity, emotional outbursts, and social inappropriateness. Three theories have been proposed to explain the disordered behavior subsequent to orbital damage in humans. These include the *somatic marker hypothesis*, put forth by Damasio and colleagues (Bechera et al., 1994; see Chapter 22); *impaired linking, of reward and punishment*, proposed by Rolls (Rolls et al., 1994; see Chapter 23); and *emotional disinhibition* accompanied by enhanced central nervous system responsivity recently proposed by Rule and colleagues (Rule et al., 1999; Shimamura, 2000).

For example, Damasio and colleagues have shown that patients with orbital PFC lesions elicit inappropriate emotional responses and abnormal galvanic skin responses (GSR) in a gambling task in which subjects must inhibit high-risk gambles (Bechera et al., 1997). These authors propose that damage in the ventromedial PFC impairs generation of a somatic state that can be used as a guide to control behavior. This proposal is supported by reduced anticipatory GSRs in patients with ventromedial damage. In another study, a group of patients with lateral PFC damage and a group with orbital PFC damage were studied in working memory and theory of mind (TOM) tasks. *Theory of mind* refers to a person's ability to infer another person's or group of people's internal mental state, and is viewed as one of the highest forms of social abilities. A double dissociation was observed. Lateral PFC patients had difficulties with working memory but were not impaired on TOM tasks. Orbital PFC patients were normal on working memory tasks but failed TOM tasks (Stone et al., 1998). This finding has been replicated and extended to indicate some potential importance of the right frontal region in another cohort of lateral- and orbital-lesioned patients (Stuss et al., 2001a). Taken together, these findings are consistent with the notion that this brain region is intricately involved in the analysis, monitoring, and control of emotionally laden stimuli and social interchange.

PHYSIOLOGY

Functional neuroimaging currently has had difficulty with imaging orbital PFC because of susceptibility artifacts from nearby sinuses, and a limited number of studies have been published (i.e., Schoenbaum et al., 1998; No-

bre et al., 1999; Elliott et al., 2000). Recent studies indicate success with neuroimaging of orbital regions (O'Doherty et al., 2001; see Chapter 23). As noted in the Neuropsychology section, three theories have been proposed to explain the disordered behavior subsequent to orbital PFC damage in humans, and all are supported by physiological data. The somatic marker hypothesis (Bechera et al., 2000) proposes that ventromedial orbital PFC or the right sensory cortical damage impairs generation of an appropriate somatic feeling needed to guide behavior (Tranel, & Damasio, 1994; Bechera et al., 1997; see Chapter 22). The somatic marker hypothesis is supported by a decreased GSR, a peripheral autonomic measure of orienting, in patients with orbital PFC damage. Another view proposes impairments in linking of reward and punishment (Rolls et al., 1994), and is supported by results from single-unit, PET, and some fMRI research (Elliott et al., 2000; see Chapter 23). A third theory, the dynamic filtering hypothesis, has also been proposed to explain some components of the orbital PFC behavioral syndrome (Rule et al., 1999; Shimamura, 2000). This theory posits that orbital PFC patients are unable to inhibit responses to certain emotional and social stimuli, and is supported by enhanced ERP measures of orienting to novel emotionally laden stimuli in these patients. The enhanced central nervous system response to emotional auditory and somatosensory stimuli in orbital PFC patients is in accord with the disinhibited, impulsive behavior observed after orbital PFC damage in humans and monkeys (Butter et al., 1969, 1970; Dias et al., 1997; Roberts and Wallis, 2000). Interestingly, Macaque monkeys with orbitofrontal lesions fail to habituate to novel auditory and visual stimuli (Butter et al., 1970). Importantly, these findings suggest regional specificity within the prefrontal cortex. Event-related potentials to novel emotional stimuli are disinhibited in patients with orbital PFC lesions, whereas patients with lateral PFC lesions show decreased novelty responses to these same stimuli (Knight & Scabini, 1998). These results indicate that orbital patients may have an excessive central nervous response to irrelevant stimuli. Direct connections from orbitofrontal cortex to posterior parietal cortex (area 7A) have been identified (Cavada et al., 2000). Orbitofrontal cortex could be exerting inhibitory control over novelty-related activity in the temporal–parietal region via these fibers. Loss of this control might contribute to the disinhibited behavior so frequently observed in these patients. Elements of all three notions of orbital function are likely correct and a more complete concept of orbital contributions to social and emotional behavior is likely to emerge in the ensuing years.

CASE REPORT, THE ORBITAL PREFRONTAL SYNDROME: PATIENT J.L.

A case study exemplifies the effects of orbital PFC lesions. Patient J.L. was seen in neurological consultation on the inpatient psychiatric service in 1988. He was admitted to the psychiatric service after an altercation at an intersection where he got into a cursing and shoving match with a driver who cut him off as he was crossing a street. J.L. was a 42-year-old accountant with a masters degree at the time of evaluation. He had been in excellent health until an accident at a party 13 years previously where he fell off a third floor balcony and sustained a severe coup injury to his frontal lobe. The CT scanning revealed extensive bilateral damage to his orbital PFC. Both the ventromedial and lateral portions of the orbital PFC were destroyed. J.L. developed grand mal seizures after the accident, which were well controlled with dilantin. Clinical and experimental neuropsychological evaluation revealed a double dissociation between cognitive and social function. Lateral PFC was spared and all tests showed that cognitive function related to lateral PFC was intact. For instance, J.L.'s IQ remained at a pre-morbid level of 128. Clinical and experimental tests of memory, including measures of source and metamemory, were intact. Attention capacity and working memory were excellent. In contrast to his excellent cognitive performance, since the incident, J.L. has had prominent problems in emotional and social control. He has gotten into numerous street altercations, and has been arrested several times. He is socially inappropriate and notes that he "comes on too strong" to women. Woman laboratory personnel where patient J.L. has been tested report that he is constantly coming on to them. When queried further, he reports that he might ask a woman to marry him after 1–2 days of knowing her. When asked if he thought this behavior was appropriate, patient J.L. responded no. Importantly, patient J.L. knows his behavior is inappropriate but is unable to control it. J.L. is also unable to handle the financial resources that accrued as a settlement for his accident and required a conservator to manage his affairs. During the interview, J.L. often laughed inappropriately. His neurological examination was normal, including testing of language, attention, memory, and perception. He admitted to obsessive–compulsive behaviors such as counting the numbers on car license plates. Testing of working memory was normal, but J.L. failed theory of mind tests, which require the ability of a person to infer another person's mental or emotional state.

Discussion of Patient J.L.

Patient J.L. manifests the typical orbital PFC syndrome of intact executive control of cognitive processes and severely impaired executive control of social and emotional behavior (see Chapters 22 and 23). His IQ was superior and he scored well in all conventional tests of attention, memory, and language. Yet he was severely impaired in his everyday social behavior and in making appropriate life decisions, as in managing his financial affairs. Remarkably, when queried about the appropriate social or emotional response or the proper decision regarding personal affairs, patient J.L. was able to respond correctly. His problems became evident when he had to implement on-line behavior. Explication of this apparent paradox of knowledge versus failure to implement such knowledge is a great challenge for the future.

WHERE ARE WE GOING

What will the future bring to our understanding of prefrontal function? Given the vast expansion of PFC in humans, explication of the function of this brain region appears to be fundamental for a complete understanding of human cognition in both health and disease. Advances have been made in multiple domains. Cognitive psychology has provided a welcome addition to the classic neuropsychological approach, and new areas of behavioral theory and analysis have enriched our understanding of PFC function. We believe that the next decade will witness an even greater implementation of sophisticated cognitive theory to prefrontal research. Approaches drawn from the discipline of social cognition and from the study of behaviors such as decision making and reality monitoring are certain to provide a broader and ecologically valid approach to understanding PFC function. This fusion of theory and experiment will provide important new insights into the role of orbital frontal cortex in social behavior. This book has provided different views on the nature of orbital frontal function in humans. We expect that by 2010 we will have a more integrated view of how this vast expanse of prefrontal cortex enables the social being.

One area likely to receive increasing attention is the contribution of PFC to the evaluation and implementation of context in behavior. The notion of context has been broadly applied to seemingly diverse areas, including probability learning, social regulation, and novelty detection. For instance, in the social domain, a behavior in one situation might be very appropriate while the same behavior could be quite counterproductive in another situation. Humans are able to fluidly draw on prior experience to set and implement the appropriate context for the current situation. Similarly, in the area of novelty processing, the effects of local context are extremely powerful. For instance, the occurrence of a visual fractal in a stream of common visual objects would elicit a powerful novelty response to the fractal. However, the occurrence of a common object in a stream of fractals would also elicit a powerful novelty response. Research on the role of PFC in application of context-dependent parameters to behavior may prove critical for understanding the role of PFC in mental flexibility.

Single-unit studies in monkeys have been crucial in developing new models of PFC function. The classic ideas of segregation of

function have been challenged by findings that PFC neurons are more plastic than traditional views might suggest. The concept of rapid learning and plasticity of PFC neurons is in accord with the neurological literature, which reports profound alterations in mental flexibility in patients with PFC damage. This single-unit research dovetails nicely with the explosion of insights drawn from fMRI research. Novel insights into segregation versus integration of function in subregions of PFC have fueled the debate. We now enjoy a powerful interplay between human and monkey research that heralds major advances in the understanding of cognitive processes. We certainly believe that by 2010 there will be a clearer answer to the question of segregation versus overlapping of function in prefrontal cortex. We predict that, as in many scientific controversies, the final answer will blend data drawn from both camps.

The way in which these executive processes are implemented at a neural level is perhaps the greatest challenge for a true understanding of PFC function. We certainly hope that work during the next decade will fill in the crucial gaps in our understanding of this central aspect of human cognition. The notion that engagement of parallel inhibition and excitation can be a useful construct for understanding PFC function is receiving support from single-unit, lesion, ERP, and functional neuroimaging research. Advances in the fusion of these experimental approaches may provide new insights into both the temporal and spatial aspects of PFC-dependent executive control. Consideration of the neuropharmacology of PFC function will be necessary for a complete understanding of prefrontal function, and we hope this volume has focused attention on this needed part of the frontal lobe riddle.

The nature of the neural code both at the local single-unit level and the systems interaction level is, of course, central to a complete picture of PFC function. How do single units in a subregion of PFC interact to produce the needed output signal to other brain regions? Are neurons concerned with inhibition intertwined with those involved in excitation? What is the nature of the output signal from PFC to other neural regions? Is it a coherent burst of neural activity, such as a gamma oscillation? These questions are only beginning to be addressed, but they promise great insights into the ways in which PFC implements executive control.

What else might be discussed at a conference on the frontal lobes in 2010? Certainly we are in the middle of an explosion of new methods to image the human brain, and this exponential progress is likely to continue. Fusion of electrophysiological and functional magnetic resonance methods promises new insights into the temporal–spatial dynamics of human cognition. Optical imaging techniques have developed that may improve temporal and spatial resolution. Perhaps as important, optical techniques can be used to image infants, extending the field of imaging to the gamut of human development. We wouldn't be surprised if the next decade yields novel information on the development of the frontal lobe from infancy to adulthood.

Finally, why bother with all this fuss about the prefrontal cortex? Is it because scientists deserve to study what fascinates them? Certainly that fascination brings and keeps many researchers to the frontal lobe table. However, that is not the true reason why we spend our time studying prefrontal cortex. Rather, we know that this brain region holds the key to understanding normal and disordered cognition, with profound implications for both the individual and society.

REFERENCES

Ackerly, S.S. & Benton, A.L. (1947). Report of a case of bilateral frontal lobe defect. *Research Publications–Association for Research in Nervous and Mental Disease, 27*, 479–504.

Ahlo, K., Woods, D.L., Algazi, A., Knight, R.T., & Naatanen, R. (1994). Lesions of frontal cortex diminish the auditory mismatch negativity. *Electroencephalography and Clinical Neurophysiology, 91*, 353–362.

Alain, C., Woods, D.L., & Knight, R.T. (1998). A distributed cortical network for auditory sensory memory in humans. *Brain Research, 812*, 23–37.

Alexander, G.E., Newman, J.D., & Symmes, D. (1976). Convergence of prefrontal and acoustic inputs upon neurons in the superior temporal gyrus of the awake squirrel monkey. *Brain Research, 116*, 334–338.

Anderson, S.W., Bechera, A., Damasio, H., Tranel, D., & Damasio, A.R. (1999). Impairments in social and moral behavior related to early damage in human prefrontal corex. *Nature Neuroscience, 2*, 1032–1037.

Asaad, W.F., Rainer, G., & Miller, E.K. (1998). Neural activity in the primate prefrontal cortex during associative learning. *Neuron, 21*, 1399–407.

Baddeley, A. & Wilson, B. (1988). Frontal amnesia and the dysexecutive syndrome. *Brain and Cognition, 7*, 212–230.

Bahramali, H., Gordon, E., Lim, C.L., Li, W., Lagapoulus, J., Rennie, C., & Meares, R.A. (1997). Evoked related potentials with and without an orienting reflex. *Neuroreport, 8*, 2665–2669.

Barcelo, F. & *Knight, R.T.* (2000). Prefrontal lesions alter context dependent value of novel stimuli during visual attention. *Soc. Neuroscience 26*:2233.

Barcelo, F. & Knight, R.T. (in press). Prefrontal lesions alter context dependent value of novel stimuli during visual attention. *Society of Neuroscience Abstracts*.

Barcelo, F. & Knight, R.T. (in press). Both random and perseverative errors underlie WCST deficits in prefrontal patients. *Neuropsychologia*.

Barcelo, P., Suwazono, S., & Knight, R.T. (2000). Prefrontal modulation of visual processing in humans. *Nature Neuroscience, 3*, 399–403.

Barch, D.M., Braver, T.S., Sabb, F.W., & Noll, D.C. (2000). Anterior cingulate and the monitoring of response conflict: evidence from an fMRI study of verb generation. *Journal of Cognitive Neuroscience, 12*, 298–309.

Bartus, R.T. & Levere, T.E. (1977). Frontal decortication in Rhesus monkeys: a test of the interference hypothesis. *Brain Research, 119*, 233–248.

Bechera, A., Damasio, A.R., Damasio, H., & Anderson, S.W. (1994). Insensitivity to future consequences floowing damage to human prefrontal cortex. *Cogniton, 50*, 7–15.

Bechera, A., Damasio, H., Tranel, D., & Damasio, A.R. (1997). Deciding advantageously before knowing the advantageous strategy. *Science, 275*, 1293–1295.

Bechera, A., Damasio, H., Tranel, D., & Anderson, S.W. (1998). Dissociation of working memory from decision making within the human prefrontal cortex. *Journal of Neuroscience, 18*, 428–37.

Bechera, A., Damasio, H., & Damasio, A.R. (2000). Emotion, decision making and the orbitofrontal cortex. *Cerebral Cortex, 10*, 295–307.

Benjamin, J., Li, L., Patterson, C., Greenberg, B.D., Murphy, D.L., & Hamer, D.H. (1996). Population and familial association between the D4 dopamine receptor gene and measures of novelty seeking. *Nature Genetics, 12*, 81–84.

Botvinick, M., Nystrom, L.E., Fissell, K., Carter, C.S., & Cohen, J.D. (1999). Conflict monitoring versus selection-for-action in anterior cingulate cortex. *Nature, 402(6758)*, 179–81.

Brutkowski, S. (1965). Functions of prefrontal cortex in animals. *Physiolological Review, 45*, 721–746.

Büchel, C. & Friston, K.J. (1997). Modulation of connectivity in visual pathways by attention: cortical interactions evaluated with structural equation modeling and fMRI. *Cerebral Cortex, 7*, 768–778.

Butter, C.M., McDonald, A., & Snyder, D.R. (1969). Orality, preference behavior, and reinforcement value of nonfood object in monkeys with orbital frontal lesions. *Science, 164(3885)*, 1306–1307.

Butter, C.M., Snyder, D.R., & McDonald, J.A. (1970). Effects of orbital frontal lesions on aversive and aggressive behaviors in Rhesus monkeys. *Journal of Comparative and Physiological Psychology, 72*, 32–144.

Carter, C.S., Botvinick, M.M., & Cohen, J.D. (1999). The contribution of the anterior cingulate cortex to executive processes in cognition. *Reviews in the Neurosciences, 10*, 49–57.

Cavada, C., Company, T., Tejedor, J., Cruz-Rizzolo, R.J., & Reinoso-Suarez, F. (2000). The anatomical connections of the Macaque monkey orbitofrontal cortex. *Cerebral Cortex, 10*, 220–242.

Chao, L.L. & Knight, R.T. (1995). Human prefrontal lesions increase distractibility to irrelevant sensory. *NeuroReport, 6*, 1605–1610.

Chao, L.L. & Knight, R.T. (1998). Contribution of human prefrontal cortex to delay performance. *Journal of Cognitive Neuroscience, 10*, 167–177.

Chawla, D., Rees, G., & Friston, K.J. (1999). The physiological basis of attentional modulation in extrastriate visual areas. *Nature Neuroscience, 2*, 671–676.

Clark, V.P., Fannon, S., Lai, S., Benson, R., & Bauer, L. (2000). Responses to rare visual target and distractor stimuli using fMRI. *Journal of Neurophysiology, 83*, 3133–3138.

Cohen, J.D., Braver, S.B., & O'Reilly, R.C. (1996). A computational approach to prefrontal cortex, cognitive control and schizophrenia: recent developmenmts and current challenges. *Philosophical Transactions of the Royal Society of London Series B, 351*, 1515–1527.

Cohen, J.D., Botvinivk, M., & Carter, C.S. (2000). Anterior cingulate and prefrontal cortex: who's in control? *Nature Neuroscience, 3*, 421–423.

Comerchero, M.D. & Polich, J. (1998). P3a, perceptual distinctiveness, and stimulus modality. *Cognitive Brain Resarch, 7*, 41–48.

Comerchero, M.D. & Polich, J. (1999). P3a and P3b from typical auditory and visual stimuli. *Clinical Neurophysiology, 110*, 24–30.

Corbetta, M. (1998). Frontoparietal cortical networks for directing attention and the eye to visual locations: identical, independent, or overlapping neural systems? *Proceedings of the National Academy of Sciences USA, 95*, 831–838.

Courchesne, E., Hillyard, S.A., & Galambos, R. (1975). Stimulus novelty, task relevance, and the visual evoked potential in man. *Electroencephalography and Clinical Neurophysiology, 39*, 131–143.

Courtney, S.M., Petit, L., Maisog, J.M., Ungerleider, L.G., & Haxby, J.V. (1998). An area specialized for spatial working memory in human frontal cortex. *Science, 279*, 1347–1351.

Daffner, K.R., Mesulam, M.-M., Holcomb, P.J., Calvo, V., Acar, D., Chabrerie, A., Kikinis, R., Jolesz, F.A., Rentz, D.M., Scinto, L.F. (2000a). Disruption of attention to novel events after frontal lobe injury in humans. *Journal of Neurology, Neurosurgery and Psychiatry, 68*, 18–24.

Daffner K.R., Mesulam, M.M., Scinto, L.F., Acar, D., Calvo, V., Faust, R., Chabrerie, A., Kennedy, B., & Holcomb, P. (2000b). The central role of the prefrontal cortex in directing attention to novel events. *Brain, 123*, 927–39.

Daffner, K.R., Mesulam, M.-M., Scinto, L.F., Calvo, V., West, W.C., & Holcomb, P. (2000c). The influence of stimulus deviance on electrophysiologic and behavioral response to novel events. *Journal of Cognitive Neuroscience, 12*, 393–406.

Damasio, A.S. (1985). The frontal lobes. In: K.M. Heilman & E. Valenstein (Eds.), *Clinical Neuropsychology, 2nd* ed. (pp. 339–374). New York: Oxford University Press.

Desimome, R. (1998). Visual attention mediatd by biased competition in extrastriate cortex. *Philosophical Transactions of the Royal Society of London. Series B: Biological Sciences, 353*, 1245–1255.

D'Esposito, M. & Postle, B.R. (1999). The dependence of span and delayed-response performance on prefrontal cortex. *Neuropsychologia, 37*, 1303–1315.

D'Esposito, M., Detre, J.A., Alsop, D.C., Shin, R.K., Atlas, S., & Grossman, M. (1995). The neural basis of the central executive system of working memory. *Nature, 378*, 279–281.

D'Esposito, M., Postle, B.R., Ballard, D., & Lease, J. (1999a). Maintenance versus manipulation of information held in working memory: an event-related fMRI study. *Brain and Cognition, 41*, 66–86.

D'Esposito, M., Postle, B.R., Jonides, J., & Smith, E.E. (1999b). The neural substrate and temporal dynamics of interference effects in working memory as revealed by event-related functional MRI. *Proceedings of the National Academy of Science USA, 96*, 7514–7519.

Dias, R., Robbins, T.W., & Roberts, A.C. (1997). Dissociable forms of inhibitory control within prefrontal cortex with an analog of the Wisconsin Card Sort Test: restriction to novel situations and independence from "on-line" processing. *Journal of Neuroscience, 17*, 9285–9297.

Downar, J., Crawley, A.P., Mikulis, D.J., & Davis, K.D. (2000). A multimodal cortical network for the detection of changes in the sensory environment. *Nature Neuroscience, 3*, 277–283.

Dronkers, N.F., Redfern, B.B., & Knight, R.T. (2000). The neural architecture of language disorders. In M. Gazzaniga (Ed.), *The New Cognitive Neurosciences* (pp. 949–958). Cambridge, MA: MIT Press.

Duncan, J. & Owen, A.M. (2000). Common regions of the human frontal lobe recruited by diverse cognitive demands. *Trends in Neuroscience, 10*, 475–483.

Ebstein, R.P., Novic, O., Umansky, R., Prie, B., Osher, V., Blaine, D., Bennett, E.R., Nemanov, L., Katz, M., & Belmaker, R.H. (1996). Dopamine D4 receptor (D4DR) exon III polymorphism associated with the human personality trait of novelty seeking. *Nature Genetics, 12*, 78–80.

Edinger, H.M., Siegel, A., & Troiano, R. (1975). Effect of stimulation of prefrontal cortex and amygdala on diencephalic neurons. *Brain Research, 97*, 17–31

Elliott, R., Dolan, R.J., & Frith, C.D. (2000). Dissociable

functions in the medial and lateral orbitofrontal cortex: evidence from human neuroimaging studies. *Cerebral Cortex, 10,* 308–317.

Escera, C., Alho, K., Winkler, I., & Naatanen, R. (1998). Neural mechanisms of involuntary attention to acoustic novelty and change. *Journal of Cognitive Neuroscience, 10,* 590–604.

Eslinger, P.J. & Damasio, A.R. (1985). Severe disturbance of higher cognition after bilateral frontal lobe ablation: patient EVR. *Neurology, 35,* 1731–1741.

Falkenstein, M., Hoormann, J., Christ, S., & Hiohnsbein, J. (2000). ERP components on reaction errors and their functional significance: a tutorial. *Biological Psychology, 51(2–3),* 87–107.

Funahashi, S., Bruce, C.J., & Goldman-Rakic, P.S. (1993). Dorsolateral prefrontal lesions and oculomotor delayed-response performance: evidence for mnemonic "scotomas". *Journal of Neuroscience, 13,* 1479–1497.

Fuster, J.M. (1989). *The Prefrontal Cortex: Anatomy, Physiology, and Neuropsychology of the Frontal Lobe,* 2nd ed. New York: Raven Press.

Fuster, J.M., Brodner, M., & Kroger, J.K. (2000). Cross-modal and cross-temporal associations in neurons of frontal cortex. *Nature, 405,* 347–351.

Galambos, R. (1956). Suppression of auditory nerve activity by stimulation of efferent fibres to the cochlea. *Journal of Neurophysiology 19,* 424–437.

Gehring, W.J., & Knight, R.T. (2000). Prefrontal-cingulate interactions in action monitoring. *Nature Neuroscience, 3,* 516–520.

Gehring, W.J., Goss, B., Coles, M.G.H., Meyer, D.E., & Donchin, E. (1993). A neural system for error detection and compensation. *Psychological Science, 4,* 385–390

Godfrey, O. & Rousseaux, M. (1997). Novel decision making in patients with prefrontal or posterior brain damage. *Neurology, 49,* 695–701.

Goldberg, E., Podell, K., & Lovell, M. (1994). Lateralization of frontal lobe functions and cognitive novelty. *Journal of Neuropsychiatry and Clinical Neuroscience, 6,* 371–378.

Goldstein, K. (1944). Mental changes due to frontal lobe damage. *Journal of Psychology, 17,* 187–208.

Grady, C.L., Van Meter, J.W., Maisog, J.M., Pietrini, P., Krasuski, J., & Rauschecker, J.P. (1997). Attention-related modulation of activity in primary and secondary auditory cortex. *NeuroReport, 8,* 2511–2516.

Grafman, J., Jonas, B., & Salazar, A. (1990). Wisconsin Card Sorting Test performance based on location and size of neuroanatomical lesion in Vietnam veterans with penetrating head injury. *Perceptual and Motor Skills, 71,* 1120–1122.

Grafman, J., Vance, S.C., Weingartner, H., Slazar, A.M., & Amin, D. (1993). The effects of lateralized frontal lesions on mood regulation. *Brain, 109,* 1127–1148.

Guillery, R.W., Feig, S.L., & Lozsadi, D.A. (1998). Paying attention to the thalamic reticular nucleus. *Trends in Neuroscience, 21,* 28–32.

Guitton, D., Buchtel, H.A., & Douglas, R.M. (1985). Frontal lobe lesions in man cause difficulties in suppressing reflexive glances and in generating goal-directed saccades. *Experimental Brain Research, 58,* 455–472.

Halgren, E., Marinkovic, K., & Chauvel, P. (1998). Generators of the late cognitive potential in auditory and visual oddball tasks. *Electroencephalography and Clinical Neurophysiology, 106,* 156–164.

Harrington, D.L., Haaland, K.Y., & Knight, R.T. (1998). Cortical networks underlying mechanisms of time perception. *Journal of Neuroscience, 18,* 1085–1095, 1998.

Hartikainen, K.M., Ogawa, K.H., Soltani, M., Pepitone, M., & Knight, R.T. (2000). Altered emotional influence on visual attention subsequent to orbitofrontal damage in humans. *Society for Neuroscience Abstract.* 26:2023

Hebb, D.O. & Penfield, W. (1940). Human behavior after extensive bilateral removals from the frontal lobes. *Archives of Neurology and Psychiatry, 4,* 421–438.

Heinze, H.J., Mangun, G.R., Burchert, W., Hinrichs, H., Scholz, M., Munte, T.F., Gos, A., Scherg, M., Johannes, S., Hundeshagen, H., Gazzaniga, M.S., & Hillyard, S.A. (1994). Combined spatial and temporal imaging of brain activity during visual selective attention in humans. *Nature, 372,* 543–546.

Hillyard, S.A. & Anllo-Vento, L. (1998). Event-related brain potentials in the study of visual selective attention. *Proceedings of the National Academy of Sciences USA, 95,* 781–787.

Hillyard, S.A., Hink, R.F., Schwent, U.L., & Picton, T.W. (1973). Electrical signs of selective attention in the human brain. *Science, 182,* 177–180.

Hopfinger, J.P., Buonocore, M.H., & Mangun, G.R. (2000). The neural mechanisms of top-down attentional control. *Nature Neuroscience, 3,* 284–291.

Jacobsen, C.F. (1935). Functions of frontal association areas in primates. *Archives of Neurology and Psychiatry, 33,* 558–569.

Janowsky, J.S., Shimamura, A.P., & Squire, L.R. (1989a). Memory and metamemory: comparisons between patients with frontal lobe lesions and amnesic patients. *Psychobiology, 17,* 3–11.

Janowsky, J.S., Shimamura, A.P., & Squire, L.R. (1989b). Source memory impairment in patients with frontal lobe lesions. *Neuropsychologia, 27,* 1043–1056.

Johnson, M.K. & Raye, C.L. (1981). Reality monitoring. *Psychological Review, 88,* 67–85.

Jonides, J., Smith, E.E., Koeppe, R.A., Awh, E., Minoshima, S., & Mintun, M.A. (1993). Spatial working memory in humans as revealed by PET. *Nature, 363,* 623–625.

Jonides, J., Smith, E.E., Marshuetz, C., Koeppe, R.A., & Reuter-Lorenz, P.A. (1998). Inhibition of verbal working memory revealed by brain activation. *Proceedings of the National Academy of Sciences USA, 95,* 8410–8413.

Kahneman, D. & Miller, D.T. (1986). Norm theory: comparing reality to its alternatives. *Psychological Review, 93,* 136–153.

Kahneman, D. & Varey, C.A. (1990). Propensities and counterfactuals: the loser that almost won. *Journal of Personality and Social Psychology, 59,* 1101–1110.

Karis, D., Fabiani, M., & Donchin, E. (1984). "P300" and

memory: individual differences in the Von Restorff effect. *Cognitive Psychology, 16,* 177–216.

Kastner, S., Pinsk, M.A., de Weerd, P., Desimone, R., & Ungerleider, L.G. (1999). Increased activity in human visual cortex during directed attention in the absence of visual stimulation. *Neuron, 22,* 751–761.

Katayama, J. & Polich, J. (1998). Stimulus context determines P3a and P3b. *Psychophysiology, 35,* 23–33.

Kertesz, A. & Dobrolowski, S. (1981). Right-hemisphere deficits, lesion size and location. *Journal of Clinical Neurophysiology, 3,* 283–299.

Kiehl, K.A., Liddle, P.F., & Hopfinger, J.B. (2000). Error processing and the anterior cingulate: an event-related fMRI study. *Psychophysiology, 37,* 216–223.

Kiehl, K.A., Laurens, K.R., Duty, T.L., Forster, B.B., & Liddle, P.F. (in press). An event-related fMRI study of a visual and auditory oddball task, *Journal of Psychophysiology.*

Klüver, H. & Bucy, P.C. (1939). Preliminary analysis of functions of the temporal lobes in monkeys. *Archives of Neurology and Psychiatry, 42,* 979–1000.

Kimble, D.P., Bagshaw, M.H., & Pribram, K.H. (1965). The GSR of monkeys during orienting and habituation after selective partial ablations of the cingulate and frontal cortex. *Neuropsychology, 3,* 121–128.

Knight, R.T. (1984). Decreased response to novel stimuli after prefrontal lesions in man. *Electroencephalography and Clinical Neurophysiology, 59,* 9–20.

Knight, R.T. (1991). Evoked potential studies of attention capacity in human frontal lobe lesions. In: H. Levin, H. Eisenberg, & F. Benton (Eds.), *Frontal Lobe Function and Dysfunction* (pp. 139–153). Oxford: Oxford University Press.

Knight, R.T. (1996). Contribution of human hippocampal region to novelty detection. *Nature, 383,* 256–259.

Knight, R.T. (1997). Distributed cortical network for visual attention. *Journal of Cognitive Neuroscience, 9,* 75–91.

Knight, R.T. & Grabowecky, M. (2000). Prefrontal ortex, time and consciousness. In: M. Gazzaniga (Ed.), *The New Cognitive Neurosciences* (pp. 1319–1339). Cambridge, MA: MIT Press.

Knight, R.T. & Scabini, D. (1998). Anatomic bases of event-related potentials and their relationship to novelty detection in humans. *Journal of Clinical Neurophysiology, 15,* 3–13.

Knight, R.T., Hillyard, S.A., Woods, D.L., & Neville, H.J. (1981). The effects of frontal cortex lesions on event-related potentials during auditory selective attention. *Electroencephalography and Clinical Neurophysiology, 52,* 571–582.

Knight, R.T., Scabini, D., & Woods, D.L. (1989a). Prefrontal cortex gating of auditory transmission in humans. *Brain Research, 504,* 338–342.

Knight, R.T., Scabini, D., Woods, D.L., & Clayworth, C.C. (1989b). Contribution of the temporal–parietal junction to the auditory P3. *Brain Research, 502,* 109–116.

Knight, R.T., Staines, W.R., Swick, D., & Chao, L.L. (1998). Prefrontal cortex regulates inhibition and excitation in distributed neural networks. *Acta Psychologia, 101,* 159–178.

Konishi, S., Naakjima, K., Uchida, I., Kaneyama, M., Nakahara, K., Sekihara, K., & Miyashita, Y. (1998). Transient activation of inferior prefrontal cortex during cognitive set shifting. *Nature Neuroscience, 1,* 80–84.

Kraus, N., Ozdamar, O., & L. Stein (1982). Auditory middle latency responses (MLRs) in patients with cortical lesions. *Electroencephalography and Clinical Neurophysiology 54,* 275–287.

Leuders, H., Leser, R.P., Harn, J., Dinner, D.S. & G. Klem (1983). Cortical somatosensory evoked potentials in response to hand stimulation. *Journal of Neurosurgery 58,* 885–894.

Lhermitte, F. (1986). Human autonomy and the frontal lobes. Part II: patient behavior in complex and social situations: the "environmental dependency syndrome". *Annals of Neurology, 19,* 335–343.

Lhermitte, F., Pillon, B., & Serdaru, M. (1986). Human anatomy and the frontal lobes. Part I: Imitation and utilization behavior: a neuropsychological study of 75 patients. *Annals of Neurology, 19,* 326–334.

Linden, D.E.J., Prvulovic, D., Formisano, E., Vollinger, M., Zanella, F.E., Goebel, R., & Dierks, T. (1999). The functional neuroanatomy of target detection: and fMRI study of visual and auditory oddball tasks. *Cerebral Cortex, 9,* 815–823.

London, E.D., Ernst, M., Grant, S., Bonson, K., & Weinstein, A. (2000). Orbitofrontal cortex and human drug abuse: functional imaging. *Cerebral Cortex, 10,* 334–342.

Luck, S.J., Chelazzi, L., Hillyard, S.A., & Desimone, R. (1997). Neural mechanisms of spatial selective attention in areas V1, V2, and V4 of macaque visual cortex. *Journal of Neurophysiology, 77,* 24–42.

Luria, A.R. (1966). *Higher Cortical Functions in Man.* New York: Basic Books.

Luu, P., Flaisch, T., & Tucker, D.M. (2000). Medial frontal cortex in action monitoring. *Journal of Neuroscience, 20,* 464–469.

Malmo, R.R. (1942). Interference factors in delayed response in monkeys after removal of frontal lobes. *Journal of Neurophysiology, 5,* 295–308.

Mangels, J., Gershberg, F.B., Shimamura, A., & Knight, R.T. (1996). Impaired retrieval from remote memory in patients with frontal lobe damage. *Neuropsychology, 10,* 32–41.

Mangun, G.R. (1995). Neural mechanisms of visual selective attention. *Psychophysiology, 32,* 4–18.

Martinez, A., Anllo-Vento, L., Sereno, M.I., Frank, L.R., Buxton, R.B., Dubowitz, D.J., Wong, E.C., Hinrichs, H., Heinze, H.J., & Hillyard, S.A. (1999). Involvement of striate and extrastriate visual cortical areas in spatial attention. *Nature Neuroscience, 2,* 364–369.

McAndrews, M.P. & Milner, B. (1991). The frontal cortex and memory for temporal order. *Neuropsychologia, 29,* 849–859.

McCarthy, G., Luby, M., Gore, J., & Goldman-Rakic, P.S. (1997). Infrequent events transiently activate human prefrontal and parietal cortex as measured by functional MRI. *Journal of Neurophysiology, 77,* 1630–1634.

McDonald, A.W., Cohen, J.D., Stenger, V.A., & Carter, C.S. (2000). Dissociating the role of the dorsolateral prefrontal and anterior cingulate cortex in cognitive control. *Science, 288,* 1835–1838.

McIntosh, A.R., Grady, C.L., Ungerleider, L.G., Haxby, J.V., Rapoport, S.I., & Horwitz, B. (1994). Network analysis of cortical visual pathways mapped with PET. *Journal of Neuroscience, 14,* 655–666.

Menon, K., Ford, J.M., Lim, K.O., Glover, G.H., & Pfefferbaum, A. (1997). A combined event-related fMRI and EEG evidence for temporal–parietal activation during target detection. *NeuroReport, 8,* 3029–3037.

Mesulam, M.-M. (1981). A cortical nerwork for directed attention and unilateral neglect. *Annals of Neurology, 10,* 309–325.

Mesualam, M.-M. (1998). From sensation to cognition. *Brain, 121,* 1013–52.

Miller, E.K. (1999). The prefrontal cortex: complex neural properties for complex behavior. *Neuron, 22,* 15–17.

Milner, B. (1971). Interhemispheric differences in the localization of psychological processes in man. *British Medical Bulletin, 27,* 272–277.

Milner, B. & Petrides, M. (1984). Behavioural effects of frontal-lobe lesions in man. *Trends in Neurosciences, 7,* 403–407.

Milner, B., Petrides M., & Smith, M.L. (1985). Frontal lobes and the temporal organization of memory. *Human Neurobiology, 4,* 137–142.

Moscovich, M. (1989). Confabulation and the frontal systems: strategic versus associative retrieval in neuropsychological theories of memory. In: H.L. Roediger III & F.I.M. Craik (Eds.), *Varieties of Memory and Consciousness: Essays in Honour of Endel Tulving* (pp. 133–160). Hillsdale, NJ: Lawrence Erlbaum Associates.

Muller, N.G. Machado, L., & Knight, R.T. (in press). Contribution of subregions of the prefrontal cortex to working memory. Evidence from brain lesions in humans. *Journal of Cognitive Neuroscience.*

Nielsen-Bohlman, L. & Knight, R.T. (1999). Prefrontal cortical involvement in visual working memory. *Cognitive Brain Research, 8,* 299–310.

Nobre, A.C., Coull, J.T., Frith, C.D., & Mesualm, M.-M. (1999). Orbitofrontal cortex is activated during breaches of expectation in tasks of visual attention. *Nature Neuroscience, 2,* 11–12.

O'Doherty, J., Rolls, E.T., Francis, S., Botwell, R., & McGlone, F. (2001). Representation of pleasant and adversive taste in the human brain. *Journal of Neurophysiology, 85* 1315–1321.

Opitz, B., Mecklinger, A., Friederici, A.D., & von Cramon, D.Y. (1999a). The functional neuroanatomy of novelty processing: integrating ERP and fMRI results. *Cerebral Cortex, 9,* 379–391.

Opitz, B., MecKlinger, A., Vob Cramon, D.Y., & Krugel, F. (1999b). Combining electrophysiological and hemodynamic measures of the auditory oddball. *Psychophysiology, 36,* 142–147.

Owen, A.M., Stern, C.E., Look, R.B., Tracey, I., Rosen, B.R., & Petrides, M. (1998). Functional organization of spatial and nonspatial working memory processing within the human lateral frontal cortex. *Proceedings National Academy Sciences USA, 95,* 7721–7726.

Pape, S.W. (1937). A proposed mechanism of emotion. *Archives of Neurology and Psychiatry 38,* 725–743.

Peterson, B.S., Skudlarski, P., Gatenby, J.C., Zhang, H., Anderson, A.W., & Gore, J.C. (1999). An fMRI study of Stroop word–color interference: evidence for cingulate subregions subserving multiple distributed attentional systems. *Biological Psychiatry, 45,* 1237–1258.

Petrides, M. & Milner, B. (1982). Deficits on subject-ordered tasks after frontal- and temporal-lobe lesions in man. *Neuropsychologia, 20,* 249–262.

Prabhakaran, V., Narayanan, K., Zhao, Z., & Gabrieli, J.D. (2000). Integration of diverse information in working memory within the frontal lobe. *Nature Neuroscience, 3,* 85–90.

Price, B.H., Daffner, K.R., & Mesalum, M.-M. (1990). The comportmental learning disabilities of early frontal lobe damage. *Brain, 113,* 1383–1393.

Raichle, M.E., Fiez, J.A., Videen, T.O., MacLeod, A.M., Pardo, J.V., Fox, P.T., & Petersen, S.E. (1994). Practice-related changes in human brain functional anatomy during non-motor learning. *Cerebral Cortex, 4,* 8–26.

Rainer, G. & Miller, E.K. (2000). Effects of visual experience on the representation of objects in the prefrontal cortex. *Neuron, 27,* 179–189.

Rainer, G., Asaad, W.F., & Miller, E.K. (1998a). Memory fields of neurons in the primate prefrontal cortex. *Proceedings of the National Academy of Sciences, USA, 95,* 15008–15013.

Rainer, G., Asaad, W.F., & Miller, E.K. (1998b). Selective representation of relevant information by neurons in the primate prefrontal cortex. *Nature, 393,* 577–579.

Rajkowska, G. & Goldman-Rakic, P.S. (1995a). Cytoarchitechtonic definition of prefrontal areas in the normal human cortex: I. Remapping of areas 9 and 46 using quantitative criteria. *Cerebral Cortex, 5,* 307–322.

Rajkowska, G. & Goldman-Rakic, P.S. (1995b). Cytoarchitechtonic definition of prefrontal areas in the normal human cortex: II. Variability in locations of areas 9 and 46 and relationship to the Talairach coordinate system. *Cerebral Cortex, 5,* 323–337.

Rao, S.C., Rainer, G., & Miller, E. (1997). Integration of what and where in the primate prefrontal cortex. *Science, 276,* 821–824.

Rees, G., Frackowiak, R., & Frith, C. (1997). Two modulatory effects of attention that mediate object categorization in human cortex. *Science 275,* 835–838.

Richer, F., Decary, A., Lapierre, M., Rouleau, I., Bouvier, G., & Saint-Hilaire, J. (1993). Target detection deficits in frontal lobectomy. *Brain and Cognition, 21,* 203–211.

Roberts, A.C. & Wallis, J.D. (2000). Inhibitory control and affective processing in the prefrontal cortex: neuropsychological studies in the common marmoset. *Cerebral Cortex, 10,* 252–262.

Rolls, E.T., Hornak, J., Wade, D., & McGrath, J. (1994). Emotion-related learning in patients with social and emotional changes associated with frontal lobe damage. *Journal of Neurology, Neurosurgery and Psychiatry, 57,* 1518–1524.

Romanski, L.M., Tian, B., Fritz, J., Mishkin, M., Goldman-Rakic, P.S., & Rauschecker, J.P. (1999). Dual streams of auditory afferents target multiple domains in the primate prefrontal cortex. *Nature Neuroscience, 2,* 1131–1136.

Rossi, A.F., Rotter, P.S., Desimone, R., & Ungerleider, L.G. (1999). Prefrontal lesions produce impairments in feature-cued attention. *Society for Neuroscience Abstracts, 29,* 2.

Rule, R., Shimamura, A., & Knight, R.T. (1999). Electrophysiological evidence of disinhibition after orbitofrontal damage in humans. *Society for Neuroscience Abstracts, 25,* 893.

Schacter, D.L., Harbluk, J.L., & McLachlan, D.R. (1984). Retrieval without recollection: an experimental analysis of source amnesia. *Journal of Verbal Learning and Verbal Behavior, 23,* 593–611.

Schoenbaum, G., Chiba, A.A., & Gallagher, M. (1998). Orbitofrontal cortex and basolateral amygdala encode expected outcomes during learning. *Nature Neuroscience, 1,* 155–159.

Shallice, T. (1988). *From Neuropsychology to Mental Structure.* Cambridge, UK: Cambridge University Press.

Shammi, P. & Stuss, D.T. (1999). Humour appreciation: a role of the right frontal lobe. *Brain, 122,* 657–666.

Shimamura, A. (2000). The role of prefrontal cortex in dynamic filtering. *Psychobiology, 28,* 207–218.

Shimamura, A.P. & Squire, L.R. (1987). A neuropsychological study of fact memory and source amnesia. *Journal of Experimental Psychology: Learning, Memory, and Cognition, 13,* 464–473.

Shimamura, A.P., Janowsky, J.S., & Squire, L.R. (1990). Memory for the temporal order of events in patients with frontal lobe lesions and amnesic patients. *Neuropsychologia, 28,* 803–813.

Shimamura A.P., Gershberg, F.B., Jurica, P.J., Mangels, J.A., & Knight, R.T. (1992). Intact implicit memory in patients with focal frontal lobe lesions. *Neuropsychologia, 30,* 931–937.

Shimamura, A.P., Jurica, P.J., Mangels, J.A., Gershberg, F.B., & Knight, R.T. (1995). Susceptibility to memory interference effects following frontal lobe damage: findings from tests of paired-associate learning. *Journal of Cognitive Neuroscience, 7,* 144–152.

Skinner, J.E. & Yingling, C.D. (1977). Central gating mechanisms that regulate event-related potentials and behavior. In: J.E. Desmedt (Ed.), *Progress in Clinical Neurophysiology.* Vol 1 (pp. 30–69). Basel: S Karger.

Sokolov, E.N. (1963). Higher nervous functions: the orienting reflex. *Annual Review of Physiology, 25,* 545–580.

Somers, D.C., Dale, A.M., Seiffert, A.E., & Tootell, R.B. (1999). Functional MRI reveals spatially specific attentional modulation in human primary visual cortex. *Proceedings of the National Academy of Sciences USA, 96,* 1663–1668.

Steinmetz, P.N., Roy, A., Fitzgerald, P.J., Hsiao, S.S., Johnson, K.O., & Niebur, E. (2000). Attention modulates synchronized neuronal firing in primate somatosensory cortex. *Nature, 404,* 187–189.

Stern, C.E., Corkin S., Gonzalez, R.G., Guimares, A.R., Baker, J.R., Jennings, P.J., Carr, C.A., Sugiura, R.M., Vedantham, V., & Rosene, B.R. (1996). The hippocampal formation participates in novel picture encoding: evidence from functional magnetic resonance imaging. *Proceedings of the National. Academy of Sciences USA, 93,* 8660–8665.

Stone, V.E., Baron-Cohen, S., & Knight, R.T. (1998). Does frontal lobe damage produce theory of mind impairment? *Journal of Cognitive Neuroscience, 10,* 640–656.

Stuss, D.T. (1991). Self, awareness, and the frontal lobes: a neuropsychological perspective. In: J. Strauss & G.R. Goethals (Eds.), *The Self: Interdisciplinary Approaches* (pp. 255–278). New York: Springer-Verlag.

Stuss, D.T. & Alexander, M.P. (2000). The anatomical basis of affective behavior, emotion and self-awareness: a specific role of the right frontal lobe. In: G. Hatano, N. Okada, & H. Tanabe (Eds.), *Affective Minds. The 13th Toyota Conference* (pp. 13–25). Amsterdam: Elsevier.

Stuss, D.T., & Benson, D.F. (1984). Neuropsychological studies of the frontal lobes. *Psychological Bulletin, 95,* 3–28.

Stuss, D.T. & D.F. Benson. (1986). *The Frontal Lobes.* New York: Raven Press.

Stuss, D.T., Delgado, M., & Guzman, D.A. (1987). Verbal regulation in the control of motor impersistence: a proposed rehabilitation procedure. *Journal of Neurologic Rehabilitation, 1987, 1,* 19–24.

Stuss, D.T., Alexander, M.P., Palumbo, C.L., Buckle, L., Sayer, L., & Pogue, J. (1994). Organizational strategies of patients with unilateral or bilateral frontal lobe injury in word list learning tasks. *Neuropsychology, 8,* 355–373.

Stuss, D.T., van Reekum, R., & Murphy, K.J. (2000). Differentiation of states and causes of apathy. In: J. Borod (Ed.), *The Neuropsychology of Emotion* (pp. 340–363). New York: Oxford University Press.

Stuss, D.T., Gallup, G.G., Jr., & Alexander, M.P. (2001a). The frontal lobes are necessary for theory of mind. *Brain, 124,* 279–286.

Stuss, D.T., Picton, T.W., & Alexander, M.P. (2001b). Consciousness, self-awareness and the frontal lobes. In: S.P. Salloway, P.F. Malloy, & J.D. Duffy (Eds.), *The Frontal Lobes and Neuropsychiatric Illness* (pp. 101–109). Washington, D.C: American Psychiatric Publishing.

Sutherling, W.W., Crandall, P.H., Darcey, T.M., Becker, D.P., Levesque, M.F., D.S. Barth (1988). The magnetic and electric fields agree with intracranial localizations of somatosensory cortex. *Neurology 38,* 1705–1714.

Suwazono, S., Machado, L., & Knight, R.T. (2000). Predictive value of novel stimuli modifies visual event-related potentials and behavior. *Clinical Neurophysiology, 111,* 29–39.

Tomita, H., Ohbayashi, M., Nakahara, K., Hasegawa, I., & Miyashita, Y. (1999). Top-down signal from prefrontal cortex in executive control of memory retrieval. *Nature, 401,* 699–703.

Tranel, D. & Damasio, H. (1994). Neuroanatomical correlates of electrodermal skin conductance responses. *Psychophysiology, 31,* 427–438.

Tsuchiya, H., Yamaguchi, S., & Kobayashi, S. (2000). Impaired novelty detection and frontal lobe dysfunction in Parkinson's disease. *Neuropsychologia, 38,* 645–654.

Tulving, E., Markowitsch, H., Kapur, S., Habib, R., & Houle, S. (1994). Novelty encoding networks in the human brain: positron emission tomography data. *NeuroReport, 5*, 2525–2528.

Tulving, E., Markowitsch, H.J., Craik, F.I.M., Habib, R., & Houle, S. (1996). Novelty and familiarity activations in PET studies of memory encoding and retrieval. *Cerebral Cortex, 6*, 71–79.

Verleger, R., Heide, W., Butt, C., & Kompf, D. (1994). Reduction of P3b potentials in patients with temporo-parietal lesions. *Cognitive Brain Research, 2*, 103–116.

Vidal, F., Hasbroucq, T., Grapperon, J., & Bonnet, M. (2000). Is the 'error negativity' specific to errors? *Biological Psychology, 51(2–3)*, 109–128.

Volkow, N.D. & Fowler, J.S. (2000). Addiction, a disease of compulsion and drive: involvement of the orbitofrontal cortex. *Cerebral Cortex, 10*, 318–325.

Von Restorff, H. (1933). Über die Wirkung von Bereischsbildungen im Spurenfeld. *Psychlogische Forschung, 18*, 299–342.

Webster, M.J., Bachevalier, J., & Ungerleider, L.G. (1994). Connections of inferior temporal areas TEO and TE with parietal and frontal cortex in macaque monkeys. *Cerebral Cortex, 5*, 470–483.

Wheeler, M.A., Stuss, D.T., & Tulving, E. (1995). Frontal lobe damage produces episodic memory impairment. *Journal of the International Neuropsychological Society, 1*, 525–536.

Wilson, F.A.W., Scalaidhe, S.P.O., & Goldman-Rakic, P.S. (1993). Dissociation of object and spatial processing in primate prefrontal cortex. *Science, 260*, 1955–1958.

Woldorff, M.G. & S.A. Hillyard (1991). Modulation of early auditory processing during selective listening to rapidly presented tones. *Electroencephalograph and Clinical Neurophysioliology (Limerick), 79*, 170–191.

Woldorff, M.G., Gallen, C.C., Hampson, S.A., Hillyard, S.A., Pantev, C., Sobel, D., & Bloom, F.E. (1993). Modulation of early sensory processing in human auditory cortex during auditory selective attention. *Proceedings of the National Academy of Sciences USA, 90*, 8722–8726.

Woldorff, M.G., Fox, P.T., Matzke, M., Lancaster, I.L., Veeraswamy, S., Zamarripa, F., Seaboldt, M., Glass, T., Gao, J.H., Martin, C.C., & Jerabek, P. (1997). Retinotopic organization of early visual spatial attention: effects as revealed by PET and ERP data. *Human Brain Mapping, 5*, 280–286.

Woods, D.L. & S.A. Hillyard (1978). Attention at the cocktail party: Brainstem evoked responses reveal no peripheral gating. In: D.A. Otto (Eds.), *Multidisciplinary Perspectives in Event-related Brain Potential Research.* (pp. 230–233) Washington, D.C.: U.S. Government Printing Office.

Woods, D.L. & Knight, R.T. (1986). Electrophysiological evidence of increased distractibility after dorsolateral prefrontal lesions. *Neurology, 36*, 212–216.

Wood, C.C., Spencer, D.D., Allison, T., McCarthy, G., Williamson, P.D. & W.B. Goff (1988). Localization of human sensorimotor cortex during surgery by cortical surface recording of somatosensory evoked potentials. *Journal of Neurosurgery 68*, 99–111.

Yago, E. & Knight, R.T. (2000). Tonic and phasic prefrontal modulation of extrastriate processing during visual attention. *Soc. Neuroscience, 26:*2232.

Yamaguchi, S. & Knight, R.T. (1990). Gating of somatosensory inputs by human prefrontal cortex. *Brain Research, 521*, 281–288.

Yamaguchi, S. & Knight, R.T. (1991). Anterior and posterior association cortex contributions to the somatosensory P300. *Journal of Neuroscience, 11*, 2039–2054.

Yamaguchi, S. & Knight, R.T. (1992). Effects of temporal–parietal lesions on the somatosensory P3 to lower limb stimulation. *Electroencephalography and Clinical Neurophysiology, 84*, 139–148.

Yingling, C.D. & Skinner, J.E. (1977). Gating of thalamic input to cerebral cortex by nucleus reticularis thalami. In: J.E. Desmedt (Ed.), *Progress in Clinical Neurophysiology*, Vol. I (pp. 70–96). Basel: S. Karger.

Yoshiura, T., Zhong, J., Shibata, D.K., Kwok, W.E., Shrier, D.A., & Numaguchi, Y. (1999). Functional MRI study of auditory and visual oddball tasks. *NeuroReport, 10*, 1683–1688.

Index